Molecular Biology of Picornaviruses

Molecular Biology of Picornaviruses

EDITED BY

Bert L. Semler
Department of Microbiology and Molecular Genetics,
College of Medicine, University of California, Irvine, CA 92697-4025

Eckard Wimmer
Department of Molecular Genetics and Microbiology,
School of Medicine, State University of New York at Stony Brook, Stony Brook, NY 11794

ASM PRESS   WASHINGTON, D.C.

Copyright © 2002 ASM Press
American Society for Microbiology
1752 N Street, N.W.
Washington, DC 20036-2904

Library of Congress Cataloging-in-Publication Data

Molecular biology of picornaviruses / edited by Bert L. Semler and
Eckard Wimmer.
   p. ; cm.
Includes bibliographical references and index.
   ISBN 1-55581-210-4
   1. Picornaviruses.   2. Picornavirus infections.
   [DNLM: 1. Molecular Biology.   2. Picornaviridae.   3.
Picornaviridae—genetics.   4. Picornaviridae Infections.   5.
Poliomyelitis—prevention & control.   6. Poliovirus. QW 168.5.P4 M7182
2002]   I. Semler, Bert L.   II. Wimmer, Eckard.
   QR410.M654 2002
   579.2'572—dc21
                                                    2002008979

All Rights Reserved
Printed in the United States of America

10 9 8 7 6 5 4 3 2 1

Address editorial correspondence to: ASM Press, 1752 N St., N.W., Washington, DC
20036-2904, U.S.A.

Send orders to: ASM Press, P.O. Box 605, Herndon, VA 20172, U.S.A.
Phone: 800-546-2416; 703-661-1593
Fax: 703-661-1501
Email: books@asmusa.org
Online: www.asmpress.org

The Editors would like to dedicate this book to the memory of our colleague,
Donald F. Summers,
a true pioneer in the study of picornavirus molecular biology
and one of our real-life heroes in science.

Contents

Contributors xi
Preface xix

HISTORICAL PERSPECTIVE

1. History of Poliomyelitis and Poliomyelitis Research   3
   HANS J. EGGERS

TAXONOMY

2. Molecular and Biological Basis of Picornavirus Taxonomy   17
   GLYN STANWAY, TAPANI HOVI, NICK J. KNOWLES, AND TIMO HYYPIÄ

VIRION STRUCTURE

3. Picornavirus Structure Overview   27
   MICHAEL G. ROSSMANN

4. Antibody Interactions with Rhinovirus   39
   THOMAS J. SMITH

5. Antigenic Variation in Foot-and-Mouth Disease Virus   51
   DAVID J. ROWLANDS AND FRED BROWN

VIRUS ENTRY

6. Cellular Receptors of Picornaviruses: an Overview   61
   ELIZABETH RIEDER AND ECKARD WIMMER

7. Poliovirus Receptors and Cell Entry   71
   JAMES M. HOGLE AND VINCENT R. RACANIELLO

8. Interaction of Major Group Rhinoviruses with Their Cellular Receptor, ICAM-1   85
   RICHARD J. KUHN AND MICHAEL G. ROSSMANN

9. Human Rhinovirus Minor Group Receptors   93
   DIETER BLAAS

10. Receptors for Coxsackieviruses and Echoviruses   107
    JEFFERY M. BERGELSON

11. Foot-and-Mouth Disease Virus-Receptor Interactions: Role in Pathogenesis and Tissue Culture Adaptation   115
    BARRY BAXT, SHERRY NEFF, ELIZABETH RIEDER, AND PETER W. MASON

VIRAL GENOMES

12. Picornavirus Genome: an Overview   127
    VADIM A. AGOL

13. Alignments and Comparative Profiles of Picornavirus Genera   149
    ANN C. PALMENBERG AND JEAN-YVES SGRO

INITIATION OF TRANSLATION

14. Initiation of Translation of Picornavirus RNAs: Structure and Function of the Internal Ribosome Entry Site   159
    ELLIE EHRENFELD AND NATALYA L. TETERINA

15. Proteins Involved in the Function of Picornavirus Internal Ribosomal Entry Sites   171
    RICHARD J. JACKSON

PROTEOLYTIC PROCESSING

16. Processing Determinants and Functions of Cleavage Products of Picornavirus Polyproteins   187
    LOUIS E.-C. LEONG, CHRISTOPHER T. CORNELL, AND BERT L. SEMLER

17. Structure and Function of Picornavirus Proteinases   199
    TIM SKERN, BERNHARD HAMPÖLZ, ALBA GUARNÉ, IGNACIO FITA, ERNST BERGMANN, JENS PETERSEN, AND MICHAEL N. G. JAMES

18. The Aphtho- and Cardiovirus "Primary" 2A/2B Polyprotein "Cleavage"   213
    MARTIN D. RYAN, GARRY LUKE, LORRAINE E. HUGHES, VANESSA M. COWTON, EDWIN TEN DAM, XUEJUN LI, MICHELLE L. L. DONNELLY, AMIT MEHROTRA, AND DAVID GANI

VIRAL RNA REPLICATION

19. Possible Unifying Mechanism of Picornavirus Genome Replication   227
    ANIKO V. PAUL

20. Role of Cellular Structures in Viral RNA Replication   247
    DENISE EGGER, RAINER GOSERT, AND KURT BIENZ

21. Poliovirus RNA-Dependent RNA Polymerase (3D^{pol}): Structure, Function, and Mechanism   255
    CRAIG E. CAMERON, DAVID W. GOHARA, AND JAMIE J. ARNOLD

22. Picornavirus Genetics: an Overview   269
    VADIM A. AGOL

23. Error Frequencies of Picornavirus RNA Polymerases: Evolutionary Implications for Virus Populations   285
    ESTEBAN DOMINGO, ERIC BARANOWSKI, CRISTINA ESCARMÍS, FRANCISCO SOBRINO, AND JOHN J. HOLLAND

SHUTOFF OF HOST CELL TRANSLATION AND TRANSCRIPTION

24. Picornavirus Proteinase-Mediated Shutoff of Host Cell Translation: Direct Cleavage of a Cellular Initiation Factor   301
    ERNST KUECHLER, JOACHIM SEIPELT, HANS-DIETER LIEBIG, AND WOLFGANG SOMMERGRUBER

25. Poliovirus-Mediated Shutoff of Host Translation: an Indirect Effect   313
    MIGUEL ZAMORA, WILFRED E. MARISSEN, AND RICHARD E. LLOYD

26. Effects of Picornavirus Proteinases on Host Cell Transcription   321
    ASIM DASGUPTA, PADMAJA YALAMANCHILI, MELODY CLARK, STEVEN KLIEWER, LEE FRADKIN, SHERYL RUBINSTEIN, SAUMITRA DAS, YUHONG SHEN, MARY K. WEIDMAN, RAJEEV BANERJEE, UTPAL DATTA, MEGAN IGO, PALLOB KUNDU, BHASWATI BARAT, AND ARNOLD J. BERK

27. Effects of Viral Replication on Cellular Membrane Metabolism and Function   337
    LUIS CARRASCO, ROSARIO GUINEA, ALICIA IRURZUN, AND ÁNGEL BARCO

PATHOGENICITY

28. Clinical Significance, Diagnosis, and Treatment of Picornavirus Infections   357
    HARLEY A. ROTBART

29. Determinants of Poliovirus Pathogenesis   367
    MATTHIAS GROMEIER AND AKIO NOMOTO

30. Poliovirus Vaccines: Molecular Biology and Immune Response   381
    P. D. MINOR AND J. ALMOND

31. Immunology of the Coxsackieviruses   391
    NORA M. CHAPMAN, CHARLES J. GAUNTT, AND STEVE TRACY

32. Pathogenesis of Coxsackievirus B Infections   405
    REINHARD KANDOLF, HANS-CHRISTOPH SELINKA, AND KARIN KLINGEL

33. Hepatitis A Virus Pathogenesis and Attenuation   415
    ROBERT H. PURCELL AND SUZANNE U. EMERSON

34. Pathogenesis of Theiler's Murine Encephalomyelitis Virus-Induced Disease   427
    RAYMOND P. ROOS

35. Persistent Infections by Picornaviruses   437
    FLORENCE COLBÈRE-GARAPIN, ISABELLE PELLETIER, AND LAURENT OUZILOU

CELL-FREE SYNTHESIS AND CELL-FREE GENETICS OF POLIOVIRUS

36. Cell-Free Genetics of Poliovirus   451
    ROHIT DUGGAL

37. Poliovirus RNA Replication and Genetic Complementation in Cell-Free Reactions   461
    DAVID J. BARTON, B. JOAN MORASCO, LUCIA EISNER SMERAGE, AND JAMES B. FLANEGAN

GLOBAL ERADICATION OF POLIOVIRUS

38. Global Eradication of Poliovirus: History and Rationale   473
    WALTER R. DOWDLE AND STEPHEN L. COCHI

39. The Mechanism of Poliovirus Eradication   481
    OLEN M. KEW AND MARK A. PALLANSCH

Color plates   following p. 156

Index   493

Contributors

VADIM A. AGOL
M. P. Chumakov Institute of Poliomyelitis & Viral Encephalitides, Russian Academy of Medical Sciences, Moscow Region 142782, and M. V. Lomonosov Moscow State University, Moscow 119899, Russia

J. ALMOND
Research and Development (France), Aventis Pasteur SA, Campus Mérieux, 1541 Ave. Marcel Mérieux, 69280 Marcy-L'Etoile, France

JAMIE J. ARNOLD
Department of Biochemistry and Molecular Biology, Pennsylvania State University, University Park, PA 16802

RAJEEV BANERJEE
Department of Microbiology, Immunology, and Molecular Genetics, UCLA School of Medicine, and The Molecular Biology Institute, University of California, Los Angeles, Los Angeles, CA 90095-1747

ERIC BARANOWSKI
Centro de Biología Molecular "Severo Ochoa," Universidad Autónoma de Madrid, Cantoblanco, 28049 Madrid, Spain

BHASWATI BARAT
Department of Microbiology, Immunology, and Molecular Genetics, UCLA School of Medicine, and The Molecular Biology Institute, University of California, Los Angeles, Los Angeles, CA 90095-1747

ÁNGEL BARCO
Center for Neurobiology and Behavior, Columbia University, 722 West 68th St., 6th Floor, New York, NY 10032

DAVID J. BARTON
Department of Microbiology and Molecular Biology Program, University of Colorado Health Sciences Center, Denver, CO 80262, and Department of Biochemistry and Molecular Biology, College of Medicine, University of Florida, Gainesville, FL 32610-0245

BARRY BAXT
U.S. Department of Agriculture, Agricultural Research Service, Plum Island Animal Disease Center, P.O. Box 848, Greenport, NY 11944-0848

JEFFREY M. BERGELSON
Division of Immunologic and Infectious Diseases, Children's Hospital of Philadelphia, Abramson 1202, 3516 Civic Center Blvd., Philadelphia, PA 19104-4318

ERNST BERGMANN
CIHR Group in Protein Structure and Function, Department of Biochemistry, University of Alberta, Edmonton, Alberta T6G 2H7, Canada

ARNOLD J. BERK
Department of Microbiology, Immunology, and Molecular Genetics, UCLA School of Medicine, and The Molecular Biology Institute, University of California, Los Angeles, Los Angeles, CA 90095-1747

KURT BIENZ
Institute for Medical Microbiology, Petersplatz 10, University of Basel, CH-4003 Basel, Switzerland

DIETER BLAAS
Institute of Medical Biochemistry, VBC, University of Vienna, Dr. Bohr Gasse 9/3, A-1030 Vienna, Austria

FRED BROWN
Plum Island Animal Disease Center, P.O. Box 848, Greenport, NY 11944

CRAIG E. CAMERON
Department of Biochemistry and Molecular Biology, Pennsylvania State University, University Park, PA 16802

LUIS CARRASCO
Centro de Biología Molecular "Severo Ochoa," Universidad Autónoma de Madrid, Cantoblanco, 28049 Madrid, Spain

NORA M. CHAPMAN
Department of Pathology and Microbiology, University of Nebraska Medical Center, 600c South 42nd St., Omaha, NE 68198-6495

MELODY CLARK
Department of Microbiology, Immunology, and Molecular Genetics, UCLA School of Medicine, and The Molecular Biology Institute, University of California, Los Angeles, Los Angeles, CA 90095-1747

STEPHEN L. COCHI
Vaccine Preventable Disease Eradication Division, National Immunization Program, Centers for Disease Control and Prevention, 1600 Clifton Rd., MS/E-05, Atlanta, GA 30333

FLORENCE COLBÈRE-GARAPIN
Groupe de Génétique Virale-Unité NRSN, Département de Virologie, Institut Pasteur, 25, rue du Dr. Roux, 75724 Paris Cedex 15, France

CHRISTOPHER T. CORNELL
Department of Microbiology and Molecular Genetics, College of Medicine, University of California, Irvine, CA 92697-4025

VANESSA M. COWTON
Centre for Biomolecular Sciences, School of Biology, University of St. Andrews, Biomolecular Sciences Building, North Haugh, St. Andrews, Fife KY16 9ST, Scotland

SAUMITRA DAS
Department of Microbiology, Immunology, and Molecular Genetics, UCLA School of Medicine, and The Molecular Biology Institute, University of California, Los Angeles, Los Angeles, CA 90095-1747

ASIM DASGUPTA
Department of Microbiology, Immunology, and Molecular Genetics, 43-144 CHS, UCLA School of Medicine, 10833 Le Conte Ave., and The Molecular Biology Institute, University of California, Los Angeles, Los Angeles, CA 90095-1747

UTPAL DATTA
Department of Microbiology, Immunology, and Molecular Genetics, UCLA School of Medicine, and The Molecular Biology Institute, University of California, Los Angeles, Los Angeles, CA 90095-1747

ESTEBAN DOMINGO
Centro de Biología Molecular "Severo Ochoa," Universidad Autónoma de Madrid, Cantoblanco, 28049 Madrid, Spain

MICHELLE L. L. DONNELLY
Marie Curie Research Institute, The Chart, Oxted, Surrey RH8 0TL, United Kingdom

WALTER R. DOWDLE
World Health Organization, The Task Force for Child Survival and Development, Suite 400, 750 Commerce Dr., Decatur, GA 30030

ROHIT DUGGAL
Agouron Pharmaceuticals, 10777 Science Center Dr., San Diego, CA 92121

DENISE EGGER
Institute for Medical Microbiology, Petersplatz 10, University of Basel, CH-4003 Basel, Switzerland

HANS J. EGGERS
Institute of Virology, University of Cologne, Fuerst-Puckler-Str. 56, 50935 Cologne, Germany

ELLIE EHRENFELD
Laboratory of Infectious Diseases, National Institute of Allergy and Infectious Diseases, National Institutes of Health, Bldg. 50, Room 6120, MSC 8011, Bethesda, MD 20892-8011

SUZANNE U. EMERSON
Hepatitis Viruses and Molecular Hepatitis Sections, Laboratory of Infectious Diseases, National Institute of Allergy and Infectious Diseases, National Institutes of Health, Bldg. 7/202, 7 Center Dr., MSC 0740, Bethesda, MD 20892-0740

CRISTINA ESCARMÍS
Centro de Biología Molecular "Severo Ochoa," Universidad Autónoma de Madrid, Cantoblanco, 28049 Madrid, Spain

IGNACIO FITA
Centre d'Investigació i Desenvolupament (CSIC), Jordi Girona Salgado 18-26, E-08034 Barcelona, Spain

JAMES B. FLANEGAN
Department of Biochemistry and Molecular Biology, College of Medicine, University of Florida, Gainesville, FL 32610-0245

LEE FRADKIN
Department of Microbiology, Immunology, and Molecular Genetics, UCLA School of Medicine, and The Molecular Biology Institute, University of California, Los Angeles, Los Angeles, CA 90095-1747

DAVID GANI
The School of Chemistry, The University of Birmingham, Edgbaston, Birmingham B15 2TT, United Kingdom

CHARLES J. GAUNTT
Department of Microbiology, University of Texas Health Science Center at San Antonio, San Antonio, TX 78284-7758

DAVID W. GOHARA
Department of Biochemistry and Molecular Biology, Pennsylvania State University, University Park, PA 16802

RAINER GOSERT
Institute for Medical Microbiology, Petersplatz 10, University of Basel, CH-4003 Basel, Switzerland

MATTHIAS GROMEIER
Department of Microbiology, Duke University Medical Center, Durham, NC 27710

ALBA GUARNÉ
Centre d'Investigació i Desenvolupament (CSIC), Jordi Girona Salgado 18-26, E-08034 Barcelona, Spain

ROSARIO GUINEA
Centro de Biología Molecular "Severo Ochoa," Universidad Autónoma de Madrid, Cantoblanco, 28049 Madrid, Spain

BERNHARD HAMPÖLZ
Institute of Medical Biochemistry, Vienna Bio Center, University of Vienna, Dr. Bohr-Gasse 9/3, A-1030 Vienna, Austria

JAMES M. HOGLE
Department of Biochemistry and Molecular Pharmacology, Harvard Medical School, Boston, MA 02115

JOHN J. HOLLAND
Department of Biology and Center for Molecular Genetics, University of California, San Diego, La Jolla, CA 92093-1006

TAPANI HOVI
Enterovirus Laboratory, KTL, Mannerheimintie 166, 00300 Helsinki, Finland

LORRAINE E. HUGHES
Centre for Biomolecular Sciences, School of Biology, University of St. Andrews, Biomolecular Sciences Building, North Haugh, St. Andrews, Fife KY16 9ST, Scotland

TIMO HYYPIÄ
Department of Virology, Haartman Institute, University of Helsinki, P.O. Box 21, 00014 Helsinki, Finland

MEGAN IGO
Department of Microbiology, Immunology, and Molecular Genetics, UCLA School of Medicine, and The Molecular Biology Institute, University of California, Los Angeles, Los Angeles, CA 90095-1747

ALICIA IRURZUN
Centro de Biología Molecular "Severo Ochoa," Universidad Autónoma de Madrid, Cantoblanco, 28049 Madrid, Spain

RICHARD J. JACKSON
Department of Biochemistry, University of Cambridge, 80 Tennis Court Rd., Cambridge CB2 1GA, United Kingdom

MICHAEL N. G. JAMES
CIHR Group in Protein Structure and Function, Department of Biochemistry, University of Alberta, Edmonton, Alberta T6G 2H7, Canada

REINHARD KANDOLF
Department of Molecular Pathology, University Hospital of Tübingen, Liebermeisterstr. 8, D-72076 Tübingen, Germany

OLEN M. KEW
Division of Viral and Rickettsial Diseases, National Center for Infectious Diseases, Centers for Disease Control and Prevention, 1600 Clifton Rd., Mailstop G-10, Atlanta, GA 30333

STEVEN KLIEWER
Department of Microbiology, Immunology, and Molecular Genetics, UCLA School of Medicine, and The Molecular Biology Institute, University of California, Los Angeles, Los Angeles, CA 90095-1747

KARIN KLINGEL
Department of Molecular Pathology, University Hospital of Tübingen, Liebermeisterstr. 8, D-72076 Tübingen, Germany

NICK J. KNOWLES
Institute for Animal Health (IAH), Pirbright Laboratory, Ash Road, Pirbright, Woking, Surrey GU24 0NF, United Kingdom

ERNST KUECHLER
Institute of Medical Biochemistry, University of Vienna, Dr. Bohr-Gasse 9/3, Vienna, A-1030, Austria

RICHARD J. KUHN
Department of Biological Sciences, Purdue University, West Lafayette, IN 47907-1392

PALLOB KUNDU
Department of Microbiology, Immunology, and Molecular Genetics, UCLA School of Medicine, and The Molecular Biology Institute, University of California, Los Angeles, Los Angeles, CA 90095-1747

LOUIS E.-C. LEONG
Invitrogen Corp., 1600 Faraday Ave., Carlsbad, CA 92008

XUEJUN LI
Centre for Biomolecular Sciences, School of Biology, University of St. Andrews, Biomolecular Sciences Building, North Haugh, St. Andrews, Fife KY16 9ST, Scotland

HANS-DIETER LIEBIG
Institute of Medical Biochemistry, University of Vienna, Dr. Bohr-Gasse 9/3, Vienna, A-1030, Austria

RICHARD E. LLOYD
Department of Molecular Virology and Microbiology, Baylor College of Medicine, One Baylor Plaza, Houston, TX 77030

GARRY LUKE
Centre for Biomolecular Sciences, School of Biology, University of St. Andrews, Biomolecular Sciences Building, North Haugh, St. Andrews, Fife KY16 9ST, Scotland

B. JOAN MORASCO
Department of Biochemistry and Molecular Biology, College of Medicine, University of Florida, Gainesville, FL 32610-0245

WILFRED E. MARISSEN
Department of Molecular Virology and Microbiology, Baylor College of Medicine, One Baylor Plaza, Houston, TX 77030

PETER W. MASON
U.S. Department of Agriculture, Agricultural Research Service, Plum Island Animal Disease Center, P.O. Box 848, Greenport, NY 11944-0848

AMIT MEHROTRA
The School of Chemistry, The University of Birmingham, Edgbaston, Birmingham B15 2TT, United Kingdom

P. D. MINOR
Division of Virology, NIBSC, Blanche Lane, South Mimms, Potters Bar, Herts EN6 3QG, United Kingdom

SHERRY NEFF
U.S. Department of Agriculture, Agricultural Research Service, Plum Island Animal Disease Center, P.O. Box 848, Greenport, NY 11944-0848

AKIO NOMOTO
Department of Microbiology, Graduate School of Medicine, University of Tokyo, Tokyo 113-0033, Japan

LAURENT OUZILOU
Groupe de Génétique Virale-Unité NRSN, Département de Virologie, Institut Pasteur, 25, rue du Dr. Roux, 75724 Paris Cedex 15, France

MARK A. PALLANSCH
Division of Viral and Rickettsial Diseases, National Center for Infectious Diseases, Centers for Disease Control and Prevention, 1600 Clifton Rd., Mailstop G-17, Atlanta, GA 30333

ANN C. PALMENBERG
Institute for Molecular Virology, University of Wisconsin-Madison, 1525 Linden Dr., Madison, WI 53706

ANIKO V. PAUL
Department of Molecular Genetics and Microbiology, State University of New York at Stony Brook, Stony Brook, NY 11790

ISABELLE PELLETIER
Groupe de Génétique Virale-Unité NRSN, Département de Virologie, Institut Pasteur, 25, rue du Dr. Roux, 75724 Paris Cedex 15, France

JENS PETERSEN
Astra Zeneca, R & D Molndal, S-431 83 Molndal, Sweden

ROBERT H. PURCELL
Hepatitis Viruses and Molecular Hepatitis Sections, Laboratory of Infectious Diseases, National Institute of Allergy and Infectious Diseases, National Institutes of Health, Bldg. 7/202, 7 Center Dr., MSC 0740, Bethesda, MD 20892-0740

VINCENT R. RACANIELLO
Department of Microbiology, Columbia University College of Physicians & Surgeons, 701 W. 168th St., New York, NY 10032

ELIZABETH RIEDER
Department of Molecular Genetics and Microbiology, School of Medicine, State University of New York at Stony Brook, Stony Brook, NY 11794

RAYMOND P. ROOS
Department of Neurology/MC2030, University of Chicago Medical Center, 5841 S. Maryland Ave., Chicago, IL 60637

MICHAEL G. ROSSMANN
Department of Biological Sciences, Purdue University, West Lafayette, IN 47907-1392

HARLEY A. ROTBART
University of Colorado Health Sciences Center, 4200 E. 9th Ave., Box C227, Denver, CO 80262

DAVID J. ROWLANDS
Division of Microbiology, School of Biochemistry and Molecular Biology, The Old Medical School, University of Leeds, Leeds LS2 9JT, United Kingdom

SHERYL RUBINSTEIN
Department of Microbiology, Immunology, and Molecular Genetics, UCLA School of Medicine, and The Molecular Biology Institute, University of California, Los Angeles, Los Angeles, CA 90095-1747

MARTIN D. RYAN
Centre for Biomolecular Sciences, School of Biology, University of St. Andrews, Biomolecular Sciences Building, North Haugh, St. Andrews, Fife KY16 9ST, Scotland

JOACHIM SEIPELT
Institute of Medical Biochemistry, University of Vienna, Dr. Bohr-Gasse 9/3, Vienna, A-1030, Austria

HANS-CHRISTOPH SELINKA
Department of Molecular Pathology, University Hospital of Tübingen, Liebermeisterstr. 8, D-72076 Tübingen, Germany

BERT L. SEMLER
Department of Microbiology and Molecular Genetics, College of Medicine, University of California, Irvine, CA 92697-4025

JEAN-YVES SGRO
Institute for Molecular Virology, University of Wisconsin-Madison, 1525 Linden Dr., Madison, WI 53706

YUHONG SHEN
Department of Microbiology, Immunology, and Molecular Genetics, UCLA School of Medicine, and The Molecular Biology Institute, University of California, Los Angeles, Los Angeles, CA 90095-1747

TIM SKERN
Institute of Medical Biochemistry, Vienna Bio Center, University of Vienna, Dr. Bohr-Gasse 9/3, A-1030 Vienna, Austria

LUCIA EISNER SMERAGE
Department of Biochemistry and Molecular Biology, College of Medicine, University of Florida, Gainesville, FL 32610-0245

THOMAS J. SMITH
Donald Danforth Plant Science Center, 975 N. Warson Rd., St. Louis, MO 63132

FRANCISCO SOBRINO
Centro de Biología Molecular "Severo Ochoa" and CISA-INIA, 28130 Valdeolmos, Madrid, Spain

WOLFGANG SOMMERGRUBER
Boehringer Ingelheim Austria, A-1121 Vienna, Austria

GLYN STANWAY
Department of Biological Sciences, Central Campus, University of Essex, Colchester C04 3SQ, United Kingdom

EDWIN TEN DAM
Centre for Biomolecular Sciences, School of Biology, University of St. Andrews, Biomolecular Sciences Building, North Haugh, St. Andrews, Fife KY16 9ST, Scotland

NATALYA L. TETERINA
Laboratory of Infectious Diseases, National Institute of Allergy and Infectious Diseases, National Institutes of Health, Bldg. 50, Room 6120, MSC 8011, Bethesda, MD 20892-8011

STEVE TRACY
Department of Pathology and Microbiology, University of Nebraska Medical Center, 600c South 42nd St., Omaha, NE 68198-6495

MARY K. WEIDMAN
Department of Microbiology, Immunology, and Molecular Genetics, UCLA School of Medicine, and The Molecular Biology Institute, University of California, Los Angeles, Los Angeles, CA 90095-1747

ECKARD WIMMER
Department of Molecular Genetics and Microbiology, School of Medicine, State University of New York at Stony Brook, Stony Brook, NY 11794

PADMAJA YALAMANCHILI
Department of Microbiology, Immunology, and Molecular Genetics, UCLA School of Medicine, and The Molecular Biology Institute, University of California, Los Angeles, Los Angeles, CA 90095-1747

MIGUEL ZAMORA
Department of Molecular Virology and Microbiology, Baylor College of Medicine, One Baylor Plaza, Houston, TX 77030

Preface

Animal virology began with foot-and-mouth-disease virus (FMDV). This infectious entity was discovered by Friedrich Loeffler and Paul Frosch in 1898 as a "filterable agent" causing foot-and-mouth disease, an enduring curse in agriculture even today. Because of its highly contagious nature, Loeffler began to conduct all research with FMDV in northern Germany on the small island of Riems in 1908, thereby establishing the first animal virus research institute ("Forschungsanstalt für Tierseuchen") in the world.

In 1909, Karl Landsteiner and Edwin Popper succeeded in infecting two Old World monkeys with a filtrate of spinal cord material from a polio victim who had died of the terrible human disease called poliomyelitis. The monkeys developed a disease syndrome resembling that of the human disease. Landsteiner and Popper thus not only identified a virus as the cause of poliomyelitis, but also established an animal model for the study of this agent.

FMDV and poliovirus, of course, are picornaviruses. Immediately after their discovery, they were intensely studied because of the dreaded diseases they cause. In the succeeding decades, a large number of viruses have been discovered with physical properties similar to those of FMDV and poliovirus. Collectively, these viruses are classified as members of the family *Picornaviridae*.

Research on picornaviruses has yielded numerous landmark discoveries, often with an impact on virology and even biology in general. Such discoveries include the growth of these viruses in cultured human cells, development of inactivated and attenuated vaccines to prevent paralytic poliomyelitis, the demonstration that genomic RNA is infectious, the discovery of receptor-mediated determinants of susceptibility to picornavirus infection, demonstration of the first RNA-dependent RNA polymerase activity of an animal virus, the discovery of polyproteins as precursors to viral polypeptides, the discovery of virally encoded proteinases mediating polyprotein processing, the first chemical structure of the genome of an autonomously replicating RNA virus [including a 5'-linked protein and 3'-terminal poly(A)], the demonstration that a cDNA copy of a picornavirus genome could produce infectious virus, the first resolution of the three-dimensional structures of animal viruses at the atomic level, the discovery of internal ribosome entry to initiate translation on uncapped picornavirus RNAs, and the production of infectious virus in cell-free extracts programmed only with purified viral RNA.

These and numerous other remarkable studies have placed picornavirus research at the forefront of discovery in molecular virology. However, the precise details of molecular events of picornavirus replication, such as virion uncoating, translation initiation, viral RNA replication, virus assembly, and the many layers of virus-host interactions (including mechanisms of pathogenesis) remain to be elucidated. This is well documented in many chapters of this volume. It is our hope that the contributions to this volume will provide not only a summary of the many significant accomplishments in picornavirus research but also a road map of the path to future exciting discoveries for this amazing group of simple but elegant animal viruses.

In the not-too-distant future, a major payoff of picornavirus research may include the worldwide eradication of poliovirus as an agent of human disease. Such a remarkable event will mark the sunset to decades of research on wild-type polioviruses as infectious agents and will signal a new era in picornavirus research, with a challenge to develop novel models of picornavirus pathogenesis while continuing to provide experimental systems and analytical tools to address the many unsolved mechanistic questions of the picornavirus infectious cycle. Considering that human picornaviruses alone cause an estimated 6 billion infections per year in humans, inflicting misery, debilitation, and even death, these viruses will remain a challenge to humankind.

We would like to thank all authors for their excellent contributions (and their patience!) and the editorial staff at ASM Press, particularly Eleanor S. Tupper and Jeff Holtmeier, for their help in bringing this book to fruition.

Bert Semler
Irvine, California

Eckard Wimmer
Stony Brook, New York

HISTORICAL PERSPECTIVE

History of Poliomyelitis and Poliomyelitis Research

HANS J. EGGERS

1

Ἐκ μέρους γιγνώσκομεν (1 Corinthians 13:9), translated by Martin Luther, "Unser Wissen ist Stückwerk" ("for we know in part").

OLD RECORDS

Poliomyelitis, in all probability, is an infection associated with mankind since ancient times. This assumption is based on biomedical considerations, and on case descriptions in history, compatible with the diagnosis "poliomyelitis." A well-known example is that of the doorkeeper (not priest) "Ram," 18th Egyptian dynasty (1550–1333 B.C.), exhibiting on a stela a "pes equinus" and an atrophic right leg, possible consequences of a previous poliovirus infection (141). Of the several descriptions of infantile lameness in history, I mention the Scottish novelist, poet, historian, and biographer Sir Walter Scott, who in his second year of life (1773) was apparently stricken by poliomyelitis with paresis, atrophy, and retardation of growth of his right leg. But with energy he overcame this disability in a fulfilled life of many talents, achievements, travels, and service for society. Like F. D. Roosevelt later, he fought helplessness with motivation and stamina.

Michael Underwood, Licentiate in Midwifery in London, is usually credited as giving the first scientific description of poliomyelitis in *A Treatise on the Diseases of Children* (137), published in 1789, the year of the French Revolution. He deplores that diseases of children are neglected too much. In the chapter "Debility of the Lower Extremities" (see the title of Heine's book, vide infra), he describes a disease compatible with poliomyelitis. Underwood notices that it is not a common disorder, attacking chiefly children 1 to 4 or 5 years old. Apparently, Underwood saw late forms of the disease, and, "when both (legs) have been paralytic, nothing has seemed to do any good but irons to the legs...."

Heine, according to his own testimony, was stimulated to look more closely at the disease of suddenly occurring paralysis of the lower extremities by a publication on paralysis in childhood by the 28-year-old British physician John Badham (5), who asked himself the following questions:

1. What is the cause of paralysis in these 2-year-old children?
2. What is (in modern terms) the pathogenesis of this paralysis?
3. What treatment will be useful?

Before I address Heine's seminal work, a remark on the nomenclature of the disease is necessary. Paul (100) listed some of the suggested names that will appear in due course in this short essay. The designation "poliomyelitis anterior infantum resp. adultrum" was introduced in 1873 by the German professor of internal medicine (in Freiburg and Strasbourg), Adolf Kussmaul (56).

JACOB HEINE DESCRIBES SPINAL INFANTILE PARALYSIS

After this "pre"-history of poliomyelitis research, its true beginning has to be dated with the publication of Heine's book in 1840, *Beobachtungen über Lähmungszustände der untern Extremitäten und deren Behandlung* (60) (*Observations on States of Lameness of the Lower Extremities and Their Treatment*), and the second edition of this monograph in 1860 with the conspicuously changed title, *Spinale Kinderlähmung. Monographie von Jac. v. Heine* (61) (*Spinal Infantile Paralysis. Monograph by Jac. v. Heine* [Heine had been ennobled in the meantime]). Heine's critical observations and interpretations cannot be overestimated. His findings may be grossly summarized as follows:

1. In contrast to other forms of paralysis known at the time, Heine characterized the syndrome of the flaccid, atrophic, spinal form of paralysis in childhood. He emphasized the—as a rule—intact tactile sensibility. Obviously, Heine did not describe all manifestations of the etiologic entity poliomyelitis, but he was the first to create order in the chaos of manifold paralytic conditions in childhood reported so far. Heine was also aware of the fact that not only the lower extremities might be stricken (as the title

Hans J. Eggers ■ Institute of Virology, University of Cologne, Fuerst-Pueckler-Str. 56, 50935 Cologne, Germany.

of the first edition seems to suggest), but also the arms or the trunk.

2. As an orthopedist, Heine was concerned with the therapy of the late, "chronic" sequelae of poliomyelitis, but his detailed case descriptions document that by taking very careful histories he likewise recognized the "acute" stage of the disease. Children, 6 to 36 months old, thus far healthy and well shaped, suddenly suffer from various acute symptoms such as fever, irritation, convulsion, vomiting, and diarrhea. More frequently, however, these signs are lacking; there may be only slight fever. Then, suddenly, overnight, the child is paralyzed, lying weak and pale in bed, looking around as if awakening from a deep sleep. Mostly, the legs are paralyzed (see title of Heine's first edition), or only one leg. More rarely, one arm or shoulder is affected. The functions of bladder and rectum are not permanently impaired, if at all. The paretic condition may subside later, in part or to a large extent. Mental functions or functions of the sense organs are undisturbed.

3. Heine concluded from his clinical observations that the cause of the sudden flaccid paralysis should be localized in the spinal cord. He regretted the lack of data from pathology. Apparently, it was difficult for Heine to have access to autopsy findings, not at least, because he held the view—as did most of his contemporaries—of a low lethality of the disease. Furthermore, the histopathologic techniques for the study of diseases of the nervous system were not well developed at the time.

4. As already indicated, Heine had to deal with the late sequelae of the disease (in 1860 he reported on 158 cases), in particular, muscular atrophy, cessation of bone development, and lower temperature of the affected limb, ultimately leading to severe impairments and deformities.

Heine presents in his book (61) 29 superb illustrations with descriptions of orthopedic treatments and remarkable improvements of movement and independence of his patients.

Not surprisingly, Heine's orthopedic hospital in Bad Cannstadt (near Stuttgart, Germany), which he opened in 1829 at the age of 29 years, soon gained recognition, and patients from all over the world came to consult him.

DUCHENNE DE BOULOGNE: ELECTRICAL METHODS

After Heine, a very useful clinical finding was reported by Duchenne de Boulogne (36), viz., early loss of the faradic irritability of muscles later permanently paralyzed, in contrast to those that may recover. Duchenne de Boulogne, on the basis of his electrical diagnosis, pointed, like Heine, to the spinal affection of the disease. His discovery was supplemented by Wilhelm Erb's study of the "degeneration reaction" of nerves and muscles treated with galvanic current (44), originally described by Salomon (123). The clinical literature of the time details electrical investigations to define the extent of paralyses and to permit a well-defined prognosis, also in respect to rehabilitation (see also Seeligmüller [127]). However, electrical treatment did not appear useful for therapy, as already stated by Heine in 1860.

As mentioned, initially an anatomical lesion accounting for the symptoms of infantile paralysis could not be detected in the spinal cord, but the thesis of the spinal origin rested on deductions from clinical and electrical investigations. This constellation markedly influenced the clinical literature. In 1851, the well-known pediatrician F. Rilliet from Geneva published a paper, "De la paralysie essentielle chez les enfants" (106) (On idiopathic paralysis of children), in which he argued that an anatomical cause of paralysis could not be detected, and, therefore, the disease should be classified as "essential": "La paralysie est toute la maladie" (Paralysis is the whole disease), a diagnosis by exclusion. This dictum became widely known in the medical literature because Rilliet's paper was reprinted in the influential textbook by Rilliet and Barthez, Traité des Maladies des Enfants, and demotivated further search for anatomical lesions. Furthermore, the term "essential paralysis," that is, even by "careful investigation of the nervous system no material lesion of the nervous centers or its ramifications can be detected," led to a blurring of the clinical picture so well described by Heine and Duchenne de Boulogne, insofar that now, for example, even affections of the peripheral nervous system were classified as essential paralysis.

CHARCOT AND NEUROPATHOLOGY

A breakthrough in the comprehension of poliomyelitis, viz., clinical disease and pathology, was possible by progress achieved in neuropathology and neuropathologic techniques. Three key papers were published in 1870 in the same volume of the Archives de Physiologie Normale et Pathologique by Charcot and Joffroy (21), Vulpian (139), and Parrot and Joffroy (99). In the first two cases, poliomyelitic paralyses had occurred years before the patients came to autopsy due to other diseases. But in each case the necropsy findings were correlated with carefully taken clinical histories and symptoms. Furthermore, the great reputation of Charcot helped pave the way for acceptance of these significant findings. Charcot and Joffroy reported a woman who had suffered from poliomyelitis at the age of 7 years, and who died from pulmonary tuberculosis 33 years later. Interpreting the sections of the spinal cord (cervical, dorsal, and lumbar), the authors conclude that the site of affection is the gray substance of the anterior horns with loss of the motoneurons, leading to paralysis of the corresponding muscles and ultimately to muscular atrophy.

Vulpian's patient suffered from acute poliomyelitis when she was ca. 7 years old, with atrophy of the right leg and impairment of growth of this limb. The autopsy carefully performed ca. 24 h after death revealed in sections of the dorsolumbar region of the spinal cord a reduction of the right side, microscopically a dramatic loss of nerve cells in the anterior horn, substituted by connective tissue. Vulpian's case allows a better correlation between the localization of paralysis and the site of lesions in the spinal cord than that of Charcot and Joffroy. The latter authors also refer to a case of poliomyelitis with paralysis of both legs, autopsied 47 years after the acute episode, and published by Cornil in 1863 (29). The spinal cord revealed atrophy of the white portion of the spinal cord and some atrophy of the gray matter. But Cornil considered the gray matter essentially unaltered. Charcot and Joffroy state in their discussion that in the section presented by Cornil, no nerve cells are recognizable. Thus Cornil's work inadvertently confirmed the thesis of Charcot, Joffroy, and Vulpian, and, thereby, Heine's original proposal.

The third case mentioned, reported by Charcot's colleagues Parrot and Joffroy, concerned a 3-year-old boy who died in the course of a measles infection acquired during his stay in the children's hospital for treatment of a paraplegia, apparently due to poliomyelitis acquired some time ago. The autopsy confirmed again Charcot's and Vulpian's work, namely, loss of nerve cells in the anterior horns of the spinal cord. The careful investigation revealed, in addition, a spotty distribution of nerve cell necrosis. Most important, the authors noted inflammatory changes, not only where motoneurons had disappeared, but also in sections with apparently intact nervous tissue. These changes were limited to the anterior horns.

The immediate cause of the loss of the motoneurons in the anterior horn of the spinal cord remained unknown. Around 1860 to 1880 poliomyelitis was hardly considered an infectious disease, and the majority of autopsies concerned patients who had been affected by the acute disease a long time before death due to a different illness. Thus, Charcot, in his "Leçons sur les maladies du système nerveux" (20) (Lectures on the diseases of the nervous system), in 1867, considered spinal infantile paralysis a primary disease of the motoneurons of the spinal cord, leading to paralysis and atrophy of the corresponding muscles. The irritation will secondarily affect the neuroglia and adjacent anterior horns, resulting in a subacute inflammation. In essence, Charcot regarded poliomyelitis a systemic disease of the nervous system.

Necropsies perfomed early after onset of disease have rarely been reported after the initial French communications. Thus, in his review of 1880, Seeligmüller (127) (see above) could list in the literature only 12 "relatively early" cases, ranging from 2 to 24 months after onset of paralysis. This was the beginning of a largely fruitless scientific battle, namely, whether—as expressed by Charcot—the initial event in poliomyelitis might be a primary disease of the ganglion cells, the "parenchymatous" view, or whether the disease began in the neuroglia, the "interstitial" view. Nevertheless, I quickly hasten to state that in the vast literature on this problem, mostly produced by pathologists and extending from 1870 over more than six decades, several shrewd considerations are to be found.

Important progress concerning the nature of the disease was already made in 1871 by Roger and Damaschino (110), reporting on three cases. The first case had been autopsied as soon as 2 months after onset of the illness. The authors concluded that infantile spinal paralysis consisted of a myelitis of the anterior gray horns with ensuing atrophy of the corresponding nerves and muscles.

Presumably one of the first cases with careful examination of the spinal cord of a patient within days after onset of disease was reported by Drummond in 1886 (35). It concerned a girl age 5 who was in her usual health at breakfast, but then felt sick, vomited, and in the afternoon was found feverish and in grave condition, dying the same day of respiratory failure. At necropsy, the anterior gray horns between the third and fourth cervical nerves in particular seemed affected by "red softening," and this portion of the cord was studied microscopically. Scattered, minute hemorrhages, congestion with free leukocytes, and swollen neuroglia were seen. The changes were most prominent in the anterior gray horns. The large ganglionic cells were swollen, granular, and ill-defined, and the majority had lost their nuclei. These changes were limited to portions of the spinal cord, and outside the affected area, the normal state returned. Drummond stresses the fact that the anterior horns were most abundantly affected, but the anterolateral white columns and part of the posterior horns were not completely free. He also wanted "to set at rest the question ... whether the inflammation is parenchymatous or interstitial," for it was obvious that several elements were affected, though the "brunt would appear to fall on the large [ganglionic] cells."

In my judgment, one of the most thoughtful pathologic-anatomical contributions before the discovery of the etiologic agent of poliomyelitis has come from Forssner and Sjövall in Stockholm (54). They discuss Schwalbe's dictum (126) that the causal relationship of parenchymatous and interstitial processes cannot be resolved by morphologic studies. They point to the spotty distribution of lesions in the central nervous system (see also references 35 and 99), the significance of correlation of clinical course and anatomy, the inclusion of study of the meninx, and the sequence of neuronal cell death and neuronophagia. Neuronophagia occurs only after irreversible damage of the nerve cells. Interstitial changes, according to their interpretation, take place subsequently. On the basis of the autopsy of two cases of poliomyelitis acuta, review of the literature, and the unknown etiologic agent, they caution against jumping to conclusions about the causal sequence of events. They also wonder about the exclusive localization of the disease in the central nervous system, since systemic symptoms like fever strongly suggest a general infection. Because the authors' cases concerned adults (16 and 23 years old), they point to the fact that there is no difference between the infantile and adult forms of poliomyelitis, a conclusion already drawn by Duchenne de Boulogne (36), Gombault (57), and Erb (44).

MEDIN'S OBSERVATIONS AND THEIR CLINICAL IMPACT

Up to the second half of the 19th century, poliomyelitis apparently became manifest almost exclusively in the sporadic form. But after 1850, a most notable change took place in that smaller and larger outbreaks of the disease were observed. It is the historic merit of the Swedish pediatrician Karl Oskar Medin (88) to have studied in detail the Stockholm poliomyelitis epidemic in 1887 with 44 paralytic cases in children. The epidemic emerging between August 9 and September 23 (with a few cases already in May to July) allowed Medin to recognize clinical forms of the disease that, in the absence of knowledge about the etiology, had so far escaped attention (see below). Medin suggests that during the last 50 years before 1887 probably no epidemic of poliomyelitis occurred in Stockholm. For clinicians, the epidemic form was so unusual it promoted the hypothesis that sporadic and epidemic forms of poliomyelitis were different diseases. Later, isolation of the etiologic agent and serologic protection tests settled this question (see below).

Medin mentions in his 1890 paper (published 1891) a few other reports of epidemic occurrence of poliomyelitis.

Bergenholtz observed, in 1881, 13 (according to Wickman, 18) cases in Umeå, North Sweden. Colmer of Springfield, La., in the fall of 1841, was consulted by parents of a child, about 1 year old, who was recovering slowly from an attack of "hemiplegia." The parents told Colmer that 8 to 10 cases of a similar nature had occurred in the area of West Feliciana, La., where the family was residing. Cordier (28), in the fall of 1886, collected data on an outbreak of poliomyelitis in June and July 1885 with 13 cases, located in the neighborhood of Lyon, and postulated the disease to be infectious, perhaps via the respiratory tract.

An early, apparently epidemic outbreak in St. Helena was reported by Sir Charles Bell (7) in the third edition of his famous book, *The Nervous System of the Human Body*, published in 1844. A lady, the wife of the English clergyman of St. Helena, consulted Bell about her child "who had one leg much wanted in its growth." She mentioned an illness preceding this affection and reported an "epidemic fever" spreading on the island among children about 3 to 5 years of age. All children "who had the fever were similarly affected with a want of growth in some part of their body or limbs!" (case 183).

After Medin's presentation in 1890, several epidemics of poliomyelitis were described, e.g., the extensive Vermont epidemic of 1894 with 132 cases, published by Caverly in 1894 and 1896 (18, 19); the Vienna epidemic of 1898 with 42 cases (referred to by Zappert et al. [143]); and 54 cases occurring in the Bratsberg region in Norway in 1899 (80). Many more could be cited, but the important point is that now—at least in European countries and the United States—the epidemiologic characteristics of poliomyelitis changed dramatically and that detailed descriptions of the clinical course and various clinical forms could be given, among which the pioneering work of Medin stands out.

Medin described the various symptoms during the fever phase and its relation to the affections of the central nervous system, with somnolence, dyspepsia, sometimes vomiting and diarrhea, and mostly obstipation. Restlessness and pain in various parts of the body were seen often. The irregular fever rarely exceeded 39°C. The frequent somnolence Medin interpreted as functional disturbance of the cerebral cortex. Besides the characteristic spinal form, Medin described bulbar, encephalitic, polyneuritic, and atactic forms.

Since Medin listed all cranial nerves from III (oculomotorius) to XII (hypoglossus) as affected, we would subclassify the bulbar form into various classes of involvement of the brain system (e.g., bulbo-pontine).

An encephalitic form of poliomyelitis had already been described by Adolf Strümpell in 1884 and 1885 (129, 130). He postulated a disease entity of the spinal (poliomyelitis acuta) and encephalitic (poliencephalitis acuta) form, since they had in common an affection of motoneurons; thus a division would be artificial. Strümpell also postulated a unified etiology with different localizations by the same or very closely related, probably infectious, agents.

Independently, Pierre Marie (87) put forward a similar suggestion as to a relatedness of poliomyelitis and a cerebral form, the latter occurring en suite of "infectious disease." However, the good clinical descriptions of Marie are hardly compatible with the diagnosis "poliomyelitis," in particular, since infections such as pertussis and mumps preceded the disease.

Medin also elaborated on the age distribution, the development of pareses with the possibility of complete remission, and lethality (3 of 44; a further death was due to diphtheria). Medin referred to the pathologic anatomy of the disease (carried out by Rissler [107]) showing all signs of an acute infectious disease with affection of the whole organism. Medin, however, was uncertain about the contagiosity of poliomyelitis. The participants of the X International Medical Congress in Berlin (1890), where Medin presented his findings, recognized the fundamental nature of Medin's contribution.

WICKMAN'S EPIDEMIOLOGICAL INVESTIGATIONS

A pupil of Medin, unfortunately not his successor as professor of pediatrics in Stockholm, Ivar Wickman (142) made further paramount discoveries concerning the epidemiology and clinical manifestations of poliomyelitis. Wickman had painstakingly studied a further devastating poliomyelitis epidemic in Scandinavia in 1905, i.e., still before the etiologic agent of the disease had been discovered, with 1,031 victims. Wickman, like Medin and others before him, described the seasonal occurrence of the disease in the late summer and early fall, with a dramatic peak of about 370 cases in August.

Wickman's original observation was a recognition of the large percentage of abortive and nonparalytic cases, and their relevance for the spread of the infection by direct contact from person to person. Before Wickman, the thesis of poliomyelitis infection by direct contact had been highly controversial, despite some observations of spread in families (see also Medin). Caverly, having carefully studied the 1894 epidemic in Vermont with 132 cases, stated "it is very certain that it was non-contagious." The reason for this assertion was that he did not find a single instance in which more than one member of a family had the disease. Wickman, in contrast to Caverly and many other researchers, meticulously tracked the spread of infections in small parishes, e.g., in Traestena with about 500 inhabitants, mostly living in isolated, widely dispersed homes. Forty-nine persons became ill, 26 of them with significant paralysis. As a common source for radial spread of the infections, Wickman identified Traestena's school with diseased and, most important, apparently healthy children. Sometimes, family visits, carefully documented, caused the spread of the infection.

Before Wickman, cases of poliomyelitis in older children and adults had occasionally been reported (e.g., see Forssner and Sjövall, Gombault, and Erb above) in contrast to previous assumptions about the disease as almost exclusively affecting young children (e.g., Heine). Wickman, however, reported that 21.4% of the victims were older than 14 years, an age distribution not known before epidemic poliomyelitis had emerged around 1880.

LANDSTEINER AND POPPER: DISCOVERY OF THE ETIOLOGIC AGENT

Wickman's important research has only rarely been appreciated, perhaps due to the more or less simultaneous discovery of the etiologic agent by Karl Landsteiner and Erwin Popper in November/December 1908 (78). The history of the etiology of poliomyelitis is a history of errors. Before the age of microbiology, incidental events like "cooling" and dentition were frequently incriminated. George Colmer in 1843 (22) stated: "... and the cause seemed to be the same in all—, namely *teething*." Heine most critically elaborated on pathophysiologic processes, considering disturbances of the development of the central nervous system in the young children by congestion or other irritations. Bell (7) closed his above-cited statement apodictically: "This deserves to be inquired into."

At the beginning of microbiology there shortly prevailed a "coccus era," when several investigators were prejudiced by a supposed parallelism between poliomyelitis and epidemic meningitis (see also Flexner, below).

However, all in all, bacteriological findings were negative; likewise, attempts to transmit an agent to the usual laboratory animals, such as rabbits, guinea pigs, or mice, failed. Landsteiner and Popper (78) injected intraperitoneally into two Old World monkeys (*Cynocephalus hamadryas* and *Macacus rhesus*) a suspension of spinal cord from a 9-year-old boy who had succumbed to severe poliomyelitis after 4 days of illness. The two monkeys, in good condition, had been available from previous experiments with syphilis. The inoculated material, which was bacteriologically sterile, yielded negative results when injected into rabbits, guinea pigs, and mice. The two monkeys, however, exhibited lesions in the spinal cord, medulla, pons, and brain stem that were indistinguishable from those observed in cases of human poliomyelitis. The rhesus monkey developed complete flaccid paralysis of both legs. Landsteiner and Popper were unable to passage the agent, but this was achieved soon afterward and independently in 1909 by Römer (111), Flexner and Lewis (50), Leiner and von Wiesner (81), and Landsteiner and Levaditi (77). In this context it should be added that the same authors observed a marked resistance of the monkeys to a challenge of virus, even if given intracerebrally, on recovery from a previous infection. These authors (see summary by Römer [111]) independently also demonstrated in a neutralization test virus-specific antibodies in the serum of monkeys convalescent from experimental poliomyelitis. Subsequently, with tests in monkeys, Netter and Levaditi (96) reported the neutralizing substances in the serum of patients having recovered from paralytic disease up to 3 years ago. Among other things, they pointed to the possibility of retrospective diagnosis, the identity of experimental simian and natural human infection, and the identity of the classic sporadic and the epidemic forms of the disease.

A note on the speed of publication in the comparatively slow nonelectronic early 20th century may be of interest. Popper's patient died on November 18, 1908, and Landsteiner reported on the successful transmission of the agent to monkeys and the histopathologic changes in the session of the k. k. Gesellschaft der Aerzte in Wien held in Vienna, Austria, on December 18, 1908. The proceedings of the session were published in the *Wiener klinische Wochenschrift* in issue 52, in 1908.

FLEXNER AND THE YOUNG SWEDISH INVESTIGATORS

As early as 1910, Flexner and Lewis (51) had cautiously suggested that poliovirus gained access to the central nervous system via the nasopharyngeal mucosa, where the virus of patients and healthy carriers had been demonstrated (49). This hypothesis was supported by experiments with monkeys performed by Flexner's group (48) and by Leiner and von Wiesner (82): swabs containing poliovirus were introduced into the nose and rubbed vigorously over the upper nasal mucous membrane, with ensuing clinical poliomyelitis. Likewise, Flexner and Lewis assumed that the virus left the body from the meninges by way of the lymphatics of the nasal and pharyngeal mucosa, through the cribriform plate (52). The authors supported their argument by pointing to the close similarities between epidemic poliomyelitis and meningococcal meningitis (51). Neustädter and Thro (97), in addition, thought to have proven that dust in the rooms of poliomyelitis patients contained the virus, and thus gained access to the nasopharynx. They, like Flexner and Lewis (51), recommended disinfection of the secretions of the nasal and buccal cavities for prophylaxis. Flexner's views on the neurotropism of poliovirus and on its entry into the body by the nasal route (47) dominated poliovirology so that other experimental evidence was more or less neglected for about 25 years until the 1930s.

In particular, the exciting results published in 1912 by a young Swedish team consisting of Carl Kling, Wilhelm Wernstedt, and Alfred Pettersson (73, 74, 103, 128) were essentially disregarded: the authors had demonstrated poliovirus in fatal and nonfatal cases of poliomyelitis, not only, as expected, from the oropharynx, nose, and trachea, but also from the small intestine. Virus was furthermore demonstrated in abortive cases and in healthy families with no known direct contact with poliomyelitis cases. Thus, virological studies strongly supported the epidemiological studies of Wickman and several other investigators. The Swedish authors considered the number of "healthy carriers" four to five times more frequent than patients with manifest symptoms. The combined epidemiologic and virologic studies led to the practical conclusion that quarantine measures for prevention of spread of the infection would be useless.

Kling et al. hypothesized that the intestine might be an important source for the spread of poliovirus infection. Besides their virological findings, they implicated the seasonal distribution (late summer and fall) and the analogy to cholera, dysentery, and typhoid fever.

Although influential investigators like Flexner were fully aware of the results of the Swedish group (Flexner attended the 1912 congress [47]; see also reference 49), the presence of poliovirus in the intestines and its pathogenic significance were not seriously pursued. Besides Flexner's views, methodologic criticism also was not wholly unfounded. Sabin and Ward (120, 121) rightly pointed out that Kling et al. often used criteria for the presence of virus that were later found not acceptable. Furthermore, Kling et al. isolated the virus not only from the washings of the small intestine in fatal cases of poliomyelitis but also found the virus in washings from the mouth, nose, pharynx, and trachea (see above). These findings could not elucidate the origin of the virus; for example, its presence in the washings of the small intestine was at the time also interpreted as representing virus that had been swallowed.

Experiments in rhesus monkeys (83) and cynomolgus monkeys (17, 72) demonstrated the possibility of poliovirus infections via the gut and not involving the olfactory pathway, but it remained questionable whether these studies were relevant for elucidation of poliovirus infections of humans.

Finally, in the late 1930s, incontrovertible evidence was brought forth for the presence of virus in the stools of patients with paralytic or nonparalytic poliomyelitis and in contacts as well (59, 68, 76, 133, 134). This important finding, however, again threw little light on the essential nature of the human disease, since there was as yet no indication that the virus in the stools did not have its origin in swallowed secretions (see above).

SABIN'S EARLY CONTRIBUTION ON PATHOGENESIS

The definitive report by Albert Sabin and Robert Ward (121) in 1941 on the natural history of human poliomyelitis settled important issues. By meticulous technique (the authors themselves performed necropsies on fatal poliomyelitis cases), they proved that the virus is distributed predominantly in two systems: (i) certain regions of the nervous system and (ii) the alimentary tract.

Presence of virus in the walls of the alimentary tract appeared to be primary localization and portal of entry. Virus was absent in the nasal mucosa, olfactory bulbs, and anterior perforated substance, which suggested that neither the respiratory tract nor the olfactory pathway is of significance in cases of natural human poliomyelitis (see above). In line with these results were the pathology studies by Cowie et al. (30) during the Michigan poliomyelitis epidemic of 1931 with 1,132 cases reported: the authors were unable to demonstrate changes in the olfactory nerves. Similar results were obtained by Smith (quoted by Sabin and Olitsky [119]). Analogous findings were reported in experiments with chimpanzees by Howe and Bodian (69). Thus, ultimately, an old dogma with epidemiologic and preventive implications could be abandoned (see also Harmon [59]).

The distribution of virus in the central nervous system is limited to certain areas and is not as indiscriminately disseminated as viruses (e.g., equine encephalomyelitis) that can invade through the blood vessels.

In this connection I may return to the once intensely debated question of the primary attack of poliovirus in the central nervous system (see above). Studies in experimental animals allowed the earliest histopathologic changes to be defined. Among others, the investigations of Fairbrother and Hurst (46), Bodian (9, 12), and Sabin and Ward (120) (who tried to define criteria for the diagnosis of poliomyelitis in monkeys) are particularly telling in that they leave no longer any doubt that primarily the neuronal cells are attacked, with cellular changes and associated development of high concentration of virus in the absence of inflammatory exudate. Thus, it was concluded that the involvement of ganglion cells is the result of virus multiplication and not of an inflammatory process, which only follows as response to nerve cell injury. Similar changes in human cases have been found in patients who died early during the disease. A very good pictorial document of the series of events can be found in plate 38 of Sabin and Ward's paper (120). These authors address also the histopathology of abortive and paralytic poliomyelitis and stress the point that the host does not need all its anterior horn nerve cells for apparently normal function. This certainly bears on the question of transitory paralysis in that an apparently normal function can be carried on with fewer than the normal number of nerve cells, and may not be a consequence of a postulated receding edema or other inflammatory changes.

It is now evident how Charcot could picture poliomyelitis as a systemic disease of the central nervous system (see above): he saw only the residues many years after the acute stage and was impressed by the selective loss of motoneurons in the anterior horns of the spinal cord.

BURNET AND MACNAMARA DISCOVER TYPE DIVERSITY

One high point of poliovirus research was the finding in 1931 by the Australians Frank M. Burnet and Jean Macnamara (16) that there existed antigenic differences between strains of poliovirus. So far, a complete similarity of the different strains had been assumed. The Australian authors compared the famous Rockefeller MV strain (see below) with a local strain isolated in Melbourne and found striking differences in cross-immunity experiments and neutralization tests in monkeys. The report was greeted with skepticism, since it came from unknown investigators on a remote continent. But in light of the ill-fated vaccine trials in the mid-1930s (13, 75), the significance of this finding was realized by Hammon, Francis, and Rivers (8).

Finally, the problem of the immunological types of poliovirus was settled by the comprehensive experiments organized and conducted by the Committee on Typing of the National Foundation for Infantile Paralysis (NFIP) in the 1940s (27).

PHILANTHROPIC ORGANIZATIONS

A brief note on philanthropic and granting agencies and their significance for poliomyelitis research in the United States is in order. In 1921, the New York lawyer Franklin Delano Roosevelt was stricken with poliomyelitis, but despite his severe disability, he in 1933 took office as President of the United States, and as a political figure, became a symbol of hope for countless victims of the disease. The nation was mobilized to provide support for all aspects of poliomyelitis: patients' care, informing the public, and finance research. On Roosevelt's birthday, January 30, Birthday Balls were held to raise funds; the President's Birthday Ball Commission in 1938 was followed by the NFIP. Critical for success was the feeling that the entire nation was involved to fight and eradicate a single, terrible disease.

Behind such organizations able and motivated individuals will lead to success, financially and scientifically. I will mention only Paul deKruif, author of *Microbe Hunters*; Basil O'Connor, Roosevelt's partner in the New York law firm; and Thomas Milton Rivers, eminent scientist of the Rockefeller Institute for Medical Research, the leading scientific spirit of the NFIP. It is fair to add that in many countries similar organizations were instrumental in supporting the fight against poliomyelitis.

POLIOVIRUS ADAPTED TO THE MOUSE

A further highlight of poliovirus research was the adaptation of the Lansing strain of poliovirus to mice by the persistent efforts of Charles Armstrong in 1939 (4). This meant that at least one strain of poliovirus was available for research and clinical epidemiological purposes in an animal far less expensive than the monkey.

Some years earlier Maurice Brodie et al. (14) had tried with ingenious techniques to multiply poliovirus in mice in support of Brodie's vaccine trials, but with the vaccine failures this work was neglected. All the more must Armstrong's persistence be admired. In this context it should be mentioned that Max Theiler (132)—in analogy to his work on yellow fever—performed more than 80 serial mouse passages with the Lansing strain and observed a dramatic attenuation—a term used first by John Kolmer of Philadelphia in connection with poliomyelitis vaccines—of the virus after intracerebral inoculation of rhesus monkeys, reducing the rate of paralysis from 100 to 0%. Rapid passages, this time in cell culture, led to the attenuated type 3 Sabin vaccine strain.

Important issues of the pathogenesis of poliomyelitis have not been settled, despite a vast amount of brilliant experimental work and sophisticated arguments (11, 12, 45, 66, 115). It has early been obvious to many investigators (88, 102, 107, 129) that poliomyelitis is a general infection of the whole body. Rissler (107), in addition to his admirable work on the neuropathology of the disease, called attention to the involvement of the intestinal mucosa and the spleen. Robertson (109) carried out six comprehensive autopsies on cases occurring in the Minnesota epidemic of 1909 and pointed to his finding of a "general toxemia": the parenchyma of the heart, liver, and kidneys was the seat of cloudy swelling, and invariably the lymph nodes and spleen showed the "customary reaction to the presence of a toxin in the general circulation." Besides pathological studies on fatal human cases (121), experimental animal work appeared imperative, but the limitations of studies in rhesus and cynomolgus monkeys to elucidate the natural history of poliovirus infections were obvious to many investigators.

BODIAN: CHIMPANZEES AS USEFUL RESEARCH ANIMALS

A chance observation in Cologne, Germany, led to the use of chimpanzees in poliomyelitis research, first by Howe and Bodian (69). There had been two cases of poliomyelitis with paralysis in chimpanzees in the Cologne zoo studied by the pediatrician Dr. Grimm of the Abraham von Oppenheim Kinderhospital. One of the chimpanzees died 4 weeks later from a respiratory infection, and autopsy by Walter Müller (92) revealed that the histopathological lesions in the central nervous system corresponded exactly to the clinical neurological findings. Mainly by the work of Howe and Bodian, it became clear that investigations with chimpanzees offered a suitable model for elucidation of the pathogenesis of poliomyelitis in humans. With added information from Sabin's investigations (reviewed by Sabin [117]), it was apparent that susceptibilities of various parts of the central nervous system and the alimentary tract in chimpanzees and humans were fairly similar, at least as compared to that of rhesus monkeys.

Bodian's work (11, 12) in poliovirus-infected chimpanzees resulted in a scheme illustrating the primary sites of viral implantation and multiplication and the pathways of viral spread in the body. The ingested virus was considered to multiply primarily in lymphatic tissues (tonsils, Peyer's patches), and secondarily in deep cervical and mesenteric lymph nodes. By the hemal route virus reaches a limited number of target organs, the most important being the central nervous system.

HORSTMANN: VIREMIA

With the recognition of the gut as the primary site of infection and multiplication (see above), regardless of whether the mucosa itself or lymphatic structures, the central question arose: how does the virus spread in the body and reach the central nervous system? Search for poliovirus in the blood of humans early on had been negative. Very rarely, virus had been recovered (1910–1914) from the blood of monkeys experimentally infected (reviewed by Ward et al. [140]). The breakthrough came with the studies in chimpanzees and humans by Dorothy Horstmann at Yale and by Bodian (reviewed by Horstmann et al. [67]). A crucial point was to try isolation during the incubation period, well before onset of paralysis, since patients with signs of central nervous involvement already had significant levels of circulating neutralizing antibodies.

The finally well-established viremia, however, could be interpreted differently from that of Bodian; e.g., Sabin considered viremia as means to amplify virus in various extraneural tissues from where poliovirus subsequently reached the central nervous system via neural, axonal spread (115). This complex issue has so far not been settled. Unquestionably, poliovirus can reach the central nervous system by the neural route, as already shown by Leiner and v. Wiesner (82), who were able to protect the monkey by clamping the virus-inoculated nervus ischiadicus, as done later analogously by Nathanson and Bodian (93). Several investigators around the turn of the century envisioned great similarities between poliomyelitis and rabies. The experiences of the tragic "Cutter incident" in 1955 also lent support to neural spread of poliovirus in the body (94). Some of the pros and cons of the relevant arguments as to the spread of poliovirus in humans are to be found in the above cited references on pathogenesis and in a review by Eggers (39).

Concerning the sites of poliovirus replication in extraneural organs besides the gut, little attention has been paid to cardiac lesions and symptoms, though from early on clinicians were confronted with cardiovascular complications in poliomyelitis patients. Certainly, the question arose whether cardiovascular symptoms were due to central nervous regulatory disturbances, to hypoxia, or to replication of poliovirus in the myocardium itself. Pathologists mostly did not question the specificity of poliomyocarditis (1, 86, 109, 124, and many others), but indisputable virus isolation from the heart of poliomyelitis cases has not been reported. Mice inoculated with various type 2 (or chimeric) poliovirus strains exhibit virus replication in the myocardium and characteristic histopathologic changes with loss of cross-striation and nuclear pycnosis in the myocardiocytes, and cellular infiltrates (39, 42). In view of the unquestionable cardiotropism of enteroviruses in humans (coxsackievirus, echovirus), these findings with polioviruses are not surprising.

Two additional remarks on pathogenetic problems of poliomyelitis seem in order. In the early literature the meninges have often been considered the portal of virus entry into the central nervous system. Sabin (112) rectifies this view: the cells present in the meninges actually represent an overflow from the perivascular spaces and are thus secondary to neuronal damage rather than the result of a true meningitis. The so-called signs of meningeal irritation are accordingly properly regarded as earliest signs of neuronal damage.

A further point is the finding that virus activity, nerve cell changes, and inflammatory reactions are localized in certain regions of the central nervous system, as expected from the different sensitivities of various neuronal regions (see above) in the same host and different species. Furthermore, well known from general virology, the virus variant is of utmost importance as already shown, e.g., in studies with "pantropic," "neurotropic" (93), and "attenuated" virus strains (117, 132). Nevertheless, a pattern of distribution of lesions of poliomyelitis in the central nervous system has been worked out since the classic investigations of Harbitz and Scheel (58), Bodian (10), and many others.

ENDERS', WELLER'S, AND ROBBINS' SEMINAL DISCOVERY

Very early (1910) attempts were made to replicate poliovirus in tissue culture or even in cell-free media (53, 84, 85). But as Sabin and Olitsky stated in their famous paper in 1936 (118), "there is no unequivocal evidence that the virus of poliomyelitis has as yet been successfully cultivated outside the body." In fact, the "globoid bodies" of Flexner and Noguchi (53) as the supposed etiologic agent of poliomyelitis so many years after Landsteiner's and Popper's discovery have been a most unfortunate research project.

Sabin and Olitsky (118) used various carefully dissected tissues of 3- to 4-month-old human embryos, e.g., brain and cord, lungs, kidney, liver, and spleen. The virus was the above-mentioned MV (mixed virus) strain of the Rockefeller Institute, a virus mixture prepared by Amoss in 1914 and kept for decades through numerous intracerebral passages in monkeys (114). The authors found that the virus multiplied readily only in the presence of nervous tissue, as evidenced by experiments in monkeys, with inclusion of neutralization tests. The experiments appeared interesting at the time, but of little practical value, and with the unfortunate choice of the highly neurotropic MV variant again apparently confirming the selective tropism of polioviruses for nervous tissue.

Despite this depressing failure and in view of the mounting evidence of the extraneural multiplication of poliovirus (see above), John Enders and his young collaborators Thomas Weller and Frederick Robbins made further attempts to cultivate poliovirus in vitro, in particular after Weller's successful cultivation of mumps virus in vitro. Enders and coworkers (43) demonstrated the dramatic replication of Lansing virus (testable in mice) in human embryonic cultures composed chiefly of skin, muscle, and connective tissue from the arms and legs, in cultures of human embryonic intestine, and in those of nervous tissue. It was Robbins who first recognized differences in cell morphology between virus-inoculated and control cultures (A. B. Sabin, personal communication, 1958), an obviously most important observation. Enders coined the term "cytopathic effects."

The implications of this famous paper, published in *Science* on January 28, 1949, were enormous and well recognized by the authors, but surprisingly not by all colleagues in poliomyelitis research, at least initially. Enders et al. readily demonstrated the multiplication of all three poliovirus types in various primate tissues, not least in nonnervous tissues, and showed that large amounts of virus could be propagated in vitro, that cultures most sensitive to the isolation of virus could be obtained in abundant amounts, and that precise quantitation of infectious virus could easily be achieved. Furthermore, besides Gilbert Dalldorf's and Grace Sickles' (31) isolation in newborn mice of coxsackieviruses, another major group of enteroviruses pathogenic for humans, the soon to be recognized potential of cell culture techniques led to the discovery of echoviruses, likewise important agents of human disease. Cooperative studies of active researchers in the field led to early definition of prototypes of enteroviruses on a serological basis, thus avoiding much confusion and duplication of work (24–26, 89). In particular, it was realized that no single property related to pathogenicity can be used to classify viruses (40).

The cell culture technique also allowed epidemiological studies so far impossible: this concerned virus isolation and seroepidemiological investigations.

EPIDEMIOLOGICAL INVESTIGATIONS AFTER WICKMAN

On epidemiological grounds, Wernstedt in 1912 (see Pettersson's report in Washington [103]) had already argued that substantial immunization of large segments of the population might take place by mild abortive cases and "virus carriers." This, conversely, would explain the apparent isolated, "sporadic" paralytic cases. He used the metaphor of a mountain range masked by fog with only certain peaks visible (a forerunner of the iceberg picture). Wernstedt came to the conclusion that the epidemiologic pattern of poliovirus infections was similar to that of measles, except certainly the obviously different manifestation rates.

First hints of widespread seropositivity in normal adults were obtained by Anderson and Frost (3), and a definite statement of seroconversion by abortive infection with protective antibody amounts was given by Peabody et al. (102).

Later, after Armstrong's discovery, more extensive and quantitative neutralization tests with type 2 could be done in mice. Thus, Turner et al. (135, 136) surveyed the immune status of different age groups in Baltimore, considering also the sociologic stratum of the population. Well known became the investigations of Paul et al. (101) demonstrating the early infection of children living under primitive sanitary conditions, e.g., in Cairo, Egypt, as compared to the more gradual acquaintance of type 2 neutralizing antibodies in children and adults in Miami, Fla., or in Iceland. In summary, the vast majority of the world population was shown to acquire poliomyelitis antibodies without recognizable clinical manifestations, but dependent on social (historic, geographic) circumstances.

As to age incidence, it has been observed that paralysis in young children is generally less severe than that in older age groups, and the incidence of nonparalytic poliomyelitis was found to be higher among children under 5 years of age than among older individuals. A quantitative study addressing this aspect was carried out by Melnick and Ledinko in Winston-Salem, N.C. (90), calculating the number of clinically recognized cases per thousand subclinical infections as 10 for the 1- to 2-year age group, 14 for the 3- to 4-year age group, 16 for the 5- to 9-year age group, and 11 for the 10- to 14-year age group. These results, however, demonstrate that the paralytic attack rate in nonimmune children and adolescents is not sufficiently different to account for the commonly observed mildness of the infection during the first years of age. Nevertheless, Gunnar Olin has shown in careful long-term (1905–1950) epidemiological studies in Sweden that with increasing age the probability of a serious clinical course is higher than in younger children (98). A reasonable interpretation of this phenomenon is not at hand, and has been analyzed by Burnet (15), Sabin (113), Horstmann (65), and Nathanson and Martin (95). It should be stressed in this context that a comprehensive explanation for the epidemicity of poliomyelitis during the last 120 years is lacking, too. The interactions of virus (virulence, contagiosity) and host (age, innate [genetic] resistance, immunity) appear very complex.

VACCINES

At the close of the 20th century, younger clinicians and virologists will not be able to appreciate the threat of poliomyelitis before 1954 (i.e., the prevaccine era), a disease annually crippling more than half a million people of all ages around the globe (in the United States alone about 21,000 paralytic cases were reported each year [89]), and often leading to death after a torturous agony (78, 110, 142). The work of Enders et al. paved the way for the two kinds of effective poliovirus vaccines, the inactivated poliovirus vaccine associated with Jonas E. Salk (122) and the live oral vaccine of Albert B. Sabin (116, 117), ultimately licensed in preference to other developments. The achievements of Hilary Koprowski and Herald Cox, however, should not be forgotten (108). Nevertheless, without the pioneering work of Enders, Weller, and Robbins, no potent vaccine against poliomyelitis could have been developed.

MOLECULAR VIROLOGY

Last but not least, the seminal paper of Enders et al. was the starting point of modern poliovirology. And it launched the scientific revolution rightly called molecular virology. In view of the multitude of highpoints, it is impossible to report justly the often interwoven achievements of polio- and picornavirology during the last 50 years. Fortunately, this will be the subject of many chapters of this book. I shall try to list a few landmarks.

The plaque assay of Dulbecco and Vogt (37) (first reported for WEE virus) permitted precise and practical quantitation of virus infectivity so far possible only in bacteriophage systems. Defining the nutritional requirements of cultured cells (38) allowed biochemical experiments in virus-infected cells with determination of, e.g., the kinetics of viral RNA and protein synthesis (32, 33). Earlier, Schaffer and Schwerdt (125) reported crystallization of purified MEF-1 (type 2) virus. Refinement of x-ray crystallography culminated in the elucidation of the three-dimensional structure of poliovirus (and other picornaviruses) at the 2.9 Å resolution level (63).

In line with earlier work on tobacco mosaic virus, it was shown that isolated picornaviral RNA was infectious for cultured cells (2, 23). This experiment proved that RNA of the virus particle could act as messenger RNA, and was further extended to demonstrate that infectious RNA does transcend the restricted host range barriers of picornaviruses, which led to the concept of specific cell receptors for the virus particle (64) and culminated in the discovery of receptor families for picornaviruses. In the replication cycle of picornaviruses several essential characteristics were discovered: (i) the RNA-dependent RNA polymerase (6, 55), (ii) the base-pairing mechanism during viral RNA replication, the "replicative form" (91), and (iii) the proteolytic cleavage of the large polyprotein synthesized by viral RNA (70, 131).

A further highlight in poliovirus research was the sequence analysis of the viral RNA in 1981 (71, 105). Combined with previous knowledge the genetic organization of picornaviral RNA was established. Recombination with poliovirus was first achieved by Hirst (62), and particularly by Nada Ledinko in Hirst's laboratory (79). Such studies were rendered difficult by the high mutation rates (average number of mutations per replication) of picornaviruses, on the order of 10^{-3} to 10^{-4} (41). Later on, using the same strategy by measuring reversion from viral drug dependence to independence, but now also taking into consideration the target size for the reversion, de la Torre et al. (34) arrived at similar figures. The observed phenomena were later viewed as intrinsic to the replication of RNA viruses, leading to the concept of "quasispecies" populations, i.e., "mutant swarms."

Genetic studies of poliovirus were made ultimately more feasible by the highly significant discovery that full-length cDNA clones produced progeny virus after transfection (104), and the use of T7 RNA polymerase to prepare full-length transcripts of the cDNA in vitro (138).

Having looked at some aspects of the long history of poliomyelitis, one of the dreadful plagues of mankind, and the ultimate triumphs of medical and basic virus research, we hope that continued efforts and vigilance will lead to eradication of the disease and save us from epidemics of newly emerging virulent picornavirus variants, such as coxsackievirus A7 or enterovirus 71 (89).

I am deeply grateful to my teachers Sven Gard, Wilson Smith, Albert Sabin, and Igor Tamm, who not only introduced me to virology, but made me personally meet most noted virologists living in the second half of the 20th century. Thomas Müller of our institute, never tired, helped me secure the ocean of literature on poliomyelitis. The staff of Bureau U. A. R. T. intelligently and cheerfully typed my drafts. I have made all efforts to do justice to the many investigators in the field of poliomyelitis, though knowing that this is impossible. John Paul's book and not least monographs of the early 20th century (Römer, Wickman, Seeligmüller, etc.) have been valuable sources.

REFERENCES

1. **Abramson, H. L.** 1918. Pathologic report of forty-three cases of acute poliomyelitis. *Arch. Intern. Med.* **22:**312–330.
2. **Alexander, H. E., G. Koch, I. M. Mountain, K. Sprunt, and O. Van Damme.** 1958. Infectivity of ribonucleic acid of poliovirus on HeLa cell monolayers. *Virology* **5:**172–173.
3. **Anderson, J. F., and W. H. Frost.** 1911. Abortive cases of poliomyelitis. *JAMA* **56:**663–667.
4. **Armstrong, C.** 1939. Successful transfer of the Lansing strain of poliomyelitis virus from the cotton rat to the white mouse. *Public Health Rep.* **54:**2302–2305.
5. **Badham, J.** 1835–1836. Paralysis in childhood. Four remarkable cases of suddenly induced paralysis in the extremities, occurring in children, without any apparent cerebral or cerebro-spinal lesion. *London Med. Gaz.* **17:**215–218.
6. **Baltimore, D., H. J. Eggers, R. M. Franklin, and I. Tamm.** 1963. Poliovirus-induced RNA polymerase and the effects of virus-specific inhibitors on its production. *Proc. Natl. Acad. Sci. USA* **49:**843–849.
7. **Bell, C.** 1844. *The Nervous System of the Human Body*, 3rd ed. Henry Renshaw, London, United Kingdom.
8. **Benison, S.** 1967. *Tom Rivers. Reflections on a Life in Medicine and Science*. The M. I. T. Press, Cambridge, Mass.
9. **Bodian, D.** 1948. The virus, the nerve cell, and paralysis; a study of experimental poliomyelitis in the spinal cord. *Bull. Johns Hopkins Hosp.* **83:**1–107.
10. **Bodian, D.** 1949. Poliomyelitis: pathologic anatomy, p. 62–84. In *Poliomyelitis: Papers and Discussions Presented at the First International Poliomyelitis Conference*. Lippincott, Philadelphia, Pa.
11. **Bodian, D.** 1955. Emerging concept of poliomyelitis infection. *Science* **122:**105–108.
12. **Bodian, D.** 1958. Some physiologic aspects of poliovirus infections, p. 23–56. In *The Harvey Lectures 1956–1957*, Series 52. Academic Press, New York, N.Y.
13. **Brodie, M., and W. H. Park.** 1936. Active immunization against poliomyelitis. *Am. J. Public Health* **26:**119–125.
14. **Brodie, M., S. A. Goldberg, and P. Stanley.** 1935. Transmission of the virus of poliomyelitis to mice. *Science* **81:**319–320.
15. **Burnet, F. M.** 1940. The epidemiology of poliomyelitis, with special reference to the Victorian epidemic of 1937–38. *Med. J. Aust.* **27:**325–335.
16. **Burnet, F. M., and J. Macnamara.** 1931. Immunological differences between strains of poliomyelitis virus. *Br. J. Exp. Pathol.* **12:**57–61.
17. **Burnet, F. M., A. V. Jackson, and E. G. Robertson.** 1939. Poliomyelitis: 3. The use of Macacus cynomolgus as an experimental animal. *Aust. J. Exp. Biol. Med. Sci.* **17:**375–391.
18. **Caverly, C. S.** 1894. History of an epidemic of acute nervous disease of unusual type. *Med. Rec.* **46:**673–677.
19. **Caverly, C. S.** 1896. Notes of an epidemic of acute anterior poliomyelitis. *JAMA* **26:**1–5.
20. **Charcot, J. M.** 1874. *Klinische Vorträge über Krankheiten des Nervensystems (Autorisierte Übersetzung)*. Verlag der J. B. Metzler'schen Buchhandlung, Stuttgart, Germany.

21. **Charcot, J. M., and A. Joffroy.** 1870. Cas de paralysie infantile spinale avec lésions des cornes antérieures de la substance grise de la moelle épinière. *Arch. Physiol. Norm. Pathol.* **3:**134–152.
22. **Colmer, G.** 1843. Paralysis in teething children. *Am. J. Med. Sci.* **5:**248.
23. **Colter, J. S., H. H. Bird, A. W. Moyer, and R. A. Brown.** 1957. Infectivity of ribonucleic acid isolated from virus-infected tissues. *Virology* **4:**522–532.
24. **Committee on Enteroviruses.** 1962. Classification of human enteroviruses. *Virology* **16:**501–504.
25. **Committee on the ECHO Viruses.** 1955. Enteric cytopathogenic human orphan (ECHO) viruses. *Science* **122:**1187–1188.
26. **Committee on the Enteroviruses.** 1957. The enteroviruses. *Am. J. Public Health* **47:**1556–1566.
27. **Committee on Typing of the National Foundation for Infantile Paralysis.** 1951. Immunologic classification of poliomyelitis viruses. *Am. J. Hyg.* **51:**191–274.
28. **Cordier, S.** 1888. Relation d'une épidémie de paralysie atrophique de l'infance. *Lyon Méd.* **57:**5–12; 48–53.
29. **Cornil, V.** 1863. Paralysie infantile; cancer des seins; autopsie: altérations de la moelle épinière, des nerfs et des muscles; généralisation du cancer. *Compt. Rend. Soc. Biol., Paris* **5:**187–192.
30. **Cowie, D. M., J. P. Parsons, and K. Lowenberg.** 1934. Clinico-pathologic observations on infantile paralysis: report of 125 acute cases with special reference to the therapeutic use of convalescent and adult blood transfusions: the possible relation of blood group to the severity of the disease. *Ann. Intern. Med.* **8:**521–551.
31. **Dalldorf, G., and G. M. Sickles.** 1948. An unidentified, filtrable agent isolated from the feces of children with paralysis. *Science* **108:**61–62.
32. **Darnell, J. E., and L. Levintow.** 1960. Poliovirus protein: source of amino acids and time course of synthesis. *J. Biol. Chem.* **235:**74–77.
33. **Darnell, J. E., L. Levintow, M. M. Thoren, and J. L. Hooper.** 1961. The time course of synthesis of poliovirus RNA. *Virology* **13:**271–279.
34. **de la Torre, J. C., E. Wimmer, and J. J. Holland.** 1990. Very high frequency of reversion to guanidine resistance in clonal pools of guanidine-dependent type 1 poliovirus. *J. Virol.* **64:**664–671.
35. **Drummond, D.** 1886. On the nature of the spinal lesion in polio-myelitis anterior acuta, or infantile paralysis. *Brain* **8:**14–20.
36. **Duchenne de Boulogne, G. B. A.** 1855. De l'Électrication Localisée et de Son Application à la Physiologie, à la Pathologie et à la Thérapeutique. J.-B. Baillière, Paris, France.
37. **Dulbecco, R., and M. Vogt.** 1954. Plaque formation and isolation of pure lines with poliomyelitis virus. *J. Exp. Med.* **99:**167–182.
38. **Eagle, H.** 1955. Nutritional needs of mammalian cells in tissue culture. *Science* **122:**501–505.
39. **Eggers, H. J.** 1993. Considerations and experiments on the pathogenesis of enterovirus disease, p. 499–515. *In* W. Doerfler and P. Böhm (ed.), *Virus Strategies.* VCH Verlagsgesellschaft, Weinheim, Germany.
40. **Eggers, H. J., and A. B. Sabin.** 1959. Factors determining pathogenicity of variants of ECHO 9 virus for newborn mice. *J. Exp. Med.* **110:**951–967.
41. **Eggers, H. J., and I. Tamm.** 1965. Coxsackie A 9 virus: mutation from drug dependence to drug independence. *Science* **148:**97–98.
42. **Eggers, H. J., and T. Mertens.** 1987. Viruses and myocardium: notes of a virologist. *Eur. Heart J.* **8**(Suppl. J.):129–133.
43. **Enders, J. F., T. H. Weller, and F. C. Robbins.** 1949. Cultivation of the Lansing strain of poliomyelitis virus in cultures of various human embryonic tissues. *Science* **109:**85–87.
44. **Erb, W.** 1875. Ueber acute Spinallähmung (poliomyelitis anterior acuta) bei Erwachsenen und über verwandte spinale Erkrankungen. *Arch. Psychiatrie und Nervenkrankheiten* **5:**758–791.
45. **Faber, H. K.** 1955. *The Pathogenesis of Poliomyelitis.* Charles C Thomas, Springfield, Ill.
46. **Fairbrother, R. W., and E. W. Hurst.** 1930. The pathogenesis of, and propagation of the virus in, experimental poliomyelitis. *J. Pathol.* **33:**17–45.
47. **Flexner, S.** 1912. The mode of infection in epidemic poliomyelitis, p. 591–595. *Transactions Fifteenth International Congress on Hygiene and Demography*, Washington, Sept. 25–28, 1912, Joint Session of Sections I and V, Sept. 26, 1912.
48. **Flexner, S., and P. F. Clark.** 1912/13. A note on the mode of infection of epidemic poliomyelitis. *Proc. Soc. Exp. Biol. Med.* **10:**1–2.
49. **Flexner, S., P. F. Clark, and F. R. Fraser.** 1913. Epidemic poliomyelitis. Fourteenth note: passive human carriage of the virus of poliomyelitis. *JAMA* **60:**201–202.
50. **Flexner, S., and P. A. Lewis.** 1909. The transmission of acute poliomyelitis in monkeys. *JAMA* **53:**1639.
51. **Flexner, S., and P. A. Lewis.** 1910. Epidemic poliomyelitis in monkeys. A mode of spontaneous infection. *JAMA* **54:**535.
52. **Flexner, S., and P. A. Lewis.** 1910. Experimental epidemic poliomyelitis in monkeys. *J. Exp. Med.* **12:**227–255.
53. **Flexner, S., and H. Noguchi.** 1913. Experiments on the cultivation of the microorganism causing epidemic poliomyelitis. *J. Exp. Med.* **18:**461–485.
54. **Forssner, G., and Sjövall, E.** 1907. Ueber die Poliomyelitis acuta samt einem Beitrag zur Neuronophagiefrage. *Z. Klin. Med.* **63:**1–30.
55. **Franklin, R. M., and D. Baltimore.** 1962. Patterns of macromolecular synthesis in normal and virus-infected mammalian cells. *Cold Spring Harbor Symp. Quant. Biol.* **27:**175–194.
56. **Frey, A.** 1874. Ein Fall von subacuter Lähmung Erwachsener—wahrscheinlich Poliomyelitis anterior subacuta. *Berl. Klin. Wochenschr.* **11:**549–551; 566–568.
57. **Gombault, M.** 1873. Note sur un cas de paralysie spinale de l'adulte, suivi d'autopsie. *Arch. Physiol. Norm. Pathol.* **5:**80–88.
58. **Harbitz, F., and O. Scheel.** 1907. Pathologisch-anatomische Untersuchungen über akute Poliomyelitis und verwandte Krankheiten von den Epidemien in Norwegen 1903–1906, p. 1–220. *Videnskabs–Selskabets Skrifter, I. Math.-naturv. Klasse No. 5.* Jacob Dybwad, Christiania, Norway.
59. **Harmon, P. H.** 1937. The use of chemicals as nasal sprays in the prophylaxis of poliomyelitis in man. *JAMA* **109:**1061.
60. **Heine, J.** 1840. *Beobachtungen über Lähmungszustände der untern Extremitäten und deren Behandlung.* Franz Heinrich Köhler, Stuttgart, Germany.
61. **Heine, J. v.** 1860. *Spinale Kinderlähmung, 2. umgearbeitete und vermehrte Auflage.* J. G. Cotta'scher Verlag, Stuttgart, Germany.
62. **Hirst, G.** 1962. Genetic recombination with Newcastle disease virus, poliovirus and influenza. *Cold Spring Harbor Symp. Quant. Biol.* **27:**303–309.
63. **Hogle, J. M., M. Chow, and D. J. Filman.** 1985. Three-dimensional structure of poliovirus at 2.9 Å resolution. *Science* **229:**1358–1365.
64. **Holland, J. J., and L. C. McLaren.** 1959. The mammalian cell-virus relationship. II. Adsorption, reception and

eclipse of poliovirus by HeLa cells. *J. Exp. Med.* **109:**487–504.
65. **Horstmann, D. M.** 1955. Poliomyelitis: severity and type of disease in different age groups. *Ann. N.Y. Acad. Sci.* **61:**956–967.
66. **Horstmann, D. M.** 1957. Poliomyelitis: problems in pathogenesis and immunization. *Yale J. Biol. Med.* **30:**81–100.
67. **Horstmann, D. M., R. W. McCollum, and A. D. Mascola.** 1954. Viremia in human poliomyelitis. *J. Exp. Med.* **99:**355–369.
68. **Howe, H. A., and D. Bodian.** 1940. Untreated human stools as a source of poliomyelitis virus. *J. Infect. Dis.* **66:**198–201.
69. **Howe, H. A., and D. Bodian.** 1941. Poliomyelitis in the chimpanzee: a clinical-pathologic study. *Bull. Johns Hopkins Hosp.* **69:**149–169.
70. **Jacobsen, M., and D. Baltimore.** 1968. Polypeptide cleavage on the formation of poliovirus proteins. *Proc. Natl. Acad. Sci. USA* **61:**77–84.
71. **Kitamura, N., B. L. Semler, P. G. Rothberg, G. R. Larsen, C. J. Adler, A. J. Dorner, E. A. Emini, R. Hanecak, J. J. Lee, S. van der Werf, C. W. Anderson, and E. Wimmer.** 1981. Primary structure, gene organization, polypeptide expression of poliovirus RNA. *Nature* **291:**547–553.
72. **Kling, C., C. Levaditi, and G. Hornus.** 1934. Comparaison entre les diverse modes de contamination du singe par le virus poliomyélitique (voies digestive et nasopharyngée). *Bull. Acad. Méd., Paris* **111:**709–716.
73. **Kling, C., W. Wernstedt, and A. Pettersson.** 1912. Recherches sur le mode de propagation de la paralysie infantile épidémique (maladie de Heine-Medin). Premier mémoire. *Z. Immunitätsforsch.* **12:**316–323.
74. **Kling, C., W. Wernstedt, and A. Pettersson.** 1912. Recherches sur le mode de propagation de la paralysie infantile épidémique (maladie de Heine-Medin). Deuxième mémoire. *Z. Immunitätsforsch.* **12:**657–670.
75. **Kolmer, J. A.** 1936. Vaccination against acute anterior poliomyelitis. *Am. J. Public Health* **26:**126–135.
76. **Kramer, S. D., A. G. Gilliam, and J. G. Molner.** 1939. Recovery of the virus of poliomyelitis from the stools of healthy contacts in an institutional outbreak. *Public Health Rep.* **54:**1914–1922.
77. **Landsteiner, K., and C. Levaditi.** 1909. La transmission de la paralysie infantile aux singes. *Compt. Rend. Soc. Biol. Paris* **67:**592–594.
78. **Landsteiner, K., and E. Popper.** 1909. Uebertragung der Poliomyelitis acuta auf Affen. *Z. Immunitätsforsch.* **2:**377–390.
79. **Ledinko, N.** 1963. Genetic recombination with poliovirus type 1. Studies of crosses between a normal horse serum-resistant mutant and several guanidine-resistant mutants of the same strain. *Virology* **20:**107–119.
80. **Leegard, C.** 1914. Die akute Poliomyelitis in Norwegen. *Deutsche Z. Nervenheilkunde* **53:**145–262.
81. **Leiner, C., and R. v. Wiesner.** 1909. Experimentelle Untersuchungen über Poliomyelitis acuta anterior. *Wiener Klin. Wochenschr.* **22:**1698–1701.
82. **Leiner, C., and R. v. Wiesner.** 1910. Experimentelle Untersuchungen über Poliomyelitis acuta. *Wiener Med. Wochenschr.* **60:**2482–2487.
83. **Leiner, C., and R. v. Wiesner.** 1910. Experimentelle Untersuchungen über Poliomyelitis acuta anterior II. *Wiener Klin. Wochenschr.* **23:**91–94.
84. **Levaditi, C.** 1910. Essais de culture du parasite de la paralysie infantile. *Presse Méd.* **20:**44.
85. **Levaditi, C.** 1913. Virus de la poliomyélite et culture des cellules in vitro. *Compt. Rend. Soc. Biol., Paris* **75:**202–205.
86. **Ludden, T. E., and J. E. Edwards.** 1949. Carditis in poliomyelitis. An anatomic study of thirty-five cases and review of the literature. *Am. J. Pathol.* **25:**357–381.
87. **Marie, P.** 1885. Hémiplégie cérébrale infantile et maladies infectieuses. *Progr. Méd.* **13:**167–169.
88. **Medin, O.** 1891. Ueber eine Epidemie von spinaler Kinderlähmung. *Verhandl. d. 10. Int. Med. Kongr. 1890*, 2. Abt. **6:**37–47.
89. **Melnick, J. L.** 1997. Poliovirus and other enteroviruses, p. 583–663. *In* A. S. Evans and R. A. Kaslow (ed.), *Viral Infections of Humans*, 4th ed. Plenum, New York, N.Y.
90. **Melnick, J. L., and N. Ledinko.** 1953. Development of neutralizing antibodies against the three types of poliomyelitis virus during an epidemic period. The ratio of inapparent infection to clinical poliomyelitis. *Am. J. Hyg.* **58:**207–222.
91. **Montagnier, L., and F. K. Sanders.** 1963. Replicative form of encephalomyocarditis virus ribonucleic acid. *Nature* **199:**664–667.
92. **Müller, W.** 1935. Spontane Poliomyelitis beim Schimpansen. *Monatsschr. Kinderheilkunde* **63:**134–137.
93. **Nathanson, N., and D. Bodian.** 1961. Experimental poliomyelitis following intramuscular virus infection. I. The effect of neural block on a neurotropic and pantropic strain. *Bull. Johns Hopkins Hosp.* **108:**308–319.
94. **Nathanson, N., and A. D. Langmuir.** 1963. The Cutter incident. Poliomyelitis following formaldehyde inactivated poliovirus vaccination in the United States during the spring of 1955. *Am. J. Hyg.* **78:**16–81.
95. **Nathanson, N., and J. R. Martin.** 1979. The epidemiology of poliomyelitis: enigmas surrounding its appearance, epidemicity, and disappearance. *Am. J. Epidemiol.* **110:**672–692.
96. **Netter, A., and C. Levaditi.** 1910. Action microbicide exercée par le sérum des malades atteints de paralysie infantile sur le virus de la poliomyélite aiguë. *Compt. Rend. Soc. Biol., Paris* **68:**617–619.
97. **Neustädter, M., and W. C. Thro.** 1912. Experimentelle Poliomyelitis acuta. *Deutsche Med. Wschrft.* **38:**693–695.
98. **Olin, G.** 1952. The epidemiologic pattern of poliomyelitis in Sweden from 1905 to 1950, p. 367–375. *In Poliomyelitis: Papers and Discussions Presented at the Second International Poliomyelitis Conference*. Lippincott, Philadelphia, Pa.
99. **Parrot, J., and A. Joffroy.** 1870. Note sur un cas de paralysie infantile. *Arch. Physiol. Norm. Pathol.* **3:**309–316.
100. **Paul, J. R.** 1971. *A History of Poliomyelitis*. Yale University Press, New Haven, Conn.
101. **Paul, J. R., J. L. Melnick, and J. T. Riordan.** 1952. Comparative neutralizing antibody patterns to Lansing (type 2) poliomyelitis virus in different populations. *Am. J. Hyg.* **56:**232–251.
102. **Peabody, F. W., G. Draper, and A. R. Dochez.** 1912. *A Clinical Study of Acute Poliomyelitis. Monographs of The Rockefeller Institute for Medical Research*, no. 4. The Rockefeller Institute for Medical Research, New York.
103. **Pettersson, A.** 1912. Ueber die Verbreitungsweise der epidemischen Kinderlähmung und die Verhütung ihrer Verbreitung, p. 595–600. *Transactions Fifteenth International Congress on Hygiene and Demography*, Washington, Sept. 25–28, 1912, Joint Session of Sections I and V, Sept. 26, 1912.
104. **Racaniello, V. R., and D. Baltimore.** 1981. Cloned poliovirus complementary DNA is infectious in mammalian cells. *Science* **214:**916–919.
105. **Racaniello, V. R., and D. Baltimore.** 1981. Molecular cloning of poliovirus cDNA and determination of the complete nucleotide sequence of the viral genome. *Proc. Natl. Acad. Sci. USA* **78:**4887–4891.

106. **Rilliet, F.** 1851. De la paralysie essentielle chez les enfants. *Gazette Méd. de Paris*, Année 21, Sér. 3, T. **6:**681–685; 704–707.
107. **Rissler, J.** 1888. Zur Kenntniss der Veränderungen des Nervensystems bei Poliomyelitis anterior acuta. *Nordiskt Medicinskt Arkiv* **20:**1–61.
108. **Robbins, F. C.** 1988. Polio—Historical, p. 98–114. *In* S. A. Plotkin and E. A. Mortimer (ed.), *Vaccines*. W. B. Saunders Co., Philadelphia, Pa.
109. **Robertson, H. E., and A. J. Chesley.** 1910. Pathology and bacteriology of acute anterior poliomyelitis. *Arch. Intern. Med.* **6:**233–269.
110. **Roger, H., and M. Damaschino.** 1871. Recherches anatomo-pathologiques sur la paralysie spinale de l'enfance. *Compt. Rend. Soc. Biol., Paris*, séance du 7 octobre: 49–93.
111. **Römer, P. H.** 1911. *Die epidemische Kinderlähmung (Heine-Medinsche Krankheit)*. Julius Springer, Berlin, Germany.
112. **Sabin, A. B.** 1942. Pathology and pathogenesis of human poliomyelitis. *JAMA* **120:**506–511.
113. **Sabin, A. B.** 1951. Paralytic consequences of poliomyelitis infection in different parts of the world and in different population groups. *Am J. Public Health* **41:**1215–1230.
114. **Sabin, A. B.** 1954. Noncytopathogenic variants of poliomyelitis viruses and resistance to superinfection in tissue culture. *Science* **120:**357.
115. **Sabin, A. B.** 1956. Pathogenesis of poliomyelitis. *Science* **123:**1151–1157.
116. **Sabin, A. B.** 1959. Present position of immunization against poliomyelitis with live virus vaccines. *Br. Med. J.* **1:**663–680.
117. **Sabin, A. B.** 1985. Oral poliovirus vaccine: history of its development and use and current challenge to eliminate poliomyelitis from the world. *J. Infect. Dis.* **151:**420–436.
118. **Sabin, A. B., and P. K. Olitsky.** 1936. Cultivation of poliomyelitis virus in vitro in human embryonic nervous tissue. *Proc. Soc. Exp. Biol. Med.* **34:**357–359.
119. **Sabin, A. B., and P. K. Olitsky.** 1937. The olfactory bulbs in experimental poliomyelitis. Their pathologic condition as an indicator of the portal of entry of the virus. *JAMA* **108:**21–24.
120. **Sabin, A. B., and R. Ward.** 1941. Nature of non-paralytic and transitory paralytic poliomyelitis in rhesus monkeys inoculated with human virus. *J. Exp. Med.* **73:**757–770.
121. **Sabin, A. B., and R. Ward.** 1941. The natural history of human poliomyelitis. I. Distribution of virus in nervous and non-nervous tissues. *J. Exp. Med.* **73:**771–793.
122. **Salk, J. E.** 1959. Poliomyelitis control, p. 499–518. *In* T. M. Rivers and F. L. Horsfall, Jr. (ed.), *Viral and Rickettsial Infections of Man*. 3rd ed. J. B. Lippincott, Philadelphia, Pa.
123. **Salomon, G.** 1868. Zur Diagnose und Therapie einiger Lähmungsformen im kindlichen Alter. *Jahrb. Kinderheilk.* **1:**370–390.
124. **Saphir, O.** 1945. Visceral lesions in poliomyelitis. *Am. J. Pathol.* **21:**99–109.
125. **Schaffer, F. L., and C. E. Schwerdt.** 1955. Crystallization of purified MEF-1 poliomyelitis virus particles. *Proc. Natl. Acad. Sci. USA* **41:**1020–1023.
126. **Schwalbe, E.** 1902. Untersuchung eines Falles von Poliomyelitis acuta infantum im Stadium der Reparation. *Beitr. Pathol. Anat. Allg. Pathol.* **32:**485–525.
127. **Seeligmüller, A.** 1880. Spinale Kinderlähmung. *In* C. Gerhardt (ed.), *Handbuch der Kinderkrankheiten, Fünfter Band, Erste Abtheilung, Zweite Hälfte*. Verlag der H. Laupp'schen Buchhandlung, Tübingen, Germany.
128. **State Medical Institute of Sweden.** 1912. Investigations on epidemic infantile paralysis. *Report to the XV International Congress on Hygiene and Demography, Washington, 1912*. Nordiska Bokhandeln, Stockholm, Sweden.
129. **Strümpell, A.** 1884. Ueber die Ursachen der Erkrankungen des Nervensystems. *Deutsch. Archiv Klin. Med.* **35:**1–17.
130. **Strümpell, A.** 1885. Ueber die acute Encephalitis der Kinder (Poliomyelitis acuta, cerebrale Kinderlähmung). *Jahrb. Kinderheilk.* **22:**173–178.
131. **Summers, D. F., and J. V. Maizel, Jr.** 1968. Evidence of large precursor proteins in poliovirus synthesis. *Proc. Natl. Acad. Sci. USA* **59:**966–971.
132. **Theiler, M.** 1941. Studies on poliomyelitis. *Medicine* **20:**443–462.
133. **Trask, J. D., A. J. Vignec, and J. R. Paul.** 1938. Poliomyelitis virus in human stools. *JAMA* **111:**6–11.
134. **Trask, J. D., J. R. Paul, and A. J. Vignec.** 1940. I. Poliomyelitic virus in human stools. *J. Exp. Med.* **71:**751–763.
135. **Turner, T. B., D. H. Hollander, S. Buckley, U. Pettikokko, and C. P. Winsor.** 1950. Age incidence and seasonal development of neutralizing antibodies to Lansing poliomyelitis virus. *Am. J. Hyg.* **52:**323–347.
136. **Turner, T. B., L. E. Young, and E. Starbuck Maxwell.** 1945. The mouse adapted Lansing strain of poliomyelitis virus. IV. Neutralizing antibodies in the serum of healthy children. *Am. J. Hyg.* **42:**119–127.
137. **Underwood, M.** 1789. *A Treatise on the Diseases of Children*. J. Mathews, London, United Kingdom.
138. **van der Werf, S., J. Bradley, E. Wimmer, F. W. Studier, and J. J. Dunn.** 1986. Synthesis of infectious poliovirus RNA by purified T 7 RNA polymerase. *Proc. Natl. Acad. Sci. USA* **83:**2330–2334.
139. **Vulpian, A.** 1870. Cas d'atrophie musculaire graisseuse datant de l'enfance. Lésions des cornes antérieures de la substance grise de la moelle épinière. *Arch. Physiol. Norm. Pathol.* **3:**316–325.
140. **Ward, R., D. M. Horstmann, and J. L. Melnick.** 1946. The isolation of poliomyelitis virus from human extraneural sources. IV. Search for virus in the blood of patients. *J. Clin. Invest.* **25:**284–286.
141. **Westendorf, W.** 1992. Erwachen der Heilkunst. *Die Medizin im alten Ägypten*. Artemis & Winkler, Munich, Germany.
142. **Wickman, I.** 1911. *Die akute Poliomyelitis bzw. Heine-Medinsche Krankheit*. Julius Springer, Berlin, Germany.
143. **Zappert, C., R. von Wiesner, and K. Leiner.** 1911. *Studien über die Heine-Medinsche Krankheit (Poliomyelitis acuta)*. Franz Deuticke, Leipzig, Germany.

TAXONOMY

Molecular and Biological Basis of Picornavirus Taxonomy

GLYN STANWAY, TAPANI HOVI, NICK J. KNOWLES, AND TIMO HYYPIÄ

2

Humans have always sought to make sense of the world by grouping items on the basis of shared properties. As is the case with all virus families, attempts have been made to classify members of *Picornaviridae* for a number of years. Originally, this was on the basis of shared pathogenic properties in humans and animals, together with biophysical properties (6). Such is the correlation between some of these properties and genetic relationships that this somewhat simplistic approach produced results surprisingly consistent with current classification. For instance, of over 30 viruses classified as echoviruses in the *Enterovirus* genus (5), 28 are closely related and are still classified together, now as members of the *Human enterovirus B* (HEV-B) species of this genus (15, 20, 29). However, something of its limitation can be seen from the fact that two other echoviruses proved to be quite distinct and now constitute a different genus, *Parechovirus*, of *Picornaviridae*, while early in classification one was defined as a rhinovirus and one was found to be a reovirus (35, 38). The original classification of hepatitis A virus (HAV) as an enterovirus and the subsequent need to reclassify it as the type member of a new genus, *Hepatovirus*, as sequence data became available, are another example of the limitations of this classical approach (6, 20). As the information available has increased, primarily through the accumulation of large amounts of sequence data, but also through structural analysis and receptor identification, the emphasis in classification has changed to a system based on phylogenetic properties, which more accurately reflect evolutionary history and the details of the virus replication mechanisms.

Classification is important because it provides the framework for understanding the properties of a virus. For instance, implicit in the current classification of a virus as an *Enterovirus* species member is that the virus has a 5′ untranslated region (UTR) of a particular general form and function, a 2A protein that is related to the chymotrypsin group of proteases, no leader protein, and a 3′ UTR containing at least two stem-loops, which interact to form a tertiary structure (20). It does not necessarily tell us about other fundamental biological properties, such as which receptor the virus recognizes, nor does it define the pathogenic properties of the virus. Thus, there may be only partial overlap with a key aspect of classification from the clinical perspective, that of facilitating an understanding of the disease process, leading to ways of diagnosing and treating disease. However, as diagnosis becomes increasingly based on sequence properties, due to the speed and sensitivity of PCR and other nucleic acid-based procedures, and as we understand the molecular basis of pathogenicity more clearly, it is probable that there will be a convergence of these aspects.

The current taxonomic situation is summarized in Table 1. Picornaviruses have traditionally been defined in terms of serotypes, grouped into genera. Recently, a radical change has been introduced with the advent of the concept of a picornavirus species, generally consisting of several serotypes (20). This classification has evolved in response to developments in our understanding of the biological and genetic properties of picornaviruses, which has accelerated greatly over the past few years. Here we examine some of the properties that can be used to group, or differentiate between, picornaviruses and some of the complications that arise from attempting to classify viruses, which are potentially highly plastic in terms of sequence and even genome organization.

PATHOGENESIS OF PICORNAVIRUS INFECTIONS

Animal Models

Animal models have been used extensively to subgroup picornaviruses, particularly enteroviruses (5, 6, 24). Enteroviruses were originally classified as poliovirus (PV), coxsackievirus A (CVA), coxsackievirus B (CVB), and echovirus on the basis of their pathogenicity in experimental

---

Glyn Stanway ■ Department of Biological Sciences, University of Essex, Colchester, C04 3SQ, United Kingdom. *Tapani Hovi* ■ Enterovirus Laboratory, KTL, Mannerheimintie 166, 00300 Helsinki, Finland. *Nick J. Knowles* ■ Institute for Animal Health (IAH), Pirbright Laboratory, Ash Road, Pirbright, Woking, Surrey, GU24 0NF, United Kingdom. *Timo Hyypiä* ■ Department of Virology, Haartman Institute, University of Helsinki, P.O. Box 21, 00014 Helsinki, Finland.

TABLE 1 Current classification of *Picornaviridae*

Genus	Species (and abbreviation)	Serotypes[a]
Enterovirus	Poliovirus	PV serotypes 1, 2, 3
	Human enterovirus A (HEV-A)	CVA serotypes 2, 3, 4, 5, 6, 7, 8, 10, 12, 14, 16; EV-71
	Human enterovirus B (HEV-B)	CVB serotypes 1, 2, 3, 4, 5, 6; CVA9
		Echovirus (E) serotypes 1, 2, 3, 4, 5, 6, 7, 9, 11, 12, 13, 14, 15, 16, 17, 18, 19, 20, 21, 24, 25, 26, 27, 29, 30, 31, 32, 33; EV-69; SVDV
	Human enterovirus C (HEV-C)	CVA serotypes 1, 11, 13, 15, 17, 18, 19, 20, 21, 22, 24
	Human enterovirus D (HEV-D)	EV-68, EV-70
	Bovine enterovirus (BEV)	BEV-1, BEV-2
	Porcine enterovirus A (PEV-A)	PEV-8
	Porcine enterovirus B (PEV-B)	PEV-9, PEV-10
Rhinovirus	Human rhinovirus A (HRV-A)	HRV serotypes 1, 2, 7, 9, 11, 15, 16, 21, 29, 36, 39, 49, 50, 58, 62, 65, 85, 89
	Human rhinovirus B (HRV-B)	HRV serotypes 3, 14, 72
Cardiovirus	Encephalomyocarditis virus (EMCV)	EMCV
	Theilovirus (ThV)	TMEV, VHEV
Aphthovirus	Foot-and-mouth disease virus (FMDV)	FMDV serotypes O, A, C, Asia1, SAT-1, SAT-2, SAT-3
	Equine rhinitis A virus	ERAV
Hepatovirus	Hepatitis A virus	HAV
	Avian encephalomyelitis-like virus[b] (AEV)	AEV
Parechovirus	Human parechovirus (HPeV)	HPeV-1, HPeV-2
Erbovirus	Equine rhinitis B virus (ERBV)	ERBV
Kobuvirus	Aichi virus (AiV)	AiV
Teschovirus	Porcine teschovirus (PTV)	PTV serotypes 1, 2, 3, 4, 5, 6, 7, 8, 9, 10, 11

[a] PV, poliovirus; CVA, CVB, coxsackievirus A, B; E, echovirus; SVDV, swine vesicular disease virus (a variant of CVB5); EV, enterovirus; BEV, bovine enterovirus; PEV, porcine enterovirus; HRV, human rhinovirus (several HRV serotypes have not yet been assigned to a species); EMCV, encephalomyocarditis virus; TMEV, Theiler's murine encephalomyelitis virus; VHEV, Vilyuisk human encephalomyelitis virus; FMDV, foot-and-mouth disease virus; ERAV, equine rhinitis A virus; HAV, hepatitis A virus; AEV, avian encephalomyelitis-like virus; HPeV, human parechovirus; ERBV, equine rhinitis B virus; AiV, Aichi virus; PTV, porcine teschovirus.

[b] Tentative species of *Hepatovirus* genus.

animals. Polioviruses cause a disease resembling human poliomyelitis in other primates (24). Coxsackieviruses are mouse pathogens, and they were discriminated into A and B subgroups on the basis of the disease observed in newborn mice: CVAs cause flaccid paralysis while CVBs cause spastic paralysis. This is due to the involvement of the central nervous system by the CVB infection whereas CVAs replicate in the muscle tissue (17). Currently, it is not known if receptor specificity of the viruses in newborn mice corresponds to that in humans. While PVs and CVBs are genetically rather uniform subgroups, CVAs have now been shown to have members in three different species (11 serotypes belong to human enterovirus A [HEV-A], CVA9 is a member of HEV-B, and 11 serotypes belong to HEV-C) (26). Therefore, there has been a conflict between the classical subgroup division based on the pathogenesis in experimental animals and genetic classification of human enteroviruses.

Clinical Manifestations

In humans, PVs cause a paralytic disease that can be often clinically recognized as poliomyelitis (24). However, paralysis is only a rare complication of PV infection, which is usually asymptomatic or causes a mild febrile illness. Human hand-foot-and-mouth disease, a vesicular rash, is known to be frequently caused by members of the HEV-A species (in particular by CVA16 and HEV71), and it represents a clinically recognized illness associated with a restricted number of enterovirus serotypes (10). Some simian enteroviruses are genetically closely related to HEV-A (30), but there is currently no information on whether they can be transmitted to humans. The members of the large HEV-B group cause a great variety of diseases varying from exanthemas to carditis and infections of the central nervous system, but the most frequent consequence of infection is mild respiratory infection (10). There is no clear association between clinical manifestations and individual virus serotypes in the group. HEV-C contains viruses that utilize the same cellular receptor as members of the major receptor group of human rhinoviruses (HRVs), and both these virus groups are responsible for respiratory infections (e.g., common cold) (8).

Among other human pathogens, human parechoviruses appear to cause mainly gastroenteritis and respiratory infections, but also infections of the central nervous system and myocarditis cases have been reported (19, 39). In spite of the remarkable differences in the molecular characteristics of parechoviruses when compared to enteroviruses, the clinical illnesses caused by these two picornavirus groups are rather similar (10). HAV is an exception when compared with other human picornaviruses, as it affects mainly the liver, like several hepatitis viruses from other families (21).

Receptors

Because cellular receptors are essential in the initiation of the viral infection cycle, they also play a key role in tissue tropism (8). However, there are additional determinants, for instance, those recognized by tissue-specific factors in the picornavirus genome, which are important in the pathogenetic process (2). All three polioviruses utilize a cellular receptor that is a member of the immunoglobulin superfamily (8), whereas CVBs use another member of this superfamily (coxsackievirus-adenovirus receptor, CAR) to enter the host cell (8). Some CVBs also recognize decay-accelerating factor (DAF), and this property may have effects on the clinical pathogenicity of infection. Also, echoviruses, which are genetically closely related to CVBs and cause highly similar clinical diseases, can utilize DAF in the recognition of the host cells. However, there are exceptional serotypes among the members of the HEV-B subgroup in this respect. Echovirus 1 does not interact with DAF but recognizes $\alpha 2\beta 1$ integrin on the cell surface, and CVA9 and echovirus 9 (Barty strain) can attach to $\alpha v\beta 3$ integrin. It is of interest that in genetic comparisons these three viruses do not significantly differ from other members of HEV-B (26). Other picornaviruses have also been reported to attach to cell surface integrins. These include human parechovirus 1, which reacts with $\alpha v\beta 1/3$ integrin, and foot-and-mouth disease virus (FMDV), which reacts with $\alpha v\beta 3$ and obviously also with other combinations of integrin subunits (8, 18, 30). In addition to picornaviruses, members of other virus groups, including adenoviruses and hantaviruses, are known to interact with cell surface integrins.

Members of the major HRV receptor group recognize intercellular adhesion molecule 1 (ICAM-1), which is also a member of the immunoglobulin superfamily, as do HEV-C members (8). However, members of the minor HRV receptor group, which are responsible for a similar disease, recognize cell surface molecules in the low-density lipoprotein (LDL)-receptor family. Moreover, these two rhinovirus receptor subgroups do not follow the genetic division of HRVs (20).

In conclusion, it is notable that picornaviruses use cell surface receptors with wide structural and functional variability in their attachment and entry in the host cells. Genetically different viruses can use the same receptor (e.g., $\alpha v\beta 3$ integrin is recognized by human parechovirus 1, FMDV, and some enteroviruses as well as adenoviruses and hantaviruses). On the other hand, closely related picornaviruses appear to utilize different molecules (e.g., HRVs interact with ICAM-1 and LDL receptors). For these reasons, the receptor specificities of picornaviruses can only be considered as minor criteria in classification.

ANTIGENIC PROPERTIES AS CLASSIFICATION CRITERIA: DO WE STILL NEED SEROTYPES?

Background: the Numerous Serotypes of Picornaviruses

The immune response of the infected host animals is an important factor limiting picornavirus transmission in host populations, thus influencing virus ecology and epidemiology of infection (24). Protection against a systemic secondary infection is generally considered to be based mainly on neutralizing serum antibodies. This is best exemplified by the high efficacy of passively administered immunoglobulin against HAV in humans (21). Early studies on immunity to poliovirus in monkeys revealed that an experimental infection by a given virus strain protected the animals against a subsequent infection by the homologous virus and also against some but not all heterologous poliovirus strains. Similar observations had been made on FMDV. Initially, serotypes were defined as groups of virus strains capable of providing mutual cross-protection in vivo. Later on, and especially after development of cell culture techniques, the tedious and expensive in vivo tests were replaced by the neutralization test in cell culture, or, in some cases, by in vitro assays based on complement fixation and hemagglutination inhibition. The current number of established picornavirus serotypes is very high, especially among the two closely related genera, enteroviruses and rhinoviruses (Table 1).

Identification of the serotype of a virus isolate is not always a simple and straightforward operation because of two phenomena, cross-reactivity between and antigenic variation within individual serotypes. A given field isolate may show a variable degree of reactivity with antisera raised against one or more heterologous prototype strains. This phenomenon appears to vary according to the genus and even depending on the species within some genera. The three types of PV are classical examples of easily distinguishable enterovirus serotypes, whereas definite cross-reactivity is readily demonstrable between, for example, several established CVA serotypes (24). PVs are also an example of antigenically stabile picornaviruses. Although intraserotypic antigenic variation can be demonstrated between field strains, the strains used in the persistently highly effective poliovirus vaccines were isolated at least 50, and some more than 60, years ago (24). All field isolates of PV can be identified using a single set of three antisera raised against the prototype strains, one for each serotype, even though the current strains are known to segregate into several defined genetic lineages, or genotypes, within each serotype (32). This situation is completely different from that of FMDV, where continuing antigenic variation may severely compromise the efficacy of vaccines. Antigenic variation also complicates diagnosis of enterovirus infections; some recent field isolates are not easily neutralized by antisera raised against the prototype strains isolated in 1950s. Sometimes the strains are prime strains, i.e., even though not neutralized by the prototype antisera, they in turn can induce antibodies that are capable of neutralizing the prototype strains as well as the immunogen. In some other cases, antigenic divergence may be expressed in both ways. This complex situation might become understandable by examining the nature of antigenic sites and patterns of evolution.

Antigenic Sites in Capsid Proteins

Amino acids, making up what are conventionally referred to as neutralization antigenic sites, have been identified by analyzing substitutions in breakthrough mutants, selected in cell culture with the aid of neutralizing monoclonal antibodies. This approach may not be able to detect sites that are strictly conserved and do not allow amino acid substitutions (23), but even so, has revealed 3 to 4 independent antigenic sites (12). In addition to polioviruses, some FMDV and HRV serotypes have been most extensively studied in this sense. Because the overall three-dimensional structure and the spatial relations of various capsid protein motifs appear to be well conserved among picornaviruses, it is assumed that antigenic sites in other picornaviruses are located in related positions. This view is partially supported by peptide scanning analyses of some *Human enterovirus B* serotypes (31). Peptide scanning can be used to rapidly screen linear antibody binding epitopes, several of which appear to overlap with sites identified in the classical way (33). The capsid protein 1D or VP1 appears to carry most of the antigenic sites, but VP2, VP3, and possibly even VP4 also contribute. For the recently introduced genomic sequence-based enterovirus identification, the sequence of VP1 appears to be the best choice providing exclusive serotype identification (26).

In spite of all this detailed knowledge, the structural and genetic counterparts of serotype identity are not understood in depth (12). It is possible that the immunological serotype identity is a polythetic property, and several different antigenic sites might contain serotype-specific determinants, each of which can be occasionally masked by the intraserotypic variation resulting from mutations selected under immunological pressure. For the serotype identity of a given strain, perhaps only one serotype-specific motif is sufficient, and it may be different for different field strains within a serotype.

The Benefit of Continuing To Define Serotype

The existence of distinct serotypes within a picornavirus species reflects long-lasting interactions between the corresponding virus and host populations and reveals successful avenues in virus evolution within the ecological niche acquired. The International Committee on Taxonomy of Viruses does not make official decisions about taxonomic positions of virus strains beyond the species level, where the definitions largely rely on phylogenetic analyses of genetic relationships. The genomic sequence is, of course, the most unequivocal determinant of the identity of a virus strain, and methods for generating partial genomic sequences are becoming easier to exploit and less expensive to use. In principle, sequencing can also be used for identifying the serotype. Still, for laboratories dealing with large numbers of strains, e.g., in epidemiological studies, conventional serotyping may be more feasible, and the guaranteed availability of standardized reagents necessary for this procedure is desirable. For practical serotyping, polyclonal antisera are clearly preferable over monoclonal antibodies.

PICORNAVIRUS GENOME ORGANIZATION

As the sequences of numerous picornaviruses have become available, they have shown that there is essentially one common genome organization (Fig. 1) (20, 35). The single-stranded RNA genome of around 6,500 to 9,500 nucleotides contains a single open reading frame, encoding a

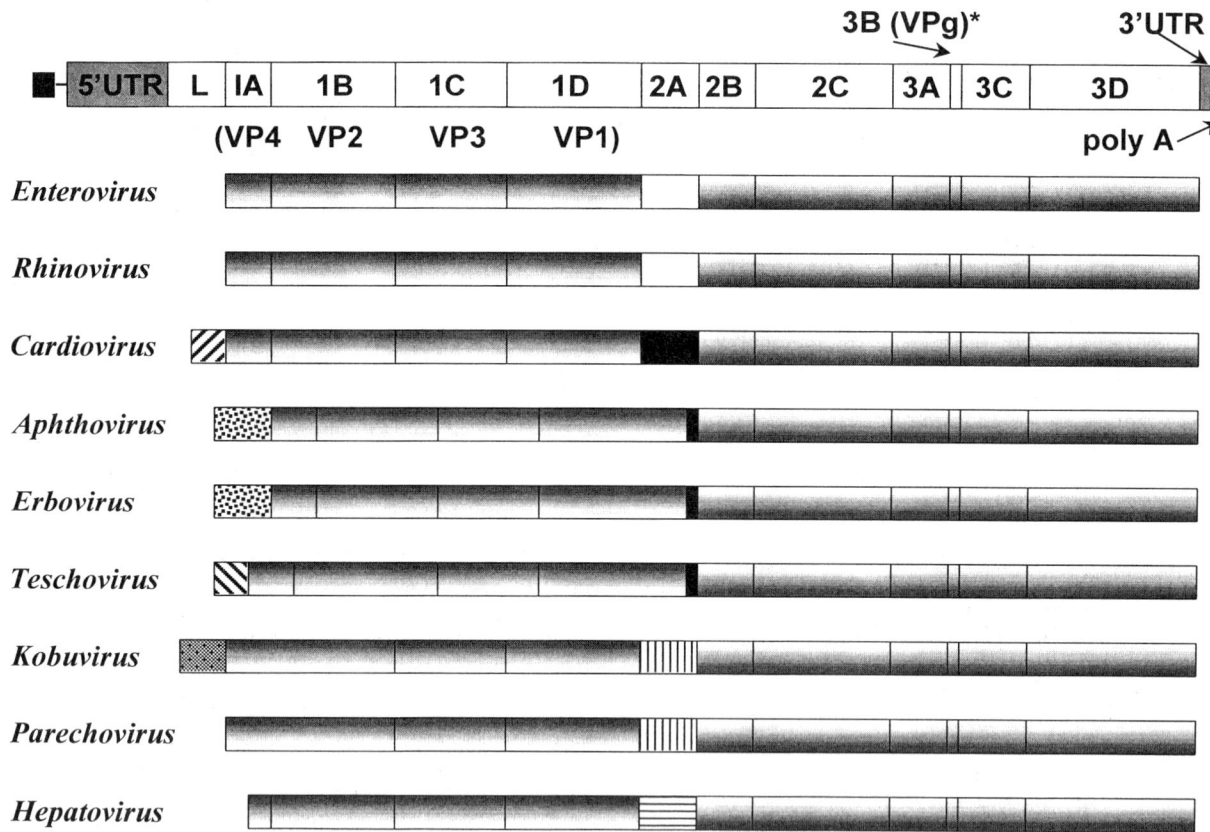

FIGURE 1 Genome structure of a typical picornavirus, together with a schematic representation of the polyproteins encoded by each genus. Most picornaviruses encode four structural proteins (1A-1D), also called VP4, VP2, VP3, and VP1). However, it appears that members of the genera *Parechovirus* and *Kobuvirus* do not undergo the cleavage of VP0 to VP4 and VP2 and so there are only three structural proteins. The main differences in terms of genome organization are the L protein and 2A. At least four (the *Aphthovirus* and *Erbovirus* L proteins are distantly related) different types of L protein are found in the five genera that have a protein at this locus. There are also four structurally diverse protein types at the 2A locus. In the figure, for both L and 2A, similar structural types of proteins are shaded in the same way. *Note that one of the two *Aphthovirus* species, FMDV, encodes three tandem copies of VPg.

polyprotein of around 2,200 amino acids. This is preceded by a 5' UTR that is quite long, typically making up around 10% of the genome, and followed by a much shorter 3' UTR (0.5 to 1.5% of the genome) and a poly(A) tract. The presence of VPg, a protein of just over 20 amino acids covalently attached to the 5' terminus of the RNA, is another important characteristic of picornaviruses. The polyprotein is cleaved into 10 to 12 proteins, depending on the picornavirus in question, through a cascade of proteolytic events brought about by virus-encoded proteases (27, 36). However, despite this consistent genome structure, there are notable differences that can help in defining the taxonomic identity of picornaviruses (Table 2).

5' UTR

Two distinct forms of the 5' UTR, originally defined in terms of internal ribosomal entry site (IRES) structure, have been identified among picornaviruses, which reflects fundamental, but relatively subtle, differences in translation initiation strategy (7, 40). The type 1 5' UTR is seen in only enteroviruses and rhinoviruses, while several picornaviruses have a type 2 5' UTR. Hepatoviruses have a variant form of this (called here type 2'), while two genera have not been studied thoroughly. In addition to correlating with genera, 5' UTR structure can also be one of the criteria defining species. For example, subgroups of the type 1 5' UTR can be identified and all members of the *Human enterovirus* A and B species have a CVB-like 5' UTR and all *Human enterovirus* C and D species members have PV-like 5' UTRs (16, 29).

L

The other major differences are observed in terms of protein structure and function (Fig. 1). Some picornaviruses encode an L protein at the N terminus of their polyprotein and these exhibit great diversity, as in each genus with an L protein this is structurally distinct. The exceptions are *Aphthovirus*, where L is a papain-like protease, and *Erbovirus*, whose L protein is somewhat related but may not have all the features necessary for protease activity (36, 42).

2A

The protein encoded at the 2A locus differs dramatically among picornaviruses, and several distinct forms have been identified (14). These are the chymotrypsin-like cysteine protease of the *Enterovirus* and *Rhinovirus* genera, the extremely short (17-amino-acid) protein of *Aphthovirus*, *Teschovirus*, and *Erbovirus* genera, which exhibit a characteristic NPGP motif at the 2A/2B boundary, and the recently defined H-box/NC proteins of the *Parechovirus* and *Kobuvirus* genera (14, 27, 36). The *Cardiovirus* 2A is much longer than that of the other NPGP proteins but has an equivalent region at its C terminus. The *Hepatovirus* 2A is a distinct type of protein.

Capsid Proteins

There are several relatively minor differences in capsid proteins between picornaviruses, largely affecting the termini and particular loops between β strands. These are also seen in three-dimensional structure terms, through major differences in surface topology, particularly in canyon morphology (1, 11, 34). An additional major difference is the absence of VP0 cleavage seen in the *Parechovirus* and *Kobuvirus* genera, meaning that these viruses have only three structural proteins (38, 43). An additional distinguishing feature is myristoylation of VP4, which appears to be critical for members of several picornavirus genera but does not occur in the *Parechovirus* and *Hepatovirus* genera (4, 38).

Thus, most of the genera defined to date exhibit some differences in genome organization (Table 2, Fig. 1), the notable exception being *Rhinovirus* and *Enterovirus*, which are identical by these criteria. The differences between *Aphthovirus* and *Erbovirus* genera are also relatively subtle as they involve only the L protein. A further complication is avian encephalomyelitis virus, currently assigned as a tentative *Hepatovirus*. This has a distinct 5' UTR type, and although it is most closely related to the *Hepatovirus* HAV, throughout most of the rest of the genome, it has an H-box/NC 2A protein rather than a *Hepatovirus*-like 2A (14). Notwithstanding these caveats, genome organization correlates well with classification and can often be an important characteristic to take into account.

GENETIC RELATIONSHIPS

To provide biologically important insights, taxonomy should ultimately be based on genetic relationships, which in turn reflect the evolutionary history of the viruses. Vast amounts of picornavirus sequence information are now available, and this is invaluable to taxonomy. As serotype is still a main criterion for defining the identity of a picornavirus and this is determined by capsid protein sequences, it makes sense to use the P1 region in phylogeny (20). Current picornavirus species definitions also look to the generally more conserved 2C plus 3CD regions. As shown in Fig. 2, where representatives of each species are analyzed, the results from comparisons of these regions agree well. It can be seen that most genera constitute distinct lineages; indeed, this is the major current criterion used for defining a genus. The exceptions are *Enterovirus* and *Rhinovirus*, which overlap, particularly in the P1 comparisons. Although distinct, there is a definite clustering of the genera *Aphthovirus*, *Cardiovirus*, *Erbovirus*, and *Teschovirus* in these comparisons, which is often, but not always, reflected in similarities in other genomic features such as 5' UTR and 2A type.

EVOLUTIONARY ASPECTS

Like other RNA viruses, picornaviruses have a high mutation rate, due to the lack of proofreading activity during

TABLE 2 Main distinguishing features of the genomes of picornavirus genera

Genus	5' UTR type	L	2A
Enterovirus	1	Absent	Chymotrypsin-like
Rhinovirus	1	Absent	Chymotrypsin-like
Cardiovirus	2	A	NPGP
Aphthovirus	2	B (papain-like)	NPGP
Erbovirus	2	B'	NPGP
Teschovirus	?	C	NPGP
Kobuvirus[a]	?	D	H-box/NC
Parechovirus[a,b]	2	Absent	H-box/NC
Hepatovirus[b]	2'	Absent	?

[a]VP0 cleavage does not occur in these viruses.
[b]VP4 does not appear to be myristoylated in these viruses.

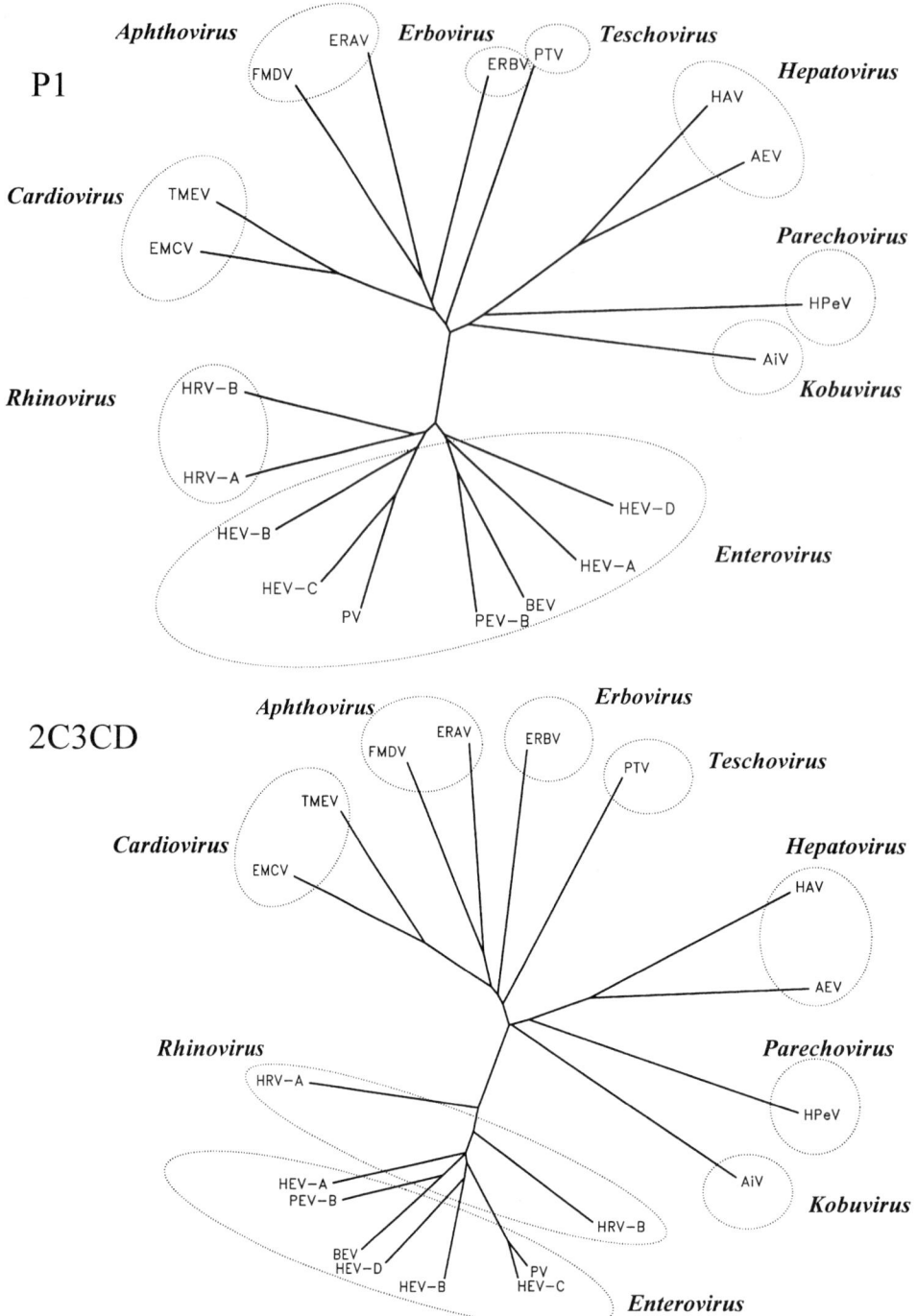

FIGURE 2 Phylogenetic trees expressing the relationship between a representative of each picornavirus species, based on amino acid identities of the P1 or 2C plus 3CD proteins. Sequences were compared using the program ClustalW and the trees were drawn using the program Treedraw (41). Abbreviations are as given in Table 1. Species names within each genus are enclosed by dotted lines.

genome replication. Approximately one mutation is generated per newly synthesized genome, giving rise to quasispecies, a diverse collection of virus mutants (13). This leads to a capability to adapt rapidly to environmental changes. Different parts of the viral genome represent distinct functions, which also have evolutionary consequences. The untranslated regions contain initiation sites for RNA synthesis; the IRES in the 5′ UTR is responsible for the initiation of translation; the capsid region codes for proteins that mediate the attachment and entry of the virion into the host cells and are also directly exposed to the host immune system, whereas the nonstructural region codes for the proteins needed in the replication. The need to maintain the secondary structures in the untranslated regions, in particular in the 5' UTR, significantly restricts the rate at which mutations are fixed in the population. The requirement to interact with the cellular receptor(s), together with the need for structural conservation of polypeptides, also causes restrictions in capsid mutations. This region is, however, the most diverse part of the genome, largely due to the variation in the loop regions of viral proteins. The polypeptides coded by the nonstructural region are relatively well conserved, which can be understood on the basis of their vital functions, interactions with other viral and cellular macromolecules, and the apparent lack of selection pressure caused by antibodies.

Although the high mutation rate does not usually cause any significant problems in picornavirus classification, recombination events complicate the genetic classification scheme. Recombination has been shown to occur among polioviruses (3, 9), and evidence of intraspecies recombination has also been reported in other genetic clusters of enteroviruses (37). The fact that there are only two genetic groups found in the 5' UTR of the enterovirus genome instead of the four clusters in other parts of the genome could also be explained by early recombination (37). Further studies are needed to illuminate how common these events are in currently circulating picornaviruses. In conclusion, these evolutionary aspects need to be carefully considered when classification-based genetic properties of picornaviruses will be further developed and compared with previously used classification principles.

PROBLEMS IN TAXONOMY

Picornaviridae is a large and complex family. The accumulation of mutations, potential recombination within the family, and acquisition of host sequences during evolution mean that there may not always be convenient divisions between viruses to make their taxonomy unambiguous (13, 37). The close similarity between the *Enterovirus* and *Rhinovirus* genera has already been mentioned and presents one type of problem. These viruses can be distinguished by physical properties, such as acid stability and buoyant density, and rhinoviruses form a coherent group in terms of pathogenicity, yet the division into *Enterovirus* and *Rhinovirus* genera is barely justified in terms of genome organization (Fig. 1) or genetic grouping (Fig. 2). However, the clinical and biological properties of rhinoviruses seem to be sufficiently distinct to warrant the continuation of two separate genera. Avian encephalomyelitis virus presents another interesting dilemma. This is clearly most closely related to HAV (*Hepatovirus* genus) in terms of P1 and 2C3CD identities (Fig. 2), but it has a divergent 5' UTR and a different type of 2A (related to that of genera *Parechovirus* and *Kobuvirus*, rather than *Hepatovirus*) (Fig. 1) (14, 22). At present it is considered as a member of a tentative *Hepatovirus* species (20), but this could change if these genomic differences came to be weighed more heavily in the decision process, and a new genus may be necessary. Finally, Ljungan virus is a somewhat similar case. This recently identified virus is a divergent relative of human parechoviruses (genus *Parechovirus*), but the 5' UTR is slightly less related to that of parechoviruses than that of other genera (25). At present it seems appropriate to consider it as a member of a new species of genus *Parechovirus*, but again this could change if other significant differences emerge.

CONCLUSION

Ever-increasing molecular information on picornaviruses has enabled genuine relationships between members to be established and has provided a rational basis for taxonomy. Although this does not always allow simple classification decisions, it is clear that the current taxonomy highlights issues of importance in research and may become increasingly important in epidemiology and clinical practice.

REFERENCES

1. **Acharya, R., E. Fry, D. Stuart, G. Fox, D. Rowlands, and F. Brown.** 1989. The three-dimensional structure of foot-and-mouth disease virus at 2.9 Å resolution. *Nature* **337:**709–716.
2. **Andino, R., N. Böddeker, D. Silvera, and A. V. Gamarnik.** 1999. Intracellular determinants of picornavirus replication. *Trends Microbiol.* **7:**76–82.
3. **Cammack, N., A. Phillips, G. Dunn, V. Patel, and P. D. Minor.** 1988. Intertypic genomic rearrangements of poliovirus strains in vaccines. *Virology* **167:**507–514.
4. **Chow, M., J. F. E. Newman, D. Filman, J. M. Hogle, D. J. Rowlands, and F. Brown.** 1987. Myristoylation of picornavirus capsid protein VP4 and its structural significance. *Nature* **327:**482–486.
5. **Committee on the ECHO Viruses.** 1955. Enteric cytopathogenic human orphan (ECHO) viruses. *Science* **122:**1187–1188.
6. **Cooper, P. D., V. I. Agol, H. L. Bachrach, F. Brown, Y. Ghendon, A. J. Gibbs, H. H. Gillespie, K. Lonberg-Holm, B. Mandel, J. L. Melnick, S. B. Mohanty, R. C. Povey, R. R. Rueckert, F. L. Schaffer, and D. A. J. Tyrrell.** 1978. Picornaviridae: second report. *Intervirology* **10:**165–180.
7. **Ehrenfeld, E., and B. L. Semler.** 1995. Anatomy of the poliovirus internal ribosome entry site. *Curr. Top. Microbiol. Immunol.* **203:**65–83.
8. **Evans, D. J., and J. W. Almond.** 1998. Cell receptors for picornaviruses as determinants of cell tropism and pathogenesis. *Trends Microbiol.* **6:**198–202.
9. **Furione, M., S. Guillot, D. Otelea, J. Balanant, A. Candrea, and R. Crainic.** 1993. Polioviruses with natural recombinant genomes isolated from vaccine-associated paralytic poliomyelitis. *Virology* **196:**199–208.
10. **Grist, N. R., E. J. Bell, and F. Assaad.** 1978. Enteroviruses in human disease. *Prog. Med. Virol.* **24:**114–157.
11. **Hogle, J. M., M. Chow, and D. J. Filman.** 1985. Three-dimensional structure of poliovirus at 2.9 Å resolution. *Science* **229:**1358–1365.
12. **Hogle, J. M., and D. J. Filman.** 1989. 3-dimensional structure of a viral antigen. *Adv. Vet. Sci. Comp. Med.* **33:**65–91.
13. **Holland, J., and E. Domingo.** 1998. Origin and evolution of viruses. *Virus Genes* **16:**13–21.
14. **Hughes, P. J., and G. Stanway.** 2000. The 2A proteins of three picornaviruses are related to each other and to the H-rev 107 family of proteins involved in the control of cell proliferation. *J. Gen. Virol.* **81:**201–207.
15. **Huttunen, P., J. Santti, T. Pulli, and T. Hyypiä.** 1996. The major echovirus subgroup is genetically coherent and related to coxsackie B viruses. *J. Gen. Virol.* **77:**715–725.
16. **Hyypiä, T., T. Hovi, N. J. Knowles, and G. Stanway.** 1997. Classification of enteroviruses based on molecular and biological properties. *J. Gen. Virol.* **78:**1–11.
17. **Hyypiä, T., M. Kallajoki, M. Maaronen, G. Stanway, R. Kandolf, P. Auvinen, and H. Kalimo.** 1993. Pathogenic differences between coxsackie A and B virus infections in newborn mice. *Virus Res.* **27:**71–78.

18. **Jackson, T., D. Sheppard, M. Denyer, W. Blakemore, and A. M. Q. King.** 2000. The epithelial integrin alpha v beta 6 is a receptor for foot-and-mouth disease virus. *J. Virol.* **74:**4949–4956.
19. **Joki-Korpela, P., and T. Hyypiä.** 1998. Diagnosis and epidemiology of echovirus 22 infections. *Clin. Infect. Dis.* **27:**129–136.
20. **King, A. M. Q., F. Brown, P. Christian, T. Hovi, T. Hyypiä, N. J. Knowles, S. M. Lemon, P. D. Minor, A. C. Palmenberg, T. Skern, and G. Stanway.** 2000. *Picornaviridae*, p. 657–673. *In* M. H. V. Van Regenmortel, C. M. Fauquet, D. H. L. Bishop, C. H. Calisher, E. B. Carsten, M. K. Estes, S. M. Lemon, J. Maniloff, M. A. Mayo, D. J. McGeoch, C. R. Pringle, and R. B. Wickner (ed.), *Virus Taxonomy. Seventh Report of the International Committee on the Taxonomy of Viruses.* Academic Press, New York, N.Y.
21. **Lemon, S. M., and B. H. Robertson.** 1993. Current perspectives in the virology and molecular biology of hepatitis A virus. *Semin. Virol.* **4:**285–296.
22. **Marvil, P., N. J. Knowles, A. P. A. Mockett, P. Britton, T. D. K. Brown, and D. Cavanagh.** 1999. Avian encephalomyelitis virus is a picornavirus and is most closely related to hepatitis A virus. *J. Gen. Virol.* **80:**653–662.
23. **Mateu, M. G.** 1995. Antibody recognition of picornaviruses and escape from neutralization—a structural view. *Virus Res.* **38:**1–24.
24. **Melnick, J. L.** 1996. Enteroviruses: polioviruses, coxsackieviruses, echoviruses, and newer enteroviruses, p. 655–712. *In* B. N. Fields, D. M. Knipe, P. M. Howley, et al. (ed.), *Fields Virology.* Lippincott-Raven Publishers, Philadelphia, Pa.
25. **Niklasson, B., L. Kinnunen, B. Hornfeldt, C. Benemar, J. Horling, O. Hedlund, L. Matskova, T. Hyypiä, and G. Winberg.** 1999. A new picornavirus isolated from bank voles (*Clethrionomys glareolus*). *Virology* **255:**86–93.
26. **Oberste, M. S., K. Maher, D. R. Kilpatrick, and M. A. Pallansch.** 1999. Molecular evolution of the human enteroviruses: correlation of serotype with VP1 sequence and application to picornavirus classification. *J. Virol.* **73:**1941–1948.
27. **Palmenberg, A. C.** 1990. Proteolytic processing of the picornaviral polyprotein. *Ann. Rev. Microbiol.* **44:**603–623.
28. **Pöyry, T., L. Kinnunen, T. Hovi, and T. Hyypiä.** 1999. Relationships between simian and human enteroviruses. *J. Gen. Virol.* **80:**635–638.
29. **Pöyry, T., L. Kinnunen, T. Hyypiä, B. Brown, C. Horsnell, T. Hovi, and G. Stanway.** 1996. Genetic and phylogenetic clustering of enteroviruses. *J. Gen. Virol.* **77:**1699–1717.
30. **Pulli, T., E. Koivunen, and T. Hyypiä.** 1997. Cell-surface interactions of echovirus 22. *J. Biol. Chem.* **272:**21176–21180.
31. **Pulli, T., H. Lankinen, M. Roivainen, and T. Hyypiä.** 1998. Antigenic sites of coxsackievirus A9. *Virology* **240:**202–212.
32. **Rico-Hesse, R., M. A. Pallansch, B. K. Nottay, and O. M. Kew.** 1987. Geographic distribution of wild poliovirus type 1 genotypes. *Virology* **160:**311–322.
33. **Roivainen, M., A. Närvänen, M. Korkolainen, M.-L. Huhtala, and T. Hovi.** 1991. Antigenic regions of poliovirus type 3/Sabin capsid proteins recognized by human sera in the peptide scanning technique. *Virology* **180:**99–107.
34. **Rossmann, M. G., E. Arnold, J. W. Erickson, E. A. Frankenberger, J. P. Griffith, H. J. Hect, J. E. Johnson, G. Kamer, M. Luo, A. G. Mosser, R. R. Rueckert, B. Sherry, and G. Vriend.** 1985. Structure of a human common cold virus and functional relationship to other picornaviruses. *Nature* **317:**145–153.
35. **Rueckert, R. R.** 1996. Picornaviridae: the viruses and their replication, p. 609–654. *In* B. N. Fields, D. M. Knipe, P. M. Howley, et al. (ed.), *Fields Virology.* Lippincott-Raven Publishers, Philadelphia, Pa.
36. **Ryan, M. D., and M. Flint.** 1997. Virus encoded proteinases of the picornavirus super-group. *J. Gen. Virol.* **78:**699–723.
37. **Santti, J., T. Hyypiä, L. Kinnunen, and M. Salminen.** 1999. Evidence of recombination among enteroviruses. *J. Virol.* **73:**8741–8749.
38. **Stanway, G., and T. Hyypiä.** 1999. Parechoviruses. *J. Virol.* **73:**5249–5254.
39. **Stanway, G., P. Joki-Korpla, and T. Hyypiä.** 2000. Human parechoviruses—biological and clinical significance. *Rev. Med. Virol.* **10:**57–69.
40. **Stewart, S. R., and B. L. Semler.** 1997. RNA determinants of picornavirus cap-independent translation initiation. *Semin. Virol.* **8:**242–255.
41. **Thompson, J. D., D. G. Higgins, and T. J. Gibson.** 1994. CLUSTAL W: improving the sensitivity of progressive multiple sequence alignment through sequence weighting, position-specific gap penalties and weight matrix choice. *Nucleic Acids Res.* **22:**4673–4680.
42. **Wutz, G., H. Auer, N. Nowotny, B. Grosse, T. Skern, and E. Kuechler.** 1996. Equine rhinovirus serotype-1 and serotype-2—relationship to each other and to aphthoviruses and cardioviruses. *J. Gen. Virol.* **77:**1719–1730.
43. **Yamashita, T., K. Sakae, H. Tsuzuki, Y. Suzuki, N. Ishikawa, N. Takeda, T. Miyamura, and S. Yamazaki.** 1998. Complete nucleotide sequence and genetic organization of Aichi virus, a distinct member of the *Picornaviridae* associated with acute gastroenteritis in humans. *J. Virol.* **72:**8408–8412.

VIRION STRUCTURE

Picornavirus Structure Overview

MICHAEL G. ROSSMANN

3

The three-dimensional, near atomic resolution structures of rhino-, entero- (polio- and coxsackie-), parecho-, and cardioviruses have been determined by X-ray crystallography (Table 1). In many cases, structures have also been determined, often using the lower resolution cryo-electron microscopy (cryo-EM) technique, of picornaviruses in complex with their cellular receptors, neutralizing antibodies, antiviral compounds, or other, biologically significant ligands. In addition, structures have been determined of viruses that closely resemble picorna virions and almost certainly have evolved from a common primordial ancestor. These include insect picornaviruses and plant comoviruses. At a slightly greater evolutionary distance are the plant and insect viruses with triangulation lattices of $T = 3$ (17). Even more distantly related are a great many other viruses that utilize the same structural motif, an eight-stranded, antiparallel, β-barrel ("jelly-roll"), for their major capsid protein.

CAPSID STRUCTURE

Picornavirus capsids are assembled (91) from 60 protomers, each composed of four structural proteins, viral protein 1 (VP1), VP2, VP3, and VP4 (Fig. 1). The first three of these proteins have molecular weights of around 30 kDa and form the external surface of the icosahedral shell. The small VP4, in conjunction with the amino termini of VP1 (about 70 residues in rhino- and enteroviruses) and VP2, forms an interface between the capsid and the internal RNA genome. These residues are disordered in immature virions in which VP0 has yet to be cleaved (10) into VP4 and VP2. The virions contain a single, positive strand of RNA consisting of about 7,000 bases. The total molecular weight of an infectious virion is roughly 8.5 kDa.

The viral protein VP0 is cleaved into its components VP4 and VP2 in the final stages of assembly (81). This maturation step is catalyzed by the juxtaposition of catalytically active amino acid residues in the assembled capsid (47), possibly aided by the entry of RNA into the capsid (5). Similar maturation cleavages occur in many viruses, a process best studied for the insect RNA nodaviruses (122).

The insect cricket paralysis virus utilizes the amino end of VP3 (instead of VP2 as in mammalian picornaviruses) to generate the essential VP4, while otherwise maintaining the same gene order.

Both X-ray crystallography and cryo-EM depend on icosahedral symmetry for determining the structure of simple viruses. Therefore, in general, it is only the icosahedrally symmetric protein shell of virions whose structure can be established clearly. Most of the time, there is little information about RNA structure. However, occasionally, some of the secondary structure of the genome assumes the symmetry of the enveloping capsid, revealing extensive segments of ordered nucleic acid, as in cowpea mosaic virus (CpMV) (24) and satellite tobacco mosaic virus (61). Nevertheless, picornaviruses have generally shown little tendency for RNA ordering, although there is a conserved tryptophan residue in VP2 (residue 56 in human rhinovirus 16 [HRV16] and HRV14) that frequently nucleates the association of one or two RNA bases.

Both the tertiary fold of the VP1, VP2, and VP3 polypeptide chains and their quaternary organization within picornavirus capsids are similar to many $T = 3$ plant and insect viruses (Table 1, Fig. 1 and 2). In the $T = 3$ viruses, the three quasi-equivalent subunits A, C, and B have identical amino acid sequences but differ slightly in their geometrical environments. In picornaviruses, the amino acid sequences in the three major capsid proteins bear no obvious similarity, but nevertheless have similar folds and are related by a pseudo-threefold axis forming a "$P = 3$" icosahedral surface lattice. Many of the $T = 3$ virus capsid proteins have basic amino termini that are internal and are associated with the genomic RNA. Although the amino termini of the picornavirus subunits are not especially basic, these termini, together with VP4, are internal, are partly disordered, and form a protein layer separating the external capsid of 180 β-barrels from the internal RNA. Conversely, the carboxy termini of the major VPs of picornaviruses and the $T = 3$ viruses are exposed on the capsid surface.

Metal ions have been identified on the symmetry axes in many icosahedral viruses. However, a specific site for Ca

---

Michael G. Rossmann ■ Department of Biological Sciences, Purdue University, West Lafayette, IN 47907-1392.

TABLE 1 Picornavirus structures (primary structural reports)

Virus	Event	Reference
Rhinoviruses	Cations in HRVs	118
HRV14	First structure determination of any picornavirus	87
	First structure of an antiviral complex with a capsid	98
	Other antiviral complexes	7–9, 20, 21, 35, 116, 117
	Refined structure	6
	Structure at acid pH	34
	Drug-resistant mutants	40
	Cryo-EM complexes with neutralizing Fabs and antibodies (Abs)	23, 99, 100
	First crystal structure of a virus complexed with an Fab	97
	Cryo-EM of complex with ICAM-1	57
HRV16	Structure of a clinically interesting virus	78
	Cryo-EM of complex with ICAM-1	11, 57, 79
	Complex with antiviral compounds	20, 38
	Refined structure	39
HRV3	Structure of virus and complex with antiviral compounds	119
HRV1A	First structure of a minor receptor-group rhinovirus	55
	Complexes with antiviral compounds	56
HRV2	Detailed structure of a minor receptor-group rhinovirus	108
	Fab fragment from a neutralizing Ab complexed with viral peptide	105–107
	Cryo-EM of Ab complexed with virus	44, 45
Enteroviruses (polio)		
PV1	First poliovirus structure	51
	Sites of neutralizing epitopes	80
	Cryo-EM complex with poliovirus receptor	13, 42, 114
	Neutralizing Fab fragment complexed with viral peptide	113
	Mutants that overcome receptor defects	112
	Complexes with antiviral compounds	48
	Cryo-EM studies of cell entry intermediates	12
PV2	Structure	64
	Mouse-adapted type 2/3 chimera	115
PV3	Structure and structural recognition of pocket factor	29
	Complex with antiviral compounds	10, 37, 49
Enteroviruses (coxsackie)		
CBV3	First coxsackievirus structure	76
CAV9	Structure	43
CAV21	Cryo-EM of virus complexed with ICAM-1	113a
Other entero- and parechoviruses		
Bovine enterovirus	Structure	101
Echovirus 1	Structure	30
Cardioviruses		
Mengo virus	First cardiovirus structure	74
	Mengovirus at different pH values	55
	Refined structure	59
Theiler's murine encephalomyelitis virus	Structure of BeAn strain	72
	Structure of DA strain	36
	Structure of GDVII strain	73
	Role of sialic acid as a cell receptor	120, 121
Aphthoviruses		
FMDV O(1)	First aphthovirus structure	3
	Conformational changes in the major antigenic loop	82
	Role of an oligosaccharide as a cell surface receptor	33
	Structure of RGD in antigenic loop controlled by S-S bonds	70
	Structure of RGD in antigenic loop complexed with Fab	109
	Structural comparisons with O(1) variant G67	62
	Complex with oligosaccharide receptor	33
	RGD-specific binding to purified integrin	53
FMDV C	Cryo-EM structure of Fab-virus complex	46, 110
	Structure and antigenic surface	63
FMDV A22	Correlation of the structure of the GH loop with cell adaption	28
Insect picornaviruses		
Cricket paralysis virus	Structure	104

(Continued on next page)

TABLE 1 (Continued)

Virus	Event	Reference
$P = 3$ plant comoviruses		
Cowpea mottle virus	Cryo-EM Fab complex with virus	84
	Capsid and RNA structure	24
	Chimeric virus structure	69
	Refined structure	67
Red clover mottle virus	Structure	68
$T = 3$ plant viruses		
Tomato bushy stunt virus	Structure	41
Southern bean mosaic virus	Structure	2
Cowpea chlorotic mottle virus	Structure	102
Cucumber mosaic virus	3.2-Å structure	96
Tobacco ringspot virus	Structure	18
Brome mosaic virus	Cryo-EM studies	60
Sesbania mosaic virus	Structure	14, 77
Physalis mottle virus	Structure	103
$T = 3$ insect viruses		
Black beetle virus	Refined structure	111
Turnip yellow mosaic virus	Structure	16
	Cryo-EM studies of full and empty particles	15

or Zn is frequently observed on the fivefold axes of picornaviruses (Color Plate 1, following p. 156) (39, 118). Ions in such central coordinating sites will undoubtedly help stabilize the virions. It may be significant, therefore, that the occupancy of the Ca ion-binding site in HRV14 is affected by the binding of stabilizing antiviral compounds (54) (see below) into a hydrophobic pocket in VP1.

EVOLUTION

Conservation of three-dimensional structure is almost invariably greater than conservation of amino acid homology (86). Thus, structural comparisons can be used to trace divergent evolution over longer time spans than is possible by amino acid sequence comparisons. Structural similarities can be measured and used to assess the probability of divergence, providing benchmarks to which other comparisons can be related (75). Thus, the similarity of picornavirus gene sequences, gene order, and structures, including insect (104) and plant picorna-like viruses (25), makes it probable that all these viruses had a common ancestor. The similarity between picornavirus and many $T = 3$ plant (1, 41) and insect (93) virus structures makes it likely that at least the structural component of the picornavirus genome is the result of triplication of the capsid protein gene while also retaining the gene order for a large component of their genomes (Fig. 2). At an even earlier time, there may have occurred the divergence from a gene able to express the eight-stranded, β-barrel motif, common to numerous animal, plant, insect, and bacterial viruses (66, 88).

ASSEMBLY

Assembly of picornaviruses proceeds from 6S protomers of VP1, VP3, and VP0, via 14S pentamers of five 6S protomers, to mature virions. The final step involves inclusion of the RNA into empty capsids or partially assembled shells with simultaneous cleavage of VP0 into VP2 and VP4. Conversely, in vitro disassembly, produced by mild denaturation, proceeds via the expulsion of VP4 followed by RNA (91). The amino and carboxy ends of VP1 and VP3 are intertwined with each other, and VP0 is intertwined with VP1 and VP3, which strongly suggests that the 6S protomer is as shown in Fig. 1. These protomers are themselves intertwined because of the fivefold β-cylinders formed by the amino ends of the VP3s and VP4s around the fivefold axes (Fig. 1 and Color Plate 1). Thus, the observed 14S pentamer assembly intermediates correlate with picornavirus structures.

Picornavirus RNA codes for only one long open reading frame. The giant precursor polyprotein is divided into three regions: P1, P2, and P3. The polyprotein is posttranslationally processed in a series of proteolytic cleavage steps to yield virion capsid proteins, as well as other noncapsid viral proteins. All cleavages, except for that of VP0, are produced by one of two virally coded specific proteases. Cleavage between the P1, P2, and P3 regions is fast, whereas the subsequent cleavage of P1, containing the structural proteins, is slower (5). The potential cleavage sites in P1, with gene order VP4-VP2-VP3-VP1 (Fig. 2), are between the β-barrel domains. The probable manner in which the carboxyl end of VP0 would be associated with the amino end of VP3 and the carboxyl end of VP3 would be associated with the amino end of VP1 within a 6S protomer can be easily visualized (5). Successive cleavages, in which the ends reposition themselves, will then direct assembly of 12S pentamers and the assembly of immature capsids. Finally, the cleavage of VP0 generates the infectious, fully assembled virion. In some picorna-like viruses, such as comoviruses, there is no cleavage between VP2 and VP3. Nevertheless, the positions of the VP2 and VP3 domains within the capsid are exactly as in other picornaviruses (Fig. 1) (71), justifying the assumption that there is no major rearrangement within the 6S protomer after cleavage into the separate proteins.

Arnold et al. (5) had suggested that cleavage of VP0 is catalyzed by a conserved serine residue in VP2 and an RNA base. Thus, catalysis could be initiated in the final stages of packaging when RNA bases are crowded close to the potential cleavage site situated on the internal face of the capsid. However, Hindiyeh et al. (47) show that, at least in polioviruses, one of the essential catalytic residues

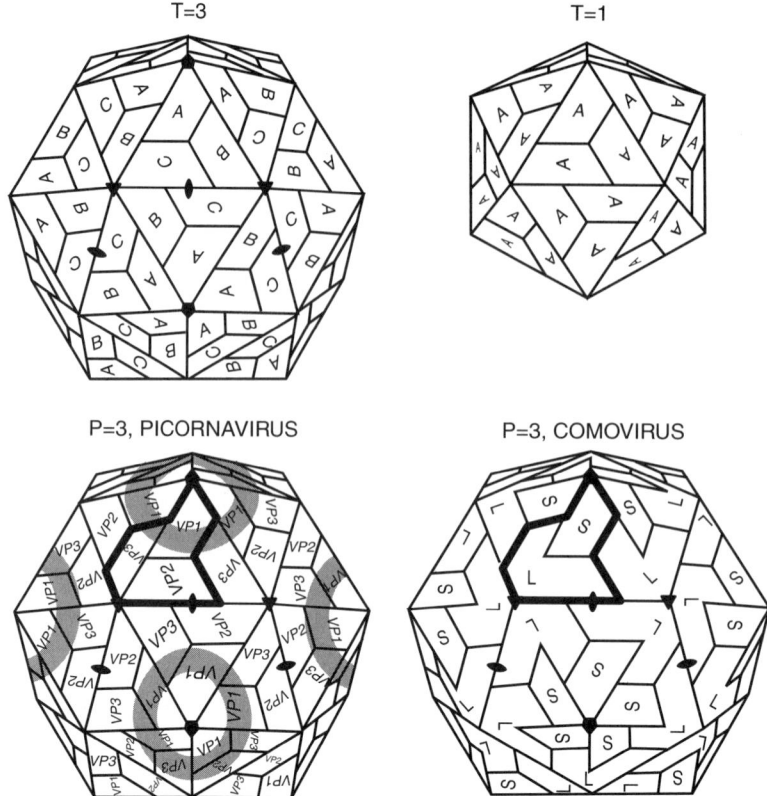

FIGURE 1 Different virion capsids with icosahedral symmetry. The $T = 1$ shell contains 60 subunits, each represented by a trapezoid that has the approximate shape of the β-barrel. All subunits in the $T = 1$ capsid are identical and are labeled A. The asymmetric unit of the $T = 3$ capsid contains subunits A, B, and C, all of which have the same amino acid sequence but are in slightly different environments. The threefold axis relating A, B, and C is not exact. This quasi-threefold axis also relates the quasi-sixfold axes (left and right vertexes of the triangle) to a fivefold axis (top vertex). Like the $T = 1$ structure, the $T = 3$ structures are formed by identical subunits with the same β-barrel fold. The $P = 3$ picornavirus shell, technically a $T = 1$ particle, is closely related to the $T = 3$ shell, being formed by 180 β-barrel domains. The three subunits, labeled VP1, VP2, and VP3, are, however, distinct proteins. The deep, canyon-like depression, the site of receptor attachment in many picornaviruses, is shaded. One 6S protomer assembly intermediate is outlined with a thick black border. The comovirus shell is very similar to the picornavirus capsid, with 180 β-barrels forming the shell. However, there are only two protein types. The large protein (labeled L) is composed of two β-barrel domains (equivalent of VP2 and VP3) covalently linked together. The small subunit (S) is a single β-barrel domain. Reprinted with permission from Rossmann and Johnson (88).

is the conserved histidine 195 of VP2. A similar autocatalytic maturation mechanism has also been recognized in the maturation of the $T = 3$ insect nodaviruses (122).

THE VIRAL PROTEINS

The β-strands that form the β-barrel structures of VP1, VP2, and VP3 are named B, C, ..., I along the polypeptide. This nomenclature was derived from the first icosahedral virus structures, tomato bushy stunt virus (41) and southern bean mosaic virus (1). In these viruses, subunit C, like VP2 in picornaviruses, has an additional, ordered β-strand at the amino end that was labeled βA. The other eight strands form a two-sided β-barrel between sheets containing the antiparallel B, I, D, and G ("BIDG") strands and the "CHEF" strands (Fig. 3). The β-barrel is wedge-shaped, with its narrow end close to the icosahedral fivefold axes in VP1 or to the pseudo-sixfold axes in VP2 and VP3 (Fig. 1). The thin edge of the wedge consists of four turns, between β-strands B and C, H and I, E and D, and F and G. The BC turn is the most external and is especially antigenic in VP1.

Sequence insertions form protrusions on VP1, VP2, and VP3, creating a deep cleft or "canyon" on the viral surface in rhino- and enteroviruses. The canyon is about 15 Å deep and 12 Å wide at its narrowest. The "south" rim of the canyon (as viewed in Fig. 1) is lined with the carboxy terminus of VP1. The "north" rim of the canyon is partially lined with the carboxy terminus of VP3. VP1 is the major contributor lining the canyon. Cardio- and aphthoviruses have their canyons partially or completely filled by an insertion following βC in cardioviruses and by an insertion

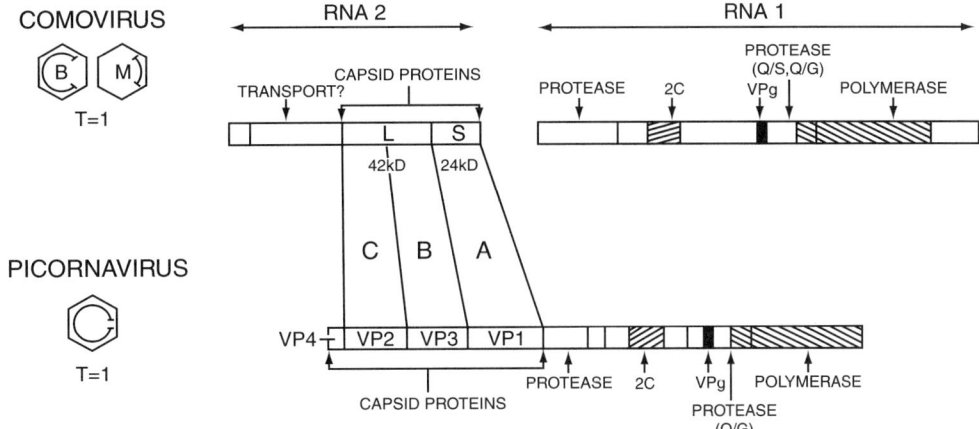

FIGURE 2 Comparison of the genome organization of CpMV and picornaviruses. RNA2 (left) and RNA1 (right) of CpMV are shown aligned with the RNA of picornaviruses. The molecular weight and function are marked for each gene product. Regions in the two genomes are shaded where the amino acid sequences had been recognized as homologous (4, 31). The 42-kDa structural protein in CpMV (L) contains β-barrel domains that correspond in location to VP2 and VP3 in picornaviruses. The 24-kDa protein in CpMV (S) corresponds to protein VP1 in picornaviruses. The letters C, B, and A indicate the positions occupied by each of these β-barrels in the $T = 3$ quasi-equivalent surface lattice. Reprinted with permission from Rossmann and Johnson (88).

between βG and βH in foot-and-mouth disease viruses (FMDVs). The canyon is the site of attachment to cellular receptors in many entero- and rhinoviruses (see below).

Various insertions between the strands that form the β-barrels of VP1, VP2, and VP3 have been identified by special names (87). The "puff" is a hypervariable, frequently antigenic region between βE and αB in VP2, forming part of the south rim of the canyon. The "foot-and-mouth loop," named for its strong antigenic properties in FMDV (although a better name is GH loop), is an insertion between βG and βH in VP1 and also forms a part of the south rim of the canyon. The "knob" is an antigenic insertion in the middle of βB of VP3. These insertions alter the surface properties of the viruses, affecting their interaction with host antibodies and potential cellular receptors. A useful way of representing these features is by means of "roadmaps" that map the surface residues and topology (Color Plate 2, following p. 156) (19, 89). These maps usually show one icosahedral asymmetric unit defined by a triangle between adjacent five-, three-, and twofold axes.

INTERACTION WITH NEUTRALIZING ANTIBODIES

The sites of binding of neutralizing monoclonal antibodies have been mapped for rhinovirus 14 (94, 95) and poliovirus 1 (80) by selecting plaques grown in the presence of the antibodies. The mutant viruses that were able to grow were mostly single mutations and could be sorted into groups that were neutralized by the same set of antibodies. The mutations were localized on the surface of the virions, showing a remarkable correspondence between the groups identified by the antibodies and the local grouping on the viral surface. Each group of mutations was found to be associated with highly exposed surface features, corresponding to the most variable amino acid sequences in a comparison of serotypes (22, 89). In particular, the BC, IH, and DE loops of VP1, the puff of VP2, and the knob of VP3 were recognized as the preferred sites of binding.

The structures of neutralizing antibody Fab fragments, complexed with virus, have been studied by cryo-EM and X-ray crystallography (Table 1). These studies have established a correlation between strong and weak neutralizing antibodies with bivalent and monovalent binding modes, respectively (23, 97).

INTERACTION WITH VIRAL RECEPTORS

The canyon was hypothesized to be the site of cellular receptor binding (87), on account of its probable inaccessi-

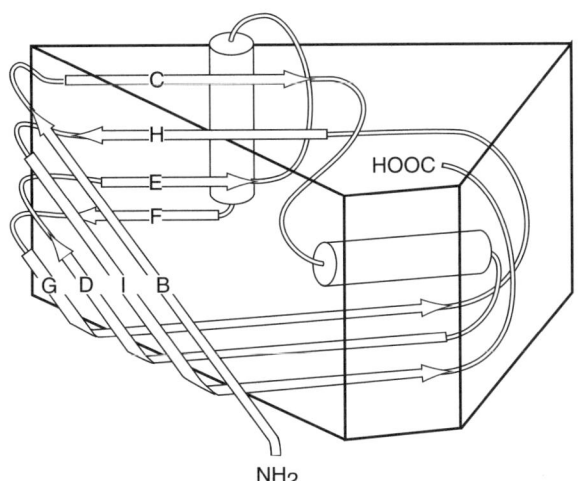

FIGURE 3 Diagrammatic representation of the polypeptide fold of one subunit of poliovirus found also in the shell-forming portion of most other viral subunit structures. Shown also is the nomenclature for the secondary structural elements βB, βC, ..., βI. Reprinted with permission from Hogle et al. (51).

bility to antibodies, thus being a site protected from the host's immune surveillance (Fig. 4). This prediction turned out to be correct for the major group of rhinoviruses (57, 79), polioviruses (13, 42, 114), and coxsackie A21 virus (113a), although the rationale of the prediction has been questioned (97). In vitro studies of virus-receptor complexes have been difficult in that the virions become unstable, forming, in succession, antigenically altered A particles and empty capsids that have lost their RNA genomes, eventually causing the capsid to completely fall apart (52). Thus, it has not yet been possible to capture the transient virus-receptor complexes long enough to permit crystallization. However, it has been possible, by careful control of temperature and incubation time, to study virus-receptor complexes by cryo-EM image reconstructions (Table 1). Armed with separate crystal structures of the cellular receptor for the major group of rhinoviruses, intercellular adhesion molecule-1 (ICAM-1), and appropriate major receptor-group rhinoviruses, it has been possible to use cryo-EM reconstructions to obtain fairly accurate analyses of virus-receptor interactions (57, 79). Similar studies of the interaction of the poliovirus receptor molecule (CD155) have lacked an accurate knowledge of the receptor molecule. Nevertheless, information on the atomic detail of the poliovirus-receptor interactions has been obtained by using homology modeling of CD155, guided by the sites of glycosylation seen in the cryo-EM densities and by mutational analyses (13, 42, 114).

It has been suggested (78, 85) that initiation of uncoating is caused by competition between receptor and a lipid-like "pocket factor" bound in a hydrophobic pocket within VP1 (see antiviral section below). Loss of this factor causes the virus to lose stability, thus giving a link between virus recognition and subsequent initiation of uncoating. The cellularly derived pocket factor would thus regulate the virion to be stable while transiting from cell to cell or host to host, but poised for infection once the virus has recognized a suitable cell (Fig. 5).

Cardioviruses have a "pit" in the position of the canyon (74), which was similarly predicted to be the site of cellular adhesion. The pit is a region of poorly ordered structure of the GH loops of VP1 and VP3. These loops achieve greater order at acidic pH. Correlation of this conformational change with infectivity, and because the pit in Theiler's virus is the site of binding to certain cell surface polysaccharides (120), gives credence to the pit being the site of receptor attachment.

Aphthoviruses have an alternative way (27) of hiding their receptor attachment sites from the host's immune system. The site of host cell binding is associated with the highly antigenic GH loop, which also contains an Arg-Gly-Asp (RGD) motif, frequently associated with binding of integrins. Indeed, an integrin has been identified as a cellular receptor for some FMDVs (53), although oligosaccharides have also been shown to bind to FMDV serotype O(1) (33). It is not surprising, therefore, that the conformation of the GH loop is highly variable, changing from being disordered to being well structured, depending on the formation of a S-S bond between the ends of the GH loop in VP1. The polymorphic conformation of this loop may be a mechanism for evading host immune surveillance (82).

There is a wide variety of cell surface molecules that are used by picornaviruses for initiating infection. For instance, a small group of rhinoviruses utilize a low-density lipoprotein receptor (50) and some coxsackieviruses utilize a decay-accelerating factor. Most of these molecules are long and slender like ICAM-1. Their shape may not only be related to their ability to find partially buried binding sites, but to their articulation, a property useful for binding to equivalent sites around the viral surface. Therefore, recruitment of additional receptor molecules that bind to a single virion will cause an increase of avidity.

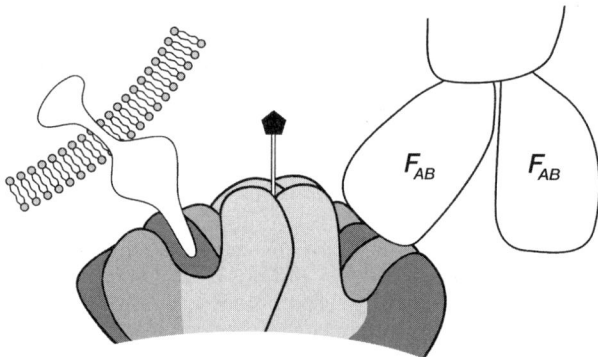

FIGURE 4 Diagrammatic representation of the canyon hypothesis. It was suggested that the canyon would be too narrow to allow the binding of a neutralizing antibody. It was also hypothesized that a receptor would be a slender molecule able to bind to the conserved amino acids lining the canyon, thereby avoiding host immune surveillance. The hypothesis was later found to be correct in as far as the site of receptor attachment and shape of the receptor molecule was concerned. However, the footprints of neutralizing antibodies and of the receptor on the viral surface were found to be partially overlapping, which gave some concern as to whether the original hypothesis was based on a correct premise, even though the basic predictions turned out to be correct for rhino- and enteroviruses.

CAPSID-BINDING ANTIVIRAL COMPOUNDS

A large variety of small, hydrophobic, flexible, organic compounds (molecular weight about 300 Da) can bind into a hydrophobic pocket within the VP1 β-barrel (Color Plate 3, following p. 156) (98). When bound, these compounds expand the previously empty pocket by raising the "roof" of the pocket, which also doubles as the "floor" of the canyon and is constructed largely from the GH loop of VP1. The presence of hydrophobic compounds, within one or more of the 60 available pockets, enhances the thermal stability of the whole virus. The change of conformation of the canyon floor can also inhibit receptor attachment in some cases (83). As a result, these compounds can inhibit both viral attachment to cells and also release of RNA into the host cell. Extensive structural studies (Table 1) of these compounds have helped to define the boundaries and chemical requirements that enhance activity against a wide spectrum of slightly different picornavirus serotypes. These studies have also elucidated the nature of drug resistance (Fig. 5) and the way in which receptor attachment can initiate viral uncoating (40, 85).

Pleconaril (Color Plate 3) is being developed as an antirhino- and antienterovirus drug by ViroPharma, Inc. (92), although the U.S. Food and Drug Administration has recently discouraged further development in light of some minor cross-reaction with other drugs in large clinical trials. Nevertheless, pleconaril has been studied in over 200

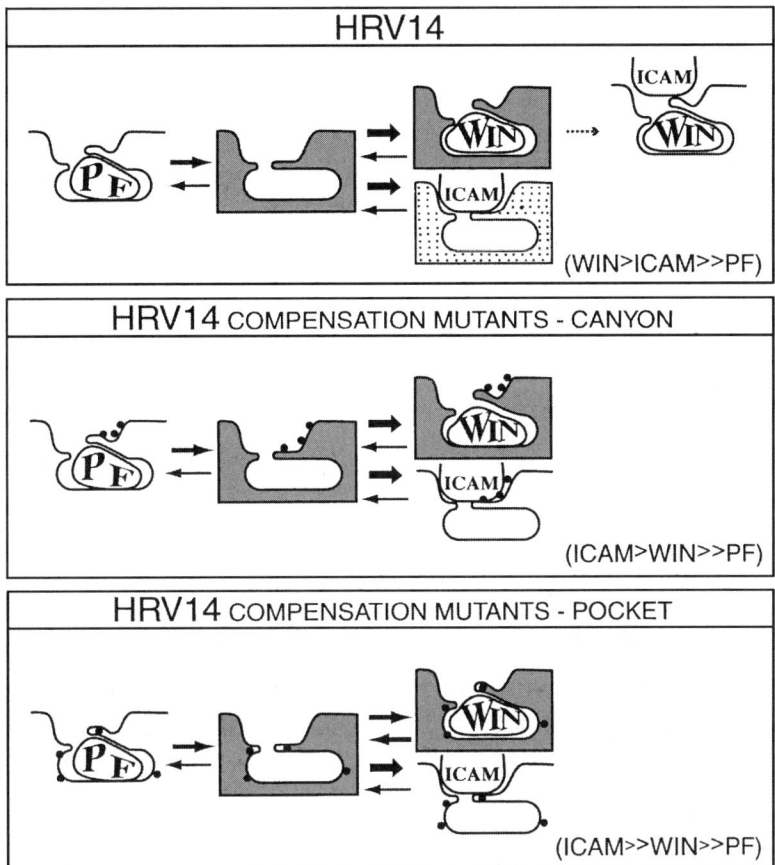

FIGURE 5 Schematic representation of the competition between receptor binding and binding of a pocket factor within the hydrophobic pocket in VP1. The structures represented in gray have been determined crystallographically, and the dotted structure in the top panel has been determined by electron microscopy. When pocket factor binds into the pocket, it deforms the canyon roof, which is also the floor of the canyon. When receptor binds into the canyon, the pocket is presumed to be empty. Thus, the effect of receptor binding is to expel the pocket factor, thereby destabilizing the virus and initiating uncoating, as shown in the top panel. For this to be able to happen, it is necessary for the affinity between the ICAM-1 receptor and the viral surface to exceed that of the antiviral compound (WIN) or pocket factor to the virus. In the middle panel are shown some of the drug-resistant compensation mutations (black spheres) that are on the floor of the canyon. They have been shown to increase the affinity of ICAM-1 for the virus (40). Thus, the binding affinity of ICAM-1 for the mutant virus would now be greater than that for the WIN compounds. Other compensation escape mutations, as shown in the bottom panel, are found lining the hydrophobic binding pocket. These have less bulk than the wild-type residues, thus reducing the affinity of the WIN compounds for the virus. Since the affinity of the receptor ICAM-1 for the virus is unchanged, the equilibrium is altered in favor of receptor binding rather than WIN compound binding. Reprinted with permission from Hadfield et al. (40).

patients with life-threatening enterovirus (neonatal sepsis, myocarditis, polio, chronic meningoencephalitis, etc.) and rhinovirus infections (pneumonia in bone marrow transplants) with impressive responses (92).

The pocket in VP1 that is utilized by these antirhino- and antienterovirus compounds is frequently found occupied by unexpected density in X-ray crystallographically derived maps. This density (pocket factor) is thought to be a fatty acid or similar hydrophobic compound with a polar head group derived from cellular components (29, 40, 78, 85). The pocket factor presumably has a stabilizing effect on the virion in the same way as do the antiviral compounds. However, the latter probably have a larger impact on the virions as they successfully compete with the pocket factor (Fig. 6). These observations have led to the suggestion that the pocket factor regulates stability (see above). The sensitive equilibrium between pocket factor and receptor binding is altered on replacing the pocket factor by better binding antiviral compounds.

The remarkable stabilizing effect of the antiviral compounds has been demonstrated by comparing the effect of proteases on the virus and on the virus complexed with one of the compounds. Surprisingly, numerous internal peptides are available to protease digestion, but these sites are protected in the presence of the antiviral compounds (65). Similar exposure of internal peptides to the viral sur-

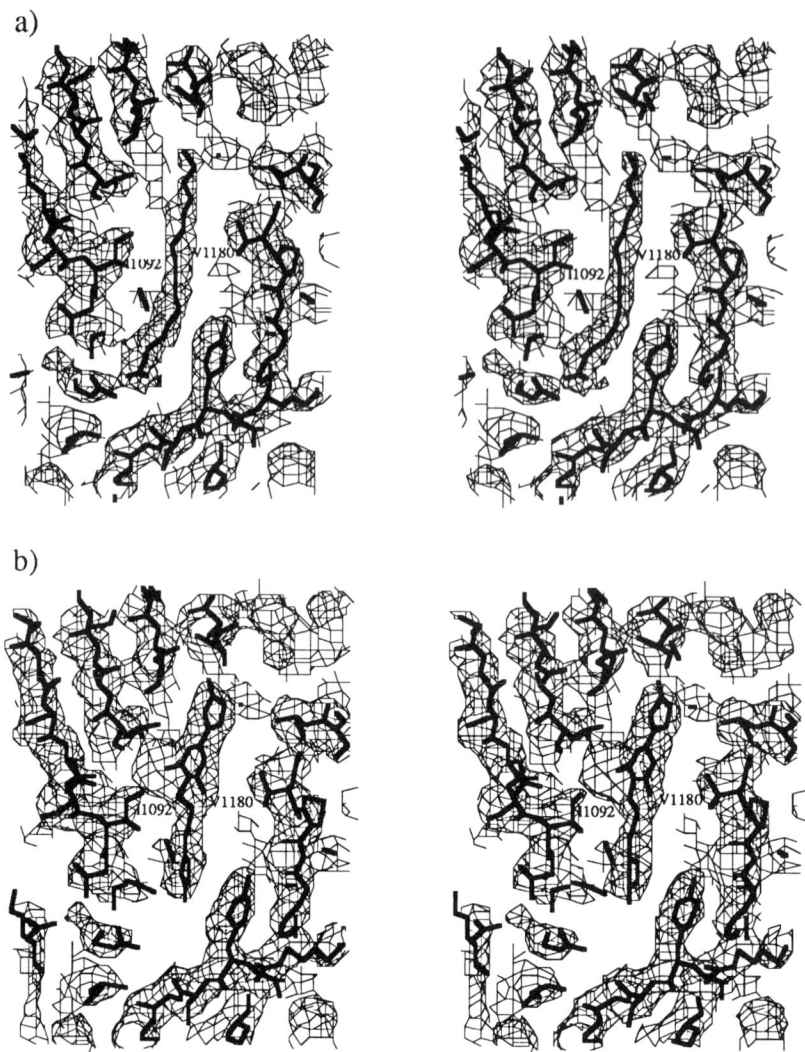

FIGURE 6 The pocket factor within the VP1 hydrophobic pocket of coxsackievirus B3 (CVB3) (76). (a) Electron density in the middle of the figure represents the pocket factor in the VP1 pocket, whereas (b) shows the VP1 pocket of CVB3 occupied by antiviral compound WIN 66393. Comparison of the two electron density maps shows clearly that the longer pocket factor has been displaced by the shorter WIN compound. The large peak is the result of an iodine atom in the antiviral compound (76). Reprinted with permission from Muckelbauer et al. (76).

face had been demonstrated by a search for antigenic regions (26). A variety of additional evidence all points to the ability of simple icosahedral viruses to be in constant flux or "breathing." This unexpected and structurally difficult-to-understand phenomenon accounts for the virus being able to externalize the internal VP4 and amino-terminal region of VP1 in the initial stages of cell entry (32).

I take this opportunity to express my deep gratitude to Roland R. Rueckert, without whose tutelage, help, and encouragement I would never have been able to gain entry into the fascinating world of picornaviruses. I also thank all the many outstanding postdoctoral fellows and graduate students who have participated in these studies during the last 20 years. Thanks also to Cheryl Towell and Sharon Wilder who helped in the preparation of this article. The work has been supported by a series of National Institutes of Health grants and an award from the Lucille P. Markey Foundation, as well as one from Purdue University.

REFERENCES

1. **Abad-Zapatero, C., S. S. Abdel-Meguid, J. E. Johnson, A. G. W. Leslie, I. Rayment, M. G. Rossmann, D. Suck, and T. Tsukihara.** 1980. Structure of southern bean mosaic virus at 2.8 Å resolution. *Nature (London)* **286:**33–39.
2. **Abad-Zapatero, C., S. S. Abdel-Meguid, J. E. Johnson, A. G. W. Leslie, I. Rayment, M. G. Rossmann, D. Suck, and T. Tsukihara.** 1981. A description of techniques used in the structure determination of southern bean mosaic virus at 2.8 Å resolution. *Acta Crystallogr.* **B37:**2002–2018.
3. **Acharya, R., E. Fry, D. Stuart, G. Fox, D. Rowlands, and F. Brown.** 1989. The three-dimensional structure of foot-and-mouth disease virus at 2.9 Å resolution. *Nature (London)* **337:**709–716.
4. **Argos, P., G. Kamer, M. J. H. Nicklin, and E. Wimmer.** 1984. Similarity in gene organization and homology be-

tween proteins of animal picornaviruses and a plant comovirus suggest common ancestry of these virus families. *Nucleic Acids Res.* **12**:7251–7267.

5. **Arnold, E., M. Luo, G. Vriend, M. G. Rossmann, A. C. Palmenberg, G. D. Parks, M. J. H. Nicklin, and E. Wimmer.** 1987. Implications of the picornavirus capsid structure for polyprotein processing. *Proc. Natl. Acad. Sci. USA* **84**:21–25.

6. **Arnold, E., and M. G. Rossmann.** 1990. Analysis of the structure of a common cold virus, human rhinovirus 14, refined at a resolution of 3.0 Å. *J. Mol. Biol.* **211**:763–801.

7. **Badger, J., S. Krishnaswamy, M. J. Kremer, M. A. Oliveira, M. G. Rossmann, B. A. Heinz, R. R. Rueckert, F. J. Dutko, and M. A. McKinlay.** 1989. Three-dimensional structures of drug-resistant mutants of human rhinovirus 14. *J. Mol. Biol.* **207**:163–174.

8. **Badger, J., I. Minor, M. J. Kremer, M. A. Oliveira, T. J. Smith, J. P. Griffith, D. M. A. Guerin, S. Krishnaswamy, M. Luo, M. G. Rossmann, M. A. McKinlay, G. D. Diana, F. J. Dutko, M. Fancher, R. R. Rueckert, and B. A. Heinz.** 1988. Structural analysis of a series of antiviral agents complexed with human rhinovirus 14. *Proc. Natl. Acad. Sci. USA* **85**:3304–3308.

9. **Badger, J., I. Minor, M. A. Oliveira, T. J. Smith, and M. G. Rossmann.** 1989. Structural analysis of antiviral agents that interact with the capsid of human rhinoviruses. *Proteins* **6**:1–19.

10. **Basavappa, R., R. Syed, O. Flore, J. P. Icenogle, D. J. Filman, and J. M. Hogle.** 1994. Role and mechanism of the maturation cleavage of VP0 in poliovirus assembly: structure of the empty capsid assembly intermediate at 2.9 Å resolution. *Protein Sci.* **3**:1651–1669.

11. **Bella, J., P. R. Kolatkar, C. W. Marlor, J. M. Greve, and M. G. Rossmann.** 1998. The structure of the two amino-terminal domains of human ICAM-1 suggests how it functions as a rhinovirus receptor and as an LFA-1 integrin ligand. *Proc. Natl. Acad. Sci. USA* **95**:4140–4145.

12. **Belnap, D. M., D. J. Filman, B. L. Trus, N. Cheng, F. P. Booy, J. F. Conway, S. Curry, C. N. Hiremath, S. K. Tsang, A. C. Steven, and J. M. Hogle.** 2000. Molecular tectonic model of virus structural transitions: the putative cell entry states of poliovirus. *J. Virol.* **74**:1342–1354.

13. **Belnap, D. M., B. M. McDermott, Jr., D. J. Filman, N. Cheng, B. L. Trus, H. J. Zuccola, V. R. Racaniello, J. M. Hogle, and A. C. Steven.** 2000. Three-dimensional structure of poliovirus receptor bound to poliovirus. *Proc. Natl. Acad. Sci. USA* **97**:73–78.

14. **Bhuvaneshwari, M., H. S. Subramanya, K. Gopinath, H. S. Savithri, M. V. Nayudu, and M. R. N. Murthy.** 1995. Structure of sesbania mosaic virus at 3 Å resolution. *Structure* **3**:1021–1030.

15. **Böttcher, B., and R. A. Crowther.** 1996. Difference imaging reveals ordered regions of RNA in turnip yellow mosaic virus. *Structure* **4**:387–394.

16. **Canady, M. A., S. B. Larson, J. Day, and A. McPherson.** 1996. Crystal structure of turnip yellow mosaic virus. *Nat. Struct. Biol.* **3**:771–781.

17. **Caspar, D. L. D., and A. Klug.** 1962. Physical principles in the construction of regular viruses. *Cold Spring Harbor Symp. Quant. Biol.* **27**:1–24.

18. **Chandrasekar, V., and J. E. Johnson.** 1998. The structure of tobacco ringspot virus: a link in the evolution of icosahedral capsids in the picornavirus superfamily. *Structure* **6**:157–171.

19. **Chapman, M. S.** 1993. Mapping the surface properties of macromolecules. *Protein Sci.* **2**:459–469.

20. **Chapman, M. S., K. H. Kim, and M. G. Rossmann.** 1993. Structural comparisons of several antiviral agents complexed with human rhinoviruses of different serotypes. *Int. Antivir. News* **1**:53–54.

21. **Chapman, M. S., I. Minor, M. G. Rossmann, G. D. Diana, and K. Andries.** 1991. Human rhinovirus 14 complexed with antiviral compound R 61837. *J. Mol. Biol.* **217**:455–463.

22. **Chapman, M. S., and M. G. Rossmann.** 1993. Structure, sequence and function correlations among parvoviruses. *Virology* **194**:491–508.

23. **Che, Z., N. H. Olson, D. Leippe, W. Lee, A. G. Mosser, R. R. Rueckert, T. S. Baker, and T. J. Smith.** 1998. Antibody-mediated neutralization of human rhinovirus 14 explored by means of cryoelectron microscopy and X-ray crystallography of virus-Fab complexes. *J. Virol.* **72**:4610–4622.

24. **Chen, Z., C. Stauffacher, Y. Li, T. Schmidt, W. Bomu, G. Kamer, M. Shanks, G. Lomonossoff, and J. E. Johnson.** 1989. Protein-RNA interactions in an icosahedral virus at 3.0 Å resolution. *Science* **245**:154–159.

25. **Chen, Z., C. V. Stauffacher, and J. E. Johnson.** 1990. Capsid structure and RNA packaging in comoviruses. *Semin. Virol.* **1**:453–466.

26. **Chow, M., R. Yabrov, J. Bittle, J. Hogle, and D. Baltimore.** 1985. Synthetic peptides from four separate regions of the poliovirus type 1 capsid protein VP1 induce neutralizing antibodies. *Proc. Natl. Acad. Sci. USA* **82**:910–914.

27. **Colman, P. M.** 1997. Virus versus antibody. *Structure* **5**:591–593.

28. **Curry, S., E. Fry, W. Blakemore, R. Abu-Ghazaleh, T. Jackson, A. King, S. Lea, J. Newman, D. Rowlands, and D. Stuart.** 1996. Perturbations in the surface structure of A22 Iraq foot-and-mouth disease virus accompanying coupled changes in host cell specificity and antigenicity. *Structure* **4**:135–145.

29. **Filman, D. J., R. Syed, M. Chow, A. J. Macadam, P. D. Minor, and J. M. Hogle.** 1989. Structural factors that control conformational transitions and serotype specificity in type 3 poliovirus. *EMBO J.* **8**:1567–1579.

30. **Filman, D. J., M. W. Wien, J. A. Cunningham, J. M. Bergelson, and J. M. Hogle.** 1998. Structure determination of echovirus I. *Acta Crystallogr.* **D54**:1261–1272.

31. **Franssen, H., J. Leunissen, R. Goldbach, G. Lomonossoff, and D. Zimmern.** 1984. Homologous sequences in non-structural proteins from cowpea mosaic virus and picornaviruses. *EMBO J.* **3**:855–861.

32. **Fricks, C. E., and J. M. Hogle.** 1990. Cell-induced conformational change in poliovirus: externalization of the amino terminus of VP1 is responsible for liposome binding. *J. Virol.* **64**:1934–1945.

33. **Fry, E. E., S. M. Lea, T. Jackson, J. W. I. Newman, F. M. Ellard, W. E. Blakemore, R. Abu-Ghazaleh, A. Samuel, A. M. Q. King, and D. I. Stuart.** 1999. The structure and function of a foot-and-mouth disease virus-oligosaccharride receptor complex. *EMBO J.* **18**:543–554.

34. **Giranda, V. L., B. A. Heinz, M. A. Oliveira, I. Minor, K. H. Kim, P. R. Kolatkar, M. G. Rossmann, and R. R. Rueckert.** 1992. Acid-induced structural changes in human rhinovirus 14: possible role in uncoating. *Proc. Natl. Acad. Sci. USA* **89**:10213–10217.

35. **Giranda, V. L., G. R. Susso, P. J. Felock, T. R. Bailey, T. Draper, D. J. Aldous, J. Suiles, F. J. Dutko, G. D. Diana, and D. C. Pevear.** 1995. Structures of four methyltetrazole-containing antiviral compounds in human rhinovirus serotype 14. *Acta Crystallogr.* **D51**:496–503.

36. **Grant, R. A., D. J. Filman, R. S. Fujinami, J. P. Icenogle, and J. M. Hogle.** 1992. Three-dimensional structure of Theiler's virus. *Proc. Natl. Acad. Sci. USA* **89**:2061–2065.

37. Grant, R. A., C. N. Hiremath, D. J. Filman, R. Syed, K. Andries, and J. M. Hogle. 1994. Structures of poliovirus complexes with anti-viral drugs: implications for viral stability and drug design. *Curr. Biol.* **4:**784–797.
38. Hadfield, A. T., G. D. Diana, and M. G. Rossmann. 1999. Analysis of three structurally related antiviral compounds in complex with human rhinovirus 16. *Proc. Natl. Acad. Sci. USA* **96:**14730–14735.
39. Hadfield, A. T., W. Lee, R. Zhao, M. A. Oliveira, I. Minor, R. R. Rueckert, and M. G. Rossmann. 1997. The refined structure of human rhinovirus 16 at 2.15 Å resolution: implication for the viral life cycle. *Structure* **5:**427–441.
40. Hadfield, A. T., M. A. Oliveira, K. H. Kim, I. Minor, M. J. Kremer, B. A. Heinz, D. Shepard, D. C. Pevear, R. R. Rueckert, and M. G. Rossmann. 1995. Structural studies on human rhinovirus 14 drug-resistant compensation mutants. *J. Mol. Biol.* **253:**61–73.
41. Harrison, S. C., A. J. Olson, C. E. Schutt, F. K. Winkler, and G. Bricogne. 1978. Tomato bushy stunt virus at 2.9 Å resolution. *Nature (London)* **276:**368–373.
42. He, Y., V. D. Bowman, S. Mueller, C. M. Bator, J. Bella, X. Peng, T. S. Baker, E. Wimmer, R. J. Kuhn, and M. G. Rossmann. 2000. Interaction of the poliovirus receptor with poliovirus. *Proc. Natl. Acad. Sci. USA* **97:**79–84.
43. Hendry, E., H. Hatanaka, E. Fry, M. Smyth, J. Tate, G. Stanway, J. Santti, M. Maaronen, T. Hyypiä, and D. Stuart. 1999. The crystal structure of coxsackievirus A9: new insights into the uncoating mechanisms of enterovirus. *Structure* **7:**1527–1538.
44. Hewat, E. A., and D. Blaas. 1996. Structure of a neutralizing antibody bound bivalently to human rhinovirus 2. *EMBO J.* **15:**1515–1523.
45. Hewat, E. A., T. C. Marlovits, and D. Blaas. 1998. Structure of a neutralizing antibody bound monovalently to human rhinovirus 2. *J. Virol.* **72:**4396–4402.
46. Hewat, E. A., N. Verdaguer, I. Fita, W. Blakemore, S. Brookes, A. King, J. Newman, E. Domingo, M. G. Mateu, and D. I. Stuart. 1997. Structure of the complex of an Fab fragment of a neutralizing antibody with foot-and-mouth disease virus: positioning of a highly mobile antigenic loop. *EMBO J.* **16:**1492–1500.
47. Hindiyeh, M., Q.-H. Li, R. Basavappa, J. M. Hogle, and M. Chow. 1999. Poliovirus mutants at histidine 195 of VP2 do not cleave VP0 into VP2 and VP4. *J. Virol.* **73:**9072–9079.
48. Hiremath, C. N., D. J. Filman, R. A. Grant, and J. M. Hogle. 1997. Ligand-induced conformational changes in poliovirus-antiviral drug complexes. *Acta Crystallogr.* **D53:**558–570.
49. Hiremath, C. N., R. A. Grant, D. J. Filman, and J. M. Hogle. 1995. The binding of the antiviral drug WIN51711 to the Sabin strain of type 3 poliovirus: structural comparison with drug binding in rhinovirus 14. *Acta Crystallogr.* **D51:**473–489.
50. Hofer, F., M. Gruenberger, H. Kowalski, H. Machat, M. Huettinger, E. Kuechler, and D. Blaas. 1994. Members of the low density lipoprotein receptor family mediate cell entry of a minor-group common cold virus. *Proc. Natl. Acad. Sci. USA* **91:**1839–1842.
51. Hogle, J. M., M. Chow, and D. J. Filman. 1985. Three-dimensional structure of poliovirus at 2.9 Å resolution. *Science* **229:**1358–1365.
52. Hoover-Litty, H., and J. M. Greve. 1993. Formation of rhinovirus-soluble ICAM-1 complexes and conformational changes in the virion. *J. Virol.* **67:**390–397.
53. Jackson, T., A. Sharma, R. Abu-Ghazaleh, W. E. Blakemore, F. M. Ellard, D. L. Simmons, J. W. I. Newman, D. I. Stuart, and A. M. Q. King. 1997. Arginine-glycine-aspartic acid-specific binding by foot-and-mouth disease virus to the purified integrin $\alpha v\beta 3$ in vitro. *J. Virol.* **71:**8357–8361.
54. Kim, K. H., P. Willingmann, Z. X. Gong, M. J. Kremer, M. S. Chapman, I. Minor, M. A. Oliveira, M. G. Rossmann, K. Andries, G. D. Diana, F. J. Dutko, M. A. McKinlay, and D. C. Pevear. 1993. A comparison of the anti-rhinoviral drug binding pocket in HRV14 and HRV1A. *J. Mol. Biol.* **230:**206–226.
55. Kim, S., U. Boege, S. Krishnaswamy, I. Minor, T. J. Smith, M. Luo, D. G. Scraba, and M. G. Rossmann. 1990. Conformational variability of a picornavirus capsid: pH-dependent structural changes of Mengo virus related to its host receptor attachment site and disassembly. *Virology* **175:**176–190.
56. Kim, S., T. J. Smith, M. S. Chapman, M. G. Rossmann, D. C. Pevear, F. J. Dutko, P. J. Felock, G. D. Diana, and M. A. McKinlay. 1989. The crystal structure of human rhinovirus serotype 1A (HRV1A). *J. Mol. Biol.* **210:**91–111.
57. Kolatkar, P. R., J. Bella, N. H. Olson, C. M. Bator, T. S. Baker, and M. G. Rossmann. 1999. Structural studies of two rhinovirus serotypes complexed with fragments of their cellular receptor. *EMBO J.* **18:**6249–6259.
58. Kraulis, P. 1991. MOLSCRIPT: a program to produce both detailed and schematic plots of protein structures. *J. Appl. Crystallogr.* **24:**946–950.
59. Krishnaswamy, S., and M. G. Rossmann. 1990. Structural refinement and analysis of Mengo virus. *J. Mol. Biol.* **211:**803–844.
60. Krol, M. A., N. H. Olson, J. Tate, J. E. Johnson, T. S. Baker, and P. Ahlquist. 1999. RNA-controlled polymorphism in the in vitro assembly of 180-subunit and novel 120-subunit virions from a single capsid protein. *Proc. Natl. Acad. Sci. USA* **96:**13650–13655.
61. Larson, S. B., S. Koszelak, J. Day, A. Greenwood, J. A. Dodds, and A. McPherson. 1993. Three-dimensional structure of satellite tobacco mosaic virus at 2.9 Å resolution. *J. Mol. Biol.* **231:**375–391.
62. Lea, S., R. Abu-Ghazaleh, W. Blakemore, S. Curry, E. Fry, T. Jackson, A. King, D. Logan, J. Newman, and D. Stuart. 1995. Structural comparison of two strains of foot-and-mouth disease virus subtype O_1 and a laboratory antigenic variant, G67. *Structure* **3:**571–580.
63. Lea, S., J. Hernández, W. Blakemore, E. Brocchi, S. Curry, E. Domingo, E. Fry, R. Abu-Ghazaleh, A. King, J. Newman, D. Stuart, and M. G. Mateu. 1994. The structure and antigenicity of a type C foot-and-mouth disease virus. *Structure* **2:**123–139.
64. Lentz, K. N., A. D. Smith, S. C. Geisler, S. Cox, P. Buontempo, A. Skelton, J. DeMartino, E. Rozhon, J. Schwartz, V. Girijavallabhan, J. O'Connell, and E. Arnold. 1997. Structure of poliovirus type 2 Lansing complexed with antiviral agent SCH48973: comparison of the structural and biological properties of the three poliovirus serotypes. *Structure* **5:**961–978.
65. Lewis, J. K., B. Bothner, T. J. Smith, and G. Siuzdak. 1998. Antiviral agent blocks breathing of the common cold virus. *Proc. Natl. Acad. Sci. USA* **95:**6774–6778.
66. Liljas, L. 1996. Viruses. *Curr. Opin. Struct. Biol.* **6:**151–156.
67. Lin, T., Z. Chen, R. Usha, C. V. Stauffacher, J. Dai, T. Schmidt, and J. E. Johnson. 1999. The refined crystal structure of cowpea mosaic virus at 2.8 Å resolution. *Virology* **265:**20–34.
68. Lin, T., A. J. Clark, Z. Chen, M. Shanks, J. Dai, L. Ying, T. Schmidt, P. Oxelfelt, G. P. Lomonossoff, and J. E. Johnson. 2000. Structural fingerprinting: subgrouping of comoviruses by structural studies of red clover mot-

tle virus to 2.4-Å resolution and comparisons with other comoviruses. *J. Virol.* **74**:493–504.
69. Lin, T., C. Porta, G. Lomonossoff, and J. E. Johnson. 1996. Structure-based design of peptide presentation on a viral surface: the structure of a plant/animal virus chimera at 2.8 Å resolution. *Folding Des.* **1**:179–187.
70. Logan, D., R. Abu-Ghazaleh, W. Blakemore, S. Curry, T. Jackson, A. King, S. Lea, R. Lewis, J. Newman, N. Parry, D. Rowlands, D. Stuart, and E. Fry. 1993. Structure of a major immunogenic site on foot-and-mouth disease virus. *Nature (London)* **362**:566–568.
71. Lomonossoff, G. P., and J. E. Johnson. 1991. The synthesis and structure of comovirus capsids. *Prog. Biophys. Mol. Biol.* **55**:107–137.
72. Luo, M., C. He, K. S. Toth, C. X. Zhang, and H. L. Lipton. 1992. Three-dimensional structure of Theiler murine encephalomyelitis virus (BeAn strain). *Proc. Natl. Acad. Sci. USA* **89**:2409–2413.
73. Luo, M., K. S. Toth, L. Zhou, A. Pritchard, and H. L. Lipton. 1996. The structure of a highly virulent Theiler's murine encephalomyelitis virus (GDVII) and implications for determinants of viral persistence. *Virology* **220**:246–250.
74. Luo, M., G. Vriend, G. Kamer, I. Minor, E. Arnold, M. G. Rossmann, U. Boege, D. G. Scraba, G. M. Duke, and A. C. Palmenberg. 1987. The atomic structure of Mengo virus at 3.0 Å resolution. *Science* **235**:182–191.
75. Matthews, B. W., and M. G. Rossmann. 1985. Comparison of protein structures. *Methods Enzymol.* **115**:397–420.
76. Muckelbauer, J. K., M. Kremer, I. Minor, G. Diana, F. J. Dutko, J. Groarke, D. C. Pevear, and M. G. Rossmann. 1995. The structure of coxsackievirus B3 at 3.5 Å resolution. *Structure* **3**:653–668.
77. Murthy, M. R. N., M. Bhuvaneswari, H. S. Subramanya, K. Gopinath, and H. S. Savithri. 1997. Structure of sesbania mosaic virus at 3 Å resolution. *Biophys. Chem.* **68**:33–42.
78. Oliveira, M. A., R. Zhao, W. Lee, M. J. Kremer, I. Minor, R. R. Rueckert, G. D. Diana, D. C. Pevear, F. J. Dutko, M. A. McKinlay, and M. G. Rossmann. 1993. The structure of human rhinovirus 16. *Structure* **1**:51–68.
79. Olson, N. H., P. R. Kolatkar, M. A. Oliveira, R. H. Cheng, J. M. Greve, A. McClelland, T. S. Baker, and M. G. Rossmann. 1993. Structure of a human rhinovirus complexed with its receptor molecule. *Proc. Natl. Acad. Sci. USA* **90**:507–511.
80. Page, G. S., A. G. Mosser, J. M. Hogle, D. J. Filman, R. R. Rueckert, and M. Chow. 1988. Three-dimensional structure of poliovirus serotype 1 neutralizing determinants. *J. Virol.* **62**:1781–1794.
81. Pallansch, M. A., O. M. Kew, B. L. Semler, D. R. Omilianowski, C. W. Anderson, E. Wimmer, and R. R. Rueckert. 1984. Protein processing map of poliovirus. *J. Virol.* **49**:873–880.
82. Parry, N., G. Fox, D. Rowlands, F. Brown, E. Fry, R. Acharya, D. Logan, and D. Stuart. 1990. Structural and serological evidence for a novel mechanism of antigenic variation in foot-and-mouth disease virus. *Nature (London)* **347**:569–572.
83. Pevear, D. C., M. J. Fancher, P. J. Felock, M. G. Rossmann, M. S. Miller, G. Diana, A. M. Treasurywala, M. A. McKinlay, and F. J. Dutko. 1989. Conformational change in the floor of the human rhinovirus canyon blocks adsorption to HeLa cell receptors. *J. Virol.* **63**:2002–2007.
84. Porta, C., G. Wang, H. Cheng, Z. Chen, T. S. Baker, and J. E. Johnson. 1994. Direct imaging of interactions between an icosahedral virus and conjugate F_{ab} fragments by cryoelectron microscopy and X-ray crystallography. *Virology* **204**:777–788.
85. Rossmann, M. G. 1994. Viral cell recognition and entry. *Protein Sci.* **3**:1712–1725.
86. Rossmann, M. G., and P. Argos. 1981. Protein folding. *Ann. Rev. Biochem.* **50**:497–532.
87. Rossmann, M. G., E. Arnold, J. W. Erickson, E. A. Frankenberger, J. P. Griffith, H. J. Hecht, J. E. Johnson, G. Kamer, M. Luo, A. G. Mosser, R. R. Rueckert, B. Sherry, and G. Vriend. 1985. Structure of a human common cold virus and functional relationship to other picornaviruses. *Nature (London)* **317**:145–153.
88. Rossmann, M. G., and J. E. Johnson. 1989. Icosahedral RNA virus structure. *Ann. Rev. Biochem.* **58**:533–573.
89. Rossmann, M. G., and A. C. Palmenberg. 1988. Conservation of the putative receptor attachment site in picornaviruses. *Virology* **164**:373–382.
90. Rotbart, H. A., and K. Kirkegaard. 1992. Picornavirus pathogenesis: viral access, attachment and entry into susceptible cells. *Semin. Virol.* **3**:483–499.
91. Rueckert, R. R. 1996. Picornaviridae: the viruses and their replication, p. 609–654. *In* B. N. Fields, D. M. Knipe, and P. M. Howley (ed.), *Fields Virology*. Lippincott-Raven Publishers, Philadelphia, Pa.
92. Schmugge, M., R. Lauener, W. Bossart, R. A. Seger, and T. Güngör. 1999. Chronic enteroviral meningo-encephalitis in X-linked agammaglobulinaemia: favourable response to anti-enteroviral treatment. *Eur. J. Pediatr.* **158**:1010–1011.
93. Schneemann, A., V. S. Reddy, and J. E. Johnson. 1998. The structure and function of nodavirus particles: a paradigm for understanding chemical biology. *Adv. Virus Res.* **50**:381–445.
94. Sherry, B., A. G. Mosser, R. J. Colonno, and R. R. Rueckert. 1986. Use of monoclonal antibodies to identify four neutralization immunogens on a common cold picornavirus, human rhinovirus 14. *J. Virol.* **57**:246–257.
95. Sherry, B., and R. Rueckert. 1985. Evidence for at least two dominant neutralization antigens on human rhinovirus 14. *J. Virol.* **53**:137–143.
96. Smith, T. J., E. Chase, T. Schmidt, and K. L. Perry. 2000. The structure of cucumber mosaic virus and comparison to cowpea chlorotic mottle virus. *J. Virol.* **74**:7578–7586.
97. Smith, T. J., E. S. Chase, T. J. Schmidt, N. H. Olson, and T. S. Baker. 1996. Neutralizing antibody to human rhinovirus 14 penetrates the receptor-binding canyon. *Nature (London)* **383**:350–354.
98. Smith, T. J., M. J. Kremer, M. Luo, G. Vriend, E. Arnold, G. Kamer, M. G. Rossmann, M. A. McKinlay, G. D. Diana, and M. J. Otto. 1986. The site of attachment in human rhinovirus 14 for antiviral agents that inhibit uncoating. *Science* **233**:1286–1293.
99. Smith, T. J., N. H. Olson, R. H. Cheng, E. S. Chase, and T. S. Baker. 1993. Structure of a human rhinovirus bivalently bound antibody complex: implications for viral neutralization and antibody flexibility. *Proc. Natl. Acad. Sci. USA* **90**:7015–7018.
100. Smith, T. J., N. H. Olson, R. H. Cheng, H. Liu, E. A. Chase, W. Lee, D. M. Leippe, A. G. Mosser, R. R. Rueckert, and T. S. Baker. 1993. Structure of human rhinovirus complexed with Fab fragments from a neutralizing antibody. *J. Virol.* **67**:1148–1158.
101. Smyth, M., J. Tate, E. Hoey, C. Lyons, S. Martin, and D. Stuart. 1995. Implications for viral uncoating from the structure of bovine enterovirus. *Nat. Struct. Biol.* **2**:224–231.

102. **Speir, J. A., S. Munshi, G. Wang, T. S. Baker, and J. E. Johnson.** 1995. Structures of the native and swollen forms of cowpea chlorotic mottle virus determined by X-ray crystallography and cryo-electron microscopy. *Structure* **3:**63–78.
103. **Sri Krishna, S., C. N. Hiremath, S. K. Munshi, D. Prahadeeswaran, M. Sastri, H. S. Savithri, and M. R. N. Murthy.** 1999. Three-dimensional structure of physalis mottle virus: implications for the viral assembly. *J. Mol. Biol.* **289:**919–934.
104. **Tate, J., L. Liljas, P. Scotti, P. Christian, T. Lin, and J. E. Johnson.** 1999. The crystal structure of cricket paralysis virus: the first view of a new virus family. *Nat. Struct. Biol.* **6:**765–774.
105. **Tormo, J., D. Blaas, N. R. Parry, D. Rowlands, D. Stuart, and I. Fita.** 1994. Crystal structure of a human rhinovirus neutralizing antibody complexed with a peptide derived from viral capsid protein VP2. *EMBO J.* **13:**2247–2256.
106. **Tormo, J., N. B. Centeno, E. Fontana, T. Bubendorfer, I. Fita, and D. Blaas.** 1995. Docking of a human rhinovirus neutralizing antibody onto the viral capsid. *Proteins* **23:**491–501.
107. **Tormo, J., E. Stadler, T. Skern, H. Auer, O. Kanzler, C. Betzel, D. Blaas, and I. Fita.** 1992. Three-dimensional structure of the Fab fragment of a neutralizing antibody to human rhinovirus serotype 2. *Protein Sci.* **1:**1154–1161.
108. **Verdaguer, N., D. Blaas, and I. Fita.** 2000. Structure of human rhinovirus serotype 2 (HRV2). *J. Mol. Biol.* **300:**1181–1196.
109. **Verdaguer, N., M. G. Mateu, D. Andreu, E. Giralt, E. Domingo, and I. Fita.** 1995. Structure of the major antigenic loop of foot-and-mouth disease virus complexed with a neutralizing antibody: direct involvement of the Arg-Gly-Asp motif in the interaction. *EMBO J.* **14:**1690–1696.
110. **Verdaguer, N., G. Schoehn, W. F. Ochoa, I. Fita, S. Brookes, A. King, E. Domingo, M. G. Mateu, D. Stuart, and E. A. Hewat.** 1999. Flexibility of the major antigenic loop of foot-and-mouth disease virus bound to a Fab fragment of a neutralising antibody: structure and neutralisation. *Virology* **255:**260–268.
111. **Wery, J. P., V. S. Reddy, M. V. Hosur, and J. E. Johnson.** 1994. The refined three-dimensional structure of an insect virus at 2.8 Å resolution. *J. Mol. Biol.* **235:**565–586.
112. **Wien, M. W., S. Curry, D. J. Filman, and J. M. Hogle.** 1997. Structural studies of poliovirus mutants that overcome receptor defects. *Nat. Struct. Biol.* **4:**666–674.
113. **Wien, M. W., D. J. Filman, E. A. Stura, S. Guillot, F. Delpeyroux, R. Crainic, and J. M. Hogle.** 1995. Structure of the complex between the Fab fragment of a neutralizing antibody for type 1 poliovirus and its viral epitope. *Nat. Struct. Biol.* **2:**232–243.
113a.**Xiao, C., C. M. Bator, V. D. Bowman, E. Rieder, Y. He, B. Hébert, J. Bella, T. S. Baker, E. Wimmer, R. J. Kuhn, and M. G. Rossmann.** 2001. Interaction of coxsackievirus A21 with its cellular receptor, ICAM-1. *J. Virol.* **75:**2444–2451.
114. **Xing, L., K. Tjarnlund, B. Lindqvist, G. G. Kaplan, D. Feigelstock, R. H. Cheng, and J. M. Casasnovas.** 2000. Distinct cellular receptor interactions in poliovirus and rhinoviruses. *EMBO J.* **19:**1207–1216.
115. **Yeates, T. O., D. H. Jacobson, A. Martin, C. Wychowski, M. Girard, D. J. Filman, and J. M. Hogle.** 1991. Three-dimensional structure of a mouse-adapted type 2/type 1 poliovirus chimera. *EMBO J.* **10:**2331–2341.
116. **Zhang, A., R. G. Nanni, T. Li, G. F. Arnold, D. A. Oren, A. Jacobo-Molina, R. L. Williams, G. Kamer, D. A. Rubenstein, Y. Li, E. Rozhon, S. Cox, P. Buontempo, J. O'Connell, J. Schwartz, G. Miller, B. Bauer, R. Versace, P. Pinto, A. Ganguly, V. Girijavallabhan, and E. Arnold.** 1993. Structure determination of antiviral compound SCH 38057 complexed with human rhinovirus 14. *J. Mol. Biol.* **230:**857–867.
117. **Zhang, A., R. G. Nanni, D. A. Oren, E. J. Rozhon, and E. Arnold.** 1992. Three-dimensional structure-activity relationships for antiviral agents that interact with picornavirus capsids. *Semin. Virol.* **3:**453–471.
118. **Zhao, R., A. T. Hadfield, M. J. Kremer, and M. G. Rossmann.** 1997. Cations in human rhinoviruses. *Virology* **227:**13–23.
119. **Zhao, R., D. C. Pevear, M. J. Kremer, V. L. Giranda, J. Kofron, R. J. Kuhn, and M. G. Rossmann.** 1996. Human rhinovirus 3 at 3.0 Å resolution. *Structure* **4:**1205–1220.
120. **Zhou, L., X. Lin, T. J. Green, H. L. Lipton, and M. Luo.** 1997. Role of sialyloligosaccharide binding in Theiler's virus persistence. *J. Virol.* **71:**9701–9712.
121. **Zhou, L., Y. Luo, Y. Wu, J. Tsao, and M. Luo.** 2000. Sialylation of the host receptor may modulate entry of demyelinating persistent Theiler's virus. *J. Virol.* **74:**1477–1485.
122. **Zlotnick, A., V. S. Reddy, R. Dasgupta, A. Schneemann, W. J. Ray, Jr., R. R. Rueckert, and J. E. Johnson.** 1994. Capsid assembly in a family of animal viruses primes an autoproteolytic maturation that depends on a single aspartic acid residue. *J. Biol. Chem.* **269:**13680–13684.

Antibody Interactions with Rhinovirus

THOMAS J. SMITH

4

The purpose of this chapter is to discuss the possible mechanisms of antibody-mediated neutralization of human rhinovirus to better understand how antibodies recognize their targets and neutralize viral infectivity. Understanding these fundamental processes is crucial for future vaccine development and new antibody therapeutics. This is especially true for viruses like the human immunodeficiency virus (HIV), where the more traditional approach of using attenuated viral strains appears to be risky and insufficiently efficacious. Therefore, for this and other viruses where attenuation may not be a viable option, we need to create synthetic vaccines that present efficacious immunogenic sites. In addition, we must ascertain whether antibodies need to cause secondary structural effects in order to neutralize the virion and then incorporate this information in our vaccine design. As discussed in this chapter, we would argue that antibodies need not induce conformational changes in the virion and, therefore, vaccine development should focus on the more straightforward goal of inducing high-affinity antibodies.

BACKGROUND

Picornaviruses are among the largest of animal virus families and include polio-, rhino-, foot-and-mouth disease, coxsackie-, and hepatitis A viruses. The rhinoviruses, of which there are more than 100 serotypes, are major causative agents of the common cold in humans (48). The virus has an ~300-Å-diameter protein shell that encapsidates a single-stranded, plus-sense RNA genome of about 7,200 bases. The human rhinovirus 14 (HRV14) capsid exhibits a pseudo-$T = 3$ ($P = 3$) icosahedral symmetry and consists of 60 copies each of four viral proteins, VP1, VP2, VP3, and VP4. VP1 to -3 each have an eight-stranded antiparallel β-barrel motif and comprise most of the capsid structure (Color Plate 4, following p. 156). VP4 is smaller, has an extended structure, and lies at the RNA-capsid interface (47). An ~20-Å-deep canyon lies roughly at the junction of VP1 (forming the "north" rim) with VP2 and VP3 (forming the "south" rim) and surrounds each of the 12 icosahedral fivefold vertices. The canyon regions of HRV14 and HRV16, both major receptor group rhinoviruses, were shown to contain the binding site of the cellular receptor, intercellular adhesion molecule 1 (ICAM-1) (13, 25, 40). Four major neutralizing immunogenic (NIm) sites, NIm-IA, NIm-IB, NIm-II, and NIm-III, were identified by studies of neutralization-escape mutants with monoclonal antibodies (51, 52) and then mapped to four protruding regions on the viral surface (47).

For the weakly precipitating antibodies, 32 to 49 antibodies were bound to the monomeric species. This supports the hypothesis that these antibodies bind both Fab arms to the same virion. These numbers are slightly higher than the predicted 30 antibodies per virion, probably because, at very high antibody concentrations, some antibodies might be binding with only one Fab arm. Strongly precipitating antibodies, in contrast, demonstrated saturation numbers of 58 to 72, consistent with the model proposing that these antibodies are unlikely to bind both Fab arms to a single virion.

Antibody Neutralization of HRV14

Neutralizing monoclonal antibodies against HRV14 have been divided into three groups: strong, intermediate, and weak neutralizers (27, 37). All strongly neutralizing antibodies bind to the NIm-IA site, which was defined by natural escape mutations at residues D1091 and E1095 of VP1 on the loop between the βB and βC strands of the VP1 β-barrel (the letter designates the amino acid, the first digit identifies the viral protein, and the remaining three digits specify the sequence number).

Of the 32 HRV14-specific neutralizing antibodies, all 10 of the strongly neutralizing antibodies recognized site IA (27). As the antibody:virus ratio increased, the surviving infectivity fell by 4 to 5 logs (Fig. 1). At high antibody concentrations, the residual infectivity is due to neutralization-resistant mutants. All of these antibodies are poor viral aggregators and are proposed to bind to the virion with both Fab arms.

The Poisson formula predicts that when there is an average of one antibody per virion, then $1/e$, or about 37%, of the virions would not have an antibody bound. If one

---

Thomas J. Smith ■ Donald Danforth Plant Science Center, 975 N. Warson Rd., St. Louis, MO 63132.

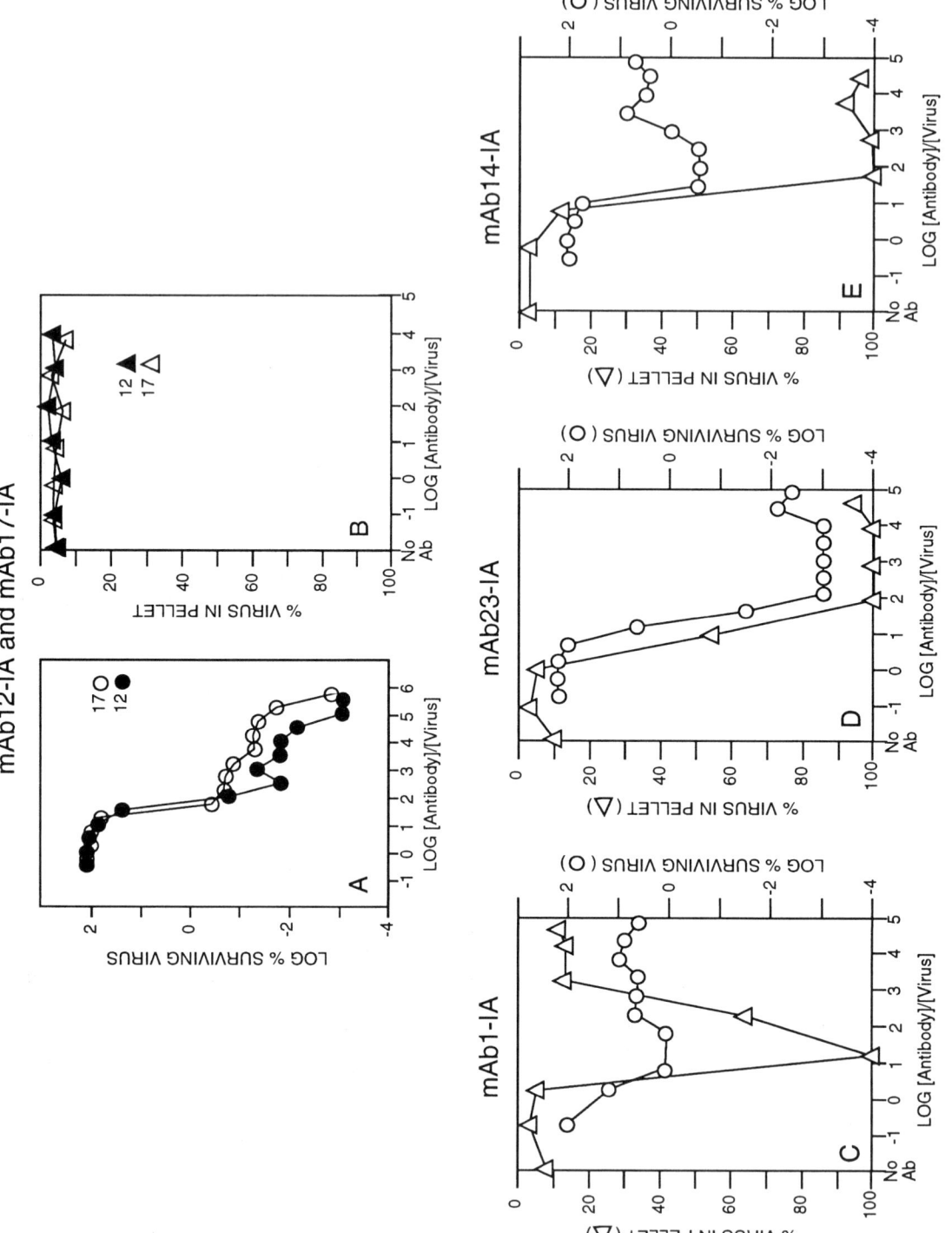

FIGURE 1 Aggregation and neutralization profiles for several NIm-IA antibodies. Panel A shows the neutralization profile of mAb17 and mAb12 at increasing concentrations of antibody. Panel B shows the amount of virus that is aggregated and pelleted upon addition of antibody. Neither of these strongly neutralizing antibodies precipitates the virions. The aggregation and neutralization profiles of other NIm-IA antibodies are shown in panels C to E. Reprinted from the *Journal of Virology* (9) with permission from publisher.

bound antibody were capable of neutralizing a virion, then the infectivity of a mixture with a ratio of one antibody per virion would be 1/e of a nonneutralized control. Therefore, the neutralization number was defined as the average number of antibodies attached per monomeric virion when the infectivity of this population has been reduced to 1/e of control infectivity. Even for these strongly neutralizing antibodies, the neutralization numbers of four neutralizing anti-HRV14 antibodies ranged from 6 to 20. None was capable of neutralizing virus with a single antibody (9, 27).

Twelve other antibodies, associated with all four antigenic sites, tended to aggregate the virions (23, 27). These precipitating antibodies proved difficult to study because (i) precipitation occurred at optimal neutralization, (ii) most of the strongly precipitating antibodies were never found associated with the monomeric virus peak except at extremely high antibody:virus input ratios, and (iii) monomeric species were very unstable. For these antibodies, the number of antibodies bound to virus at saturation could be determined, but not the neutralization stoichiometry. In contrast to the strongly neutralizing antibodies, antibodies like mAb1 only weakly inhibited plaque formation with a maximum inhibition of ~2 orders of magnitude and with a slight enhancement in neutralization at intermediate antibody:virus ratios (Color Plate 5C, following p. 156). Unlike mAb12 and mAb17, mAb1 strongly aggregated the virions over the same range of ratios in which neutralization enhancement was observed. At very high antibody:virus ratios, there was little precipitation but yet significant (~1.5 log) neutralization. Therefore, mAb1 does not neutralize HRV14 solely by precipitating it, but neutralization is enhanced by aggregation at intermediate antibody:virus ratios. Since mAb1 strongly aggregates HRV14, cannot form stable, monomeric virus:antibody species, and binds with a maximal stoichiometry of ~60 antibodies/virion, this antibody binds monovalently to the virion surface.

Ten antibodies, associated with sites IA 2 and 3, gave curves that had shapes intermediate between these two groups. As a group, the neutralization curves of these 10 antibodies formed a continuum with the other two groups, so assignment to an "intermediate" group was somewhat arbitrary. We assume that their interactions with virions had some of the characteristics of both of the other two groups. It may be that these antibodies have intermediate affinity for the capsid, and/or the orientation of the Fab arms does not predispose the antibodies to bind predominantly in either a mono- or bivalent manner. For example, mAb23-IA and mAb14-IA (Fig. 1D and E) also bind to the NIm-IA site and precipitate HRV14 over a wider range of antibody concentrations than mAb1. However, unlike mAb1, mAb23 is a strongly neutralizing antibody. This implies that bivalent binding is not a prerequisite for efficient neutralization. Instead, it suggests that the intrinsic binding of the Fab arm to HRV14 is higher in mAb23 compared to mAb1, and it is the binding strength itself (avidity or affinity) that determines neutralization efficacy. Finally, mAb14 neutralizes slightly better than mAb17 but aggregates over a wider range of antibody:virus ratios than mAb1. In this case, it may be that the binding orientation of mAb14 is better suited for interparticle cross-linking than mAb1.

It is important to note, however, that neutralization efficacy is very dependent on how the assay is performed. In the experiments discussed above, samples of HRV14 were incubated with antibody overnight and added to monolayers of HeLa cells. After incubation for 1 h at room temperature to allow for viral attachment to the cells, unbound virus-antibody complexes were washed away. In contrast, when antibody is kept in the plaque assay overlays, all three antibodies neutralize HRV14 infectivity with comparable efficacy. This difference is due to the fact that, in the latter assays, the antibody is around to inhibit secondary infections that are needed for plaque development. This demonstrates that one must be careful when assessing the efficacy of an antibody based solely on in vitro assays. While the latter assay methodology may more accurately represent in vivo conditions (where antibodies are not removed after the first round of viral attachment), the assay shown in Fig. 1 is more sensitive to differences in antibody affinities. Most important, one may have used brief incubation times and incorrectly concluded that some of the antibodies are nonneutralizing even though enzyme-linked immunosorbent assays (ELISAs) demonstrate that all antibodies react with the virus (Chase and Smith, unpublished results).

Cryo-TEM Analysis of Antibody-Virus Complexes

Using a combination of molecular biology, cryo-transmission electron microscopy (cryo-TEM), and crystallographic studies, we have examined the structures of several antibodies bound to HRV14. For these experiments, we chose to examine antibodies that react to the NIm-IA site. Whereas antibodies that bind to the NIm-IA site exhibit both strongly and weakly neutralizing properties, the other three neutralizing sites only produce weakly neutralizing, aggregating antibodies. It was thought that comparison of strongly versus weakly neutralizing antibodies would allow us to directly compare these potentially different neutralizing mechanisms without having to compensate for differing binding regions.

We have now examined the structures of three different Fab-HRV14 (Fab17, Fab12, and Fab1) complexes (9, 57) (Color Plate 5, following p. 156) and of one mAb-HRV14 (mAb17) complex (56). Both mAb17 and mAb12 are strongly neutralizing antibodies, whereas mAb1 is a weakly neutralizing antibody. What was immediately apparent was that these different antibodies had different binding orientations. Fab17 and Fab12 both bound to the NIm-IA site at a somewhat tangential orientation that placed the constant domains ($C_{H1} \cdot C_V$) of twofold related Fabs in close proximity to each other. This suggested that the intrinsic paratope-epitope interactions of these antibodies place the Fab arms in an orientation that facilitates bidentate binding to twofold related NIm-IA sites. In contrast, Fab1 binds almost vertically to the virion surface with a "twist" that made it seem unlikely that these antibodies could bind bivalently.

Since it was possible that conformational changes are only induced by mAb binding, we used cryo-TEM to determine the structure of the mAb17-HRV14 complex (56). In this complex, there was a clear connection between the Fab arms. However, the Fc region was only observed as a weak island of density above the connection. This is more than likely due to the fact that the hinge region is very flexible, causing the Fc region to be averaged away during the reconstruction procedure. These results supported the contention that strongly neutralizing antibodies bind bivalently while weakly neutralizing antibodies bind monovalently. The fact that antibodies to the other NIm sites appear to only bind monovalently suggests that the distance and orientation of the other icosahedrally related antigenic sites make it difficult for antibodies to bind with both Fab arms. This is in contrast to some antibodies to human rhinovirus 2 and calicivirus that have been suggested to undergo a great deal of contortion about the hinge region to bind bivalently (21, 59). Nevertheless, there was no evidence of changes in the capsid structure in this mAb17-HRV14 complex. Therefore, it seemed unlikely that bivalently bound antibodies are more efficacious due to induced structural changes in the capsid.

Finally, it seems likely that bivalent binding is not essential for neutralization since Fabs also neutralize the virus, although less effectively than the intact mAbs (12). The measured Fab activity was diminished in accordance with the loss in avidity. Therefore, it seemed likely that if antibodies neutralize via induction of conformational changes, then these changes must occur with Fabs. Such conformational changes were not observed with any of the studied Fabs or mAbs used for these cryo-TEM studies.

Pseudo-Atomic Models of the Fab-Virus Complexes

The density of the bound Fab molecules was asymmetric and therefore allowed for a fairly unique fit of the atomic models into the density (Color Plate 5). We were then able to test the accuracy of these early "pseudo-atomic" models using site-directed mutagenesis (57). In the Fab17-HRV14 complex, the loop of the NIm-IA site on HRV14 sits clamped in the cleft between the heavy- and light-chain hypervariable regions and forms complementary electrostatic interactions with $Lys58^H$ (on heavy chain) and $Arg91^L$ (on light chain) of Fab17. In addition, a cluster of lysines on HRV14 (K1236, K1097, K1085) interacts with two acidic residues, $Asp45^H$ and $Asp54^H$, in the CDR2 region (CDR, complementarity determining region) of the Fab heavy chain (54). These modeling results were tested using site-directed mutagenesis. Indeed, it was found that even though K1236, K1097, and K1085 were not identified as sites of naturally occurring escape mutations, they do affect antibody binding (Table 1). This is likely due to the fact that these mutations yielded poorly replicating viruses (9). Therefore, these results demonstrate two major points. First, electrostatic interactions can dominate paratope-epitope interactions. This was contrary to the prevailing dogma that, due to high entropic input, hydrophobic interactions dominate the antibody-antigen interactions. Second, the naturally occurring escape mutations are clearly only a small subset of residues crucial for antibody binding. Indeed, mutating K1097, a residue present only halfway down the canyon, is very deleterious to the virus. This latter result emphasizes that escape mutations are not necessarily the most crucial or the only residues that make contact with the antibody. Therefore, one cannot use the location of epitopes as unequivocal evidence that the convolutions in the virion surface hide crucial residues.

The three-dimensional reconstruction of the Fab1-HRV14 complex clearly differs from the other two virus-Fab reconstructions (Color Plate 5). The Fab arms of the weakly neutralizing, strongly aggregating mAb1 bind in a more radial orientation on the capsid, and they are rotated ~25° about their long axes compared to Fab12 and Fab17. In this orientation, the constant domains of the symmetry-related, bound Fab1 fragments point away from each other. Unlike mAb17 (56), a model for bivalently bound mAb1 can only be generated if the structure is forced to assume unacceptable conformations about the elbow axis region. The large separation of neighboring Fab1 molecules and the more radial orientation of the constant region in Fab1 presumably favors monovalent binding. Though the hinge region of antibodies is known to be highly flexible (59, 61), the distance between icosahedral, twofold-related NIm-IA sites is sufficiently large so the relatively small difference between Fab17 and Fab1 binding orientations produces a profound effect on binding valency. Notably, an antibody/foot-and-mouth disease virus (FMDV) complex has a similar distance constraint on bivalent binding (22).

It is interesting to note that although Fab17 and Fab1 have disparate binding orientations, they share some key residues that maintain electrostatic interactions (9). The cluster of basic groups in the cleft between Fab17 heavy and light chains that interact with D1091 and E1095 are also found in Fab1. In addition, the D55 and D57 in Fab17 that form important interactions with a cluster of basic groups on the HRV14 surface (e.g., K1097 and R1094) are also found in the CDR2 loop of Fab1. The important difference is that the two homologous Asp residues in Fab1 are three residues upstream from where they are located in Fab17. This places these acidic groups in a counterclockwise position on the paratope relative to Fab17. This apparent dominance of charged groups on the binding orientation of the Fab can be best explained by the fact that the coulombic interactions will be felt at a much longer distance than any other chemical interactions. In this way, the docking of the Fab may be directed and optimized by the charged residues.

Crystal Structure of the Fab17-HRV14 Complex

The above studies consistently demonstrated that antibodies do not induce conformational changes in the virion upon binding. This has been also shown in the reconstructions of virus-Fab complexes of cowpea mosaic virus (43, 63), canine parvovirus (67), FMDV (22), Sindbis virus (55), Ross River virus (55), and HRV2 (21). However, all of these cryo-TEM studies are limited to 20- to 30-Å resolution where relatively small conformational changes may not be observable. To address this problem, we crystallized and determined the crystal structure of the Fab17-HRV14 complex. Again, as noted above, previous results clearly demonstrate that if conformational changes are associated with neutralization, they should be observed in this structure.

Using the atomic models for Fab17, HRV14, and the pseudo-atomic model of the complex, we determined the structure of the Fab17-HRV14 complex to 4-Å resolution (Color Plate 6, following p. 156). The first observation was that the pseudo-atomic model created using the cryo-TEM electron density was a fairly accurate representation of the

TABLE 1 Residual infectivity (% of residual plaques) of HRV14 wild-type and mutant viruses after treatment with NIm-IA antibodies

Antibody	LP1(WT)	K1085E	K1236E	K1097Q	K1097E
mAb1	0.0021	0.032	0.0088	0.0054	0.27
mAb3	0.0064	0.060	0.014	0.011	83
mAb4	0.0031	0.045	0.0082	0.0059	0.44
mAb6	0.0045	0.050	0.014	0.012	71
mAb7	0.0064	0.063	0.014	0.015	106
mAb14	0.0	0.0	0.0	0.0	0.19
mAb17	0.0190	0.052	0.016	3.1	87
mAb20	0.0000	0.003	0.0013	0.00066	0.018

actual structure. When the Fab17 model was placed into the cryo-TEM density, the limited resolution was insufficient to justify adjustments to the model to improve the paratope-epitope interactions. This was clearly the root of most of the error in the cryo-TEM fitting process. Indeed, the CDR3 of Fab17 moves by ~5 Å to better accommodate the epitope, which places the Fab closer to the surface and further down into the canyon than previously modeled. Interestingly, Fab17 binds poorly to peptides representing the NIm-IA loop. Our recent Fab17-peptide crystallographic studies suggest that this may be, in part, due to the fact that the peptide is insufficient to induce conformational changes in the paratope cleft that are necessary to accommodate the βB-βC loop (J. Wu and T. Smith, unpublished results).

This structure also clearly showed that there were no significant changes in the virion due to Fab binding. The only observable changes were localized in a few side chains on the βB-βC loop on which the naturally occurring escape mutations lie. D1091 and E1095 rotate slightly to form salt bridges with the basic residues in the paratope cleft and K1097 and R1094 rotate to better interact with D55 and D57. There were not, however, any significant changes in the NIm-IA loop itself. This result is not entirely surprising since none of the crystallographic structures of antigen-Fab complexes determined to date have demonstrated large antibody-induced conformational changes.

The resolution of this Fab17-HRV14 structure permits us to analyze the antibody-virus interactions more quantitatively. First, it is quite apparent that, in contradiction to the "canyon hypothesis," Fab17 penetrates into the canyon region (Color Plate 6). It is able to do this by binding somewhat on its side, with the V_H domain making extensive interactions with the north and south walls of the canyon. The hypervariable residues contact the entire north wall, the bottom of the canyon, and part of the lower south wall (Table 2). The framework residues contact the upper south wall only. The vast majority of these interactions are via either charged or polar residues. This clearly demonstrates that antibodies are much more facile at recognizing crevasses in viral surfaces than originally thought.

Interestingly, there is a great deal of contact between the framework region of Fab17 and the upper, south wall of the canyon (Color Plate 6). This kind of extensive framework interaction has never been previously observed. Both Fab17 and Fab12 bind in nearly identical orientations. From the small number of basic changes, and because these two antibodies came from the same mouse, it seemed likely that they came from the same progenitor cell and their sequences now differed due to affinity maturation. While some changes in framework residues have been suggested to indirectly affect antibody binding, it seems rather fortuitous that three amino acid differences cluster about the framework-south wall contact region. These potential interactions are currently under examination using an ScFv version of Fab17.

Shown in Color Plate 7 are the locations of the various NIm sites and the contact areas mapped onto the viral surface. Color Plate 7A elucidates a number of features of the antigenic surface of HRV14. First, it is striking how small the NIm-IA epitope is compared to the other antigenic sites. The simplest explanation for this is that these residues may be the only ones that can be mutated without having significant effects on viral replication and therefore the only ones to appear during the selection process. This is consistent with our finding that mutating residues adjacent to the NIm-IA site are deleterious to the virus (9). Another interesting feature is that there is a large ridge between the NIm-II and NIm-III sites. If surface exposure is the most important criterion for antibody recognition, it seems rather curious that this region is not a major epitope. It may be that the NIm-II and NIm-III antibodies recognize portions of this ridge, but that mutations in this region are not tolerated. It is hoped our ongoing analysis of these antibody-virus complexes will clarify this issue. Finally, it is interesting to note the depth of the depression at the icosahedral twofold axis that is nearly as deep as the canyon and is an extremely thin part of the capsid.

Color Plate 8B, following p. 156, shows the area of HRV14 contacted by Fab17. As noted above, the hypervariable region contacts the canyon region nearest the fivefold axis and the bottom portion of the canyon (Color Plates 6 and 7; Table 2). The framework region of the VH domain contacts the upper portion of the south canyon wall nearest the NIm-II site. Again, it is striking to see the size of the epitope as determined by natural escape mutations versus the actual area contacted by Fab17. The area of the HRV14 surface, to which Fab17 binds, directly overlaps the contact surface of the receptor, ICAM-1. From the cryo-TEM structure of the ICAM-1-HRV14 complex, it has been suggested that ICAM-1 interacts with the south canyon wall (40). This area of contact is immediately adjacent to the NIm-II site and about two-thirds of which is encompassed by the Fab17 contact area. Therefore, it appears that the canyon does not, in fact, adequately hide the ICAM-1-binding surface from antibody recognition.

Color Plate 7C, following p. 156, is a representation of the results from a paper published shortly after the structure of HRV14 had been determined (34). In this study, polyclonal serum was raised against two peptides representing portions of VP1 and VP3, 1147–1162 and 3126–3141. This immune serum was able to neutralize HRV14 and several other rhinovirus serotypes as well as react in an ELISA. The serum raised to the VP1 peptide was more efficacious than the VP3 peptide. These results are interesting for several reasons. The region represented by the VP1 peptide lies under the NIm-IA site and extends down into the canyon. This area does not overlap with the NIm-IA site but does slightly overlap with the Fab17-IA contact area. Perhaps these antibodies are a variation of the V_H-dominant NIm-IA binding antibodies and bind to a different portion of the canyon floor. The second peptide region lies near the NIm-II site and on the rim of the pit at the twofold

TABLE 2 Fab17-HRV14 contacts

Residue type	Area (Å²)	% Total
Acidic (D, E)	96	11
Base (H, K, R)	142	17
Polar (N, Q, S, T)	187	22
Small (A, G)	61	7
Hydrophobic (C, I, L, M, P, V)	23	3
Aromatic polar (W, Y)	336	38
Total	845	
North wall contacts (CDR)	532	63
South wall contacts	313	37
Hypervariable (CDR) contacts	103	12
Framework contacts	207	24

axis. This region is also fairly deep in the viral depressions. There are several possible reasons for these results. As suggested by the relatively low affinity, these antibodies may be cross-reacting with other antigenic sites. Alternatively, it may be that by using these peptides, they were able to circumvent the normally immunodominant NIm sites. If true, then this suggests that far more of the virus is visible to the immune response than previously thought. In light of the structural results, it would be interesting to revisit these studies with monoclonal or ScFv library methodology to try to verify the binding location for these antibodies.

One unexpected result in this structure was that density was observed in the "drug pocket" (Color Plate 8). Although such density is coincident with the binding location of the WIN drugs, it had never been observed before with HRV14. However, density has been observed in the structures of other viruses, and it has been suggested that it represents a "pocket factor" that plays some role in the viral replication cycle. The major difference in HRV14 preparation between these two crystals is the polyethylene glycol (PEG) 400 that was added as a cryoprotectant. This strongly suggests that the pocket factor found in the HRV14-Fab complex came from PEG 400. Since there has been no direct evidence that pocket factors are derived from the host cell, these results further suggest that pocket factors found in the other viruses might also be compounds used in purification or crystallization. These results have led us to propose that the canyon is not used to avoid immune surveillance but rather to promote facile changes in the capsid upon receptor binding.

Mechanism of Antibody-Mediated Neutralization

In the context of these structural results, we can now re-evaluate the previously proposed neutralization mechanisms.

Aggregation

Aggregation is conceptually the simplest method of neutralization. In this mechanism, the loss of infectivity is due to the reduction of the number of independent infectious units. Aggregation and neutralization have been shown to have a direct, linear relationship in several studies that showed residual infectivity of antibody-bound virion dimers and trimers isolated from sucrose gradients was approximately one-half and one-third, respectively, of the native virions (23, 58). It has been suggested that aggregation and neutralization occur concomitantly and that virus:antibody ratios in vivo favor aggregation (4, 6, 58).

These studies on HRV14 strongly suggest that aggregation is not a major factor in neutralization. First, antibodies that bind bivalently to virions do not induce aggregation over antibody:virus ratios that range several orders of magnitude, yet such antibodies are strong neutralizers (9). Second, antibodies that are strong aggregators neutralize virus even at antibody:virus concentrations that do not favor aggregation (Fig. 1). Neutralization for aggregating antibodies is often optimal at ratios where immunoprecipitation is greatest. In this circumstance, neutralization may be enhanced within a narrow range of antibody:virus ratios that favors precipitation. This enhancement may result from a decrease of independent infectious particles or from avidity effects (apparent increase in affinity due to multivalent binding of antibodies) caused by antibodies bound bivalently to neighboring particles in the large immunocomplexes. Though aggregation probably does not play a significant role in vitro, it may facilitate innate immunological responses such as opsonization in vivo.

Virion Stabilization

Rhinoviruses are unstable at pHs below 6.0 (48). Twelve different monoclonal antibodies that bound to the NIm-1A site were shown to be capable of stabilizing HRV14 infectivity at pH 5.0, and three of these stabilized at pH 4.5 (9, 26). Four antibodies, binding to other NIm sites, could not protect HRV14 from inactivation after incubation at pH 5.0. Fab fragments of one of the NIm-IA antibodies, mAb17-IA, did not protect viral infectivity at pH 5.0 even if present at a concentration of 200 Fab molecules per virion, suggesting that bivalent binding of the antibody was necessary for pH stabilization. However, mAbI-1A, a strong aggregator and therefore unlikely to bind bivalently, was also able to protect the virions against low pH effects. Therefore, bivalent binding may not be necessary for stabilization. We propose that antibodies to this site stabilize the virion, perhaps by binding down in the canyon region. In this way, antibody avidity or the antibody-binding site is a more important determinant for stabilization than bivalent binding per se. Furthermore, antibodies to all four NIm sites prevent cellular attachment (12), thereby blocking infectivity prior to possible stabilization effects. Therefore, this stabilization effect also appears to not be related to abrogation of cellular attachment.

It is important to note that no escape mutation has yet been observed that prevents neutralization without affecting antibody binding. If capsid stabilization or destabilization was a significant determinant of neutralization, it seems likely that some escape mutations, distal to the antibody-binding site, could abrogate these effects. Such compensatory mutations are clearly possible as made evident by some drug resistance mutants that are distal to the WIN-binding pocket (20, 38, 39). These drugs stabilize the capsid upon binding. While some drug resistance mutations lie within the drug-binding cavity, a number are found quite distal to the bound drug. In addition, such a mechanism seems to be a rather undependable way for animals to attack the virion. For example, the large flexible receptor-binding loop in FMDV seems to be the perfect way to structurally isolate the antigenic site from the capsid. If induction of structural changes or stabilization is required for neutralization, FMDV should be able to completely evade antibody neutralization—yet it does not. Such stabilization is even more unlikely in the more complex, multilayered viruses. For all of these reasons, we argue that capsid stabilization may occur but is not a major mechanism of neutralization.

Induction of Conformational Changes

Prior to these structural studies, the prime mechanism of neutralization was thought to be the alteration of the conformation of the virus coat. This hypothesis was supported by observations suggesting that antiserum neutralized virus with one-hit kinetics (16) and that the pI of picornaviruses dropped from 7 to 4 upon treatment with antiserum (31). These observations led to the hypothesis that the binding of a single antibody molecule caused a concerted conformational change in the virus capsid leading to loss of infectivity and a change in the surface charge. For picornaviruses, the shift in pI after antibody binding has been duplicated in several laboratories (12, 17) although the causal relationship between the pI shift and neutralization has been questioned (6, 23). If it could be shown that a single antibody is sufficient to neutralize infectivity, then the proposed process of antibody-induced conformational changes would be strongly supported. However, when the number of antibodies required for neutralization of unaggregated virions was carefully quantified, no monoclonal antibodies were found to be capable of neutralization at a ratio of one antibody per virion (23, 27). These measurements are not without debate because there has been one report of single-antibody-mediated neutralization using polyclonal antibodies (64). However, this latter study used polyclonal serum rather than monoclonal antibodies.

Several laboratories reported that antibodies specific for protein sequences buried inside the virus capsid are capable of precipitation (45) or neutralization (29). Those investigators hypothesize that the virus "breathes," exposing residues normally buried. It was suggested that antibodies reacting with these previously buried residues might trap the virus in a noninfectious conformation. However, the dominant epitopes only map to the external portions of the virions. Therefore, while these studies clearly demonstrate a remarkable flexibility in the capsid structure, these epitopes only appear when synthetic antigen is injected into the animal.

Finally, some poliovirus-specific monoclonal antibodies have been found to mediate RNA release from virions when binding at low ionic strength or elevated temperatures (5, 14). The authors of these studies speculated that virus neutralization by such antibodies may be activated by fever. In these cases, it is possible that the virus is undergoing conformational changes due to the high temperatures and low ionic strength and the antibodies are binding to these altered forms. This has shown to be the case with some antibodies to Sindbis virus (36).

The crystal structure of the Fab17-HRV14 complex clearly demonstrated that efficacious neutralization does not require large conformational changes in the capsid (54). Instead, large conformational changes in the paratope region of Fab17 permit the Fab to better accommodate the epitope without inducing structural changes in the virion (54). Furthermore, antibodies to the four different antigenic sites that were tested (mAbs 13, 17, 21, 28, 29, 33, 34, 35) did cause apparent changes in the pI of the capsid (12). However, it seems unlikely that such dissimilar antibodies, which bind to disparate epitopes, would all cause the same conformational change in the capsid. Antibodies might cause conformational changes in protein structure upon binding, but such changes would more likely be expected to occur on flexible portions of the viral structure. Indeed, binding affinity is proportional to the sum of all chemical interactions at the paratope-epitope interface. Subtracted from this sum would be the energy required to induce conformational changes upon binding. Therefore, antibody-induced conformational changes on less flexible regions would require a greater cost in binding energy, thereby potentially diminishing antibody affinity. For these reasons, we believe that induced conformational changes play little or no significant role in the mechanism of antibody neutralization.

Abrogation of Cellular Attachment

A representative series of antibodies that bound to each of the four NIm sites of HRV14 were tested for their ability to block cell attachment (12). The investigators found that a monoclonal antibody (mAb34) to the NIm-IA site reduced attachment to HeLa cell membranes in a dose-dependent fashion. Antibody-induced aggregation of virus by antibodies binding to other sites made the precipitation-based assay uninformative. However, high concentrations of papain-derived Fab fragments of these antibodies were shown to block attachment to HeLa membranes. At high concentrations, the Fab fragments also decreased the pI of HRV14 from 7.0 to values between 2.0 and 3.6.

In the case of mAb17, 16 antibodies per virion were required to inhibit attachment by 90%. In addition, 14 antibodies per virion were required to neutralize 90% of the input infectivity (26). This result suggests that, for at least this antibody, inhibition of attachment may be the primary mechanism of neutralization. Competition between receptor and NIm-IA antibody binding might simply be explained as a steric hindrance effect. NIm-II is immediately adjacent to the ICAM-binding region, and the $\sim$600-to-900-Å^2 contact region of NIm-II antibodies probably overlaps the ICAM site or at least hinders attachment to ICAM. However, NIm-III is quite distal ($\sim$40-Å away) to the receptor-binding region, yet NIm-III antibodies also compete with receptor binding (12). Hence, antibody competition with receptor may merely be a consequence of the bulkiness of an antibody molecule and not necessarily due to direct overlap with the ICAM-binding region.

Significance of In Vitro Neutralization Mechanisms In Vivo

Taken together, results of many studies with HRV14 suggest that neutralization in vitro may occur by a much simpler mechanism than previously envisioned: the presence of antibodies bound to the surface of HRV14 is sufficient to block attachment to virus receptors. For poliovirus and rhinovirus, interactions with their receptors appear to be essential for the proper release of the genomic RNA into the cytoplasm of the host cell. When antibody-poliovirus complexes enter cells, the viral RNA is quickly digested (30). In contrast, FMDV-antibody complexes are infectious if allowed to enter cells via artificially expressed Fc receptors (32). Therefore, these two viruses have different roles for their receptor-virus interactions; rhinovirus and poliovirus require the receptor to initiate uncoating whereas FMDV just needs its receptor to deliver the virus to cytoplasm. In both cases, antibodies can block normal receptor entry, and therefore infection, quite effectively. Thus, a simple steric model (antibody binding blocks receptor binding) is sufficient to explain the neutralization behavior of many antibodies to these viruses. Binding of some antibodies might cause secondary effects to viral capsids (14, 16, 29, 66), but these effects seem to be dispensable for neutralization, and, perhaps more important, antibodies that induce such effects would not be exclusively selected for during B-cell clonal expansion. This is because B-cell proliferation is simply driven by the strength of the interaction between the antigen and surface immunoglobulins and independent of potential secondary effects of antibody binding.

It is important to note, however, that the in vitro mechanisms we have described may not represent the primary mode by which antibodies protect animals from viral infections. For example, some antibodies against Sindbis (49) and FMDV (35) that are not efficacious in vitro still protect animals from viral challenge. Also, nonneutralizing antibodies against the neuraminidase (NA) of influenza affect disease progression in vivo (50). Hence, the primary role of antibodies in vivo may be to act synergistically with other components of the immune system. Vaccine design strategies might, therefore, benefit by focusing on the production of high-affinity antibodies rather than on a particular in vitro neutralization property. This has been shown to be true for a number of antibodies to viruses larger and more complex than the picornaviruses, such as HIV, where antibody neutralization efficacy is directly proportional to binding affinity and does not depend on which epitope is recognized (41).

CANYON HYPOTHESIS

When the high-resolution structure of influenza virus N9 NA was solved, it was noted that the conserved residues involved in sialic acid binding were located in a crevasse. The investigators suggested that such architecture might have several functional implications (11). Analogous to most enzymes, a cavity or pocket-like structural feature may have evolved to facilitate contact with receptor. It was further noted that a concave morphological feature like that occurring on the NA spike would also offer some protection against binding of host antibodies to functionally important residues. However, even if some of the conserved residues were accessible to antibodies, the quaternary structure of the NA spike required antibody contacts with some of the variable loops at the top of the sialic acid-binding site. Influenza virus could, therefore, escape antibody binding without any need to alter crucial portions of its NA spike.

The X-ray structure of HRV14 exhibited some of the same crevasse-like features as NA (47). In HRV14, a 20-Å-deep and 20-Å-wide canyon encircles each of the icosahedral fivefold axes (Color Plate 4). These dimensions and the knowledge that the sites of escape mutations map to the canyon rim led to the hypothesis that the canyon region is involved in receptor binding (46, 47). It was also suggested that HRV evolved this quaternary structure as a means to protect conserved residues necessary for receptor recognition (47). However, the X-ray structure of the HRV14-Fab complex demonstrated that antibodies bind into deep recesses of virion surfaces and contact conserved residues (54). Furthermore, it was predicted that the receptor-binding regions of all viruses that replicate in mammals would be hidden in deep convolutions of the capsid surface. This is a reasonable and necessary thesis if antibody response is a major factor in viral evolution. Again, the two major points of this thesis are that (i) all viruses will have receptor-binding regions in convoluted portions of the capsid and (ii) conserved residues necessary for receptor binding will be hidden from antibodies. The results from several virus systems argue that these hypotheses are probably not correct.

FMDV

The Arg-Gly-Asp (RGD) sequence in FMDV that probably interacts with the integrin receptor is highly exposed on the βG-βH loop in VP1 (1). The residues flanking the RGD motif residues vary with serotypes. This led investigators to suggest that FMDV can use "camouflage" to hide crucial residues "in plain sight." According to this hypothesis, crucial residues might be exposed to antibodies but simply do not change in response to antibodies since doing so will be lethal to the virus. The exposed nature of these residues has been further demonstrated by structural studies that show these conserved residues make extensive interactions with a neutralizing antibody (60). Furthermore, the functional overlap between antibody and receptor binding is made evident by the fact that adaptation of FMDV to different growth conditions often leads to changes in antigenicity (15, 44). Perhaps even more important, these results demonstrate that antigenic drift can be independent of host immunity.

The position of the secondary receptor, heparin, was recently elucidated (18). Heparin sulfate has been suggested to be involved in a two-step attachment process where low-affinity interactions with heparin sulfate at one site are followed by high-affinity binding to an integrin receptor via the RGD sequence (24). Like the RGD sequence, this oligosaccharide binding site is not only exposed but is also part of one of the antigenic sites (18). Therefore, it is very clear that FMDV is exactly contrary to what was predicted by the canyon hypothesis.

Alphaviruses

Anti-idiotypic antibodies to a neutralizing antibody were found to compete with virus for cell receptors (62). This suggests that not only is the crucial receptor-binding region on the virus exposed to antibodies, but it can also be mimicked by anti-idiotypic antibodies. In our cryo-TEM studies, this region was shown to lie on the outermost tip of the trimeric viral spikes (55). In these studies, a similar virus, Ross River virus, was also examined. An antibody was used that binds to an epitope immediately adjacent to residues that change upon adaptation to different hosts. Therefore, it seems likely that these antibodies also recognize a portion of the spikes involved in receptor recognition. Indeed, while these antibodies bound in a different orientation than that observed in the Fab-Sindbis complex, the contact area was identical and highly exposed.

Influenza Virus

As described above, the sialic acid-binding site in the NA spike of influenza lies in a depression on its spike. Whereas the residues within this deep depression are conserved, the residues about the rim vary with serotype. This suggests that conserved residues are hidden from antibody recognition. However, subsequent studies demonstrated that about one-third of the conserved binding region in this depression is contacted by a neutralizing antibody (3). To explain how viruses might evade antibody attack while leaving conserved residues immunologically exposed, Colman has proposed that this capability may reflect the potential for different proteins to recognize identical protein surfaces (10). In this way, receptors and antibodies can bind to overlapping areas of the viral surface but can exhibit differing sensitivities to mutations at these contact surfaces.

Poliovirus

Similar to human rhinovirus, poliovirus has a deep canyon about the icosahedral fivefold axes and escape mutations are located on top of the canyon. However, in contradiction to the canyon hypothesis, there is a direct link between the receptor-binding site and the serotypic determinants in poliovirus. It has been shown that upper, exposed regions of the poliovirus canyon are crucial for receptor interactions, but residues at the bottom of the poliovirus canyon are not. In fact, changes at the top of the canyon that affect antibody-neutralizing sites also alter receptor-virus interactions (19). Yielding similar conclusions, other studies showed that mutations at the north and south walls of the canyon overcome deleterious defects in the poliovirus receptor. These mutations, which are quite distal to the canyon floor, lie very close to the antigenic sites and appear to represent destabilizing mutations (65). These results are further evidence that the canyon plays a pivotal role in capsid structural homeostasis and conservation of canyon residues is probably due to viability issues rather than accessibility to antibodies. Indeed, it has been noted that if the canyon exists solely to assist in hiding the receptor-binding site, then one would expect to see far more than the three poliovirus serotypes (19). It was also noted that some RNA viruses have been shown to diverge antigenically in the absence of the immune system, thereby questioning the idea that antibodies are the only selective pressure driving antigenic diversification. Finally, the cryo-TEM structure of the poliovirus-receptor complex (2, 68) clearly shows that some of the mutation sites that affect serotype-specific binding to mutant receptors lie within the receptor contact area (19).

CONCLUSIONS

In a 1937 review, Burnet et al. (7) concluded that antibody neutralization was reversible and required more than one antibody. Studies over the next six decades have both supported and challenged these results. In several recent papers on the more complex viruses (8, 41), it is clear that antibody neutralization is directly proportional to antibody binding. It has been further shown that the antibody:virus ratio for this neutralization is, in fact, proportional to the surface area of the pathogen (42).

We have shown that, while antibodies might induce conformational changes, strongly neutralizing antibodies do not need to cause structural changes. Instead, we have found that increasing the valency of antibody binding can increase the neutralization efficacy and this is most likely due to an increase in antibody avidity. At least for this system, it appears that the main effect of antibody in vitro is the abrogation of cellular attachment. In vivo, it is likely that components of innate immunity play a synergistic role in neutralization. If this is true, then the development of vaccines is greatly simplified in that one needs only to elicit antibodies that can recognize the native virions and not be concerned with antibody-mediated induction of secondary effects. Clearly, in the laboratory, one should focus on the induction of strongly neutralizing antibodies. However, this property appears to be mostly dependent on antibody avidity and recognition of the infectious particle.

These results also suggest that the canyon did not evolve in response to immunological pressure. We would argue that the canyon has evolved to interact with receptor and to facilitate subsequent conformational changes that facilitate injection of viral genome into the host cell. This is supported by our recent mass spectroscopic analysis of HRV14 trypsin digestion products that demonstrated that the canyon and the drug-binding cavity play a role in capsid dynamics (28). We conclude that the drug-binding region is an empty cavity beneath the canyon that affords the region the necessary conformational flexibility to respond to receptor binding. Empty cavities keep proteins at a higher energy state where it will take less energy to cause structural changes (33). Indeed, a direct relationship between protein stability and function has been demonstrated in T4 lysozyme (53). Therefore, we propose that the major evolutionary force in all viruses is the recognition of a receptor and subsequent conformational processes that facilitate genome release. This will increase the efficiency of the infection process that allows the virus to spread to naïve hosts.

REFERENCES

1. **Acharya, R., E. Fry, E. Stuart, G. Fox, E. Rowlands, and F. Brown.** 1989. The three-dimensional structure of foot-and-mouth disease virus at 2.9 Å resolution. *Nature* **327:**709–716.
2. **Belnap, D. M., B. M. McDermott, D. J. Filman, N. Cheng, B. L. Trus, H. J. Zuccola, V. R. Racaniello, J. M. Hogle, and A. C. Steven.** 2000. Three-dimensional structure of poliovirus receptor bound to poliovirus. *Proc. Natl. Acad. Sci. USA* **97:**73–78.
3. **Bizebard, T., B. Gigant, P. Rigolet, B. Rasmussen, O. Diat, P. Bosecke, S. A. Wharton, J. J. Skehel, and M. Knossow.** 1995. Structure of influenza virus haemagglutinin complexed with a neutralizing antibody. *Nature* **376:**92–94.
4. **Brioen, P., D. Dekegel, and A. Boeyé.** 1983. Neutralization of poliovirus by antibody-mediated polymerization. *Virology* **127:**463–468.
5. **Brioen, P., B. Rombaut, and A. Boeyé.** 1985. Hit-and-run neutralization of poliovirus. *J. Gen. Virol.* **66:**2495–2499.
6. **Brioen, P., A. A. M. Thomas, and A. Boeyé.** 1985. Lack of quantitative correlation between the neutralization of poliovirus and the antibody-mediated pI shift of the virions. *J. Gen. Virol.* **66:**609–613.
7. **Burnet, F. M., E. V. Keogh, and D. Lush.** 1937. The immunological reactions of the filterable viruses. *Aust. J. Exp. Biol. Med. Sci.* **15:**227–368.
7a. **Burton, D. R., E. O. Saphire, and P. W. H. I. Parren.** 2001. A model for neutralization of viruses based on antibody coating of the virion surface, p. 109–143. *In* D. R. Burton (ed.), *Current Topics in Microbiology and Immunology.* Springer-Verlag, New York, N.Y.
8. **Burton, D. R., R. A. Williamson, and P. W. Parren.** 2000. Antibody and virus: binding and neutralization. *Virology* **270:**1–3.
9. **Che, Z., N. H. Olson, D. Leippe, W.-M. Lee, A. Mosser, R. R. Rueckert, T. S. Baker, and T. J. Smith.** 1998. Antibody-mediated neutralization of human rhinovirus 14 explored by means of cryo-electron microscopy and X-ray crystallography of virus-Fab complexes. *J. Virol.* **72:**4610–4622.
10. **Colman, P. M.** 1997. Virus versus antibody. *Structure* **5:**591–593.
11. **Colman, P. M., J. N. Varghese, and W. G. Laver.** 1983. Structure of the catalytic and antigenic sites in influenza virus neuraminidase. *Nature (London)* **303:**41–44.
12. **Colonno, R. J., P. L. Callahan, D. M. Leippe, and R. R. Rueckert.** 1989. Inhibition of rhinovirus attachment by neutralizing monoclonal antibodies and their Fab fragments. *J. Virol.* **63:**36–42.
13. **Colonno, R. J., J. H. Condra, S. Mizutani, P. L. Callahan, M. E. Davies, and M. A. Murcko.** 1988. Evidence for the direct involvement of the rhinovirus canyon in receptor binding. *Proc. Natl. Acad. Sci. USA* **85:**5449–5453.
14. **Delaet, I., and A. Boeye.** 1993. Monoclonal antibodies that disrupt poliovirus only at fever temperatures. *J. Virol.* **67:**5299–5302.
15. **Diez, J., M. Davila, C. Escarmis, M. G. Mateu, J. Dominguez, J. J. Perez, E. Giralt, J. A. Melero, and E. Domingo.** 1990. Unique amino acid substitutions in the capsid proteins of foot-and-mouth disease virus from a persistent infection in cell culture. *J. Virol.* **64:**5519–5528.
16. **Dulbecco, R., M. Vogt, and A. G. R. Strickland.** 1956. A study of the basic aspects of neutralization of two animal viruses, western equine encephalitis and poliomyelitis virus. *Virology* **2:**162–205.

17. Emini, E. A., P. Ostapchuk, and E. Wimmer. 1983. Bivalent attachment of antibody onto poliovirus leads to conformational alteration and neutralization. *J. Virol.* **48:** 547–550.
18. Fry, E. E., S. M. Lea, T. Jackson, J. W. I. Newman, F. M. Ellard, W. E. Blakemore, R. Abu-Ghazaleh, A. Samuel, A. M. Q. King, and D. I. Stuart. 1999. The structure and function of a foot-and-mouth disease virus—oligosaccharide receptor complex. *EMBO J.* **18:** 543–554.
19. Harber, J., G. Bernhardt, H. H. Lu, J. Y. Sgro, and E. Wimmer. 1995. Canyon rim residues, including antigenic determinants, modulate serotype-specific binding of polioviruses to mutants of the poliovirus receptor. *Virology* **214:** 559–570.
20. Heinz, B. A., R. R. Rueckert, D. A. Shepard, F. J. Dutko, M. A. McKinlay, M. Francher, M. G. Rossmann, J. Badger, and T. J. Smith. 1989. Genetic and molecular analysis of spontaneous mutants of human rhinovirus 14 resistant to an antiviral compound. *J. Virol.* **63:** 2476–2485.
21. Hewat, E. A., and D. Blaas. 1996. Structure of a neutralizing antibody bound bivalently to human rhinovirus 2. *EMBO J.* **15:** 1515–1523.
22. Hewat, E. A., N. Verdaguer, I. Fita, W. Blakemore, S. Brookes, A. King, J. Newman, E. Domingo, M. G. Mateu, and D. I. Stuart. 1997. Structure of the complex of an Fab fragment of a neutralizing antibody with foot-and-mouth disease virus: positioning of a highly mobile antigenic loop. *EMBO J.* **16:** 1492–1500.
23. Icenogle, J., H. Shiwen, G. Duke, S. Gilbert, R. Rueckert, and J. Anderegg. 1983. Neutralization of poliovirus by a monoclonal antibody: kinetics and stoichiometry. *Virology* **127:** 412–425.
24. Jackson, T., F. M. Ellard, R. Abu-Ghazaleh, S. M. Brookes, W. E. Blakemore, A. H. Corteyn, D. I. Stuart, J. W. I. Newman, and A. M. Q. King. 1996. Efficient infection of cells in culture by type O foot-and-mouth disease virus requires binding to cell surface heparan sulfate. *J. Virol.* **70:** 5282–5287.
25. Kolatkar, P. R., J. Bella, N. H. Olson, C. M. Bator, T. S. Baker, and M. G. Rossmann. 1999. Structural studies of two rhinovirus serotypes complexed with fragments of their cellular receptor. *EMBO J.* **18:** 6249–6259.
26. Lee, W. M. 1992. Human rhinovirus 14: synthesis and characterization of a molecular cDNA clone which makes highly infectious transcripts. Ph.D. Thesis. Department of Biochemistry, University of Wisconsin, Madison.
27. Leippe, D. M. 1991. Stoichiometry of picornavirus neutralization by murine monoclonal antibodies. Ph.D. thesis. University of Wisconsin, Madison.
28. Lewis, J. K., B. Bothner, T. J. Smith, and G. Siuzdak. 1998. Antiviral agent blocks breathing of the common cold virus. *Proc. Natl. Acad. Sci. USA* **95:** 6774–6778.
29. Li, Q., A. G. Yafal, Y. M. H. Lee, J. Hogle, and M. Chow. 1994. Poliovirus neutralization by antibodies to internal epitopes of VP4 and VP1 results from reversible exposure of the sequences at physiological temperatures. *J. Virol.* **68:** 3965–3970.
30. Mandel, B. 1967. The interaction of neutralized poliovirus with HeLa cells. II. Elution, penetration, uncoating. *Virology* **31:** 247–259.
31. Mandel, B. 1976. Neutralization of poliovirus: a hypothesis to explain the mechanism and the one-hit character of the neutralization reaction. *Virology* **69:** 500–510.
32. Mason, P. W., B. Baxt, F. Brown, J. Harber, A. Murdin, and E. Wimmer. 1993. Antibody-complexed foot-and-mouth disease virus, but not poliovirus, can infect normally insusceptible cells via the Fc receptor. *Virology* **192:** 568–577.
33. Matthews, B. W. 1993. Structural and genetic analysis of protein folding and stability. *Curr. Opin. Struct. Biol.* **3:** 589–593.
34. McCray, J., and G. Werner. 1987. Different rhinovirus serotypes neutralized by antipeptide antibodies. *Nature* **329:** 736–738.
35. McCullough, K. C., F. De Simone, E. Brocchi, L. Capucci, J. R. Crowther, and U. Kihm. 1992. Protective immune response against foot-and-mouth disease. *J. Virol.* **66:** 1835–1840.
36. Meyer, W. J., S. Gidwitz, V. K. Ayers, R. J. Schoepp, and R. E. Johnston. 1992. Conformational alteration of Sindbis virion glycoproteins induced by heat, reducing agents, or low pH. *J. Virol.* **66:** 3504–3513.
37. Mosser, A. G., D. M. Leippe, and R. R. Rueckert. 1989. Neutralization of picornaviruses: support for the pentamer bridging hypothesis, p. 155–167. *In* B. L. Semler and E. Ehrenfeld (ed.), *Molecular Aspects of Picornavirus Infection and Detection.* American Society for Microbiology, Washington, D.C.
38. Mosser, A. G., and R. R. Rueckert. 1993. WIN 51711-dependent mutants of poliovirus type 3: evidence that virions decay after release from cells unless drug is present. *J. Virol.* **67:** 1246–1254.
39. Mosser, A. G., J. Y. Sgro, and R. R. Rueckert. 1994. Distribution of drug resistance mutations in type 3 poliovirus identifies three regions involved in uncoating functions. *J. Virol.* **68:** 8193–8201.
40. Olson, N. H., P. R. Kolatkar, M. A. Oliveira, R. H. Cheng, J. M. Greve, A. McClelland, T. S. Baker, and M. G. Rossmann. 1993. Structure of a human rhinovirus complexed with its receptor molecule. *Proc. Natl. Acad. Sci. USA* **90:** 507–511.
41. Parren, P. W., I. Mondor, D. Naniche, H. J. Ditzel, P. J. Klasse, D. R. Burton, and Q. J. Sattentau. 1998. Neutralization of human immunodeficiency virus type 1 by antibody to gp120 is determined primarily by occupancy of sites on the virion irrespective of epitope specificity. *J. Virol.* **72:** 3512–3519.
42. [See reference 7a.]
43. Porta, C., R. H. Cheng, Z. Chen, T. S. Baker, and J. E. Johnson. 1994. Direct imaging of interactions between an icosahedral virus and conjugate Fab fragments by cryoelectron microscopy and X-ray crystallography. *Virology* **204:** 777–788.
44. Rieder, E., B. Baxt, and P. W. Mason. 1994. Animal-derived antigenic variants of foot-and-mouth disease virus type A12 have low affinity for cells in culture. *J. Virol.* **68:** 5296–5299.
45. Roivainen, M., L. Piirainen, T. Rysa, A. Narvanen, and T. Hovi. 1993. An immunodominant N-terminal region of VP1 protein of poliovirion that is buried in crystal structure can be exposed in solution. *Virology* **195:** 762–765.
46. Rossmann, M. G. 1989. The canyon hypothesis. *J. Biol. Chem.* **264:** 14587–14590.
47. Rossmann, M. G., E. Arnold, J. W. Erickson, E. A. Frankenberger, J. P. Griffith, H. J. Hecht, J. E. Johnson, G. Kamer, M. Luo, A. G. Mosser, R. R. Rueckert, B. Sherry, and G. Vriend. 1985. Structure of a human common cold virus and functional relationship to other picornaviruses. *Nature (London)* **317:** 145–153.
48. Rueckert, R. R. 1996. Picornaviridae and their replication, p. 609–654. *In* B. N. Fields and D. M. Knipe (ed.), *Fundamental Virology.* Raven Press, New York, N.Y.
49. Schmaljohn, A. L., E. D. Johnson, J. M. Dalrymple, and G. A. Cole. 1982. Nonneutralizing monoclonal antibodies can prevent lethal alphavirus encephalitis. *Nature* **297:** 70–72.

50. Schulman, J. L. 1975. Immunology of influenza, p. 373–393. *In* E. D. Kilbourne (ed.), *The Influenza Viruses and Influenza*. Academic Press, New York, N.Y.
51. Sherry, B., A. G. Mosser, R. J. Colonno, and R. R. Rueckert. 1986. Use of monoclonal antibodies to identify four neutralization immunogens on a common cold picornavirus, human rhinovirus 14. *J. Virol.* **57:**246–257.
52. Sherry, B., and R. R. Rueckert. 1985. Evidence for at least two dominant neutralization antigens on human rhinovirus 14. *J. Virol.* **53:**137–143.
53. Shoichet, B. K., W. A. Baase, R. Kuroki, and B. W. Matthews. 1995. A relationship between protein stability and protein function. *Proc. Natl. Acad. Sci. USA* **92:**452–456.
54. Smith, T. J., E. S. Chase, T. J. Schmidt, N. H. Olson, and T. S. Baker. 1996. Neutralizing antibody to human rhinovirus 14 penetrates the receptor-binding canyon. *Nature (London)* **383:**350–354.
55. Smith, T. J., R. H. Cheng, N. H. Olson, P. Peterson, E. Chase, R. J. Kuhn, and T. S. Baker. 1995. Putative receptor binding sites on alphaviruses as visualized by cryo-electron microscopy. *Proc. Natl. Acad. Sci. USA* **92:**10648–10652.
56. Smith, T. J., N. H. Olson, R. H. Cheng, E. S. Chase, and T. S. Baker. 1993. Structure of a human rhinovirus-bivalently bound antibody complex: implications for virus neutralization and antibody flexibility. *Proc. Natl. Acad. Sci. USA* **90:**7015–7018.
57. Smith, T. J., N. H. Olson, R. H. Cheng, H. Liu, E. Chase, W. M. Lee, D. M. Leippe, A. G. Mosser, R. R. Rueckert, and T. S. Baker. 1993. Structure of human rhinovirus complexed with Fab fragments from a neutralizing antibody. *J. Virol.* **67:**1148–1158.
58. Thomas, A. A. M., P. Brioen, and A. Boeyé. 1985. A monoclonal antibody that neutralizes poliovirus by cross-linking virions. *J. Virol.* **54:**7–13.
59. Thouvenin, E., S. Laurent, M. F. Madelaine, D. Rasschaert, J. F. Vautherot, and E. A. Hewat. 1997. Bivalent binding of a neutralising antibody to a calicivirus involves the torsional flexibility of the antibody hinge. *J. Mol. Biol.* **270:**238–246.
60. Verdaguer, N., M. G. Mateu, D. Andreu, E. Giralt, E. Domingo, and I. Fita. 1995. Structure of the major antigenic loop of foot-and-mouth disease virus complexed with a neutralizing antibody: direct involvement of the Arg-Gly-Asp motif in the interaction. *EMBO J.* **14:**1690–1696.
61. Wade, R. H., J. C. Taveau, and J. N. Lamy. 1989. Concerning the axial rotational flexiblity of the Fab regions of immunoglobulin G. *J. Mol. Biol.* **206:**349–356.
62. Wang, K.-S., A. L. Schmaljohn, R. J. Kuhn, and J. H. Strauss. 1991. Antiidiotypic antibodies as probes for the Sindbis virus receptor. *Virology* **181:**694–702.
63. Wang, P., C. Porta, Z. Chen, T. S. Baker, and J. E. Johnson. 1992. Identification of a Fab interaction site (footprint) on an icosahedral virus by cryo-electron microscopy and X-ray crystallography. *Nature* **355:**275–278.
64. Wetz, K., P. Willingmann, H. Zeichhardt, and K. O. Habermehl. 1986. Neutralization of poliovirus by polyclonal antibodies requires binding of a single IgG molecule per virion. *Arch. Virol.* **91:**207–220.
65. Wien, M. W., S. Curry, D. J. Filman, and J. M. Hogle. 1997. Structural studies of poliovirus mutants that overcome receptor defects. *Nat. Struct. Biol.* **4:**666–674.
66. Wien, M. W., D. J. Filman, E. A. Stura, S. Guillot, F. Delpeyroux, R. Crainic, and J. M. Hogle. 1995. Structure of the complex between the Fab fragment of a neutralizing antibody for type 1 poliovirus and its viral epitope. *Nat. Struct. Biol.* **2:**232–243.
67. Wikoff, W. R., G. Wang, C. R. Parrish, R. H. Cheng, M. L. Strassheim, T. S. Baker, and M. G. Rossmann. 1994. The structure of a neutralized virus: canine parvovirus complexed with neutralizing antibody fragment. *Structure* **2:**595–607.
68. Yongning, H., V. D. Bowman, S. Mueller, C. M. Bator, J. Bella, X. Peng, T. S. Baker, E. Wimmer, R. J. Kuhn, and M. G. Rossmann. 2000. Interaction of the poliovirus receptor with poliovirus. *Proc. Natl. Acad. Sci. USA* **97:**79–84.

Antigenic Variation in Foot-and-Mouth Disease Virus

DAVID J. ROWLANDS AND FRED BROWN

5

Antigenic variation in foot-and-mouth disease (FMD) is important for both practical and fundamental reasons. In the first place, it has considerable importance in the control of the disease by vaccination because vaccines providing protection against one of the seven serotypes afford no protection against viruses belonging to the other six serotypes. Equally important, the wide spectrum of antigenic variation within the serotypes provides similar control problems.

The second reason is the opportunity that antigenic variation provides for studying the immunochemistry of the virus. Because foot-and-mouth disease virus (FMDV) is a relatively simple molecule, which has been studied in considerable detail, the important antigenic sites have been identified and peptides corresponding to one of these sites have been shown to provide protection against challenge infection. Consequently, this work has provided the opportunity to study the structural differences between antigenic variants and possibly design peptides that will give a wider spectrum of protection within a serotype. It is of particular interest that a major antigenic feature of the virus is coincident with the cell receptor-binding motif. This provides us with the intriguing challenge of trying to understand how the apparently conflicting requirements of maintaining receptor-binding specificity while allowing antigenic variation to occur in the same structural feature are resolved.

DISCOVERY OF SEROTYPES

The discovery of serotypes stemmed from the observation that animals in the field could become infected on more than one occasion. In 1922, Vallee and Carre in France provided results from cross-immunity experiments with the strain that was prevalent in that country at that time and a second strain thought to have come from Germany. These strains were labeled O (from the department of Oise) and A (from Allemagne), respectively. This finding was confirmed by Waldmann and Trautwein in Germany with strains they labeled A and B and a third they called C. The confusion that arose when it was shown that the O was the same as the German workers' A, and the French workers' A was the same as the German workers' B, can be imagined. Following discussions at the Office International des Epizooties in Paris, the three strains were named Valle O, Valle A, and Waldmann C, but they are now known simply as O, A, and C.

Serotyping was a tedious and costly exercise in those days, relying on cross-immunity tests in animals. It was fortunate that Waldmann and Pepe had found in 1920 that the guinea pig could be infected with the virus, so this species could be used in most cases instead of the more costly cattle. In addition, the virus is not transmitted naturally between guinea pigs so the chances of cross-infection, which occurs only too readily between cattle and pigs, could be avoided.

Three more serotypes from outbreaks occurring in Africa were added to the list in the late 1940s and early 1950s. These strains, known as SAT 1 (Southern African territories 1), SAT 2, and SAT 3, were found in Bechuanaland and Rhodesia. Not surprisingly, reexamination, by complement fixation, of isolates that had been sent to the Pirbright Laboratory in the 1930s showed that these serotypes were among the collection. By methods available in the 1930s they had been regarded as atypical of the three well-established O, A, and C serotypes.

The last serotype to be discovered is Asia 1, found in a sample from Pakistan. Since this was discovered in 1954 and the extensive examination of viruses occurring worldwide at the World Reference Laboratory at Pirbright has not found any evidence for other serotypes, it seems reasonable to conclude that no more will be found.

Until recently the seven serotypes of FMDV were alone classified within the genus *Aphthoviridae*. However, analysis of the genome sequence of equine rhinitis virus clearly shows that this virus too belongs within the genus and it is now included as a separate species. It shares a number of important features with the FMDVs although there are also significant differences. The extent to which its anti-

---

David J. Rowlands ■ Division of Microbiology, School of Biochemistry and Molecular Biology, University of Leeds, Leeds LS2 9JT, United Kingdom. *Fred Brown* ■ Plum Island Animal Disease Center, P.O. Box 848, Greenport, NY 11944.

genic properties parallel those of the FMDVs remains to be determined.

VARIATION WITHIN SEROTYPES

Control of the disease by vaccination has been entirely dependent on the recognition of the different serotypes. This has been highly successful in western Europe and several countries in South America and resulted in the elimination of the disease from these areas. Vaccination was abandoned as a consequence of the eradication of endemic FMD, since important trading advantages may be accrued from achieving a disease-free status and this is currently impossible while vaccination is being employed to control infection. The major outbreaks of FMD both in South America and Europe (especially the United Kingdom) during 2001 serve as salutary reminders of the vigilance that must be exercised in the prevention of this highly contagious disease. Occasionally, however, even when a country is apparently protected against the disease by vaccination, outbreaks can still occur, and there are several well-documented cases. The first to be reported were those in several countries in western Europe in 1965 to 1966 when the comprehensive vaccination programs that had been in operation for several years were unable to control the outbreak of the disease caused by a virus of serotype O. This was the result of the introduction of a virus distinct from that being used to prepare the vaccine.

A similar situation occurred in the Middle East in 1965 when a virus of serotype A emerged that differed so much from that in the vaccines being used in western Europe that it was considered for some time that the new virus belonged to a different serotype. A vaccine prepared from the outbreak virus contained the situation.

However, these situations could have been anticipated from the work done by Trautwein and Waldmann in Germany and Bedson and the Maitlands in England in the late 1920s. These two groups had shown that antigenic variation occurred within serotypes. Although the differences between the isolates were quantitative, they were real, and later events were to show that these differences are important. For example, in the very early days of experimental vaccines, it was shown quite clearly that an effective killed vaccine prepared in the Pirbright Laboratory against a virus of serotype A isolated in Kent, England, in 1932 was ineffective against the serotype A virus causing widespread outbreaks in Mexico during 1946 to 1954.

PRACTICAL CONSIDERATIONS

Successful vaccination depends on the producers being able to grow the appropriate viruses to high titer and in large amounts. Usually between 1 and 10 μg of virus, after appropriate inactivation, are required to evoke protective levels of neutralizing antibodies against the homologous virus. This level of production is sometimes difficult to achieve immediately when a virus is received from a field outbreak. Adaptation to an appropriate tissue culture system can sometimes result in the selection of antigenic variants that do not "fit" with the outbreak strain. The derivation of appropriate strains for vaccination purposes is currently an empirical process, and adaptation and characterization of appropriate viruses can be a protracted and uncertain procedure. Adapted virus strains can differ remarkably in their immunogenicity and the degree of cross-protection afforded against a range of field strains. In the face of new outbreaks of the disease, the suitability of available vaccines is measured by determining the serological cross-reaction between the outbreak virus and that from which the vaccine was prepared, and in general this approach has worked well.

ANTIGENIC STRUCTURE OF FMDV

Early indications of the importance of the structural integrity of the virus particle in determining its antigenic characteristics came from studies of the immunogenic potential of the virus or its subunits. FMDV is readily denatured by heat or mild acid conditions into three components: the RNA genome; an aggregate of the small internal protein, VP4; and soluble pentameric 12S subunits comprising five copies of each of the remaining capsid proteins, VP1 to 3. The ability of this mixture, or of purified 12S subunits alone, to induce virus-reactive neutralizing antibodies was very much reduced compared to that in intact virus particles (10, 37). Furthermore, adsorption of antivirus antiserum with an excess of 12S subunits failed to remove detectable levels of neutralizing activity, indicating an important qualitative difference between the antigenic characteristics of the assembled virus and its component subunits (39). Clearly, the antigenic structure of the 12S structural subunit is dramatically different from that of the intact virus particle. However, the uncleaved structural protein precursor, P1, produced in insect cells by expression from recombinant baculovirus was found to be antigenically similar to native virus particles (41), suggesting that the processing cleavages convert the precursor protein into a potentially unstable form.

A study of the effects of proteolysis on the immunogenic properties of the virus provided the first indications that there are multiple antigenic determinants on the surface of the particle and that these differ in their relative importance for inducing virus-neutralizing antibodies. Trypsin treatment of the virus resulted in limited cleavage of the capsid proteins but had dramatic effects on its biological properties. Infectivity was reduced by two or three orders of magnitude due to a greatly reduced ability of the virus to attach to cells (39, 48). The ability of trypsin-treated virus particles to induce protective antibody responses was also diminished, although the treated particles were still able to adsorb the majority of the antibodies from anti-FMDV antisera (39). However, the trypsinized particles did not adsorb measurable amounts of the virus-neutralizing activity from such antisera, implying that a particularly important antigenic site had been destroyed. It also transpired that the early immunoglobulin M (IgM) antibody responses were directed almost exclusively to an antigenic feature of the virus that was destroyed by trypsin (11). When negatively stained samples of virus-IgM complexes were examined by electron microscopy, it was apparent that the sites recognized by these antibodies were relatively small in number and evenly distributed around the particles.

The special significance of the VP1 protein in determining the antigenic characteristics of the virus became apparent when it was demonstrated that the isolated protein, either purified from virus particles or expressed by recombinant techniques, could induce virus-neutralizing and protective immune responses, albeit at low levels (2, 23, 30). As sequence data became available, it was possible to compare the structural proteins of antigenically distinguishable viruses. These studies identified regions of VP1 protein that were more variable in sequence than the remainder of the protein. This was a valuable clue as to the location of antigenic sites since it was to be expected that these would be characterized by a high degree of variation (7, 42). Biochemical analysis of the proteins of trypsin-treated virus showed that one of them, VP1, had been cleaved into two smaller fragments but that the remainder were unaltered as assessed by sodium dodecyl sulfate-polyacrylamide gel electrophoresis. Comparison of the terminal amino acid sequences of the trypsin-derived fragments, as determined biochemically, with the full sequence of the protein, as deduced from nucleotide sequencing, allowed the identification of the residues sensitive to trypsin cleavage (42). These were, for FMDV serotype O1, arginine at 138 and lysine at 154 and arginine at 200 near the C terminus of the molecule. Thus, trypsin cleavage had removed a small segment of 15 amino acids from the central portion of the VP1 and 13 amino acids from the C terminus. The investigators also identified the cleavage sites of VP1 of cyanogen bromide and of mouse submaxillary gland protease and, by combining this evidence with the results of immunogenicity experiments using purified fragments derived from VP1, they predicted the location of the antigenic determinants on the protein (Fig. 1). Together, these results suggested the presence of dominant epitope(s) at one or both of these positions in VP1 and that this may be coincident with an important receptor-binding site on the virus particle. Sequence comparisons showed that the region of VP1 between residues approximately 140 to 160 was highly variable both in sequence and length between different serotypes and strains of the virus, again suggesting the possibility that it contained an antigenically important feature. This region has subsequently become known as antigenic site 1 or A.

The rather precise location of a major neutralizing antibody-inducing epitope within the sequence of VP1 encouraged the investigation of synthetic versions of the site as potential immunogens. These studies were remarkably successful, and it was soon established that a synthetic peptide representing residues 141 to 160 of the protein could be used to induce the production of antibodies that neutralized the virus in vitro (9, 35). More important, the synthetic vaccine was able to induce protective immunity in the guinea pig laboratory model for FMD.

Although the peptide alone was capable of inducing a protective response, its immunogenicity was rather low. However, the immune response was markedly improved following conjugation to a carrier molecule, such as keyhole limpet hemocyanin, cosynthesis as part of more complex peptide structure, or expression of the critical sequence genetically fused to other proteins. Fusion to virus proteins capable of assembling into virus-like particles, such as the core protein of hepatitis B virus, was particularly effective (18). More recently the use of retropeptides constructed from D amino acids to avoid in vivo degradation by proteolysis has produced promising results (45).

These studies established that there is a major antigenic site on FMDV particles that has an important role in the induction of protective immunity and has the characteristics of a linear epitope, i.e., it lies within a contiguous sequence of amino acids and does not involve interaction with other features on the virus surface. This finding had obvious implications for the development of novel chemically synthesized vaccines and the generality of the observation was investigated by studying other serotypes of the virus. It was found that, in contrast to results obtained with representative viruses of serotypes A, O, and C, a peptide representing the equivalent region of the serotype A12 virus failed to induce a measurable neutralizing response against the virus. Further investigations revealed that the

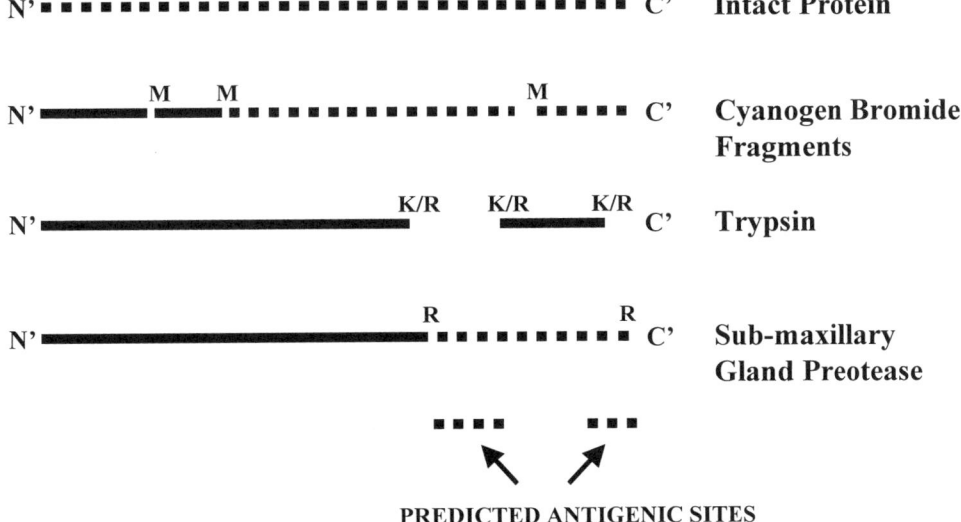

FIGURE 1 Identification of antigenic determinants on the VP1 protein of FMDV, serotype O1. The abilities of purified intact protein and enzymatically or chemically cleaved fragments to elicit virus-neutralizing antibodies in mice were determined. The precise locations of the cleavage points were ascertained by direct sequencing and comparison with the amino acid sequence predicted from the nucleic acid sequence. The fine location of the sites was deduced by comparing the active and nonactive fragments. Modified from reference 42.

virus sample that was used to test the antipeptide antiserum was, in fact, a mixture containing three variants, which differed from the published sequence at specific positions within the amino acid sequence 141 to 160 (38). Subsequently, several other variant sequences have been identified in individual viruses cloned from the same parent stock, all with changes at the same two positions in the sequences, i.e., residues 148 and 153.

These observations illustrate a fundamental shortcoming of the use of single peptides as potential vaccine candidates. The sequence variability of the virus is such that the immune pressure exerted by an immune response directed against such a restricted antigenic feature is likely to rapidly select neutralization-resistant variants. Contrary to these predictions, early results obtained with synthetic peptide vaccines representing the site 1 of serotype O1 virus showed that the antipeptide serum was more cross-reactive against variant viruses in in vitro neutralization tests than antivirus serum. Moreover, attempts to select neutralization-resistant mutants with the polyclonal serum failed (34). However, field trials of candidate synthetic peptide vaccines have shown that the theoretical drawback to the simple synthetic vaccine approach of rapid selection of neutralization-resistant viruses is a reality in practice (43). Also, a number of trials have shown that the straightforward correlation between protection against virulent virus challenge and the level of neutralizing antibody induced by synthetic peptide vaccines that is seen in the guinea pig model does not necessarily apply to target species such as cattle and pigs (14). The rapid selection of antigenic variants is clearly one aspect of this problem, but there appear to be other correlates of immune protection that are not well understood at present.

Although the antigenic site 1 is often the most immunodominant feature of the virus (27), the use of monoclonal antibodies to select resistant mutants has demonstrated the presence of other neutralization and non-neutralization sites on the particle. A total of five non-overlapping neutralization sites have been described for serotype O1 virus, and several sites have been described for serotype C and A viruses (12, 22, 29). The precise number of sites seen is likely to be a feature of the monoclonal antibody panels used to identify them, but it is important to note that the virus has more antigenic features on its surface than just the much studied linear site 1. In common with other picornaviruses, most of the antigenic sites, other than site 1, are formed by the juxtaposition of residues from different parts of the same protein or from different proteins at the particle surface. For serotype O1 virus (Fig. 2) site 1 lies within amino acids 135 and 165 of VP1 with a contribution from 218 toward the C terminus. Site 2 involves residues 70 to 77 (the B-C loop) and 130 to 137 (the E-F loop) of VP2. Site 3 is located at 43 to 48 (the B-C loop) of VP1 and site 4 is at 147 to 148 of VP3. Site 5 is apparently a second distinct site in the VP1 G-H loop (12). In addition to the VP1 G-H loop of serotype A, residue 618 in the H-I loop and adjacent to the B-C loop has been implicated (6, 44). Serotype C virus is broadly similar to serotype O virus as assessed by the location of monoclonal antibody-selected escape mutations (24), but the sites are denoted alphabetically. In some cases these sites contribute significantly to the immune response to the virus. In serotype C, for example, site D comprises residues from VP2 and VP3 and vies with site A for immunodominance.

The identification of antigenic sites on the virus surface is typically made through the selection of neutralization-

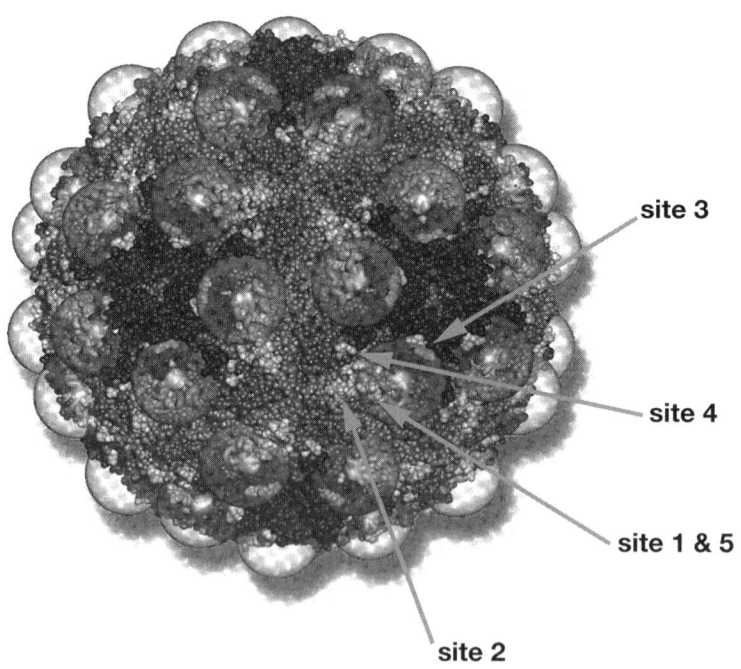

FIGURE 2 Space-filling model of FMDV, serotype O1, showing the location of antibody-selected mutations (indicated in white) that define the antigenic sites. The transparent balloons show the potential space occupancy of the major antigenic site, site 1, associated with the mobile G-H loop of VP1. Arrows indicate the individual antigenic sites. Figure generously supplied by E. Fry and D. Stuart, Oxford, United Kingdom.

resistant mutants selected in the presence of monoclonal antibodies. Cross-resistance analyses involving panels of monoclonal antibodies and panels of resistant viruses are used to map the mutations into nonoverlapping sites. These sites are obviously biologically relevant in the sense that antibodies recognizing them are, by definition, capable of neutralizing the virus in in vitro assays, but the extent to which they contribute to protective immune responses is unclear. In fact, it has been shown that a serotype O1 virus that has been multiply selected for resistance to antibodies to all of the five sites recognized for this virus is resistant to neutralization by polyclonal bovine antiserum. Despite these antigenic differences, the virus was still capable of inducing protective immune responses against the parent virus in guinea pigs, suggesting that virus neutralization as assessed by in vitro assays is not the only factor involved in protective immunity (16).

MOLECULAR STRUCTURE OF FMDV

The studies summarized above identified a specific region of VP1 as being of special significance for both the antigenic properties of the virus and its ability to bind to receptors on susceptible cells. A clue to the receptor-binding specificity of the virus emerged from the comparative analyses of virus sequences, from which it was clear that within the antigenic site sequence there is a highly conserved triplet, arginine-glycine-aspartic acid (RGD) (32). This sequence is the signature of the ligands for many integrin receptor proteins. A number of investigations involving the use of peptides in competition binding experiments and also site-directed mutagenesis of the viral RGD motif have confirmed that it is intimately involved in receptor recognition (5, 8, 17, 25). However, there is some controversy (and variation?) regarding the specific integrin molecule(s) used by the virus in vivo (3, 8, 21).

Given the important biological properties associated with this region of VP1, the initial description of the structure of the virus, as deduced from X-ray crystallography, was rather disappointing (1) (Fig. 2). The sequence corresponding to antigenic site A was found to comprise the loop linking the G and H strands of the VP1 β-barrel, and hence is known as the G-H loop, but this region was too disordered in the crystals to allow its structure to be determined. However, the rationale for its immunogenic importance could be guessed at since, although the overall structure of the virus surface is rather smooth and featureless, the VP1 G-H loop was clearly a major, if disordered, dominating feature. The location of the receptor-binding domain of the virus on this exposed loop rather than within a depression on the virus surface, as appears to be the case with other members of the picornavirus family, also has important consequences for the process of attachment and uncoating.

Careful study of the structure of the first strain of FMDV to be solved, serotype O1BFS, showed that there was a disulfide bond linking a cysteine residue at position 120 in VP2 to Cys 134 at the base of the G-H loop of VP1 (33). Furthermore, the electron density profile showed that this bond was present in at least two conformations and was unequally distributed between them. This disulfide bond serves to maintain the G-H loop in a protruding and disordered conformation at the surface of the virus particle, in contrast to the more commonly perceived role of disulfide bonds of stabilizing structure. Under reducing conditions the VP1 G-H loop collapses onto the surface of the particle such that its structure can be readily determined (33). Under these conditions it was seen to be predominantly helical in structure, with the RGD motif located at the turn linking the two helical domains (Fig. 3). The RGD is in the "open" conformation as seen in other RGD-containing proteins that are known to function as ligands for integrin receptors. It is thought that the structure of the loop as seen under reducing conditions is representative of its internal structure when present in the oxidized state and that the disorder that prevents the determination of its structure from native virus crystals is a consequence of flexion at its base. Although the disulfide bond at the base of the G-H loop of serotype O1 virus is not seen in other serotypes of the virus, the loop is disordered with respect to the remainder of the particle in all of the FMDV structures that have been determined (1, 13, 24). It is likely, therefore, that the flexibility of the loop plays an important biological role, probably in the process of attachment and/or penetration. In fact, recent evidence suggests that virus attachment is compromised when the loop is in the collapsed state (A. M. Q. King, personal communication).

The precise relationships between the G-H loop and the remainder of the particle also influence the fine specificity of its antigenic structure in ways that are not fully understood. This became apparent during a study of neutralization-resistant mutants selected with monoclonal antibodies against serotype O1 virus. Although there was good evidence that these antibodies recognized epitopes within the VP1 G-H loop, the amino acid substitutions present in the resistant viruses were located at positions close to but not within the loop. Determination of the crystal structure of the variant viruses showed that the distribution of electron density between the two visible orientations of the disulfide bond (referred to above) that links the base of the VP1 G-H loop to VP2 was reversed compared to that of the parental virus (33). It thus appears

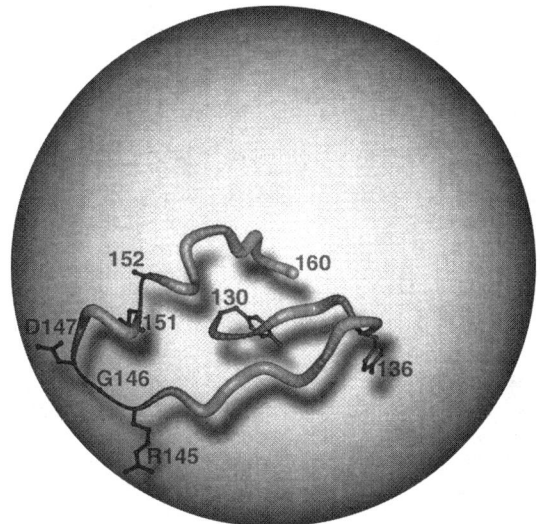

FIGURE 3 Model of the antigenic site 1 (the VP1 G-H loop) of FMDV, serotype O1, as determined from the crystal structure of reduced virus. The RGD residues that are key components of the receptor-binding properties of the sequence are shown at the bend joining the helical regions of the loop. Figure generously supplied by E. Fry and D. Stuart, Oxford, United Kingdom.

that subtle alterations in the preferred orientation of the loop with respect to the remainder of the virus particle can have far-reaching effects on recognition by antibody and possibly other functions such as receptor recognition.

The conformation of the VP1 G-H loop as seen in crystals of reduced virus is very similar to that of synthetic peptides representing the loop sequence when complexed with the Fab fragments of neutralizing antibodies (15, 20, 31, 46). Moreover, the conformations of the specificity-determining pockets of such antibodies were shown to alter from the apo-form to acquire induced fits to accommodate the antigenic peptides (15, 47). This provides further evidence that the structure of the loop as seen in the reduced virus crystals is representative of its conformation in the native structure. The same overall conformation of the VP1 G-H loop has also been seen in the crystal structures of complexes of monoclonal antibody Fab fragments and peptides representing multiple substituted sequences. It appears, therefore, that the secondary, and possibly tertiary, aspects of the structure of the VP1 G-H loop sequence are necessarily conserved to maintain virus viability.

ANTIGENIC STRUCTURE AND RECEPTOR BINDING

All of the available evidence suggests that the VP1 G-H loop is both a major antigenic determinant and the receptor-binding feature of the virus. In fact, the RGD motif involved in integrin binding is also involved in the binding of many neutralizing antibodies although, of course, the specificity of such antibodies is additionally influenced by residues outside the RGD triplet. Comparison of the abilities of multiple substituted synthetic peptides representing the G-H loop sequence to compete with virus for binding to cells in culture demonstrated the key involvement of the RGD residues and also of Leu residues at positions +1 and +4 downstream of the RGD (28).

The prime function of the loop is to recognize and bind the cell receptor as a prelude to endocytosis. Uncoating of the virus appears to be solely as a result of the acidification that occurs following endocytosis. All isolates of FMDV are highly susceptible to acid-mediated inactivation and are disrupted at pH values between 6.5 and 6.8, and this highly conserved feature is probably essential to the entry process adopted by the virus. As a consequence of the acid-induced uncoating mechanism for cell entry, it is possible to infect cells by alternative routes. This has been demonstrated by engineering a cell infection pathway that relies on Fc receptors. It has been shown that, in contrast to poliovirus, the infectivity of FMDV particles complexed with neutralizing antibodies can be restored if they are allowed to bind to cells bearing Fc receptors (26). The subsequent endocytosis and acidification are all that is needed to permit delivery of the nucleic acid to the cytoplasm and so initiate an infection. Similarly, it has been found that selective adaptation of the virus to replicate in cells in vitro can result in the evolution of alternative modes of attachment and entry. Acquisition of the ability to bind to heparin sulfate at cell surfaces has been seen in FMDV, as it has in other tissue culture-adapted viruses (4, 40). In addition, an alternative entry pathway involving neither integrin nor heparin sulfate has been reported (4). Although it is possible to alter or dispense with the role (and antigenic properties) of the VP1 G-H loop by in vitro manipulation (36), it is likely that there are other constraints that prevent this from occurring in the field.

A full understanding of the functional constraints on the structure of the VP1 G-H loop on one hand and the conformational freedom that is compatible with its function on the other could be of great value for further exploration of the potential for synthetic vaccines. Will it be possible to create rational mixtures of peptide sequences so that the rapid selection of variant viruses can be avoided?

CONCLUSIONS

Antigenic variation is somewhat of a hallmark of FMDV and is of major importance in disease control strategies that rely on vaccination. Antigenic change can be rapidly selected for in in vitro experiments and there is genetic evidence that positive selection acts on the capsid protein genes in the field (19). Although the seven distinct serotypes that comprise the FMDVs are not evenly distributed throughout the parts of the world affected by the disease, they overlap sufficiently to complicate the formulation of vaccine cocktails. In addition to interserotype differences, there is significant antigenic variation within the different serotypes and it is usual to tailor vaccine blends to match the characteristics of local strains.

Through a combination of biochemical, virological, immunological, and structural approaches our understanding of the fundamental basis for antigenic variation in FMDV has advanced greatly in the past two or three decades. However, many detailed explanations of the phenomenon remain elusive. In addition, the relationship between the antigenic properties of the virus, as measured by in vitro techniques such as antibody-binding assays and neutralization tests, and the in vivo protection afforded by vaccination in relevant species needs to be better understood. Improved conventional vaccines should result from such advances, and it might even be possible to achieve the Holy Grail of an effective synthetic vaccine.

REFERENCES

1. **Acharya, R., E. Fry, D. Stuart, G. Fox, D. Rowlands, and F. Brown.** 1989. The 3-dimensional structure of foot-and-mouth-disease virus at 2.9-Å resolution. *Nature* **337:** 709–716.
2. **Bachrach, H. L., D. M. Moore, P. D. McKercher, and J. Polatnick.** 1975. Immune and antibody responses to an isolated capsid protein of foot and mouth disease virus. *J. Immunol.* **115:**1636–1641.
3. **Baranowski, E., C. M. Ruiz-Jarabo, and E. Domingo.** 2001. Evolution of cell recognition by viruses. *Science* **292:**1102–1105.
4. **Baranowski, E., C. M. Ruiz-Jarabo, N. Sevilla, D. Andreu, E. Beck, and E. Domingo.** 2000. Cell recognition by foot-and-mouth disease virus that lacks the RGD integrin-binding motif: flexibility in aphthovirus receptor usage. *J. Virol.* **74:**1641–1647.
5. **Baxt, B., and Y. Becker.** 1990. The effect of peptides containing the arginine-glycine-aspartic acid sequence on the adsorbtion of foot-and-mouth disease virus to tissue culture cells. *Virus Genes* **4:**73–83.
6. **Baxt, B., V. Vakharia, D. M. Moore, A. J. Franke, and D. O. Morgan.** 1989. Analysis of neutralizing antigenic sites on the surface of type A12 foot-and-mouth disease virus. *J. Virol.* **63:**2143–2151.
7. **Beck, E., G. Feil, and K. Strohmaier.** 1983. The molecular basis of the antigenic variation of foot-and-mouth disease virus. *EMBO J.* **2:**555–559.
8. **Berinstein, A., M. Roivainen, T. Hovi, P. Mason, and B. Baxt.** 1995. Antibodies to the vitronectin receptor (in-

tergrin avb3) inhibit binding and infection of foot and mouth disease virus to cultured cells. *J. Virol.* **69**:2664–2666.
9. Bittle, J. L., R. A. Houghten, H. Alexander, T. M. Shinnick, J. G. Sutcliffe, R. A. Lerner, D. J. Rowlands, and F. Brown. 1982. Protection against foot and mouth disease by immunization with a chemically synthesized peptide predicted from the viral nucleotide sequence. *Nature* **298**:30–33.
10. Brown, F. 1995. Antibody recognition and neutralization of foot-and-mouth disease virus. *Semin. Virol.* **6**:243–248.
11. Brown, F., and C. J. Smale. 1970. Demonstration of three specific sites on the surface of foot-and-mouth disease virus by antibody complexing. *J. Gen. Virol.* **7**:115–127.
12. Crowther, J. R., S. Farias, W. C. Carpenter, and A. R. Samuel. 1993. Identification of a fifth neutralizable site on type O foot-and-mouth disease virus following characterization of single and quintuple monoclonal antibody escape mutants. *J. Gen. Virol.* **74**(Pt. 8):1547–1553.
13. Curry, S., E. Fry, W. Blakemore, R. Abu-Ghazaleh, T. Jackson, A. King, S. Lea, J. Newman, D. Rowlands, and D. Stuart. 1996. Perturbations in the surface structure of A22 Iraq foot-and-mouth disease virus accompanying coupled changes in host cell specificity and antigenicity. *Structure* **4**:135–145.
14. Di Marchi, R., G. Brooke, C. Gale, V. Cracknell, T. Doel, and N. Mowat. 1986. Protection of cattle against foot and mouth disease virus by a synthetic peptide. *Science* **232**:639–641.
15. Domingo, E., N. Verdaguer, W. F. Ochoa, C. M. Ruiz-Jarabo, N. Sevilla, E. Baranowski, M. G. Mateu, and I. Fita. 1999. Biochemical and structural studies with neutralizing antibodies raised against foot-and-mouth disease virus. *Virus Res.* **62**:169–175.
16. Dunn, C. S., A. R. Samuel, L. A. Pullen, and J. Anderson. 1998. The biological relevance of virus neutralisation sites for virulence and vaccine protection in the guinea pig model of foot-and-mouth disease. *Virology* **247**:51–61.
17. Fox, G., N. Parry, P. V. Barnett, B. McGinn, D. J. Rowlands, and F. Brown. 1989. The cell attachment site on foot-and-mouth disease virus includes the amino acid sequence RGD (arginine-glycine-aspartic acid). *J. Gen. Virol.* **70**:625–637.
18. Francis, M. J., and B. E. Clarke. 1989. Peptide vaccines based on enhanced immunogenicity of peptide epitopes presented with T cell determinants or hepatitis B core protein. *Methods Enzymol.* **178**:659.
19. Haydon, D. T., A. D. Bastos, N. J. Knowles, and A. R. Samuel. 2001. Evidence for positive selection in foot-and-mouth disease virus capsid genes from field isolates. *Genetics* **157**:7–15.
20. Hewat, E. A., N. Verdaguer, I. Fita, W. Blakemore, S. Brookes, A. King, J. Newman, E. Domingo, M. G. Mateu, and D. I. Stuart. 1997. Structure of the complex of an Fab fragment of a neutralizing antibody with foot-and-mouth disease virus: positioning of a highly mobile antigenic loop. *EMBO J.* **16**:1492–1500.
21. Jackson, T., D. Sheppard, M. Denyer, W. Blakemore, and A. M. Q. King. 2000. The epithelial integrin avb6 is a receptor for foot-and-mouth disease virus. *J. Virol.* **74**:4949–4956.
22. Kitson, J. D., D. McCahon, and G. J. Belsham. 1990. Sequence analysis of monoclonal antibody resistant mutants of type O foot and mouth disease virus: evidence for the involvement of the three surface exposed capsid proteins in four antigenic sites. *Virology* **179**:26–34.
23. Kleid, D. G., D. G. Yansura, B. Small, D. Dowbenko, D. Moore, M. J. Grubman, P. D. McKercher, D. O. Morgan, B. H. Robertson, and H. L. Bachrach. 1981. Cloned viral protein vaccine for foot and mouth disease; response in cattle and swine. *Science* **214**:1125–1129.
24. Lea, S., J. Hernandez, W. Blakemore, E. Brocchi, S. Curry, E. Domingo, E. Fry, R. Abu-Ghazaleh, A. King, J. Newman, D. Stuart, and M. G. Mateu. 1994. The structure and antigenicity of a type C foot-and-mouth disease virus. *Structure* **2**:123–139.
25. Mason, P., E. Rieder, and B. Baxt. 1994. RGD sequence of foot-and-mouth disease virus is essential for infecting cells via the natural receptor but can be bypassed by an antibody-dependent enhancement pathway. *Proc. Natl. Acad. Sci. USA* **91**:1932–1936.
26. Mason, P. W., B. Baxt, F. Brown, J. Harber, A. Murdin, and E. Wimmer. 1993. Antibody-complexed foot-and-mouth-disease virus, but not poliovirus, can infect normally unsusceptible cells via the Fc receptor. *Virology* **192**:568–577.
27. Mateu, M. G., J. A. Camarero, E. Giralt, D. Andreu, and E. Domingo. 1995. Direct evaluation of the immunodominance of a major antigenic site of foot-and-mouth disease virus in a natural host. *Virology* **206**:298–306.
28. Mateu, M. G., M. L. Valero, D. Andreu, and E. Domingo. 1996. Systematic replacement of amino acid residues within an Arg-Gly-Asp-containing loop of foot-and-mouth disease virus and effect on cell recognition. *J. Biol. Chem.* **271**:12814–12819.
29. McCahon, D., J. R. Crowther, G. J. Belsham, J. D. Kitson, M. Duchesne, P. Have, R. H. Meloen, D. O. Morgan, and F. De Simone. 1989. Evidence for at least four antigenic sites on type O foot-and-mouth disease virus involved in neutralization; identification by single and multiple site monoclonal antibody-resistant mutants. *J. Gen. Virol.* **70**(Pt. 3):639–645.
30. Meloen, R., D. J. Rowlands, and F. Brown. 1979. Comparison of the antibodies elicited by the individual structural polypeptides of foot and mouth disease virus and poliovirus. *J. Gen. Virol.* **45**:761–763.
31. Ochoa, W. F., S. G. Kalko, M. G. Mateu, P. Gomes, D. Andreu, E. Domingo, I. Fita, and N. Verdaguer. 2000. A multiply substituted G-H loop from foot-and-mouth disease virus in complex with a neutralizing antibody: a role for water molecules. *J. Gen. Virol.* **81**:1495–1505.
32. Palmenberg, A. C. 1989. Sequence alignments of picornaviral capsid proteins, p. 211–241. *In* B. L. Semler and E. Ehrenfeld (ed.), *Molecular Aspects of Picornavirus Infection and Detection*. American Society for Microbiology, Washington, D.C.
33. Parry, N., G. Fox, D. Rowlands, F. Brown, E. Fry, R. Acharya, D. Logan, and D. Stuart. 1990. Structural and serological evidence for a novel mechanism of antigenic variation in foot-and-mouth disease virus. *Nature* **347**:569–572.
34. Parry, N. R., E. J. Ouldridge, P. V. Barnett, B. E. Clarke, M. J. Francis, J. D. Fox, D. J. Rowlands, and F. Brown. 1989. Serological prospects for peptide vaccines against foot-and-mouth disease virus. *J. Gen. Virol.* **70**(Pt. 11):2919–2930.
35. Pfaff, E., M. Mussgay, H. O. Bohm, G. E. Schulz, and H. Schaller. 1982. Antibodies against a preselected peptide recognize and neutralize foot and mouth disease virus. *EMBO J.* **1**:869–874.
36. Rieder, E., A. Berinstein, B. Baxt, A. Kang, and P. W. Mason. 1996. Propagation of an attenuated virus by design: engineering a novel receptor for a noninfectious foot-and-mouth disease virus. *Proc. Natl. Acad. Sci. USA* **93**:10428–10433.
37. Rowlands, D. J. 1993. Progress towards peptide vaccines for foot-and-mouth disease, p. 54–86. *In* R. Panday, S.

Hogland, and G. Prasad (ed.), *Veterinary Vaccines.* Springer-Verlag, New York, N.Y.

38. **Rowlands, D. J., B. E. Clarke, A. R. Carroll, F. Brown, B. H. Nicholson, J. L. Bittle, R. A. Houghten, and R. A. Lerner.** 1983. Chemical basis of antigenic variation in foot-and-mouth disease virus. *Nature* **306:**694–697.

39. **Rowlands, D. J., D. V. Sangar, and F. Brown.** 1971. Relationship of the antigenic structure of foot-and-mouth disease virus to the process of infection. *J. Gen. Virol.* **13:**85–93.

40. **Sa-Carvalho, D., E. Rieder, B. Baxt, R. Rodarte, A. Tanuri, and P. W. Mason.** 1997. Tissue culture adaptation of foot-and-mouth disease virus selects viruses that bind to heparin and are attenuated in cattle. *J. Virol.* **71:**5115–5123.

41. **Saiz, J. C., J. Cairo, M. Medina, D. Zuidema, C. Abrams, G. J. Belsham, E. Domingo, and J. M. Vlak.** 1994. Unprocessed foot-and-mouth disease virus capsid precursor displays discontinuous epitopes involved in viral neutralization. *J. Virol.* **68:**4557–4564.

42. **Strohmaier, K., R. Franze, and K. H. Adam.** 1982. Location and characterization of the antigenic portion of the FMDV immunizing protein. *J. Gen. Virol.* **59:**295–306.

43. **Taboga, O., C. Tami, E. Carrillo, J. I. Nunez, A. Rodriguez, J. C. Saiz, E. Blanco, M. L. Valero, X. Roig, J. A. Camarero, D. Andreu, M. G. Mateu, E. Giralt, E. Domingo, F. Sobrino, and E. L. Palma.** 1997. A large-scale evaluation of peptide vaccines against foot-and-mouth disease: lack of solid protection in cattle and isolation of escape mutants. *J. Virol.* **71:**2606–2614.

44. **Thomas, A. A., R. J. Woortmeijer, W. Puijk, and S. J. Barteling.** 1988. Antigenic sites on foot-and-mouth disease virus type A10. *J. Virol.* **62:**2782–2789.

45. **Van Regenmortel, M. H., G. Guichard, N. Benkirane, J. P. Briand, S. Muller, and F. Brown.** 1998. The potential of retro-inverso peptides as synthetic vaccines. *Dev. Biol. Stand.* **92:**139–143.

46. **Verdaguer, N., M. G. Mateu, D. Andreu, E. Giralt, E. Domingo, and I. Fita.** 1995. Structure of the major antigenic loop of foot-and-mouth disease virus complexed with a neutralizing antibody: direct involvement of the Arg-Gly-Asp motif in the interaction. *EMBO J.* **14:**1690–1696.

47. **Verdaguer, N., M. G. Mateu, J. Bravo, E. Domingo, and I. Fita.** 1996. Induced pocket to accommodate the cell attachment Arg-Gly-Asp motif in a neutralizing antibody against foot-and-mouth-disease virus. *J. Mol. Biol.* **256:**364–376.

48. **Wild, T. F., and F. Brown.** 1967. Nature of the inactivating action of trypsin on foot-and-mouth disease virus. *J. Gen. Virol.* **1:**247–250.

VIRUS ENTRY

Cellular Receptors of Picornaviruses: an Overview

ELIZABETH RIEDER AND ECKARD WIMMER

6

The most surprising result of studies focused on early events in animal virus infection is the diversity of cell surface proteins serving as receptors. It amounts to a seemingly random mode by which a virus has chosen its doorman for cell entry. In 1994, we had already written about this phenomenon (78), and even a deluge of new data has not introduced any measure of order into the chaos. To us, there is no apparent reason why one viral species would select entity A as receptor while its very close relative may have chosen the totally different entity B (compare the intercellular adhesion molecule 1 [ICAM-1] receptor for human rhinovirus [HRV] 14 and the low-density lipoprotein [LDL] receptor for HRV2). On the other hand, two viruses belonging to two entirely different families, say, the small RNA coxsackievirus B and the large DNA adenovirus 2, have chosen the same small cell surface protein as receptor (CAR) (4, 72). Perhaps *Retroviridae* assembled the most diverse menu of cellular receptors (68). But picornaviruses too have shown a great deal of ingenuity in selecting receptors (Fig. 1 and Table 1).

DEFINITION OF A VIRAL RECEPTOR

In principle, every cell surface protein capable of binding a virus may be called a viral receptor. If this definition is accepted, one must determine whether binding to the receptor will also lead to infection. Quite often, this is not the case. Two examples may be cited. First, encephalomyocarditis virus (EMCV) binds to glycophorin A, an interaction responsible for the agglutination of human erythrocytes (2). The binding of EMCV to glycophorin A, however, does not lead to an infection. For cell entry and replication, EMCV has chosen the vascular cell adhesion molecule 1 (VCAM-1), an entity entirely different from glycophorin A (31). Second, CD55, also known as decay-accelerating factor (DAF), can function as binding protein for several echo- and coxsackieviruses (Table 1; see below). Binding of an enterovirus to DAF covaries with agglutination of human erythrocytes. However, in many cases, docking to DAF does not lead to a productive infection. For example, coxsackievirus A21 (CVA21), a C-cluster enterovirus, can bind to Chinese hamster ovary (CHO) cells expressing human DAF, but this interaction does not lead to an infection (62). On the other hand, C-cluster coxsackieviruses use human ICAM-1 as a receptor and this interaction leads to infection, even of mouse cells expressing human ICAM-1 (61). Available evidence suggests that DAF enhances CVA21 infection of HeLa cells but that DAF is not essential in this process. These considerations indicate the involvement of "accessory factors" that appear to affect the efficiency of infection (see below).

One may ask the question: Where is the block in viral uptake after the CVA21 has docked to DAF at the surface of the rodent cell? For an infection to occur, the interaction between virus and receptor must lead to uncoating and release of the viral genome. In the case of enteroviruses, which are remarkably resistant entities to low pH or proteolytic enzymes, the cell-surface interaction must trigger destabilization, either catalyzed by the receptor or by an accessory factor. Therefore, unlike aphthoviruses, enteroviruses need specific cell surface proteins for uncoating. Foot-and-mouth disease virus (FMDV) falls apart at the low pH inside late endosomes. Any pathway (for example, transport by artificial receptors, see below) bringing FMDV into the low pH endosomal compartment can lead to a productive infection.

RECEPTOR IDENTITY

The cellular receptors for picornaviruses that have been identified so far are depicted in Fig. 1. Most receptors belong to the immunoglobulin (Ig) superfamily or the integrin receptor family. Considering the many unresolved puzzles concerning enterovirus entry, and the steady expansion of picornavirus genera, we can anticipate the number of picornavirus receptors will increase significantly in the future.

Integrins are noncovalently linked, heterodimeric molecules, consisting of a variety of α and β subunits. The cellular function of integrins includes binding extracellular

---

Elizabeth Rieder and Eckard Wimmer ■ Department of Molecular Genetics and Microbiology, School of Medicine, State University of New York at Stony Brook, Stony Brook, NY 11794.

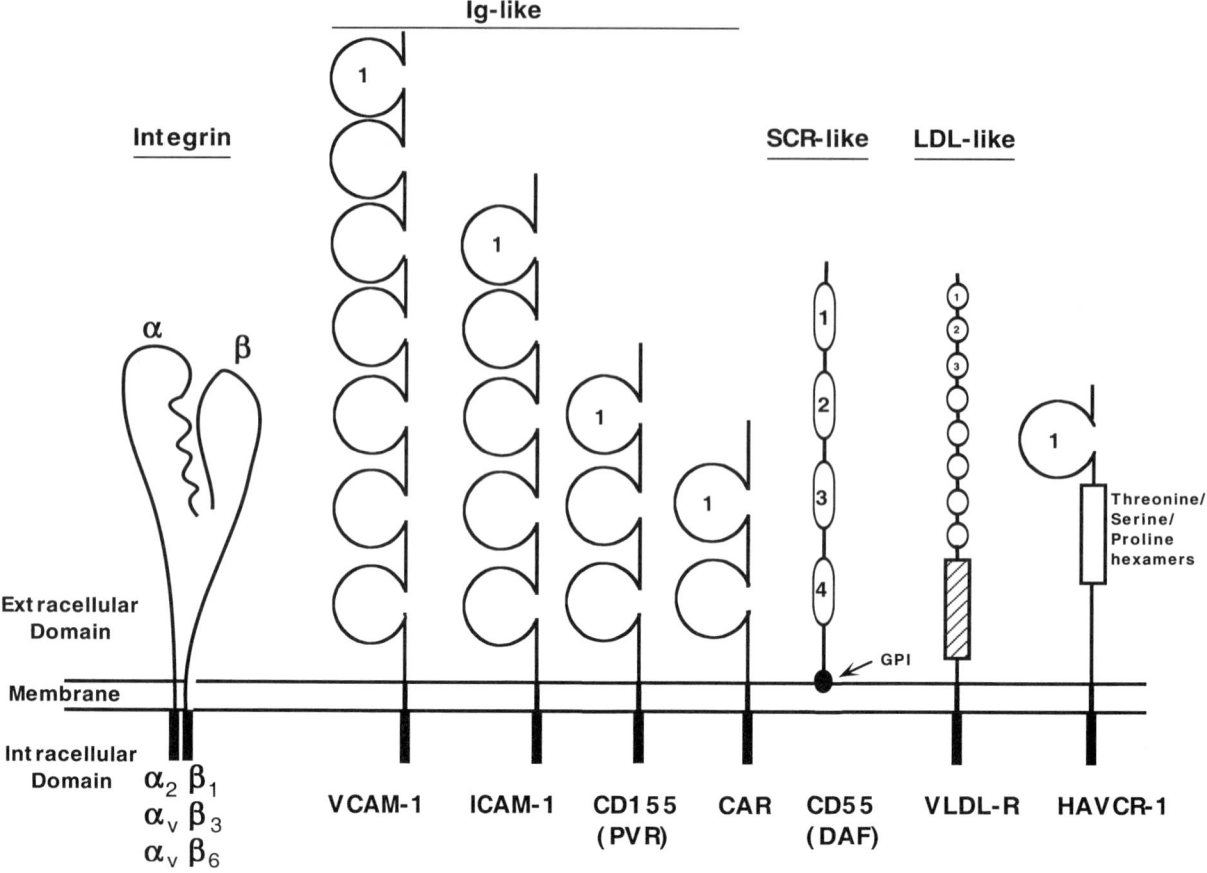

FIGURE 1 Classes of molecules that serve as cell receptor for picornaviruses. The structure shown for the integrins family is a generic representation. Abbreviations: PVR, poliovirus receptor; CAR, coxsackievirus-adenovirus receptor; DAF, decay-accelerating factor; GPI, glycosylphosphatidylinositol; HAVCR-1, hepatitis A virus cellular receptor type 1; ICAM-1, intercellular adhesion molecule type 1; VCAM-1, vascular cell adhesion molecule type 1; VLDL-R, very-low-density lipoprotein receptor. Other molecules of the LDL receptor gene superfamily also serve as receptor for minor group human rhinoviruses (see chapter 9). Adapted from Wimmer (78). Numbers indicate domains implicated in virus binding.

matrix proteins, cell-cell interactions, and signal transduction (18, 33). Integrins involved in picornavirus docking include $\alpha_2\beta_1$ (= VLA-2), a collagen and laminin receptor, and $\alpha_v\beta_3$ and $\alpha_v\beta_6$, which function as vitronectin receptors. Binding of the natural ligand requires both polypeptide chains while picornaviruses appear to bind to only one of the subunits: echovirus 1 to the α chain of $\alpha_2\beta_1$ (8), and CVA9 and FMDV to the β chain of $\alpha_v\beta_3$ (46). A trademark of many (but by far not of all) integrins is the recognition of an Arg-Gly-Asp (RGD) motif and, indeed, the virions of FMDV or CVA9 display RGD motifs essential for the docking process. The $\alpha_2\beta_1$ integrin, on the other hand, does not recognize an RGD motif and, accordingly, the interaction between echoviruses 1 and 8 and receptor is RGD independent (see chapters 10 and 11).

VCAM-1 is an important adhesion molecule promoting lymphocyte migration (11). Enhanced expression of VCAM-1 on vascular endothelial cells (VEC) adjacent to infection sites augments inflammatory cell migration into the affected tissue. VCAM is a receptor for EMCV.

ICAM-1 is a cell surface molecule whose cellular function is to bind to leukocyte function-associated antigen 1, thereby providing adhesion between leukocytes and endothelial cells. ICAM-1 functions as receptor for the major receptor group HRVs and C-cluster coxsackieviruses (C-CVAs) (Table 1).

CD155 ("cluster of differentiation 155") (see reference 16), also referred to as Pvr, is an Ig-like glycoprotein whose gene is expressed in four splice variants (CD155α, CD155β, CD155γ, and CD155δ). All four isotypes have identical extracellular domains (V-C2-C2), but the isotypes CD155β and CD155γ are secreted. The two type 1, single-span isotypes CD155α and CD155δ, glycoproteins that differ only in their intracellular domains, function as poliovirus receptors (38, 44, 79; see chapter 7). The cellular functions of CD155 are slowly being understood. In CD155/β-gal tg mice, the promoter of the CD155 gene is active in the developing neural tube and neuroretina (22), an observation suggesting a function in central nervous system (CNS) development during embryogenesis. Indeed, the anatomical distribution of CD155 promoter activity during the development of the CNS matches that of transacting factors previously identified to regulate CD155 transcription activity (66, 67). Recently, it has been reported

TABLE 1 Overview of disease syndromes and receptors[a] of six genera of *Picornaviridae*

Genus	Clusters[b]	Receptor[c]	Accessory factors[d]	References[e]	Major syndromes[f]
Enterovirus	**A**				
	Coxsackieviruses A 2, 3, 5, 7, 8, 10, 12, 14, 16	ND			Herpangina, hand-foot-and-mouth disease, respiratory disease, meningitis, poliomyelitis (CVA7)
	Enterovirus 71	ND			Hand-foot-and-mouth disease, meningitis, paralysis
	B				
	Coxsackievirus A9	$\alpha_v\beta_3$; alt. receptor likely	β_2-m, MAP-70	75	(See A-CVAs), poliomyelitis
	Coxsackieviruses B1–6	HCAR		54, 74	Myocarditis, pleurodynia
	Coxsackieviruses B1, 3, 5	DAF (=CD55)	$\alpha_v\beta_6$	4, 71, 72	Meningitis, respiratory disease, neonatal infections
	Echoviruses 1, 8	VLA-2 (=$\alpha_2\beta_1$)		1, 60	Meningitis, encephalitis
	Echoviruses 3, 6, 7, 11, 12, 13, 19, 21, 24, 25, 29, 30, 33	DAF	β_2-m, CD59	5, 19, 76, 77	Pleurodynia, exanthema
	Echovirus 6	Heparan sulfate?		20	
	Enterovirus 69	ND			
	C				
	Polioviruses 1–3	CD155 (Pvr)		44	Poliomyelitis (meningitis)
	Coxsackieviruses A13, 17, 18, 20, 21, 24	ICAM-1		12, 61[g]	Common cold, infantile diarrhea
	Coxsackievirus A21			62	
	Coxsackievirus 24v[h]	ICAM-1, second receptor?	DAF		Acute hemorrhagic conjunctivitis
	D				
	Enteroviruses 70 (68)	DAF		37	Acute hemorrhagic conjunctivitis
	E				
	Bovine enterovirus types 1 and 2	ND			Diarrhea (cattle)
Parechovirus	Human echovirus types 22 and 23	$\alpha_v\beta_3$		73	Respiratory disease, encephalitis
Rhinovirus	Major receptor group rhinov. (>90 serotypes)	ICAM-1		21, 69, 70	Common cold
	Minor receptor group rhinov. (>10 serotypes)	LDL receptor related		29	Common cold
Hepatovirus	Hepatitis A virus	HAVcr-1		36, 65	Type A hepatitis
Aphthovirus	Foot-and-mouth disease virus FMDV A12	$\alpha_v\beta_3$, $\alpha_v\beta_6$		9, 35	Foot-and-mouth disease (cloven-footed livestock)
	Strains of FMDV O$_1$	Heparan sulfate		34	
Cardiovirus	Encephalomyocarditis virus, mengovirus	VCAM-1		31	Encephalitis, myocarditis
	Theiler's murine encephalomyelitis virus	Sialylated glycophorin		2	
	Vilyuisk virus	ND			

[a]Receptors: the molecules listed are sufficient to dock a virion to the cell surface, but they are not necessarily competent to initiate an infectious cycle. Receptors in bold letters are likely to be essential and sufficient for infectivity. Abbreviations: $\alpha_v\beta_3$, $\alpha_v\beta_6$, $\alpha_2\beta_1$, integrins ($\alpha_v\beta_3$, $\alpha_v\beta_6$, vitronectin receptors; $\alpha_2\beta_1$ = VLA-2, a collagen and laminin receptor); DAF, decay-accelerating factor (CD55); CD155, poliovirus receptor (Pvr); ICAM-1, intercellular adhesion molecule 1; HCAR, human coxsackievirus B and adenovirus 2 receptor; VCAM, vascular cell adhesion molecule; HAVcr-1, receptor for hepatitis A virus; β_2-m, β_2-microglobulin, a component of MHC class I; MAP-70, a protein of the MHC class I; CD59, complement control protein. Italics denote a nonhuman pathogen; ND, not determined.

[b]Clusters of enteroviruses refer to groups of enteroviruses arranged predominantly according to genotypic kinship (33a; chapter 2). Poliovirus was added to the C-cluster because of its close relationship to the C-cluster coxsackieviruses A. More clusters including mainly animal enteroviruses have been proposed.

[c]Receptors may be specific for specific serotypes. For details, see text.

[d]Accessory factors are defined here as proteins that enhance infectivity. In some cases, blocking an accessory factor by monoclonal antibodies may block infection. This, however, may be restricted to specific virus-cell pairing (e.g., infectivity of some echoviruses on RD cells, but not on HeLa cells, can be blocked with monoclonal antibodies to β_2-m).

[e]Numbers in this column refer to references describing the identification of receptors.

[f]List of human syndromes adapted from reference 22a. Common syndromes in humans caused predominantly by one and/or other member(s) of the cluster, but member viruses of other clusters or even genera may cause the same syndrome.

[g]Rieder and Wimmer, unpublished data.

[h]Coxsackievirus A24v is a genetic variant of coxsackievirus A24.

that the ectodomain of CD155 mediates cell-to-matrix contacts by specifically binding to vitronectin (39). Both CD155 and vitronectin colocalize to follicular dendritic cells and B cells inside the germinal centers of secondary lymphoid tissue (tonsils), a site known to be a target of poliovirus infection. Finally, the C-terminal tails of both membrane-bound splice variants of CD155 (CD155α and CD155δ) interact with Tctex, a small protein of the dynein motor complex, an observation suggesting a role of CD155 in intracellular (retrograde axonal?) transport (45).

Humans are the only natural hosts for poliovirus. Monkeys, however, can be experimentally infected because they express receptors homologous to CD155. Koike et al. (38) have shown that, in contrast to human CD155, monkey poliovirus receptors (mCD155) of African green monkey cells are encoded by the two related genes AGMα1 and AGMα2 (African green monkey receptor). The predicted gene products mCD155α1 and mCD155δ1 (for AGMα1) and mCD155α2 (for AGMα2) are integral membrane glycoproteins that serve as poliovirus receptors (38). Secreted splice variants of AGMα1 and AGMα2 have not been detected (38, 79).

CAR, the coxsackievirus B and adenovirus 2 receptor, is expressed in many human tissues. Unlike CD155, CAR has been reported to have cell adhesion function (30). The precise physiological function of CAR that is highly conserved between primates and rodents remains obscure. However, CAR is also expressed during embryonic development in the central and peripheral nervous system (71), an observation somewhat reminiscent of the expression of CD155.

DAF (CD55) is a member of the regulator of the complement activity protein family and protects the cell from autologous lysis (41). In contrast to all other known picornavirus receptors, DAF is anchored to the cell surface by glycosylphosphatidylinositol. DAF carries short consensus sequences (SCRs) that mediate virus binding (see chapter 10 and below). DAF can function as receptor or accessory protein for a large number of B-, C-, and D-cluster enteroviruses (Table 1). A receptor function of DAF leading to productive infection, however, has only been demonstrated for echovirus 7 (49).

LDL receptor family represents a complex menu of different cell surface proteins of widely differing sizes (up to 600 kD). Their extracellular domains, of which that of the very-low-density lipoprotein receptor (VLDL-R) is depicted in Fig. 1, can interact with numerous ligands. The receptors carry "A-repeats" to which the minor group HRVs attach (see chapter 9).

HAVcr-1, hepatitis A virus cellular receptor-1, is a class I integral membrane glycoprotein of unknown natural function. Its N-terminal Ig-like domain functions to dock the virion (65).

Heparan sulfate, a ubiquitous cell surface glycosaminoglycan (also known as GAG), consists of sulfated polysaccharides covalently linked to a protein core. Heparan sulfate has been implicated in receptor function for certain strains of FMDV (34) and clinical isolates of echovirus 6 (20). Interestingly, heparan sulfate is also a receptor for alpha herpesviruses (64).

CAN A SINGLE PICORNAVIRUS USE MORE THAN ONE RECEPTOR?

The question of how many different receptors can be utilized by a single picornavirus is complex (see discussion in chapter 10). To be sure, there are purist picornaviruses using only one receptor for cell entry. For example, it appears that polioviruses and the major receptor group HRVs use *only* CD155 and ICAM-1, respectively. This monogamous relationship may be governed by the desire of the virus to be rapidly uncoated without need for any further help. Poliovirus pays dearly for its impatience because CD155 can render the virus inactive before it has a chance to enter the cell (by converting the virion to A particle; see below). Thus, the particle to infectious unit ratio is highly unfavorable (100 to 1, or worse). Nevertheless, only CD155 seems to be able to dock and unlock the stable poliovirion (see chapter 7). Experimental evidence suggests that the N-terminal domain (the V domain) of CD155 is essential and sufficient to fulfill this role (59). Failure to identify a second receptor for a virus, however, does not preclude the possibility that more that one receptor (or accessory factor) exists.

In contrast to poliovirus and major receptor group HRVs, many picornaviruses have been shown to be able to use more than one receptor. Four examples may be cited:

Coxsackievirus A9

CVA9 can use the vitronectin receptor $\alpha_v\beta_3$, where the attachment to this receptor is mediated by an RGD triplet mapping to the C terminus of VP1. Treatment of CVA9 with trypsin or intestinal fluid cleaves the capsid protein VP1, thereby removing the RGD motif. Although the trypsin-treated CVA9 can no longer utilize $\alpha_v\beta_3$ it is nevertheless able to infect green monkey kidney cells via an unknown second receptor. This second receptor is presumably also expressed on rhabdomyosarcoma cells (RD cells) that lack integrin $\alpha_v\beta_3$; RD cells are readily infected by trypsin-cleaved CVA9 (52–54).

Coxsackieviruses B

For lack of expression of CAR, the prototype Nancy strain of CVB3 (CVB3-N) cannot infect RD cells. CVB3-N, however, can be adapted to productively infect RD cells, yielding strain CVB3-RD. It has subsequently been shown that CVB3-RD uses DAF (CD55) as a receptor (7, 58, and references therein) although DAF alone may not be sufficient to induce an infectious cycle. Interestingly, CVB-RD retained its ability to bind CAR, that is, binding to CAR or DAF is not mutually exclusive. All CVB serotypes can be grown in human fibroblasts (25 and references therein) that are deficient in CAR (27). Perhaps because of its acquired affinity to DAF, CVB-RD grows exceptionally well in human fibroblasts.

Interestingly, the affinity of CVB3 isolates to CAR or DAF appears to be strongly influenced by the amino acid sequences in the capsid protein VP1 (58 and references therein). Indeed, different affinities to receptors, governed by capsid sequences, are the most likely explanation for the profound differences CVBs display in their pathogenic profiles as, for example, febrile illness, infectious myocarditis, or pancreatitis (6, 7, 43, 58, and references therein). It should be noted, however, that different affinities to CAR and/or DAF alone can hardly explain the diversity of CVB-induced pathogenesis. As mentioned, RD cells lacking CAR support CVB-RD infection via the DAF receptor. Whereas CHO cells expressing CAR can be infected with CVB3-RD, CHO cells expressing DAF cannot. This observation is reminiscent of the inability of DAF-expressing CHO cells to support infection with CVA21 (see above). It appears, therefore, that DAF alone may be unable to serve as receptor to initiate an infectious cycle and that DAF may be in need of an accessory factor(s) that is missing on CHO cells.

Echoviruses

The productive interaction between echoviruses (other than echoviruses 1 and 8) and host cell receptors is particularly complex and is, for the most part, not understood. Whereas DAF plays a major role in virus docking (5, 48, 76), either a second receptor or an accessory factor seems necessary for viral proliferation. Recently, heparan sulfate has been suggested to be such second receptor (20).

FMDVs

Most laboratory strains of FMDV can use the vitronectin receptor ($\alpha_v\beta_3$) as cellular receptor for cell entry (9). The interaction is mediated via an RGD motif exposed in a surface protrusion of the virion. Exceptions include laboratory strains of serotype O_1 FMDV that are unable to bind to $\alpha_v\beta_3$ in spite of carrying the RGD motif. These strains of serotype O_1 FMDV use heparan sulfate as receptor (34). The difference in receptor utilization not only yields host range phenotypes in vitro, but it has also a profound effect on pathogenesis in animals. Briefly, serotype O_1 FMDV strains using heparan sulfate are highly attenuated in cattle. However, when selected to acquire affinity to bind $\alpha_v\beta_3$ by passage through cattle, serotype O_1 FMDV strains regain virulence while concomitantly losing affinity to heparan sulfate (57). Recently, a second integrin ($\alpha_v\beta_6$) has been identified to function as receptor for FMDV (35). This is particularly interesting since $\alpha_v\beta_6$ is an integrin expressed on epithelial cells, the first target cells in infection in cattle.

An intriguing experiment has been reported by Rieder et al. (50), who fused the antigen-binding domain of an FMDV-specific antibody with ICAM-1 such that the fusion protein, once expressed in cells void of a bona fide FMDV receptor, could function as an artificial cell surface receptor. Cells expressing such artificial receptors were infected independently of the RGD pathway. This experiment showed that integrins or heparan sulfate molecules, although functioning as natural receptors, are not essential for the process of FMDV uncoating (see below; for details, see chapter 11).

ACCESSORY FACTORS

We define accessory factors, first, as cellular molecules that, subsequent to virus docking, are indispensable for the infection to proceed. In this case, these essential accessory factors are often referred to as "secondary receptors." Second, accessory factors may serve to enhance the efficiency of infection, or they may play an essential role in uptake of a virus with some tissue culture cells but not with all.

The most thoroughly studied examples of an obligatory role of an accessory factor are (i) human immunodeficiency virus, requiring CD4 for attachment and a chemokine receptor for penetration (14), and (ii) adenovirus type 2, requiring CAR for attachment and either nectin $\alpha_v\beta_3$ or nectin $\alpha_v\beta_5$ for penetration (47). For picornavirus uptake, such a stringent requirement for a second protein has yet to be established, with the possible exception of $\alpha_v\beta_3$-dependent infection by CVA9 (see below). Nevertheless, several cell surface entities have been reported to enhance the infectivity of enteroviruses under special circumstances.

DAF enhances the efficiency of uptake of CVA21 although this virus can infect cells lacking DAF (62; E. Rieder and E. Wimmer, unpublished data). Moreover, monoclonal antibodies directed to the site of the DAF domain (SCR1) that mediates CVA21 binding will significantly inhibit infection of Hep-2 cells but not of HeLa cells (62). Currently, these interesting phenomena remain largely unexplained.

β_2-Microglobulin (β_2-m), a component of major histocompatibility complex (MHC) class I, has been indirectly implicated in the infection of RD cells by certain echoviruses. Anti-β_2-m antibodies block infection of RD cells without inhibiting virus binding (77). However, infection of HeLa cells by many echoviruses is not blocked by anti-β_2-m antibodies, suggesting that the effect is unique to RD cells.

A stringent requirement for β_2-m has been reported for the $\alpha_v\beta_3$-dependent infection by CVA9 of different tissue culture cells: green monkey kidney cells, RD cells, or genetically modified CHO cells (75). Anti-β_2-m antibodies (a mixture of two different antibodies) were found to completely block infection while hardly interfering with CVA9 binding to $\alpha_v\beta_3$. The data suggest that a step after binding of CVA9 to $\alpha_v\beta_3$ requires the presence of β_2-m to proceed to uncoating.

MAP-70 is another protein of MHC class I. It has recently been implicated to play a role as accessory factor in CVA9 infection (74).

CD59, a complement control protein, has been suggested to function as accessory factor for several echoviruses (particularly echovirus 7) in infections of RD cells (19).

Integrin $\alpha_v\beta_6$ has been reported to enhance coxsackievirus B1 lytic infection of human colon cancer cells (1).

The significance of these different accessory factors in the life cycle of picornaviruses is not yet known. We consider it likely, however, that they may play an important role in tissue-specific pathogenesis (see below).

THE SITES OF ATTACHMENT ON VIRIONS AND RECEPTORS

Much progress has been made to map the sites on virions and receptors that interact in the docking process.

Ig-Like Receptors

Picornaviruses using Ig-like receptors bind to the N-terminal domain of the polypeptide chain. With the exception of EMCV/VCAM-1, this has been demonstrated for ICAM-1, CD155 (reviewed recently by Rossmann et al. [56]; see chapters 7 and 8), CAR (24), and HAVcr-1 (36, 65). The experiments included genetic analyses of mutated or truncated receptor polypeptides or structural analyses employing cryo-electron microscopy and X-ray crystallography. As shown in Table 2, the very closely related C-cluster enteroviruses (polioviruses and C-CVAs) use different receptors, whereas the more distantly related major group HRVs and C-CVAs share the same receptor.

Where do the receptors attach at the surface of the virions? For the major group rhinoviruses, the C-cluster enteroviruses (poliovirus, C-cluster coxsackieviruses) and coxsackieviruses B, the N-terminal domains of the Ig-like proteins penetrate into the viral canyon surrounding the fivefold axis (55). There are large differences, however, in the orientation of receptor molecules within the respective canyons. The V domain of CD155, in comparison to the

TABLE 2 Sites of attachment on virions and receptors

Virus	Taxonomy	Receptor[a]	Orientation in the canyon
PV	C-cluster enterovirus/CD155	(V*-C-C-)	More tangential; southwest
CVA21	C-cluster enterovirus/ICAM-1	(C*-C-C-C-C-)	More radial; east-southeast
HRV	Genus rhinovirus/ICAM-1	(C*-C-C-C-C-)	More radial; southeast
CVB3	B-cluster enterovirus/CAR	(C*-C)	Two CARs form dimers bridging two canyons

[a]V, V domain; C, C domain; * indicates N-terminal binding domain.

C domains of the other receptors, contains two extra β strands (C' and C", 32 residues) that significantly increase the size of the domain. On the basis of mutational studies of CD155, it was originally proposed that the V domain places itself tangentially into the canyon (like a sausage in a bun) (10). This more tangential orientation was directly demonstrated by cryo-electron microscopy (3, 23, 80).

As has been mentioned before, poliovirus and C-CVAs belong to the same, closely related cluster of enteroviruses (see chapter 2). Considering the fact that the N-terminal domains of their Ig-like receptors (CD155 and ICAM-1) insert themselves into the respective viral canyons, the following question may be raised: To what extent must the C-CVA canyon be mutated to accommodate binding of CD155? This is of interest because a receptor switch of a C-CVA from ICAM-1 to CD155 is likely to signal the evolution of a new poliovirus (51). (Note that a previous suggestion that C-CVAs may have evolved by recombination between polioviruses and HRVs [32] is not supported by recent phylogenetic considerations.)

All structural studies of CD155 or ICAM-1 with virions by cryo-electron microscopy have been carried out by employing the ecto domain (or fragments thereof) of the receptor molecules. Of special interest is a recent report describing the interaction of full-length CAR (ecto domain-transmembrane domain-cytoplasmic domain in the presence of detergent) with the CVB3 virion by cryo-electron microscopy (24). While domain 1 intrudes into the canyon, the transmembrane domain, in association with a detergent, forms a membrane-like structure. It is appealing to speculate that this structure may resemble the native receptor-virion interaction involving CD155 and ICAM-1 and respective viruses.

LDL-Like Receptors

Structurally, the major receptor group and minor group HRVs are so similar that it is difficult to comprehend why these viruses would have selected entirely different receptors. Results of site-directed mutagenesis experiments suggest that the LDL-like receptors do not bind at a site similar to that of ICAM-1 (15). This was supported by high-resolution analyses of the HRV16-ICAM-1 and HRV14-ICAM-1 complexes that, combined with an analysis of structure of the HRV2 virion, identified residues in the HRV2 canyon preventing insertion of domain 1 of ICAM-1 into the HRV2 canyon (see chapters 3 and 8). The nature of the binding of the VLDL to HRV2 has been determined recently, making use of the first three ligand binding repeats (Fig. 1). Interestingly, the VLDL receptor binds to the star-shaped dome on the fivefold axis (26; see chapter 9).

Integrins

Picornaviruses have selected either the α or β chain of the heterodimeric integrin receptor for attachment. Briefly, echoviruses 1 and 8 bind to the I domain of the α chain of $\alpha_2\beta_1$ (VLA-2) (see chapter 10), while CVA9 and FMDVs bind to the β chain of $\alpha_v\beta_3$ (see chapter 11).

DAF

The polypeptide chain of DAF consists of four SCRs, some of which are involved in virus binding. It came as a surprise, however, that there is no uniform pattern by which enteroviruses bind DAF. CVA21, a C-cluster enterovirus, and E70, a D-cluster enterovirus (see references 62 and 37, respectively), attach to SRC1. The other DAF-binding enteroviruses that belong to cluster B have chosen different binding domains: CVB that was adapted to proliferation in RD cells (CVB-RD) binds to SCR2 (7); CVB1, -3, and -6 and hemagglutinating echoviruses bind to SCR3 (48, 63). The site of attachment on the virion of any of these viruses has not been determined.

THE CONSEQUENCE OF VIRAL ATTACHMENT TO THE RECEPTOR

Attachment to a cellular receptor alone is of very little use for a virus. It is the molecular events following attachment that matter. In most virus-receptor interactions, these events are poorly understood. Among picornaviruses, poliovirus and major group HRVs are notable exceptions.

Poliovirus and the major receptor group rhinoviruses have evolved to produce, after attachment to their respective receptors, the so-called A particles (see chapter 7). These particles were discovered in the 1960s, and many of the early studies have adequately described properties and parameters of their generation (see review in reference 13). These particles are subviral particles that have lost the small capsid polypeptide VP4. It is likely but not universally accepted that A particles are intermediates of uncoating in a pathway that can be summarized as follows:

$$160S \text{ virion } [(VP1-4)_{60}RNA]$$
$$\Rightarrow 130S \text{ A particle } [(VP1-3)_{60}RNA] + VP4$$
$$\Rightarrow 80S \text{ particle } [(VP1-3)_{60}] + RNA$$

Importantly, A particles, although resistant to RNase, are quite unstable to proteolytic enzymes and detergents (in contrast to poliovirus, they fall apart in 1% sodium dodecyl sulfate); and they are significantly more hydrophobic than the parental virion (17, 40).

Recent papers have produced a plausible hypothesis that may explain how the interaction of the receptors with major group HRVs and poliovirus leads to uncoating (reviewed in chapters 7 and 8). Nonpolio enteroviruses produce A particles, just like poliovirus, through the interaction with receptors (42, 49, 61). There is little known about these events. Nevertheless, production of A particles in a virion-receptor-binding assay is seen as the crucial test of uncoating of a nonpolio enterovirus.

RECEPTORS AND PATHOGENESIS

Pathogenesis is determined by (i) tissue tropism, (ii) spread of the virus to target tissues, and (iii) virulence (which we define as the ability of the virus to replicate and kill cells of the target tissue). Of these, tissue tropism depends most strongly, and often exclusively, on the cellular receptor. Picornaviruses cause a bewildering array of disease syndromes, some of which are listed in Table 1. In some cases, a comparison of receptor usage and clinical syndrome can co-vary with the disease: the receptor of C-CVAs and major group HRVs is ICAM-1. Although these viruses belong to different genera, they cause the common cold. However, C-CVAs but not the HRVs can cause infantile diarrhea. The restriction of HRVs to upper respiratory tissue may relate to the instability of HRVs to low pH (preventing them from passing unharmed through the stomach) and a ts phenotype of replication.

Poliovirus causes mild enteric infections that remain mostly unnoticed. Rarely (1% probability) does the virus find its way into the CNS where it targets motor neurons and cells of the meningi. The tropism for motor neurons is astounding and remains to be explained: Why does the virus cause little if any damage to the huge number of cells in the brain parenchyma other than motor neurons (astrocytes, oligodendrocytes, microglia cells, sensory neurons, etc.)? Is the expression of CD155 in these cells below a critical threshold to allow viral entry? Or is this a matter of cell-internal restriction? Or the absence of an accessory protein? In any event, tumor cells arising from astrocytes and oligodendrocytes (human glioma) express adequate levels of CD155, and they are readily infected and destroyed by poliovirus (21a).

As mentioned, the intracellular domains of CD155 α and δ can bind Tctex-1, a subunit of the dynein motor complex (45). Dynein motor complexes have been shown to be involved in retrograde transport in axons along the microtubules. It is intriguing to speculate that poliovirus moves from the neuromuscular junction to the cell body of a motor neuron via retrograde axonal transport, mediated by CD155/Tctex-1 interaction (45). Once in the cell body, the virus would then replicate and destroy motor neuron function, an event leading to poliomyelitis.

A particular challenge is posed by the perplexing number of disease syndromes caused by B-cluster enteroviruses, particularly CVBs. This cluster of enteroviruses, more than any group of picornaviruses, seems to have developed the ability to bind to different receptors and accessory proteins. As pointed out above, it has been suggested that subtle changes in the capsid proteins of a viral variant may modify the affinity for a receptor or for accessory protein, thereby modifying tissue tropism and pathogenesis.

CVA9, en route to the intestinal tract, most likely undergoes cleavage of VP1, thereby losing its affinity to $\alpha_v\beta_3$ (see above; 53). The alternative receptor for this modified CVA9 is not known, but its properties are likely to direct the virus to a tissue distinct from the tissue targeted by the native CVA9 particle.

Surprisingly, the receptor(s) of the A-cluster enteroviruses has not yet been determined even though this cluster includes common pathogens like CVA16 and, notably, the dangerous enterovirus 71 (28). Both CVA16 and enterovirus 71 cause a hand-foot-and-mouth syndrome, similar to the foot-and-mouth diseases caused by FMDV and, more rarely, CVA9. It would make sense if CVA16 and enterovirus 71 also use $\alpha_v\beta_3$ as receptor, just like FMDV and CVA9. However, neither CVA16 nor enterovirus 71 displays an RGD motif at the surface of their respective virions. It follows that all we know is that we know very little.

We are indebted to Barry Baxt, Jeffrey Bergelson, Dieter Blass, David Evans, Sally Hover, Tapani Hovi, Timo Hyppiä, and Merja Roivainen for illuminating discussions. Work reported from this laboratory was supported by grants from the National Institutes of Health.

NOTE ADDED IN PROOF

EV68 and HRV87 have been determined to be the same serotype, presenting features of both entero- and rhinoviruses, by using DAF as receptor (S. Blomqvist, C. Savolainen, L. Raman, M. Roivainen, and T. Hovi, Europic/America 2002, abstr. A38).

REFERENCES

1. **Agrez, M. V., D. R. Shafren, X. Gu, K. Cox, D. Sheppard, and R. D. Barry.** 1997. Integrin alpha v beta 6 enhances coxsackievirus B1 lytic infection of human colon cancer cells. *Virology* **239**:71–77.
2. **Allaway, G. P., and A. T. Burness.** 1986. Site of attachment of encephalomyocarditis virus on human erythrocytes. *J. Virol.* **59**:768–770.
3. **Belnap, D. M., B. M. McDermott, Jr., D. J. Filman, N. Cheng, B. L. Trus, H. J. Zuccola, V. R. Racaniello, J. M. Hogle, and A. C. Steven.** 2000. Three-dimensional structure of poliovirus receptor bound to poliovirus. *Proc. Natl. Acad. Sci. USA* **97**:73–78.
4. **Bergelson, J. M., J. A. Cunningham, G. Droguett, E. A. Kurt-Jones, A. Krithivas, J. S. Hong, M. S. Horwitz, R. L. Crowell, and R. W. Finberg.** 1997. Isolation of a common receptor for coxsackie B viruses and adenoviruses 2 and 5. *Science* **275**:1320–1323.
5. **Bergelson, J. M., M. Chan, K. R. Solomon, N. F. St. John, H. Lin, and R. W. Finberg.** 1994. Decay-accelerating factor (CD55), a glycosylphosphatidylinositol-anchored complement regulatory protein, is a receptor for several echoviruses. *Proc. Natl. Acad. Sci. USA* **91**:6245–6249.
6. **Bergelson, J. M., J. F. Modlin, W. Wieland-Alter, J. A. Cunningham, R. L. Crowell, and R. W. Finberg.** 1997. Clinical coxsackievirus B isolates differ from laboratory strains in their interaction with two cell surface receptors. *J. Infect. Dis.* **175**:697–700.
7. **Bergelson, J. M., J. G. Mohanty, R. L. Crowell, N. F. St. John, D. M. Lublin, and R. W. Finberg.** 1995. Coxsackievirus B3 adapted to growth in RD cells binds to decay-accelerating factor (CD55). *J. Virol.* **69**:1903–1906.
8. **Bergelson, J. M., M. P. Shepley, B. M. Chan, M. E. Hemler, and R. W. Finberg.** 1992. Identification of the integrin VLA-2 as a receptor for echovirus 1. *Science* **255**:1718–1720.
9. **Berinstein, A., M. Roivainen, T. Hovi, P. W. Mason, and B. Baxt.** 1995. Antibodies to the vitronectin receptor (integrin alpha V beta 3) inhibit binding and infection of

foot-and-mouth disease virus to cultured cells. *J. Virol.* **69:** 2664–2666.

10. **Bernhardt, G., J. Harber, A. Zibert, M. deCrombrugghe, and E. Wimmer.** 1994. The poliovirus receptor: identification of domains and amino acid residues critical for virus binding. *Virology* **203:**344–356.

11. **Carlos, T. M., B. R. Schwartz, N. L. Kovach, E. Yee, M. Rosso, L. Osborn, G. Chi-Rosso, B. Newman, R. Lobb, and J. M. Harlan.** 1990. Vascular cell adhesion molecule-1 mediates lymphocyte adherence to cytokine-activated cultured human endothelial cells. *Blood* **76:** 965–970.

12. **Colonno, R. J.** 1986. Cell surface receptors for picornaviruses. *Bioessays* **5:**270–274.

13. **Crowell, R. L., D. L. Krah, J. Mapoles, and B. J. Landau.** 1983. Methods for assay of cellular receptors for picornaviruses. *Methods Enzymol.* **96:**443–452.

14. **Doms, R. W.** 2001. Chemokine receptors and HIV entry. *AIDS* **15**(Suppl. 1)**:**S34–S35.

15. **Duechler, M., S. Ketter, T. Skern, E. Kuechler, and D. Blaas.** 1993. Rhinoviral receptor discrimination: mutational changes in the canyon regions of human rhinovirus types 2 and 14 indicate a different site of interaction. *J. Gen. Virol.* **74:**2287–2291.

16. **Freistadt, M. S., and K. E. Eberle.** 1997. CD155 (poliovirus receptor) workshop panel report, p. 1075–1077. *VI International Workshop and Conference on Human Leucocyte Differentiation Antigens.* Garland, Cambridge, United Kingdom.

17. **Fricks, C. E., and J. M. Hogle.** 1990. Cell-induced conformational change in poliovirus: externalization of the amino terminus of VP1 is responsible for liposome binding. *J. Virol.* **64:**1934–1945.

18. **Gonzalez-Amaro, R., and F. Sanchez-Madrid.** 1999. Cell adhesion molecules: selectins and integrins. *Crit. Rev. Immunol.* **19:**389–429.

19. **Goodfellow, I. G., R. M. Powell, T. Ward, O. B. Spiller, J. W. Almond, and D. J. Evans.** 2000. Echovirus infection of rhabdomyosarcoma cells is inhibited by antiserum to the complement control protein CD59. *J. Gen. Virol.* **81**(Pt. 5)**:**1393–1401.

20. **Goodfellow, I. G., A. B. Sioofy, R. M. Powell, and D. J. Evans.** 2001. Echoviruses bind heparan sulfate at the cell surface. *J. Virol.* **75:**4918–4921.

21. **Greve, J. M., G. Davis, A. M. Meyer, C. P. Forte, S. C. Yost, C. W. Marlor, M. E. Kamarck, and A. McClelland.** 1989. The major human rhinovirus receptor is ICAM-1. *Cell* **56:**839–847.

21a. **Gromeier, M., S. Lachmann, M. R. Rosenfeld, P. H. Gutin, and E. Wimmer.** 2000. Intergenetic poliovirus recombinants for the treatment of malignant glioma. *Proc. Natl. Acad. Sci. USA* **97:**6803–6808.

22. **Gromeier, M., D. Solecki, D. D. Patel, and E. Wimmer.** 2000. Expression of the human poliovirus receptor/CD155 gene during development of the central nervous system: implications for the pathogenesis of poliomyelitis. *Virology* **273:**248–257.

22a. **Gromeier, M., E. Wimmer, and A. E. Gorbalenya.** 1999. Genetics, pathogenesis, and evolution of picornaviruses, p. 287–343. *In* E. Domingo, R. G. Webster, and J. J. Holland (ed.), *Origin and Evolution of Viruses.* Academic Press, Inc., New York, N.Y.

23. **He, Y., V. D. Bowman, S. Mueller, C. M. Bator, J. Bella, X. Peng, T. S. Baker, E. Wimmer, R. J. Kuhn, and M. G. Rossmann.** 2000. Interaction of the poliovirus receptor with poliovirus. *Proc. Natl. Acad. Sci. USA* **97:**79–84.

24. **He, Y., P. R. Chipman, J. Howitt, C. M. Bator, M. A. Whitt, T. S. Baker, R. J. Kuhn, C. W. Anderson, P. Freimuth, and M. G. Rossmann.** 2001. Interaction of coxsackievirus B3 with the full-length coxsackievirus-adenovirus receptor. *Nat. Struct. Biol.* **10:**874–878.

25. **Heim, A., C. Brehm, M. Stille-Siegener, G. Muller, S. Hake, R. Kandolf, and H. R. Figulla.** 1995. Cultured human myocardial fibroblasts of pediatric origin: natural human interferon-alpha is more effective than recombinant interferon-alpha 2a in carrier-state coxsackievirus B3 replication. *J. Mol. Cell Cardiol.* **27:**2199–2208.

26. **Hewat, E. A., E. Neumann, J. F. Conway, R. Moser, B. Ronacher, T. C. Marlovits, and D. Blaas.** 2000. The cellular receptor to human rhinovirus 2 binds around the 5-fold axis and not in the canyon: a structural view. *EMBO J.* **19:**6317–6325.

27. **Hidaka, C., E. Milano, P. L. Leopold, J. M. Bergelson, N. R. Hackett, R. W. Finberg, T. J. Wickham, I. Kovesdi, P. Roelvink, and R. G. Crystal.** 1999. CAR-dependent and CAR-independent pathways of adenovirus vector-mediated gene transfer and expression in human fibroblasts. *J. Clin. Invest.* **103:**579–587.

28. **Ho, M.** 2000. Enterovirus 71: the virus, its infections and outbreaks. *J. Microbiol. Immunol. Infect.* **33:**205–216.

29. **Hofer, F., M. Gruenberger, H. Kowalski, H. Machat, M. Huettinger, E. Kuechler, and D. Blass.** 1994. Members of the low density lipoprotein receptor family mediate cell entry of a minor-group common cold virus. *Proc. Natl. Acad. Sci. USA* **91:**1839–1842.

30. **Honda, T., H. Saitoh, M. Masuko, T. Katagiri-Abe, K. Tominaga, I. Kozakai, K. Kobayashi, T. Kumanishi, Y. G. Watanabe, S. Odani, and R. Kuwano.** 2000. The coxsackievirus-adenovirus receptor protein as a cell adhesion molecule in the developing mouse brain. *Brain Res. Mol. Brain Res.* **77:**19–28.

31. **Huber, S. A.** 1994. VCAM-1 is a receptor for encephalomyocarditis virus on murine vascular endothelial cells. *J. Virol.* **68:**3453–3458.

32. **Hughes, P. J., C. North, P. D. Minor, and G. Stanway.** 1989. The complete nucleotide sequence of coxsackievirus A21. *J. Gen. Virol.* **70:**2943–2952.

33. **Hynes, R. O.** 1992. Integrins: versatility, modulation, and signaling in cell adhesion. *Cell* **69:**11–25.

33a. **Hyypiä, T., T. Hovi, N. J. Knowles, and G. Stanway.** 1997. Classification of enteroviruses based on molecular and biological properties. *J. Gen. Virol.* **78:**1–11.

34. **Jackson, T., F. M. Ellard, R. A. Ghazaleh, S. M. Brookes, W. E. Blakemore, A. H. Corteyn, D. I. Stuart, J. W. Newman, and A. M. King.** 1996. Efficient infection of cells in culture by type O foot-and-mouth disease virus requires binding to cell surface heparan sulfate. *J. Virol.* **70:**5282–5287.

35. **Jackson, T., D. Sheppard, M. Denyer, W. Blakemore, and A. M. King.** 2000. The epithelial integrin $\alpha v \beta 6$ is a receptor for foot-and-mouth disease virus. *J. Virol.* **74:** 4949–4956.

36. **Kaplan, G., A. Totsuka, P. Thompson, T. Akatsuka, Y. Moritsugu, and S. M. Feinstone.** 1996. Identification of a surface glycoprotein on African green monkey kidney cells as a receptor for hepatitis A virus. *EMBO J.* **15:** 4282–4296.

37. **Karnauchow, T. M., S. Dawe, D. M. Lublin, and K. Dimock.** 1998. Short consensus repeat domain 1 of decay-accelerating factor is required for enterovirus 70 binding. *J. Virol.* **72:**9380–9383.

38. **Koike, S., H. Horie, I. Ise, A. Okitsu, M. Yoshida, N. Iizuka, K. Takeuchi, T. Takegami, and A. Nomoto.** 1990. The poliovirus receptor protein is produced both as membrane-bound and secreted forms. *EMBO J.* **9:**3217–3224.

39. **Lange, R., X. Peng, E. Wimmer, M. Lipp, and G. Bernhardt.** 2001. The poliovirus receptor cd155 mediates cell-to-matrix contacts by specifically binding to vitronectin. *Virology* **285:**218–227.

40. **Lonberg-Holm, K., L. B. Gosser, and E. J. Shimshick.** 1976. Interaction of liposomes with subviral particles of

41. **Lublin, D. M., and J. P. Atkinson.** 1989. Decay-accelerating factor: biochemistry, molecular biology, and function. *Annu. Rev. Immunol.* **7:**35–58.
42. **McGeady, M. L., and R. L. Crowell.** 1981. Proteolytic cleavage of VP1 in 'A' particles of coxsackievirus B3 does not appear to mediate virus uncoating by HeLa cells. *J. Gen. Virol.* **55:**439–450.
43. **Mena, I., C. Fischer, J. R. Gebhard, C. M. Perry, S. Harkins, and J. L. Whitton.** 2000. Coxsackievirus infection of the pancreas: evaluation of receptor expression, pathogenesis, and immunopathology. *Virology* **271:**276–288.
44. **Mendelsohn, C. L., E. Wimmer, and V. R. Racaniello.** 1989. Cellular receptor for poliovirus: molecular cloning, nucleotide sequence, and expression of a new member of the immunoglobulin superfamily. *Cell* **56:**855–865.
45. **Mueller, S., X. Cao, R. Welker, and E. Wimmer.** 2002. Interaction of the poliovirus CD155 with the dynein light chain Tctex-1 and its implication for poliovirus pathogenesis. *J. Biol. Chem.* **277:**7897–7904.
46. **Neff, S., P. W. Mason, and B. Baxt.** 2000. High-efficiency utilization of the bovine integrin $\alpha v\beta 3$ as a receptor for foot-and-mouth disease virus is dependent on the bovine beta(3) subunit. *J. Virol.* **74:**7298–7306.
47. **Nemerow, G. R.** 2000. Cell receptors involved in adenovirus entry. *Virology* **274:**1–4.
48. **Powell, R. M., V. Schmitt, T. Ward, I. Goodfellow, D. J. Evans, and J. W. Almond.** 1998. Characterization of echoviruses that bind decay accelerating factor (CD55): evidence that some haemagglutinating strains use more than one cellular receptor. *J. Gen. Virol.* **79:**1707–1713.
49. **Powell, R. M., T. Ward, D. J. Evans, and J. W. Almond.** 1997. Interaction between echovirus 7 and its receptor, decay-accelerating factor (CD55): evidence for a secondary cellular factor in A-particle formation. *J. Virol.* **71:**9306–9312.
50. **Rieder, E., A. Berinstein, B. Baxt, A. Kang, and P. W. Mason.** 1996. Propagation of an attenuated virus by design: engineering a novel receptor for a noninfectious foot-and-mouth disease virus. *Proc. Natl. Acad. Sci. USA* **93:**10428–10433.
51. **Rieder, E., A. E. Gorbalenya, C. Xiao, V. He, T. S. Baker, R. J. Kuhn, M. G. Rossmann, and E. Wimmer.** 2001. Will the polio niche remain vacant? *Dev. Biol.* **105:**111–122.
52. **Roivainen, M., T. Hyypia, L. Piirainen, N. Kalkkinen, G. Stanway, and T. Hovi.** 1991. RGD-dependent entry of coxsackievirus A9 into host cells and its bypass after cleavage of VP1 protein by intestinal proteases. *J. Virol.* **65:**4735–4740.
53. **Roivainen, M., L. Piirainen, and T. Hovi.** 1996. Efficient RGD-independent entry process of coxsackievirus A9. *Arch. Virol.* **141:**1909–1919.
54. **Roivainen, M., L. Piirainen, T. Hovi, I. Virtanen, T. Riikonen, J. Heino, and T. Hyypia.** 1994. Entry of coxsackievirus A9 into host cells: specific interactions with alpha v beta 3 integrin, the vitronectin receptor. *Virology* **203:**357–365.
55. **Rossmann, M. G., E. Arnold, J. W. Erickson, E. A. Frankenberger, J. P. Griffith, H. J. Hecht, J. E. Johnson, G. Kamer, M. Luo, A. G. Mosser, R. Rueckert, B. Sherry, and G. Vriend.** 1985. Structure of a human common cold virus and functional relationship to other picornaviruses. *Nature* **317:**145–153.
56. **Rossmann, M. G., J. Bella, P. R. Kolatkar, Y. He, E. Wimmer, R. J. Kuhn, and T. S. Baker.** 2000. Cell recognition and entry by rhino- and enteroviruses. *Virology* **269:**239–247.
57. **Sa-Carvalho, D., E. Rieder, B. Baxt, R. Rodarte, A. Tanuri, and P. W. Mason.** 1997. Tissue culture adaptation of foot-and-mouth disease virus selects viruses that bind to heparin and are attenuated in cattle. *J. Virol.* **71:**5115–5123.
58. **Schmidtke, M., H. C. Selinka, A. Heim, B. Jahn, M. Tonew, R. Kandolf, A. Stelzner, and R. Zell.** 2000. Attachment of coxsackievirus B3 variants to various cell lines: mapping of phenotypic differences to capsid protein VP1. *Virology* **275:**77–88.
59. **Selinka, H. C., A. Zibert, and E. Wimmer.** 1991. Poliovirus can enter and infect mammalian cells by way of an intercellular adhesion molecule 1 pathway. *Proc. Natl. Acad. Sci. USA* **88:**3598–3602.
60. **Shafren, D. R., R. C. Bates, M. V. Agrez, R. L. Herd, G. F. Burns, and R. D. Barry.** 1995. Coxsackieviruses B1, B3, and B5 use decay accelerating factor as a receptor for cell attachment. *J. Virol.* **69:**3873–3877.
61. **Shafren, D. R., D. J. Dorahy, S. J. Greive, G. F. Burns, and R. D. Barry.** 1997. Mouse cells expressing human intercellular adhesion molecule-1 are susceptible to infection by coxsackievirus A21. *J. Virol.* **71:**785–789.
62. **Shafren, D. R., D. J. Dorahy, R. A. Ingham, G. F. Burns, and R. D. Barry.** 1997. Coxsackievirus A21 binds to decay-accelerating factor but requires intercellular adhesion molecule 1 for cell entry. *J. Virol.* **71:**4736–4743.
63. **Shafren, D. R., D. J. Dorahy, R. F. Thorne, T. Kinoshita, R. D. Barry, and G. F. Burns.** 1998. Antibody binding to individual short consensus repeats of decay-accelerating factor enhances enterovirus cell attachment and infectivity. *J. Immunol.* **160:**2318–2323.
64. **Shieh, M. T., D. WuDunn, R. I. Montgomery, J. D. Esko, and P. G. Spear.** 1992. Cell surface receptors for herpes simplex virus are heparan sulfate proteoglycans. *J. Cell Biol.* **116:**1273–1281.
65. **Silberstein, E., G. Dveksler, and G. G. Kaplan.** 2001. Neutralization of hepatitis A virus (HAV) by an immunoadhesin containing the cysteine-rich region of HAV cellular receptor-1. *J. Virol.* **75:**717–725.
66. **Solecki, D., G. Bernhardt, M. Lipp, and E. Wimmer.** 2000. Identification of a nuclear respiratory factor-1 binding site within the core promoter of the human polio virus receptor/CD155 gene. *J. Biol. Chem.* **275:**12453–12462.
67. **Solecki, D., E. Wimmer, M. Lipp, and G. Bernhardt.** 1999. Identification and characterization of the cis-acting elements of the human CD155 gene core promoter. *J. Biol. Chem.* **274:**1791–1800.
68. **Sommerfelt, M. A.** 1999. Retrovirus receptors. *J. Gen. Virol.* **80:**3049–3064.
69. **Staunton, D. E., V. J. Merluzzi, R. Rothlein, R. Barton, S. D. Marlin, and T. A. Springer.** 1989. A cell adhesion molecule, ICAM-1, is the major surface receptor for rhinoviruses. *Cell* **56:**849–853.
70. **Tomassini, J. E., D. Graham, C. M. DeWitt, D. W. Lineberger, J. A. Rodkey, and R. J. Colonno.** 1989. cDNA cloning reveals that the major group rhinovirus receptor on HeLa cells is intercellular adhesion molecule 1. *Proc. Natl. Acad. Sci. USA* **86:**4907–4911.
71. **Tomko, R. P., C. B. Johansson, M. Totrov, R. Abagyan, J. Frisen, and L. Philipson.** 2000. Expression of the adenovirus receptor and its interaction with the fiber knob. *Exp. Cell Res.* **255:**47–55.
72. **Tomko, R. P., R. Xu, and L. Philipson.** 1997. HCAR and MCAR: the human and mouse cellular receptors for subgroup C adenoviruses and group B coxsackieviruses. *Proc. Natl. Acad. Sci. USA* **94:**3352–3356.
73. **Triantafilou, K., M. Triantafilou, Y. Takada, and N. Fernandez.** 2000. Human parechovirus 1 utilizes integrins alphavbeta3 and alphavbeta1 as receptors. *J. Virol.* **74:**5856–5862.
74. **Triantafilou, M., K. Triantafilou, and K. M. Wilson.** 2000. A 70 kDa MHC class I associated protein (MAP-

70) identified as a receptor molecule for coxsackievirus A9 cell attachment. *Hum. Immunol.* **61**:867–878.

75. **Triantafilou, M., K. Triantafilou, K. M. Wilson, Y. Takada, N. Fernandez, and G. Stanway.** 1999. Involvement of beta2-microglobulin and integrin alphavbeta3 molecules in the coxsackievirus A9 infectious cycle. *J. Gen. Virol.* **80**:2591–2600.

76. **Ward, T., P. A. Pipkin, N. A. Clarkson, D. M. Stone, P. D. Minor, and J. W. Almond.** 1994. Decay-accelerating factor CD55 is identified as the receptor for echovirus 7 using CELICS, a rapid immuno-focal cloning method. *EMBO J.* **13**:5070–5074.

77. **Ward, T., R. M. Powell, P. A. Pipkin, D. J. Evans, P. D. Minor, and J. W. Almond.** 1998. Role for beta2-microglobulin in echovirus infection of rhabdomyosarcoma cells. *J. Virol.* **72**:5360–5365.

78. **Wimmer, E.** 1994. Introduction, p. 1–13. *In* E. Wimmer (ed.), *Cellular Receptors for Animal Viruses*. Cold Spring Harbor Press, Cold Spring Harbor, N.Y.

79. **Wimmer, E., J. J. Harber, J. A. Bibb, M. Gromeier, H.-H. Lu, and G. Bernhardt.** 1994. The poliovirus receptor, p. 101–127. *In* E. Wimmer (ed.), *Cellular Receptors for Animal Viruses*. Cold Spring Harbor Press, Cold Spring Harbor, N.Y.

80. **Xing, L., K. Tjarnlund, B. Lindqvist, G. G. Kaplan, D. Feigelstock, R. H. Cheng, and J. M. Casasnovas.** 2000. Distinct cellular receptor interactions in poliovirus and rhinoviruses. *EMBO J.* **19**:1207–1216.

Poliovirus Receptors and Cell Entry

JAMES M. HOGLE AND VINCENT R. RACANIELLO

7

Poliovirus is an ideal model for understanding how nonenveloped viruses enter cells and initiate infection. Poliovirus has been studied for many years, first as a serious disease pathogen, and subsequently as a model system for the replication of RNA viruses, and both the virus (Fig. 1) and its cellular receptor (Fig. 2) are readily studied by reverse genetics and structural characterization (reviewed in reference 55). As a result, poliovirus and its cell entry pathway are well characterized biochemically and genetically.

The study of entry of a wide variety of viruses reveals common themes that are the consequence of a central problem faced by all viruses in the passage from cell to cell or from host to host. To withstand the rigors of the extracellular environment, the virion must be stable to a variety of insults such as extremes of pH, ionic strength, temperature, and the presence of proteases. However, once the virion reaches its target cell, it must undergo structural changes that allow it to cross a membrane and deliver the genome to the appropriate compartment of the cell to initiate replication. For many viruses the solution to this problem involves a link between the final stages of assembly and the initiation of cell entry, an attractive model since it emphasizes the role of the virion as an intermediate (linking assembly and entry) in a cycle.

The final stage of assembly for many viruses involves proteolytic processing of a virion protein. By first folding the protein as a precursor, and subsequently introducing a covalent alteration, the global free-energy form of the precursor need not be the global free-energy state for the final product. However, the lowest energy form of the protein (for an enveloped virus) or the intact virus (for the nonenveloped viruses) may not be accessible due to energy barriers. The protein or virus particle is then kinetically trapped in a metastable state. When the virus encounters the appropriate trigger (such as receptor-coreceptor binding, acidification of an endosome), the protein (or virion) is released from a metastable state and proceeds to a lower energy state, which exposes hydrophobic sequences that allow it to attach to membranes. For enveloped viruses, membrane attachment facilitates fusion of the viral envelope with the cell membrane. For nonenveloped viruses, the hydrophobic sequences must either generate a pore or disrupt a cellular membrane to facilitate entry.

The entry of influenza A virus into cells is perhaps the best characterized example of this sequence of events. The cellular receptor, sialic acid, plays a single role, namely, to concentrate virus at the surface of susceptible cells, and the trigger that releases the hemagglutinin from its metastable state is acidification of the endosome. Although the hemagglutinin of influenza A virus is the only glycoprotein for which the metastable and fusogenic forms have been characterized structurally (10, 72), similar conformational changes have been proposed for other viral envelope glycoproteins, based on structures of analogues of the fusogenic form (3, 11, 23, 43, 44, 70, 71, 75). Recent studies on the mechanism of poliovirus entry into cells suggest that very similar mechanisms may also occur during entry of nonenveloped viruses.

THE POLIOVIRUS REPLICATION CYCLE

Receptor Binding

The replication cycle is initiated when poliovirus encounters the poliovirus receptor (Pvr), a transmembrane glycoprotein with three extracellular immunoglobulin (Ig)-like domains (Fig. 2). The cellular function of Pvr is not known, but related proteins in humans and mice, Nectin-1 and Nectin-2, are homophilic adhesion proteins that interact with the actin skeleton through a cytoplasmic protein called afadin (66). Mice lacking Nectin-2 have defects in spermatogenesis (9), and Pvr, Nectin-1, and Nectin-2 are coreceptors for alphaherpesviruses (63). Several lines of evidence suggest that the first (N-terminal) Ig-like domain of Pvr is responsible for virus binding and infection. Cells expressing a membrane-bound form of domain 1 alone or as chimera with other Ig-like proteins are susceptible to infection with poliovirus (38, 47, 60, 61). This functionality is independent of the cytoplasmic domain or the nature of the transmembrane anchor, suggesting that

---

James M. Hogle ■ Department of Biochemistry and Molecular Pharmacology, Harvard Medical School, Boston, MA 02115. *Vincent R. Racaniello* ■ Department of Microbiology, Columbia University College of Physicians & Surgeons, New York, NY 10032.

72 ■ VIRUS ENTRY

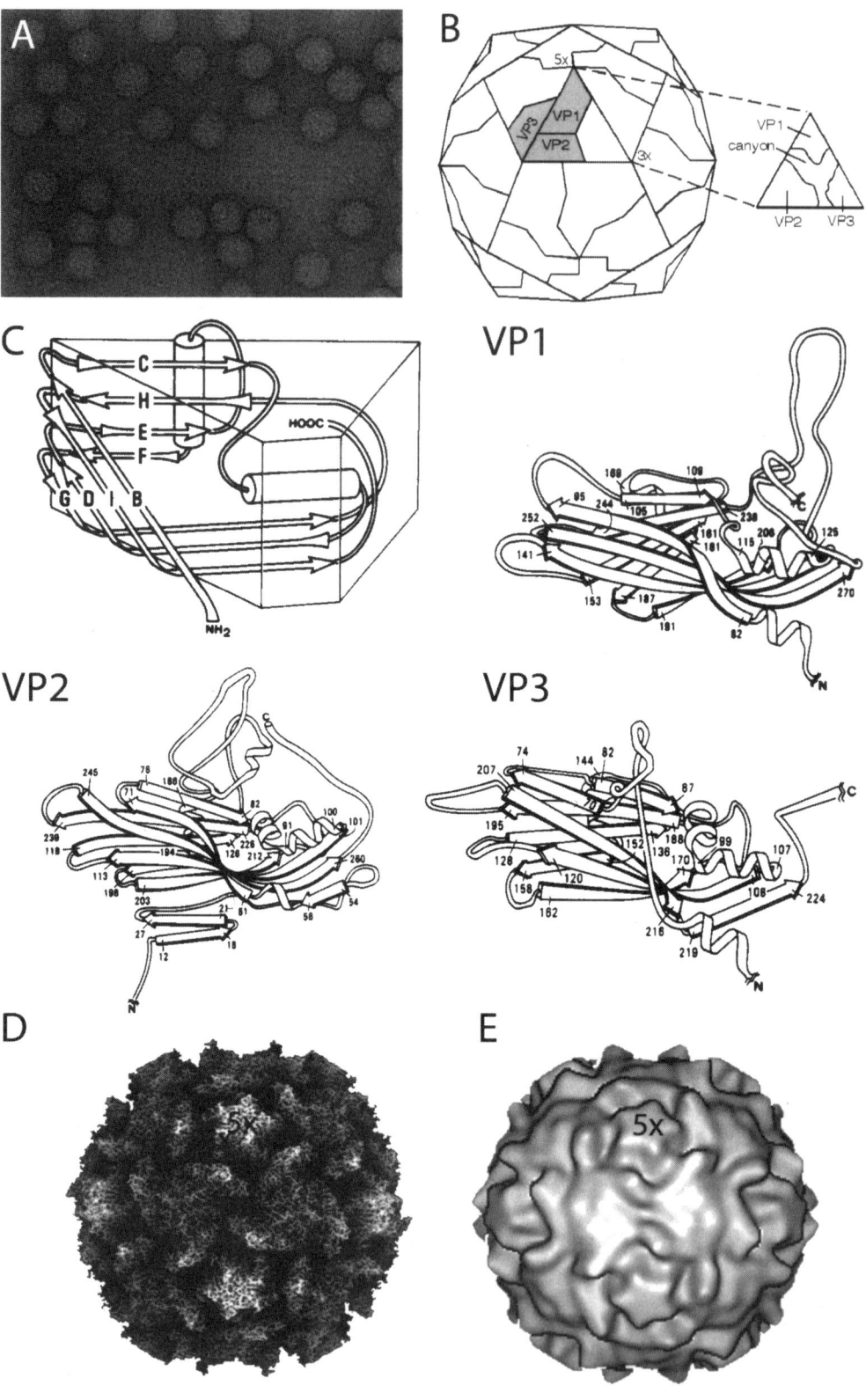

intracellular signaling is not critical for the ability of Pvr to function as a receptor. Furthermore, amino acid changes in the first Ig-like domain of Pvr effect virus binding (1, 8, 48).

The Site of Cell Entry

Characterization of the entry mechanism of poliovirus is complicated by the relatively high particle-to-PFU ratio (ranging from 10^2 to 10^3). When virus or viral-derived particles are detected in a given compartment during entry, it is not clear whether the particles are involved in productive or nonproductive events. As a result, classical biochemical and electron microscopic studies on poliovirus entry have led to contradictory findings. Early experiments with monensin and lysosomotropic amines suggested that poliovirus entry requires acidification (42). However, subsequent studies with bafilomycin A1, which blocks acidification of endosomes, demonstrated that poliovirus entry does not require low pH (54). The contradictory results of the earlier studies, in which the effect of lysosomotropic amines on infectious progeny were measured, were probably due to inhibition of later events in infection, such as viral RNA replication. More recently, dominant negative mutants of dynamin have also been used to examine the route of entry of poliovirus into cells. Dynamin is a large G-protein that plays a key role in "pinching off" coated vesicles to form coated pits during clathrin-mediated endocytosis. Expression of a dominant negative dynamin mutant abrogates infection of cells by rhinovirus 14 but not poliovirus (20). Infection of cells by poliovirus is therefore not dependent on either low pH or clathrin-mediated endocytosis.

Structural Alterations Associated with Cell Entry

When poliovirus is bound at physiological temperatures to cells expressing Pvr, irreversible conformational changes in the virus occur that result in production of the altered or A particle (24, 35). The native to A particle conversion can also be induced by solubilized Pvr (36) or the soluble ectodomain of Pvr in the absence of cells (2, 46, 76). The A particle differs from the native particle in sedimentation rate (135S versus 160S for the native virion) and antigenicity (19). In contrast to the virion, which is soluble and stable to proteases, the A particle is sensitive to proteases and is highly hydrophobic (27). Myristoyl-VP4 and the N-terminal extension of the capsid protein VP1, both of which are in the interior of the native virion, are external in the A particle (27), and the exposed amino-terminal extension of VP1, which is predicted to form an amphipathic helix, has been shown to make the A particle capable of attaching to liposomes (27). Insertion of the N terminus of VP1 (and perhaps the myristoyl group of VP4) into the membrane may facilitate cell entry either by disrupting a membrane or by forming a pore through which the RNA is extruded.

Transient and reversible exposure of VP4 and the N-terminal extension of VP1 occurs when the virus is at physiological temperatures (but not room temperature) in a process that has been termed "breathing" (40). Breathing provides striking evidence for the dynamic nature of the poliovirus capsid and suggests that the virus is primed to undergo the more extensive, concerted, and irreversible changes associated with receptor binding.

In a typical experimental infection, a significant fraction (from 10 to 90% depending on conditions) of the A particle subsequently elutes from cells in what is thought to represent an abortive infection (24, 35). However, the A particle is also the predominant cell-associated form of the virus early in infection (within the first 20 to 30 min) (22, 41). At later times postinfection the levels of A particles begin to decrease. Although there is no direct proof of a product precursor relationship in vivo, the timing of the disappearance of the A particle is correlated with the appearance of a second altered form of the virus that has lost its RNA and now sediments at 80S (27). The trigger for conversion to the 80S form is not known, but it does not require receptor. Although there is still considerable controversy concerning the role of the two particles, the A particle may be an intermediate in the cell entry pathway, and the 80S empty particle may be the final protein product that accumulates after the RNA is released into the cytoplasm to initiate translation and replication.

Is the A Particle a Cell Entry Intermediate?

Several lines of evidence suggest that the A particle is an intermediate in the entry of poliovirus into cells. Compounds that bind to the capsid and stabilize the virion, preventing the virion to A particle conversion, have significant antiviral activity (28). Several properties of the A particle, including kinetics of appearance and disappearance, and the ability of the A particle to attach to (27) and to form channels in membranes (67), are consistent with a role in both entry and release. The A particle is infectious, although Pvr is not required for its infectivity (18). The low efficiency of infection with the A particle —nearly four orders of magnitude lower than that of virions—can be significantly enhanced by preincubating the A particles with non-neutralizing antibodies and infecting cells expressing the Fc receptor (32). These findings suggest that the low infectivity of the A particle is largely attrib-

---

FIGURE 1 Structural features of poliovirus. (A) Electron micrograph of negatively stained poliovirus, magnification ×270,000. Courtesy of N. Cheng and D. M. Belnap, NIH. (B) Schematic of the poliovirus capsid, showing the arrangement of VP1, VP2, and VP3; VP4 is on the interior. The biological protomer (gray) is not the same as the icosahedral asymmetric subunit (triangle at right). (C) Diagram of the wedge-like structure formed by eight β-strands of each capsid protein. Also shown are ribbon diagrams of poliovirus VP1, VP2, and VP3. Adapted from J. M. Hogle et al., *Science* 229:1358–1365, 1985, with permission. (D) Model of poliovirus type 1, based on X-ray crystallographic structure determined at 2.9 Å (31). The model is highlighted by radial depth cuing so that portions of the model farthest from the center are bright. The fivefold axis of symmetry (5×) is characterized by a star-shaped mesa. Surrounding the fivefold axis is the canyon, which is the receptor-binding site. At the threefold axis is a propeller-shaped feature. (E) Model of poliovirus type 1 (20 Å), made by image reconstruction from cryo-electron microscopy data. The star-shaped mesa, canyon, and propeller are visible.

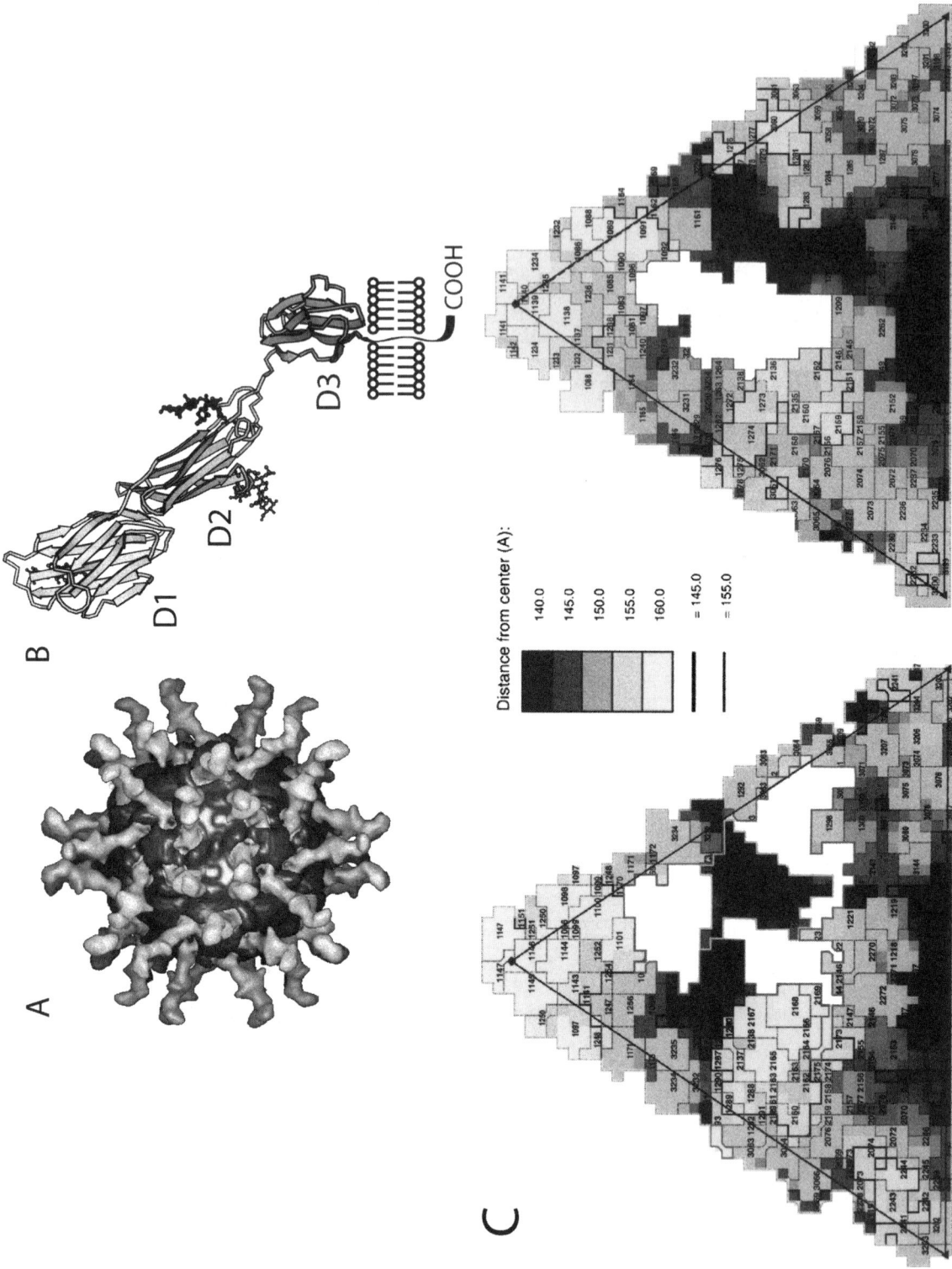

FIGURE 2 Interaction of poliovirus with its cellular receptor, Pvr. (A) Image reconstruction of poliovirus type 1 and a soluble form of Pvr (7). Only domain 1 of Pvr binds in the canyon of the virus; there are 60 receptor-binding sites on the viral capsid. (B) Model of Pvr produced from homology modeling and the density map from cryo-electron microscopy data of the virus-receptor complex (7). Ig-like domains are labeled. Carbohydrate side chains have been modeled on domains 1 and 2. (C) "Roadmap" view of poliovirus 1 (left) and rhinovirus 14 (right). The corresponding triangular area of the capsid surface, bounded by a fivefold and two threefold icosahedral symmetry axes, is shown. The radial distances of surface residues from the virion center are coded by different shades of gray. Receptor footprints (Pvr on poliovirus, ICAM-1 on rhinovirus 14) are white.

utable to the lack of a receptor to bring the particle to high concentration at the cell surface.

The role of the A particle as an intermediate in poliovirus entry has been questioned, based on the observation that poliovirus can replicate in cells at 25°C without detectable A particle formation (21). Although this observation raises an important caveat concerning the role of the A particle in entry, the failure to observe an intermediate in a steady-state process in cell entry does not necessarily imply that the intermediate does not exist. In a steady-state process, an intermediate is expected to accumulate to appreciable levels only if a rate-limiting step in the pathway occurs downstream of the putative intermediate. The accumulation of the A particle at 37°C but not at 25°C could be explained if the rate-limiting step in the cell entry process at physiological temperatures is downstream of the A particle (e.g., RNA release). At 25°C the conversion of virus to A particles becomes rate limiting, and the A particle would not accumulate because it would be used as quickly as it is produced. The results of experiments in which the kinetics of RNA release are determined at 37 and 25°C after infection with virions or 135S particles are consistent with this hypothesis (32).

In Vitro Production of Altered Particles

The conversion of native virions to A particles and the conversion of A particles to 80S particles can be induced in the absence of receptor by warming the particle in hypotonic buffers in the presence of millimolar levels of calcium ions. Like the receptor-mediated conversion of native virus to A particles, the thermal-mediated conversion is inhibited by the capsid-binding antiviral agents (69). The temperature required to convert the A particle to 80S is significantly higher than the temperature required for the conversion of native virion to A particle, and a direct precursor-product relationship between the A particle and the 80S particle has been demonstrated (Curry, Hiremath, and Hogle, unpublished data). In the absence of calcium, the native virion is converted directly to the 80S particle, suggesting that calcium is required to stabilize the A particle. Depletion of calcium at some stage during the normal entry process may therefore serve as a trigger for RNA release. The ability to recapitulate these conformational alterations by warming the virion provides a convenient assay system for studying the kinetics of the virion to A particle conversion as a function of temperature and has led to four important observations (68, 69).

1. The virion is kinetically trapped. The dependence on high temperature for Pvr-independent conversion of native virus to A particles suggests that there is a high activation energy for this step, consistent with a model in which the virus is kinetically trapped in a metastable state. The kinetics of the thermal-induced virion to A particle conversion as a function of temperature support this model. The rate of the conversion displays a very steep temperature dependence and is consistent with an activation energy barrier of ~140 kcal/mol.

2. The receptor facilitates conversion by lowering the activation barrier. The dependence of Pvr-independent conversion on elevated temperature suggests that the receptor might facilitate the conversion at physiological temperature by lowering the activation barrier. Analysis of the kinetics of the receptor-mediated conversion as a function of temperature confirms that Pvr produces a significant enhancement of the rate, such that the rate becomes biologically relevant at physiological temperatures. The data also demonstrate that Pvr lowers the activation barrier for the reaction by nearly 50 kcal/mol. Pvr therefore acts much like a classical transition state catalyst.

3. Capsid-binding antiviral agents stabilize virus via entropic effects. As a corollary to the original proposal that receptor would facilitate conversion by lowering the activation barrier, we proposed that the capsid-binding antiviral agents that prevent the conversion at physiological temperatures would stabilize the virions by raising the activation barrier of conversion (12). A model based on this prediction suggests that the antiviral agents act like a peg to make the capsid structurally rigid. Surprisingly, kinetic studies of the thermal-mediated transition show that the capsid-binding antiviral agents have no effect on the activation barrier (an enthalpic term) and suggest that the drugs act via entropic stabilization of the virion. These experimental studies are consistent with computational studies of rhinovirus that show that capsid-binding drugs increase rather than decrease the compressibility of the virus, providing a higher density of low-energy states to the virion (64).

4. The receptor-catalyzed reaction proceeds through an activated intermediate. Although inhibition of Pvr-independent conversion of virions to A particles by capsid-binding antiviral drugs is mediated through entropic effects, the inhibition of the Pvr-mediated pathway includes both enthalpic and entropic contributions. These results can only be explained if the receptor-mediated pathway proceeds via an intermediate not present in the receptor-independent pathway. By analogy with classic enzyme kinetic models, we propose that this intermediate represents an activated receptor virus complex in which the virus (and possibly receptor) has undergone conformational changes to switch from an initial complex to a "tight-binding" complex (68). This proposal is also consistent with the finding of two affinities of poliovirus for Pvr, with the low-affinity site dominating at low temperature and the prevalence of the high-affinity site increasing with higher temperature (46). In contrast to classic models in enzymology in which tight-binding complexes are "slow-binding" (the result of the enzyme closing down on the substrate) where a reduction in k_{on} is more than compensated for by a very large reduction in k_{off}, the tight-binding mode for the Pvr-poliovirus complex is characterized by a significant increase in k_{on}, which more than compensates for a small increase in k_{off}. This observation suggests that the tight-binding mode for the Pvr-poliovirus complex results from opening of the receptor-binding site on the virus, making it more accessible to Pvr.

Assembly

Upon release into the cytoplasm, the single open reading frame of the viral RNA is translated to produce a polyprotein that is processed cotranslationally by viral proteases to yield the viral proteins. The polyprotein is myristoylated at its N terminus. An early cotranslational cleavage of the polyprotein by the viral 2A^{pro} protease releases a precursor protein P1 from the N terminus of the polyprotein. The P1 protein contains all of the capsid protein sequences. Subsequent cleavage of P1 by the viral protease 3CD^{pro} produces the capsid proteins VP1 and VP3 and the immature capsid protein myristoyl-VP0. This cleavage is associated with the assembly of the proteins into a pentameric intermediate, which spontaneously forms empty capsids containing 60 copies each of VP0, VP3, and VP1. The empty capsids and pentamers are apparently in equilibrium within the cell, and it has not been possible to determine whether RNA is encapsidated by pentamers or by insertion into the preformed empty capsids. Regardless, the encapsidation appears to be tightly linked to RNA replication as there is an absolute dependence of encapsidation on de novo synthesis of progeny RNA (52). Encapsidation may lead to the formation of a precursor called the provirion that contains the RNA and 60 copies each of VP0, VP3, and VP1. Processing of the immature protein myristoyl-VP0 to yield myristoyl-VP4 and VP2 is associated with encapsidation of the RNA. There is no known protease requirement for this cleavage, and it is thought to be autocatalytic, depending only on the capsid proteins themselves and perhaps the viral RNA. Cleavage of VP0 to form the virion is associated with a significant increase in the stability of the particle (5).

SNAPSHOTS OF THE CELL ENTRY PATHWAY

We have attempted to obtain structural "snapshots" of stable intermediates in the poliovirus cell entry pathway and to couple the structural information with the results of genetic, biophysical, and biochemical observations to fill in the gaps in the pathway. The structural snapshots begin with the virus structure, which has been determined at high resolution by X-ray crystallographic methods, and also includes a high-resolution structure of the empty capsid assembly intermediate and low-resolution structures of the virus-receptor complex, the A particle, and the 80S particle.

The Virion

The protein shell of the poliovirus capsid is composed of 60 copies of the four capsid proteins VP1, VP2, VP3, and VP4 arranged on an icosahedral surface (Fig. 1B). The three large capsid proteins (VP1, VP2, and VP3) share a common fold (an eight-stranded β-barrel) (Fig. 1C) (31) that is also seen in a number of other plant, insect, and animal viruses (58). The β-barrel cores of the capsid proteins are decorated with unique loops connecting the β-strands and unique C-terminal and rather long N-terminal extensions. The β-barrel cores of the proteins make up the closed shell of the virus with the narrow end of VP1 packing around the fivefold axes and the narrow end of VP2 and VP3 alternating around the threefold axes.

The shape of the structure formed by the cores alone is very similar among all picornaviruses. The outer surface of the shell is decorated by the connecting loops and C-terminal extensions, which confer unique surface structure to each virus. The outer surface of the virus is dominated by star-shaped mesas at the fivefold axes and a threefold propeller-like structure (Fig. 1D, E). These prominent surface features are punctuated by depressions surrounding the fivefold axes and crossing the twofold axes. The depressions surrounding the star-shaped mesa at the fivefold axes are joined to form a moat-like canyon, which is the site of receptor attachment in poliovirus and some rhinoviruses (Fig. 2).

At the base of the canyon there is an opening into the hydrophobic core of capsid protein VP1 (Fig. 3). In poliovirus, other enteroviruses, and most rhinoviruses, the hydrophobic pocket is occupied by a fatty acid-like ligand or "pocket factor" that has been modeled as sphingosine, palmitate, or other shorter-chain fatty acids (25, 26, 37, 51, 62). The results of genetic analyses suggest that the pocket factor may regulate the thermal stability of the virion (50). The hydrophobic pocket is also the binding site for the capsid-binding antiviral agents.

The N-terminal extensions of VP1, VP2, and VP3, together with VP4, decorate the inner surface of the protein shell, forming an elaborate network that contributes substantially to the protein-protein interactions stabilizing the protein shell. A particularly striking feature of this network is an interaction formed by five copies of the N terminus of VP3 as they intertwine around the fivefold axis to form cylindrically parallel β-sheets. This "β-tube" is cradled by five copies of the myristoyl moiety at the N terminus of VP4 and is flanked on its inner surface by five copies of a short three-stranded β-sheet consisting of two strands from the N terminus of VP4 and one strand that is believed to represent residues from the extreme N terminus of VP1. The β-tube forms a plug on the inner surface of the shell that blocks a solvent-filled channel separating the five copies of VP1 as they pack around the fivefold axis (Fig. 3).

The Empty Capsid Assembly Intermediate

An intermediate consisting of 60 copies of VP0, VP3, and VP1 and sedimenting at 73S accumulates to low levels in cells infected with some picornaviruses (reviewed in reference 59). When properly isolated, this particle is antigenically indistinguishable from virus and can be completely dissociated to assemble competent 14S pentamers by treatment at slightly alkaline pH (pH 8.3). The 73S particles are very unstable and readily converted to a faster sedimenting, nondissociable particle with altered antigenicity by exposure to room temperature or extremes of ionic strength. Levels of the 73S empty capsid can be increased significantly by adding to cells at 2 to 3 h postinfection millimolar levels of guanidine, an inhibitor of RNA replication. The outer surface and the protein shell of the 73S empty capsid intermediate and the native virion are virtually identical (5). However, the network formed by the VP4 and the N-terminal extensions of the other capsid proteins is almost completely disrupted. With the exception of the N-terminal extension of VP3 (including the β-tube) and the N terminus of VP4, the peptide segments contributing to the internal network are either rearranged or completely disordered in 73S empty capsids. The disruption of the network abrogates interactions between pentamers, accounting for the ability to dissociate 73S capsids into pentamers. Disruption of the network also eliminates extensive contacts between VP1, VP2, and VP3 within a protomer (the copies derived from proteolysis of the capsid precursor P1) and between protomers in the pentamer. The loss of these critical interactions may explain the decreased stability of the 73S empty capsid compared to the native virus. Conversely, the additional stabilizing interactions provided by the network as it forms subsequent to VP0 cleavage is expected to play a critical role in locking the virus in its metastable state.

One portion of the network that is ordered in the empty capsids, but in a position substantially different from that observed in the virus, is the region spanning the scissile bond of VP0 (corresponding to the C terminus of VP4 and the N terminus of VP2 in the virion). In the empty capsids the peptide segment spanning the scissile bond is located nearly 25 Å away from the site occupied by the C terminus of VP4 and the N terminus of VP2 in the virion. The amino acids spanning the scissile bond pass over the top of a depression or pocket in the inner surface of the protein shell, below the interface between VP2 and VP3 from a single protomer. In the virion this depression is filled with

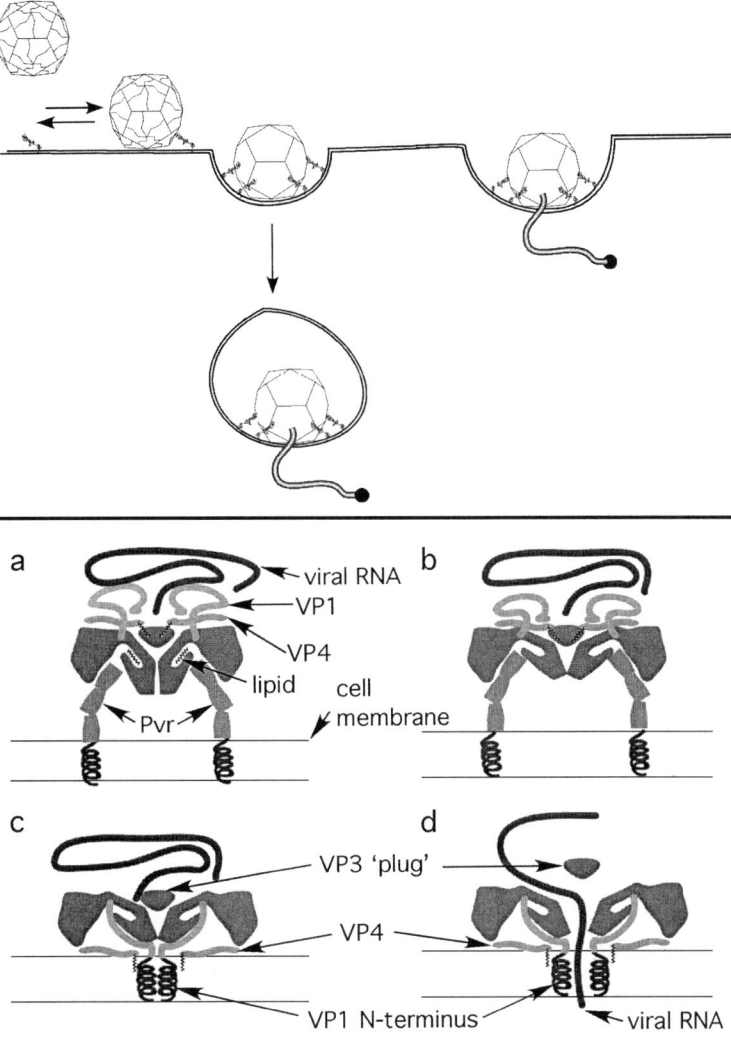

FIGURE 3 Models for poliovirus entry into cells. (Top) Overview. The 160S native virion binds to the cell receptor, Pvr, and at temperatures greater than 33°C is converted to the A particle. The viral RNA (curved line) might exit the particle from the plasma membrane or from within vesicles, although clathrin-mediated endocytosis is not required for poliovirus entry. (Bottom) Hypothetical mechanism for translocation of poliovirus RNA across the cell membrane. (a) Cross section of the initial virus-receptor complex. The viral RNA is in the capsid, and lipid occupies the hydrophobic pocket. (b) Docking of the receptor in the canyon leads to loss of the lipid in the hydrophobic pocket, allowing the capsid to undergo conformational changes including the externalization of VP4 and the N terminus of VP1. (c) Five copies of the N terminus of VP1 insert into the membrane and form a channel by a mechanism that may be facilitated by myristoyl-VP4. (d) Later in the entry process VP1 moves away from the fivefold axis, the five amphipathic helices rotate, and the internal plug formed by the N termini of VP3 moves, resulting in the formation of a channel through which the viral RNA may pass.

a loop of the N-terminal extension of VP1 (residues 44–56), which is covered on the inner surface by residues from the C terminus of VP4. Interactions of this loop of VP1 with the inner surface of VP2 and VP3 would be expected to contribute significantly to the stability of the capsid. Without these contacts, the interactions between VP2 and VP3 within a protomer are restricted to a thin band at the outer edge of the interface joining their β-barrel cores. Alterations in this loop of VP1, together with changes on the inner surface of the core of VP2 and residues that contact VP2 in the C-terminal half of VP4, cause a wide variety of phenotypes, including alteration of thermal stability, resistance to or dependence on capsid-binding drugs, mouse adaptation, and resistance to neutralization by soluble Pvr (reviewed in reference 12). These findings suggest that these amino acids play an important role in regulating structural transitions of the virus during cell entry.

In the empty capsid, amino acids spanning the scissile bond block access to the N terminus of VP1, suggesting that cleavage of VP0 is absolutely required for the completion of this portion of the network. This observation leads to a model in which the cleavage and subsequent rearrangement of VP4 and the N-terminal extensions of VP1 and VP2 are responsible for locking the virus in the metastable state. Some of the last segments of the network to be put in place (VP4 and the N terminus of VP1) are externalized reversibly when the virus "breathes" and irreversibly in receptor-mediated conformational rearrangements early in the entry process, consistent with the suggestion that cleavage and reorganization may also prime the virus for conformational changes required for cell entry. Analysis of thermal-induced conformational changes in the empty capsid demonstrates that exposure of sequences corresponding to VP4 cannot take place unless VP0 is cleaved (4). This process can be viewed as analogous to setting a mousetrap.

The Virus Receptor Complex

Structures of picornavirus-receptor complexes that have been solved at low resolution (15 to 25 Å) by image reconstruction analysis of cryo-electron micrographs include rhinoviruses 14 and 16 and coxsackievirus A21 bound to intercellular adhesion molecule 1 (ICAM-1) (39, 53, 73), poliovirus 1 (Mahoney) bound to Pvr (7, 29, 74), and rhinovirus 2 bound to the LDL receptor (30). Both Pvr and ICAM-1, Ig-like molecules with three and five domains, respectively, bind in the canyon of their cognate viruses, in agreement with the results of mutational analyses (13–15). However, the footprints of the receptors on the virus surface and the geometry of approach of the receptor to the virus surface differ greatly. ICAM-1 approaches the canyon of rhinoviruses and coxsackievirus A21 radially with only the far end of the first (membrane distal) domain contacting the virus. In contrast, Pvr approaches the virus surface more tangentially (Fig. 2). The far end of domain 1 contacts the base of the canyon, and one lateral surface of domain 1 contacts VP3 and the C terminus of VP1 in the southeast corner of the "roadmap" representation shown in Fig. 2. The greater area of contact of Pvr on poliovirus (1,300 $Å^2$) compared with ICAM-1 on rhinovirus (900 $Å^2$) might account for the greater association rate (k_{on}) reported for the poliovirus-Pvr complex (46, 74). There is no evidence for significant conformational changes in poliovirus (13), coxsackievirus, or rhinovirus upon receptor attachment. However, the complexes were prepared at low temperatures and may therefore represent only the initial binding mode.

The structure of poliovirus bound to Pvr has been solved independently in three different laboratories. Although the reconstructions are very similar, the orientation of domain 1 in the models differs significantly. At least two of the models must be wrong, a sobering reminder of the difficulty of building models at relatively low resolution.

Not all picornavirus receptors interact with canyons on the virus surface. The receptor for minor group rhinoviruses, VLDL-R, binds at the top of the star-shaped mesa at the fivefold axis, interacting primarily with residues from the BC and the HI loop of VP1 (30). Both the Arg-Gly-Asp (RGD) sequence of VP1 that is the binding site for the integrin receptor for foot-and-mouth disease virus (45) and a high-affinity heparan sulfate binding site used by cell culture-adapted strains of this virus (34) are highly exposed on the surface of the virus.

Why is the receptor-binding site for poliovirus and for major group rhinoviruses located in a deep invagination in the virus surface, while the receptor-binding sites for minor group rhinoviruses and FMDV are located on highly exposed surfaces? The answer may rest in differences in the roles played by the receptors for these different viruses. Both rhinovirus 2 and FMDV require acidification for productive cell entry, and the receptors for these viruses act only as a "hook" to increase the concentration of virus at the surface of the target cell. In contrast, the receptors for poliovirus and the major group rhinoviruses also act as an "unzipper," by triggering conformational changes that are necessary for subsequent events in entry. To induce such changes, receptor binding must provide sufficient energy to overcome the kinetic barrier that holds the virus in its native conformation. Since the binding energy is roughly proportional to the area of contact between virus and receptor, a virus whose receptor served the dual function of hook and unzipper should have a larger area of contact with its receptor than a virus whose receptor served only as a hook. There are two ways to increase the area of contact between a virus and a receptor: by using a large receptor that envelops a significant portion of the virus or by having the receptor bind in a deep depression in the virus surface.

Structures of Two Putative Cell Entry Intermediates

Structures of the A particle and the 80S empty particle solved at low resolution (22 to 23 Å) by cryo-electron microscopy (6) differ significantly from either a low-resolution surface generated from the high-resolution model of the virion or a reconstruction of the virion at comparable resolution. The effects of the structural alterations are especially apparent when viewing the star-shaped mesa or the three-bladed propeller down the fivefold or threefold axes, respectively (Fig. 4). The 135S and 80S particles are somewhat (~4%) larger than native virus.

Models for the coat protein subunits have been docked into the resulting reconstructions and refined using methods that are analogous to the approaches used to refine high-resolution crystallographic structures. Due to the limited resolution, the modeling and refinement have assumed that the individual capsid proteins move as rigid bodies. Despite this approximation, the models exhibit a remarkable fit to the reconstruction density, with the exception of several large loops (e.g., the GH loop of VP1) and VP4 and the N-terminal extension of VP1 that are known to be reorganized and either fully (VP4) or partially (N terminus of VP1) externalized in the altered particles.

Comparison of the models suggests that the virion to A particle transition is accompanied by shifts in all three of the major capsid proteins (VP1, VP2, and VP3). In the model for the A particle the subunits of VP1 have undergone a movement much like the opening of an umbrella, with the tips of the subunits at the fivefold axes serving as a pivot and the wide end of the subunit (that forms the north wall and part of the base of the canyon) moving radially outward. VP2 and VP3 undergo a similar movement, in this case with the narrow ends of the subunit pivoting about the threefold axes and the wide ends pivoting outward radially. VP1, VP3, and VP2 also undergo significant tangential reorientation (in the plane of the virus surface) with the tangential shifts of VP2 being largest. As a result of the umbrella-like motions, the base of the canyon is moved outward appreciably, giving the particle a much more angular appearance, especially when viewed down the twofold axes. In this view both the models and

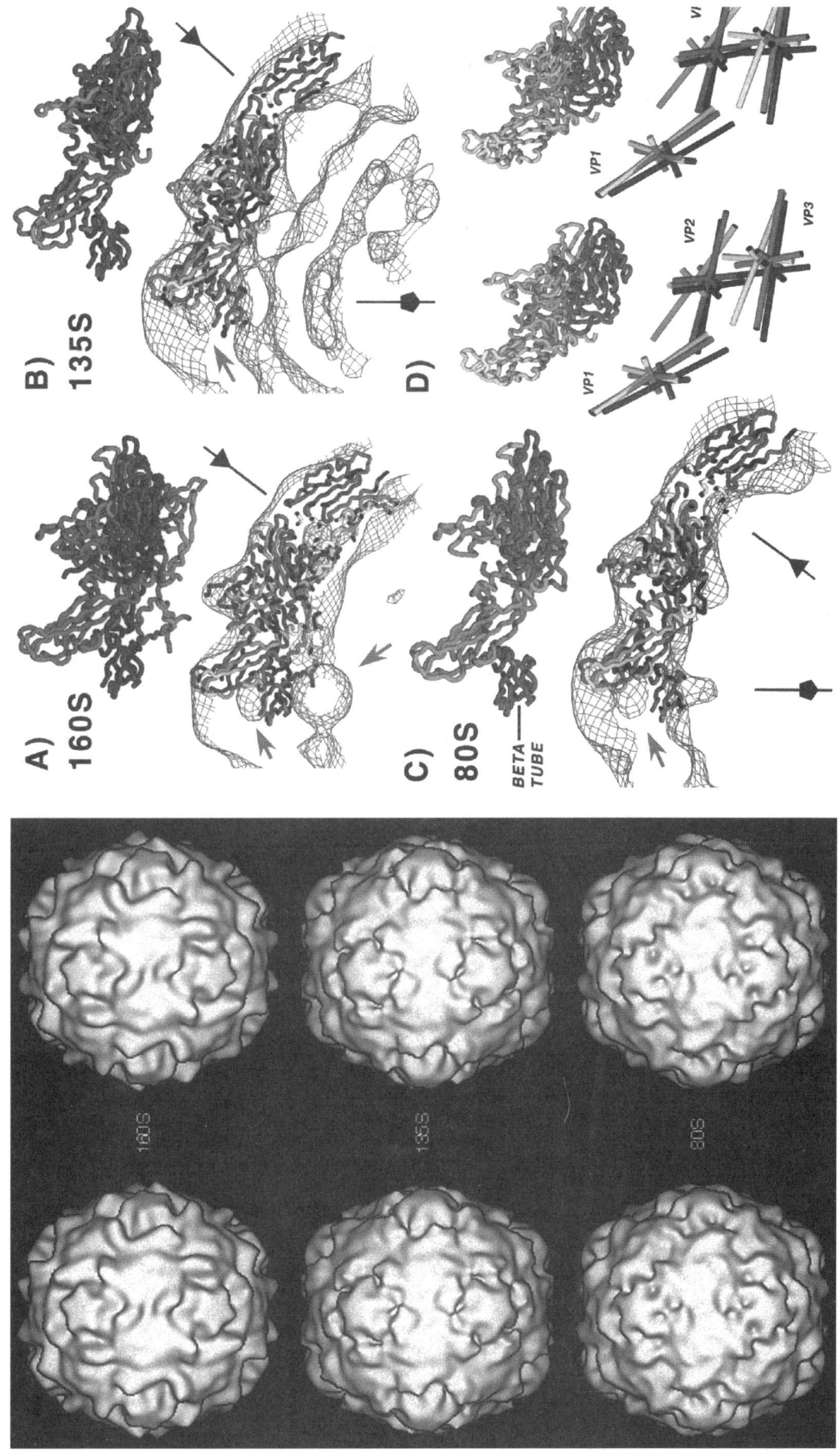

FIGURE 4 Structures of poliovirus A (135S) and 80S particles. Stereo views of reconstructions of the 160S, 135S, and 80S particles (6) are shown in the left panel. Pseudo-atomic models for each of the forms of the virus were derived by fitting the atomic model of the capsid proteins derived from X-ray crystallographic studies of the 160S particle (31) to the low-resolution reconstruction density, treating each of the capsid proteins, VP1, VP2, and VP3, as rigid bodies. The models for the capsid proteins of one protomer for (A) the 160S particle, (B) the 135S particle, and (C) the 80S particles and their fit to the reconstruction densities are shown in the panel on the right. The fivefold axis (pentagons) and threefold axis (triangles) are indicated. In (D) the individual capsid proteins for the 160S particle (dark gray), 135S particle (light gray), and 80S particle (intermediate gray) are represented as simple stick models. Note that there is significant density in all three reconstructions that corresponds to the VP3 β-tube plug at the fivefold axes (gray arrows).

the reconstructions take on a distinctly hexagonal appearance, in sharp contrast to the virion, which appears roughly spherical in all views. The movement of VP1 also opens gaps at the base of the canyon between fivefold related copies of VP1. The separation is apparent in the reconstructions (the density is noticeably thinner) but is not sufficient to result in the appearance of "holes" in the density at 22-Å resolution.

In the models for the 80S particle the subunits have undergone a partial reversal of the structural rearrangements that characterized the virion to A particle transition (Fig. 4). The orientations of VP2 and VP3 in the 80S particle are very similar to their orientations in the virion. In contrast, the orientation of VP1 remains similar to that seen in the A particle.

Based on analogies with several other viruses, it has been proposed that VP4 and the N terminus of VP1 exit the virion via a channel at the fivefold axes during the N to A transition (57). The model is attractive since it would place five copies of the N terminus of VP1 (which is predicted to form an amphipathic helix) in a position where they could interact and insert into the membrane to form a helical channel. However, as discussed above, this channel is plugged at its base on the inside surface of the virion by a "plug" consisting of a β-tube formed as five copies of the N terminus of VP3 interdigitate around the fivefold axis (Fig. 3). In all three reconstructions (virion, A particle, and 80S) there is clear density indicating that the VP3 plug occludes the channel. Moreover, there is no space in the channel in either the A particle or 80S particle reconstruction for five copies of that portion of the N terminus of VP1 which must remain after the extreme N-terminal segment has been externalized.

An alternative model for the egress of VP4 and the N terminus of VP1 is based on analogy with structurally related plant viruses that undergo a significant (~10%) expansion when exposed to slightly basic pH in the presence of chelators of divalent cations (33). Structures of the expanded state of tomato bushy stunt virus and cowpea chlorotic mottle virus (56, 65) reveal that expansion is characterized by a coordinated rotation and outward movement of the subunits that are analogous to VP2 and VP3 along the threefold axes, and rotation and outward movement of the subunits analogous to VP1 along the fivefold axes. These coordinated movements result in the opening of large holes at the interfaces between the capsid protein subunits, at positions that are structurally analogous to the base of the canyon in the picornaviruses. In the case of the tomato bushy stunt virus, it has been shown that the amino-terminal domains of two of the capsid protein subunits exit through this pore upon expansion. The extrusion of the N-terminal domains is reversible if the particles are "shrunk" by gradually lowering the pH, but the N terminus is trapped outside if the particle is "shrunk" by rapid acidification.

Mutations in the interfaces of poliovirus that are analogous to the interfaces that are disrupted during expansion of the plant viruses have been shown to have a variety of effects on viral stability, on the ability of the virus to recognize suboptimal receptors, and on the sensitivity of the virus to neutralization by soluble receptor (14–17, 25, 49). Although the capsid protein movements are less pronounced in the virion to A particle transition of poliovirus than in the expansion of the plant viruses, the umbrella-like movements of VP1, VP2, and VP3 result in significant gaps between the models for the subunits at the base of the canyon in positions that are entirely analogous to the larger openings seen in the plant viruses. Inspection of the reconstruction density in the vicinity of the gaps (which are located where the N-terminal extension of VP1 leaves the β-barrel core and enters the interior of the virion) suggests that the N-terminal extension of VP1 may exit through this gap and proceed up the outer surface of the mesa at the fivefold axis (Fig. 3). This model is attractive as it would locate five copies of the presumed amphipathic helix at the N terminus of VP1 close together such that they could form a fivefold helical bundle once inserted into the membrane.

A notable feature of the reconstructions of the A particle and the 80S particle is the lack of openings in the viral surface that would be large enough to allow the facile extrusion of VP4 and the N-terminal extensions of VP1 in the N to A transition or the RNA in the A to 80S transition. Given the large shift in sedimentation coefficient (135S for the A particle versus 160S for the virion), we had anticipated a much more significant expansion (on the order of 10 to 15%). We, therefore, postulate that there are additional, as yet undetected, intermediates in the pathway between the virion and the A particle, and between the A particle and the 80S particle. Such particles should be sufficiently expanded to create openings for the release of the VP4 and the N terminus of VP1 during the native to altered particle transition, and release of RNA during the A particle to 80S transition. The additional intermediate in the native to altered particle pathway would be analogous to the expanded form of plant viruses, and the A particle would correspond to the quenched form of the expanded plant virus in which the N-terminal arm is trapped outside the particle. The transient and reversible externalization of the N terminus of VP1 that occurs when the virus "breathes" may indicate a reversible equilibrium between the virion and the new intermediate that is analogous to the expansion and slow acidification transition that returns the N-terminal arm to the inside of the particle in the plant viruses.

The nature of the intermediate linking the A particle and the 80S particle is less clear. Nonetheless, some factor must dictate that the RNA be released from a unique site in an otherwise icosahedrally symmetric particle, lest the RNA and protein shell be tied in an inextricable knot. In the course of a natural infection one factor that could influence which site is chosen for RNA release could be the presence of membrane near one surface of the virus. However, the presence of membrane is not a necessary factor, since the RNA is efficiently released in the absence of membranes in vitro. Other factors that could regulate which of many otherwise equivalent sites is used could be steric factors (e.g., the proximity of a specific structure in the viral RNA, including perhaps the genome-linked protein VPg) or kinetic factors (e.g., a very slow initiation, followed by rapid release at the first initiation site that is established). Because the structures observed to date are symmetric, they tell us little about the site of release. The only clues from the structures that may indicate the site of RNA release are differences in the density of the RNA in the reconstructions of the virion and the A particle. The density in the interior region of the virion provides a view of the icosahedrally averaged structure of the linear genome. The appearance of the average RNA structure differs in the virion and the A particle, with the RNA making a closer approach to the fivefold axis in the A particle.

A WORKING MODEL FOR POLIOVIRUS CELL ENTRY

On the basis of structural, genetic, and biochemical evidence available to date, we propose a working model for the cell entry of poliovirus, related enteroviruses, and major group rhinoviruses (Fig. 3). The first step in the entry pathway is the formation of an initial binding complex with the receptor. The formation of this complex requires no significant conformational alterations in either the virus or the receptor, and would be the predominant and perhaps only form of the complex when binding is done at low temperatures. The published virus-receptor structures likely represent this form of the complex. At physiological temperatures the formation of this initial complex may cause conformational changes in the virus (and perhaps the receptor), leading to tight binding.

In one model for the tight-binding complex, most of the initial contacts between virus and receptor involve the south wall of the canyon; subsequent structural changes in the virus cause VP1 to move away from the fivefold axis, pinching the canyon such that the receptor makes bridging contacts with both the north and south walls of the canyon, and opening the channel (57). Because pinching the canyon results in more extensive contacts with the receptor, the receptor should have a slow on rate and a much slower off rate. This prediction is contradicted by kinetic data for both poliovirus-Pvr and rhinovirus-ICAM-1 binding, which show that the tight complex is characterized by a fast off rate and a much faster on rate (46). The model also predicts that VP4 and the N terminus of VP1 are released through the newly opened fivefold channel, which is inconsistent with the structure of the A particle.

We propose an alternative model in which the transition from the initial binding complex to the tight-binding complex is characterized by movements of VP1, VP2, and VP3 that mimic the umbrella-like movements of the virion to A particle transition. Consistent with the kinetic data, these movements would open the receptor-binding site, providing for a faster association rate for binding additional receptors. This tight-binding site is detectable at room temperature but may be transient at physiological temperature. At physiological temperatures binding of multiple receptors destabilizes the particles, resulting in the release of the pocket factor as the particle begins to expand to form the first transient state, which permits the externalization of VP4 and the N terminus of VP1. Once these peptide segments are externalized, the particle undergoes a partial reversal of the expansion to form the A particle. At some time in this process, five copies of the N terminus of VP1 insert into the membrane by a mechanism that may be facilitated by the myristoyl group at the N terminus of VP4. The membrane-associated portions of VP1 then associate to form a channel composed of five amphipathic helices, each with its hydrophobic surface facing the membrane and its hydrophilic surface facing the interior of the channel. Later in the entry process a trigger results in a second round of expansion. In this expansion the wide end of VP1, VP2, and VP3 may serve as the pivot points for an umbrella-like movement of VP1 away from the fivefold axis, coupled with a rotation of the five amphipathic helices, and a movement of the internal plug formed by the N termini of VP3 to form a large channel through which RNA is released. After the RNA has been released the particle shrinks to form the 80S structure.

REFERENCES

1. Aoki, J., S. Koike, I. Ise, Y. Sato-Yoshia, and A. Nomoto. 1994. Amino acid residues on human poliovirus receptor involved in interaction with poliovirus. *J. Biol. Chem.* **269**:8431–8438.
2. Arita, M., S. Koike, J. Aoki, H. Horie, and A. Nomoto. 1998. Interaction of poliovirus with its purified receptor and conformational alteration in the virion. *J. Virol.* **72**:3578–3586.
3. Baker, K. A., R. E. Dutch, R. A. Lamb, and T. S. Jardetsky. 1999. Structural basis for paramyxovirus-mediated membrane fusion. *Mol. Cell* **3**:309–319.
4. Basavappa, R., A. Gomez-Yafal, and J. M. Hogle. 1998. The poliovirus empty capsid specifically recognizes the poliovirus receptor and undergoes some, but not all, of the transitions associated with cell entry. *J. Virol.* **72**:7551–7556.
5. Basavappa, R., R. Syed, O. Flore, J. P. Icenogle, D. J. Filman, and J. M. Hogle. 1994. Role and mechanism of the maturation cleavage of VP0 in poliovirus assembly: structure of the empty capsid assembly intermediate at 2.9 Å resolution. *Protein Sci.* **3**:1651–1669.
6. Belnap, D. M., D. J. Filman, B. L. Trus, N. Cheng, F. P. Booy, J. F. Conway, S. Curry, C. N. Hiremath, S. K. Tsang, A. C. Steven, and J. M. Hogle. 2000. Molecular tectonic model of virus structural transitions: the putative cell entry states of poliovirus. *J. Virol.* **74**:1342–1354.
7. Belnap, D. M., B. M. McDermott, Jr., D. J. Filman, N. Cheng, B. L. Trus, H. J. Zuccola, V. R. Racaniello, J. M. Hogle, and A. C. Steven. 2000. Three-dimensional structure of poliovirus receptor bound to poliovirus. *Proc. Natl. Acad. Sci. USA* **97**:73–78.
8. Bernhardt, G., J. A. Bibb, J. Bradley, and E. Wimmer. 1994. Molecular characterization of the cellular receptor for poliovirus. *Virology* **199**:105–113.
9. Bouchard, M. J., Y. Dong, B. M. McDermott, Jr., D. H. Lam, K. R. Brown, M. Shelanski, A. R. Bellve, and V. R. Racaniello. 2000. Defects in nuclear and cytoskeletal morphology and mitochondrial localization in spermatozoa of mice lacking nectin-2, a component of cell-cell adherens junctions. *Mol. Cell Biol.* **20**:2865–2873.
10. Bullough, P. A., F. M. Hughson, J. J. Skehel, and D. C. Wiley. 1994. Structure of influenza haemagglutinin at the pH of membrane fusion. *Nature* **371**:37–43.
11. Chan, D. C., D. Fass, J. M. Berger, and P. S. Kim. 1997. Core structure of gp41 from the HIV envelope glycoprotein. *Cell* **89**:263–273.
12. Chow, M., R. Basavappa, and J. M. Hogle. 1997. The role of conformational transitions in poliovirus pathogenesis, p. 157–186. *In* W. Chiu, R. Garcea, and R. Burnette (ed.), *Structural Biology of Viruses*. Oxford University Press, Oxford, United Kingdom.
13. Colonno, R., J. Condra, S. Mizutani, P. Callahan, M.-E. Davies, and M. Murcko. 1988. Evidence for the direct involvement of the rhinovirus canyon in receptor binding. *Proc. Natl. Acad. Sci. USA* **85**:5449–5453.
14. Colston, E., and V. R. Racaniello. 1994. Soluble receptor-resistant poliovirus mutants identify surface and internal capsid residues that control interaction with the cell receptor. *EMBO J.* **13**:5855–5862.
15. Colston, E. M., and V. R. Racaniello. 1995. Poliovirus variants selected on mutant receptor-expressing cells identify capsid residues that expand receptor recognition. *J. Virol.* **69**:4823–4829.
16. Couderc, T., N. Guédo, V. Calvez, I. Pelletier, J. Hogle, F. Colbère-Garapin, and B. Blondel. 1994. Substitutions in the capsids of poliovirus mutants selected in human neuroblastoma cells confer on the Mahoney type 1 strain

a phenotype neurovirulent in mice. *J. Virol.* **68:**8386–8391.
17. **Couderc, T., J. Hogle, H. Le Blay, F. Horaud, and B. Blondel.** 1993. Molecular characterization of mouse-virulent poliovirus type 1 Mahoney mutants: involvement of residues of polypeptides VP1 and VP2 located on the inner surface of the capsid protein shell. *J. Virol.* **67:**3808–3817.
18. **Curry, S., M. Chow, and J. M. Hogle.** 1996. The poliovirus 135S particle is infectious. *J. Virol.* **70:**7125–7131.
19. **De Sena, J., and B. Mandel.** 1977. Studies on the in vitro uncoating of poliovirus II. Characteristics of the membrane-modified particle. *Virology* **78:**554–566.
20. **DeTulleo, L., and T. Kurchhausen.** 1998. The clathrin endocytic pathway in viral infection. *EMBO J.* **17:**4585–4593.
21. **Dove, A. W., and V. R. Racaniello.** 1997. Cold-adapted poliovirus mutants bypass a postentry replication block. *J. Virol.* **71:**4728–4735.
22. **Everaert, L., R. Vrijsen, and A. Boeyé.** 1989. Eclipse products of poliovirus after cold-synchronized infection of HeLa cells. *Virology* **171:**76–82.
23. **Fass, D., S. C. Harrison, and P. S. Kim.** 1996. Retrovirus envelope domain at 1.7 angstrom resolution. *Nat. Struct. Biol.* **3:**465–469.
24. **Fenwick, M. L., and P. D. Cooper.** 1962. Early interactions between poliovirus and ERK cells. Some observations on the nature and significance of the rejected particles. *Virology* **18:**212–223.
25. **Filman, D. J., R. Syed, M. Chow, A. J. Macadam, P. D. Minor, and J. M. Hogle.** 1989. Structural factors that control conformational transitions and serotype specificity in type 3 poliovirus. *EMBO J.* **8:**1567–1579.
26. **Filman, D. J., M. W. Wien, J. A. Cunningham, J. M. Bergelson, and J. M. Hogle.** 1998. Structure determination of echovirus 1. *Acta Crystallogr. D Biol. Crystallogr.* **54:**1261–1272.
27. **Fricks, C. E., and J. M. Hogle.** 1990. The cell-induced conformational change of poliovirus: externalization of the amino terminus of VP1 is responsible for liposome binding. *J. Virol.* **64:**1934–1945.
28. **Grant, R. A., C. N. Hiremath, D. J. Filman, R. Syed, K. Andries, and J. M. Hogle.** 1994. Structures of poliovirus complexes with anti-viral drugs: implications for viral stability and drug design. *Curr. Biol.* **4:**784–797.
29. **He, Y., V. D. Bowman, S. Mueller, C. M. Bator, J. Bella, X. Peng, T. S. Baker, E. Wimmer, R. J. Kuhn, and M. G. Rossmann.** 2000. Interaction of the poliovirus receptor with poliovirus. *Proc. Natl. Acad. Sci. USA* **97:**79–84.
30. **Hewat, E. A., E. Neumann, J. F. Conway, R. Moser, B. Ronacher, T. C. Marlovits, and D. Blaas.** 2000. The cellular receptor to human rhinovirus 2 binds around the 5-fold axis and not in the canyon: a structural view. *EMBO J.* **19:**6317–6325.
31. **Hogle, J. M., M. Chow, and D. J. Filman.** 1985. Three-dimensional structure of poliovirus at 2.9 Å resolution. *Science* **229:**1358–1365.
32. **Huang, Y., J. M. Hogle, and M. Chow.** 2000. Is the 135S poliovirus particle an intermediate during cell entry? *J. Virol.* **74:**8757–8761.
33. **Incardona, N. L., and P. Kaesberg.** 1964. A pH-induced structural change in bromegrass mosaic virus. *Biophys. J.* **4:**11–21.
34. **Jackson, T., F. M. Ellard, R. A. Ghazaleh, S. M. Brookes, W. E. Blakemore, A. H. Corteyn, D. I. Stuart, J. W. Newman, and A. M. Q. King.** 1996. Efficient infection of cells in culture by type O foot-and-mouth disease virus requires binding to cell surface heparan sulfate. *J. Virol.* **70:**5282–5287.
35. **Joklik, W. K., and J. E. Darnell.** 1961. The absorption and early fate of purified poliovirus in HeLa cells. *Virology* **13:**439–447.
36. **Kaplan, G., M. S. Freistadt, and V. R. Racaniello.** 1990. Neutralization of poliovirus by cell receptors expressed in insect cells. *J. Virol.* **64:**4697–4702.
37. **Kim, S., T. J. Smith, M. S. Chapman, M. G. Rossmann, D. C. Pevear, F. J. Dutko, P. J. Felock, G. D. Diana, and M. A. McKinlay.** 1989. Crystal structure of human rhinovirus serotype 1A (HRV1A). *J. Mol. Biol.* **210:**91–111.
38. **Koike, S., I. Ise, and A. Nomoto.** 1991. Functional domains of the poliovirus receptor. *Proc. Natl. Acad. Sci. USA* **88:**4104–4108.
39. **Kolatkar, P. R., J. Bella, N. H. Olson, C. M. Bator, T. S. Baker, and M. G. Rossmann.** 1999. Structural studies of two rhinovirus serotypes complexed with fragments of their cellular receptor. *EMBO J.* **18:**6249–6259.
40. **Li, Q., A. G. Yafal, Y. H. Lee, J. Hogle, and M. Chow.** 1994. Poliovirus neutralization by antibodies to internal epitopes of VP4 and VP1 results from reversible exposure of these sequences at physiological temperature. *J. Virol.* **68:**3965–3970.
41. **Lonberg-Holm, K., L. B. Goser, and J. C. Kauer.** 1975. Early alteration of poliovirus in infected cells and its specific inhibition. *J. Gen. Virol.* **27:**329–342.
42. **Madshus, I. H., S. Olsnes, and K. Sandvig.** 1984. Mechanism of entry into the cytosol of poliovirus type 1: requirement for low pH. *J. Cell. Biol.* **98:**1194–1200.
43. **Malashkevich, V. N., D. C. Chan, C. T. Chutkowksi, and P. S. Kim.** 1998. Crystal structure of the simian immunodeficiency virus (SIV) gp41 core: conserved helical interactions underlie the broad inhibitory activity of gp41 peptides. *Proc. Natl. Acad. Sci. USA* **95:**9134–9139.
44. **Malashkevich, V. N., B. J. Schneider, M. L. McNally, M. A. Milhollen, J. X. Pang, and P. S. Kim.** 1999. Core structure of the envelope glycoprotein GP2 from Ebola virus at 1.9-Å resolution. *Proc. Natl. Acad. Sci. USA* **96:**2662–2667.
45. **Mason, P. W., E. Rieder, and B. Baxt.** 1994. RGD sequence of foot-and-mouth disease virus is essential for infecting cells via the natural receptor but can be bypassed by an antibody-dependent enhancement pathway. *Proc. Natl. Acad. Sci. USA* **91:**1932–1936.
46. **McDermott, B. M., Jr., A. H. Rux, R. J. Eisenberg, G. H. Cohen, and V. R. Racaniello.** 2000. Two distinct binding affinities of poliovirus for its cellular receptor. *J. Biol. Chem.* **275:**23089–23096.
47. **Morrison, M. E., and V. R. Racaniello.** 1992. Molecular cloning and expression of a murine homolog of the human poliovirus receptor gene. *J. Virol.* **66:**2807–2813.
48. **Morrison, M. E., Y. Yuan-Jing, M. W. Wien, J. W. Hogle, and V. R. Racaniello.** 1994. Homolog scanning mutagenesis reveals poliovirus receptor residues important for virus binding and replication. *J. Virol.* **68:**2578–2588.
49. **Moss, E. G., and V. R. Racaniello.** 1991. Host range determinants located on the interior of the poliovirus capsid. *EMBO J.* **10:**1067–1074.
50. **Mosser, A. G., and R. R. Rueckert.** 1993. WIN 51711-dependent mutants of poliovirus type 3: evidence that virions decay after release from cells unless drug is present. *J. Virol.* **67:**1246–1254.
51. **Muckelbauer, J. K., M. Kremer, I. Minor, G. Diana, F. J. Dutko, J. Groarke, D. C. Pevear, and M. G. Rossmann.** 1995. The structure of coxsackievirus B3 at 3.5 Å resolution. *Structure* **3:**653–667.
52. **Nugent, C. I., K. L. Johnson, P. Sarnow, and K. Kirkegaard.** 1999. Functional coupling between replication and packaging of poliovirus replicon RNA. *J. Virol.* **73:**427–435.

53. Olson, N. H., P. R. Kolatkar, M. A. Oliveira, R. H. Cheng, J. M. Greve, A. McClelland, T. S. Baker, and M. G. Rossmann. 1993. Structure of a human rhinovirus complexed with its receptor molecule. *Proc. Natl. Acad. Sci. USA* **90:**507–511.
54. Pérez, L., and L. Carrasco. 1993. Entry of poliovirus into cells does not require a low-pH step. *J. Virol.* **67:**4543–4548.
55. Racaniello, V. R. 2001. Picornaviridae: the viruses and their replication, p. 685–722. In P. Howley and D. Knipe (ed.), *Fields Virology*, 4th ed., vol. 1. Lippincott Williams & Wilkins, Philadelphia, Pa.
56. Robinson, I. K., and S. C. Harrison. 1982. Structure of the expanded state of tomato bushy stunt virus. *Nature* **297:**563–568.
57. Rossmann, M. G., J. Bella, P. R. Kolatkar, Y. He, E. Wimmer, R. J. Kuhn, and T. S. Baker. 2000. Cell recognition and entry by rhino- and enteroviruses. *Virology* **269:**239–247.
58. Rossmann, M. G., and J. E. Johnson. 1989. Icosahedral RNA virus structure. *Annu. Rev. Biochem.* **58:**533–573.
59. Rueckert, R. R. 1976. On the structure and morphogenesis of picornaviruses. *Compr. Virol.* **6:**131–200.
60. Selinka, H.-C., A. Zibert, and E. Wimmer. 1992. A chimeric poliovirus/CD4 receptor confers susceptibility to poliovirus on mouse cells. *J. Virol.* **66:**2523–2526.
61. Selinka, H.-C., A. Zibert, and E. Wimmer. 1991. Poliovirus can enter and infect mammalian cells by way of an intercellular adhesion molecule 1 pathway. *Proc. Natl. Acad. Sci. USA* **88:**3598–3602.
62. Smyth, M., J. Tate, E. Hoey, C. Lyons, S. Martin, and D. Stuart. 1995. Implications for viral uncoating from the structure of bovine enterovirus. *Struct. Biol.* **2:**224–231.
63. Spear, P. G., R. J. Eisenberg, and G. H. Cohen. 2000. Three classes of cell surface receptors for alphaherpesvirus entry. *Virology* **275:**1–8.
64. Speelman, B., B. R. Brooks, and C. B. Post. 2001. Molecular dynamics simulations of human rhinovirus and an antiviral compound. *Biophys J.* **80:**121–129.
65. Speir, J. A., S. Munshi, G. Wang, T. S. Baker, and J. E. Johnson. 1995. Structures of the native and swollen forms of cowpea chlorotic mottle virus determined by X-ray crystallography and cryo-electron microscopy. *Structure* **3:**63–78.
66. Takahashi, K., H. Nakanishi, M. Miyahara, K. Mandel, K. Satoh, A. Satoh, H. Nishioka, J. Aoki, A. Nomoto, A. Mizoguchi, and Y. Takai. 1999. Nectin/PRR: an immunoglobulin-like cell adhesion molecule recruited to cadherin-based adherens junctions through interaction with Afadin, a PDZ domain-containing protein. *J. Cell. Biol.* **145:**539–549.
67. Tosteson, M. T., and M. Chow. 1997. Characterization of the ion channels formed by poliovirus in planar lipid membranes. *J. Virol.* **71:**507–511.
68. Tsang, S., B. M. McDermott, V. R. Racaniello, and J. M. Hogle. 2001. A kinetic analysis of the effect of poliovirus receptor on viral uncoating: the receptor as a catalyst. *J. Virol.* **75:**4984–4989.
69. Tsang, S. K., P. Danthi, M. Chow, and J. M. Hogle. 2000. Stabilization of poliovirus by capsid-binding antiviral drugs is due to entropic effects. *J. Mol. Biol.* **296:**335–340.
70. Weissenhorn, W., A. Dessen, L. J. Calder, S. C. Harrison, J. J. Skehel, and D. C. Wiley. 1999. Structural basis for membrane fusion by enveloped viruses. *Mol. Membr. Biol.* **16:**3–9.
71. Weissenhorn, W., A. Dessen, S. C. Harrison, J. J. Skehel, and D. C. Wiley. 1997. Atomic structure of the ectodomain from HIV-1 gp41. *Nature* **387:**426–430.
72. Wilson, I. A., J. J. Skehel, and D. C. Wiley. 1981. Structure of the haemagglutinin membrane glycoprotein of influenza virus at 3 Å resolution. *Nature* **289:**366–373.
73. Xiao, C., C. M. Bator, V. D. Bowman, E. Rieder, Y. He, B. Hebert, J. Bella, T. S. Baker, E. Wimmer, R. J. Kuhn, and M. G. Rossmann. 2001. Interaction of coxsackievirus A21 with its cellular receptor, ICAM-1. *J. Virol.* **75:**2444–2451.
74. Xing, L., K. Tjarnlund, B. Lindqvist, G. G. Kaplan, D. Feigelstock, R. H. Cheng, and J. M. Casasnovas. 2000. Distinct cellular receptor interactions in poliovirus and rhinoviruses. *EMBO J.* **19:**1207–1216.
75. Zhao, X., M. Singh, V. N. Malashkevich, and P. S. Kim. 2000. Structural characterization of the human respiratory syncytial virus fusion protein core. *Proc. Natl. Acad. Sci. USA* **97:**14172–14177.
76. Zibert, A., H. C. Selinka, O. Elroy-Stein, and E. Wimmer. 1992. The soluble form of two N-terminal domains of the poliovirus receptor is sufficient for blocking viral infection. *Virus Res.* **25:**51–61.

Interaction of Major Group Rhinoviruses with Their Cellular Receptor, ICAM-1

RICHARD J. KUHN AND MICHAEL G. ROSSMANN

8

The first step in the virus life cycle is the interaction between the virus and the cellular receptor. This initial interaction is probably the most significant determinant of pathogenesis. For picornaviruses, the best studied virus-receptor interaction has been that of the major group rhinoviruses and their cellular receptor, intercellular adhesion molecule-1 (ICAM-1, CD54). The first atomic structure of an animal virus, rhinovirus 14 (HRV14), was solved in 1985 (35). An unusual feature found in rhinovirus was a surface depression, or canyon, 12 Å deep and between 12 and 15 Å wide that surrounded the fivefold axis. The base of the canyon consisted of conserved amino acid residues, whereas more variable residues could be found at the top of the canyon (37). The region surrounding the canyon was also found to be the binding site of neutralizing monoclonal antibodies (39). These observations prompted the suggestion that the canyon might serve as the receptor-binding site, being protected from antibody surveillance by steric restrictions (33, 35). The canyon hypothesis predicted the receptor molecule to be sufficiently narrow to penetrate the canyon and contact the conserved residues at its base. Several years following the structure determination of rhinovirus, the receptor for the major group of rhinoviruses was identified as ICAM-1 (12, 43). This molecule is a member of the immunoglobulin (Ig) superfamily of cell adhesion molecules and consists of five Ig-like extracellular domains. Subsequent studies employing cryo-electron microscopy (cryo-EM) and complexes of rhinovirus and ICAM-1 showed that the canyon is the binding site for the cellular receptor, as had been predicted (28). Nevertheless, Smith et al. (40; see also chapter 4, this volume) question the validity of the canyon hypothesis, preferring to suggest that the canyon evolved not in response to immune surveillance by the host, but as a requirement for the virus to display a region on its surface complementary to the shape of the cellular receptor.

The atomic structures of numerous picornaviruses have now been solved, and although there are several exceptions, many of them have depressions surrounding their fivefold vertices (for a review see chapter 3 in this volume). In addition, cryo-EM of virus-receptor complexes from poliovirus (with Pvr or CD155, the poliovirus receptor) (3, 16, 46), coxsackievirus A21 (CVA21) (with ICAM-1) (45), and coxsackievirus B3 (with the coxsackievirus-adenovirus receptor, CAR) (17) all demonstrate binding of their respective receptors into their canyons. In all three cases, the cellular receptor is an Ig superfamily member that has an extended shape that fits well within the canyon. The minor group rhinoviruses, defined by their failure to use ICAM-1 as a cellular receptor, use instead members of the low-density lipoprotein (LDL)-receptor family, including the very-low-density lipoprotein (VLDL) receptor (19, 24). Hewat et al. (18) have demonstrated with cryo-EM that the minor group rhinovirus HRV2 binds to the VLDL receptor on a small star-shaped dome present on the icosahedral fivefold axis of the virus. This is in spite of the fact that the minor group rhinoviruses also have a well-defined canyon surrounding their fivefold axes. Thus, although not universally used, the canyon is an important physical feature that many picornaviruses have utilized for attachment to their cognate cellular receptors (34). Those viruses that utilize canyon-binding receptors are destabilized upon receptor binding, whereas viruses that utilize receptors that bind in regions other than the canyon are not destabilized by binding. It, therefore, should be informative to examine the features of a receptor and a virus that use this canyon strategy for attachment and entry. In this chapter, we will look at a well-studied example of this interaction at a structural level, the interaction of the major group rhinoviruses with their cellular receptor, ICAM-1.

STRUCTURE OF ICAM

ICAM-1 is expressed on many cells involved in the immune and inflammatory response (41). Although its level of expression is normally low, cytokine stimulation can lead to enhanced levels required for adhesion of leukocytes to endothelial cells at sites of infection. This adhesion is mediated by ICAM-1 binding to its normal cellular ligands, leukocyte function-associated antigen-1 (LFA-1, CD11a/CD18) and macrophage-1 antigen (Mac-1, CD11b/CD18), both members of the integrin family of membrane proteins.

Richard J. Kuhn and Michael G. Rossmann ■ Department of Biological Sciences, Purdue University, West Lafayette, IN 47907-1392.

In addition to ICAM-1's role in binding the major group of human rhinoviruses, ICAM-1 has also been shown to serve as a receptor for coxsackieviruses A13, A18, and A21 (10) and for the malarial parasite, *Plasmodium falciparum* (4).

ICAM-1 is a type I membrane protein and consists of five Ig-like domains located on the extracellular side of the membrane, a transmembrane domain, and a short cytoplasmic domain (Fig. 1) (42). The protein is highly glycosylated, having four asparagine-linked sites on domain D2, and two on D3 and D4. Several close relatives of ICAM-1 have been identified and are named ICAM-2, -3, and -4. They share sequence identity with ICAM-1, similar adhesive properties mediated by LFA-1 binding, and yet are incapable of supporting rhinovirus infection (12, 43). Molecular genetic and structural studies have demonstrated that rhinoviruses bind to domain D1 of ICAM-1 (26–28, 30).

The atomic structures of several forms of the N-terminal two domains of ICAM-1 (D1D2) have been solved (2, 8, 22). Problems were originally encountered because of the high degree of glycosylation present on D2, but were overcome by either removal of three of the four sites or expression of the protein in a cell line that had a modified pathway for carbohydrate addition. Subsequently, the structure of a fully glycosylated form of the D1D2 domains of the protein was reported using molecular replacement (22). Despite these different crystal forms of the D1D2 ICAM-1, there was limited variability of the elbow angle that relates the orientation of the two domains with respect to one another. This restriction would prove useful in the fitting of the ICAM-1 structure into cryo-EM density maps of virus-receptor complexes.

The structure of the D1D2 domains of ICAM-1 has been solved to 2.2-Å resolution (Color Plate 9, following p. 156) (2). The two-domain structure is ~75 Å long and 20 Å in diameter, and the domains are related by a 150° elbow angle. Domain 1 is an intermediate Ig-type domain whereas domain 2 is a constant 2 Ig-type domain. The Ig superfamily members have folds that have been divided into V, C1, C2, and I, with I being intermediate between the V and C folds (15). It is defined as a β-sandwich domain with one sheet containing ABED strands and the other sheet containing A'GFCC' strands. Both ICAM-1 and ICAM-2 lack the C' strand in domain 1 (Color Plate 9) and have very similar folds with a root mean square difference of only 1.2 Å between 82 superimposed C_α atoms (2, 7). Thus, a comparison between the structures of ICAM-1 and -2 domain 1 could be useful to discern the determinants of rhinovirus binding.

ICAM-RHINOVIRUS COMPLEXES

A major tenet of the canyon hypothesis suggested that the receptor would bind in the crevice that surrounds each of the fivefold vertices (32). This was supported by molecular genetic studies in which residues that line the floor of the canyon in HRV14 were mutated and the resulting virus particles had altered levels of receptor binding (11). Furthermore, it was shown that a series of drugs could enter a hydrophobic pocket located under the canyon floor through a pore at the base of the canyon (1, 21, 29, 40). These drugs interfered with virus uncoating or attachment and suggested that alterations in the canyon induced by drug binding affected receptor interactions. Confirmation of the binding of ICAM-1 into the canyon came from cryo-EM studies of HRV16 complexed with the amino-terminal two domains of ICAM-1 (Color Plate 10a, following p. 156) (28). The electron density values for D1D2 were nearly identical to those of the virus, indicating a nearly complete saturation of all of the 60 available binding sites on the virion. ICAM-1 binds in the central region of the canyon and has greater contact with the so called "south" side of the canyon rather than the "north" face (Color Plate 10b; north refers to the side of the canyon closest to the fivefold axis whereas south refers to the side further away from the fivefold axis). Complexes of HRV16 and D1D2 have a radius of 215 Å to the tip of the distal domain of ICAM-1. Since HRV16 has a 150-Å radius and the length of the two-domain ICAM-1 is 75 Å, the receptor penetrates approximately 10 Å into the canyon. In agreement with mutational studies, contact between the virus and the receptor occurs exclusively through D1 (25, 26).

In contrast with the fairly stable complex of HRV16 with ICAM-1, complexes of the receptor with HRV14 did not last long even at 4°C and resulted in the breakdown of the virus particles (14, 20). It was possible, however, to obtain a cryo-EM reconstruction of HRV14 with its receptor as shown on the left side of Color Plate 10a, although the occupancy of ICAM-1 in the density was determined to be reduced relative to its binding in HRV16 (22). Remarkably, the two HRV-ICAM-1 complexes look similar in shape and orientation. There is a slight 10° difference in their binding angle, reflecting minor differences in the interaction between the two viruses and ICAM-1.

Several other HRV16-ICAM-1 complexes have been solved using cryo-EM and image reconstruction technology (22). A modified form of ICAM-1, lacking three of the four glycosylation sites on D2, was found to bind in exactly the same position as the native D1D2, but its occupancy was only 70% that of the native D1D2. This difference in occupancy suggests that the removal of carbohydrate moieties influences the binding of the receptor to the virus. The reason for this occupancy difference is not known, but there is a small variation in density between the two forms of D1D2. This variation, which occurs near the virus surface, is not compatible with a glycosylation site and thus might reflect an alteration in the orientation of D1D2 binding between the two complexes. A larger ICAM-1, containing all five of the extracellular Ig domains, was also complexed with HRV16 and its structure determined with cryo-EM techniques (22). In this study, D3 demonstrated

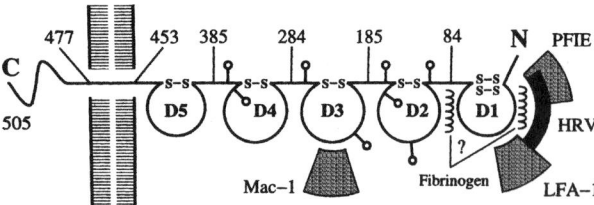

FIGURE 1 A diagram of an ICAM-1 molecule showing sites of glycosylation (lollipops) and the approximate location of binding sites of LFA-1, Mac-1, the major group of human rhinoviruses, fibrinogen, and *P. falciparum*-infected erythrocytes (PFIE). Ig-like domains are numbered D1 through D5. Amino acid residues are given by the number above the schematic. Reprinted from the *Proceedings of the National Academy of Sciences, U.S.A.* (2) with permission of the publisher.

lower occupancy than D1 and D2 whereas density for D4 and D5 was lacking. This was attributed to increased flexibility of those domains and loss of icosahedral order. However, more recent studies using a mutant five-domain ICAM-1 binding to HRV16 or native five-domain ICAM-1 binding to coxsackievirus A21 have shown all five domains in their respective reconstructions (45). In these studies, the number of particles used in the reconstructions was far greater than those used in the former studies. In addition, the coherence of the microscope's electron beam was better and probably contributed to the visualization of the five domains. Thus, the five-domain ICAM-1 molecule is more rigid than previously thought.

The glycosylation sites of D2 were obvious in the cryo-EM reconstructions. They appeared as four "lumps" emanating from the density ascribed to D2 (22). The nature of these lumps was confirmed by creating a difference density map between the complexes containing the fully glycosylated versus the partially glycosylated D1D2 molecules. In this difference map, three sites appeared whereas the last site, common to both molecules, disappeared. These positional markers were then used to facilitate the placement of the X-ray crystal structure of ICAM-1 D1D2 into the cryo-EM density maps for the HRV14 and HRV16 complexes. These reconstructions were then refined as rigid bodies in reciprocal space with respect to difference maps obtained by subtraction of the HRV contribution from the cryo-EM reconstructed density of the complexes. The refined fits of the ICAM-1 models into the cryo-EM density maps were consistent with the predicted positions of the glycosylation sites. The quality of the fit for both the HRV14 and HRV16 reconstructions was similar, and the elbow angle for D1 and D2 between the two complexes was no greater than 5 Å. The root mean square difference in equivalent C_α positions for the HRV14 and HRV16 complexes was 3.3 Å, corresponding to a 6.8° orientation difference between these two structures.

The footprints of ICAM-1 on the viral surfaces of HRV16 and HRV14 were determined by using distance matrix and buried surface analyses (22). The calculated area of contact between ICAM-1 and either HRV14 or HRV16 is 990 Å^2. Residues that become less exposed to solvent upon complex formation (assuming a probe radius of 1.4 Å) are shown as roadmaps in Fig. 2 (9, 22). Loops BC and FG of D1 contact both VP1 and VP3, whereas loop DE only contacts VP1 (Color Plate 9 and Table 1). Loop CD abuts a large area of VP2 on the south wall of the canyon and strands βC and βD make additional contacts with some VP1 and VP2 residues. The footprint of ICAM-1 on HRV14 is shifted slightly with respect to the footprint on HRV16. In both complexes, the ICAM-1 footprint includes several of the residues that define the deepest regions in the canyon (Fig. 2). Residues Lys1095–Leu1100 and Val1210–Leu1217 in HRV16 define the "roof" of the hydrophobic drug-binding pocket in VP1 (viral residues are numbered sequentially, starting at 1000, 2000, 3000, and 4000 for the polypeptide chains VP1, VP2, VP3, and VP4, respectively). Of these residues, only Asp1213 makes contact with ICAM-1. Equivalent residues in HRV14, Asp1101–Leu1106 and Val1217–Met1224, are all outside the ICAM-1 footprint when the pocket is closed, and none of the residues are closer than 4 Å to any ICAM-1 residue. When the pocket is filled with an antiviral compound, then only His1220 becomes part of the ICAM-1 footprint. Nevertheless, mutations at residues Lys1101, Val1217, His1220, and Ser1223, in the roof of the hydrophobic pocket in HRV14, all modify the ability of the virus to bind to HeLa cell membranes (11). This lack of structural interaction between residues in the floor of the canyon and ICAM-1 may be because the observed cryo-EM structure represents an initial recognition complex that is succeeded in a second step by a closer contact required to initiate uncoating. As illustrated in Table 1, a major component of the ICAM-1 and HRV interaction is through electrostatic interactions. Although HRV14 and HRV16 differ in their complementary amino acid residue numbers to ICAM-1, they maintain the character of the amino acid side chain. The same cannot be said for the minor group HRVs, thus providing some basis for their alternative receptor specificity.

ICAM as a Receptor for Rhinovirus and Other Picornaviruses

ICAM-1 has been conclusively shown to be the sole cellular receptor molecule for the major group HRVs (12, 44). This specificity extends to ICAM-1 of primate origin but not to other mammals, and solely to ICAM-1, not ICAM-2, ICAM-3, or others (30). Since the X-ray crystal structure of ICAM-2 has been solved (7), it is possible to compare its structure with that of ICAM-1 to identify residues or regions that might explain this specificity. A comparison of the distance between superimposed, equivalent C_α atoms between the D1 domains of ICAM-1 and ICAM-2 shows three short regions where there is a substantial difference

TABLE 1 Rhinovirus-ICAM charge complementarity

ICAM-1		Major group[a]		Minor group by homology to HRV16	
Site	Residue	HRV16	HRV14	HRV2	HRV1a
BC loop	D26	R1277	K1280 K1283	V	V
BG loop	K29	D1213 D3181	D3179	N G	D N
βC	E34	K2164	K2143	L	R
βE	K50	VP3-COOH	—	—	—
FG loop	D71	R1277 K3086	K1283	V R	V K

[a]See text for an explanation of HRV amino acid nomenclature.

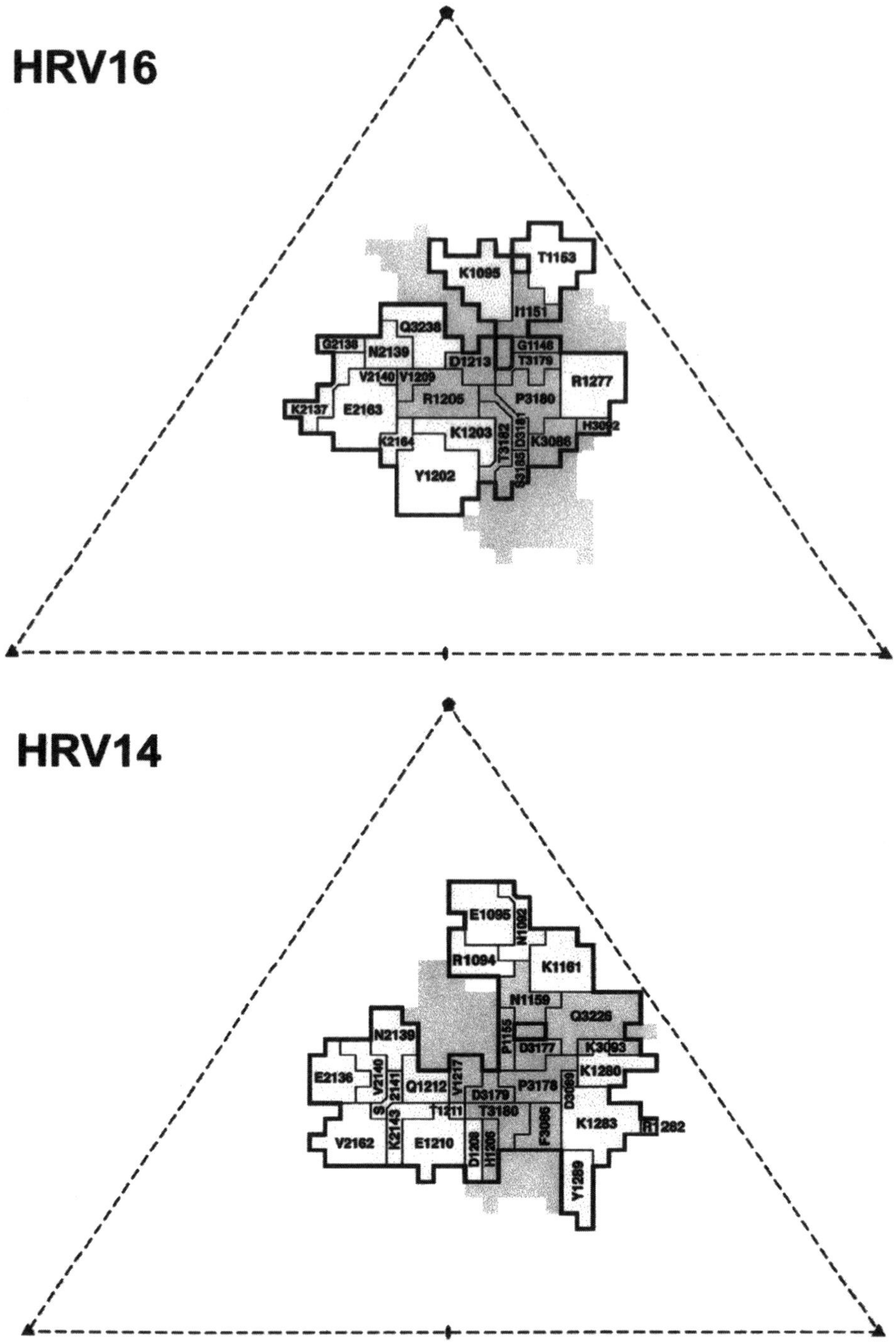

HRV16

HRV14

FIGURE 2 Roadmap representation (9) showing the amino acids within the ICAM-1 footprint (thick outline) on the surface of (A) HRV16 and (B) HRV14. The figure shows one icosahedral asymmetric unit with a fivefold axis at the top and threefold axes to the left and right at the bottom. Residues closer than 145 Å to the viral center, shaded in gray, outline the central and deepest region of the canyon. Reprinted from the EMBO Journal (22) with permission of the publisher.

in structure (2). These regions correspond to the BC, DE, and FG loops that were identified in the cryo-EM studies as being the sites of binding for HRV14 and HRV16. By far, the largest conformational changes between the two ICAM D1s occur at those sites where ICAM-1 interacts with HRVs, consistent with the fact that ICAM-1 but not ICAM-2 serves as a receptor.

Many distinct cellular receptors have been identified for the picornavirus family of viruses. Although there are some exceptions, many of the receptors belong to families of cell surface adhesion molecules (see chapter 6, this volume). Numerous members of the Ig superfamily have been shown to serve as picornavirus receptors. In each case in which an Ig superfamily receptor has been examined by cryo-EM in complex with its cognate virus, the receptor has been shown to bind with its distal amino-terminal domain in the canyon (36). Virus-receptor complexes that have been solved in this manner include HRV14, HRV16, CVA21 with ICAM-1, PV1 with CD155 (Pvr), and CVB3 with HCAR. Despite having the receptor bind in approximately the same location in the canyon for each of these complexes, the orientation of the long axis of the receptor and the residues of the virus and receptor involved in the footprint are different. This is evident by examining the residues involved in binding D1 of ICAM-1 for HRV14 and HRV16 (Fig. 2 and Table 1). Similarly, residues of ICAM-1 D1 binding to HRV14 and HRV16 differ from those binding to CVA21 (Color Plate 9b) (45). Two factors that contribute to the binding interface and the orientation of the bound receptor are the complementarity of amino acid residues and the surface contour of the canyon. Not only are residues on the floor of the canyon important for this binding, but also residues that line the rim, most notably the south rim, that presumably provide stable support for the long and slender receptor. In the case of the poliovirus receptor, the protein lies more tangential to the surface of the virus than with ICAM-1 and the HRVs (3, 16, 46) and probably occurs because of the wider canyon present in poliovirus.

ICAM-1 has been reported to bind to LFA-1 in the form of a dimer (31). The crystallographic structures that have been reported also show the D1 domain of ICAM-1 involved in dimer contacts, although different interfaces have been reported (2, 8). The transmembrane domain of ICAM-1 contains a dimerization motif, and thus it is likely that ICAM-1 is present as a dimer on the cell surface. A critical residue on D1, Glu 34, implicated in binding to LFA-1, lies on the opposite face from the proposed dimer interface. It is now clear from genetic and structural studies that the binding sites for LFA-1, HRV, and *P. falciparum*-infected erythrocytes are distinct. Whether the dimeric form of ICAM-1 binds to HRV and is required for proper function remains unanswered. However, due to steric constraints, it is unlikely that an ICAM dimer could bind bivalently to the virus, although binding one monomer to the virus could influence binding of the second monomer. In addition, experiments using soluble monomeric forms of ICAM-1 have established its capability for binding and inducing conformational changes in the virion that lead to disassembly (5, 20) and thus the dimer is unlikely to be required for rhinovirus entry.

Mechanisms of ICAM-Induced Entry

The entry pathway for the major group HRVs has not been established, and different viruses within this group may turn out to enter through different routes (38). It is clear, however, that the interaction of the major group rhinoviruses HRV14 and HRV16 with ICAM-1 can be sufficient to induce changes in the virion structure that can lead to particle disassembly and RNA release. Studies with the major group HRV3 employing surface plasmon resonance and soluble ICAM-1 demonstrated two classes of binding sites that differ in affinity and association rate constants (6). The nature of these binding events is unclear, but two possible explanations might be that (i) there are two physically distinct binding sites due to local differences in the canyon, for example, the presence of pocket factor in the hydrophobic pocket under the canyon; or (ii) the binding of ICAM-1 to virus and subsequent conformational changes is a two-step process that involves differential binding affinities. The association of ICAM-1 with HRV3 was slow compared with other protein-protein interactions, suggesting that the receptor may have a difficult time penetrating the canyon and making the correct contacts. This hypothesis was further supported by surface plasmon resonance experiments comparing the association of HRV3 and HRV16 with ICAM-1 and the association of poliovirus with CD155 (46). Poliovirus-receptor association was faster, suggesting that the receptor-binding site might be better accessible in the poliovirus canyon compared with the rhinovirus canyon.

As was mentioned previously, and discussed in greater detail in chapter 3, a hydrophobic pocket lies beneath the canyon floor. This pocket has been shown to be the binding site for a number of antiviral agents that inhibit the replication of HRVs and other picornaviruses (1, 21, 29, 40). Upon binding of the antiviral compound, many major group HRVs have reduced attachment to cells. In the crystal structures of several picornaviruses, this pocket is occupied by a small lipid-like molecule termed "pocket factor" (34). It has been suggested that pocket factors contribute to the stability of the virus. Furthermore, it has been hypothesized that binding of ICAM-1 to rhinovirus causes displacement of the pocket factor by depressing the canyon floor, resulting in destabilization of the virus and facilitating uncoating. However, the failure of ICAM-1 to contact the residues that constitute the roof of the hydrophobic pocket (i.e., floor of the canyon) in rhinovirus raises questions as to the mechanism by which the receptor induces conformational changes in the virus.

A two-step mechanism that takes these observations into account has been proposed for the ICAM-1-induced uncoating of rhinoviruses (Fig. 3) (22). The initial recognition and binding event of ICAM-1 to HRV is represented by the cryo-EM complexes that have been previously described. In this first step, the D1 domain of ICAM-1 penetrates deep in the canyon, with virus interactions predominantly on the south wall of the canyon. In a subsequent step, the receptor moves slightly to allow the north wall, as well as the south wall, to bind to D1. The resulting conformational change in the virion is envisaged to move VP1 away from the fivefold axis, thereby opening a channel at the pentamer vertex through which the amino termini of VP1 and VP4, and eventually RNA, can escape. This model is consistent with the kinetic data suggesting two binding states, although alternative routes for the externalization of these viral components are also possible. The presence of an antiviral drug in the pocket would inhibit the second step of binding by either failing to be displaced upon ICAM-1 binding or by inhibiting the second "sliding" step of ICAM-1 deeper into the canyon and altering the conformation of VP1.

A static model that describes this uncoating process is probably an oversimplification. Recent data suggest that rhinoviruses "breathe," allowing buried sequences such as VP4 and the amino termini of VP1 to be periodically exposed, possibly at the pentamer vertex (23). These results are consistent with the proposed model. As more receptor molecules bind the virus, displacing the pocket factor and destabilizing the particle, breathing may be progressively stimulated until irreversible uncoating occurs. Not surprisingly, binding of the antiviral compounds in the pocket decreases the amount of breathing.

Although the last few years have seen significant progress in our understanding of the molecular events that surround the attachment of the cellular receptor to rhi-

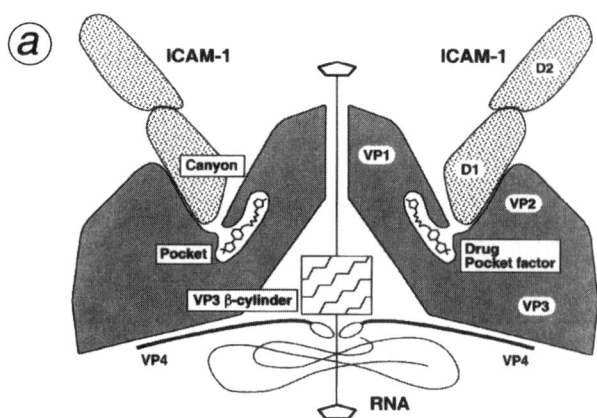

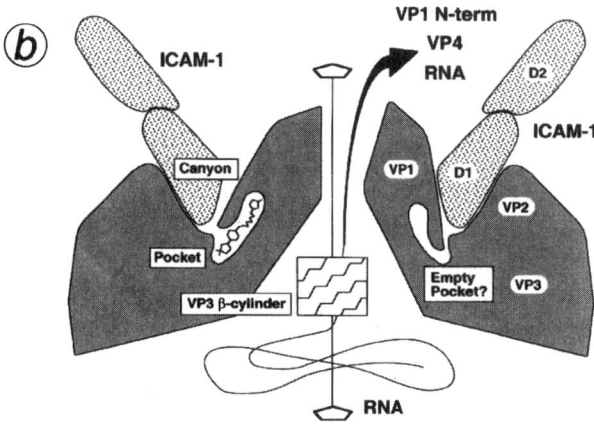

FIGURE 3 Schematic representation of a proposed two-step binding mechanism between ICAM-1 and major group HRVs. ICAM-1 is represented only as a two-domain fragment. (a) The first (observed) step corresponds to the cryo-EM reconstructions of HRV-ICAM-1 complexes in which ICAM-1 binds primarily to the floor and south wall of the canyon. (b) The second (hypothesized) step involves a conformational change in the virus surface, shown only on the right-hand side of the diagram. Probably both walls of the canyon bind to domain D1 of ICAM-1 and, in so doing, open up the fivefold channel. This requires conformational flexibility of VP1, which forms a large part of both the north and south walls of the canyon, and probably also an empty hydrophobic pocket in VP1. Opening of the pentamer vertex, induced by the binding of one or more ICAM-1 molecules, may facilitate externalization of VP4 and other internal viral components, including RNA. Reprinted from the *EMBO Journal* (22) with permission of the publisher.

novirus, significant gaps still persist that will require additional efforts until the complete picture will emerge.

REFERENCES

1. Badger, J., I. Minor, M. J. Kremer, M. A. Oliveira, T. J. Smith, J. P. Griffith, D. M. A. Guerin, S. Krishnaswamy, M. Luo, M. G. Rossmann, M. A. McKinlay, G. D. Diana, F. J. Dutko, M. Fancher, R. R. Rueckert, and B. A. Heinz. 1988. Structural analysis of a series of antiviral agents complexed with human rhinovirus 14. *Proc. Natl. Acad. Sci. USA* **85:**3304–3308.
2. Bella, J., P. R. Kolatkar, C. W. Marlor, J. M. Greve, and M. G. Rossmann. 1998. The structure of the two amino-terminal domains of human ICAM-1 suggests how it functions as a rhinovirus receptor and as an LFA-1 integrin ligand. *Proc. Natl. Acad. Sci. USA* **95:**4140–4145.
3. Belnap, D. M., B. M. McDermott, Jr., D. J. Filman, N. Cheng, B. L. Trus, H. J. Zuccola, V. R. Racaniello, J. M. Hogle, and A. C. Steven. 2000. Three-dimensional structure of poliovirus receptor bound to poliovirus. *Proc. Natl. Acad. Sci. USA* **97:**73–78.
4. Berendt, A. R., D. L. Simmons, J. Tancey, C. I. Newbold, and K. Marsh. 1989. Intercellular adhesion molecule-1 is an endothelial cell adhesion receptor for *Plasmodium falciparum*. *Nature (London)* **347:**57–59.
5. Casasnovas, J. M., J. K. Bickford, and T. A. Springer. 1998. The domain structure of ICAM-1 and the kinetics of binding to rhinovirus. *J. Virol.* **72:**6244–6246.
6. Casasnovas, J. M., and T. A. Springer. 1995. Kinetics and thermodynamics of virus binding to receptor. Studies with rhinovirus, intercellular adhesion molecule-1 (ICAM-1), and surface plasmon resonance. *J. Biol. Chem.* **270:**13216–13224.
7. Casasnovas, J. M., T. A. Springer, J. Liu, S. C. Harrison, and J. Wang. 1997. Crystal structure of ICAM-2 reveals a distinctive integrin recognition surface. *Nature (London)* **387:**312–315.
8. Casasnovas, J. M., T. Stehle, J. Liu, J. Wang, and T. A. Springer. 1998. A dimeric crystal structure for the N-terminal two domains of intercellular adhesion molecule-1. *Proc. Natl. Acad. Sci. USA* **95:**4134–4139.
9. Chapman, M. S. 1993. Mapping the surface properties of macromolecules. *Protein Sci.* **2:**459–469.
10. Colonno, R. J., P. L. Callahan, and W. J. Long. 1986. Isolation of a monoclonal antibody that blocks attachment of the major group of human rhinoviruses. *J. Virol.* **57:**7–12.
11. Colonno, R. J., J. H. Condra, S. Mizutani, P. L. Callahan, M. E. Davies, and M. A. Murcko. 1988. Evidence for the direct involvement of the rhinovirus canyon in receptor binding. *Proc. Natl. Acad. Sci. USA* **85:**5449–5453.
12. Greve, J. M., G. Davis, A. M. Meyer, C. P. Forte, S. C. Yost, C. W. Marlor, M. E. Kamarck, and A. McClelland. 1989. The major human rhinovirus receptor is ICAM-1. *Cell* **56:**839–847.
13. [See reference 12.]
14. Greve, J. M., C. P. Forte, C. W. Marlor, A. M. Meyer, H. Hoover-Litty, D. Wunderlich, and A. McClelland. 1991. Mechanisms of receptor-mediated rhinovirus neutralization defined by two soluble forms of ICAM-1. *J. Virol.* **65:**6015–6023.
15. Harpaz, Y., and C. Chothia. 1994. Many of the immunoglobulin superfamily domains in cell adhesion molecules and surface receptors belong to a new structural set which is close to that containing variable domains. *J. Mol. Biol.* **238:**528–539.
16. He, Y., V. D. Bowman, S. Mueller, C. M. Bator, J. Bella, X. Peng, T. S. Baker, E. Wimmer, R. J. Kuhn, and M. G. Rossmann. 2000. Interaction of the poliovirus receptor with poliovirus. *Proc. Natl. Acad. Sci. USA* **97:**79–84.
17. He, Y. N., P. R. Chipman, J. Howitt, C. M. Bator, M. A. Whitt, T. S. Baker, R. J. Kuhn, C. W. Anderson, P. Freimuth, and M. G. Rossmann. 2001. Interaction of coxsackievirus B3 with the full length coxsackievirus-adenovirus receptor. *Nat. Struct. Biol.* **8:**874–878.
18. Hewat, E. A., E. Neumann, J. F. Conway, R. Moser, B. Ronacher, T. C. Marlovits, and D. Blaas. 2000. The cellular receptor to human rhinovirus 2 binds around the 5-fold axis and not in the canyon: a structural view. *EMBO J.* **19:**6317–6325.

19. Hofer, F., M. Gruenberger, H. Kowalski, H. Machat, M. Huettinger, E. Kuechler, and D. Blaas. 1994. Members of the low density lipoprotein receptor family mediate cell entry of a minor-group common cold virus. *Proc. Natl. Acad. Sci. USA* **91**:1839–1842.
20. Hoover-Litty, H., and J. M. Greve. 1993. Formation of rhinovirus-soluble ICAM-1 complexes and conformational changes in the virion. *J. Virol.* **67**:390–397.
21. Kim, K. H., P. Willingmann, Z. X. Gong, M. J. Kremer, M. S. Chapman, I. Minor, M. A. Oliveira, M. G. Rossmann, K. Andries, G. D. Diana, F. J. Dutko, M. A. McKinlay, and D. C. Pevear. 1993. A comparison of the anti-rhinoviral drug binding pocket in HRV14 and HRV1A. *J. Mol. Biol.* **230**:206–226.
22. Kolatkar, P. R., J. Bella, N. H. Olson, C. M. Bator, T. S. Baker, and M. G. Rossmann. 1999. Structural studies of two rhinovirus serotypes complexed with fragments of their cellular receptor. *EMBO J.* **18**:6249–6259.
23. Lewis, J. K., B. Bothner, T. J. Smith, and G. Siuzdak. 1998. Antiviral agent blocks breathing of the common cold virus. *Proc. Natl. Acad. Sci. USA* **95**:6774–6778.
24. Marlovits, T. C., C. Abrahamsberg, and D. Blaas. 1998. Very-low-density lipoprotein receptor fragment shed from HeLa cells inhibits human rhinovirus infection. *J. Virol.* **72**:10246–10250.
25. Martin, S., J. M. Casasnovas, D. E. Staunton, and T. A. Springer. 1993. Efficient neutralization and disruption of rhinovirus by chimeric ICAM-1/immunoglobulin molecules. *J. Virol.* **67**:3561–3568.
26. McClelland, A., J. deBear, S. C. Yost, A. M. Meyer, C. W. Marlor, and J. M. Greve. 1991. Identification of monoclonal antibody epitopes and critical residues for rhinovirus binding in domain 1 of ICAM-1. *Proc. Natl. Acad. Sci. USA* **88**:7993–7997.
27. Ockenhouse, C. F., R. Betageri, T. A. Springer, and D. E. Staunton. 1992. *Plasmodium falciparum*-infected erythrocytes bind ICAM-1 at a site distinct from LFA-1, Mac-1, and human rhinovirus. *Cell* **68**:63–69.
28. Olson, N. H., P. R. Kolatkar, M. A. Oliveira, R. H. Cheng, J. M. Greve, A. McClelland, T. S. Baker, and M. G. Rossmann. 1993. Structure of a human rhinovirus complexed with its receptor molecule. *Proc. Natl. Acad. Sci. USA* **90**:507–511.
29. Pevear, D. C., F. J. Fancher, P. J. Feloc, M. G. Rossmann, M. S. Miller, G. Diana, A. M. Treasurywala, M. A. McKinlay, and F. J. Dutko. 1989. Conformational change in the floor of the human rhinovirus canyon blocks adsorption to HeLa cell receptors. *J. Virol.* **63**:2002–2007.
30. Register, R. B., C. R. Uncapher, A. M. Naylor, D. W. Lineberger, and R. J. Colonno. 1991. Human-murine chimeras of ICAM-1 identify amino acid residues critical for rhinovirus and antibody binding. *J. Virol.* **65**:6589–6596.
31. Reilly, P. L., J. R. Woska, Jr., D. D. Jeanfavre, E. McNally, R. Rothlein, and B. J. Bormann. 1995. The native structure of intercellular adhesion molecule-1 (ICAM-1) is a dimer. Correlation with binding to LFA-1. *J. Immunol.* **155**:529–532.
32. Rossmann, M. G. 1989. The canyon hypothesis. *Vir. Immunol.* **2**:143–161.
33. Rossmann, M. G. 1989. The canyon hypothesis. Hiding the host cell receptor attachment site on a viral surface from immune surveillance. *J. Biol. Chem.* **264**:14587–14590.
34. Rossmann, M. G. 1994. Viral cell recognition and entry. *Protein Sci.* **3**:1712–1725.
35. Rossmann, M. G., E. Arnold, J. W. Erickson, E. A. Frankenberger, J. P. Griffith, H.-J. Hecht, J. E. Johnson, G. Kamer, M. Luo, A. G. Mosser, R. R. Rueckert, B. Sherry, and G. Vriend. 1985. Structure of human cold virus and functional relationship to other picornaviruses. *Nature (London)* **317**:145–153.
36. Rossmann, M. G., J. Bella, P. R. Kolatkar, Y. He, E. Wimmer, R. J. Kuhn, and T. S. Baker. 2000. Cell recognition and entry by rhino- and enteroviruses. *Virology* **269**:239–247.
37. Rossmann, M. G., and A. C. Palmenberg. 1988. Conservation of the putative receptor attachment site in picornaviruses. *Virology* **164**:373–382.
38. Schober, D., P. Kronenberger, E. Prchla, D. Blaas, and R. Fuchs. 1998. Major and minor receptor group human rhinoviruses penetrate from endosomes by different mechanisms. *J. Virol.* **72**:1354–1364.
39. Sherry, B., A. G. Mosser, R. J. Colonno, and R. R. Rueckert. 1986. Use of monoclonal antibodies to identify four neutralization immunogens on a common cold picornavirus, human rhinovirus 14. *J. Virol.* **57**:246–257.
40. Smith, T. J., M. J. Kremer, M. Luo, G. Vriend, E. Arnold, G. Kamer, M. G. Rossmann, M. A. McKinlay, G. D. Diana, and M. J. Otto. 1986. The site of attachment in human rhinovirus 14 for antiviral agents that inhibit uncoating. *Science* **233**:1286–1293.
41. Springer, T. A. 1990. Adhesion receptors of the immune system. *Nature (London)* **346**:425–434.
42. Staunton, D. E., S. D. Marlin, C. Stratowa, M. L. Dustin, and T. A. Springer. 1988. Primary structure of ICAM-1 demonstrates interaction between members of the immunoglobulin and integrin supergene families. *Cell* **52**:925–933.
43. Staunton, D. E., V. J. Merluzzi, R. Rothlein, R. Barton, S. D. Marlin, and T. A. Springer. 1989. A cell adhesion molecule, ICAM-1, is the major surface receptor for rhinoviruses. *Cell* **56**:849–853.
44. [See reference 43.]
45. Xiao, C., C. M. Bator, V. D. Bowman, E. Rieder, Y. N. He, B. Hebert, J. Bella, T. S. Baker, E. Wimmer, R. J. Kuhn, and M. G. Rossmann. 2001. Interaction of coxsackievirus A21 with its cellular receptor, ICAM-1. *J. Virol.* **75**:2444–2451.
46. Xing, L., K. Tjarnlund, B. Lindqvist, G. G. Kaplan, D. Feigelstock, R. H. Cheng, and J. M. Casasnovas. 2000. Distinct cellular receptor interactions in poliovirus and rhinoviruses. *EMBO J.* **19**:1207–1216.

Human Rhinovirus Minor Group Receptors

DIETER BLAAS

9

More than 25 years ago Lonberg-Holm and colleagues demonstrated that out of 11 human rhinovirus serotypes investigated, HRV3, -5, -10, -14, -15, -39, -41, and -51 competed for the same binding site on HeLa cells whereas HRV1A, -1B, and -2 were found to recognize other sites on the cell surface (59, 60). The division of rhinoviruses into two subgroups based on competition for cellular receptors was subsequently extended to 24 serotypes and the picture of a "minor group" (including HRV1A, -1B, -2, -44, and -49) and a "major group" including the remaining 19 serotypes started to emerge (1). A monoclonal antibody (MAb), isolated from a mouse immunized with HeLa cell membranes, was then shown to strongly inhibit attachment and replication of 78 HRV serotypes out of 88 tested (22). The number of HRVs belonging to the major and to the minor receptor group was thus again extended to 78 and 10 serotypes, respectively.

Subsequently, the antibody was used for the purification by immunoaffinity chromatography of a membrane protein that bound major group rhinoviruses (98); sequence analysis of tryptic peptides, cDNA cloning, and sequencing finally revealed that the human rhinovirus major group receptor is identical with the intercellular adhesion molecule 1 (ICAM-1, CD-54). The identity of ICAM-1 with the major group viral receptor was confirmed by transfection of receptor-negative Vero cells. Upon transfection with an ICAM-1 cDNA clone that had been identified in a HeLa cell cDNA λ-library by hybridization with oligonucleotides derived from the peptide sequences, the cells acquired binding activity for virus as well as for the MAb, which also blocked viral infection (97).

ICAM-1 was originally defined with MAbs inhibiting lymphocyte adhesion to the integrin lymphocyte function-associated molecule 1 (LFA-1). This interaction plays an important role in immune reactions (85). The extracellular N-terminal portion of ICAM-1 is composed of five immunoglobulin-like domains, thus classifying this receptor as a member of the immunoglobulin supergene family. Two other laboratories showed that ICAM-1-specific MAbs inhibited infection of HeLa cells with HRV14 and arrived at the same conclusions by similar methodologies (37, 91).

On the basis of inhibition of attachment by the antibody isolated in the group of Richard Colonno, it was finally determined that 91 of the 102 different serotypes bind ICAM-1 (99). Of the remaining 11 serotypes, all but one (HRV87) could be shown to compete for another, at that time unknown, receptor molecule.

In contrast to major group HRVs, which are highly specific for human ICAM-1 (80) and only bind to cells of human or primate origin, minor group HRVs attach to cells derived from a large number of species (99); indeed, only mouse M4 cells, in which the low-density lipoprotein receptor (LDLR) (51) and the low-density lipoprotein receptor-related protein (LRP) (104) had been knocked out, do not bind minor group HRVs (Reithmayer et al., in press). Nevertheless, most cell lines are refractive to infection as replication of HRVs is restricted to primate cells, and rhinoviruses could only be adapted to grow in mouse cells by a time-consuming procedure (107, 108). Therefore, the absence of replication in a given cell line is not necessarily indicative of the absence of a viral receptor; it might also be due to the lack of cellular functions required for viral replication to occur. The ubiquitous presence of minor group HRV receptors was taken to indicate that it was evolutionarily strongly conserved; this was then confirmed by the discovery of its identity with the LDLR and the existence of several closely related molecules with virus-binding activity (see below).

IDENTIFICATION OF THE MINOR GROUP RHINOVIRUS RECEPTOR

Early experiments aimed at isolating MAbs blocking viral infection of HeLa cells with the minor group virus HRV2 failed, despite the screening of more than 10,000 hybridoma clones obtained from mice immunized with HeLa cell membranes. Therefore, purification of the virus-binding activity from detergent-solubilized cell membranes was carried out by conventional biochemical methods. First experiments indicated that radiolabeled HRV2 could bind to detergent extracts of HeLa cell membranes immobilized to nitrocellulose sheets (69). These dot blot experiments had

---

Dieter Blaas ■ Institute of Medical Biochemistry, VBC, University of Vienna, Dr. Bohr Gasse 9/3, A-1030 Vienna, Austria.

also shown that solubilization even with the strong anionic detergent sodium dodecyl sulfate (SDS) preserved virus-binding activity to some extent. HeLa cell membrane proteins were thus separated on polyacrylamide gels containing SDS in the absence of reducing agents and electrophoretically transferred to nitrocellulose membranes. Incubation with radiolabeled virus revealed for the first time specific binding of HRV2 to a protein with an apparent molecular mass of about 120 kDa under nonreducing conditions (68). Some high-molecular-mass bands were also seen, which were at that time assumed to be aggregation products derived from the viral receptor. The specificity of the attachment reaction was assessed by various means. Incubation of the samples with dithiothreitol prior to application to the gel led to complete loss of binding, indicating the requirement of intact disulfide bridges within the receptor molecule. Furthermore, in accordance with the early observation of the requirement of Ca ions for cell attachment of HRV2 (60), the presence of EDTA during incubation of the nitrocellulose membranes also abolished virus binding. Heating of the virus to 56°C for 10 min (57) or to 50°C for 15 min (58) has been shown to result in a conformational change of the capsid and concomitant release of the genomic RNA. At the same time, the capacity to attach to HeLa cells is lost (58); this treatment also resulted in loss of binding to the immobilized protein. The data were thus taken as a strong indication for the 120-kDa protein being identical with the minor group rhinovirus receptor.

First attempts at purifying the receptor protein from detergent extracts (69) revealed rapid loss of activity upon column chromatography. We therefore thought of other means of solubilizing virus-binding activity from the cell surface. Proteases or phospholipases have been used previously to sever the intact extracellular domain of membrane proteins from their transmembrane domain or from a glycosylphosphatidylinositol (GPI) anchor, respectively. Cells were thus incubated with various hydrolytic enzymes such as trypsin, papain, or phospholipase-C at 34°C, and the supernatants were examined for the presence of eventually released receptor fragments still active in virus binding. Unexpectedly, the only incubation that resulted in substantial virus-binding activity in the cell supernatant was the control incubation with buffer alone (46). Virus overlay blots revealed that the majority of the virus-binding activity in the supernatant migrated with an apparent molecular mass of about 84 kDa, suggesting its originating from cleavage of the 120-kDa protein. The time course (shown in Fig. 1) implied that the virus-binding activity was degraded or inactivated upon incubations exceeding 40 min. As no activity was recovered when EGTA was present during the incubation of the cells with buffer, it was assumed that a Ca^{++}-dependent proteinase cleaved the receptor off the cell surface upon incubation at 34°C. From this it appeared likely that release of the activity would also take place under conditions of cell propagation in tissue culture; this turned out to be indeed the case. Therefore, we started purification from about 200 liters of spent tissue culture medium by pressure dialysis, ion-exchange chromatography, lectin affinity chromatography, and ammonium sulfate precipitation. The activity of the virus-binding material was followed throughout by ligand blotting with radioactive HRV2; this method proved extremely useful for the assessment of purification and revealed that the 120-kDa protein was predominantly enriched, with the 84-kDa protein being only a minor

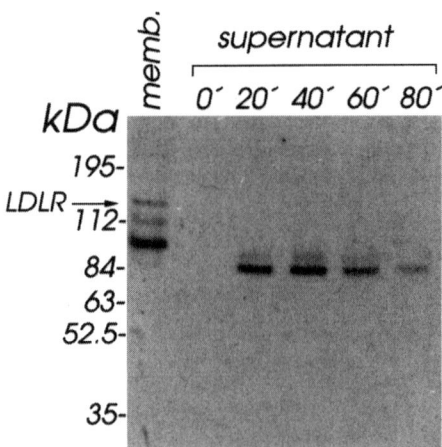

FIGURE 1 Virus-binding activity is released from HeLa cells upon incubation in PBS. Rhino-HeLa cells grown in T-flasks were suspended in PBS and incubated at 37°C. At the times indicated, cell supernatants from individual flasks were saved, an S80 extract was prepared, and the supernatants were concentrated to 50 μl by centrifugation dialysis in Centricon tubes. The retained material was analyzed by SDS-8% polyacrylamide gel electrophoresis under nonreducing conditions followed by electrophoretic transfer of the proteins to PVDF membranes. As a control, HeLa cell membrane proteins from about 5×10^6 cells were also analyzed in parallel. Virus-binding activity was detected by incubation of the blot with [^{35}S]methionine-labeled HRV2 (70) followed by autoradiography. Reproduced from the *Journal of Virology* (63) with permission of the publisher.

component that was largely lost during purification. Finally, the protein was resolved by polyacrylamide gel electrophoresis under nonreducing conditions, and the band found to be active in virus binding was electroeluted. Whereas the activity migrated with an apparent molecular mass of 120 kDa under nonreducing conditions, an M_r of 160 kDa was found upon incubation with β-mercaptoethanol, suggesting extensive disulfide bridging of the native protein. Some 20 μg of electrophoretically pure protein was then cleaved with trypsin, the peptides were separated by high-pressure liquid chromatography, and selected peptides were subjected to automated N-terminal protein sequencing. The amino acid sequences of all peptides were found to be present in the human LDLR.

The spent tissue culture medium, which had originally been used for purification of the virus-binding activity, had not been subjected to high-speed centrifugation (47). We thus assume that LDLR was rather purified from shed membrane fragments. Traces of an LDLR fragment could also be detected in the supernatant of HeLa cells incubated in phosphate-buffered saline (PBS) at 37°C (63), and release of small membrane fragments is not uncommon for cells maintained in tissue culture and is well documented for HeLa cells (27).

Identification of LDLR as receptor for minor group HRVs thus added a novel protein family to those used by picornaviruses for cell entry (47). LDLR is strongly conserved through evolution. It thus came by chance that one of the amino acid residues sequenced differs between the human and the bovine receptor (AA 613 is valine in the human and isoleucine in the bovine LDLR precursor protein), allowing researchers to unambiguously identify the purified protein as human and to exclude the bovine serum present in the growth medium as the source of this peptide.

The LDLR Gene Superfamily

A structural hallmark of members of the LDLR family is various numbers of incomplete direct repeats of about 40 amino acids containing six cysteines each (106), which are all involved in disulfide bridges (14). Ca ions are required for the maintenance of the structural integrity of these repeats (6, 13, 29, 31, 72). These ligand-binding repeats or "complement type-A repeats" (from their similarity to a sequence in the C-9 component of complement [30]) are involved in the interaction with multiple ligands. As depicted in Fig. 2, different numbers and arrangements of the complement type-A repeats are present in LDLR (7 repeats) (106), the very-low-density lipoprotein receptor (VLDLR; 8 repeats) (95), the LDLR-related protein or α_2-macroglobulin receptor (LRP; 2+8+10+11 repeats) (42, 56, 93), and gp330 or megalin (7+8+10+11 repeats) (86). The latter two receptors are very large polypeptides with a relative molecular mass of more than 600 kDa. LRP is the only member of the family that is composed of two subunits arising from furin cleavage during transit of the precursor molecule through the Golgi. The smaller subunit (84 kDa) is anchored in the membrane and remains noncovalently associated with the large subunit (515 kDa), which contains the complement type-A repeats (for a recent review on this receptor family see reference 36). The ligand-binding domain is followed (or interspersed in the case of LRP and megalin) by regions with similarity to epidermal growth factor (EGF) precursor; a region that is heavily O-glycosylated is present in some but not all of the receptors and precedes the transmembrane segment. In the case of VLDLR alternative splicing has been found to result in two forms of the molecule, one with an O-glycosylated region and one without (50, 61). Finally, all receptors possess a short C-terminal cytoplasmic domain, which contains typical internalization signals responsible for clustering of the receptors in coated pits (20).

Whereas the physiologic function of LDLR proper is the maintenance of serum cholesterol homeostasis by binding and internalizing lipids assembled with apolipoprotein-B or apolipoprotein-E, other members of the family are multifunctional receptors that bind a multitude of structurally and functionally unrelated ligands (94). These include proteinase-proteinase inhibitor complexes, lipoprotein lipase, lipoproteins, and Pseudomonas exotoxins among many others. Furthermore, they are involved in brain development (34), and a small protein with only one repeat serves as a receptor for Rous sarcoma virus of subgroup A (8).

LDLR expression is subject to a stringent control. In the presence of high concentrations of cholesterol it is down-regulated, whereas lack of cholesterol increases expression of the receptor. In vitro this property can be used to modulate the number of receptor molecules on the cell surface (26). Under normal tissue culture conditions the presence of lipids in bovine serum is usually sufficient to substantially suppress the expression of LDLR; addition of cholesterol/25-hydroxy cholesterol leads to further decrease of receptor expression whereas growth of the cells in delipidated serum results in strong up-regulation of receptor expression. Impaired expression of LDLR is associated with various forms of familial hypercholesterolemia (FH) that usually result in premature arteriosclerosis and myocardial infarction. A great number of naturally occurring mutations and deletions in the LDLR gene have been characterized (44; http://www.umd.necker.fr:2004/).

To obtain additional evidence for LDLR being involved in virus interaction, we assayed virus internalization and

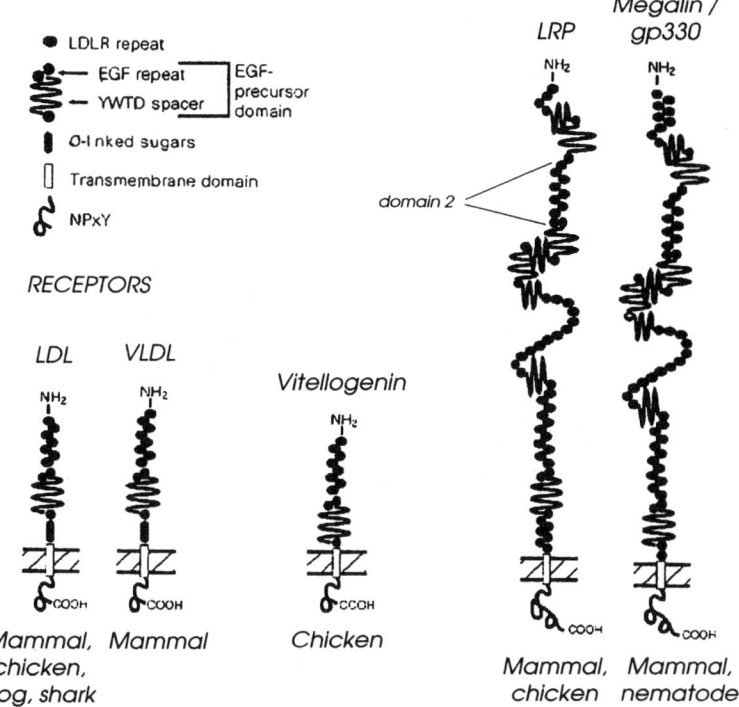

FIGURE 2 Structural features of various members of the LDL superfamily.

replication under conditions of cholesterol-mediated suppression of LDLR expression. For comparison, the same experiments were carried out with cells grown in delipidated serum. Viral internalization and production of viral progeny closely followed the level of LDLR expression (47). By the same token, fibroblasts from a patient with FH showed a reduction of internalization of radiolabeled HRV2 to about 7% with respect to virus internalization into wild-type cells. Unexpectedly, however, upon challenge of FH fibroblasts with HRV2, virus yield was only reduced to about 20% when compared to the control cells. This was taken to indicate that LDLR was not the only receptor allowing for HRV entry into the host cell. LRP appeared to be a likely candidate for a second viral receptor, and use of gradient polyacrylamide gels for the separation of fibroblast cell membrane proteins prior to ligand blots with radiolabeled virus indeed revealed the presence of a virus-binding activity with a migration behavior similar to that of LRP. This activity was present in both wild-type cells and FH fibroblasts whereas binding to the band corresponding to LDLR was only seen in wild-type cells and (Fig. 3). This agreed well with the previously observed binding of virus to high-molecular-weight material collected at the top of the gels that had been thought to arise from aggregates (see above).

For additional confirmation of LRP as a viral receptor, we made use of the receptor-blocking activity of a polypeptide of about 39 kDa that had been found to copurify with LRP; it was originally thought to be a third subunit of the receptor and was consequently called receptor-associated protein (RAP) (56). However, more recently, RAP was found to contain an endoplasmic reticulum retention signal sequence at its C terminus. It was shown to function as a specific chaperone aiding in folding and preventing aggregation between receptors and ligands during their common biosynthetic pathway (16, 17, 73, 103). At physiologic pH RAP exhibits a very high affinity toward LRP, megalin, and VLDLR and has been used in many studies as a specific inhibitor of receptor function (40, 67, 103). This competitor indeed inhibited viral infection of FH cells, thus confirming that LDLR and LRP were functional minor group human rhinovirus receptors.

In the course of a project aimed at producing MAbs directed against the ligand-binding domain of the chicken ovarian VLDLR (OVR, see below), the specific single-chain antibody scFv7 was isolated; this antibody was found to cross-react with bovine LDLR and human LRP in Western blots and had a somewhat lower affinity toward LDLR as determined by plasmon surface resonance techniques (45). Infection of FH fibroblasts with HRV2 was inhibited by this antibody, indicating that the virus binds to or close to a structure that is recognized by the virus. Nevertheless, in accordance with results of studies of several groups on inhibition of internalization of ligands binding to LRP and/or LDLR, total inhibition of infection was achieved neither with RAP nor with the single-chain antibody.

Other Human Rhinovirus Minor Group Receptors

An important criterion for the specificity of a viral receptor is the capability of a soluble version of the protein to inhibit viral infection by competition with the receptors present on the cell surface. Purification of amounts of LDLR or of LRP large enough to carry out cell-protection experiments appeared tedious, and expression of these proteins in bacteria was expected to be difficult due to the large number of disulfide bridges present in the native proteins. We thus chose to use another system for cell-protection assays. A homologue of mammalian VLDLR is expressed in hen ovaries where it is responsible for the transport of huge amounts of vitellogenin into the growing oocyte (92). This protein, termed ovarian vitellogenin/very-low-density lipoprotein receptor (OVR), can be easily prepared in comparatively large amounts, and it turned out to indeed bind HRV2 on ligand blots; by using solubilized purified OVR as a model, it was then demonstrated that at least this member of the LDLR superfamily protects HeLa cells against infection with the minor group rhinovirus HRV2 (39). However, OVR is not involved in viral infection since HRVs do not replicate in birds.

The virus-binding activity purified from spent tissue culture supernatants migrated with an apparent relative molecular mass of about 120 kDa on SDS-polyacrylamide gels whereas the protein isolated from the supernatant of cells incubated at 37°C in PBS migrated with an M_r of 84 kDa (46, 47). As antibodies against several members of the LDLR supergene family became available, we thus decided to reinvestigate the issue to resolve this discrepancy. The material released from HeLa cells upon incubation with buffer turned out to be a fragment derived from the splicing variant of VLDLR, which lacks the O-linked glycosylation domain. We also showed that material enriched on a glutathione S-transferase-RAP column inhibited virus infection of HeLa cells. Moreover, expression of a soluble fragment of human VLDLR consisting only of the eight ligand-binding repeats and a C-terminally appended hexahistidine tag in insect Sf9 cells allowed the unequivocal demonstration of binding of human VLDLR to HRV2 and protection of HeLa cells against infection (63). From these findings we concluded that the smaller splicing variant of

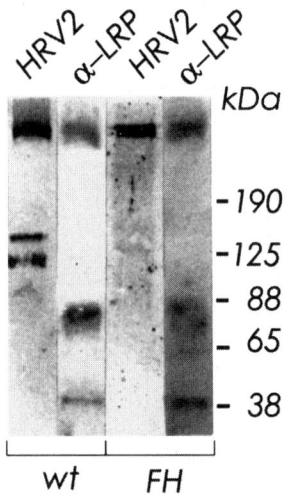

FIGURE 3 LDLR and LRP bind HRV2 on virus overlay blots. Cell membranes from wild-type human fibroblasts (wt) and from fibroblasts from a patient with FH were solubilized under nonreducing conditions and proteins were separated on a 4 to 12% gradient polyacrylamide gel in the presence of SDS. Polypeptides were electrophoretically transferred to a nitrocellulose membrane, and virus-binding activity was revealed by incubation with ^{35}S-methionine-labeled HRV2 followed by autoradiography. The two subunits of LRP (515 kDa and 84 kDa) and the tightly associated RAP (39 kDa) were visualized with antiserum against LRP (α-LRP). Modified from reference 47 with permission of the publisher.

VLDLR is being expressed in HeLa cells and is easily shed from the cell surface; it can also serve as a functional receptor for minor group HRVs (to be published elsewhere).

MINIMAL STRUCTURE REQUIREMENTS FOR VIRAL RECOGNITION

The interaction between ICAM-1 and major group viruses has been well characterized. Amino acid residues involved in binding were identified by systematic replacement of selected residues in the human protein for those present at the equivalent positions in the (nonbinding) mouse homologue (80, 89). The two N-terminal domains of human ICAM-1 could be expressed in bacteria and were necessary and sufficient for binding and cell protection (66). The site of interaction of ICAM-1 with major group HRVs had long been assumed to lie in the canyon, a crevice encircling the fivefold axes of icosahedral symmetry (84). Using an infectious cDNA clone of HRV14, Colonno and colleagues introduced mutations within the canyon region and noticed substantial changes in the attachment behavior and plaque size of the mutant viruses as compared to wild type (23). This was taken to indicate that the canyon was indeed involved in receptor binding. Based on the known three-dimensional structures of immunoglobulin constant domains, a model of the amino-terminal domain of ICAM-1 was then built and docked onto the atomic structure of HRV14 in an orientation consistent with the mutational data (35). Finally, the structure of a complex between recombinant soluble ICAM-1 and HRV16 was solved at about 20-Å resolution by cryo-electron microscopy image reconstruction techniques (77). The structure revealed binding of the receptor into the canyon and thus essentially confirmed the canyon hypothesis (83) put forward by Michael Rossmann 8 years earlier (84).

The structure of the building blocks of LDLR is completely different from that of ICAM-1. Although highly suggestive, we believed that the canyon did not necessarily need to be the site of attachment of LDLR to minor group viruses; indeed, cryo-electron microscopy of complexes between HRV2 and a recombinant VLDLR shows that the binding site is close to but not in the canyon (43; see below).

To determine the minimal structure requirements of LDLR for viral recognition and the LDLR-binding site on the viral capsid, we thus started to express soluble truncated LDLR in insect Sf9 cells. First, a recombinant baculovirus encoding a receptor fragment containing the entire ligand-binding domain with its seven complement type-A repeats was constructed. To achieve efficient secretion, the native signal sequence was replaced by the melittin leader peptide and a hexa-his tag was appended at the C terminus to allow one-step affinity purification. Expression was set under the control of the polyhedrin promoter, making use of pVT_Bac_His2 (64), a derivative of pVT_Bac (96). Upon infection of Sf9 insect cells, this recombinant LDLR fragment (termed $rLDLR_{1-7}h$) was released into the tissue culture supernatant and could be purified by Ni^{2+}-nitrilotriacetic acid (NTA) chelate chromatography. However, whereas $rLDLR_{1-7}h$ migrated as a single band upon SDS-polyacrylamide gel electrophoresis under reducing conditions, the material was largely heterogeneous when β-mercaptoethanol was omitted from the sample buffer. This is consistent with the results of ligand blots, which revealed that only a small proportion of the receptor was present as a monomer in an active, virus-binding conformation. Nevertheless, the material was strongly protecting HeLa cells from infection with various minor group HRVs. As seen in Fig. 4, only 0.08 μl of recombinant baculovirus-infected Sf9 cell supernatant (corresponding to material released from about 150 Sf9 cells) was sufficient to prevent cell damage by 500 50% tissue culture infective doses ($TCID_{50}$) of HRV1A, HRV29, HRV30, and to some extent HRV47. Preincubation of virus with larger amounts of the Sf9 cell supernatant prior to challenge of HeLa cells resulted in a completely undamaged cell layer. Recombinant soluble LDLR did not protect against infection with the major group rhinovirus HRV14 (64).

To define the region necessary and required for interaction with minor group rhinoviruses, soluble minireceptors composed of various numbers of ligand-binding repeats were then produced using the Bac-to-Bac cloning and expression system (Fig. 5). The minireceptors were found to be secreted into the cell supernatant and were easily purified by Ni^{++}-NTA chelate chromatography. As already seen for $rLDLR_{1-7}h$, single well-resolved bands appeared upon analysis by polyacrylamide gel electrophoresis under reducing conditions, whereas the material turned out to be heterogeneous when separated under nonreducing conditions (Fig. 6). This was taken to indicate the presence of a population of molecules with many disulfide bonds incorrectly formed intra- or intermolecularly. Note that for a receptor fragment encompassing only three complement type-A repeats there are 34,459,425 ways for the 18 cysteines to combine in disulfide bridges; consequently, 42 cysteines, as present in the ligand-binding domain of LDLR, could form more than 10^{25} different isomers (3). Ligand affinity chromatography was thus used for selective enrich-

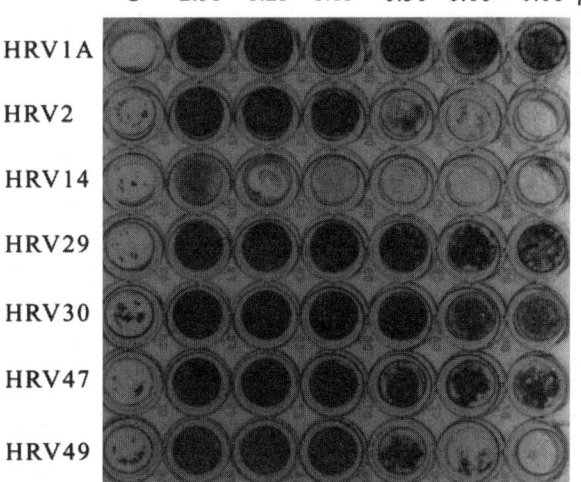

FIGURE 4 Recombinant soluble LDLR protects HeLa cells against infection with minor receptor group HRVs. Supernatants from Sf9 cells infected with recombinant baculovirus carrying the cDNA encoding the ligand-binding domain of human LDLR with a C-terminal hexa-his tag ($rLDLR_{1-7}h$) were incubated for 150 min at 34°C with 500 $TCID_{50}$ of the respective HRV. HeLa cells grown in microtiter plates were then challenged with the mixtures, and incubation was continued for an additional 3 days. Cells remaining attached to the plastic as a result of no cytopathic effect were then stained with amido black. Reproduced from reference 64 with permission of the publisher.

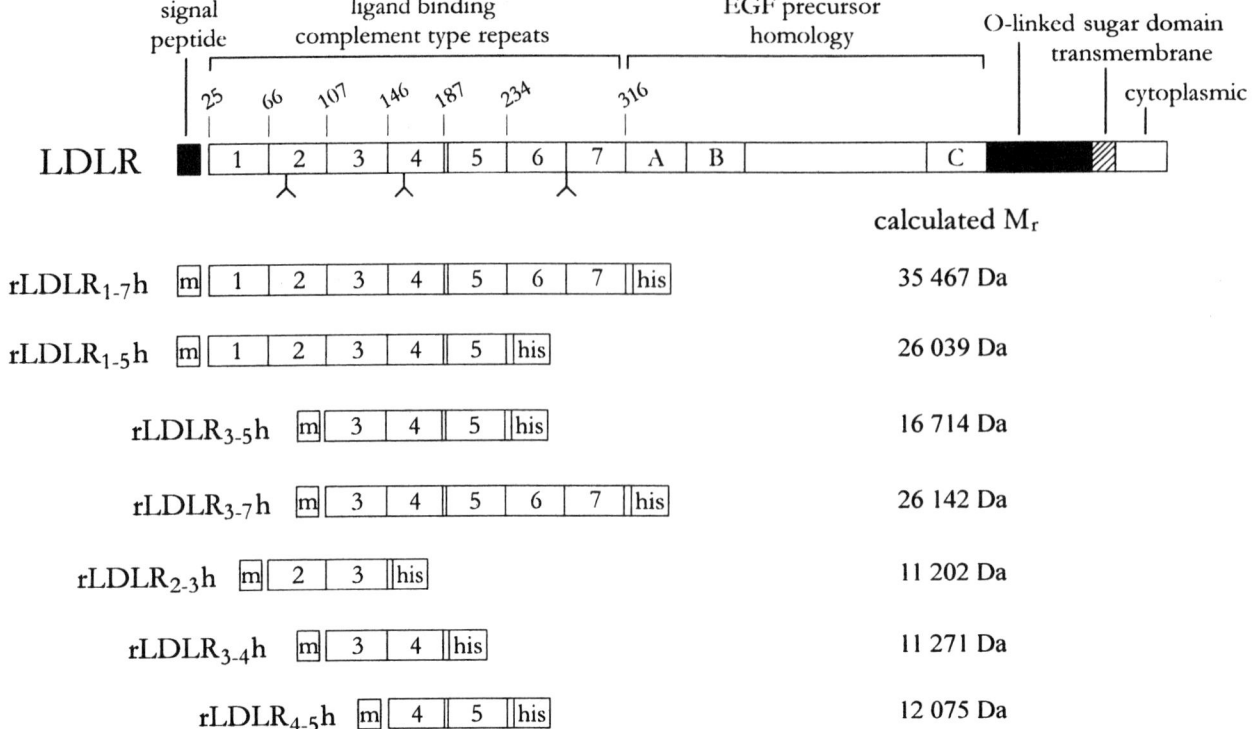

FIGURE 5 Structure of recombinant LDL minireceptors expressed in Sf9 cells. Reproduced from reference 62 with permission of the publisher.

ment of that fraction of material that was present in a native-like conformation.

Rabbit beta-migrating VLDL (β-VLDL) binds strongly to various members of the LDLR family (52, 102) and had been used previously for ligand affinity purification of OVR (7). A similar method was thus employed for the purification of recombinant soluble minireceptors expressed in insect Sf9 cells (62). Recombinant receptors that had been enriched by metal chelate chromatography on a Ni^{++}-NTA column were subjected to β-VLDL column chromatography. Minireceptors containing more than two complement type-A repeats (rLDLR$_{1-7}$h, rLDLR$_{1-5}$h, rLDLR$_{3-7}$h, and rLDLR$_{3-5}$h) were found to be retained on the column and were eluted with a high-pH buffer. Minireceptors with only two repeats (rLDLR$_{2-3}$h, rLDLR$_{3-4}$h, and rLDLR$_{4-5}$h) were not retained, indicating lack of interaction with β-VLDL. These proteins could thus not be purified further and were used as such in all binding assays. Analysis of the retained proteins by SDS-polyacrylamide gel electrophoresis under nonreducing conditions revealed that single species were enriched and migrated as homogeneous bands, indicating that the majority of the incorrectly folded material was inactive in ligand binding and had been removed by the affinity chromatography. On a virus overlay blot all minireceptors (including those containing only two complement type-A repeats) were found to be active in virus binding (62). Apparently, two contiguous complement type-A repeats of LDLR are sufficient for virus recognition whereas β-VLDL requires the presence of at least three repeats. More equivalent binding sites are present on the viral surface as compared to the number of binding sites on β-VLDL; this might result in an increase of the avidity toward the receptors immobilized on the PVDF membrane at high concentration (see also below). It should be kept in mind that the individual ligand-binding repeats are not identical in sequence, and fragments encompassing different numbers and combinations of the repeats will certainly not bind with the same affinity.

LDL Minireceptors Protect HeLa Cells against Infection with the Minor Group Virus HRV2

Recombinant LDL minireceptors purified over β-VLDLR columns were subjected to a cell-protection assay under conditions similar to that described above. Cells challenged with virus that had been preincubated with the soluble minireceptors were further grown for 5 days; cells remaining attached to the plastic as a consequence of lacking cytopathic effect were then stained with amido black. The stain was solubilized in 1 M NaOH and A_{560} was determined with a microplate reader. The values were taken as a measure for the integrity of the monolayer and hence for cell protection. The values determined from cells challenged with virus that had been preincubated with medium from Sf9 cells infected with wild-type baculovirus were taken as 0% protection, and those from cells incubated with no virus were taken as 100% protection. From these data a minimal inhibitory concentration (MIC_{50}) was defined as that concentration of the respective minireceptor affording 50% protection of the cells against viral damage under the given experimental conditions (5). Interestingly, the strongest cell protection (MIC_{50} = 0.3 μg/ml) was seen for rLDLR$_{3-7}$h and not for rLDLR$_{1-7}$h, which encompasses the entire ligand-binding domain (Fig. 7). This might be due to the presence of dimers in this particular preparation that are expected to either interact more strongly with single virions or to promote aggregation (see below).

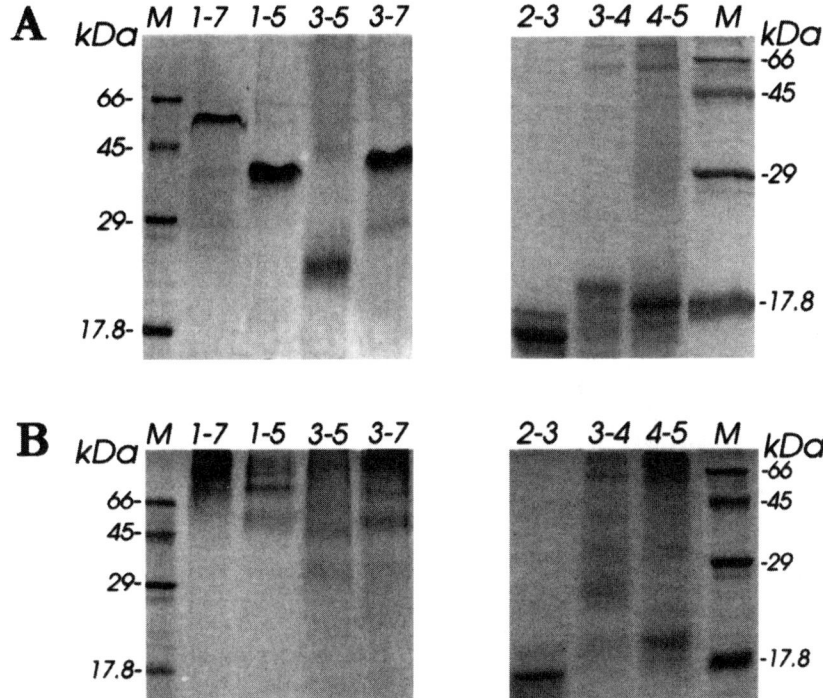

FIGURE 6 Polyacrylamide gel electrophoretic analysis of recombinant soluble LDL minireceptors expressed in insect Sf9 cells. Tissue culture supernatants from recombinant baculovirus-infected insect Sf9 cells were passed over a Ni^{2+}-NTA Sepharose column, and the material retained was eluted with ammonia and analyzed under reducing (A) and under nonreducing (B) conditions on 12% polyacrylamide gels in the presence of SDS. Numbers refer to the repeats present in the minireceptor. The gels were stained with Coomassie brilliant blue. Reproduced from reference 62 with permission of the publisher.

Mechanism of Cell Protection

Receptor derivatives might inhibit virus infection by various mechanisms. In most cases soluble receptors compete for the membrane receptors present on the cell surface. However, for major group HRVs, recombinant soluble ICAM-1 not only binds to the virus and thus competes for cell surface ICAM-1, but it also induces structural changes in the viral capsid upon attachment. The native form of the virus, which sediments at 150S, loses its innermost capsid protein VP4 and becomes more extended (resulting in a decrease of the sedimentation constant to about 135S). Depending on the serotype, the modification may even go further; the genomic RNA is released and a subviral particle sedimenting at 80S remains (19, 38). This modification is strongly temperature dependent and has been shown for HRV3 to not occur below 20°C (48).

Similar structural changes are also induced by low pH or heating to a temperature exceeding 50°C, resulting in 135S and 80S subviral particles (55, 57, 58). Receptor and/or low pH thus appear to be driving forces for the modifications occurring during the infectious pathway in vivo that ultimately result in transfer of the RNA into the cytosol (9, 87). Binding of ICAM-1 inside the canyon most probably leads to physical strain, resulting in destabilization of the capsid (18, 54). Viral neutralization is increased upon artificial dimerization of the molecule by fusing two C-terminally truncated ICAM-1 molecules with the constant heavy-chain regions of an immunoglobulin molecule (65). The reason for this increase in viral neutralization has, however, not been investigated. It might be related to bivalent binding of the chimeric molecule to a single virion or to aggregation of multiple virions.

In the case of minor group viruses, no such uncoating process has been observed upon interaction with OVR (39) or with purified recombinant soluble LDLR fragment r-$LDLR_{1-7}h$ (64). Whereas OVR gave rise to virus-receptor complexes that sedimented somewhat behind native virus, LDLR appeared to induce aggregation of the viral particles. However, upon dissociation of virus and receptor by chelating Ca ions with EDTA, infectivity was restored (64). This is reminiscent of the situation with echovirus 7, which is also neutralized by its receptor (DAF, CD55) without giving rise to 135S subviral particles; neutralization is thus completely reversible as well (78). As long as a homogeneous soluble LDLR preparation devoid of any dimers or oligomers is not available, it will be difficult to identify the exact mechanism of cell protection.

The Receptor-Binding Site

Recently, fragments of the VLDLR fused to maltose-binding protein were produced in bacteria and folded into a conformation active in virus binding (82). These recombinant proteins were subsequently shown to attach to HRV2 in solution in a stoichiometric manner (74, 75). Virus-receptor complexes were analyzed by cryo-electron microscopy (43), and image reconstruction revealed that the receptor fragments bound to the star-shaped mesa at the fivefold axes of icosahedral symmetry and not within

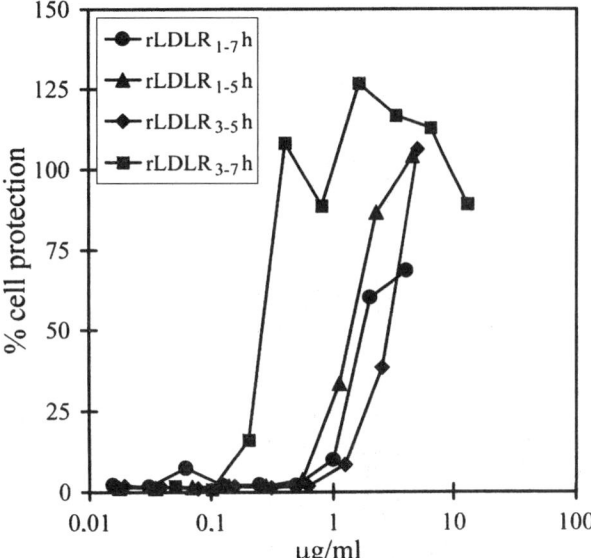

FIGURE 7 LDL minireceptors expressed in insect Sf9 cells protect HeLa cells against infection with minor group viruses. LDL receptor fragments were purified by Ni^{2+}-NTA and β-VLDL column chromatography from supernatants of Sf9 cells infected with recombinant baculoviruses carrying the cDNA encoding various combinations of ligand-binding complement type-A repeats fused to a C-terminal hexa-his tag. The purified proteins were incubated at the concentrations shown for 1.5 h at 34°C with 100 $TCID_{50}$ of HRV2. HeLa cells grown in microtiter plates were challenged with the mixtures and incubation was continued for 5 days. Cells remaining attached to the plastic as a result of lacking cytopathic effect were then stained with amido black. The stain was dissolved in NaOH and A_{560} was determined. Values measured for cells infected in the presence of wild-type baculovirus-infected Sf9 supernatant were taken as 0% protection; the values from cells grown in the absence of HRV2 were taken as 100% protection. The minimal inhibitory concentration affording 50% cell protection was determined by interpolation. Reproduced from reference 62 with permission of the publisher.

the canyon (Fig. 8). The receptor footprint covers the BC and the HI loop of VP1. This challenges the canyon hypothesis and shows that sites that are solvent exposed and visible to the immune system can also be used for receptor attachment to human rhinoviruses. The molecular basis of the interaction between 10 minor group HRV serotypes with largely divergent sequences within their BC and HI loops with one type of receptor is currently not understood.

The Way into the Cell
Shortly after binding to cell surface receptors, HRVs are internalized into coated vesicles and delivered to endosomes (10, 15, 79, 87). This process is slower for the major group virus HRV14 than for the minor group virus HRV2 (60), most probably because ICAM-1 lacks internalization signals and should therefore not be actively incorporated into coated pits. Internalization might thus be accounted for by the natural turnover of this membrane receptor (2). Moreover, it was shown that ICAM-1 lacking the intracellular C-terminal domain or having the transmembrane and cytoplasmic domain replaced by a GPI anchor is able to promote viral infection of transfected COS cells (90).

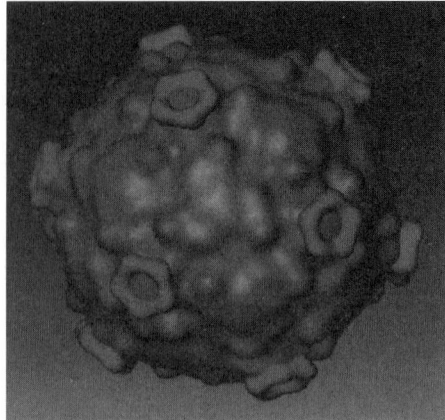

FIGURE 8 Cryo-electron microscopy image reconstruction of a complex between HRV2 (main body) and VP1–3 (protrusions) as seen down a threefold symmetry axis. Five receptor molecules bind close to the fivefold axes to the star-like mesa and cover the BC and the HI loops of VP1. Due to the close vicinity of the symmetry related sites, the receptor molecules appear to touch each other, giving rise to a ring-like appearance (density map from reference 43).

These results are difficult to reconcile with recent data from De Tulleo and Kirchhausen (28); using HeLa cells overexpressing nonfunctional dynamin, which arrests clathrin-coated pit budding, these investigators showed that HRV14 infection requires a functional clathrin-dependent endocytosis pathway. This might indicate the involvement of a putative coreceptor that directs ICAM-1 into clathrin-coated pits; it is also conceivable that internalization of ICAM-1 is somehow triggered by the clustering induced upon binding of the multivalent viral ligand.

Although LDLR mutants with truncated cytoplasmic tails were identified in patients with FH, it was not investigated whether these mutant cells are impaired with respect to infection with minor group HRVs; however, interpretation of such experiments would be difficult as one has to take into account the presence of LRP, which also functions as viral receptor.

Whereas HRV14, and possibly other less stable major group HRVs (48), can be uncoated in the presence of the specific vesicular H^+-ATPase inhibitor bafilomycin A1, i.e., in an environment with neutral pH in vivo (9, 87), minor group viruses are strictly dependent on the low pH for infection to occur (70, 79), with the receptor only functioning as a vehicle for cell entry.

OPEN QUESTIONS
Although the receptors responsible for minor group HRV infection have been identified and structural elements interacting with the virus are known, the contact site between receptors and HRVs has not yet been determined at the molecular level. Cocrystals of VLDLR fragments and HRV2 have been obtained, but low occupancy has so far precluded the determination of the X-ray structure. Selection for virus variants resistant against neutralization by any one of the receptors and identification of the changed amino acid residues might yield clues for the identification of those amino acids directly involved in the interaction. In the case of the major group virus HRV39, variants re-

quiring about a fivefold higher concentration of soluble ICAM-1 for neutralization have been isolated. However, the nature of the mutations and the basis of resistance have not been elucidated. It is thus not clear whether they are located at the site of receptor binding or are rather at the interface between the subunits and thereby influence uncoating (4). Site-directed mutagenesis of amino acid residues exposed in the canyon of HRV14 was carried out previously and allowed the identification of amino acids involved in receptor recognition (23). Similar experiments were also done with HRV2. Amino acids conserved within minor group HRVs and within major group HRVs but differing between the two groups were mutated in this study. However, the mutations were either without effect or lethal. The low transfection efficiency of in vitro transcribed full-length HRV2 RNA prevented the identification of the step in viral infection that was affected by the mutations (32).

The C termini of the ligand-binding repeats of LDLRs contain negatively charged amino acid residues. These are involved in the coordination of the Ca ion (33) but are also thought to contribute to the interaction with positive charges present on the surface of the ligands (41, 105). It is thus tempting to speculate that charge clusters on the viral surface are involved in receptor binding; the data of the mutagenesis study mentioned above (32) favor this idea, as the change of the surface-exposed tripeptide sequences $TEK_{1222-1224}$ conserved in all minor group viruses for the corresponding sequences present in the major group viruses HRV14, -39, and -89 (NEH, TNQ, and TSN, respectively) was lethal. Comparisons of the electrostatic surface potentials of major group viruses and minor group viruses with known structure also indicate the presence of positive charge clusters close to the fivefold axes of icosahedral symmetry on the surface of HRV1A and HRV2 that are at least different from those of HRV3, HRV14, and HRV16. However, whether these basic amino acid residues at the viral surface are indeed interacting with the receptors will only be known when the structure of the complex at high resolution becomes available.

Nuclear magnetic resonance (NMR) analysis and X-ray crystallography recently revealed the unusual folding pattern of recombinant single ligand-binding repeats and the spatial arrangement of the C-terminal acidic amino acid residues around the caged Ca ion (6, 21, 24, 31, 49). Single repeats are inactive in binding any of the various ligands, except for the conformation-dependent MAb IgG-C7 (25). NMR analysis of concatemers of two contiguous repeats has shown the virtual absence of mutual interaction (11, 71). It is thus unlikely that individual repeats need to contact each other's surfaces to form a binding site.

Analysis of the three-dimensional structures of so far five different HRV serotypes, the major group viruses HRV3, HRV14, and HRV16 and the minor group viruses HRV1A and HRV2 (53, 76, 84, 100, 101, 109), and extensive comparison between all available capsid protein sequences could so far not explain the divergent evolution of HRVs toward use of structurally different receptors. Furthermore, most of the amino acid residues involved in interaction between major group viruses and ICAM-1 are also present in minor group viruses (12) although HRV2 fails to attach to ICAM-1. The natural mutation rate of picornaviruses is in the range of 10^{-4} to 10^{-5} (88). As viral challenge of HeLa cells, whose ICAM-1 was blocked with a MAb, failed to result in infection despite the virus being used at a very high multiplicity of infection (98), exchange of single amino acid residues in HRV14 appears to be insufficient to enable the use of a different receptor. These results have to be interpreted with caution, however, as ICAM-1 might also be necessary in a step of the viral life cycle different from endocytosis. Nevertheless, we recently succeeded in adapting the major group virus HRV89 to grow in cells devoid of ICAM-1 and thus using another receptor whose nature is so far unknown (81). This demonstrates the great plasticity of rhinoviruses and indicates that a change in receptor usage might not be as uncommon as previously thought. Nevertheless, the mutants did not acquire characteristics of a minor group virus. These findings call for caution with polioviruses as these dangerous pathogens might also be able to switch receptors under strong selection pressure.

Experiments aimed at determining whether minor group viruses can be adapted to exploit another receptor for cell entry are more difficult to perform due to the unavailability of human cells lacking LDLR, LRP, and VLDLR altogether.

The use of more than one receptor by minor group viruses as compared to only one by major group viruses has clearly complicated the determination of these proteins. Analysis of the molecular details of the site of interaction between minor group viruses and any of their receptors is eagerly awaited; it will certainly add to the understanding of infection strategies and viral evolution.

A number of students have contributed to the work on the minor group rhinovirus receptor. Their names are found in the publications referenced here; I wish to explicitly acknowledge their contributions to the field. I thank T. Skern for critically reading the manuscript. The work presented here was funded by grants from the Austrian Science Foundation and by the Austrian Science Ministry.

REFERENCES

1. **Abraham, G., and R. J. Colonno.** 1984. Many rhinovirus serotypes share the same cellular receptor. *J. Virol.* **51:** 340–345.
2. **Almenar Queralt, A., A. Duperray, L. A. Miles, J. Felez, and D. C. Altieri.** 1995. Apical topography and modulation of ICAM-1 expression on activated endothelium. *Am. J. Pathol.* **147:**1278–1288.
3. **Anfinsen, C. B., and H. A. Scheraga.** 1975. Experimental and theoretical aspects of protein folding. *Adv. Protein Chem.* **29:**205–300.
4. **Arruda, E., C. E. Crump, and F. G. Hayden.** 1994. In vitro selection of human rhinovirus relatively resistant to soluble intercellular adhesion molecule-1. *Antimicrob. Agents Chemother.* **38:**66–70.
5. **Arruda, E., C. E. Crump, S. D. Marlin, V. J. Merluzzi, and F. G. Hayden.** 1992. In vitro studies of the anti-rhinovirus activity of soluble intercellular adhesion molecule-1. *Antimicrob. Agents Chemother.* **36:**1186–1191.
6. **Atkins, A. R., I. M. Brereton, P. A. Kroon, H. T. Lee, and R. Smith.** 1998. Calcium is essential for the structural integrity of the cysteine-rich, ligand-binding repeat of the low-density lipoprotein receptor. *Biochemistry* **37:**1662–1670.
7. **Barber, D. L., E. J. Sanders, R. Aebersold, and W. J. Schneider.** 1991. The receptor for yolk lipoprotein deposition in the chicken oocyte. *J. Biol. Chem.* **266:** 18761–18770.
8. **Bates, P., J. A. Young, and H. E. Varmus.** 1993. A receptor for subgroup A Rous sarcoma virus is related to the low density lipoprotein receptor. *Cell* **74:**1043–1051.

9. **Bayer, N., E. Prchla, M. Schwab, D. Blaas, and R. Fuchs.** 1999. Human rhinovirus HRV14 uncoats from early endosomes in the presence of bafilomycin. *FEBS Lett.* **463**:175–178.
10. **Bayer, N., D. Schober, E. Prchla, R. F. Murphy, D. Blaas, and R. Fuchs.** 1998. Effect of bafilomycin A1 and nocodazole on endocytic transport in HeLa cells: implications for viral uncoating and infection. *J. Virol.* **72**:9645–9655.
11. **Beglova, N., C. L. North, and S. C. Blacklow.** 2001. Backbone dynamics of a module pair from the ligand-binding domain of the LDL receptor. *Biochemistry* **40**:2808–2815.
12. **Bella, J., P. R. Kolatkar, C. W. Marlor, J. M. Greve, and M. G. Rossmann.** 1998. The structure of the two amino-terminal domains of human ICAM-1 suggests how it functions as a rhinovirus receptor and as an LFA-1 integrin ligand. *Proc. Natl. Acad. Sci. USA* **95**:4140–4145.
13. **Bieri, S., A. R. Atkins, H. T. Lee, D. J. Winzor, R. Smith, and P. A. Kroon.** 1998. Folding, calcium binding, and structural characterization of a concatemer of the first and second ligand-binding modules of the low-density lipoprotein receptor. *Biochemistry* **37**:10994–11002.
14. **Bieri, S., J. T. Djordjevic, N. L. Daly, R. Smith, and P. A. Kroon.** 1995. Disulfide bridges of a cysteine-rich repeat of the LDL receptor ligand-binding domain. *Biochemistry* **34**:13059–13065.
15. **Blaas, D., and R. Fuchs.** 1999. Early steps in rhinoviral infection, p. 485–503. *In* S. G. Pandalai (ed.), *Recent Research Developments in Virology*, vol. 1. Transworld Research Network, Kerala, India.
16. **Bu, G. J., H. J. Geuze, G. J. Strous, and A. L. Schwartz.** 1995. 39 kDa receptor-associated protein is an ER resident protein and molecular chaperone for LDL receptor-related protein. *EMBO J.* **14**:2269–2280.
17. **Bu, G. J., and S. Rennke.** 1996. Receptor-associated protein is a folding chaperone for low density liporeceptor-related protein. *J. Biol. Chem.* **271**:22218–22224.
18. **Casasnovas, J. M.** 2000. The dynamics of receptor recognition by human rhinoviruses. *Trends Microbiol.* **8**:251–254.
19. **Casasnovas, J. M., and T. A. Springer.** 1994. Pathway of rhinovirus disruption by soluble intercellular adhesion molecule 1 (ICAM-1): an intermediate in which ICAM-1 is bound and RNA is released. *J. Virol.* **68**:5882–5889.
20. **Chen, W. J., J. L. Goldstein, and M. S. Brown.** 1990. NPXY, a sequence often found in cytoplasmic tails, is required for coated pit-mediated internalization of the low density lipoprotein receptor. *J. Biol. Chem.* **265**:3116–3123.
21. **Clayton, D., I. M. Brereton, P. A. Kroon, and R. Smith.** 2000. Three-dimensional NMR structure of the sixth ligand-binding module of the human LDL receptor: comparison of two adjacent modules with different ligand binding specificities. *FEBS Lett.* **479**:118–122.
22. **Colonno, R. J., P. L. Callahan, and W. J. Long.** 1986. Isolation of a monoclonal antibody that blocks attachment of the major group of human rhinoviruses. *J. Virol.* **57**:7–12.
23. **Colonno, R. J., J. H. Condra, S. Mizutani, P. L. Callahan, M. E. Davies, and M. A. Murcko.** 1988. Evidence for the direct involvement of the rhinovirus canyon in receptor binding. *Proc. Natl. Acad. Sci. USA* **85**:5449–5453.
24. **Daly, N. L., J. T. Djordjevic, P. A. Kroon, and R. Smith.** 1995. Three-dimensional structure of the second cysteine-rich repeat from the human low-density lipoprotein receptor. *Biochemistry* **34**:14474–14481.
25. **Daly, N. L., M. J. Scanlon, J. T. Djordjevic, P. A. Kroon, and R. Smith.** 1995. Three-dimensional structure of a cysteine-rich repeat from the low-density lipoprotein receptor. *Proc. Natl. Acad. Sci. USA* **92**:6334–6338.
26. **Davis, C. G., J. L. Goldstein, T. C. Sudhof, R. G. Anderson, D. W. Russell, and M. S. Brown.** 1987. Acid-dependent ligand dissociation and recycling of LDL receptor mediated by growth factor homology region. *Nature* **326**:760–765.
27. **De Broe, M. E., R. J. Wieme, G. N. Logghe, and F. Roels.** 1977. Spontaneous shedding of plasma membrane fragments by human cells in vivo and in vitro. *Clin. Chim. Acta* **81**:237–245.
28. **De Tulleo, L., and T. Kirchhausen.** 1998. The clathrin endocytic pathway in viral infection. *EMBO J.* **17**:4585–4593.
29. **Dirlam Schatz, K. A., and A. D. Attie.** 1998. Calcium induces a conformational change in the ligand binding domain of the low density lipoprotein receptor. *J. Lipid Res.* **39**:402–411.
30. **DiScipio, R. G., M. R. Gehring, E. R. Podack, C. C. Kan, T. E. Hugli, and G. H. Fey.** 1984. Nucleotide sequence of cDNA and derived amino acid sequence of human complement component C9. *Proc. Natl. Acad. Sci. USA* **81**:7298–7302.
31. **Dolmer, K., W. Huang, and P. G. W. Gettins.** 1998. Characterization of the calcium site in two complement-like domains from the low-density lipoprotein receptor-related protein (LRP) and comparison with a repeat from the low-density lipoprotein receptor. *Biochemistry* **37**:17016–17023.
32. **Duechler, M., S. Ketter, T. Skern, E. Kuechler, and D. Blaas.** 1993. Rhinoviral receptor discrimination: mutational changes in the canyon regions of human rhinovirus types 2 and 14 indicate a different site of interaction. *J. Gen. Virol.* **74**:2287–2291.
33. **Fass, D., S. Blacklow, P. S. Kim, and J. M. Berger.** 1997. Molecular basis of familial hypercholesterolaemia from structure of LDL receptor module. *Nature* **388**:691–693.
34. **Gilmore, E. C., and K. Herrup.** 2000. Cortical development: receiving reelin. *Curr. Biol.* **10**:R162–166.
35. **Giranda, V. L., M. S. Chapman, and M. G. Rossmann.** 1990. Modeling of the human intercellular adhesion molecule-1, the human rhinovirus major group receptor. *Proteins* **7**:227–233.
36. **Gliemann, J.** 1998. Receptors of the low density lipoprotein (LDL) receptor family in man. Multiple functions of the large family members via interaction with complex ligands. *Biol. Chem.* **379**:951–964.
37. **Greve, J. M., G. Davis, A. M. Meyer, C. P. Forte, S. C. Yost, C. W. Marlor, M. E. Kamarck, and A. McClelland.** 1989. The major human rhinovirus receptor is ICAM-1. *Cell* **56**:839–847.
38. **Greve, J. M., C. P. Forte, C. W. Marlor, A. M. Meyer, H. Hoover-Litty, D. Wunderlich, and A. McClelland.** 1991. Mechanisms of receptor-mediated rhinovirus neutralization defined by two soluble forms of ICAM-1. *J. Virol.* **65**:6015–6023.
39. **Gruenberger, M., R. Wandl, J. Nimpf, T. Hiesberger, W. J. Schneider, E. Kuechler, and D. Blaas.** 1995. Avian homologs of the mammalian low-density lipoprotein receptor family bind minor receptor group human rhinovirus. *J. Virol.* **69**:7244–7247.
40. **Hardy, M. M., J. Feder, R. A. Wolfe, and G. J. Bu.** 1997. Low density lipoprotein receptor-related protein modulates the expression of tissue-type plasminogen activator in human colon fibroblasts. *J. Biol. Chem.* **272**:6812–6817.

41. Haridas, M., B. F. Anderson, H. M. Baker, G. E. Norris, and E. N. Baker. 1994. X-ray structural analysis of bovine lactoferrin at 2.5 A resolution. *Adv. Exp. Med. Biol.* **357:**235–238.

42. Herz, J., U. Hamann, S. Rogne, O. Myklebost, H. Gausepohl, and K. K. Stanley. 1988. Surface location and high affinity for calcium of a 500-kd liver membrane protein closely related to the LDL-receptor suggest a physiological role as lipoprotein receptor. *EMBO J.* **7:**4119–4127.

43. Hewat, E. A., E. Neumann, J. F. Conway, R. Moser, B. Ronacher, T. C. Marlovits, and D. Blaas. 2000. The cellular receptor to human rhinovirus 2 binds around the 5-fold axis and not in the canyon: a structural view. *EMBO J.* **19:**6317–6325.

44. Hobbs, H. H., M. S. Brown, and J. L. Goldstein. 1992. Molecular genetics of the LDL receptor gene in familial hypercholesterolemia. *Hum. Mutat.* **1:**445–466.

45. Hodits, R. A., J. Nimpf, D. M. Pfistermueller, T. Hiesberger, W. J. Schneider, T. J. Vaughan, K. S. Johnson, M. Haumer, E. Kuechler, G. Winter, and D. Blaas. 1995. An antibody fragment from a phage display library competes for ligand binding to the low density lipoprotein receptor family and inhibits rhinovirus infection. *J. Biol. Chem.* **270:**24078–24085.

46. Hofer, F., B. Berger, M. Gruenberger, H. Machat, R. Dernick, U. Tessmer, E. Kuechler, and D. Blaas. 1992. Shedding of a rhinovirus minor group binding protein—evidence for a Ca^{2+}-dependent process. *J. Gen. Virol.* **73:**627–632.

47. Hofer, F., M. Gruenberger, H. Kowalski, H. Machat, M. Huettinger, E. Kuechler, and D. Blaas. 1994. Members of the low density lipoprotein receptor family mediate cell entry of a minor-group common cold virus. *Proc. Natl. Acad. Sci. USA* **91:**1839–1842.

48. Hoover-Litty, H., and J. M. Greve. 1993. Formation of rhinovirus-soluble ICAM-1 complexes and conformational changes in the virion. *J. Virol.* **67:**390–397.

49. Huang, W., K. Dolmer, and P. G. W. Gettins. 1999. NMR solution structure of complement-like repeat CR8 from the low density lipoprotein receptor-related protein. *J. Biol. Chem.* **274:**14130–14136.

50. Iijima, H., M. Miyazawa, J. Sakai, K. Magoori, M. R. Ito, H. Suzuki, M. Nose, Y. Kawarabayasi, and T. T. Yamamoto. 1998. Expression and characterization of a very low density lipoprotein receptor variant lacking the O-linked sugar region generated by alternative splicing. *J. Biochem.* **124:**747–755.

51. Ishibashi, S., M. S. Brown, J. L. Goldstein, R. D. Gerard, R. E. Hammer, and J. Herz. 1993. Hypercholesterolemia in low density lipoprotein receptor knockout mice and its reversal by adenovirus-mediated gene delivery. *J. Clin. Invest.* **92:**883–893.

52. Kamps, J. A. A. M., and T. J. C. Vanberkel. 1992. Complete down-regulation of low-density-lipoprotein-receptor activity in the human hepatoma cell line HepG2 by beta-migrating very-low-density lipoprotein and non-lipoprotein cholesterol—different cellular regulatory pools of cholesterol. *Eur. J. Biochem.* **206:**973–978.

53. Kim, S., T. J. Smith, M. S. Chapman, M. G. Rossmann, D. C. Pevear, F. J. Dutko, P. J. Felock, G. D. Diana, and M. A. McKinlay. 1989. Crystal structure of human rhinovirus serotype-1A (Hrv1A). *J. Mol. Biol.* **210:**91–111.

54. Kolatkar, P. R., J. Bella, N. H. Olson, C. M. Bator, T. S. Baker, and M. G. Rossmann. 1999. Structural studies of two rhinovirus serotypes complexed with fragments of their cellular receptor. *EMBO J.* **18:**6249–6259.

55. Korant, B. D., K. Lonberg-Holm, J. Noble, and J. T. Stasny. 1972. Naturally occurring and artificially produced components of three rhinoviruses. *Virology* **48:**71–86.

56. Kristensen, T., S. K. Moestrup, J. Gliemann, L. Bendtsen, O. Sand, and L. Sottrup Jensen. 1990. Evidence that the newly cloned low-density-lipoprotein receptor related protein (LRP) is the alpha 2-macroglobulin receptor. *FEBS Lett.* **276:**151–155.

57. Lonberg-Holm, K., and J. Noble Harvey. 1973. Comparison of in vitro and cell-mediated alteration of a human rhinovirus and its inhibition by sodium dodecyl sulfate. *J. Virol.* **12:**819–826.

58. Lonberg-Holm, K., and F. H. Yin. 1973. Antigenic determinants of infective and inactivated human rhinovirus type 2. *J. Virol.* **12:**114–123.

59. Lonberg-Holm, K., R. L. Crowell, and L. Philipson. 1976. Unrelated animal viruses share receptors. *Nature* **259:**679–681.

60. Lonberg-Holm, K., and B. D. Korant. 1972. Early interaction of rhinoviruses with host cells. *J. Virol.* **9:**29–40.

61. Magrane, J., M. Reina, R. Pagan, A. Luna, R. P. Casaroli Marano, B. Angelin, M. Gafvels, and S. Vilaro. 1998. Bovine aortic endothelial cells express a variant of the very low density lipoprotein receptor that lacks the O-linked sugar domain. *J. Lipid Res.* **39:**2172–2181.

62. Marlovits, T. C., C. Abrahamsberg, and D. Blaas. 1998. Soluble LDL minireceptors—minimal structure requirements for recognition of minor group human rhinovirus. *J. Biol. Chem.* **273:**33835–33840.

63. Marlovits, T. C., C. Abrahamsberg, and D. Blaas. 1998. Very-low-density lipoprotein receptor fragment shed from HeLa cells inhibits human rhinovirus infection. *J. Virol.* **72:**10246–10250.

64. Marlovits, T. C., T. Zechmeister, M. Gruenberger, B. Ronacher, H. Schwihla, and D. Blaas. 1998. Recombinant soluble low density lipoprotein receptor fragment inhibits minor group rhinovirus infection in vitro. *FASEB J.* **12:**695–703.

65. Martin, S., J. M. Casasnovas, D. E. Staunton, and T. A. Springer. 1993. Efficient neutralization and disruption of rhinovirus by chimeric ICAM-1/immunoglobulin molecules. *J. Virol.* **67:**3561–3568.

66. Martin, S., A. Martin, D. E. Staunton, and T. A. Springer. 1993. Functional studies of truncated soluble intercellular adhesion molecule-1 expressed in *Escherichia coli*. *Antimicrob. Agents Chemother.* **37:**1278–1285.

67. Medh, J. D., G. L. Fry, S. L. Bowen, M. W. Pladet, D. K. Strickland, and D. A. Chappell. 1995. The 39-kDa receptor-associated protein modulates lipoprotein catabolism by binding to LDL receptors. *J. Biol. Chem.* **270:**536–540.

68. Mischak, H., C. Neubauer, B. Berger, E. Kuechler, and D. Blaas. 1988. Detection of the human rhinovirus minor group receptor on renaturing Western blots. *J. Gen. Virol.* **69:**2653–2656.

69. Mischak, H., C. Neubauer, E. Kuechler, and D. Blaas. 1988. Characteristics of the minor group receptor of human rhinoviruses. *Virology* **163:**19–25.

70. Neubauer, C., L. Frasel, E. Kuechler, and D. Blaas. 1987. Mechanism of entry of human rhinovirus 2 into HeLa cells. *Virology* **158:**255–258.

71. North, C. L., and S. C. Blacklow. 2000. Evidence that familial hypercholesterolemia mutations of the LDL receptor cause limited local misfolding in an LDL-A module pair. *Biochemistry* **39:**13127–13135.

72. North, C. L., and S. C. Blacklow. 2000. Solution structure of the sixth LDL-A module of the LDL receptors. *Biochemistry* **39:**2564–2571.

73. **Obermoeller, L. M., Z. Chen, A. L. Schwartz, and G. Bu.** 1998. Ca2+ and receptor-associated protein are independently required for proper folding and disulfide bond formation of the low density lipoprotein receptor-related protein. *J. Biol. Chem.* **273:**22374–22381.
74. **Okun, V. M., R. Moser, D. Blaas, and E. Kenndler.** 2001. Complexes between monoclonal antibodies and receptor fragments with a common cold virus: determination of stoichiometry by capillary electrophoresis. *Anal. Biochem.* **73:**3900–3906.
75. **Okun, V. M., R. Moser, B. Ronacher, E. Kenndler, and D. Blaas.** 2001. VLDL receptor fragments of different lengths bind to human rhinovirus HRV2 with different stoichiometry. An analysis of virus-receptor complexes by capillary electrophoresis. *J. Biol. Chem.* **276:**1057–1062.
76. **Oliveira, M. A., R. Zhao, W. M. Lee, M. J. Kremer, I. Minor, R. R. Rueckert, G. D. Diana, D. C. Pevear, F. J. Dutko, M. A. McKinlay, and M. G. Rossmann.** 1993. The structure of human rhinovirus 16. *Structure* **1:**51–68.
77. **Olson, N. H., P. R. Kolatkar, M. A. Oliveira, R. H. Cheng, J. M. Greve, A. McClelland, T. S. Baker, and M. G. Rossmann.** 1993. Structure of a human rhinovirus complexed with its receptor molecule. *Proc. Natl. Acad. Sci. USA* **90:**507–511.
78. **Powell, R. M., T. Ward, D. J. Evans, and J. W. Almond.** 1997. Interaction between echovirus 7 and its receptor, decay accelerating factor (Cd55): evidence for a secondary cellular factor in A particle formation. *J. Virol.* **71:**9306–9312.
79. **Prchla, E., E. Kuechler, D. Blaas, and R. Fuchs.** 1994. Uncoating of human rhinovirus serotype 2 from late endosomes. *J. Virol.* **68:**3713–3723.
80. **Register, R. B., C. R. Uncapher, A. M. Naylor, D. W. Lineberger, and R. J. Colonno.** 1991. Human-murine chimeras of ICAM-1 identify amino acid residues critical for rhinovirus and antibody binding. *J. Virol.* **65:**6589–6596.
81. **Reischl, A., M. Reithmayer, G. Winsauer, R. Moser, I. Gösler, and D. Blaas.** 2001. Viral evolution toward change in receptor usage: adaptation of a major group human rhinovirus to grow in ICAM-1 negative cells. *J. Virol.* **75:**9312–9319.
82. **Ronacher, B., T. C. Marlovits, R. Moser, and D. Blaas.** 2000. Expression and folding of human very-low-density lipoprotein receptor fragments: neutralization capacity toward human rhinovirus HRV2. *Virology* **278:**541–550.
83. **Rossmann, M. G.** 1989. The canyon hypothesis. Hiding the host cell receptor attachment site on a viral surface from immune surveillance. *J. Biol. Chem.* **264:**14587–14590.
84. **Rossmann, M. G., E. Arnold, J. W. Erickson, E. A. Frankenberger, J. P. Griffith, H. J. Hecht, J. E. Johnson, G. Kamer, M. Luo, A. G. Mosser, R. R. Rueckert, B. Sherry, and G. Vriend.** 1985. Structure of a human common cold virus and functional relationship to other picornaviruses. *Nature* **317:**145–153.
85. **Rothlein, R., M. L. Dustin, S. D. Marlin, and T. A. Springer.** 1986. A human intercellular adhesion molecule (ICAM-1) distinct from LFA-1. *J. Immunol.* **137:**1270–1274.
86. **Saito, A., S. Pietromonaco, A. K. C. Loo, and M. G. Farquhar.** 1994. Complete cloning and sequencing of rat gp330/"megalin," a distinctive member of the low density lipoprotein receptor gene family. *Proc. Natl. Acad. Sci. USA* **91:**9725–9729.
87. **Schober, D., P. Kronenberger, E. Prchla, D. Blaas, and R. Fuchs.** 1998. Major and minor-receptor group human rhinoviruses penetrate from endosomes by different mechanisms. *J. Virol.* **72:**1354–1364.
88. **Sherry, B., and R. Rueckert.** 1985. Evidence for at least two dominant neutralization antigens on human rhinovirus 14. *J. Virol.* **53:**137–143.
89. **Staunton, D. E., M. L. Dustin, H. P. Erickson, and T. A. Springer.** 1990. The arrangement of the immunoglobulin-like domains of ICAM-1 and the binding sites for LFA-1 and rhinovirus. *Cell* **61:**243–254.
90. **Staunton, D. E., A. Gaur, P. Y. Chan, and T. A. Springer.** 1992. Internalization of a major group human rhinovirus does not require cytoplasmic or transmembrane domains of ICAM-1. *J. Immunol.* **148:**3271–3274.
91. **Staunton, D. E., V. J. Merluzzi, R. Rothlein, R. Barton, S. D. Marlin, and T. A. Springer.** 1989. A cell adhesion molecule, ICAM-1, is the major surface receptor for rhinoviruses. *Cell* **56:**849–853.
92. **Stifani, S., R. George, and W. J. Schneider.** 1988. Solubilization and characterization of the chicken oocyte vitellogenin receptor. *Biochem. J.* **250:**467–475.
93. **Strickland, D. K., J. D. Ashcom, S. Williams, W. H. Burgess, M. Migliorini, and W. S. Argraves.** 1990. Sequence identity between the alpha 2-macroglobulin receptor and low density lipoprotein receptor-related protein suggests that this molecule is a multifunctional receptor. *J. Biol. Chem.* **265:**17401–17404.
94. **Strickland, D. K., M. Z. Kounnas, and W. S. Argraves.** 1995. LDL receptor-related protein: a multiligand receptor for lipoprotein and proteinase catabolism. *FASEB J.* **9:**890–898.
95. **Takahashi, S., Y. Kawarabayasi, T. Nakai, J. Sakai, and T. Yamamoto.** 1992. Rabbit very low density lipoprotein receptor: a low density lipoprotein receptor-like protein with distinct ligand specificity. *Proc. Natl. Acad. Sci. USA* **89:**9252–9256.
96. **Tessier, D. C., D. Y. Thomas, H. E. Khouri, F. Laliberte, and T. Vernet.** 1991. Enhanced secretion from insect cells of a foreign protein fused to the honeybee melittin signal peptide. *Gene* **98:**177–183.
97. **Tomassini, E., T. Graham, C. DeWitt, D. Lineberger, J. Rodkey, and R. Colonno.** 1989. cDNA cloning reveals that the major group rhinovirus receptor on HeLa cells is intercellular adhesion molecule 1. *Proc. Natl. Acad. Sci. USA* **86:**4907–4911.
98. **Tomassini, J. E., and R. J. Colonno.** 1986. Isolation of a receptor protein involved in attachment of human rhinoviruses. *J. Virol.* **58:**290–295.
99. **Uncapher, C. R., C. M. Dewitt, and R. J. Colonno.** 1991. The major and minor group receptor families contain all but one human rhinovirus serotype. *Virology* **180:**814–817.
100. **Verdaguer, N., D. Blaas, and I. Fita.** 2000. Structure of human rhinovirus serotype 2 (HRV2). *J. Mol. Biol.* **300:**1179–1194.
101. **Verdaguer, N., T. C. Marlovits, J. Bravo, D. I. Stuart, D. Blaas, and I. Fita.** 1999. Crystallization and preliminary X-ray analysis of human rhinovirus serotype 2 (HRV2). *Acta Crystallogr. D Biol. Crystallogr.* **55:**1459–1461.
102. **Willnow, T. E..** 1999. The low-density lipoprotein receptor gene family: multiple roles in lipid metabolism. *J. Mol. Med.* **77:**306–315.
103. **Willnow, T. E., S. A. Armstrong, R. E. Hammer, and J. Herz.** 1995. Functional expression of low density lipoprotein receptor-related protein is controlled by receptor-associated protein in vivo. *Proc. Natl. Acad. Sci. USA* **92:**4537–4541.

104. **Willnow, T. E., and J. Herz.** 1994. Genetic deficiency in low density lipoprotein receptor-related protein confers cellular resistance to Pseudomonas exotoxin A. Evidence that this protein is required for uptake and degradation of multiple ligands. *J. Cell Sci.* **107:**719–726.
105. **Wilson, C., M. R. Wardell, K. H. Weisgraber, R. W. Mahley, and D. A. Agard.** 1991. Three-dimensional structure of the LDL receptor-binding domain of human apolipoprotein E. *Science* **252:**1817–1822.
106. **Yamamoto, T., C. G. Davis, M. S. Brown, W. J. Schneider, M. L. Casey, J. L. Goldstein, and D. W. Russell.** 1984. The human LDL receptor: a cysteine-rich protein with multiple Alu sequences in its mRNA. *Cell* **39:**27–38.
107. **Yin, F. H., and N. B. Lomax.** 1986. Establishment of a mouse model for human rhinovirus infection. *J. Gen. Virol.* **67:**2335–2340.
108. **Yin, F. H., and N. B. Lomax.** 1983. Host range mutants of human rhinovirus in which nonstructural proteins are altered. *J. Virol.* **48:**410–418.
109. **Zhao, R., D. C. Pevear, M. J. Kremer, V. L. Giranda, J. A. Kofron, R. J. Kuhn, and M. G. Rossmann.** 1996. Human rhinovirus 3 at 3.0 angstrom resolution. *Structure* **4:**1205–1220.

Receptors for Coxsackieviruses and Echoviruses

JEFFREY M. BERGELSON

10

Studies in the late 1950s demonstrated that homogenates of particular tissues could adsorb picornaviruses, including some echoviruses and coxsackieviruses, and correlated virus adsorption with susceptibility to infection (23). These results led to the idea that tissue-specific expression of receptors was an important determinant of virus host range and tissue tropism. Receptors for group B coxsackieviruses (CVB) were found to be protease sensitive and associated with the plasma membrane, suggesting that they were integral membrane proteins (68, 69). An erythrocyte receptor for echovirus 7 (EV7) was partially purified, shown to inhibit attachment by EV7 and EV19, as well as CVB3, and found to contain protein, lipid, and carbohydrate (40). These results are interesting in light of more recent observations that all three of these viruses bind to CD55, a red cell glycoprotein with a glycolipid membrane anchor. However, the identity of the receptors was only determined within the past 10 years.

COXSACKIEVIRUS B RECEPTORS

Our understanding of the receptors for CVBs is largely based on work by Richard Crowell and his colleagues, beginning in the 1960s, and culminating in the identification of two receptor molecules within the past 5 years. Attachment-interference studies, in which saturation of cellular receptors by one virus was found to prevent attachment of a related virus, identified several picornavirus receptor families, whose members were likely to share receptors (13). All six CVB serotypes were found to compete with each other for attachment, but not with the three poliovirus serotypes, which defined a second receptor family. Group A coxsackieviruses (CVA) appeared to bind receptors distinct from the CVB receptor, but CVA21 was found to compete with the major group of human rhinoviruses (whose receptor was subsequently identified as intercellular adhesion molecule 1 [ICAM-1]) (21). The unexpected observation that adenovirus type 2 competed with CVB3 for an attachment site on HeLa cells led to the suggestion that these genetically and structurally distinct viruses bound to a common receptor (32).

Other work suggested that CVBs could bind to at least two receptors. CVB3 was found to associate in a detergent-stable complex with a 45- to 50-kDa cellular protein (34) and with a protein of approximately the same size on virus overlay blots (26). A monoclonal antibody raised against this protein blocked infection by all six CVB serotypes (25), suggesting that the 45-kDa protein—now identified as CAR, the coxsackievirus and adenovirus receptor—is the group-specific receptor. However, CVB3 adapted to growth in rhabdomyosarcoma (RD) cells (48) bound to an additional 70-kDa protein on overlay blots (26, 38), and a monoclonal antibody that recognized this second protein blocked infection by prototype strains of CVB1, -3, and -5 (but not CVB2, -4, or -6) (12). This antibody was also found to inhibit infection by echovirus 6 (12). Following the recognition that echovirus 6 and other echoviruses bind to decay-accelerating factor (DAF) (see below), the 70-kDa protein was also identified as DAF.

DAF (CD55)

DAF is expressed on many cell types and functions to protect cells from lysis by autologous complement (33). Unlike proteins that are anchored in the membrane by a hydrophobic transmembrane domain, DAF is linked directly to the outer leaflet of the cell membrane by a glycolipid (glycosylphosphatidylinositol [GPI]) anchor. Rodent cells transfected with human DAF cDNA bind some but not all strains of CVB3, as well as some strains of CVB1 and CVB5 (6, 53). Anti-DAF antibodies block infection by CVB1, CVB3, and CVB5, but not by CVB2, CVB4, or CVB6 (12, 53). Although DAF-transfected rodent cells may bind virus, they do not become productively infected (6, 53). Because such cells produce virus when transfected with viral RNA (53), it appears that DAF-transfected cells are deficient in some early postattachment function, perhaps in virus internalization or uncoating.

DAF is a member of a family of complement regulatory proteins composed of homologous short consensus repeat

---

Jeffrey M. Bergelson ■ Division of Immunologic and Infectious Diseases, Children's Hospital of Philadelphia, Abramson 1202, 3615 Civic Center Boulevard, Philadelphia, PA 19104-44318.

(SCR) domains. DAF is composed of four SCR domains, with an additional membrane-proximal mucin-like domain that is heavily glycosylated on serine and threonine residues (Fig. 1). Experiments with SCR deletion mutants and with monoclonal antibodies that recognize individual DAF SCR domains indicate that SCRs 1 and 4 are not required for attachment of CVB3-RD and suggest that virus binds primarily to SCR2, and possibly to SCR3 (6). Antibody blockade suggests that SCR3 is important for attachment of another DAF-binding isolate (56). In contrast, poliovirus and rhinovirus attachment to cells involves the insertion of the receptor N-terminal domain into a canyon or depression on the virus surface. It is clear that CVB3 interaction with DAF must involve a different spatial relationship between virus and receptor.

As is discussed below, a number of other enteroviruses also interact with DAF. In general, these are viruses recognized to be capable of agglutinating human erythrocytes. The prototype CVB3-Nancy strain studied by Crowell and coworkers does not agglutinate, but the CVB3-RD strain, which binds DAF, does agglutinate red cells (48).

CAR

As described above, a 45- to 50-kDa protein was proposed to be the group-specific receptor for all six CVB serotypes. Antibodies to this protein were used to isolate a cDNA clone that encodes a receptor for CVBs and for adenoviruses 2 and 5 (4, 60). Other investigators independently isolated a coxsackievirus-binding protein that proved to be the coxsackievirus and adenovirus receptor (CAR) (11).

CAR is a 46-kDa cell surface glycoprotein composed of an extracellular portion (containing two immunoglobulin [Ig]-like domains), a typical hydrophobic transmembrane region, and a 107-amino-acid-long cytoplasmic domain. Rodent cells transfected with CAR cDNA gain the capacity to bind virus and—unlike DAF transfectants—to become infected. The murine CAR homologue also functions as a receptor, consistent with the susceptibility of mice to infection by CVBs (5, 60). The murine and human proteins are very similar (91% amino acid identity within the extracellular domain, 77% within the transmembrane domain, and 95% identity within the cytoplasmic domain). Two forms of the protein have been identified, differing only at the C terminus, and most likely resulting from alternative RNA splicing. Both CVB3 (21a) and adenovirus (10, 19) interact with CAR's membrane-distal (N-terminal) Ig-like domain. CAR homologues have been identified in a variety of other mammalian species (17) as well as in the zebrafish (62).

Consistent with the original observation that all six CVB serotypes compete for a single receptor, CAR has been shown to mediate infection by laboratory and clinical isolates belonging to all six serotypes (35), including viruses like CVB3-RD that also interact with DAF. No tested CVB3 isolate fails to interact with CAR. In addition, human CAR functions in infection by swine vesicular disease virus, a porcine pathogen that is genetically related to CVB5 (35).

CAR is a novel protein whose function remains uncertain. CAR expression on transfected cells facilitates homotypic cell adhesion (11a, 24). Consistent with this, CAR's N-terminal Ig-like domain forms a homodimer; residues involved in homodimerization are more highly conserved in evolution than are other residues in the extracellular domain, suggesting that the capacity for dimerization may be related to CAR's function (62). In nonpolarized cells, CAR is concentrated at cell-cell contacts, and in polarized epithelial cells it is absent from the apical cell surface and concentrated at intercellular tight junctions (11a, 41, 42, 63). There is evidence suggesting that CAR-mediated intercellular interactions may be involved in regulating cell proliferation (39b).

The evolutionary conservation of the cytoplasmic domain suggests that CAR may interact with other intracel-

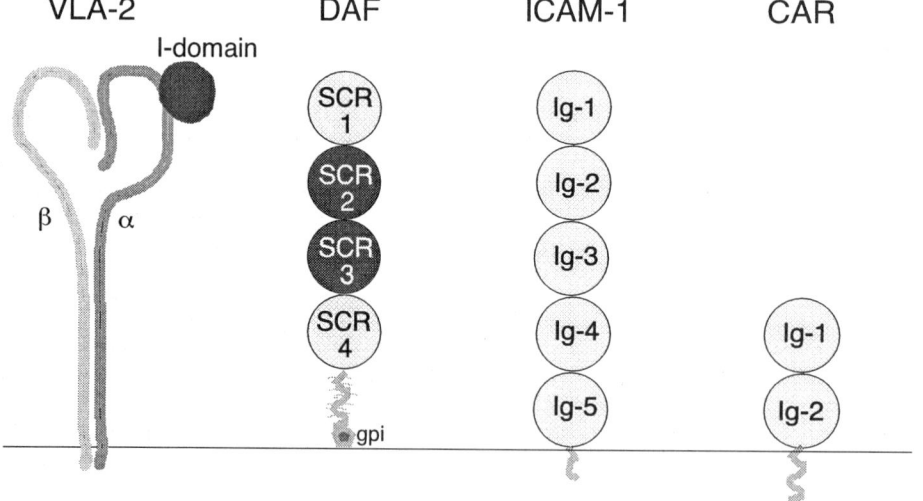

FIGURE 1 Receptors for echoviruses and coxsackieviruses. Each of these proteins has been shown by cDNA transfection to mediate virus attachment or infection. EV1 and EV8 interact directly with the I domain within the α subunit of the integrin VLA-2. CVB3-RD interacts with SCR domain 2 (and possibly SCR3) of DAF. Other viruses may interact with other DAF SCR domains (see text). CVA21 interacts with ICAM-1, and CVB interact with CAR. These viruses are likely to interact with the distal Ig-like domains of their receptors.

lular proteins. However, deletion of the cytoplasmic domain or expression of CAR as a GPI-anchored protein lacking both cytoplasmic and transmembrane domains does not eliminate its function as a receptor, indicating that only the extracellular domain is required for virus infection (64). It thus appears that the failure of DAF to support virus infection does not result from the fact that it is a GPI-anchored rather than a transmembrane protein.

Virus Structure in Relation to Receptor Attachment

The structure of CVB3 has been determined by X-ray crystallography (39). The structure is remarkable not only for the presence of a canyon at the fivefold axis—similar to depressions seen in rhinovirus (51) and poliovirus (22)—but for an additional deep depression at the twofold axis. An amino acid residue thought to be important in interaction with DAF (serine 151 of VP2) (31) projects into the depression at the twofold axis, suggesting that the twofold axis may be the site of interaction with DAF. CAR's N-terminal domain inserts into the canyon with the rest of the molecule projecting orthogonally from the virus surface (21a). Because DAF's N-terminal SCR domain is not involved in virus attachment, it seems likely that DAF lies "sideways" or tangential to the virus surface.

Other Proteins Possibly Involved in CVB Attachment and Entry

A 100-kDa HeLa cell protein, distinct from DAF and CAR, and with sequence similarity to human nucleolin, was found to bind all six coxsackievirus serotypes on virus overlay blots (14). So far, neither transfection experiments introducing this protein into a receptor-negative cell line nor antibody-blocking experiments demonstrating its involvement in virus attachment to the cell surface have been performed. At this time, the evidence is insufficient to be certain that the 100-kDa nucleolin homologue functions in coxsackievirus attachment or infection.

Expression of another protein, the integrin $\alpha v \beta 6$, enhances the susceptibility of intestinal epithelial cells to infection by CVB1 (1). The effect depends on the presence of an intact $\beta 6$ cytoplasmic domain. Although the mechanism is uncertain, $\alpha v \beta 6$ had no effect on virus attachment, suggesting that the effect on these cells—which express both DAF and CAR—is related to some postattachment event in infection. The αv integrins have been shown to facilitate internalization of adenoviruses expressing the sequence Arg-Gly-Asp (RGD) within a capsid protein (67). CVB1 capsid proteins do not contain an RGD sequence, but it is possible that $\alpha v \beta 6$ is involved in virus internalization or uncoating. However, because $\alpha v \beta 6$ is not expressed on HeLa cells, which are quite susceptible to CVB1 infection, it cannot be essential for virus infection.

What Are the Functions of the Multiple Receptors?

Despite considerable progress in our understanding of coxsackievirus-receptor interactions, a number of earlier observations remain puzzling, and many questions remain, particularly about the role for DAF in virus infection.

It is clear that attachment to DAF is not essential for coxsackievirus infection, either in vitro or in vivo: CAR-transfected CHO cells, which do not express DAF, are readily infected; and although murine DAF does not bind virus (57), mice are susceptible to infection. Nonetheless, a number of coxsackievirus and other enterovirus isolates—including low-passage clinical isolates—bind to human DAF. Enteroviruses grouped in separate phylogenetic clusters interact with DAF, possibly at different sites within the DAF molecule (as determined by inhibition with SCR-specific monoclonal antibodies or attachment to DAF deletion mutants); this may suggest that the DAF-binding phenotype has evolved independently in different virus strains because it confers some selective advantage within the host (45). Although CAR is absent from the apical surface of polarized epithelial cells, DAF is often abundant on the apical surface. Interaction with DAF on the apical surface of polarized epithelial cells in vitro facilitates infection by DAF-binding CVB (J. T. C. Shieh and J. M. Bergelson, submitted for publication). It is thus possible that DAF is important for virus interaction with mucosal surfaces in vivo.

The observation that CAR-transfected rodent cells become infected, while DAF-transfected CHO cells do not, suggests that DAF cannot perform some postattachment function essential for virus infection. Contact of poliovirus and rhinovirus with their receptors leads to alterations in the virus capsid (A particle formation) that are believed to initiate the uncoating process. In both instances, the receptors belong to the Ig superfamily and bind in the viral canyon. It is not yet known whether CAR, an Ig family member, binds to the CB canyon; however, as discussed above, there is evidence that DAF does not. One possibility, which has not yet been tested, is that CAR interaction in the canyon is sufficient to trigger viral uncoating (and thus to permit infection), whereas DAF attachment outside the canyon does not destabilize the virus particle.

Under certain circumstances, DAF appears to mediate infection by another virus, CVA21, even in the absence of the primary receptor, ICAM-1 (52). It is not known whether DAF expression, in the absence of CAR, is ever sufficient for infection by CVBs. The prototype DAF-binding isolate, CVB3-RD, was selected for its ability to grow in RD cells, which express very little if any CAR, and chimeric viruses were used to map the RD phenotype to a region within VP2, which differed at only two residues (V108 and S151) from the prototype Nancy strain. These residues are present in an independent hemagglutinating isolate (56); however, despite its capacity to bind DAF, this isolate does not replicate in RD cells, suggesting that DAF binding and RD cell replication are separable phenotypes. Although RD cells were reported to express no surface CAR detectable by labeled antibody, cells received from Richard Crowell's laboratory express CAR mRNA detectable by PCR (R. J. Kaner and J. M. Bergelson, unpublished observation); significant levels of surface CAR were reported to appear on RD cells after multiple passages (56). It is possible that RD cells in different laboratories differ in their expression of CAR, and thus in their susceptibility to infection by DAF-binding strains; very low levels of CAR expression may be sufficient to permit infection once virus has been concentrated at the virus surface by attachment to DAF.

Attachment of CVB1, -3, and -5 to HeLa cells is 100-fold more rapid than attachment of CVB2, -4, and -6 (13), which do not bind DAF and are not inhibited by DAF antibodies. It is possible that this reflects more rapid attachment to CAR by the odd-numbered than by the even-numbered serotypes. However, our own preliminary observations indicate that both CVB3 and CVB4 attach slowly to CAR on transfected CHO cells, whereas CVB3 but not CVB4 attaches rapidly to HeLa cells. Another possible explanation for the rapid binding of odd-numbered serotypes is that the abundant DAF on HeLa cells may participate in the attachment of viruses that do not bind measurably to DAF in isolation. Anti-DAF antibodies inhibit attachment to HeLa cells by viral isolates that do not bind measurably to DAF (6). Although no direct interaction between CAR and DAF has been demonstrated on the cell surface, formation of a CAR-DAF complex might account both for inhibition of virus attachment by DAF antibodies, as well as for the apparent increased avidity of odd-numbered viruses for HeLa cells. Structural studies and kinetic analysis of virus interaction with the two receptors, as well as biochemical demonstration of CAR interaction with DAF, will be important for understanding the role of DAF in virus infection.

CVA RECEPTORS

There are 23 CVA serotypes. Early experiments demonstrated that a number of these bound to receptors distinct from those used by polioviruses and CVBs (13). CVA21 was found to compete for the receptor used by the major group of human rhinoviruses (32), subsequently identified as ICAM-1 (21, 58, 59), and an anti-ICAM monoclonal antibody was found to protect HeLa cells against infection by CVA13, -18, and -21 (116).

ICAM-1 and DAF

Recent experiments confirm that ICAM-1 is in fact a receptor for CVA21 (54). CVA21 also binds to DAF, but whereas ICAM-1-transfected rodent cells are susceptible to infection, DAF-transfected cells are not (55). This appears similar to the situation with CVB3, CAR, and DAF. However, RD cells, which express DAF but not ICAM-1, can be infected if DAF is first cross-linked with antibodies (52); the mechanism by which this occurs is not clear. A monoclonal antibody that recognizes DAF SCR1 blocks virus attachment, suggesting that CVA21 may interact with the N-terminal domain.

αv Integrins and MHC-I-Associated Proteins

The identification of the sequence RGD in a capsid protein (VP1) of CVA9 suggested that this virus might interact with integrin molecules, some of which recognize RGD motifs within their natural ligands. Consistent with this, RGD-containing peptides were found to inhibit CVA9 infection (49), and antibodies recognizing the αv and $\beta 3$ integrin subunits also inhibited infection (50). CVA9 binds directly to $\alpha v \beta 3$ (50), and its binding to CHO cells is enhanced by expression of $\alpha v \beta 3$ (61). The RGD motif is exposed on the virus surface, and susceptible to removal by proteolytic enzymes. Protease-treated virus loses its capacity to interact with $\alpha v \beta 3$ but remains fully infectious and capable of binding to cells in an RGD-independent manner, suggesting that this virus enters cells by both integrin-dependent and integrin-independent routes.

As has been observed with infection by some echoviruses, infection by CVA9 is inhibited by antibodies that recognize β_2-microglobulin (61). Although virus does not bind directly to β_2-microglobulin or to major histocompatibility complex (MHC) class I molecules, virus does bind to an MHC-associated heat shock protein, glucose-regulated 78-kDa protein (GRP78) (60a). Interaction between virus-associated GRP78 and MHC-I appears important for a postattachment event in virus infection.

ECHOVIRUSES

VLA-2

Monoclonal antibodies that protected HeLa cells from infection were used to identify an integrin molecule, VLA-2, as a receptor for EV1 (7). Integrins are heterodimeric glycoproteins composed of α and β subunits. Several antibodies that recognized the 150-kDa $\alpha 2$ subunit of VLA-2, a collagen and laminin receptor, blocked EV1 attachment, whereas antibodies to the 130-kDa $\beta 1$ subunit were less effective (2, 7). Transfection of the human $\alpha 2$ subunit into human or hamster cells expressing $\beta 1$ rendered these cells susceptible to virus attachment and infection (7, 8).

Virus attaches to a 200-amino-acid region (the I domain) within the $\alpha 2$ subunit, and the isolated I domain, synthesized in bacteria, is capable of binding virus (9, 29). The binding site for collagen and laminin is also located within the I domain, and some anti-VLA-2 monoclonal antibodies that recognize epitopes within the I domain block both virus attachment and interaction with collagen (2, 9). However, analysis of site-specific mutants indicates that the binding sites for collagen and virus are not identical (15, 30). The crystal structures of both the I domain (16) and of EV1 (18) have been determined, but the structure of the virus-receptor complex has not yet been completed.

DAF

There are 30 EV serotypes. Of 21 echoviruses tested, only EV1 and EV8 are inhibited by anti-VLA-2 antibodies. Radiolabeled EV1 and EV8 compete with each other, but not with EV7, for an attachment site on HeLa cells; EV1 and EV8, but not EV6 or EV7, bind hamster cells transfected with human VLA-2. Thus it appears that only EV1 and EV8 bind to VLA-2. These two viruses were originally thought to be distinct serologically, but subsequently were reclassified as a single serotype. Sequence analysis indicates that their capsid proteins are 94% identical at the amino acid level, and much more closely related to each other than to other echoviruses whose sequences have been determined (39a).

To identify receptors for other EVs, two groups of investigators generated monoclonal antibodies that protected cells from infection by EV7 (3, 45, 65). These antibodies were shown to identify human DAF, and cells transfected with human DAF become capable of binding EV7. Echoviruses 3, 6, 7, 11, 12, 13, 19, 21, 24, 25, 29, 30, and 33 have been found to interact with DAF, based on inhibition of infection by anti-DAF monoclonal antibodies or by soluble DAF. Enterovirus 70 also attaches to DAF, and, unlike many DAF-binding picornaviruses, appears to interact primarily with SCR1 (27, 28). Like the DAF-binding coxsackieviruses, DAF-binding echoviruses and enterovirus 70 have the capacity to agglutinate human red cells.

As is the case for coxsackieviruses, despite echovirus attachment to DAF, infection of DAF-transfected rodent cells is inefficient at best, with little or no virus produced (65) and only a few cells expressing viral antigen in an immunofocal assay (43). Although EV7 is converted to A particles after contact with HeLa cells, it has been reported that EV7 is not converted after contact with soluble DAF (44). This has led to the suggestion that A particle formation requires an additional cellular factor present on HeLa cells. The absence of such a factor may account for the inefficient infection observed in DAF-transfected rodent cells.

Although EV6 and EV7 both interact with DAF, removal of DAF from the surface of human RD cells prevents attachment of EV7, but not of some strains of EV6 (43). These results suggest that EV6 may also bind to an second, unidentified receptor. It is possible that many—if not all—of the DAF-binding enteroviruses require interaction with a second cell surface protein for efficient infection.

Other Molecules Involved in Echovirus Attachment and Entry

αv Integrins

Like CVA9, EV22 (now classified as parechovirus 1) contains an RGD sequence within VP1, and the two viruses compete for an attachment site on some cell types (50). However, based on partial inhibition of infection by anti-αv and anti-$\beta 1$ antibodies, it has been suggested that EV22 interacts with the integrin $\alpha v \beta 1$ (46).

Unidentified 44-kDa Molecule

Infection by a variety of echovirus serotypes, as well as by CVA9, was reportedly inhibited by a monoclonal antibody to a 44-kDa cell surface protein (36, 37). The antibody was not shown to inhibit virus attachment, nor has the protein been identified.

β_2-Microglobulin and CD59

Antibodies to β_2-microglobulin inhibit infection of RD cells by a variety of echoviruses (66), including EV6 and EV7, which are known to bind DAF, as well as EV1 which binds to VLA-2. Anti-β_2-microglobulin antibodies do not inhibit virus attachment, suggesting that the block to infection occurs at some postattachment step. Infection of HeLa cells is not inhibited by anti-β_2-microglobulin antibodies, and cells deficient in β_2-microglobulin can be infected, so β_2-microglobulin is not essential for infection.

It has been suggested that β_2-microglobulin and the associated 44-kDa MHC class I protein are components of a virus-receptor complex and may be involved in virus entry once attachment has occurred. Antibodies to CD59, a complement-regulatory protein, also inhibit EV7 infection of RD cells without blocking virus attachment (20), and it has been proposed that this protein is also a component of the complex. However, no direct evidence from transfection experiments is available to support a role for β_2-microglobulin or CD59 in virus infection.

FINAL COMMENTS

Attachment to a receptor permits virus to be concentrated at the cell surface; for picornaviruses, subsequent events in infection must include disruption of the viral capsid and delivery of viral RNA to a cytoplasmic compartment. Our understanding of these postattachment events is still not satisfactory. For some picornaviruses, a single receptor molecule may serve multiple functions during early infection (47). In contrast, viruses such as CVA21, EV7, and CVB3 may interact with multiple receptor molecules, and these interactions may have different functions in the pathway leading to infection. In the past few years there has been remarkable progress in the identification of picornavirus receptor molecules; the next challenge will be to define the mechanisms by which a viral genome is transported into a cell.

Work was supported by grants from the National Institutes of Health (AI 35667 and HL 54734) and by an Established Investigator Award from the American Heart Association. Susan Coffin, Robert Finberg, and Tauni Ohman provided helpful comments on the manuscript.

REFERENCES

1. Agrez, M. V., D. R. Shafren, X. Gu, K. Cox, D. Sheppard, and R. D. Barry. 1997. Integrin $\alpha v \beta 6$ enhances coxsackievirus B1 lytic infection of human colon cancer cells. *Virology* **239:**71–77.
2. Bergelson, J. M., B. M. C. Chan, R. W. Finberg, and M. E. Hemler. 1993. The integrin VLA-2 binds echovirus 1 and extracellular matrix ligands by different mechanisms. *J. Clin. Invest.* **92:**232–239.
3. Bergelson, J. M., M. Chan, K. Solomon, N. F. St. John, H. Lin, and R. W. Finberg. 1994. Decay-accelerating factor, a glycosylphosphatidylinositol-anchored complement regulatory protein, is a receptor for several echoviruses. *Proc. Natl. Acad. Sci. USA* **91:**6245–6248.
4. Bergelson, J. M., J. A. Cunningham, G. Droguett, E. A. Kurt-Jones, A. Krithivas, J. S. Hong, M. S. Horwitz, R. L. Crowell, and R. W. Finberg. 1997. Isolation of a common receptor for coxsackie B viruses and adenoviruses 2 and 5. *Science* **275:**1320–1323.
5. Bergelson, J. M., A. Krithivas, L. Celi, G. Droguett, M. S. Horwitz, T. Wickham, R. L. Crowell, and R. W. Finberg. 1998. The murine CAR homologue (mCAR) is a receptor for coxsackie B viruses and adenoviruses. *J. Virol.* **72:**415–419.
6. Bergelson, J. M., J. G. Mohanty, R. L. Crowell, N. F. St. John, D. M. Lublin, and R. W. Finberg. 1995. Coxsackievirus B3 adapted to growth in RD cells binds to decay-accelerating factor (CD55). *J. Virol.* **69:**1903–1906.
7. Bergelson, J. M., M. P. Shepley, B. M. C. Chan, M. E. Hemler, and R. W. Finberg. 1992. Identification of the integrin VLA-2 as a receptor for echovirus 1. *Science* **255:**1718–1720.
8. Bergelson, J. M., N. St. John, S. Kawaguchi, M. Chan, H. Stubdal, J. Modlin, and R. W. Finberg. 1993. Infection by echoviruses 1 and 8 depends on the $\alpha 2$ subunit of human VLA-2. *J. Virol.* **67:**6847–6852.
9. Bergelson, J. M., N. F. St. John, S. Kawaguchi, R. Pasqualini, F. Berdichevsky, M. E. Hemler, and R. W. Finberg. 1994. The I domain is essential for echovirus 1 interaction with VLA-2. *Cell Adhesion Commun.* **2:**455–464.
10. Bewley, M. C., K. Springer, Y.-B. Zhang, P. Freimuth, and J. M. Flanagan. 1999. Structural analysis of the mechanism of adenovirus binding to its human cellular receptor, CAR. *Science* **286:**1579–1583.
11. Carson, S. D., N. N. Chapman, and S. M. Tracy. 1997. Purification of the putative coxsackievirus B receptor from HeLa cells. *Biochem. Biophys. Res. Commun.* **233:**325–328.

11a. Cohen, C. J., J. T.-C. Shieh, R. J. Pickles, T. Okegawa, J.-T. Hsieh, and J. M. Bergelson. 2001. The coxsackievirus and adenovirus receptor is a transmembrane component of the tight junction. *Proc. Natl. Acad. Sci. USA* **98:**15191–15196.

11b. Colonno, R. J., P. L. Callahan, and W. J. Long. 1986. Isolation of a monoclonal antibody that blocks attachment of the major group of human rhinoviruses. *J. Virol.* **57:**7–12.

12. Crowell, R. L., A. K. Field, W. A. Schlief, W. L. Long, R. J. Colonno, J. E. Mapoles, and E. A. Emini. 1986. Monoclonal antibody that inhibits infection of HeLa and rhabdomyosarcoma cells by selected enteroviruses through receptor blockade. *J. Virol.* **57:**438–445.

13. **Crowell, R. L., and M. A. Landau.** 1983. Receptors in the initiation of picornavirus infections, p. 1–42. *In* H. Fraenkel-Conrat and R. R. Wagner (ed.), *Comprehensive Virology*, vol. 18. Plenum Publishing Corp., New York, N.Y.
14. **de Verdugo, U. R., H.-C. Selinka, M. Huber, B. Kramer, J. Kellerman, P. H. Hofschneider, and R. Kandolf.** 1995. Characterization of a 100-kilodalton binding protein for the six serotypes of coxsackie B viruses. *J. Virol.* **69:**6751–6757.
15. **Dickeson, S. K., N. L. Mathis, M. Rahman, J. M. Bergelson, and S. A. Santoro.** 1999. Determinants of ligand binding specificity of the $\alpha 2\beta 1$ and $\alpha 2\beta 1$ integrins. *J. Biol. Chem.* **274:**32182–32191.
16. **Emsley, J., S. L. King, J. M. Bergelson, and R. C. Liddington.** 1997. Crystal structure of the I domain from integrin $\alpha 2\beta 1$. *J. Biol. Chem.* **272:**28518–28522.
17. **Fechner, H., A. Haack, H. Wang, X. Wang, K. Eizema, M. Pauschinger, R. G. Schoemaker, R. van Veghel, A. B. Houtsmuller, H.-P. Schultheiss, J. M. J. Lamers, and W. Poller.** 1999. Expression of coxsackie adenovirus receptor and alpha v-integrin does not correlate with adenovector targeting in vivo indicating anatomical vector barriers. *Gene Ther.* **6:**1520–1535.
18. **Filman, D. J., M. W. Wien, J. A. Cunningham, J. M. Bergelson, and J. M. Hogle.** 1998. The structure determination of echovirus 1. *Acta Crystallogr. D* **54:**1261–1272.
19. **Freimuth, P., K. Springer, C. Berard, J. Hainfield, M. Bewley, and J. Flanagan.** 1999. Coxsackievirus and adenovirus receptor amino-terminal immunoglobulin V-related domain binds adenovirus type 2 and fiber knob from adenovirus type 12. *J. Virol.* **73:**1392–1398.
20. **Goodfellow, I. G., R. M. Powell, T. Ward, O. B. Spiller, J. W. Almond, and D. J. Evans.** 2000. Echovirus infection of rhabdomyosarcoma cells is inhibited by antiserum to the complement control protein CD59. *J. Gen. Virol.* **81:**1393–1401.
21. **Greve, J. M., G. Davis, A. M. Meyer, C. P. Forte, S. C. Yost, C. W. Marlor, M. E. Kamarck, and A. McClelland.** 1989. The major human rhinovirus receptor is ICAM-1. *Cell* **56:**839–847.
21a. **He, Y., P. R. Chipman, J. Howitt, C. M. Bator, M. A. Whitt, T. S. Baker, R. J. Kuhn, C. W. Anderson, P. Freimuth, and M. G. Rossmann.** 2001. Interaction of coxsackievirus B3 with the full length coxsackievirus-adenovirus receptor. *Nat. Struct. Biol.* **8:**874–878.
22. **Hogle, J. M., M. Chow, and D. J. Filman.** 1985. Three-dimensional structure of poliovirus at 2.9 Å resolution. *Science* **229:**1358–1365.
23. **Holland, J. J.** 1961. Receptor affinities as major determinants of enterovirus tissue tropism in humans. *Virology* **15:**312–326.
24. **Honda, T., H. Saitoh, M. Masuko, T. Katagiri-Abe, K. Tominaga, I. Kozakai, K. Kobayashi, T. Kominishi, Y. G. Watanabe, S. Odani, and R. Kuwano.** 2000. The coxsackievirus adenovirus receptor as a cell adhesion molecule in the developing mouse brain. *Mol. Brain Res.* **77:**19–28.
25. **Hsu, K.-H. L., K. Lonberg-Holm, B. Alstein, and R. L. Crowell.** 1988. A monoclonal antibody specific for the cellular receptor for the group B coxsackieviruses. *J. Virol.* **62:**1647–1652.
26. **Hsu, K.-H. L., S. Paglini, B. Alstein, and R. L. Crowell.** 1990. Identification of a second cellular receptor for a coxsackievirus B3 variant, CB3-RD, p. 271–277. *In* M. Brinton and F. Heinz (ed.), *New Aspects of Positive-Strand RNA Viruses*. American Society for Microbiology, Washington, D.C.
27. **Karnauchow, T. M., S. Dawe, D. M. Lublin, and K. Dimock.** 1998. Short consensus repeat domain 1 of decay-accelerating factor is required for enterovirus 70 binding. *J. Virol.* **72:**9380–9383.
28. **Karnauchow, T. M., D. L. Tolson, B. A. Harrison, E. Altman, D. M. Lublin, and K. Dimock.** 1996. The HeLa cell receptor for enterovirus 70 is decay-accelerating factor (CD55). *J. Virol.* **70:**5143–5152.
29. **King, S. L., J. A. Cunningham, R. W. Finberg, and J. M. Bergelson.** 1995. Echovirus 1 interaction with the isolated VLA-2 I domain. *J. Virol.* **69:**3237–3239.
30. **King, S. L., T. Kamata, J. A. Cunningham, J. Emsley, R. C. Liddington, Y. Takada, and J. M. Bergelson.** 1997. Echovirus 1 interaction with the human very late antigen-2 (integrin $\alpha 2\beta 1$) I domain: identification of two independent virus contact sites distinct from the metal ion-dependent adhesion site. *J. Biol. Chem.* **272:**28518–28522.
31. **Lindberg, A. M., R. L. Crowell, R. Zell, R. Kandolf, and U. Pettersson.** 1992. Mapping of the RD phenotype of the Nancy strain of coxsackievirus B3. *Virus Res.* **24:**187–196.
32. **Lonberg-Holm, K., R. L. Crowell, and L. Philipson.** 1976. Unrelated animal viruses share receptors. *Nature* **259:**679–681.
33. **Lublin, D. M., and J. P. Atkinson.** 1989. Decay-accelerating factor: biochemistry, molecular biology, and function. *Annu. Rev. Immunol.* **7:**35–57.
34. **Mapoles, J. E., D. L. Krah, and R. L. Crowell.** 1985. Purification of a HeLa cell receptor protein for group B coxsackieviruses. *J. Virol.* **55:**560–566.
35. **Martino, T. A., M. Petric, H. Weingartl, J. M. Bergelson, M. A. Opavsky, C. D. Richardson, J. F. Modlin, R. W. Finberg, K. C. Kain, N. Willis, C. J. Gauntt, and P. P. Liu.** 2000. The coxsackie-adenovirus receptor (CAR) is used by reference strains and clinical isolates representing all six serotypes of coxsackievirus group B, and by swine vesicular disease virus. *Virology* **271:**99–108.
36. **Mbida, A. D., O. G. Gaudin, O. Sabido, B. Pozzetto, and J.-C. L. Bihan.** 1992. Monoclonal antibody specific for the cellular receptor of echoviruses. *Intervirology* **33:**17–22.
37. **Mbida, A. D., B. Pozzetto, O. G. Gaudin, F. Grattard, J.-C. L. Bihan, Y. Akono, and A. Ros.** 1992. A 44,000 glycoprotein is involved in the attachment of echovirus-11 onto susceptible cells. *Virology* **189:**350–353.
38. **Mohanty, J. G., and R. L. Crowell.** 1993. Attempts to purify a second cellular receptor for a coxsackievirus B3 variant, CB3-RD from HeLa cells. *Virus Res.* **29:**305–320.
39. **Muckelbauer, J. K., M. Kremer, I. Minor, G. Diana, F. J. Dutko, J. Groarke, D. G. Pevear, and M. G. Rossmann.** 1995. The structure of coxsackievirus B3 at 3.5 Å resolution. *Structure* **3:**653–667.
39a. **Ohman, T., S. L. King, A. Krithivas, J. C. Cunningham, S. K. Dickeson, S. A. Santoro, and J. M. Bergelson.** 2001. Echoviruses 1 and 8 are genetically closely related, and bind to similar determinants within the VLA-2 I domain. *Virus Res.* **76:**1–8.
39b. **Okegawa, T., R.-C. Pong, Y. Li, J. M. Bergelson, A. I. Sagalowsky, and J.-T. Hsieh.** 2001. The mechanism of the growth inhibitory effect of coxsackie and adenovirus receptor (CAR) on human bladder cancer: a functional analysis of CAR protein structure. *Cancer Res.* **61:**6592–6600.
40. **Philipson, L., S. Bengtsson, S. Brishammar, L. Svennerholm, and O. Zetterqvist.** 1964. Purification and chemical analysis of the erythrocyte receptor for hemagglutinating enteroviruses. *Virology* **22:**580–590.
41. **Pickles, R. J., J. A. Fahrner, J. M. Petrella, R. C. Boucher, and J. M. Bergelson.** 2000. Retargeting the

coxsackievirus and adenovirus receptor to the apical surface of polarized epithelial cells reveals the glycocalyx as a barrier to adenovirus-mediated gene transfer. *J. Virol.* **74:**6050–6057.

42. **Pickles, R. J., D. McCarty, H. Matsui, P. J. Hart, S. H. Randell, and R. C. Boucher.** 1998. Limited entry of adenovirus vectors into well-differentiated airway epithelium is responsible for inefficient gene transfer. *J. Virol.* **72:**6014–6023.

43. **Powell, R. M., V. Schmitt, T. Ward, I. Goodfellow, D. J. Evans, and J. W. Almond.** 1998. Characterization of echoviruses that bind decay accelerating factor (CD55): evidence that some haemagglutinating strains use more than one cellular receptor. *J. Gen. Virol.* **79:**1707–1713.

44. **Powell, R. M., T. Ward, D. J. Evans, and J. W. Almond.** 1997. Interaction between echovirus 7 and its receptor, decay-accelerating factor (CD55): evidence for a secondary cellular factor in A-particle formation. *J. Virol.* **71:**9306–9312.

45. **Powell, R. M., T. Ward, I. Goodfellow, J. W. Almond, and D. J. Evans.** 1999. Mapping the binding domains on decay accelerating factor (DAF) for haemagglutinating enteroviruses: implications for the evolution of a DAF-binding phenotype. *J. Gen. Virol.* **80:**3145–3152.

46. **Pulli, T., E. Koivunen, and T. Hyypia.** 1997. Cell-surface interactions of echovirus 22. *J. Biol. Chem.* **272:**21176–21180.

47. **Racaniello, V. R.** 1996. The poliovirus receptor: a hook, or an unzipper? *Structure* **4:**769–773.

48. **Reagan, K. J., B. Goldberg, and R. L. Crowell.** 1984. Altered receptor specificity of coxsackie B3 after growth in rhabdomyosarcoma cells. *J. Virol.* **49:**635–640.

49. **Roivainen, M., T. Hyypia, L. Piirainen, N. Kalkkinen, G. Stanway, and T. Hovi.** 1991. RGD-dependent entry of coxsackievirus A9 into host cells and its bypass after cleavage of VP1 protein by intestinal proteases. *J. Virol.* **65:**4735–4740.

50. **Roivainen, M., L. Piirainen, T. Hovi, I. Virtanen, T. Riikinen, J. Heino, and T. Hyypia.** 1994. Entry of coxsackievirus A9 into host cells: specific interactions with alpha v beta 3 integrin, the vitronectin receptor. *Virology* **203:**357–365.

51. **Rossmann, M. G., E. Arnold, J. W. Erickson, E. A. Frankenberger, J. P. Griffith, H.-J. Hecht, J. E. Johnson, G. Kamer, M. Luo, A. G. Moser, R. R. Rueckert, B. Sherry, and G. Vriend.** 1985. Structure of a human common cold virus and functional relationship to other picornaviruses. *Nature* **317:**145–153.

52. **Shafren, D. R.** 1998. Viral cell entry induced by cross-linked decay-accelerating factor. *J. Virol.* **72:**9407–9412.

53. **Shafren, D. R., R. C. Bates, M. V. Agrez, R. L. Herd, G. F. Burns, and R. D. Barry.** 1995. Coxsackieviruses B1, B3, and B5 use decay accelerating factor as a receptor for cell attachment. *J. Virol.* **69:**3873–3877.

54. **Shafren, D. R., D. J. Dorahy, S. J. Greive, G. F. Burns, and R. D. Barry.** 1997. Mouse cells expressing human intercellular adhesion molecule-1 are susceptible to infection by coxsackievirus A21. *J. Virol.* **71:**785–789.

55. **Shafren, D. R., D. J. Dorahy, R. A. Ingham, G. F. Burns, and R. D. Barry.** 1997. Coxsackievirus A21 binds to decay-accelerating factor but requires intercellular adhesion molecule 1 for cell entry. *J. Virol.* **71:**4736–4743.

56. **Shafren, D. R., D. T. Williams, and R. D. Barry.** 1997. A decay-accelerating factor-binding strain of coxsackievirus B3 requires the coxsackievirus-adenovirus receptor protein to mediate lytic infection of rhabdomyosarcoma cells. *J. Virol.* **71:**9844–9848.

57. **Spiller, O. B., I. G. Goodefellow, D. J. Evans, J. W. Almond, and B. B. Morgan.** 2000. Echoviruses and coxsackie B viruses that use human decay-accelerating factor (DAF) as a receptor do not bind the rodent analogues of DAF. *J. Infect. Dis.* **181:**350–343.

58. **Staunton, D. E., V. J. Merluzzi, R. Rothlein, R. Barton, S. D. Marlin, and T. A. Springer.** 1989. A cell adhesion molecule, ICAM-1, is the major surface receptor for rhinoviruses. *Cell* **56:**849–853.

59. **Tomassini, J. E., D. Graham, C. M. DeWitt, D. W. Lineberger, J. A. Rodkey, and R. J. Colonno.** 1989. cDNA cloning reveals that the major group rhinovirus receptor on HeLa cells is intercellular adhesion molecule 1. *Proc. Natl. Acad. Sci. USA* **86:**4907–7911.

60. **Tomko, R. P., R. Xu, and L. Philipson.** 1997. HCAR and MCAR: the human and mouse cellular receptors for subgroup C adenoviruses and group B coxsackieviruses. *Proc. Natl. Acad. Sci. USA* **94:**3352–3356.

60a. **Triantafilou, K., D. Fradelizi, K. Wilson, and M. Triantafilou.** 2002. GRP78, a coreceptor for coxsackievirus A9, interacts with major histocompatibility complex class I molecules which mediate virus internalization. *J. Virol.* **76:**633–643.

61. **Triantafilou, M., K. Triantafilou, K. M. Wilson, Y. Takada, N. Fernandez, and G. Stanway.** 1999. Involvement of β2-microglobulin and integrin $\alpha v \beta 3$ molecules in the coxsackievirus A9 infectious cycle. *J. Gen. Virol.* **80:**2591–2600.

62. **van Raaij, M. J., E. Chouin, H. van der Zandt, J. M. Bergelson, and S. Cusack.** 2000. Dimeric structure of the coxsackievirus and adenovirus receptor D1 domain at 1.7 Å resolution. *Struct. Fold. Des.* **8:**1147–1155.

63. **Walters, R. W., T. Grunst, J. M. Bergelson, R. W. Finberg, M. W. Welsh, and J. Zabner.** 1999. Basolateral localization of fiber receptors limits adenovirus infection of airway epithelia. *J. Biol. Chem.* **274:**10219–10226.

64. **Wang, X., and J. M. Bergelson.** 1999. CAR cytoplasmic and transmembrane domains are not essential for infection by coxsackie B viruses and adenoviruses. *J. Virol.* **73:**2259–2562.

65. **Ward, T., P. A. Pipkin, N. A. Clarkson, D. M. Stone, P. D. Minor, and J. W. Almond.** 1994. Decay accelerating factor (CD55) identified as a receptor for echovirus 7 using CELICS, a rapid immuno-focal cloning method. *EMBO J.* **13:**5070–5074.

66. **Ward, T., R. M. Powell, P. A. Pipkin, D. J. Evans, P. D. Minor, and J. W. Almond.** 1998. Role for beta2-microglobulin in echovirus infection of rhabdomyosarcoma cells. *J. Virol.* **72:**5360–5365.

67. **Wickham, T. J., P. Mathias, D. A. Cheresh, and G. R. Nemerow.** 1993. Integrins $\alpha v \beta 3$ and $\alpha v \beta 5$ promote adenovirus internalization but not virus attachment. *Cell* **73:**309–319.

68. **Zajac, I., and R. L. Crowell.** 1965. Effect of enzymes on the interaction of enteroviruses with living HeLa cells. *J. Bacteriol.* **89:**574–582.

69. **Zajac, I., and R. L. Crowell.** 1965. Location and regeneration of enterovirus receptors of HeLa cells. *J. Bacteriol.* **89:**1097–1100.

Foot-and-Mouth Disease Virus-Receptor Interactions: Role in Pathogenesis and Tissue Culture Adaptation

BARRY BAXT, SHERRY NEFF, ELIZABETH RIEDER, AND PETER W. MASON

11

The first step in picornaviral infection is the interaction of the virion with a cell surface receptor. Although picornaviruses are closely related structurally and genetically, they are responsible for many different disease syndromes in both humans and animals and utilize a diverse range of cell surface molecules as receptors. It has been recognized for many years that viral receptors play a role in tissue tropism and disease pathogenesis (28, 97). While other factors, including coreceptors, intracellular factors, and the genetic background of the virus, may also determine viral pathogenicity and host range (32, 89), the fact that individual viruses within the *Picornaviridae* that cause similar disease syndromes utilize similar receptors is a strong argument for a role of receptors in disease.

Foot-and-mouth disease (FMD) is an extremely contagious viral disease of cloven-hoofed animals (cattle, pigs, sheep, goats, and many wild animals) of agricultural and economic importance. The causative agent of this disease, foot-and-mouth disease virus (FMDV), is one of the best-characterized picornaviruses and was the first filterable agent of an animal disease described (63). Although control of this disease has been aggressively pursued since the discovery of its etiologic agent, FMD continues to threaten the world's livestock production. The difficulties in controlling the disease are due, in part, to its rapid spread among animals and the speed with which infected animals begin to shed virus and display clinical signs (often less than 48 h following infection). In addition, the genetic flexibility and quasispecies nature of the virus (see chapter 23, this volume), which has given rise to seven serotypes (A, O, C, SAT1, SAT2, SAT3, and Asia1) and innumerable subtypes and variants, complicates disease control efforts.

The variety of sero- and subtypes of FMDV is accompanied by changes in amino acid residues covering a large portion of the surface of the virion (see chapter 5, this volume). However, all of the known serotypes of virus produce similar signs of infection: fever and vesicular lesions of the epithelium of the mouth, tongue, nose, muzzle, feet, and teats (19–21, 92). Thus, if pathogenesis of FMDV is dependent on utilization of a specific cellular component or components for attachment and entry, then either this component or components must exhibit multiple binding sites for the different subtypes or the subtypes must have maintained a virion structure capable of recognizing the same site on the cell surface.

In this chapter, we will examine the early events that occur upon infection of cultured cells with FMDV and define the known virus-receptor interactions. In addition, we will try to relate what is known about these early interactions to disease pathogenesis.

EARLY FMDV INTERACTIONS WITH CULTURED CELLS AND RECEPTOR SPECIFICITY AMONG SEROTYPES

Initial studies of early FMDV-cell events focused on the interactions of radioactively labeled virus with cultured cells (either BHK-21 or bovine kidney cells) or isolated plasma membranes (7, 8). By using FMDV strain A_{12}, it was shown that virus bound rapidly to both cells and plasma membranes at either 4° or 37°C and that cultured cells expressed 10^3 to 10^4 receptor sites per cell. It was further shown by cross-competition binding experiments that FMDV, poliovirus, and encephalomyocarditis virus all utilize different cellular receptors on either HeLa or BHK-21 cells (90). Examination of the fate of virus particles subsequent to adsorption revealed that, unlike the enteroviruses, which undergo a receptor-induced conformational change to an altered (A) particle lacking VP4 and displaying different sedimentation values (29, 33, 42, 55, 65), FMDV undergoes eclipse and uncoating in a single step: the mature viral particle directly dissociates to VP4, pentameric 12S subunits, and the viral genome (6–8, 25). FMDV uncoating appears to be triggered by the entry of the virus into an acidic endosome, since agents that raise the pH of intracellular endosomes and inhibit viral repli-

Barry Baxt, Sherry Neff, and Peter W. Mason ■ United States Department of Agriculture, Agricultural Research Service, Plum Island Animal Disease Center, Greenport, NY 11944-0848. *Elizabeth Rieder* ■ Department of Molecular Genetics and Microbiology, State University of New York at Stony Brook, Stony Brook, NY 11794-5222.

cation prevent uncoating (6, 23, 24). In addition, while a large percentage of bound enteroviruses can be eluted from the cell surface in the form of A particles (66), eluted FMDV virions have unaltered protein content and sedimentation characteristics (7, 23). Taken together, these studies suggest that the early interactions of FMDV with cells are fundamentally different from those of enteroviruses, many of which access their target tissues following passage through a low-pH environment, a condition incompatible with the acid lability of FMDV.

Although the binding studies cited above for FMDV type A_{12} indicated that the virus bound a single class of receptors (expressed at about 10^3 to 10^4 binding sites per cell), competition studies similar to the one shown in Fig. 1 indicated that some serotypes bound to a second class of receptors present at much higher copy number (7, 90). In Fig. 1 it can be seen that relatively small amounts of unlabeled type A or O virus could prevent the binding of radiolabeled type A virus to cells, but the converse was not true; much greater amounts of unlabeled type A and O viruses were required to prevent the binding of radiolabeled type O to cells. Similar competition binding studies performed with six of the seven serotypes indicated that all viruses share a common receptor site on cultured cells, with some serotypes binding to additional, high-copy-number sites on the cell surface (7, 90). These were the first indications that the aphthoviruses could utilize multiple receptor sites to infect cells.

ROLE OF THE VIRION'S RGD SEQUENCE IN CELL BINDING

The first step toward the identification of the cell receptor for FMDV came from investigations into the biology of a cellular adhesion molecule, fibronectin. In 1984, Pierschbacher and Ruoslahti (78) reported that an arginine-glycine-aspartic acid (RGD) sequence within fibronectin was a cellular recognition site for this molecule. In the same year, these authors reported a search of the National Biomedical Research Foundation sequence database that revealed that the RGD sequence was also found in the VP1 capsid protein of FMDV (79). This finding suggested that the RGD sequence could function in binding FMDV to cells through interaction with either the fibronectin receptor or a related cell surface molecule. Interestingly, the RGD in FMDV was subsequently proven to be involved in virus-cell binding (see below), but RGDs in the sequences of surface proteins of two other viruses, yellow fever virus

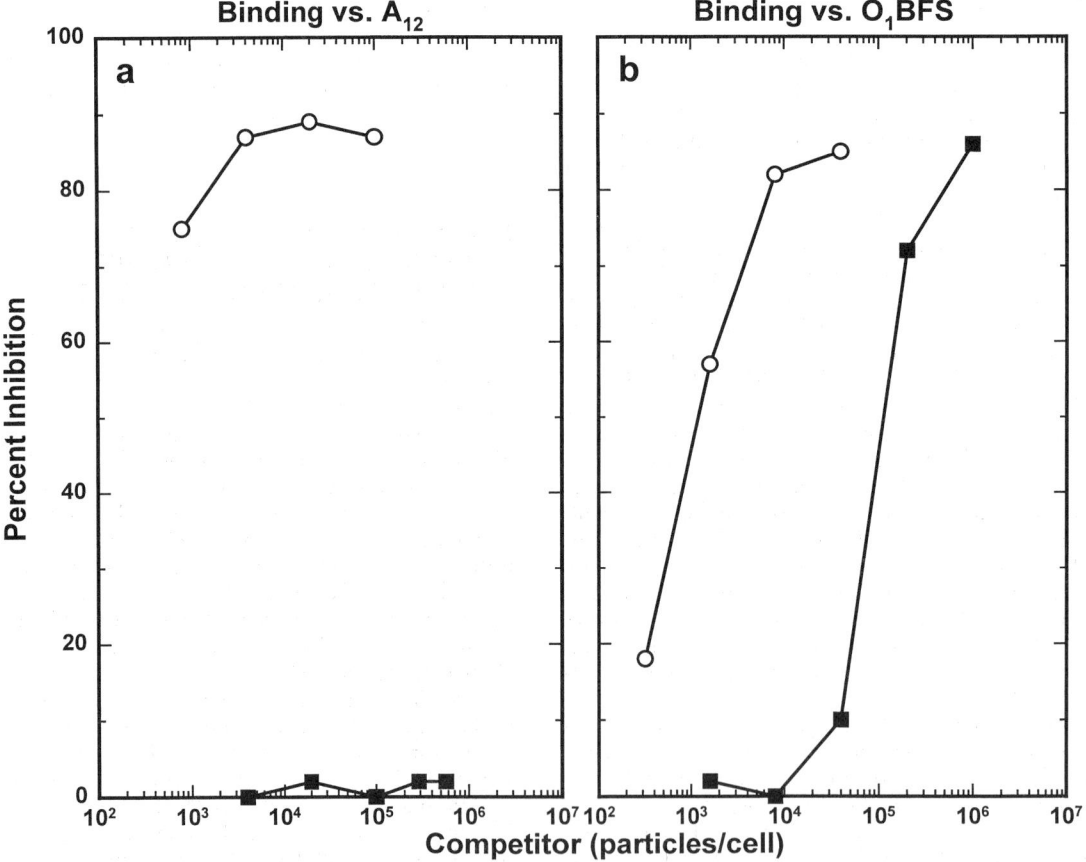

FIGURE 1 Competition binding of FMDV types A_{12} and O_1BFS. Purified ^{3}H-uridine-labeled FMDV types A_{12} (○) or O_1BFS (■), at a concentration of 1×10^3 particles/cell, were mixed with increasing concentrations of either purified unlabeled (a) type A_{12} or (b) O_1BFS and allowed to bind to BHK-21 cells for 90 min at room temperature. The level of binding was determined for labeled virus in the absence of unlabeled competitor, and the inhibition of binding of the labeled viruses by the unlabeled viruses is shown.

and Sindbis virus, which were identified by Pierschbacher and Ruoslahti in the same 1984 report (79), have not been shown to mediate attachment to cells.

While the nature of the fibronectin receptor was unknown at that time, within 2 years it was shown that it was a member of a group of transmembrane glycoproteins, consisting of two subunits in mammalian cells, that was given the name "integrin" (93). It was soon recognized that integrins formed a large family of cell surface receptors involved in cell adhesion, cell migration, thrombosis, and lymphocyte-mediated immunological interactions (49). The fibronectin-integrin interaction has been extensively characterized; analyses of attachment activities of a number of synthetic peptides that reproduce the adhesive properties of fibronectin in cell attachment in vitro indicated that the RGD plays an essential role in binding to integrins and that sequences surrounding the RGD tripeptide have minimal effect on cell attachment (77, 78).

The next observation that supported a role for the RGD in FMDV cell attachment came from a study pointing out that the sequences surrounding the RGD tripeptide were highly variable between isolates, but that the RGD itself was highly conserved (76). Structural studies showed that the RGD is located at the apex of a long flexible loop, between the G and H β strands of VP1 (G-H loop) (1, 64). Additional data for the role of an RGD-binding cell surface protein in infection came from studies showing that synthetic peptides containing the RGD sequence inhibited FMDV binding to cells (9, 37). Interestingly, differences in blocking activity of peptides with different serotypes (9), the requirement for very large amounts of peptides to efficiently inhibit binding (9, 37), and the ability of proteinases that cleave other portions of VP1 to inhibit virus binding (37) suggested that other regions of the capsid could be involved in the interaction of virus with cells in culture. By evaluating genetically engineered derivatives of FMDV, it has been possible to demonstrate that alterations in G-H loop sequences bordering the RGD can affect virus-cell interactions in vitro (59, 70, 81), and specific alterations in the loop have been associated with adaptation of animal-derived viruses to cell culture (81).

A direct demonstration for the role of the RGD sequence in the binding of FMDV to cells came from reverse genetic studies that either directly mutated or deleted this sequence from infectious cDNA clones. These studies demonstrated that in vitro transcribed viral RNAs containing these mutations or deletions yielded viral particles upon transfection into cultured cells, but these particles were noninfectious (59, 70) as a result of being unable to bind to cells (70). Viruses lacking the RGD sequence were also noninfectious in cattle but could protect these animals from challenge with live virus, demonstrating that the RGD sequence was also required for the virus to cause disease (70, 71).

IDENTIFICATION OF AN INTEGRIN AS A CELLULAR RECEPTOR FOR FMDV

Integrins are heterodimeric molecules consisting of two subunits, α and β, which interact noncovalently at the cell surface (50). The subunits are type I membrane proteins, consisting of a large N-terminal extracellular domain and smaller transmembrane and cytoplasmic domains. The functions of integrins include binding extracellular matrix proteins, cell-cell interactions, and signal transduction (40, 50). These receptors bind to their natural ligands through a ligand-binding domain made of elements of both subunits' ectodomains (36). There are 18 α and 8 β subunits which dimerize in various combinations producing 24 known mammalian integrins (51). At least eight integrins bind to RGD sequences in their natural ligands (86); all the integrins that currently have been identified as FMDV receptors are members of this subclass (see below). A number of other picornaviruses utilize integrins that do not bind to an RGD recognition site as viral receptors (see chapter 10, this volume).

The first identification of the integrin receptor for FMDV was made by comparing its receptor specificity with that of the human enterovirus, coxsackievirus A9 (CAV9), which contains a 17-amino-acid C-terminal insertion in VP1 containing an RGD sequence (26, 27). This sequence was shown to be essential for the attachment of CAV9 to monkey kidney cells (83), and the cellular receptor involved in the RGD-dependent mechanism of infection was identified as the integrin $\alpha v \beta 3$, also referred to as the "vitronectin receptor" (85). Competition binding studies between CAV9 and FMDV revealed that both viruses were using the same binding site in both monkey kidney and BHK-21 cells (11), in contrast to earlier studies showing that FMDV and poliovirus used very different receptors (90). Using a panel of anti-integrin antibodies, we showed that antibodies to the $\alpha v \beta 3$ integrin were able to inhibit both FMDV binding and plaque formation in monkey kidney cells (11), strongly suggesting that FMDV was able to utilize this integrin as a receptor in these cells. The similarities between CAV9 and FMDV interactions with their common receptor have been emphasized by the recently solved crystal structure of CAV9 (46). The CAV9 C-terminal extension of VP1, containing the RGD sequence, assumes a flexible and disordered conformation similar to the FMDV G-H loop of VP1 (1, 64). CAV9 has also been shown to utilize an RGD-independent mechanism of viral attachment to an as yet unidentified receptor found in a rhabdomyosarcoma cell line, which is probably not an integrin (47, 83, 84). The relationships of receptor usage to the pathogenesis of CAV9 infection, however, remain unclear.

The ability of $\alpha v \beta 3$ to serve as a receptor for FMDV in cells in culture was confirmed genetically using cells transfected with integrin subunit cDNAs. Specifically, K562 erythroleukemia cells transfected with cDNAs encoding human αv and $\beta 3$ subunits (12, 13), were tested for their susceptibility to infection with FMDV types A_{12} and O_1BFS (74). Susceptibility to infection was measured by either assaying for biosynthesis of FMDV proteins or evaluating the increase in viral titer over a 24-h infection period. These experiments revealed that viral proteins were only synthesized in type A_{12} infected cells transfected with $\alpha v \beta 3$ cDNAs (74), and this was accompanied by an increase in viral titer in these cells (S. Neff, P. W. Mason, and B. Baxt, unpublished data). When K562 cells were transfected with the closely related integrin, $\alpha v \beta 5$, however, neither viral proteins nor an increase in viral titer was observed (Neff et al., unpublished). These studies also suggested that the $\alpha 5 \beta 1$ integrin, which is naturally expressed in this cell line, was also unable to function as an FMDV receptor. To extend these results we performed a similar experiment with type O_1BFS and found that this virus was able to replicate in nontransfected K562 cells (74). Furthermore, antibodies to $\alpha 5 \beta 1$ were unable to inhibit viral replication, and RGD peptides were also unable to inhibit viral adsorption (Neff et al., unpublished), suggesting that this virus was not utilizing an integrin receptor. The significance of these results is discussed in the next section.

ALTERNATIVE RECEPTORS AND ALTERATION OF FMDV VIRULENCE AND HOST RANGE

Studies in our laboratory demonstrated a fundamental difference in the ability of FMDV and poliovirus to enter cells via an antibody-dependent enhancement of infection pathway (10, 68). Specifically, these studies suggested that functional receptors for FMDV are only needed to dock the virus to susceptible cells. Based on these suppositions, it seemed likely that an alternative FMDV receptor could be engineered by joining the antigen-binding domain of an FMDV-specific antibody to a cell surface receptor specific for another virus. We accomplished this task by fusing the virus-binding portion of an anti-FMDV type A_{12} monoclonal antibody, in the form of a single chain antibody (scAb) (69), to intercellular adhesion molecule 1 (ICAM-1), the receptor for the major group of human rhinoviruses (82). Interestingly, CHO cells expressing this surrogate receptor molecule supported productive infection of type A_{12} virus, while nontransfected CHO cells were resistant to infection, supporting the hypothesis that infection of cells by FMDV only requires binding of the virion to the cell surface. Moreover, as expected, this receptor was only functional for viruses carrying the epitope recognized by the scAb, and the RGD sequence was unnecessary for infection with these viruses (82). Using cells expressing this receptor, we were able to produce large amounts of serotype A viruses lacking the RGD sequence, which were shown to be noninfectious in cells normally susceptible to infection with RGD-containing viruses (82; M. Almeida, E. Rieder, and P. W. Mason, unpublished data), and unable to infect bovines (71) or swine (Almeida et al., unpublished).

Shortly after publication of the report describing the engineering of the scAb-ICAM-1 receptor, Jackson and coworkers (53) reported that serotype O_1 FMDV could utilize heparan sulfate (HS) as a coreceptor molecule. HS is a ubiquitous cell surface glycosaminoglycan (GAG) consisting of a sulfated polysaccharide covalently linked to a protein core. These investigators provided strong evidence for a role of HS in the attachment and entry of serotype O_1 FMDVs, utilizing biochemical studies (competition with heparin and treatment of cells with heparinase) and genetic evidence (use of GAG-deficient CHO cell lines) to demonstrate the importance of HS for FMDV binding and infection. Based on the existing knowledge of the conservation and importance of the RGD sequence in FMDV binding and infection of susceptible cells (see above), and the well-documented role of HS as a coreceptor for alphaherpes viruses (91, 98), it was proposed by this group that HS was a coreceptor for FMDV infection (53).

Although earlier studies had not excluded a role for a coreceptor in FMDV entry, our working hypothesis that the nature of the molecule utilized by the virus as a receptor was only dependent on its ability to bind the virion to cells argued against the existence of a coreceptor in cultured cells. Furthermore, we had shown that serotype A viruses could not infect CHO cells, which contained large amounts of HS, in the absence of the scAb-ICAM-1 receptor, suggesting that HS alone could not be utilized as a receptor for type A viruses (82). Our next set of investigations demonstrated that HS could act as an "alternative" receptor for infection in vitro, and confirmed the importance of the RGD sequence for infection in vivo. These studies (87) utilized genetically defined derivatives of a serotype O_1 virus (O_1Campos) similar to the viruses (O_1Kaufbueren and O_1BFS) utilized by Jackson et al. (53). They demonstrated that growth of virus in cell culture resulted in selection of viruses capable of growing in CHO cells, an adaptation accompanied by the selection of an arginine (R) residue at position 56 of VP3 (referred to by the nomenclature 3056R). The additional positive charge on the surface of the virion could mediate electrostatic binding to negatively charged heparin or HS. Moreover, heparin inhibited plaque formation by the 3056R viruses but had no effect on plaque formation by viruses with a "field" type histidine (H) residue in this position (3056H) (87). The cDNAs encoding the capsids of these two variants were inserted into a type A_{12} infectious cDNA clone and used to produce viruses exhibiting the phenotypes of the original variants (87).

The most interesting results of our O_1Campos studies came from the inoculation of four bovines with these genetically engineered viruses. These studies showed that the 3056H virus was highly virulent in bovines, whereas the 3056R virus was over 100,000-fold less virulent in these animals (87). However, two bovines inoculated with large amounts of the HS-binding 3056R virus eventually showed signs of FMD. The viruses isolated from vesicular lesions in these animals had lost their ability to bind heparin or replicate in CHO cells and contained amino acid substitutions either at residue 3056 (R→C) or at residue 134 in VP2 (2134K→E). Interestingly, these substituted residues, which are only 8 Å apart on the surface of the viral particle, are distant from the G-H loop RGD sequence. Moreover, both substitutions resulted in loss of positive charges on the surface of the virion, consistent with their inability to bind heparin (87).

To further characterize these virus variants and type O_1BFS, we examined their receptor utilization in wild-type and GAG-deficient CHO cells and compared them with type A_{12} and a variant of type A_{12}, which contains sequences found in virus isolated from infected bovine tongue tissue (vRM-SSP) (81). We transfected these cells with cDNAs encoding human $\alpha v\beta 3$ integrin subunits, resulting in cell lines expressing specific integrin and GAG receptors (74). The results of studies of viral replication in this panel of CHO cells are summarized in Table 1 (74). It can be seen that the tissue culture-adapted type O_1BFS and the avirulent 3056R viruses could only replicate in the cells expressing HS, independent of whether $\alpha v\beta 3$ was expressed. A 3056R virus with an RGD→KGE mutation also only replicated in the HS-expressing cells, indicating that this virus was not utilizing another RGD-dependent integrin. The A_{12}, vRM-SSP, and virulent 3056H viruses, however, could only replicate in cells expressing the $\alpha v\beta 3$ integrin, and did not need HS for replication. A 3056H virus containing an RGD→KGE mutation was unable to replicate in cells expressing either HS or the $\alpha v\beta 3$ integrin, identical to results obtained with RGD-mutated type A_{12} (70). These results indicate that virus that is virulent for its natural host utilizes the $\alpha v\beta 3$ integrin as a receptor. Thus, adaptation of type O_1 virus to tissue culture results in a loss of virulence and the acquisition of the ability to utilize HS as a primary receptor.

Interestingly, the tissue culture-adapted phenotype is related to genetic changes distant from the RGD, in amino acid residue 3056 (in VP3), and is dependent on residue 2134 (in VP2). The importance of these residues (as well

TABLE 1 Replication of FMDV in CHO cells with defined receptor specificity[a]

Virus[b]	Receptor expression			
	$HS^+/\alpha v\beta 3^+$	$HS^+/\alpha v\beta 3^-$	$HS^-/\alpha v\beta 3^+$	$HS^-/\alpha v\beta 3^-$
A_{12}	Yes[c]	No[d]	Yes	No
A_{12} vRM-SSP	Yes	No	Yes	No
O_1BFS	Yes	Yes	No	No
O_1Campos 3056R	Yes	Yes	No	No
O_1Campos 3056R-KGE	Yes	Yes	No	No
O_1Campos 3056H	Yes	No	Yes	No
O_1Campos 3056H-KGE	No	No	ND[e]	ND

[a] Adapted from data in reference 74.
[b] See text for descriptions of the viruses.
[c] Viral proteins detected in infected cells by radioimmunoprecipitation.
[d] No viral proteins detected in infected cells.
[e] Not determined.

as others near the VP2/3 interface) in binding heparin was directly supported by structural data obtained by X-ray crystallographic resolution of virus crystals infused with heparin (38). Although this work was one of the first studies to reveal the structure of a virus with a receptor molecule at the atomic level, the role of this interaction in vivo is unclear, since all of the structural data were obtained from a tissue culture-passaged type O virus, which contains the 3056R mutation that is absent from field and animal-virulent viruses (38, 87).

While changes resulting in the addition of positive charged residues to the viral surface are best characterized for type O viruses, similar changes have been found associated with cell culture-passaged type C_1 viruses (2, 3, 67) and type A24 viruses (M. Almeida, B. Baxt, and P. W. Mason, unpublished data). With the type C_1 viruses, however, variants have also been isolated that contain an RGDD→RGGD mutation and can replicate in HS-deficient CHO cells, suggesting another integrin-independent FMDV-receptor system (2), or the ability of the RGGD to bind to RGD-dependent integrins. Recently, a second integrin, which utilizes the RGD-recognition sequence, $\alpha v\beta 6$, has been identified as a receptor for FMDV (54). The significance of multiple receptor specificities will be discussed below.

MOLECULAR CLONING AND ANALYSIS OF THE BOVINE $\alpha v\beta 3$ INTEGRIN

The transfected cell studies reviewed above tested the ability of human forms of integrins to serve as receptors for FMDV. This virus, however, rarely infects humans, and FMD is not considered to be a zoonotic disease (4, 5). Therefore, we molecularly cloned cDNAs encoding the bovine homologue of the $\alpha v\beta 3$ integrin to examine virus-receptor interactions using a receptor from a susceptible host species (73). The deduced amino acid sequences of the bovine and human $\alpha v\beta 3$ subunits show extensive sequence similarities, with the putative ligand-binding domains of the bovine and human $\beta 3$ subunit possessing the least similarity of all of the integrin functional domains (93.5%) (73).

COS-1 cells transfected with either bovine, human, or mixed bovine-human subunits were infected with FMDV types A_{12}, vRM-SSP, or the O_1Campos 3056H virus. Analyses of viral protein synthesis showed that cells expressing bovine $\alpha v\beta 3$ synthesized higher levels of viral proteins than cells expressing the human integrin, and this higher level of viral replication correlated with the presence of the bovine $\beta 3$ subunit (73). Transfecting cells with engineered bovine-human chimeric $\beta 3$ subunits revealed that this increase in viral receptor efficiency of the bovine integrin was not dependent on the origin of the putative ligand-binding region, but mapped to the C-terminal one-third of the $\beta 3$ subunit ectodomain (73), which contains elements essential to the structure and function of β subunits, known as the cysteine-rich repeats (22, 34, 41, 56). Thus, amino acid changes within this region may be responsible for the increase in the receptor utilization of the bovine homologue by FMDV.

Other important functional domains of integrins include the cytoplasmic domains of the α and β subunits. These have been shown to be involved in signal transduction, ligand-binding affinity, and integrin activation (14, 15, 44, 48, 58, 75, 80, 88). We have examined the role of the cytoplasmic domains of the bovine integrin $\alpha v\beta 3$ in FMDV infection of cultured cells (72a). Truncations or additions to the cytoplasmic domains of either subunit, including removal of essentially the entire cytoplasmic domain of each subunit, had no effect on the ability of the integrin to function as an FMDV receptor. Surprisingly, infection mediated by the truncated $\alpha v\beta 3$ subunits was inhibited by the lysosomotropic agent monensin, suggesting that integrins with truncated cytoplasmic domains were internalizing the virus by a mechanism similar to that seen with wild-type integrins (6). Recently it has been shown that truncations of the cytoplasmic domain of the $\beta 5$ subunit of the $\alpha v\beta 5$ integrin interfered with adenovirus gene delivery (60, 61, 94). However, these truncations did not affect the ability of the integrin to internalize the virus into endosomes (94).

CONCLUSIONS AND FUTURE INVESTIGATIONS

While we have learned much about the early interactions of FMDV with its receptors in vitro, the role these receptors play in the pathogenesis of the disease is still unclear. Studies on the pathogenesis of FMD have shown that initial sites of viral replication are the lung and pharyngeal areas followed by rapid dissemination of the virus to the oral and pedal epithelia (19, 21, 92). Following experimental aerosol infection, the virus was detected within the first 24 h in respiratory bronchiolar epithelium, subepithelium, and interstitial areas of the lung. By 72 h, the virus was present in keratin-containing epithelial cells (keratinocytes) of the tongue, soft palate, feet, tonsils, and tracheobronchial lymph nodes (20). FMDV has also been reported to replicate in vitro in bovine keratinocytes (31).

In vitro investigations have demonstrated that field strains of FMDV can utilize at least two integrin receptors, $\alpha v \beta 3$ and $\alpha v \beta 6$, to gain entry into cultured cells (11, 54, 73, 74). However, it remains unclear which of these molecules may function in viral infection in the tissues of infected animals. Thus, the distribution of these integrins in vivo is of great interest. Although there are no published reports of the distribution of these integrins in FMD-susceptible animals, there are many studies on their distribution in humans. $\alpha v \beta 3$ is generally expressed on vascular endothelium and smooth muscle cells (18, 35, 62). In the lung, $\alpha v \beta 3$ is restricted to large-vessel endothelium (30) and could not be detected on bronchiolar epithelium (72). In addition, cultured human keratinocytes can express very low levels of $\alpha v \beta 3$ (57). In contrast, expression of $\alpha v \beta 6$ is restricted to epithelial cells (17). This integrin is poorly expressed in normal tissue, but is upregulated in development, wound repair, and malignant neoplasia (16). In normal airway and bronchial epithelium, $\alpha v \beta 6$ could not be detected, but it can be found in inflamed lung tissue and in human airway epithelial cells cultured in vitro (95, 96). In oral mucosa, $\alpha v \beta 6$ was not detected in either keratinized or nonkeratinized tissue but was strongly expressed in wounded oral mucosa, principally in suprabasal and basal epithelial cells (45). The integrin was not expressed in freshly isolated dermal keratinocytes but was expressed in keratinocytes isolated from epidermal wounds and in cultured keratinocytes (43).

While it is possible that there may be some differences in integrin expression within identical organs of different species, the published reports on the distribution of $\alpha v \beta 3$ and $\alpha v \beta 6$ in human tissues may serve as a guide for where these integrins will be found in swine and bovine. With these data, it is clear that the distribution of neither $\alpha v \beta 3$ nor $\alpha v \beta 6$ in human tissues colocalizes precisely with the animal tissues known to be affected in FMD. Thus, it is possible that these integrins are utilized in different tissues (for example, $\alpha v \beta 6$ could be utilized in the lung, and $\alpha v \beta 3$ could be utilized in disease spread and in dermal keratinocytes). Alternatively, one of the other RGD-binding integrins ($\alpha 5 \beta 1$, $\alpha 8 \beta 1$, $\alpha v \beta 1$, $\alpha v \beta 5$, $\alpha v \beta 8$) could be utilized to mediate viral infection in one or more of the target tissues of FMDV. Among these, $\alpha v \beta 5$ appears to have a distribution most consistent with the tissues affected by FMDV (it is highly expressed on normal human keratinocytes [57] and in undifferentiated human airway epithelia [39]); however, we have shown that the human homologue of $\alpha v \beta 5$ cannot function as a receptor for FMDV (Neff et al., unpublished), and antibodies to this receptor did not inhibit viral adsorption or replication in cultured cells (11, 54). However, given the differences seen between FMDV interaction with human and bovine $\alpha v \beta 3$ (73), it is possible that a bovine homologue of $\alpha v \beta 5$ could be a viral receptor, where the human homologue would not fulfill this function. Recently FMDV has been shown to bind to isolated human $\alpha 5 \beta 1$ (52), which shows a very wide tissue distribution, but studies utilizing either antibody inhibition (11, 54) or viral replication (74) have suggested that the human $\alpha 5 \beta 1$ is unable to function as a receptor for FMDV.

Application of knowledge of the detailed mechanisms of FMDV-receptor interactions in vitro to the disease in the whole animal should provide insights into viral pathogenesis and may provide new information on how to control this important disease. Thus, future research should concentrate on determining which of the RGD-binding integrins found in susceptible hosts are capable of serving as receptors for FMDV. Furthermore, the possibility that different receptors are utilized at different stages of FMD, from initial contact to spread and pathological damage of tissues, needs to be examined. In addition, analyses of tissues that express viral receptors but do not become infected may allow determination of coreceptors involved in infection and determination of whether the receptor interaction with the virus leads to additional pathology besides allowing the virus to enter and infect cells.

REFERENCES

1. **Acharya, R., E. Fry, D. Stuart, G. Fox, D. Rowlands, and F. Brown.** 1989. The three-dimensional structure of foot-and-mouth disease virus at 2.9 Å resolution. *Nature* **337:**709–716.
2. **Baranowski, E., C. M. Ruiz-Jarabo, N. Sevilla, D. Andreu, E. Beck, and E. Domingo.** 2000. Cell recognition by foot-and-mouth disease virus that lacks the RGD integrin-binding motif: flexibility in aphthovirus receptor usage. *J. Virol.* **74:**1641–1647.
3. **Baranowski, E., N. Sevilla, N. Verdaguer, C. Ruiz-Jarabo, E. Beck, and E. Domingo.** 1998. Multiple virulence determinants of foot-and-mouth disease virus in cell culture. *J. Virol.* **72:**6362–6372.
4. **Barteling, S. J., and J. Vreeswijk.** 1991. Developments in foot-and-mouth disease vaccines. *Vaccine* **9:**75–88.
5. **Bauer, K.** 1997. Foot-and-mouth disease as zoonosis, p. 95–97. *In* O.-R. Kaaden, C.-P. Czerny, and W. Eichhorn (ed.), *Viral Zoonoses and Food of Animal Origin. A Re-Evaluation of Possible Hazards for Human Health.* Springer-Verlag Wien, New York, N.Y.
6. **Baxt, B.** 1987. Effect of lysosomotropic compounds on early events in foot-and-mouth disease virus replication. *Virus Res.* **7:**257–271.
7. **Baxt, B., and H. L. Bachrach.** 1980. Early interactions of foot-and-mouth disease virus with cultured cells. *Virology* **101:**42–55.
8. **Baxt, B., and H. L. Bachrach.** 1982. The adsorption and degradation of foot-and-mouth disease virus by isolated BHK-21 cell plasma membranes. *Virology* **116:**391–405.
9. **Baxt, B., and Y. Becker.** 1990. The effect of peptides containing the arginine-glycine-aspartic acid sequence on the adsorption of foot-and-mouth disease virus to tissue culture cells. *Virus Genes* **4:**73–83.
10. **Baxt, B., and P. W. Mason.** 1995. Foot-and-mouth disease virus undergoes restricted replication in macrophage cell cultures following Fc receptor-mediated adsorption. *Virology* **207:**503–509.
11. **Berinstein, A., M. Roivainen, T. Hovi, P. W. Mason, and B. Baxt.** 1995. Antibodies to the vitronectin receptor (integrin $\alpha_v \beta_3$) inhibit binding and infection of foot-and-mouth disease virus to cultured cells. *J. Virol.* **69:**2664–2666.
12. **Blystone, S. D., I. L. Graham, F. P. Lindberg, and E. J. Brown.** 1994. Integrin $\alpha_v \beta_3$ differentially regulates adhesive and phagocytic functions of the fibronectin receptor $\alpha_5 \beta_1$. *J. Cell Biol.* **127:**1129–1137.
13. **Blystone, S. D., F. P. Lindberg, S. E. LaFlamme, and E. J. Brown.** 1995. Integrin β_3 cytoplasmic tail is necessary and sufficient for regulation of $\alpha_5 \beta_1$ phagocytosis by

$\alpha_v\beta_3$ and integrin-associated protein. *J. Cell Biol.* **130**: 745–754.
14. **Blystone, S. D., F. P. Lindberg, M. P. Williams, K. McHugh, and E. J. Brown.** 1996. Inducible tyrosine phosphorylation of the β_3 integrin requires the α_v integrin cytoplasmic tail. *J. Biol. Chem.* **271**:31458–31462.
15. **Blystone, S. D., M. P. Williams, S. E. Slater, and E. J. Brown.** 1997. Requirement of integrin β_3 tyrosine 747 for β_3 tyrosine phosphorylation and regulation of $\alpha_v\beta_3$ avidity. *J. Biol. Chem.* **272**:28757–28761.
16. **Breuss, J. M., J. Gallo, H. M. DeLisser, I. V. Klimanskaya, H. G. Folkesson, J. F. Pittet, S. L. Nishimura, K. Aldape, D. V. Landers, W. Carpenter, N. Gillett, D. Sheppard, M. A. Matthay, S. M. Albelda, R. H. Krammer, and R. Pytela.** 1995. Expression of the β_6 integrin subunit in development, neoplasia, and tissue repair suggests a role in epithelial remodeling. *J. Cell Sci.* **108**: 2241–2251.
17. **Breuss, J. M., N. Gillett, L. Lu, D. Sheppard, and R. Pytela.** 1993. Restricted distribution of β_6 messenger RNA in primate epithelial tissues. *J. Histochem. Cytochem.* **41**:1521–1527.
18. **Brooks, P. C., R. A. F. Clark, and D. A. Cheresh.** 1994. Requirement of vascular integrin $\alpha_v\beta_3$ for angiogenesis. *Science* **264**:569–571.
19. **Brown, C. C., R. F. Meyer, H. J. Olander, C. House, and C. A. Mebus.** 1992. A pathogenesis study of foot-and-mouth disease in cattle using in situ hybridization. *Can. J. Vet. Res.* **56**:189–193.
20. **Brown, C. C., M. E. Piccone, P. W. Mason, T. S.-C. McKenna, and M. J. Grubman.** 1996. Pathogenesis of wild-type and leaderless foot-and-mouth disease virus in cattle. *J. Virol.* **70**:5638–5641.
21. **Burrows, R. J., A. Mann, A. J. M. Garland, A. Grieg, and D. Goodridge.** 1981. The pathogenesis of natural and simulated natural foot-and-mouth disease virus infection in cattle. *J. Comp. Pathol.* **91**:599–609.
22. **Calvete, J. J., A. Henschen, and J. González-Rodríguez.** 1991. Assignment of disulphide bonds in human platelet GPIIIa. A disulphide pattern for the β-subunits of the integrin family. *Biochem. J.* **274**:63–71.
23. **Carrillo, E. C., C. Giachetti, and R. Campos.** 1984. Effect of lysosomotropic agents on the foot-and-mouth disease virus replication. *Virology* **135**:542–545.
24. **Carrillo, E. C., C. Giachetti, and R. Campos.** 1985. Early steps in FMDV replication: further analysis on the effects of chloroquine. *Virology* **147**:118–125.
25. **Cavanagh, D., D. J. Rowlands, and F. Brown.** 1978. Early events in the interaction between foot-and-mouth disease virus and primary pig kidney cells. *J. Gen. Virol.* **41**:255–264.
26. **Chang, K. H., P. Auvinen, T. Hyypiä, and G. Stanway.** 1989. The nucleotide sequence of coxsackievirus A9: implications for receptor binding and enterovirus classification. *J. Gen. Virol.* **70**:3269–3280.
27. **Chang, K. H., C. Day, J. Walker, T. Hyypiä, and G. Stanway.** 1992. The nucleotide sequences of wild type coxsackievirus A9 strains imply that an RGD motif in VP1 is functionally significant. *J. Gen. Virol.* **73**:621–626.
28. **Crowell, R. L., B. J. Landau, and J. Siak.** 1981. Picornavirus receptors in pathogenesis, p. 170–180. *In* K. Lonberg-Holm and L. Philipson (ed.), *Receptors and Recognition. Virus Receptors, part 2, Animal Viruses,* series B, vol. 8. Chapman and Hall, New York, N.Y.
29. **Curry, S., M. Chow, and J. M. Hogle.** 1996. The poliovirus 135S particle is infectious. *J. Virol.* **70**:7125–7131.
30. **Damjanovich, L., S. M. Albelda, S. A. Mette, and C. A. Buck.** 1992. Distribution of integrin cell adhesion receptors in normal and malignant lung tissue. *Am. J. Respir. Cell Mol. Biol.* **6**:197–206.
31. **David, D., Y. Stram, H. Yadin, Z. Trainin, and Y. Becker.** 1995. Foot-and-mouth disease virus replication in bovine skin langerhans cells under *in vitro* conditions detected by RT-PCR. *Virus Genes* **10**:5–13.
32. **Evans, D. J., and J. W. Almond.** 1998. Cell receptors for picornaviruses as determinants of cell tropism and pathogenesis. *Trends Microbiol.* **6**:198–202.
33. **Everaert, L., R. Vrijsen, and A. Boeyé.** 1989. Eclipse products of poliovirus after cold-synchronized infection of HeLa cells. *Virology* **171**:76–82.
34. **Faull, R. J., J. Wang, D. I. Leavesley, W. Puzon, G. R. Russ, D. Vestweber, and Y. Takada.** 1996. A novel activating anti-β_1 integrin monoclonal antibody binds to the cysteine-rich repeats in the β_1 chain. *J. Biol. Chem.* **271**:25099–25106.
35. **Felding-Haberman, B., and D. A. Cheresh.** 1993. Vitronectin and its receptors. *Curr. Opin. Cell Biol.* **5**:864–868.
36. **Fernández, C., K. Clark, L. Burrows, N. R. Schofield, and M. J. Humphries.** 1998. Regulation of the extracellular ligand binding activity of integrins. *Front. Biosci.* **3**: 684–700.
37. **Fox, G., N. R. Parry, P. V. Barnett, B. McGinn, D. J. Rowlands, and F. Brown.** 1989. The cell attachment site on foot-and-mouth disease virus includes the amino acid sequence RGD (arginine-glycine-aspartic acid). *J. Gen. Virol.* **70**:625–637.
38. **Fry, E. E., S. M. Lea, T. Jackson, J. W. Newman, F. M. Ellard, W. E. Blakemore, R. Abu-Ghazaleh, A. Samuel, A. M. King, and D. I. Stuart.** 1999. The structure and function of a foot-and-mouth disease virus-oligosaccharide receptor complex. *EMBO J.* **18**:543–554.
39. **Goldman, M. J., and J. M. Wilson.** 1995. Expression of $\alpha_v\beta_5$ integrin is necessary for efficient adenovirus-mediated gene transfer in the human airway. *J. Virol.* **69**: 5951–5958.
40. **González-Amaro, R., and F. Sánchez-Madrid.** 1999. Cell adhesion molecules: selectins and integrins. *Crit. Rev. Immunol.* **19**:389–429.
41. **Green, L., A. P. Mould, and M. J. Humphries.** 1998. The integrin beta subunit. *Int. J. Biochem. Cell Biol.* **30**: 179–184.
42. **Greve, J. M., C. P. Forte, C. W. Marlor, A. M. Meyer, H. Hoover-Litty, D. Wunderlich, and A. McClelland.** 1991. Mechanisms of receptor-mediated rhinovirus neutralization defined by two soluble forms of ICAM-1. *J. Virol.* **65**:6015–6023.
43. **Haapasalmi, K., K. Zhang, M. Tonnesen, J. Olerud, D. Sheppard, T. Salo, R. Kramer, R. A. Clark, V. J. Uitto, and H. Larjava.** 1996. Keratinocytes in human wounds express $\alpha_v\beta_6$ integrin. *J. Invest. Dermatol.* **106**:42–48.
44. **Haas, T. A., and E. F. Plow.** 1997. Development of a structural model for the cytoplasmic domain of an integrin. *Protein Eng.* **10**:1395–1405.
45. **Häkkinen, L., C. Hildebrand, A. Berndt, H. Kosmehl, and H. Larjava.** 2000. Immunolocalization of tenascin-C, α_9 integrin subunit, and $\alpha_v\beta_6$ integrin during wound healing in oral mucosa. *J. Histochem. Cytochem.* **48**:985–998.
46. **Hendry, E., H. Hatanaki, E. Fry, M. Smyth, J. Tate, G. Stanway, J. Santti, M. Maaronen, T. Hyypiä, and D. Stuart.** 1999. The crystal structure of coxsackievirus A9: new insights into the uncoating mechanisms of enteroviruses. *Structure* **7**:1527–1538.
47. **Hughes, P. I., C. Horsnell, and G. Stanway.** 1995. The coxsackievirus A9 RGD motif is not essential for virus viability. *J. Virol.* **69**:8035–8040.
48. **Hughes, P. E., T. E. O'Toole, J. Ylänne, S. J. Shattil, and M. H. Ginsberg.** 1995. The conserved membrane-

proximal region of an integrin cytoplasmic domain specifies ligand binding affinity. *J. Biol. Chem.* **270:**12411–12417.
49. **Hynes, R. O.** 1987. Integrins: a family of cell surface receptors. *Cell* **48:**549–554.
50. **Hynes, R. O.** 1992. Integrins: versatility, modulation, and signaling in cell adhesion. *Cell* **69:**11–25.
51. **Hynes, R. O.** 1999. Cell adhesion: old and new questions. *Trends Cell Biol.* **9:**M33–M37.
52. **Jackson, T., W. Blakemore, J. W. I. Newman, N. J. Knowles, A. P. Mould, M. J. Humphries, and A. M. Q. King.** 2000. Foot-and-mouth disease virus is a ligand for the high-affinity binding conformation of integrin $\alpha_5\beta_1$: influence of the leucine residue within the RGDL motif on selectivity of integrin binding. *J. Gen. Virol.* **81:**1383–1391.
53. **Jackson, T., F. M. Ellard, R. Abu-Ghazaleh, S. M. Brooks, W. E. Blakemore, A. H. Corteyn, D. I. Stuart, J. W. I. Newman, and A. M. Q. King.** 1996. Efficient infection of cells in culture by type O foot-and-mouth disease virus requires binding to cell surface heparan sulfate. *J. Virol.* **70:**5282–5287.
54. **Jackson, T., D. Sheppard, M. Denyer, W. Blakemore, and A. M. Q. King.** 2000. The epithelial integrin $\alpha_v\beta_6$ is a receptor for foot-and-mouth disease virus. *J. Virol.* **74:**4949–4956.
55. **Kaplan, G., M. S. Freistadt, and V. R. Racaniello.** 1990. Neutralization of poliovirus by cell receptors expressed in insect cells. *J. Virol.* **64:**4697–4702.
56. **Kashiwagi, H., Y. Tomiyama, S. Tadokoro, S. Honda, M. Shiraga, H. Mizutani, M. Handa, Y. Kurata, Y. Matsuzawa, and S. J. Shattil.** 1999. A mutation in the extracellular cysteine-rich repeat region of the β_3 subunit activates integrins $\alpha_{IIb}\beta_3$ and $\alpha_v\beta_3$. *Blood* **93:**2559–2568.
57. **Kim, J. P., K. Zhang, J. D. Chen, R. H. Kramer, and D. T. Woodley.** 1994. Vitronectin-driven human keratinocyte locomotion is mediated by the $\alpha_v\beta_5$ integrin receptor. *J. Biol. Chem.* **269:**26926–26932.
58. **Law, D. A., F. R. DeGuzman, P. Heiser, K. Ministri-Madrid, N. Kileen, and D. R. Phillips.** 1999. Integrin cytoplasmic tyrosine motif is required for outside-in $\alpha_{IIb}\beta_3$ signaling and platelet function. *Nature* **401:**808–811.
59. **Leippert, M., E. Beck, F. Weiland, and E. Pfaff.** 1997. Point mutations within the βG-βH loop of foot-and-mouth disease virus O1K affect virus attachment to target cells. *J. Virol.* **71:**1046–1051.
60. **Li, E., D. Stupack, G. M. Bokoch, and G. R. Nemerow.** 1998. Adenovirus endocytosis requires actin cytoskeleton reorganization mediated by Rho family GTPases. *J. Virol.* **72:**8806–8812.
61. **Li, E., D. Stupack, R. Klemke, D. A. Cheresh, and G. R. Nemerow.** 1998. Adenovirus endocytosis via α_v integrins requires phosphoinositide-3-OH kinase. *J. Virol.* **72:**2055–2061.
62. **Liaw, L., M. P. Skinner, E. W. Raines, R. Ross, D. A. Cheresh, S. M. Schwartz, and C. M. Giachelli.** 1995. The adhesive and migratory effects of osteopontin are mediated via distinct cell surface integrins. Role of $\alpha_v\beta_3$ in smooth muscle cell migration to osteopontin in vitro. *J. Clin. Invest.* **95:**713–724.
63. **Loeffler, F., and P. Frosch.** 1898. Berichte der Kommission zur Erforschung der Maulund klauenseuche bei dem Institut für Infektionskrankheiten in Berlin. *Zentbl. Bakteriol., Parasitenkd Infektkrankh., Abt. 1* **23:**371–391.
64. **Logan, D., R. Abu-Ghazaleh, W. Blakemore, S. Curry, T. Jackson, A. King, S. Lea, R. Lewis, J. Newman, N. Parry, D. Rowlands, D. Stuart, and F. Brown.** 1993. Structure of a major immunogenic site on foot-and-mouth disease virus. *Nature* **362:**566–568.

65. **Lonberg-Holm, K., L. B. Gosser, and J. C. Kauer.** 1975. Early alteration of poliovirus in infected cells and its specific inhibition. *J. Gen. Virol.* **27:**329–342.
66. **Lonberg-Holm, K., and N. M. Whiteley.** 1976. Physical and metabolic requirements for early interaction of poliovirus and human rhinoviruses with HeLa cells. *J. Virol.* **19:**857–870.
67. **Martínez, M., N. Verdaguer, M. G. Mateu, and E. Domingo.** 1997. Evolution subverting essentiality: dispensability of the cell attachment Arg-Gly-Asp motif in multiply passaged cell foot-and-mouth disease virus. *Proc. Natl. Acad. Sci. USA* **94:**6798–6802.
68. **Mason, P. W., B. Baxt, F. Brown, J. Harber, A. Murdin, and E. Wimmer.** 1993. Antibody-complexed foot-and-mouth disease, but not poliovirus, can infect normally insusceptible cells via the Fc receptor. *Virology* **192:**568–577.
69. **Mason, P., A. Berinstein, B. Baxt, R. Parsells, A. Kang, and E. Rieder.** 1996. Cloning and expression of a single-chain antibody fragment specific for foot-and-mouth disease virus. *Virology* **224:**548–554.
70. **Mason, P. W., E. Rieder, and B. Baxt.** 1994. RGD sequence of foot-and-mouth disease virus is essential for infecting cells via the natural receptor but can be bypassed by an antibody dependent enhancement pathway. *Proc. Natl. Acad. Sci. USA* **91:**1932–1936.
71. **McKenna, T. St. C., J. Lubroth, E. Rieder, B. Baxt, and P. W. Mason.** 1995. Receptor binding site-deleted foot-and-mouth disease (FMD) virus protects cattle from FMD. *J. Virol.* **69:**5787–5790.
72. **Mette, S. A., J. Pilewski, C. A. Buck, and S. M. Albelda.** 1993. Distribution of integrin cell adhesion receptors on normal bronchial epithelial cells and lung cancer cells in vitro and in vivo. *Am. J. Respir. Cell Mol. Biol.* **8:**562–572.
72a.**Neff, S., and B. Baxt.** 2001. The ability of the integrin $\alpha_v\beta_3$ to function as a receptor for foot-and-mouth disease virus is not dependent on the presence of complete cytoplasmic domains. *J. Virol.* **75:**527–532.
73. **Neff, S., P. W. Mason, and B. Baxt.** 2000. High efficiency utilization of the bovine integrin $\alpha_v\beta_3$ as a receptor for foot-and-mouth disease virus is dependent on the bovine β_3 subunit. *J. Virol.* **74:**7298–7306.
74. **Neff, S., D. Sá-Carvalho, E. Rieder, P. W. Mason, S. D. Blystone, E. J. Brown, and B. Baxt.** 1998. Foot-and-mouth disease virus virulent for cattle utilizes the integrin $\alpha_v\beta_3$ as its receptor. *J. Virol.* **72:**3587–3594.
75. **O'Toole, T. E., Y. Katagiri, R. J. Faull, K. Peter, R. Tamura, V. Quaranta, J. C. Loftus, S. J. Shattil, and M. H. Ginsberg.** 1994. Integrin cytoplasmic domains mediate inside-out signal transduction. *J. Cell Biol.* **124:**1047–1059.
76. **Pfaff, E., H. J. Thiel, E. Beck, K. Strohmaier, and H. Schaller.** 1988. Analysis of neutralizing epitopes on foot-and-mouth disease virus. *J. Virol.* **62:**2033–2040.
77. **Pierschbacher, M. D., E. G. Hayman, and E. Ruoslahti.** 1985. The cell attachment determinant in fibronectin. *J. Cell. Biochem.* **28:**115–126.
78. **Pierschbacher, M. D., and E. Ruoslahti.** 1984. Cell attachment activity of fibronectin can be duplicated by small synthetic fragments of the molecule. *Nature* **309:**30–33.
79. **Pierschbacher, M. D., and E. Ruoslahti.** 1984. Variants of the cell recognition site of fibronectin that retain attachment-promoting activity. *Proc. Natl. Acad. Sci. USA* **81:**5985–5988.
80. **Puzon-McLaughlin, W., T. A. Yednock, and Y. Takada.** 1996. Regulation of conformation and ligand binding function of integrin $\alpha_5\beta_1$ by the β_1 cytoplasmic domain. *J. Biol. Chem.* **271:**16580–16585.

81. **Rieder, E., B. Baxt, and P. W. Mason.** 1994. Animal-derived antigenic variants of foot-and-mouth disease virus type A_{12} have low affinity for cells in culture. *J. Virol.* **68:**5296–5299.
82. **Rieder, E., A. Berinstein, B. Baxt, A. Kang, and P. W. Mason.** 1996. Propagation of an attenuated virus by design: engineering a novel receptor for a noninfectious foot-and-mouth disease virus. *Proc. Natl. Acad. Sci. USA* **93:**10428–10433.
83. **Roivainen, M., T. Hyypiä, L. Piirainen, N. Kalkkinen, G. Stanway, and T. Hovi.** 1991. RGD-dependent entry of coxsackievirus A9 into host cells and its bypass after cleavage of VP1 protein by intestinal proteases. *J. Virol.* **65:**4735–4740.
84. **Roivainen, M., L. Piirainen, and T. Hovi.** 1996. Efficient RGD-independent entry process of coxsackievirus A9. *Arch. Virol.* **141:**1909–1919.
85. **Roivainen, M., L. Piirainen, T. Hovi, I. Virtanen, T. Riikonen, J. Heino, and T. Hyypiä.** 1994. Entry of coxsackievirus A9 into host cells: specific interactions with $\alpha_v\beta_3$ integrin, the vitronectin receptor. *Virology* **203:**357–365.
86. **Ruoslahti, E.** 1996. RGD and other recognition sequences for integrins. *Ann. Rev. Cell Dev. Biol.* **12:**697–715.
87. **Sá-Carvalho, D., E. Rieder, B. Baxt, R. Rodarte, A. Tanuri, and P. W. Mason.** 1997. Tissue culture adaptation of foot-and-mouth disease virus selects viruses that bind to heparin and are attenuated in cattle. *J. Virol.* **71:**5115–5123.
88. **Schaffner-Reckinger, E., V. Gouon, C. Melchior, S. Plançon, and N. Kieffer.** 1998. Distinct involvement of β_3 integrin cytoplasmic domain tyrosine residues 747 and 759 in integrin-mediated cytoskeletal assembly and phosphotyrosine signaling. *J. Biol. Chem.* **273:**12623–12632.
89. **Schneider-Schaulies, J.** 2000. Cellular receptors for viruses: links to tropism and pathogenesis. *J. Gen. Virol.* **81:**1413–1429.
90. **Sekiguchi, K., A. J. Franke, and B. Baxt.** 1982. Competition for cellular receptor sites among selected aphthoviruses. *Arch. Virol.* **74:**53–64.
91. **Shieh, M.-T., D. WuDunn, R. I. Montgomery, J. D. Esko, and P. Spear.** 1992. Cell surface receptors for herpes simplex virus are heparan sulfate proteoglycans. *J. Cell Biol.* **116:**1273–1281.
92. **Sutmoller, P., and J. McVicar.** 1976. Pathogenesis of foot-and-mouth disease: the lung as an additional portal of entry of the virus. *J. Hyg. (Cambridge)* **77:**235–243.
93. **Tamkun, J. W., D. W. DeSimone, D. Fonda, R. S. Patel, C. Buck, A. F. Horwitz, and R. O. Hynes.** 1986. Structure of integrin, a glycoprotein involved in the transmembrane linkage between fibronectin and actin. *Cell* **46:**271–282.
94. **Wang, K., T. Guan, D. A. Cheresh, and G. R. Nemerow.** 2000. Regulation of adenovirus membrane penetration by the cytoplasmic tail of integrin β_5. *J. Virol.* **74:**2731–2739.
95. **Wang, A., Y. Yokosaki, R. Ferrando, J. Balmes, and D. Sheppard.** 1996. Differential regulation of airway epithelial integrins by growth factors. *Am. J. Respir. Cell Mol. Biol.* **15:**664–672.
96. **Weinacker, A., R. Ferrando, M. Elliot, J. Hogg, J. Balmes, and D. Sheppard.** 1995. Distribution of integrins $\alpha_v\beta_6$ and $\alpha_9\beta_1$ and their known ligands, fibronectin and tenascin, in human airways. *Am. J. Respir. Cell Mol. Biol.* **12:**547–556.
97. **Wimmer, E.** 1994. Introduction, p. 1–13. *In* E. Wimmer (ed.), *Cellular Receptors for Animal Viruses.* Cold Spring Harbor Laboratory Press, Plainview, N.Y.
98. **WuDunn, D., and P. G. Spear.** 1989. Initial interaction of herpes simplex virus with cells is binding to heparan sulfate. *J. Virol.* **63:**52–58.

VIRAL GENOMES

Picornavirus Genome: an Overview

VADIM I. AGOL

12

The aim of this chapter is to provide an overview of the organization of the picornavirus genome. Other sections of this volume also are largely, or entirely, devoted to functions of either the viral RNA or the proteins it encodes. It seems, however, reasonable to consider the structure and functions of the picornaviral genome as an integrated system designed to ensure efficient self-reproduction. To achieve this goal, the genetic system should store information about how to synthesize the new generation of viral RNA and protein molecules endowed with the ability to assemble into virions capable of infecting new host cells. All this should be accomplished by enforcing cooperation on the part of the host cell (organism) despite a variety of antiviral defensive measures.

As any other genetic system, the picornavirus genome combines strong conservatism with remarkable plasticity, allowing it to adapt to a new environment and to survive even after relatively severe injuries. These aspects of the viral genetic organization are considered in chapter 22.

To those interested in the exciting history of the problem and the evolution of its understanding, a number of informative reviews can be recommended (99, 144, 162, 212, 231, 245, 254, 296). These reviews as well as other chapters of this volume should be consulted for additional references.

MILESTONES IN THE ELUCIDATION OF THE NATURE OF THE PICORNAVIRUS GENOME

The starting point of the picornavirus genome studies was the discovery, in 1955, that one of the viruses belonging to this group, poliovirus, is represented by a nucleoprotein containing 25 to 30% RNA (253). Shortly thereafter, the infectivity of mengovirus (56), poliovirus (8, 57), encephalomyocarditis virus (EMCV) (120), and foot-and-mouth disease virus (FMDV) (46) RNAs was demonstrated. The picornavirus genome turned out to be a single-stranded RNA (117), and its mass was estimated by ultracentrifugation and electron microscopy to be around 2.5×10^6 Da or ca. 7,500 nucleotides. The capacity of poliovirus RNA to code for protein has been documented by its translation in a cell-free system (294). The existence of four structural (169) and several nonstructural (272) poliovirus proteins has been demonstrated (the novel technique of polyacrylamide gel electrophoresis in the presence of sodium dodecyl sulfate was specially devised for the latter study). Unexpectedly, the sum of molecular mass of all of the resolved virus-specific proteins was several times greater than could have been expected judging by the size of the viral RNA (170). The paradox was correctly explained by the assumption that some of the larger virus-specific proteins were, in fact, precursors of the others, as evidenced by the results of pulse-chase experiments (116, 270). Further analysis has led to the suggestion that the entire coding potential of the poliovirus (125) and coxsackie B1 virus (142) is expressed as a single polyprotein initiated at the unique site of the viral genome. By extrapolation, all other eukaryotic mRNAs were also proposed to be monocistronic (125). On the basis of this idea, it became possible to establish the order of the regions encoding specific proteins. At a stage of efficient viral protein synthesis, further initiation of viral translation was stopped by an appropriate inhibitor and short pulses of labeled amino acids were given at different time intervals thereafter. The farther the appropriate coding sequence was from the polyprotein start site, the later should relevant viral proteins be labeled after initiation stopping (236, 271, 276).

The 3'-termini of the poliovirus (306) and mengovirus (183) RNAs were shown to be polyadenylated, whereas the 5' end of the virion RNA turned out to be covalently associated with a small virus-specific protein termed VPg (77, 159, 160). The establishment of the complete primary structure of the poliovirus RNA (143, 233) followed by sequencing of many other picornavirus RNAs (see chapter 13, this volume) was a major breakthrough in the understanding of the nature of the picornavirus genome.

Demonstration of infectivity of the poliovirus cDNA (234) heralded the advent of a new era in picornavirus genome research. Now that any region of the viral RNA can be mutated, deleted, transposed into a vector, etc., elu-

---

Vadim I. Agol ■ M. P. Chumakov Institute of Poliomyelitis & Viral Encephalitides, Russian Academy of Medical Sciences, Moscow Region 142782; and M. V. Lomonosov Moscow State University, Moscow 119899, Russia.

cidation of many long-lasting problems becomes technically feasible. Among the most important achievements of this approach are characterization (though not yet complete) of the functions of nonstructural proteins and identification of translational and replicative cis-elements of the picornaviral genome.

THE OVERALL DESIGN OF THE PICORNAVIRUS GENOME

Picornavirus genomes (Fig. 1) are represented by single-stranded RNA molecules varying in length (from 7.1 kb [human rhinovirus] to 8.2 kb [FMDV]) and base composition (204). They may be considered as composed of three parts, the 5′ untranslated region (5′ UTR) (~600 to 1,200 nucleotides [nt]), the coding region (6,500 to 7,000 nt), and the 3′ untranslated region (3′ UTR) containing a heteropolymeric segment (up to ~100 nt) and a poly(A) tail (several dozen nucleotides). Aphthovirus and some cardiovirus genomes contain an extended (up to several hundred nucleotides) internal poly(C) tract within the 5′ UTR. The noncoding regions harbor cis-elements involved in the replication and translation of viral RNA, whereas the coding segment is largely responsible for the synthesis of viral polypeptides but also contains some control cis-acting elements. Schematically, the genome should encode four major functions: (i) generation of structural and nonstructural proteins, (ii) RNA replication, (iii) virion assembly, and (iv) progeny release from the cell. The RNA sequences that encode these functions tend to cluster, but the clustering is not perfect. In fact, the "labor division" between viral proteins is not strict, and many of them are polyfunctional.

In spite of the availability of complete primary structures of many picornavirus RNAs, the number of genes they contain is not immediately obvious. In these viruses, a single polyprotein molecule is cleaved into a variety of "intermediate" and "mature" polypeptide chains, and the functions of intermediate precursors do not necessarily correspond to the sum of the functions of the final products. With this specification, one may state that there are altogether about 10 final products encoded in three subregions. Disregarding some details (see below), subregion P1 codes for capsid polypeptides VP4, VP2, VP3, and VP1 (in this order); P2 contains information for polypeptides 2A, 2B, and 2C, with various, not yet well-defined functions; and P3 encodes four polypeptides, 3A through 3D, involved primarily in polyprotein processing and viral RNA replication.

In the pages to follow, the picornavirus genetic elements will be grouped according to their functions in the viral life.

DETERMINANTS OF TRANSLATION

The part of the picornavirus genome associated with translation is composed of two functionally and spatially distinct segments: the cis-elements ensuring and controlling translation initiation, on the one hand, and the coding sequence, on the other. The organization of both of these elements was unprecedented at the time of their first characterization. Translation initiation of picornaviral RNAs is accomplished through a cap-independent mechanism involving an RNA segment hundreds of nucleotides long called the internal ribosome entry site (IRES) located within the 5′ UTR (127, 208, 285). As to the coding sequence, picornavirus RNAs have, with a single known exception (see below), only one functional open reading frame (ORF), which directs synthesis of the polyprotein precursor of all of the viral proteins (125, 142).

cis-Elements Involved in Translation Initiation

The majority of eukaryotic mRNAs possess a 5′-terminal cap structure (m^7GpppN) serving as the recognition signal for the translation initiation factor eIF-4F (through its cap-binding subunit, eIF-4E). The template/factor association leads eventually to the recruitment of the 40S ribosomal subunit as well as of other initiation factors and to the assembly of the preinitiation complex (180). By contrast, picornavirus RNAs possess no cap but are instead 5′-terminated with a polypeptide VPg (77, 159, 160), a tyrosine residue of which is linked to the 5′-terminal uridylate by a phosphodiester bond (10, 242). Intracellularly, the VPg moiety of those viral RNA molecules that are not destined for encapsidation is cleaved off by a host enzyme (11), leaving a 5′-terminal pUp group (75, 114, 191). The presence or absence of VPg does not affect the translational template activity of the viral RNA (213).

Another peculiarity of the picornaviral RNAs as translational templates is the presence, in an unusually long 5′ UTR, of multiple AUGs, some of which are in a context optimal for initiation, RNN**AUG**R (where R and N are purine and any nucleotide, respectively) (reviewed in reference 1). These facts are hardly compatible with the scanning model of eukaryotic translation stating that ribosome binds to the capped 5′ end of the template and then scans this template until the first AUG in an optimal context is encountered, at which point translation is initiated (149). Therefore, just the sequencing data accumulated early in the 1980s strongly suggested that picornaviruses should rely on another mode of translation initiation, which should be both cap independent and internal.

A key participant of this alternative mode is the IRES, the cis-element ensuring formation of a preinitiation template/ribosome complex. The existence of IRESs within the picornavirus 5′ UTR is substantiated primarily by two types

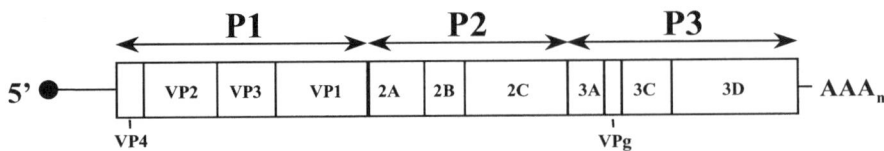

FIGURE 1 A schematic representation of the picornavirus RNA. The genomes of certain picornaviruses may have additional distinctive features, such as the presence of a poly(C) tract within the 5′ UTR (e.g., aphthoviruses and some cardioviruses), a gene encoding leader polypeptide (aphthoviruses and cardioviruses), an alternative short reading frame encoding polypeptide L* (some strains of TMEV), and three copies of the VPg-coding gene (aphthoviruses).

of experiments: (i) a template (either viral or heterologous) containing the picornavirus-derived IRES can be translated in a cap-independent manner (208), e.g., in the presence of cap inhibitors or in extracts from poliovirus-infected cells, where the cap-dependent translation initiation is suppressed due to inactivation of eIF-4G (see below); and, more convincingly, (ii) IRES-containing sequences, being placed into the intercistronic spacer of a bicistronic template, ensure expression of the downstream cistron both in vitro and in vivo (126, 127, 209, 210).

There are problems with the exact mapping of the IRES borders (1). First, assays for the IRES by transfer of truncated 5' UTR into an intercistronic spacer do not result in the all-or-none response; second, the results partly depend on the specific assay conditions (e.g., the host cells) (124). It seems reasonable to distinguish the IRES core and auxiliary cis-elements, even though the distinction between them is not always clear-cut. The IRES core may be defined as the minimal sequence ensuring a significant level of the expression of the adjoining downstream cistron of a bicistronic template. The auxiliary elements may modulate (e.g., enhance) the IRES activity. In some settings, the auxiliary elements may even become essential. Moreover, the IRES appears to be composed of discontinuous RNA segments (see reference 297), which are likely to form tertiary contacts with each other in order to acquire a functional conformation.

Computer-aided sequence comparisons, probing of single- and double-stranded RNA regions, and mutation analysis revealed that enterovirus and rhinovirus 5' UTRs may acquire a conserved (type 1) folding in spite of a more or less marked divergence in their primary structures (220, 237, 262). The genomic regions encompassing the IRES of cardio-, aphtho-, and parechoviruses possess another, but again highly conserved within the group, type of folding (type 2) (70, 84, 186, 219). The secondary structure of the hepatitis A virus (HAV) IRES is distantly reminiscent of the type 2 folding (45), but the differences are great enough to consider the HAV IRES as belonging to a separate class (type 3). Still, it was suggested that IRESs of all picornaviruses share some common traits (157).

RNA folding is intrinsically dynamic and is influenced by many variables such as local ionic conditions and, in particular, RNA-binding proteins. Theoretical calculations suggest that the conformation of type 2 IRES is relatively more stable, whereas polio- and enterovirus IRES folding in solution may significantly vary among identical molecules. To generate the functional "ribosome landing pad," interactions with specific chaperone-like RNA-binding proteins may in this case be particularly important (204).

The ultimate function of the IRES is to bind a ribosome (or its 40S subunit) in a specific orientation. It is essential to form a productive complex between the active center (P site) of the ribosome and the cognate polyprotein initiation codon. This codon is separated from the 3' border of IRESs of different picornavirus RNAs by "spacers" of different lengths, being only ~20 nt in the cardiovirus RNA and over 150 nt in the poliovirus and other enterovirus genomes (these are only approximate values due to uncertainty with the IRES 3' border). The length of the spacer does not appear to be directly related to the IRES type. Thus, in rhinoviruses, the IRES-initiator AUG distance is severalfold shorter than that in enteroviruses, in spite of the fact the IRESs of both virus groups belong to type 1. The choice of an AUG as the initiator codon is a function of its context and distance from the IRES (140, 214, 221) as well as of the IRES nature (198).

The IRES-bound ribosome appears to form a productive complex with the template only within a limited RNA segment, the starting window (221). In the Theiler's murine encephalomyelitis virus (TMEV), the starting window is a dozen nucleotides in length and is located ~17 nt downstream of the IRES. If the starting window contains an optimal-context AUG, translation begins just there. Thus, EMCV polyprotein is initiated strictly at the 11th AUG triplet regardless of the presence of another good-context AUG merely 8 nt upstream (140). If there is no AUG in the starting window, the ribosome is postulated to undertake downstream scanning of the template in search of an efficient initiator codon (221), as is perhaps the case upon poliovirus RNA translation. The optimal AUG context for the IRES-driven formation of the productive initiation complex is RNNAUGR (62, 214), similar to that for the canonical eukaryotic mRNAs (149). If the starting window AUG is within a suboptimal context and/or is located close to the 5' border of the window, it may only inefficiently serve as the initiator, and therefore initiation from the next downstream AUGs may also occur. Thus, two in-frame initiator codons are used in the case of FMDV (54) and HAV (278), whereas some TMEV strains utilize two AUGs belonging to different ORFs (147, 304).

An additional cis-acting element was postulated to exist in this area. It is composed of an oligopyrimidine stretch and an AUG separated from each other by some 20 nt (26, 128, 223). This element was named Y_n-X_m-AUG (128) or the oligopyrimidine/AUG tandem (OAT) (223). The AUG component of the OAT should not necessarily be in an optimal Kozak's context (207, 223). It is not clear, however, whether all three OAT components (the oligopyrimidine, AUG, and the spacer) function as moieties of a single recognizable template element (128, 222, 223), or whether the first two of them are separate elements and the length of the spacer actually determines the position of the AUG relative to the IRES or starting window.

Translational cis-acting elements are not confined to the IRES-initiator codon region. Another such element seems to be located within the 5'-terminal "cloverleaf" structure known to play a key role in the replication of enterovirus RNA (see below). Mutational alteration of this cloverleaf may adversely affect in vivo translation of appropriate templates (80, 261).

Possible envelopment of the 3' UTR in the control of picornavirus translation is not adequately explored (see Note Added in Proof).

trans-Acting Partners of the Viral Translational *cis*-Elements

A major function of translational cis-elements is to serve as recognition signals for the components of the protein-synthesizing machinery (ribosomes and initiation factors). Little is known, however, about specific interactions between a given cis-signal of the picornavirus RNAs and this or that trans-factor. It was hypothesized that the oligopyrimidine moiety of OAT may interact with the 3' end of the 18S ribosomal RNA mimicking the Shine-Dalgarno sequence of prokaryotic templates (26, 223; reviewed in reference 251). No direct support for this hypothesis has been reported, however. Initiation factor eIF-4G (a subunit of eIF-4F) interacts with the J-K domain of EMCV IRES (145). There is evidence for specific binding of initiation factors eIF-4B (181) and eIF-2 (250) to picornavirus IRESs.

The latter may affect selection of the initiation codon out of two functional AUGs in the FMDV RNA (281).

Translational *cis*-elements may be involved in interactions not only with ribosomes and canonical initiation factors but also with a class of host proteins. Various cellular proteins exhibit an RNA-binding activity, and in many cases this activity is sequence specific and/or secondary structure specific. Viral RNAs simply cannot avoid interactions with these ligands and should be adapted to such interactions by either exploiting them for acquiring functional conformations or resisting their potentially adverse effects. The pyrimidine tract-binding protein (PTB) (110, 112, 188), poly(C)-binding protein 2 (37, 38, 98), autoantigen La (176, 259, 275), and protein unr (119) are examples of such potentially important RNA-binding proteins (for reviews, see references 29 and 30). Removal of such proteins from cell-free extracts may result in suppression of picornavirus RNA translatability, and the defect can be relieved by the addition of the relevant protein. These observations suggest (though do not prove) that such proteins may play a role in in vivo translation under physiological conditions (see also reference 95). IRESs of different viruses may require different additional protein factors (29, 30, 119, 225, 292), and the name IRES-specific translation factors (ITAFs) was suggested (225). There is some evidence that the host dependence of the efficiency of viral translation is controlled, at least in part, by tissue-specific differences in the ITAFs' abundance (cf. 42, 225).

The function of ITAFs is not yet adequately characterized. In some cases, they may serve as bridges between the IRES *cis*-acting elements and the ribosome and/or canonical initiation factors. They also perhaps function as chaperones involved in the generation of the functional IRES structure. On the other hand, they may negatively affect the structure and function of IRESs (305).

An important question is whether there are virus-encoded proteins interacting with the translational *cis*-elements. Polypeptide 2A was reported to stimulate poliovirus RNA translation independently of its ability to suppress the host cap-dependent translation (104, 238). Moreover, certain mutations in the 5' UTR could be suppressed by appropriate 2A mutations (168, 243), suggesting a direct interaction between this protein and a *cis*-element in the noncoding RNA region. Not alternatively, stimulation of enterovirus translation by 2A may also be due to the 2A-mediated cleavage of an unidentified host protein(s) (238, 311). A similar effect may be produced by a functionally related FMDV protease Lb (238, 312). It may be noted that EMCV 2A is an RNA-binding protein (92), but 2A proteins of entero- and rhinoviruses, on the one hand, and cardioviruses, on the other, exhibit no obvious structural or functional similarity.

Another putative viral player in the control of initiation of the viral polyprotein is protein 3CD. Its binding to the 5'-terminal cloverleaf structure of the poliovirus genome exerts a suppressive effect on the initiation of translation (80). It is proposed that this effect is a part of the control of the viral translation/replication switch.

Elongation and Termination

Nearly no information is available about genetic elements, if any, controlling (modulating) postinitiation events in picornavirus RNA translation, even though the genomic organization would make a kind of internal termination quite reasonable. Indeed, partial termination of translation after the capsid protein-coding region could have been an efficient resource-saving measure, ensuring generation of capsid proteins in excess over nonstructural ones. Indirect evidence compatible with this notion was a significant delay of elongation (or even occurrence of termination) in the vicinity of the 2A/2B border of the EMCV RNA seen under some experimental conditions (273). The physiological relevance of this observation is, however, unclear. It has recently been suggested that elongation of the FMDV polyprotein may be interrupted at the 2A/2B boundary, generating thereby two primary translation products corresponding to precursors of capsid and noncapsid proteins, respectively (247). This idea is awaiting direct experimental verification.

One of the reasons for the modulations of elongation rates could be the theoretical possibility that such a modulation may influence the accuracy of protein folding. Changes in elongation rate may be caused by rare codons. In line with this hypothesis, the poliovirus ORF contains loci with a marked preference for rare codons (82). Surprisingly, the codon usage varies tremendously among different picornaviruses (266). If the proportion of G+C in the third codon position is taken as a parameter reflecting codon usage differences, the genomes of FMDV and rhinovirus fall in contrasting classes, the values of this parameter being 60 to 65% and 25 to 30%, respectively. Partly, this difference may be due to distinct temperature conditions of the growth of respective viruses (rhinoviruses multiply in the nose). However, the codon bias in the HAV ORF is close to that of rhinoviruses, suggesting that the temperature dependence of the RNA structure is not the (sole) factor responsible for the peculiarities of the codon usage in picornavirus genomes.

Additional Reading Frames

An important exception to the picornavirus single-ORF rule is a short additional reading frame within the leader (L) protein-coding region expressed in some TMEV strains (147). This alternative frame directs synthesis of the so-called L* protein, which appears to play a role in the demyelinating activity of these TMEV strains (49), probably by promoting their replication (277) and persistence in macrophages. The initiator AUG of the L* ORF lies a dozen nucleotides downstream of the relatively leaky initiator AUG of the polyprotein.

There are a number of short ORFs within the 5' UTR. Upon certain conditions, some of them can perhaps be expressed in vitro (118) but hardly to a significant extent in vivo. Evidence for a physiological role of any of the putative translation products of these ORFs is lacking.

DETERMINANTS OF POLYPROTEIN PROCESSING

The single-ORF strategy adopted by the picornaviruses demands that the primary translation product, the polyprotein, should be properly processed into final "mature" polypeptides. The processing is accomplished by two markedly different mechanisms: (i) the *cis*- and *trans*-activities of the viral proteases, and (ii) autocatalytic cleavages. The processing begins cotranslationally, and no significant amounts of the full-length viral polyprotein can normally be detected upon either in vitro or in vivo translation. Limited proteolysis gives rise, in an ordered fashion, to a variety of intermediates, whose properties do not necessarily mimic properties of their constituent parts. As a result, the functional capacity of the viral genome is significantly enhanced.

Viral Proteases

All picornaviruses encode related thiol proteases known as 3C^{pro} (94, 203). This enzyme either by itself or as a component of its precursor 3CD^{pro} (138, 307) is responsible for most of the proteolytic events in the polyprotein processing. Although some picornaviruses, e.g., cardioviruses or HAV, appear to possess only a single protease, 3C/3BC (in the case of HAV also possibly in the form of other 3C precursors; reference 229), many others have a second proteolytic enzyme. Thus, polypeptide 2A of enteroviruses and rhinoviruses (but not of other picornaviruses) is another thiol protease (2A^{pro}), which, among its other activities, is responsible for the "primary" (cotranslational) cleavage between the capsid and nonstructural protein moieties of the nascent polyprotein (284). A specific feature of aphthoviruses is a protease activity of the leader protein, L, one of the functions of which is the removal of L from the capsid protein precursor (269). This enzyme belongs to a class of serine proteases and is found in two forms, Lab and Lb (due to use of different initiation codons) (54). Properties of picornavirus proteases have recently been reviewed (247).

Autocatalytic Cleavages

Some cleavage events in the picornavirus polyprotein processing appear to occur without the involvement of any bona fide proteases. There are two different examples of this sort.

One is represented by a "rudimentary" (16 to 18 nt long) 2A of FMDV. A 19-nt-long oligopeptide spanning 2A and a few N-terminal 2B amino acid residues is able to self-cleave at the site corresponding to the 2A/2B junction (248). This oligopeptide retains its "autocatalytic" cleavage activity upon the transplantation into a heterologous protein (48, 246). C-terminal oligopeptides of a similar length derived from cardiovirus 2A (the intact EMCV and TMEV 2A have some 150 amino acid residues) also appear to express such an activity (68). Recently, it has been proposed that the cleavage at the 2A/2B boundary of FMDV and cardiovirus polyproteins may occur by an entirely different mechanism, namely, by interruption of the translation elongation followed by reinitiation (247). To accept this idea, further support is required.

The second instance of autocatalytic cleavage concerns splitting of VP0 into VP4 and VP2, which occurs at a late step of the virion maturation. This event will be briefly discussed below.

Cleavage Sites

Proteases 3C^{pro} of different picornaviruses vary in the specificity and stringency of the cleavage sites. For example, the poliovirus 3C^{pro} is strictly specific and cleaves only between Gln and Gly, whereas its HAV counterpart is more promiscuous, splitting the polyprotein between six different amino acid pairs (202).

Remarkably, the proper cleavage sites are selectively distinguished among numerous similar sequences scattered over the polyprotein. For example, poliovirus 2A^{pro} attacks only the Tyr-Gly bond between VP1 and 2A (as well as an analogous bond within 3D) but not in other places. A possible explanation is that the recognizable signal is not just the dipeptide but includes its context as well (109). Another likely factor is the tertiary structure of relevant parts of the polyprotein, the interdomain regions being relatively more susceptible (308).

Possible Involvement of Nonviral Proteases

Little is known about the susceptibility of picornavirus proteins to intracellular proteases. In principle, rapid turnover of some of these proteins might contribute to the maintenance of an optimal ratio between different products of the viral polyprotein cleavage. EMCV and HAV 3C proteases harbor specific signals recognizable by the ubiquitin-dependent proteasome system and are degraded rapidly by this system both in vivo and in vitro (86, 155, 156). It would be interesting to know whether such factors as, for example, misfolding caused by an inappropriate rate of elongation could trigger physiologically significant selective degradation of certain viral proteins.

DETERMINANTS OF REPLICATION

The viral genetic replicative elements consist of genes encoding replicative proteins and of cis-acting RNA sequences (for reviews, see references 4, 136, and 300).

Replicative Proteins

There are two picornavirus proteins directly involved in the synthesis of viral RNA, the RNA polymerase 3D^{pol} and VPg (3B), the latter serving, after being uridylylated by 3D^{pol} (206), as a primer for the initiation of both positive and negative RNA strands (189, 215).

The picornaviral RNA polymerases form a family of closely related proteins (148) with the crystal structure solved for the poliovirus enzyme (105; see also reference 200). Picornavirus 3D^{pol} polymerases are capable of carrying out only RNA-strand elongation (76) and, in their strict requirement for a primer, are distinct from the majority of the RNA-dependent RNA polymerases of other viruses. On the other hand, with respect to this property and the ability to catalyze nucleotidylylation of a viral protein, they are functionally similar to adenovirus DNA polymerases (206).

Several, or maybe even all, other nonstructural picornaviral proteins are also involved in the genome replication, directly or otherwise. They fulfill different, not yet adequately elucidated, functions, as briefly discussed below.

cis-Elements Involved in Initiation of (−) Strands

Initiation of a (−) strand demands positioning of the polymerase in close proximity to the 3′ end of a (+) strand, which is represented by a poly(A) stretch. The replicative machinery should be able to distinguish the viral poly(A) from poly(A) tails of host mRNA species. The discrimination seems to involve specific viral RNA cis-elements. A major such element, oriR, is located in the sequence separating the end of the polyprotein ORF and poly(A) and possibly includes a portion of the poly(A) tract. The primary and secondary structures of this segment vary significantly in different picornaviruses (60, 61, 224). The oriR elements of enteroviruses are represented by a multidomain quasi-globular structure maintained by tertiary ("kissing") interactions between loops of hairpin elements (178, 184, 226, 293). Mutations destabilizing this interaction result in a full or partial loss of the viral replicative potential. The mutual orientation of the oriR helical elements appears to be important for interaction with replicative trans-factors (177). The likely function of the oriR is to direct the assembly of a replicative ribonucleoprotein complex composed of viral (108) and probably host (179, 291) proteins.

Surprisingly, the replacement of enterovirus oriR by a structurally unrelated rhinovirus oriR (240) or even complete removal (282) of this seemingly essential element does not kill the virus. Thus, the oriR is not the sole determinant responsible for the (+) RNA template recognition by the replicative machinery. There are also internal replicative cis-elements in the coding region of the viral RNA (i.e., CRE; see references 89, 166, and 175 and Note Added in Proof) and even in the 5′ UTR (41, 126, 260). The latter could hardly be essential as evidenced by the viability of chimerical polioviruses having their cognate IRES replaced by structurally unrelated IRESs of EMCV or even non-picornavirus hepatitis C virus (99).

cis-Elements Involved in Initiation of (+) Strands

cis-Acting elements responsible for the initiation of the picornaviral (+) RNA strands, oriL, are entirely, or at least largely, encoded in the 5′ UTRs and vary significantly in different picornavirus groups. There is little obvious similarity between the primary structures of oriL and oriR. This fact should facilitate differential control of the (+) and (−) RNA strand synthesis. On the other hand, it demands that the replicative machinery should be able to recognize substantially different sets of cis-acting signals. Theoretically, there are three not mutually exclusive possibilities for the location of specific oriL signals: at the 3′ end of (−) strands, the 5′ end of (+) strands, and the "left" end of the double-stranded replicative form.

The oriL elements of enteroviruses and rhinoviruses correspond to a ~100-nt-long 5′-terminal cloverleaf-like segment (14, 237). It is postulated that the ribonucleoprotein complex involved in the initiation of viral (+) RNA strands is first assembled on the 5′ terminus of an already existing (+) strand and then is somehow forwarded to the 3′ end of the template (−) strand (13). The complex appears to contain precursors of the viral replicative proteins $3D^{pol}$ (3CD) and VPg (3AB) (13, 80, 81, 108, 299) as well as host proteins, e.g., poly(rC)-binding polypeptides 1 and 2 (79, 81, 205) and possibly some others. Relatively detailed, though somewhat speculative, models explaining the interplay of the cis-element and trans-factors in the initiation of (+) strands have been proposed (reviewed in references 4, 80, and 300).

The oriL elements of other picornaviruses are characterized rather poorly. It is tempting to speculate that 5′-terminal hairpins of cardiovirus (288), aphthovirus (187), and HAV (45, 152) RNAs play a role in the initiation of (+) strands, but detailed analysis of their functional significance is yet to be carried out. There is evidence that pseudoknots located downstream of the poly(C) stretch in the mengovirus (172) and FMDV (53) RNAs are essential for the replication. A roughly similarly situated locus within HAV RNA also appears to be involved in the genome replication (256). It is unknown, however, whether these elements are involved in the initiation of (+) strands.

DETERMINANTS OF ENVIRONMENTAL CONTROL AND TRAFFICKING

A set of essential functions of the picornaviral genomes aim at creating optimal conditions for viral reproduction. Among such functions are (i) rearrangements of the intracellular infrastructure, e.g., generation of membranous vesicles ensuring proper compartmentation of the virus-specific macromolecules; (ii) changes in the intracellular environment; and (iii) direct guidance (targeting) of viral components to a proper destination.

Determinants of Intracellular Structural Changes

It has long been known that infection with some picornaviruses results in a prompt rearrangement of the intracellular membrane network, namely, in generating vesicular structures believed to serve as a major, if not the only, site for the replication of the viral RNA (reviewed in reference 144). These changes appear to be triggered by virus-specific proteins encoded in the P2 region (2B, 2BC, 2C) (7, 21, 50, 96, 279, 280). The mechanism by which these proteins achieve such dramatic structural rearrangements in a matter of a few hours is unknown. The modified intracellular membranes are associated with the P2 proteins (33), most likely with their hydrophobic or amphipathic domains. The rearrangement seems to be an active process involving phospholipid synthesis (101) and components from different organelles, primarily endoplasmic reticulum but also possibly from the Golgi complex (39, 249, 252). It is proposed that the rearrangements, at least in part, could be due to the interference, by enterovirus 2B (2BC) and 3A, with intracellular membrane trafficking (21, 56, 67).

Picornavirus proteins affect also the cytoskeleton. Poliovirus and rhinovirus $3C^{pro}$ were reported to cleave microtubule-associated protein 4 (MAP-4) (133). Enterovirus $2A^{pro}$ cleaves dystrophin (17), a muscular protein known to be altered in several muscular disorders. Dystrophin degradation may contribute to pathogenesis of cardiopathy elicited by infection with some coxsackieviruses (17).

Determinants of Intracellular Environmental Changes

Picornavirus infection is accompanied by changes in the permeability of both intracellular and plasma membranes. Appropriate specific alterations occur early and late in the reproduction cycle (reviewed in reference 47). These events were studied more extensively in enterovirus (poliovirus and coxsackie B virus) models. There is evidence that 2B (or 2BC) (6, 287) and 3AB (153) may enhance permeability of endoplasmic reticulum. It is speculated that some of these proteins may generate porin-like channels (47, 287). The ionic changes may be involved in the control of the viral translation and replication. Other effects on membrane permeability may be due to activation of certain phospholipases (122), but the nature of viral proteins involved in this activation is yet to be determined.

A significant but not yet fully understood environmental change accompanying picornavirus infection consists of redistribution of host macromolecules between intracellular compartments as exemplified by the accumulation of certain nuclear proteins in the cytoplasm. Nuclear/cytoplasmic redistribution begins early in infection and appears to be selective to some extent. The distribution may result from enhanced export of nuclear proteins into the cytoplasm and their suppressed import into the nucleus (28, 101a). Among nuclear proteins known to be relocated into the cytoplasm in poliovirus-infected cells are autoantigen La (176); Sam68, a protein probably involved in mitosis (173); and nucleolin (291). Since these proteins exhibit RNA-binding properties and show preferential affinities to different segments of the viral RNA, they may well affect its translational and/or replicative activity. Redistribution of some of these proteins, e.g., La, could be due to its limited proteolysis by the viral protease 3C, resulting in the loss of a nuclear localization signal (259). However, proteolysis of nuclear proteins is not a general prerequisite for the accumulation of nuclear proteins in the cytoplasm (28). Noteworthy, certain nuclear proteins (e.g., TATA-binding protein [173], splicing factor SC-35 [176], or even mutated Sam68 [174]) did not change their location. The viral genetic determinants responsible for the redistribution of host macromolecules remain unknown.

Determinants of Trafficking Guidance

One of the essential viral genome functions is to ensure the assembly of virus-specific protein-protein and protein-RNA complexes at a proper intracellular location, which is certainly nonrandom (see reference 39). Little is known about respective genetic determinants, but certain regularities are emerging. As already mentioned, the major site of picornavirus RNA replication is membranous vesicular structures. It seems likely that viral proteins are targeted to this destination due to covalent (as precursors) or noncovalent (59, 298) association primarily with polypeptides 2B, 3A, and possibly 2C, which possess hydrophobic and/or amphipathic domains. Thus, membrane association of the replicative ribonucleoprotein complex at the 5'-terminal cloverleaf $oriL$ depends most likely on hydrophobicity of 3A. RNA-binding properties of some of the nonstructural proteins, like poliovirus 2C (19, 239), may also contribute to the generation of functional supramolecular complexes.

The mechanisms of targeting viral RNA molecules to their destinations (translation, replication, virion assembly) are unknown. Since only the VPg-linked viral RNA species are encapsidated, a role for VPg as a guide to the assembly machinery is contemplated (190).

DETERMINANTS OF ANTI-HOST OFFENSE AND DEFENSE

An important function of the viral genome is to prevent or neutralize the host defensive measures. There is a general way to achieve this goal: just to suppress important cellular functions not required for efficient viral reproduction, e.g., expression of the host genome at the levels of translation and transcription. On the other hand, picornaviruses have evolved the capacity to specifically counteract some cellular antiviral mechanisms.

Determinants of Macromolecular Shutoff

The ability to suppress host macromolecular synthesis is a characteristic, though not obligatory, trait of picornaviruses (reviewed in references 71 and 265). Cleavage of essential host translation or transcription factors by the viral proteases explains many of the shutoff phenomena. Remarkably, the cleavage sites susceptible to these enzymes, being relatively rare, are present in some key participants of the cellular synthetic machinery.

The FMDV leader protease (64) and rhinovirus and enterovirus $2A^{pro}$ (102, 164, 289) cleave and inactivate the translation initiation factor eIF-4GI (formerly p220), especially when it is complexed with eIF-4E (102). There is some evidence that poliovirus 2A may be involved in the eIF-4GI inactivation also indirectly, by stimulation of a cellular protease (43). Recently, proteolysis of a related initiation factor, eIF-4GII, was implicated in the shutoff triggered by poliovirus (97) and rhinovirus (274). Proteolysis of eIF-4GII, like that of eIF-4GI, is accomplished by $2A^{pro}$ (194). A mutation in poliovirus 2A resulting in failure to cleave eIF-4G is accomplished by a deficiency in induction of the translational shutoff (32). The poly(A)-binding protein (PABP) is another target for the poliovirus $2A^{pro}$ and $3C^{pro}$ as well as of coxsackie B virus $2A^{pro}$, and PABP destruction may contribute to the translational shutoff (134, 141).

Poliovirus $2A^{pro}$ cleaves the TATA-binding protein (301), whereas $3C^{pro}$ attacks the same transcription factor (52) as well as CREB and Oct-1 (302, 303). Transcription factors of RNA polymerase I (244) and of RNA polymerase III (51, 258) are also affected by poliovirus $3C^{pro}$. FMDV $3C^{pro}$ carries out proteolysis of histone H3 (74).

An entirely different mechanism of macromolecular shutoff involves changes in the phosphorylation status of key regulatory factors. In cardiovirus-infected cells, where no proteolysis of essential translation factors seems to occur (185), the cap-binding factor eIF-4E is inactivated due to interaction with a dephosphorylated form of its cellular inhibitor, an eIF-4E-binding protein (4E-BP1) (85). A similar mechanism may operate also in poliovirus-infected cells, thus complementing the effect of the proteolysis of initiation factors. The viral determinant(s) responsible for the dephosphorylation of 4E-BP1 is not yet identified, nor are we aware of the mechanism underlying the detachment of host mRNA from the cytoskeleton, which also appears to contribute to the translational shutoff during poliovirus infection (40).

The importance of the macromolecular shutoff for picornavirus reproduction is not completely clear. Inhibition of eIF-4G proteolysis due to mutational inactivation of poliovirus $2A^{pro}$ (32) or FMDV leader protease (217) was accompanied by strong and slight decrease in the growth potential, respectively. It seems that the inhibition of the host macromolecular synthesis is more important for some virus-host combinations than for others. Moreover, suppression of the host metabolism is not a general property of all picornaviruses. Some of them, e.g., echoviruses (310), parechoviruses (55), and HAV (63), do not trigger protein synthesis shutoff in the infected cells. The shutoff is also absent or at least markedly diminished in many cases of persistent infection triggered by different picornavirus, including such typically cytocidal agents as poliovirus.

In addition to the early host-specific shutoff, inhibition of translation of both the cellular and viral templates may occur by the end of the replicative cycle. The late inhibition is most likely caused by the phosphorylation of the α-subunit of eIF-2 due to accumulation of double-stranded RNA and activation of the double-stranded RNA-dependent protein kinase, PKR (32, 199). This phenomenon can hardly be considered as directed against host defense mechanisms but is more likely related to the cytopathic effect. Interestingly, early PKR activation, which could be detrimental to viral reproduction, is not accompanied by eIF-2 phosphorylation upon poliovirus infection (235) due to an enhanced PKR degradation caused by an unidentified viral function (35).

Determinants of Antiapoptotic Activity

Depending on the virus and specific conditions, picornavirus infection may lead to the host cell apoptotic response, which may be considered a kind of defensive antiviral measure. To counteract this defense, picornaviruses possess antiapoptotic functions (283). The existing evidence suggests that several nonstructural poliovirus proteins, 2B/2BC and

3A, appear to interfere with distinct apoptotic pathways (187a). In particular, the expression of 3A results in the depletion of the major receptor for tumor necrosis factor alpha (TNF-α) from the plasma membrane, thereby rendering the cells resistant to TNF-α-induced apoptosis. The depletion of this metabolically unstable receptor appeared to result from the lack of its adequate replenishment caused by the disruption of the Golgi-mediated trafficking (187a). On the other hand, poliovirus 2B/BC and 2C exhibit a marked suppressive antiapoptotic activity, comparable to or even exceeding that of Bcl-2, against apoptosis triggered by other stimuli (N. Neznanov and A. Gudkov, personal communication). These effects may be due to the involvement of the viral proteins in the rearrangement of the intracellular infrastructure and, not alternatively, to their interaction with the components of the host apoptotic/antiapoptotic machinery.

A protein encoded by the TMEV genome out of the polyprotein ORF, L*, exhibits an antiapoptotic effect in macrophages, thereby suppressing development of apoptosis in response to the viral infection (83). The mechanism of this effect is yet to be elucidated.

Determinants of Modulation of Immune Response

Picornavirus infections may affect production of cytokines and cytokine receptors. In particular, TMEV and coxsackie B virus infections were studied in this regard because of a significant immunological contribution to the pathogenesis of the diseases elicited by these viruses. Unfortunately, nearly nothing is known about the viral genetic determinants involved in the control of cytokine production. Inhibition by poliovirus 2BC (21) or 3A (66) of exocytotic pathways may interfere with the secretion of antiviral cytokines (e.g., beta interferon and interleukin 6 and 8) (65a), the synthesis of which is in addition suppressed due to the translational shutoff. Also, presentation of antigens on the cellular surface in the context of major histocompatibility complex class I molecules is inhibited by poliovirus 3A (63a).

DETERMINANTS OF VIRION ASSEMBLY

The general scheme of virion assembly is believed to include the following steps: (i) synthesis of the capsid protein precursor as a part of the whole polyprotein; (ii) primary cleavage liberating the precursor of the four capsid proteins (VP1 to 4), sometimes with N-terminal (leader polypeptide) or C-terminal (2A) extensions; (iii) removal of the above extra parts, if they are present (although HAV 2A does not appear to be readily cleaved off from the VP1 moiety and is likely a structural component of the virion [see reference 12]); (iv) cleavage of the precursor into VP0, VP3, and VP1, which remain in a noncovalent complex, the protomer, with one another; (v) association of protomers into pentamers; (vi) association of six pentamers into the icosahedral empty particle; (vii) packaging of the viral RNA into the empty particle; and (viii) the "maturation" cleavage of VP0 into VP4 and VP2 (15, 245). Although this scheme contains some not-well-characterized reactions, and minor variations among different picornaviruses are quite possible, it is clear that there are three types of key determinants of the assembly pathway: those controlling specific protein-protein interactions among capsid proteins, specific RNA-protein interactions between the genome and capsid proteins, as well as the determinants of the "maturation" cleavage. Only the two latter types of determinants will be briefly considered here.

Encapsidation Signals

The specificity of picornavirus RNA packaging implies the existence of specific encapsidation RNA signals and the ability of capsid proteins to recognize these signals. Surprisingly, identification of both of these types of determinants turned out to be a hard problem, which, despite strong effort by numerous investigators, is not yet solved.

The major poliovirus RNA packaging signal lies somewhere outside the capsid-coding region. Indeed, defective interfering (DI) genomes lacking this region are efficiently packaged (151). Nonetheless, unidentified signals in the 5' UTR seem to stimulate poliovirus RNA packaging (135). On the basis of some indirect arguments, it was suggested that the poliovirus RNA encapsidation signal or signals map most likely to the 2B or 3D coding regions (20).

The specificity of the genome-capsid interaction is strong (192) but not absolute. It is long known that the poliovirus RNA can be encapsidated into coxsackievirus proteins (115, 264). More recently it was reported that poliovirus RNA (or poliovirus RNA-based replicons) might be encapsidated into the rhinovirus and even mengovirus but not HAV capsid (132). On the other hand, certain poliovirus replicons exhibit a much higher specificity, failing to be efficiently encapsidated into the proteins of other enteroviruses (20, 228). The reason for the somewhat discrepant results obtained in different types of experiments is not immediately obvious, but these facts may hint at the existence of more than one packaging pathway exhibiting different levels of specificity and efficacy.

Even though VPg-lacking viral RNA species serving as translational templates are abundant in the infected cell, they are not efficiently packaged (190). This may be due to either direct participation of the VPg moiety in encapsidation or coupling between genomic RNA synthesis and its packaging. Indeed, only nascent viral RNA chains appear to be efficiently packaged (195).

Capsid protein determinants responsible for the recognition of the viral genome are yet to be characterized. There is evidence that each protein component of a pentamer (i.e., VP0, VP3, and VP1) contacts (can be cross-linked with) the viral RNA in the poliovirus replicative complexes (196, 216). Therefore, encapsidation may, in principle, start already at the pentamer level rather than at the empty particle step.

The genomic RNA and capsid proteins may be not the only virus-specific players in virion generation: mutations in the 2C-encoding gene of poliovirus may perhaps affect the assembly pathway (163, 286). The mechanism underlying this effect is unknown.

Most knowledge about picornavirus maturation is derived from experiments with poliovirus. In other systems there are certain variations on the main theme. For example, the 2A domain of HAV VP1-2A fusion polypeptide appears to play a role in the assembly of pentamers, whereas VP4 is perhaps involved in further aggregation of the capsid proteins (230).

Determinants of the Maturation Cleavage

The mechanism of the final maturation cleavage of VP0 into VP4 and VP2 occurring between Asn and Ser residues and resulting in a significant stabilization of the capsid structure (25) has not been fully elucidated (reviewed in reference 111). It was speculated that the cleavage of VP0 occurs autocatalytically by activation of a serine residue of VP2 by virion RNA (16), but this hypothesis did not find experimental support (106). The explanation of the mechanism of this cleavage should take into account that (nearly) all of the 60 copies of VP0 are undergoing this transformation practically simultaneously.

The maturation-associated VP0 cleavage is very slow in HAV (34) and particularly inefficient in parechoviruses (267).

DETERMINANTS OF VIRION RELEASE

Determinants of Lytic versus Nonlytic Infection

The picornavirus RNA, like any other viral genome, should encode function(s) ensuring externalization of the progeny virions. The simplest way to achieve this goal is just to destroy, lyse, the cell. Many, though not all, of the picornaviruses are endowed with such a capacity. The lytic or nonlytic outcome of the infection depends on both partners, the virus and the host. For example, poliovirus, famous for its cytolytic activity, grows nonlytically in undifferentiated erythroblastoid cells (165), but hemin-induced differentiation of these cells renders them susceptible to poliovirus killing (31). On the other hand, cytopathic variants of HAV, generally a nonlytic virus, can be selected (58, 290).

Surprisingly little is known about viral mechanisms involved in the pathological alterations of the infected cell ending up in its lysis. Obviously, there is no specific "cytopathic gene" in picornaviruses: mutations in several viral proteins may affect the extent of cytopathic effect (CPE) and/or its time course. Picornaviral proteins involved in the shutoff of host macromolecular synthesis are likely involved, as evidenced, for example, by modulation of the CPE development by mutations in poliovirus 2A (32). However, inhibitors of RNA and protein synthesis fail to kill uninfected cells within time intervals comparable to the length of the infectious cycle. Moreover, morphological alterations induced by such inhibitors appear to be different from those observed upon viral infections, the latter being specific for different virus-cell combinations.

Viral proteins responsible for the rearrangement of the cellular infrastructure and permeability changes also contribute to CPE development. This fact may be illustrated by the restrictions of the viral yield and cytopathic activity in Vero (though not HeLa) cells caused by a mutation in poliovirus 3A (importantly, this mutation does not appear to significantly alter accumulation of virus-specific macromolecules in the infected cell) (154).

Mutations converting a normally nonlytic HAV into a cell-killing (cytopathic) form map primarily to the P2 region but also to P3 and 5' UTR (309). Again, no coherent picture of the mechanisms responsible for the survival or death of the infected cell can be reconstructed. Thus, the actual genetic determinants of the picornavirus-induced CPE are yet to be defined.

The exit of mature virions from the cell may be accomplished also by mechanisms other than lysis, e.g., related to vesicular transport and a kind of exocytosis, as is seemingly the case with noncytopathic strains of HAV (36). Strong association of HAV progeny with cellular membranes (161) is perhaps related to this not-yet-understood mode of viral exit. It may be noted that the cell type dependence of viral progeny release is a general phenomenon and may not necessarily be correlated with the lytic/nonlytic character of the infection (268).

Determinants of Cytopathic versus Apoptotic Host Response

Picornavirus-infected cells may die of either CPE or apoptosis (283). Apoptosis serves as a host defensive response to the virus-induced stress and its biological role perhaps consists of limiting virus spread. This goal can be achieved by preventing the completion of the reproduction cycle and sequestration of at least a part of the progeny within the apoptotic bodies. In HeLa cells, poliovirus infection results in early turn-on of the apoptotic program, as a response to the damage inflicted to cellular functions by $2A^{pro}$ (23, 88), $3C^{pro}$ (22), and possibly by other viral proteins. A significant role in the activation of this program is played by virus-induced mitochondrial damage (G. A. Belov, L. I. Romanova, E. A. Tolskaya, M. S. Kolesnikova, Y. A. Lazebnik, and V. I. Agol, unpublished data). The implementation of this program, however, is interrupted by the activation of not yet well-defined viral antiapoptotic function(s) (3), which involve degradation of certain key components of the apoptotic pathway (Belov et al., unpublished). It was reported that coxsackie B3 virus capsid protein VP2 may induce apoptosis as a result of its interaction with antiapoptotic host protein siva (113).

The outcome of infection (CPE versus apoptosis) depends on the type of host cells (130, 167), the state of their differentiation (129), genetic makeup of the virus (130), and conditions of infection (2, 283). It becomes apparent that the mechanism of cell killing by the so-called cytopathic variants of HAV, generally a nonlytic agent, may at least in certain systems be related to apoptosis rather than to the canonical CPE (44, 96).

DETERMINANTS OF RNA INTERNALIZATION

The viral genome should encode structural features enabling the virion-encapsidated RNA to eventually enter new host cells. Schematically, the internalization is a two-step process. First, the virion should be fixed at the surface of the prospective host cell by interacting with viral receptors serving as "hooks" and then it should be "unzipped" to allow the release of the viral genome from the virion (see reference 232).

Different exposed cellular components, normally engaged in diverse functions, serve as receptors for different picornaviruses; in turn, different capsid structures of different picornaviruses are involved in the interactions with receptors (73, 295). There are no consensus parts of the picornavirus capsid that are responsible for the interaction with receptors. Moreover, since these parts should be specifically oriented on the outer viral surface, many other parts of the capsid structure should also be important for the receptor binding and uncoating of a picornavirus. The latter step requires destabilization of the capsid, formation of holes permitting the escape of RNA, and perhaps generation of a channel across the plasma membrane through which the RNA enters the cytoplasm. For some picornaviruses, there are plausible models of this complex rearrangement (27, 241).

INTEGRATION AND COORDINATION OF VIRAL FUNCTIONS

The viral genetic makeup should ensure generation of the appropriate building blocks (RNA and capsid proteins) in optimal ratios and locations. The capsid proteins are required in great excess over the viral RNA (with a molar ratio of at least 60:1). To achieve this goal the synthesis of viral proteins and positive and negative RNA species should be properly coordinated. This coordination involves both coupling and interference between different partial reactions of the reproductive cycle.

To serve as templates for the negative-strand synthesis, positive RNA strands should first be translated, but the viral RNA polymerase is unable to replicate the RNA molecule undergoing translation (24, 80, 193). To prevent collision of the ribosome and RNA polymerase on an RNA template, a special mechanism appears to be operative. Binding of 3CD to the oriL results in the inhibition of translation of poliovirus (+) RNA, on the one hand, and activation of the initiation of (−) strand at the oriR, on the other (80).

It is likely that oriR can be utilized for the initiation of a negative strand only once. On the other hand, a negative strand can serve for the simultaneous synthesis of multiple copies of positive strands (18). Such a design ensures preferential accumulation of positive strands required in a greater amount (for replication, translation, and virion assembly). A single RNA molecule appears to produce many copies of the polyprotein, as judged by the existence of heavy polyribosomes containing the viral RNA template (211). Therefore, the virus-specific proteins are generated in a significant excess over the viral genomes, just as is required by the reproduction strategy adopted.

The virion assembly does not appear to be a straightforward consequence of the availability of pools of capsid proteins, on the one hand, and full-length positive RNA strands, on the other. Only nascent RNA molecules appear to be encapsidated (195). The mechanism of coupling between replication and packaging is unknown. One may speculate that the encapsidation signal(s) are efficiently exposed on the nascent RNA molecules only. Another possibility could consist of different compartmentation of free and replicative intermediate-associated RNA species.

The regulatory genetic mechanisms just described are in good accord with the general sequence of events in the viral reproductive cycle: translation of the input RNA → synthesis and processing of the polyprotein → synthesis of a (−) RNA strand → synthesis of multiple copies of (+) strands → replication of the newly synthesized (+) strands and accumulation of virus-specific proteins → assembly of virions. The real time course of these reactions is, however, influenced by numerous factors, known or yet to be defined. For example, distinct kinetics of the cleavages in the P3 precursor polypeptide (3A/B/C/D) due to different susceptibilities of particular cleavage sites, as well as differences in cis and trans proteolytic activities of 3C^{pro}, may contribute to the ordered succession of replicative events.

A significant but not yet adequately explored aspect of the integration of viral functions consists of the fact that products of the picornavirus genes often perform their function not as individual entities, but rather, they are involved in multiple interactions with each other. The potential for such mutual interactions is evident from the so-called "protein linkage maps" derived by the yeast two-hybrid technique for the products of the poliovirus P2 (59) and P3 (298) genomic regions.

In addition to quantitative and temporal controls, viral functions should be properly organized within the intracellular space. However, the mechanisms responsible for the compartmentation and topological integration of the partial reaction of viral reproduction are poorly understood.

ESSENTIAL AND NONESSENTIAL GENETIC ELEMENTS

Although the picornavirus genome is relatively small and encodes only a limited number of proteins, not all of them are indispensable. Thus, the FMDV L gene is not essential, at least under certain conditions. Engineered genomes lacking this gene produced viruses with only slightly diminished growth potential (217). The TMEV proteins L (146), L* (197, 277), and 2A (182) are essential for efficient growth only in some host cells but not in others. The same is true of mengovirus L protein (313), and viable mutants of this virus with deletions in 2A are described (314). Deletions of 10 to 15 amino acid residues from HAV 2A only slightly affect the viral growth in vitro and do not abolish infectivity for marmosets (107). Removal of one or two (out of existing three) (78) of the FMDV VPg genes, while diminishing viral RNA synthesis, exhibited relatively minor effects on the yield of infectious virus (74).

There are segments in the noncoding regions of the picornavirus genomes that also can be deleted without dramatic phenotypic alterations, at least when studied in cell cultures. The segment with coordinates 184 to 228 (65) or the spacer preceding the initiator AUG$_{745}$ (87, 150) can be taken as examples of such elements in the poliovirus 5′ UTR. However, conservation of these (and other seemingly dispensable) (72, 255) genomic segments during picornavirus evolution suggests that they are functionally important under certain (e.g., natural) conditions. Indeed, removal of the IRES/AUG spacer from the poliovirus 5′ UTR is accompanied by a decrease in neurovirulence (121, 263). The same is true of the poly(C) tract of mengovirus: it is dispensable for viral growth in HeLa cells (171) but essential for viral virulence (69, 201). The possibility of deleting oriR from poliovirus RNA was already mentioned.

GENETIC BASIS OF VIRAL PHENOTYPES

Viral phenotypes reflect the qualitative and quantitative abilities of a virus to arrive at, multiply in, and impair functions of specific cells (or organism) under given conditions. While discussing genetic determinants of viral phenotypes, two aspects of the problem should be distinguished. One concerns changes in viral properties associated with specific alterations in a given part of the viral genome. This is a widely used and highly productive approach, which has yielded a good deal of the knowledge described in this chapter. On the other hand, one may be interested in the molecular basis of specific phenotypic traits of a virus, e.g., its host range, pathogenicity, etc.

A major determinant of the host range (at both the cellular and organismic levels) is the compatibility/incompatibility of the viral capsid proteins and receptors on particular cells (reviewed in references 99 and 295). For example, the strict primate specificity of poliovirus is due to the absence of appropriate receptors in other animals. The ability of certain EMCV strains to elicit diabetes in mice can be abolished by a single mutation in the capsid protein VP1, which decreases viral binding to β-cells (139). Determinants of host range may reside not only on the surface capsid proteins but also on the internal VP4 polypeptide (131).

Obviously, to fulfill their specific reproductive functions, viral proteins should often cooperate with host proteins. The compatibility between such viral and cellular counterparts also contributes to the viral host range or at least to the different levels of viral reproduction in distinct types of cells.

cis-Acting elements of the viral RNAs represent still another group of viral determinants controlling host selectivity (42, 238). Picornavirus IRESs exhibit variable requirements for the auxiliary host initiation factors (ITAFs); in turn, such factors may exhibit organ- or cell-specific distribution (225, 227). Indeed, certain alterations in the cis-acting translational elements of the 5′ UTRs are known to affect picornavirus interaction with specific cells and hence viral virulence (5, 103, 222, 226a, 227). The attenuated phenotype of Sabin strains of poliovirus is partly due to the 5′ UTR mutations (9). Similarly, the virulence of mengovirus depends on the length of the poly(C) tract in its 5′ UTR (69, 201). These cis-elements may differ from one another with regard to the stringency of their requirements for host-specific factors (42, 257).

In addition to the ability or inability to grow efficiently in specific cells, phenotypic variability among picornaviruses may reflect the capacity of particular viral proteins to elicit specific host damages. It is quite possible (though poorly documented) that some important host proteins may be cleaved by the proteases of certain but not all picornaviruses. Thus, only the viruses having either 2A or leader polypeptide-associated proteolytic activities are able to destroy such essential translation initiation factors as eIF-4G (see above).

Still another group of viral biological properties is related to their capacity to trigger various defense reactions at cellular and organismic levels (see above). For example, the ability of some TMEV strains to elicit persistent demyelinating disease is associated, at least in part, with the expression of polypeptide L* endowed with an antiapoptotic activity (83, 277).

Picornaviruses differ in the levels of cellular and humoral immune responses they trigger. This variability is obviously related to the peculiarities of the antigenic structure of the capsids, but the capacity to present antigenic determinants in a form recognizable by the immune system may also be a significant though poorly investigated factor (63a).

Physical and chemical properties of virions, for example, their resistance to elevated temperatures, low pH, or intestinal enzymes, may also contribute to the biological properties of a virus.

BRIEF EVOLUTIONARY COMMENTS

Relatedness between Genomes of Different Picornaviruses

Evolution of picornavirus genomes is based on several major mechanisms: (i) accumulation of point mutations and short deletions or insertions resulting in divergence of RNA and protein sequences; (ii) genomic changes resulting in the loss or acquisition of domains (and associated functions) in the polyprotein; and (iii) replacements of extended segments of, or entire, noncoding regions by unrelated structures with remarkable conservation of essential functions.

The amino acid sequences of cognate proteins of picornaviruses exhibit a variable level of conservation, with proteins L (leader), 2A, and VP4 being most variable, and proteins 2C, 3C, and 3D being most conserved (99). The two former proteins appear to share, in different viruses, only their position in the polyprotein, upstream of VP4 and downstream of VP1, respectively. There are no L homologues in entero- and rhinoviruses, and the leader polypeptides of only FMDV and equine rhinoviruses exhibit a protease activity. The proteins nicknamed 2A are represented by a chymotrypsin-like protease in entero- and rhinoviruses, contain a domain with an autocatalytic cleavage activity in cardio- and aphthoviruses, and exhibit no identifiable function in other picornaviruses. All the other picornavirus proteins show clear signs of structural and functional similarity. Unlike other picornaviruses, FMDV has three VPg genes.

According to a plausible model for picornavirus evolution based on the comparative analysis of the protein sequences (99), the picornaviruses are a distinct monophyletic group. At an initial stage of picornavirus evolution, parechovirus and hepatovirus branches were split from a common ancestor, followed by a bifurcation into the progenitors of entero- and rhinoviruses, on the one hand, and cardio- and aphthoviruses, on the other. This model is corroborated by the analysis of nucleotide sequences of noncoding regions. Moreover, it is not unlikely that changes in the UTRs were a major factor contributing to emergence of new genera. Remarkably, the capacity to initiate translation by the cap-independent internal mode (the IRES function) was conserved despite dramatic variability of the IRES structures.

Entero- and rhinovirus 5′ UTRs have a similar 5′-terminal cloverleaf but can be distinguished by the absence, in the latter virus group, of an extended spacer between the IRES and initiator AUG. There is ground to speculate that this spacer was created by a duplication of preexisting genetic material (218), which perhaps occurred concomitantly with the separation of enteroviruses from rhinoviruses. Rhinoviruses differ from enteroviruses not only in the 5′ UTR but also in the 3′ UTR. Further separation of enteroviruses into polio- and coxsackieviruses was also accompanied by changes in the 3′ UTR, which contains one more hairpin domain in the former group (224).

The correlation between taxonomic position and the UTR structure is, however, not always that clear-cut. For example, FMDV (an aphthovirus) and EMCV (a cardiovirus) both contain a poly(C) tract in their 5′ UTRs, whereas TMEV (another cardiovirus) does not. Different scenarios can be envisioned to interpret this fact: for example, either EMCV had acquired the poly(C) tract or TMEV had lost it after the separation of FMDV and cardioviruses.

Relatedness between Genes of Picornaviruses, Genes of Other Viruses, and Cellular Genes

Two major criteria are used for the evaluation of the kinship between genomes of different viruses, the level of amino acid conservation in functionally similar proteins and the overall genome organization (gene order). By using these criteria, a large group of viruses, in addition to the "true" picornaviruses, could be considered picorna-like. The group encompasses animal (caliciviruses), plant (como-, poty-, and sequiviruses), and some insect viruses (99). These viruses encode proteins exhibiting clear signs of sequence conservation and structural similarity to the picornavirus 2C NTP-binding proteins, 3C proteases, and 3D RNA polymerases. In addition, the order of these genes (2C/3C/3D) is the same. It is hypothesized that a "module" containing the three relevant genes was already present in the common progenitor of picorna-like viruses. The genes themselves seem to be extremely old since the characteristic amino acid motifs can be found not only in different unrelated viruses but also among cellular proteins (90, 91, 99).

It is also possible to find putative counterparts of other picornavirus proteins (and by implication, of relevant genes) among proteins of other viruses and cellular proteins. For example, such relatives could be suggested for the FMDV leader protease (93, 100). Functional, though not structural, analogues of VPg exist in some other picorna-like viruses (como-, poty-, and caliciviruses), double-strand RNA-containing viruses (birnaviruses), and DNA-containing viruses (phage φ29, adeno-, and hepadnaviruses).

An intriguing question concerns the origin of picornavirus UTRs. The IRES function is known in other viral (e.g., hepatitis C) and cellular translation templates. However, any obvious structural relatives of picornavirus IRESs have not been found outside this viral family, although there are perhaps some common motifs (158). Likewise, no counterparts of complex oriR of enteroviruses are known, but some similarities between simpler equine rhinovirus oriR and 3'-terminal structures of some other RNA viruses were reported (137).

Thus, no novel function has been invented by Nature for the picornavirus design. The genes encoding ancestors of picornavirus proteins were likely existent long before the appearance of the first picornavirus. Some of these ancient genes (predecessors of 2C, 3C, and 3D) had been assembled into a module, borrowed as such during the picornavirus "creation." Nevertheless, the real source of these genes, let alone some other viral genes as well as UTRs, is not currently even a matter for serious speculations. Fully enigmatic is the process that had led to fusion of the appropriate RNA segments into what is now the picornavirus genome.

CONCLUDING REMARKS

Some Corollaries of the Peculiar cis-Acting Elements

A major feature of the genetic organization of picornaviruses consists of the uncommon (though not unique) cap-independence of their translation templates. This property has significant biological consequences. It may greatly enhance the competitive potential of the viral RNAs relative to the cellular mRNAs. Since a single viral RNA molecule may initiate the infection, a successful competition with an enormous excess of cellular templates is certainly a great advantage.

The principles underlying functions of replicative cis-elements of picornavirus RNAs are not so well understood. We can only state that they appear to be well suited for the selective regulation of positive and negative RNA-strand synthesis. The structure of these elements should also somehow be adapted to the major distinct feature of the picornavirus replicative machinery, its dependence on protein priming.

Some Corollaries of the Peculiar Coding Organization

The existence of a single ORF is also among the most important features of the picornavirus genetic makeup. Single initiation and termination sites of translation dictate that all of the virus-specific proteins should be generated in equimolar quantities. Thus, to produce a set of the capsid proteins required for one virion (that is, 60 copies of each), an equal number of catalytic molecules of, say, $2A^{pro}$, $3C^{pro}$, or $3D^{pol}$ should be produced. Although this may appear a rather "wasteful" design, a seemingly high excess of catalytic proteins may have some functional justifications. At least certain cleavages in the polyprotein precursor occur in cis, and hence processing of each polyprotein molecule requires the presence of a built-in protease(s). It is not known whether efficient recycling of $3D^{pol}$ is in place. If it is not (for example, because 3D precursor is obligatorily required also), generation of a fresh molecule of the polymerase during each round of template translation is also a must. Not infrequently, picornaviral nonstructural proteins are functioning as oligomers, demanding an additional supply of these species.

In more general terms, it may be questioned whether material and energy savings are major selective factors in viral evolution.

Built-in Quality Controls

The picornavirus genome not merely encodes functions required for the generation of progeny virions, but it also possesses inherent capacity to coordinate these functions in an orderly and "rational" fashion. The genetic organization of picornaviruses also appears to provide several kinds of "quality controls." The viral reproduction system is permanently checking whether only intact RNA molecules are used for replication and encapsidation. Indeed, the replicative templates are inspected for the presence of their termini, oriR and oriL. These termini not only serve as recognition elements for the initiation of negative and positive RNA strands, respectively, but in addition, they may participate in more complex controls. As already mentioned, binding of appropriate host and viral proteins to oriL may affect initiation of the ($-$) strand at the oriR as well as initiation of translation. The internal replicative cis-signals also serve as quality control tools. The gross alterations in the coding region (such as changes in the reading frame, appearance of internal stop codons, deletions in the region encoding replicative proteins, etc.) are checked by coupling translation and replication and possibly by the requirement of certain replicative proteins in cis. Moreover, it is hypothesized that nucleotide misincorporation may promote RNA recombination, which helps get rid of adverse mutations and thereby serves as a substitute for the absent proofreading activity of the viral RNA polymerase. Finally, only nascent (and hence less likely having undergone degradation) RNA molecules are efficiently encapsidated.

Some Unsolved Problems

A major task in understanding genome functions left for the new century is a clear explanation of viral phenotypes. Why, for example, does poliovirus elicit acute damage to anterior horns of the spinal cord, whereas some TMEV strains trigger a chronic demyelinating disease and not vice versa? Some important steps to solve such problems have already been done, but the major breakthroughs are yet to come.

Despite spectacular achievements in the molecular biology of the picornavirus genome, as evidenced by this volume, a coherent and detailed picture of how these genomes are functioning in the intact cell to efficiently produce viral progeny is not available. Certainly, there are big gaps in our comprehension of the capacity of picornavirus genomes to counteract various defensive measures on the part of host cells or organisms.

The global eradication of poliomyelitis is on the current agenda. Other picornavirus diseases may follow this example. The success of these programs will be accompanied by imminent prohibition (or at least, severe restriction) of using relevant viruses (e.g., poliovirus, undoubtedly the best-studied picornavirus) as experimental models. We certainly should not be too lazy.

Current work in the author's laboratory is supported by grants from INTAS, The Ludwig Institute for Cancer Research, Russian Foundation for Basic Research, and the National Multiple Sclerosis Society (United States).

NOTE ADDED IN PROOF

Notable among many recent developments are data suggesting that 5′- and 3′-terminal sequences of picornavirus RNA may bind to each other via protein bridges and that this noncovalent circularization may be important for regulation of translation and replication of the viral genome (24a, 113a). Remarkably, the existence of circular molecules of double-stranded encephalomyocarditis virus RNA, which reversibly linearized upon partial denaturation, was reported long ago (3a, 240a).

Identification of the internal *cis*-acting replicative element CRE as the template for VPg uridylylation (205a, 236a) is another significant step forward.

REFERENCES

1. **Agol, V. I.** 1991. The 5′-untranslated region of picornaviral genomes. *Adv. Virus Res.* **40**:103–180.
2. **Agol, V. I., G. A. Belov, K. Bienz, D. Egger, M. S. Kolesnikova, N. T. Raikhlin, L. I. Romanova, E. A. Smirnova, and E. A. Tolskaya.** 1998. Two types of death of poliovirus-infected cells: caspase involvement in the apoptosis but not cytopathic effect. *Virology* **252**:342–353.
3. **Agol, V. I., G. A. Belov, K. Bienz, D. Egger, M. S. Kolesnikova, L. I. Romanova, L. V. Sladkova, and E. A. Tolskaya.** 2000. Competing death programs in poliovirus-infected cells: commitment switch in the middle of the infectious cycle. *J. Virol.* **74**:5534–5541.
3a. **Agol, V. I., Y. F. Drygin, L. I. Romanova, and A. A. Bogdanov.** 1970. Circular structures in preparations of the replicative form of encephalomyocarditis virus RNA. *FEBS Lett.* **8**:13–16.
4. **Agol, V. I., A. V. Paul, and E. Wimmer.** 1999. Paradoxes of the replication of picornaviral genomes. *Virus Res.* **62**:129–147.
5. **Agol, V. I., E. V. Pilipenko, and O. R. Slobodskaya.** 1996. Modification of translation control elements as a new approach to design of attenuated picornavirus strains. *J. Biotech.* **44**:119–128.
6. **Aldabe, R., R. Barco, and L. Carrasco.** 1996. Membrane permeabilization by poliovirus proteins 2B and 2BC. *J. Virol.* **71**:6214–6217.
7. **Aldabe, R., and L. Carrasco.** 1995. Induction of membrane proliferation by poliovirus proteins 2C and 2BC. *Biochem. Biophys. Res. Commun.* **206**:64–76.
8. **Alexander, H. E., G. Koch, L. M. Mountain, K. Sprunt, and O. Van Damme.** 1958. Infectivity of ribonucleic acid of poliovirus on HeLa cell monolayers. *Virology* **5**:172–173.
9. **Almond, J. W.** 1987. The attenuation of poliovirus virulence. *Annu. Rev. Microbiol.* **41**:153–180.
10. **Ambros, V., and D. Baltimore.** 1978. Protein is linked to the 5′ end of poliovirus RNA by a phosphodiester linkage to tyrosine. *J. Biol. Chem.* **253**:5263–5266.
11. **Ambros, V., R. F. Pettersson, and D. Baltimore.** 1978. An enzymatic activity in uninfected cells that cleaves the linkage between poliovirion RNA and the 5′ terminal protein. *Cell* **15**:1439–1446.
12. **Anderson, D. A., and B. C. Ross.** 1990. Morphogenesis of hepatitis A virus: isolation and characterization of subviral particles. *J. Virol.* **64**:5284–5289.
13. **Andino, R., G. E. Rieckhof, P. L. Achacoso, and D. Baltimore.** 1993. Poliovirus RNA synthesis utilizes an RNP complex formed around the 5′-end of viral RNA. *EMBO J.* **12**:3587–3598.
14. **Andino, R., G. E. Rieckhof, and D. Baltimore.** 1990. A functional ribonucleoprotein complex forms around the 5′ end of poliovirus RNA. *Cell* **63**:369–380.
15. **Ansardi, D. C., D. C. Porter, M. J. Anderson, and C. D. Morrow.** 1996. Poliovirus assembly and encapsidation of genomic RNA. *Adv. Virus Res.* **46**:1–68.
16. **Arnold, E., M. Luo, G. Vriend, M. G. Rossmann, A. C. Palmenberg, G. D. Parks, M. J. H. Nicklin, and E. Wimmer.** 1987. Implications of the picornavirus capsid structure for polyprotein processing. *Proc. Natl. Acad. Sci. USA* **84**:21–25.
17. **Badorff, C., G. H. Lee, B. J. Lamphear, M. E. Martone, K. P. Campbell, R. E. Rhoads, and K. U. Knowlton.** 1999. Enteroviral protease 2A cleaves dystrophin: evidence of cytoskeletal disruption in an acquired cardiomyopathy. *Nat. Med.* **5**:320–326.
18. **Baltimore, D., and M. Girard.** 1966. An intermediate in the synthesis of poliovirus RNA. *Proc. Natl. Acad. Sci. USA* **56**:741–748.
19. **Banerjee, R., A. Echeverri, and A. Dasgupta.** 1997. Poliovirus-encoded 2C polypeptide specifically binds to the 3′ terminal sequences of viral negative-strand RNA. *J. Virol.* **71**:9570–9578.
20. **Barclay, W., Q. Li, G. Hutchinson, D. Moon, A. Richardson, N. Percy, J. W. Almond, and D. Evans.** 1998. Encapsidation studies of poliovirus subgenomic replicons. *J. Gen Virol.* **79**:1725–1734.
21. **Barco, A., and L. Carrasco.** 1995. A human virus protein, poliovirus protein 2BC, induces membrane proliferation and blocks the exocytic pathway in the yeast *Saccharomyces cerevisiae. EMBO J.* **14**:3349–3364.
22. **Barco, A., E. Feduchi, and L. Carrasco.** 2000. Poliovirus protease 3C(pro) kills cells by apoptosis. *Virology* **266**:352–360.
23. **Barco, A., E. Feduchi, and L. Carrasco.** 2000. A stable HeLa cell line that inducibly expresses poliovirus 2A(pro): effects on cellular and viral gene expression. *J. Virol.* **74**:2383–2392.
24. **Barton, D. J., B. J. Morasco, and J. B. Flanegan.** 1999. Translating ribosomes inhibit poliovirus negative-strand RNA synthesis. *J. Virol.* **73**:10104–10112.
24a. **Barton, D. J., B. J. O'Donnell, and J. B. Flanegan.** 2001. 5′ Cloverleaf in poliovirus RNA is a *cis*-acting replication element required for negative-strand synthesis. *EMBO J.* **20**:1439–1448.
25. **Basavappa, R., R. Syed, O. Flore, J. P. Icenogle, D. J. Filman, and J. M. Hogle.** 1994. Role and mechanism of the maturation cleavage of VP0 in poliovirus assembly: structure of the empty capsid assembly intermediate at 2.9 A resolution. *Protein Sci.* **3**:1651–1669.
26. **Beck, E., S. Forss, K. Strebel, R. Cattaneo, and G. Feil.** 1983. Structure of the FMDV translation initiation site

and of the structural proteins. *Nucleic Acids Res.* **11**:7873–7885.

27. **Belnap, D. M., D. J. Filman, B. L. Trus, N. Cheng, F. P. Booy, J. F. Conway, S. Curry, C. N. Hiremath, S. K. Tsang, A. C. Steven, and J. M. Hogle.** 2000. Molecular tectonic model of virus structural transitions: the putative cell entry states of poliovirus. *J. Virol.* **74**:1342–1354.

28. **Belov, G. A., A. G. Evstafieva, Y. P. Rubtsov, O. Mikitas, A. B. Vartapetian, and V. I. Agol.** 2000. Early alteration of nucleocytoplasmic traffic induced by some RNA viruses. *Virology* **275**:244–248.

29. **Belsham, G. J., and N. Sonenberg.** 1966. RNA-protein interactions in regulation of picornavirus RNA translation. *Microbiol. Rev.* **60**:499–511.

30. **Belsham, G. J., and N. Sonenberg.** 2000. Picornavirus RNA translation: roles for cellular proteins. *Trends Microbiol.* **8**:330–335.

31. **Benton, P. A., D. J. Barrett, R. L. Matts, and R. E. Lloyd.** 1996. The outcome of poliovirus infections in K562 cells is cytolytic rather than persistent after hemin-induced differentiation. *J. Virol.* **70**:5525–5532.

32. **Bernstein, H. D., N. Sonenberg, and D. Baltimore.** 1985. Poliovirus mutant that does not selectively inhibit host cell protein synthesis. *Mol. Cell. Biol.* **5**:2913–2923.

33. **Bienz, K., D. Egger, and L. Pasamontes.** 1987. Association of polioviral proteins of the P2 genomic region with the viral replication complex and virus-induced membrane synthesis as visualized by electron microscopic immunocytochemistry and autoradiography. *Virology* **160**:220–226.

34. **Bishop, N. E., and D. A. Anderson.** 1993. RNA-dependent cleavage of VP0 capsid protein in provirions of hepatitis A virus. *Virology* **197**:616–623.

35. **Black, T. L., G. N. Barber, and M. G. Katze.** 1993. Degradation of the interferon-induced 68,000-M(r) protein kinase by poliovirus requires RNA. *J. Virol.* **67**:791–800.

36. **Blank, C. A., D. A. Anderson, M. Beard, and S. M. Lemon.** 2000. Infection of polarized cultures of human intestinal epithelial cells with hepatitis A virus: vectorial release of progeny virions through apical cellular membranes. *J. Virol.* **74**:6476–6484.

37. **Blyn, L. B., K. M. Swiderek, O. Richards, D. C. Stahl, B. L. Semler, and E. Ehrenfeld.** 1996. Poly(rC) binding protein 2 binds to stem-loop IV of the poliovirus RNA 5′ noncoding region: identification by automated liquid chromatography-tandem mass spectrometry. *Proc. Natl. Acad. Sci. USA* **93**:11115–11120.

38. **Blyn, L. B., J. S. Towner, B. L. Semler, and E. Ehrenfeld.** 1997. Requirement of poly(rC) binding protein 2 for translation of poliovirus RNA. *J. Virol.* **71**:6243–6246.

39. **Bolten, R., D. Egger, R. Gosert, G. Schaub, L. Landmann, and K. Bienz.** 1998. Intracellular localization of poliovirus plus- and minus-strand RNA visualized by strand-specific fluorescent in situ hybridization. *J. Virol.* **72**:8578–8585.

40. **Bonneau, A. M., A. Darveau, and N. Sonenberg.** 1985. Effect of viral infection on host protein synthesis and mRNA association with the cytoplasmic cytoskeletal structure. *J. Cell Biol.* **100**:1209–1218.

41. **Borman, A. M., F. G. Deliat, and K. M. Kean.** 1994. Sequences within the poliovirus internal ribosome entry segment control viral RNA synthesis. *EMBO J.* **13**:3149–3157.

42. **Borman, A. M., P. Le Mercier, M. Girard, and K. M. Kean.** 1997. Comparison of picornaviral IRES-driven internal initiation of translation in cultured cells of different origins. *Nucleic Acids Res.* **25**:925–932.

43. **Bovee, M. L., W. E. Marissen, M. Zamora, and R. E. Lloyd.** 1998. The predominant eIF4G-specific cleavage activity in poliovirus-infected HeLa cells is distinct from 2A protease. *Virology* **245**:229–240.

44. **Brack, K., W. Frings, A. Dotzauer, and A. Vallbracht.** 1998. A cytopathogenic, apoptosis-inducing variant of hepatitis A virus. *J. Virol.* **72**:3370–3376.

45. **Brown, E. A., S. P. Day, R. W. Jansen, and S. M. Lemon.** 1991. The 5′ nontranslated region of hepatitis A virus RNA: secondary structure and elements required for translation in vitro. *J. Virol.* **65**:5828–5838.

46. **Brown, F., R. F. Sellers, and D. L. Stewart.** 1958. Infectivity of ribonucleic acid from mice and tissue culture infected with the virus of foot-and-mouth disease. *Nature* **182**:535–536.

47. **Carrasco, L.** 1995. Modification of membrane permeability by animal viruses. *Adv. Virus Res.* **45**:61–112.

48. **Chaplin, P. J., E. B. Camon, B. Villarreal-Ramos, M. Flint, M. D. Ryan, and R. A. Collins.** 1999. Production of interleukin-12 as a self-processing 2A polypeptide. *J. Interferon Cytokine Res.* **19**:235–241.

49. **Chen, H.-H., W.-P. Kong, L. Zhang, P. L. Ward, and R. Roos.** 1995. A picornaviral protein synthesized out of frame with the polyprotein plays a key role in a virus-induced immune-mediate demyelinating disease. *Nat. Med.* **1**:927–931.

50. **Cho, M. W., N. L. Teterina, D. Egger, K. Bienz, and E. Ehrenfeld.** 1994. Membrane rearrangement and vesicle induction by recombinant poliovirus 2C and 2BC in human cells. *Virology* **202**:129–145.

51. **Clark, M. E., T. Hammerle, E. Wimmer, and A. Dasgupta.** 1991. Poliovirus proteinase 3C converts an active form of transcription factor IIIC to an inactive form: a mechanism for inhibition of host cell polymerase III transcription by poliovirus. *EMBO J.* **10**:2941–2947.

52. **Clark, M. E., P. M. Lieberman, A. J. Berk, and A. Dasgupta.** 1993. Direct cleavage of human TATA-binding protein by poliovirus protease 3C in vivo and in vitro. *Mol. Cell. Biol.* **2**:1232–1237.

53. **Clarke, B. E., A. L. Brown, K. M. Currey, S. E. Newton, D. J. Rowlands, and A. R. Carroll.** 1987. Potential secondary and tertiary structure in the genomic RNA of foot and mouth disease virus. *Nucleic Acids Res.* **15**:7067–7079.

54. **Clarke, B. E., D. V. Sangar, J. N. Burroughs, S. E. Newton, A. R. Caroll, and D. J. Rowlands.** 1985. Two initiation sites for foot-and-mouth disease virus polyprotein in vivo. *J. Gen. Virol.* **66**:2615–2626.

55. **Coller, B. A., N. M. Chapman, M. A. Beck, M. A. Pallansch, C. J. Gauntt, and S. M. Tracy.** 1990. Echovirus 22 is an atypical enterovirus. *J. Virol.* **64**:2692–2701.

56. **Colter, J. S., H. H. Bird, and R. A. Brown.** 1957. Infectivity of ribonucleic acid from Ehrlich ascites tumour cells infected with Mengo encephalitis. *Nature* **179**:859–860.

57. **Colter, J. S., H. H. Bird, A. W. Moyer, and R. A. Brown.** 1957. Infectivity of ribonucleic acid isolated from virus infected tissues. *Virology* **4**:522–532.

58. **Cromeans, T., M. D. Sobsey, and H. A. Fields.** 1987. Development of a plaque assay for a cytopathic, rapidly replicating isolate of hepatitis A virus. *J. Med. Virol.* **22**:45–56.

59. **Cuconati, A., W. Xiang, F. Lahser, T. Pfister, and E. Wimmer.** 1998. A protein linkage map of the P2 nonstructural proteins of poliovirus. *J. Virol.* **72**:1297–1307.

60. **Cui, T., and A. G. Porter.** 1995. Localization of binding site for encephalomyocarditis virus RNA polymerase in the 3′-noncoding region of the viral RNA. *Nucleic Acids Res.* **23**:377–382.

61. **Cui, T., S. Sankar, and A. G. Porter.** 1993. Binding of encephalomyocarditis virus RNA polymerase to the 3′-

noncoding region of the viral RNA is specific and requires the 3′-poly(A) tail. *J. Biol. Chem.* **268:**26093–26098.
62. **Davies, M., and R. J. Kaufmann.** 1992. The sequence context of the initiation codon in the encephalomyocarditis virus leader modulated efficiency of internal translation initiation. *J. Virol.* **66:**1924–1932.
63. **De Chastonay, J., and G. Siegl.** 1987. Replicative events in hepatitis A virus-infected MRC-5 cells. *Virology* **157:**268–275.
63a.**Deitz, S. B., D. A. Dodd, S. Cooper, P. Parham, and K. Kirkegaard.** 2000. MHC I-dependent antigen presentation is inhibited by poliovirus protein 3A. *Proc. Natl. Acad. Sci. USA* **97:**13790–13795.
64. **Devaney, M. A., V. N. Vakharia, R. E. Lloyd, E. Ehrenfeld, and M. J. Grubman.** 1988. Leader protein of foot-and-mouth disease virus is required for cleavage of the p220 component of the cap-binding protein complex. *J. Virol.* **62:**4407–4409.
65. **Dildine, S. L., and B. L. Semler.** 1989. The deletion of 41 proximal nucleotides reverts a poliovirus mutant containing a temperature-sensitive lesion in the 5′ noncoding region of genomic RNA. *J. Virol.* **63:**847–862.
65a.**Dodd, D. A., T. H. Gidding, Jr., and K. Kirkegaard.** 2001. Poliovirus 3A protein limits interkeukin-6 (IL-6), IL-8, and beta interferon secretion during viral infection. *J. Virol.* **75:**8158–8165.
66. **Doedens, J. R., and K. Kirkegaard.** 1995. Inhibition of cellular protein secretion by poliovirus proteins 2B and 3A. *EMBO J.* **14:**894–907.
67. **Doedens, J. R., Giddings, T. H., Jr., and K. Kirkegaard.** 1997. Inhibition of endoplasmic reticulum-to-Golgi traffic by poliovirus protein 3A: genetic and ultrastructural analysis. *J. Virol.* **71:**9054–9064.
68. **Donnelly, M. L., D. Gani, M. Flint, S. Monaghan, and M. D. Ryan.** 1997. The cleavage activities of aphthovirus and cardiovirus 2A proteins. *J. Gen. Virol.* **78:**13–21.
69. **Duke, G. M., J. E. Osorio, and A. C. Palmenberg.** 1990. Attenuation of Mengo virus through genetic engineering of the 5′ noncoding poly(C) tract. *Nature* **343:**474–476.
70. **Duke, G. M., M. A. Hoffman, and A. C. Palmenberg.** 1992. Sequence and structural elements that contribute to efficient encephalomyocarditis virus RNA translation. *J. Virol.* **66:**1602–1609.
71. **Ehrenfeld, E.** 1984. Picornavirus inhibition of host cell protein synthesis. *Comp. Virol.* **19:**177–221.
72. **Escarmis, C., J. Dopazo, M. Davila, E. L. Palma, and E. Domingo.** 1995. Large deletions in the 5′-untranslated region of foot-and-mouth disease virus of serotype C. *Virus Res.* **35:**155–167.
73. **Evans, D. J., and J. W. Almond.** 1998. Cell receptors for picornaviruses as determinants of cell tropism and pathogenesis. *Trends Microbiol.* **6:**198–202.
74. **Falk, M. M., F. Sobrino, and E. Beck.** 1992. VPg gene amplification correlates with infective particle formation in foot-and-mouth disease virus. *J. Virol.* **66:**2251–2260.
75. **Fernandez-Munoz, R., and J. E. Darnell.** 1976. Structural difference between the 5′ termini of viral and cellular mRNA in poliovirus-infected cells: possible basis for the inhibition of host protein synthesis. *J. Virol.* **18:**719–726.
76. **Flanegan, J. B., and D. Baltimore.** 1977. Poliovirus-specific primer-dependent RNA polymerase able to copy poly(A). *Proc. Natl. Acad. Sci. USA* **74:**3677–3680.
77. **Flanegan, J. B., R. F. Pettersson, V. Ambros, N. J. Hewlett, and D. Baltimore.** 1977. Covalent linkage of a protein to a defined nucleotide sequence at the 5′-terminus of virion and replicative intermediate RNAs of poliovirus. *Proc. Natl. Acad. Sci. USA* **74:**961–965.
78. **Forss, S., and H. Schaller.** 1982. A tandem repeat gene in a picornavirus. *Nucleic Acids Res.* **10:**6441–6450.
79. **Gamarnik, A. V., and R. Andino.** 1997. Two functional complexes formed by KH domain containing proteins with the 5′ noncoding region of poliovirus RNA. *RNA* **3:**882–892.
80. **Gamarnik, A. V., and R. Andino.** 1998. Switch from translation to RNA replication in a positive-stranded RNA virus. *Genes Dev.* **12:**2293–2304.
81. **Gamarnik, A. V., and R. Andino.** 2000. Interactions of viral protein 3CD and poly(rC) binding protein with the 5′ untranslated region of the poliovirus genome. *J. Virol.* **74:**2219–2226.
82. **Gavrilin, G. V., E. A. Cherkasova, G. Y. Lipskaya, O. M. Kew, and V. I. Agol.** 2000. Evolution of circulating wild poliovirus and of vaccine-derived poliovirus in an immunodeficient patient: a unifying model. *J. Virol.* **74:**7381–7390.
83. **Ghadge, G. D., L. Ma, S. Sato, J. Kim, and R. P. Roos.** 1998. A protein critical for a Theiler's virus-induced immune system-mediated demyelinating disease has a cell type-specific antiapoptotic effect and a key role in virus persistence. *J. Virol.* **72:**8605–8612.
84. **Ghazi, F., P. J. Hughes, T. Hyypia, and G. Stanway.** 1998. Molecular analysis of human parechovirus type 2 (formerly echovirus 23). *J. Gen. Virol.* **79:**2641–2650.
85. **Gingras, A. C., Y. Svitkin, G. J. Belsham, A. Pause, and N. Sonenberg.** 1996. Activation of the translational suppressor 4E-BP1 following infection with encephalomyocarditis virus and poliovirus. *Proc. Natl. Acad. Sci. USA* **93:**5578–5583.
86. **Gladding, R. L., A. L. Haas, D. L. Gronros, and T. G. Lawson.** 1997. Evaluation of the susceptibility of the 3C proteases of hepatitis A virus and poliovirus to degradation by the ubiquitin-mediated proteolytic system. *Biochem. Biophys. Res. Commun.* **238:**119–125.
87. **Gmyl, A. P., E. V. Pilipenko, S. V. Maslova, G. A. Belov, and V. I. Agol.** 1993. Functional and genetic plasticities of the poliovirus genome: quasi-infectious RNAs modified in the 5′-untranslated region yield a variety of pseudorevertants. *J. Virol.* **67:**6309–6316.
88. **Goldstaub, D., A. Gradi, Z. Bercovitch, Z. Grossman, Y. Nophar, S. Luria, N. Sonenberg, and C. Kahana.** 2000. Poliovirus 2A protease induces apoptotic cell death. *Mol. Cell. Biol.* **20:**1271–1277.
89. **Goodfellow, I., Y. Chaudhry, A. Richardson, J. Meredith, J. W. Almond, W. Barclay, and D. J. Evans.** 2000. Identification of a cis-acting replication element within the poliovirus coding region. *J. Virol.* **74:**4590–4600.
90. **Gorbalenya, A. E.** 1995. Origin of RNA viral genomes: approaching the problem by comparative sequence analysis, p. 49–66. *In* A. J. Gibbs, C. H. Calisher, and F. Garcia-Arenal (ed.), *Molecular Basis of Virus Evolution*. Cambridge University Press, Cambridge, United Kingdom.
91. **Gorbalenya, A. E., and E. V. Koonin.** 1993. Helicases: amino acid sequence comparisons and structure-function relationships. *Curr. Opin. Struct. Biol.* **3:**419–429.
92. **Gorbalenya, A. E., K. M. Chumakov, and V. I. Agol.** 1978. RNA-binding properties of nonstructural polypeptide G of encephalomyocarditis virus. *Virology* **88:**183–185.
93. **Gorbalenya, A. E., and E. J. Snyder.** 1996. Viral cysteine proteinases. *Persp. Drug. Discov. Design* **6:**65–86.
94. **Gorbalenya, A. E., Y. V. Svitkin, Y. A. Kazachkov, and V. I. Agol.** 1979. Encephalomyocarditis virus-specific polypeptide p22 is involved in the processing of the viral precursor polypeptides. *FEBS Lett.* **108:**1–5.
95. **Gosert, R., K. H. Chang, R. Rijnbrand, M. Yi, D. V. Sangar, and S. M. Lemon.** 2000. Transient expression of cellular polypyrimidine-tract binding protein stimulates

cap-independent translation directed by both picornaviral and flaviviral internal ribosome entry sites in vivo. *Mol. Cell. Biol.* **20**:1583–1595.

96. Gosert, R., D. Egger, and K. Bienz. 2000. A cytopathic and a cell culture adapted hepatitis A virus strain differ in cell killing but not in intracellular membrane rearrangements. *Virology* **266**:157–169.
97. Gradi, A., Y. V. Svitkin, H. Imataka, and N. Sonenberg. 1998. Proteolysis of human eukaryotic translation initiation factor eIF4GII, but not eIF4GI coincides with the shutoff of host protein synthesis after poliovirus infection. *Proc. Natl. Acad. Sci. USA* **95**:11089–11094.
98. Graff, J., J. Cha, B. Lawrence, and E. Ehrenfeld. 1998. Interaction of poly(rC) binding protein 2 with the 5' noncoding region of hepatitis A virus RNA and its effects on translation. *J. Virol.* **72**:9668–9675.
99. Gromeier, M., E. Wimmer, and A. E. Gorbalenya. 1999. Genetics, pathogenesis and evolution of picornaviruses, p. 287–343. *In* E. Domingo, R. G. Webster, and J. J. Holland (ed.), *Origin and Evolution of Viruses.* Academic Press, San Diego, Calif.
100. Guarne, A., J. Tormo, R. Kirchweger, D. Pfistermueller, I. Fita, and T. Skern. 1998. Structure of the foot-and-mouth disease virus leader protease: a papain-like fold adapted for self-processing and eIF4G recognition. *EMBO J.* **17**:7469–7479.
101. Guinea, R., and L. Carrasco. 1990. Phospholipid biosynthesis and poliovirus genome replication, two coupled phenomena. *EMBO J.* **9**:2011–2016.
101a. Gustin, K. E., and P. Sarnow. 2001. Effects of poliovirus infection on nucleocytoplasmic trafficking and nuclear pore complex composition. *EMBO J.* **20**:240–249.
102. Haghighat, A., Y. V. Svitkin, I. Novoa, E. Kuechler, T. Skern, and N. Sonenberg. 1996. The eF4G-eIF4E complex is the target for direct cleavage by the rhinovirus 2A proteinase. *J. Virol.* **70**:8444–8450.
103. Haller, A. A., S. R. Stewart, and B. L. Semler. 1996. Attenuation stem-loop lesions in the 5' noncoding region of poliovirus RNA: neuronal-specific translation defects. *J. Virol.* **70**:1467–1474.
104. Hambidge, S. J., and P. Sarnow. 1992. Translational enhancement of the poliovirus 5' noncoding region mediated by virus-encoded polypeptide 2A. *Proc. Natl. Acad. Sci. USA* **89**:10272–10276.
105. Hansen, J. L., A. M. Long, and S. C. Schultz. 1997. Structure of the RNA-dependent RNA polymerase of poliovirus. *Structure* **5**:1109–1122.
106. Harber, J. J., J. Bradley, C. W. Anderson, and E. Wimmer. 1991. Catalysis of poliovirus VP0 maturation cleavage is not mediated by serine 10 of VP2. *J. Virol.* **65**:326–334.
107. Harmon, S. A., S. U. Emerson, Y. K. Huang, D. F. Summers, and E. Ehrenfeld. 1995. Hepatitis A viruses with deletions in the 2A gene are infectious in cultured cells and marmosets. *J. Virol.* **69**:5576–5581.
108. Harris, K. S., W. Xiang, L. Alexander, W. S. Lane, A. V. Paul, and E. Wimmer. 1994. Interaction of the poliovirus polypeptide 3CD[pro] with the 5' and 3' termini of the poliovirus genome: identification of viral and cellular cofactors needed for efficient binding. *J. Biol. Chem.* **269**:27004–27014.
109. Hellen, C. U., C. K. Lee, and E. Wimmer. 1992. Determinants of substrate recognition by poliovirus 2A proteinase. *J. Virol.* **66**:3330–3338.
110. Hellen, C. U., T. V. Pestova, M. Literest, and E. Wimmer. 1994. The cellular polypeptide p57 (pyrimidine tract-binding protein) binds to multiple sites in the poliovirus 5' nontranslated region. *J. Virol.* **68**:941–950.
111. Hellen, C. U., and E. Wimmer. 1992. Maturation of poliovirus proteins. *Virology* **187**:391–397.
112. Hellen, C. U., G. W. Witherell, M. Schmid, S. H. Shin, T. V. Pestova, A. Gil, and E. Wimmer. 1993. A cytoplasmic 57-kDa protein that is required for translation of picornavirus RNA by internal ribosomal entry is identical to the nuclear pyrimidine tract-binding protein. *Proc. Natl. Acad. Sci. USA* **90**:7642–7646.
113. Henke, A., H. Launhardt, K. Klement, A. Stelzner, R. Zell, and T. Munder. 2000. Apoptosis in coxsackievirus B3-caused diseases: interaction between the capsid protein VP2 and the proapoptotic protein siva. *J. Virol.* **74**:4284–4290.
113a. Herold, J., and R. Andino. 2001. Poliovirus RNA replication requires genome circularization through a protein-protein bridge. *Mol. Cell* **7**:581–591.
114. Hewlett, M. J., J. K. Rose, and D. Baltimore. 1976. 5'-terminal structure of poliovirus polyribosomal RNA is pUp. *Proc. Natl. Acad. Sci. USA* **73**:327–330.
115. Holland, J. J., and C. E. Cords. 1964. Maturation of poliovirus RNA with capsid protein coded by heterologous enteroviruses. *Proc. Natl. Acad. Sci. USA* **60**:1015–1022.
116. Holland, J. J., and E. D. Kiehn. 1968. Specific cleavage of viral proteins as steps in the synthesis and maturation of enteroviruses. *Proc. Natl. Acad. Sci. USA* **60**:1015–1022.
117. Holland, J. J., L. C. McLaren, B. H. Hoyer, and J. T. Syverton. 1960. Enteroviral ribonucleic acid. *J. Exp. Med.* **112**:841–864.
118. Humphries, S., F. Knauert, and E. Ehrenfeld. 1979. Capsid protein precursor is one of two initiated products of translation of poliovirus RNA in vitro. *J. Virol.* **30**:481–488.
119. Hunt, S. L., J. J. Hsuan, N. Totty, and R. J. Jackson. 1999. unr, a cellular cytoplasmic RNA-binding protein with five cold-shock domains, is required for internal initiation of translation of human rhinovirus RNA. *Genes Dev.* **13**:437–448.
120. Huppert, J., and F. K. Sanders. 1957. An infective "ribonucleic acid" component from tumour cells infected with encephalomyocarditis virus. *Nature* **182**:515–517.
121. Iizuka, N., M. Kohara, K. Hagino-Yamagishi, S. Abe, T. Komatsu, K. Tago, M. Arita, and A. Nomoto. 1989. Construction of less neurovirulent polioviruses by introducing deletions into the 5' noncoding sequence of the genome. *J. Virol.* **63**:5354–5363.
122. Irurzun, A., L. Perez, and L. Carrasco. 1993. Enhancement of phospholipase activity during poliovirus infection. *J. Gen. Virol.* **74**:1063–1071.
123. Ishii, T., K. Shiroki, A. Iwai, and A. Nomoto. 1999. Identification of a new element for RNA replication within the internal ribosome entry site of poliovirus RNA. *J. Gen. Virol.* **80**:917–920.
124. Ishii, T., K. Shiroki, D. H. Hong, T. Aoki, Y. Ohta, S. Abe, S. Hashizume, and A. Nomoto. 1998. A new internal ribosomal entry site 5' boundary is required for poliovirus translation initiation in a mouse system. *J. Virol.* **72**:2398–2405.
125. Jacobson, M. F., and D. Baltimore. 1968. Polypeptide cleavages in the formation of poliovirus proteins. *Proc. Natl. Acad. Sci. USA* **61**:77–84.
126. Jang, S. K., M. V. Davies, R. J. Kaufman, and E. Wimmer. 1989. Initiation of protein synthesis by internal entry of ribosomes into the 5' nontranslated region of encephalomyocarditis virus RNA in vivo. *J. Virol.* **63**:1651–1660.
127. Jang, S. K., H. Krausslich, M. J. H. Nicklin, G. M. Duke, A. S. Palmenberg, and E. Wimmer. 1988. A segment of the 5' nontranslated region of encephalomyocarditis virus RNA directs internal entry of ribosomes during in vitro translation. *J. Virol.* **62**:2636–2643.

128. Jang, S. K., T. V. Pestova, C. U. Hellen, G. W. Witherell, and E. Wimmer. 1990. Cap-independent translation of picornavirus RNAs: structure and function of the internal ribosomal entry site. *Enzyme* **44**:292–309.
129. Jelachich, M. L., C. Bramlage, and H. L. Lipton. 1999. Differentiation of M1 myeloid precursor cells into macrophages results in binding and infection by Theiler's murine encephalomyelitis virus and apoptosis. *J. Virol.* **73**:3227–3235.
130. Jelachich, M. L., and H. L. Lipton. 1996. Theiler's murine encephalomyelitis virus kills restrictive but not permissive cells by apoptosis. *J. Virol.* **70**:6856–6861.
131. Jia, Q., S. Ohka, K. Iwasaki, K. Tohyama, and A. Nomoto. 1999. Isolation and molecular characterization of a poliovirus type 1 mutant that replicates in the spinal cords of mice. *J. Virol.* **73**:6041–6047.
132. Jia, X., M. Van Eden, M. G. Busch, E. Ehrenfeld, and D. F. Summers. 1998. trans-Encapsidation of a poliovirus replicon by different picornavirus capsid proteins. *J. Virol.* **72**:7972–7977.
133. Joachims, M., K. S. Harris, and D. Etchison. 1995. Poliovirus 3C mediated cleavage of microtubule-associated protein 4. *Virology* **211**:451–461.
134. Joachims, M., P. S. Van Breugel, and R. E. Lloyd. 1999. Cleavage of poly(A)-binding protein by enterovirus proteases concurrent with inhibition of translation in vitro. *J. Virol.* **73**:718–727.
135. Johansen, L. K., and C. D. Morrow. 2000. The RNA encompassing the internal ribosome entry site in the poliovirus 5′ nontranslated region enhances the encapsidation of genomic RNA. *Virology* **273**:391–399.
136. Johnson, K. L., and P. Sarnow. 1995. Viral RNA synthesis, p. 95–112. In H. A. Rotbart (ed.), *Human Enterovirus Infections*. American Society for Microbiology, Washington, D.C.
137. Jonassen, C. M., T. O. Jonassen, and B. Grinde. 1998. A common RNA motif in the 3′ end of the genomes of astroviruses, avian infectious bronchitis virus and an equine rhinovirus. *J. Gen. Virol.* **79**:715–718.
138. Jore, J., B. De Geus, R. J. Jackson, P. H. Pouwels, and B. E. Enger-Valk. 1988. Poliovirus protein 3CD is the active protease for processing of the precursor protein P1 in vitro. *J. Gen. Virol.* **69**:1627–1636.
139. Jun, H. S., Y. Kang, H. S. Yoon, K. H. Kim, A. L. Notkins, and J. W. Yoon. 1998. Determination of encephalomyocarditis viral diabetogenicity by a putative binding site of the viral capsid protein. *Diabetes* **47**:576–582.
140. Kaminski, A., M. T. Howell, and R. J. Jackson. 1990. Initiation of encephalomyocarditis virus RNA translation: the authentic initiation site is not selected by a scanning mechanism. *EMBO J.* **9**:3753–3759.
141. Kerekatte, V., B. D. Keiper, C. Badorff, A. Cai, K. U. Knowlton, and R. E. Rhoads. 1999. Cleavage of poly(A)-binding protein by coxsackievirus 2A protease in vitro and in vivo: another mechanism for host protein synthesis shutoff? *J. Virol.* **73**:709–717.
142. Kiehn, E. D., and J. J. Holland. 1970. Synthesis and cleavage of enterovirus polypeptides in mammalian cells. *J. Virol.* **5**:358–367.
143. Kitamura, N., B. L. Semler, P. G. Rothberg, C. R. Larsen, C. J. Adler, A. J. Dorner, E. A. Emini, R. Hanecak, J. J. Lee, S. van der Werf, C. W. Anderson, and E. Wimmer. 1981. Primary structure, gene organization and polypeptide expression of poliovirus RNA. *Nature* **291**:547–553.
144. Koch, F., and G. Koch. 1985. *The Molecular Biology of Poliovirus*. Springer-Verlag, Vienna, Austria.
145. Kolupaeva, V. G., T. V. Pestova, C. U. Hellen, and I. N. Shatsky. 1998. Translation eukaryotic initiation factor 4G recognizes a specific structural element within the internal ribosome entry site of encephalomyocarditis virus RNA. *J. Biol. Chem.* **273**:18599–18604.
146. Kong, W. P., G. D. Ghadge, and R. P. Roos. 1994. Involvement of cardiovirus leader in host cell-restricted virus expression. *Proc. Natl. Acad. Sci. USA* **91**:1796–1800.
147. Kong, W. P., and R. P. Roos. 1991. Alternative translation initiation site in the DA strain of Theiler's murine encephalomyelitis virus. *J. Virol.* **65**:3395–3399.
148. Koonin, E. V. 1991. The phylogeny of RNA-dependent RNA polymerases of positive-strand RNA viruses. *J. Gen. Virol.* **72**:2197–2206.
149. Kozak, M. 1989. The scanning model for translation: an update. *J. Cell Biol.* **108**:229–241.
150. Kuge, S., and A. Nomoto. 1987. Construction of viable deletion and insertion mutants of the Sabin strain of type 1 poliovirus: function of the 5′ noncoding sequence in viral replication. *J. Virol.* **61**:1478–1487.
151. Kuge, S., I. Saito, and A. Nomoto. 1986. Primary structure of poliovirus defective-interfering particle genomes and possible generation mechanisms of the particles. *J. Mol. Biol.* **192**:473–487.
152. Kusov, Y. Y., and V. Gauss-Müller. 1997. In vitro RNA binding of the hepatitis A virus proteinase 3C (HAV 3C^{pro}) to secondary structure elements within the 5′ terminus of the HAV genome. *RNA* **3**:291–302.
153. Lama, J., and L. Carrasco. 1996. Screening for membrane-permeabilizing mutants of the poliovirus protein 3AB. *J. Gen. Virol.* **77**:2109–2119.
154. Lama, J., M. A. Sanz, and L. Carrasco. 1998. Genetic analysis of poliovirus protein 3A: characterization of a non-cytopathic mutant virus defective in killing Vero cells. *J. Gen. Virol.* **79**:911–1921.
155. Lawson, T. G., L. L. Smith, A. C. Palmenberg, and R. E. Thach. 1989. Inducible expression of encephalomyocarditis virus 3C protease activity in stably transformed mouse cell lines. *J. Virol.* **63**:5013–5022.
156. Lawson, T. G., D. L. Gronros, P. E. Evans, M. C. Bastien, K. M. Michalewich, J. K. Clark, J. H. Edmonds, K. H. Graber, J. A. Werner, B. A. Lurvey, and J. M. Cate. 1999. Identification and characterization of a protein destruction signal in the encephalomyocarditis virus 3C protease. *J. Biol. Chem.* **274**:9904–9908.
157. Le, S. Y., and J. V. Maizel, Jr. 1998. Evolution of a common structural core in the internal ribosome entry sites of picornaviruses. *Virus Genes* **16**:25–38.
158. Le, S. Y., A. Siddiqui, and J. V. Maizel, Jr. 1996. A common structural core in the internal ribosome entry sites of picornavirus, hepatitis C virus, and pestivirus. *Virus Genes* **12**:135–147.
159. Lee, Y. F., A. Nomoto, B. N. Detjen, and E. Wimmer. 1977. A protein covalently linked to poliovirus genome RNA. *Proc. Natl. Acad. Sci. USA* **74**:59–63.
160. Lee, Y. F., A. Nomoto, and E. Wimmer. 1976. The genome of poliovirus is an exceptional eukaryotic mRNA. *Prog. Nucleic Acid Res. Mol. Biol.* **19**:89–96.
161. Lemon, S. M., and L. N. Binn. 1985. Incomplete neutralization of hepatitis A virus in vitro due to lipid-associated virions. *J. Gen. Virol.* **66**:2501–2505.
162. Levintow, L. 1974. The reproduction of picornaviruses. *Comp. Virol.* **2**:109–169.
163. Li, J. P., and D. Baltimore. 1990. An intragenic revertant of a poliovirus 2C mutant has an uncoating defect. *J. Virol.* **64**:1102–1107.
164. Liebig, H. D., E. Ziegler, R. Yan, K. Hartmuth, H. Klump, H. Kowalski, D. Blaas, W. Sommergruber, L. Frasel, B. Lamphear, R. Rhoads, E. Kuechler, and T. Skern. 1993. Purification of two picornaviral 2A pro-

teinases: interaction with eIF-4 gamma and influence on in vitro translation. *Biochemistry* **32:**7581–7588.
165. **Lloyd, R. E., and M. Bovee.** 1993. Persistent infection of human erythroblastoid cells by poliovirus. *Virology* **194:**200–209.
166. **Lobert, P.-E., N. Escrious, J. Ruelle, and T. Michiels.** 1999. A coding RNA sequence acts as a replication signal in cardioviruses. *Proc. Natl. Acad. Sci. USA* **96:**11560–11565.
167. **Lopez-Guerrero, J. A., M. Alonso, F. Martin-Belmonte, and L. Carrasco.** 2000. Poliovirus induces apoptosis in the human U937 promonocytic cell line. *Virology* **272:**250–256.
168. **Macadam, A. J., G. Ferguson, T. Fleming, D. M. Stone, J. W. Almond, and P. D. Minor.** 1994. Role for poliovirus protease 2A in cap independent translation. *EMBO J.* **13:**924–927.
169. **Maizel, J. V.** 1963. Evidence for multiple components in the structural protein of type 1 poliovirus. *Biochem. Biophys. Res. Commun.* **13:**483–489.
170. **Maizel, J. V., and D. F. Summers.** 1968. Evidence for differences in size and composition of the poliovirus-specific polypeptides in infected HeLa cells. *Virology* **36:**48–54.
171. **Martin, L. R., G. M. Duke, J. E. Osorio, D. J. Hall, and A. C. Palmenberg.** 1996. Mutational analysis of the mengovirus poly(C) tract and surrounding heteropolymeric sequences. *J. Virol.* **70:**2027–2031.
172. **Martin, L. R., and A. S. Palmenberg.** 1996. Tandem mengovirus 5′ pseudoknots are linked to viral RNA synthesis, not poly(C)-mediated virulence. *J. Virol.* **70:**8182–8186.
173. **McBride, A. E., A. Schlegel, and K. Kirkegaard.** 1996. Human protein Sam 68 relocalization and interaction with poliovirus RNA polymerase in infected cells. *Proc. Natl. Acad. Sci. USA* **93:**2296–2301.
174. **McBride, A. E., S. J. Taylor, D. Shalloway, and K. Kirkegaard.** 1998. KH domain integrity is required for wild-type localization of Sam68. *Exp. Cell. Res.* **241:**84–95.
175. **McKnight, K. L., and S. M. Lemon.** 1998. The rhinovirus type 14 genome contains an internally located RNA structure that is required for viral replication. *RNA* **4:**1569–1584.
176. **Meerovitch, K., Y. V. Svitkin, H. S. Lee, F. Lejbkowicz, D. J. Kenan, E. K. Chan, V. I. Agol, J. D. Keene, and N. Sonenberg.** 1993. La autoantigen enhances and corrects aberrant translation of poliovirus RNA in reticulocyte lysate. *J. Virol.* **67:**3798–3807.
177. **Melchers, W. J., J. M. Bakkers, H. J. Bruins Slot, J. M. Galama, V. I. Agol, and E. V. Pilipenko.** 2000. Crosstalk between orientation-dependent recognition determinants of a complex control RNA element, the enterovirus oriR. *RNA* **6:**976–987.
178. **Melchers, W. J. G., H. Heenderop, H. J. Bruins Slot, C. Pleij, E. V. Pilipenko, V. I. Agol, and J. Galama.** 1997. Kissing of the two predominant hairpin loops in the coxsackie B virus 3′UTR in the origin of replication required for (−) strand RNA synthesis. *J. Virol.* **71:**686–696.
179. **Mellits, K. H., J. M. Meredith, J. B. Rohll, D. J. Evans, and J. W. Almond.** 1998. Binding of a cellular factor to the 3′ untranslated region of the RNA genomes of entero- and rhinoviruses plays a role in virus replication. *J. Gen. Virol.* **79:**1715–1723.
180. **Merrick, W. C., and J. W. B. Hershey.** 1996. The pathway and mechanism of eukaryotic protein synthesis, p. 31–69. *In* J. W. Hershey, M. B. Mathews, and N. Sonenberg (ed.), *Translational Control*. Cold Spring Harbor Laboratory Press, Cold Spring Harbor, N.Y.
181. **Meyer, K., A. Petersen, M. Niepmann, and E. Beck.** 1995. Interaction of eucaryotic initiation factor eF-4B with a picornavirus internal translation initiation site. *J. Virol.* **69:**2819–2824.
182. **Michiels, T., V. Dejong, R. Rodrigus, and C. Shaw-Jacson.** 1997. Protein 2A is not required for Theiler's virus replication. *J. Virol.* **71:**9549–9556.
183. **Miller, R. L., and P. G. Plagemann.** 1972. Purification of mengovirus and identification of an A-rich segment in its ribonucleic acid. *J. Gen. Virol.* **17:**349–353.
184. **Mirmomeni, M. H., P. J. Hughes, and G. Stanway.** 1997. An RNA structure in the 3′ untranslated region of enteroviruses is necessary for efficient replication. *J. Virol.* **71:**2363–2370.
185. **Mosenkis, J., S. Daniels-McQueen, S. Janoves, R. Duncan, J. W. B. Hershey, J. A. Grifo, W. C. Merrick, and R. Thach.** 1985. Shutoff of host translation by encephalomyocarditis virus infection does not involve cleavage of the eucaryotic initiation factor 4F polypeptide that accompanies poliovirus infection. *J. Virol.* **54:**643–645.
186. **Nateri, A. S., P. J. Hughes, and G. Stanway.** 2000. In vivo and in vitro identification of structural and sequence elements of the human parechovirus 5′ untranslated region required for internal initiation. *J. Virol.* **74:**6269–6277.
187. **Newton, S. E., A. R. Carroll, R. O. Campbell, B. E. Clarke, and D. J. Rowlands.** 1985. The sequence of foot-and-mouth disease virus RNA to the 5′ side of the poly(C) tract. *Gene* **40:**331–336.
187a. **Neznanov, N., A. Kondratova, K. M. Chumakov, B. Angres, B. Zhumbayeva, V. I. Agol, and A. V. Gudkov.** 2001. Poliovirus protein 3A inhibits tumor necrosis factor (TNF)-induced apoptosis by eliminating the TNF receptor from the cell surface. *J. Virol.* **75:**10409–10420.
188. **Niepmann, M., A. Petersen, K. Meyer, and E. Beck.** 1997. Functional involvement of polypyrimidine tract-binding protein in translation initiation complexes with the internal ribosome entry site of foot-and-mouth disease virus. *J. Virol.* **71:**8330–8339.
189. **Nomoto, A., B. Detjen, R. Pozzatti, and E. Wimmer.** 1977. The location of the polio genome protein in viral RNAs and its implication for RNA synthesis. *Nature* **268:**208–213.
190. **Nomoto, A., N. Kitamura, F. Golini, and E. Wimmer.** 1977. The 5′-terminal structures of poliovirion RNA and poliovirus mRNA differ only in the genome-linked protein VPg. *Proc. Natl. Acad. Sci. USA* **74:**5345–5349.
191. **Nomoto, A., Y. F. Lee, and E. Wimmer.** 1976. The 5′ end of poliovirus mRNA is not capped with m^{7}G(5′)ppp(5′)Np. *Proc. Natl. Acad. Sci. USA* **73:**375–380.
192. **Novak, J. E., and K. Kirkegaard.** 1991. Improved method for detecting poliovirus negative strands used to demonstrate specificity of positive-strand encapsidation and the ratio of positive to negative strands in infected cells. *J. Virol.* **65:**3384–3387.
193. **Novak, J. E., and K. Kirkegaard.** 1994. Coupling between genome translation and replication in an RNA virus. *Genes Dev.* **8:**1726–1237.
194. **Novoa, I., and L. Carrasco.** 1999. Cleavage of eukaryotic translation initiation factor 4G by exogenously added hybrid proteins containing poliovirus 2Apro in HeLa cells: effects on gene expression. *Mol. Cell. Biol.* **19:**2445–2454.
195. **Nugent, C. I., K. L. Jonson, P. Sarnov, and K. Kirkegaard.** 1999. Functional coupling between replication and packaging of poliovirus replicon RNA. *J. Virol.* **73:**427–435.

196. **Nugent, C. I., and K. Kirkegaard.** 1995. RNA binding properties of poliovirus subviral particles. *J. Virol.* **69:** 13–22.
197. **Obuchi, M., J. Yamamoto, T. Odagiri, M. N. Uddin, H. Iizuka, and Y. Ohara.** 2000. L* protein of Theiler's murine encephalomyelitis virus is required for virus growth in a murine macrophage-like cell line. *J. Virol.* **74:**4898–4901.
198. **Ohlmann, T., and R. J. Jackson.** 1999. The properties of chimeric picornavirus IRESes show that discrimination between internal translation initiation sites is influenced by the identity of the IRES and not just the context of the AUG codon. *RNA* **5:**764–778.
199. **O'Neill, R. E., and V. R. Racaniello.** 1989. Inhibition of translation in cells infected with a poliovirus 2Apro mutant correlates with phosphorylation of the alpha subunit of eucaryotic initiation factor 2. *J. Virol.* **63:**5069–5075.
200. **O'Reilly, E. K., and C. C. Kao.** 1998. Analysis of RNA-dependent RNA polymerase structure and function as guided by known polymerase structures and computer predictions of secondary structure. *Virology* **252:** 287–303.
201. **Osorio, J. E., L. R. Martin, and A. C. Palmenberg.** 1996. The immunogenic and pathogenic potential of short poly(C) tract Mengo viruses. *Virology* **223:**344–350.
202. **Palmenberg, A. C.** 1990. Proteolytic processing of picornaviral polyprotein. *Annu. Rev. Microbiol.* **44:**603–623.
203. **Palmenberg, A. C., M. A. Pallansch, and R. R. Rueckert.** 1979. Protease required for processing picornaviral coat protein resides in the viral replicase gene. *J. Virol.* **32:**770–778.
204. **Palmenberg, A. C., and J.-Y. Sgro.** 1997. Topological organization of picornaviral genomes: statistical prediction of RNA structural signals. *Semin. Virol.* **8:**231–241.
205. **Parsley, T. B., J. S. Towner, L. B. Blyn, E. Ehrenfeld, and B. L. Semler.** 1997. Poly (rC) binding protein 2 forms a ternary complex with the 5′-terminal sequences of poliovirus RNA and the viral 3CD proteinase. *RNA* **3:**1124–1134.
205a. **Paul, A. V., E. Rieder, D. W. Kim, J. H. van Boom, and E. Wimmer.** 2000. Identification of an RNA hairpin in poliovirus RNA that serves as the primary template in the in vitro uridylylation of VPg. *J. Virol.* **74:**10359–10570.
206. **Paul, A. V., J. H. van Boom, D. Filippov, and E. Wimmer.** 1998. Protein-primed RNA synthesis by purified poliovirus RNA polymerase. *Nature* **393:**280–284.
207. **Pelletier, J., M. N. Flynn, G. Kaplan, V. Racaniello, and N. Sonenberg.** 1989. Mutational analysis of upstream AUG codons of poliovirus RNA. *J. Virol.* **62:** 4486–4492.
208. **Pelletier, J., G. Kaplan, V. Racaniello, and N. Sonenberg.** 1988. Cap-independent translation of poliovirus mRNA is conferred by sequence elements within the 5′ noncoding region. *Mol. Cell. Biol.* **8:**1103–1112.
209. **Pelletier, J., and N. Sonenberg.** 1988. Internal initiation of translation of eucaryotic mRNA directed by a sequence derived from poliovirus RNA. *Nature* **334:**320–325.
210. **Pelletier, J., and N. Sonenberg.** 1989. Internal binding of eucaryotic ribosomes on poliovirus RNA: translation in HeLa cell extracts. *J. Virol.* **63:**441–444.
211. **Penman, S., K. Scherrer, Y. Becker, and J. E. Darnell.** 1963. Polyribosomes in normal and poliovirus-infected HeLa cells and their relationship to messenger-RNA. *Proc. Natl. Acad. Sci. USA* **49:**654–662.
212. **Perez Bercoff, R. (ed.).** 1979. *The Molecular Biology of Picornaviruses.* Plenum Press, New York, N.Y.
213. **Perez Bercoff, P., and M. Gander.** 1978. In vitro translation of mengovirus RNA deprived of the terminally-linked (capping?) protein. *FEBS Lett.* **96:**306–312.
214. **Pestova, T. V., C. U. Hellen, and E. Wimmer.** 1994. A conserved AUG triplet in the 5′ nontranslated region of poliovirus can function as an initiation codon in vitro and in vivo. *Virology* **204:**729–737.
215. **Pettersson, R. F., V. Ambros, and D. Baltimore.** 1978. Identification of a protein linked to nascent poliovirus RNA and to the polyuridylic acid of negative-strand RNA. *J. Virol.* **27:**357–365.
216. **Pfister, T., D. Egger, and K. Bienz.** 1995. Poliovirus subviral particles associated with progeny RNA in the replication complex. *J. Gen. Virol.* **76:**63–71.
217. **Piccone, M. E., E. Rieder, P. W. Mason, and M. J. Grubman.** 1995. The foot-and-mouth disease virus leader proteinase gene is not required for viral replication. *J. Virol.* **69:**5376–5382.
218. **Pilipenko, E. V., V. M. Blinov, and V. I. Agol.** 1990. Gross rearrangements within the 5′-untranslated region of the picornaviral genomes. *Nucleic Acids Res.* **18:** 3371–3375.
219. **Pilipenko, E. V., V. M. Blinov, B. K. Chernov, T. M. Dmitrieva, and V. I. Agol.** 1989. Conservation of the secondary structure elements of the 5′-untranslated region of cardio- and aphthovirus RNAs. *Nucleic Acids Res.* **17:**5701–5711.
220. **Pilipenko, E. V., V. M. Blinov, L. I. Romanova, A. N. Sinyakov, S. V. Maslova, and V. I. Agol.** 1989. Conserved structural domains in the 5′-untranslated region of picornaviral genomes: an analysis of the segment controlling translation and neurovirulence. *Virology* **168:** 201–209.
221. **Pilipenko, E. V., A. P. Gmyl, S. V. Maslova, G. A. Belov, A. N. Sinyakov, M. Huang, T. D. K. Brown, and V. I. Agol.** 1994. Starting window, distinct element in the cap-independent internal initiation of translation on picornaviral RNA. *J. Mol. Biol.* **241:**398–414.
222. **Pilipenko, E. V., A. P. Gmyl, S. V. Maslova, E. V. Khitrina, and V. I. Agol.** 1995. Attenuation of Theiler's murine encephalomyelitis virus by modifications of the oligopyrimidine/AUG tandem, a host-dependent translational cis-element. *J. Virol.* **69:**864–870.
223. **Pilipenko, E. V., A. P. Gmyl, S. V. Maslova, Y. V. Svitkin, A. N. Sinyakov, and V. I. Agol.** 1992. A prokaryotic-like cis-element in the cap-independent internal initiation of translation on picornavirus RNA. *Cell* **68:**119–131.
224. **Pilipenko, E. V., S. V. Maslova, A. N. Sinyakov, and V. I. Agol.** 1992. Toward identification of cis-acting elements involved in the replication of enterovirus and rhinovirus RNAs: a proposal for the existence of tRNA-like terminal structures. *Nucleic Acids Res.* **20:**1739–1745.
225. **Pilipenko, E. V., T. V. Pestova, V. G. Kolupaeva, E. V. Khitrina, A. N. Poperechnaya, V. I. Agol, and C. U. Hellen.** 2000. A cell cycle-dependent protein serves as a template-specific translation initiation factor. *Genes Dev.* **14:**2028–2045.
226. **Pilipenko, E. V., K. V. Poperechny, S. V. Maslova, W. J. G. Melchers, H. J. Bruins Slot, and V. I. Agol.** 1996. Cis-element, oriR, involved in the initiation of (−) strand poliovirus RNA: a quasi-globular multidomain RNA structure maintained by tertiary ("kissing") interaction. *EMBO J.* **19:**5428–5436.
226a. **Pilipenko, E. V., E. G. Viktorova, S. T. Guest, V. I. Agol, and R. P. Roos.** 2001. Cell-specific proteins reg-

ulate viral RNA translation and virus-induced disease. *EMBO J.* **20:**6899–6908.

227. **Pilipenko, E. V., E. G. Viktorova, E. V. Khitrina, S. V. Maslova, N. Jarousse, M. Brahic, and V. I. Agol.** 1999. Distinct attenuation phenotypes caused by mutations in the translational starting window of Theiler's murine encephalomyelitis virus. *J. Virol.* **73:**3190–3196.

228. **Porter, D. C., D. C. Ansardi, J. Wang, S. McPherson, Z. Moldoveanu, and C. D. Morrow.** 1998. Demonstration of the specificity of poliovirus encapsidation using a novel replicon which encodes enzymatically active firefly luciferase. *Virology* **243:**1–11.

229. **Probst, C., M. Jecht, and V. Gauss-Muller.** 1998. Processing of proteinase precursors and their effect on hepatitis A virus particle formation. *J. Virol.* **72:**8013–8020.

230. **Probst, C., M. Jecht, and V. Gauss-Müller.** 1999. Intrinsic signals for the assembly of hepatitis A virus particles. Role of structural proteins VP4 and 2A. *J. Biol. Chem.* **274:**4527–4531.

231. **Racaniello, V. R. (ed.).** 1990. Picornaviruses. *Curr. Top. Microbiol. Immunol.* **161:**1–188.

232. **Racaniello, V. R.** 1996. The poliovirus receptor: a hook, or an unzipper? *Structure* **4:**769–773.

233. **Racaniello, V. R., and D. Baltimore.** 1981. Molecular cloning of poliovirus cDNA and determination of the complete nucleotide sequence of the viral genome. *Proc. Natl. Acad. Sci. USA* **78:**4887–4891.

234. **Racaniello, V. R., and D. Baltimore.** 1981. Cloned poliovirus complementary DNA is infectious in mammalian cells. *Science* **214:**916–919.

235. **Racaniello, V. R., and A. Dasgupta.** 1987. Activation of double-stranded RNA-activated protein kinase in HeLa cells after poliovirus infection does not result in increased phosphorylation of eucaryotic initiation factor-2. *J. Virol.* **61:**1781–1787.

236. **Rekosh, D.** 1972. Gene order of the poliovirus capsid proteins. *J. Virol.* **9:**479–487.

236a. **Rieder, E., A. V. Paul, D. W. Kim, J. H. van Boom, and E. Wimmer.** 2000. Genetic and biochemical studies of poliovirus cis-acting replication element cre in relation to VPg uridylylation. *J. Virol.* **74:**10371–10380.

237. **Rivera, V. M., J. D. Welsh, and J. Maizel.** 1988. Comparative sequence analysis of the 5' noncoding region of the enteroviruses and rhinoviruses. *Virology* **165:**42–50.

238. **Roberts, L. O., R. A. Seamons, and G. J. Belsham.** 1998. Recognition of picornavirus internal ribosome entry sites within cells; influence of cellular and viral proteins. *RNA* **4:**520–529.

239. **Rodriguez, P. L., and L. Carrasco.** 1995. Poliovirus protein 2C contains two regions involved in RNA binding activity. *J. Biol. Chem.* **270:**10105–10112.

240. **Rohll, J. B., D. H. Moon, D. J. Evans, and J. W. Almond.** 1995. The 3' untranslated region of picornavirus RNA: features required for efficient genome replication. *J. Virol.* **69:**7835–7844.

240a. **Romanova, L. I., and V. I. Agol.** 1979. Interconversion of linear and circular forms of double-stranded RNA of encephalomyocarditis virus. *Virology* **93:**574–577.

241. **Rossmann, M. G., J. Bella, P. R. Kolatkar, Y. He, E. Wimmer, R. J. Kuhn, and T. S. Baker.** 2000. Cell recognition and entry by rhino- and enteroviruses. *Virology* **269:**239–247.

242. **Rothberg, P. G., T. J. R. Harris, A. Nomoto, and E. Wimmer.** 1978. O^4-(5'uridylyl) tyrosine is the bond between the genome-linked protein and the RNA of poliovirus. *Proc. Natl. Acad. Sci. USA* **75:**4868–4872.

243. **Rowe, A., G. L. Ferguson, P. D. Minor, and A. J. Macadam.** 2000. Coding changes in the poliovirus protease 2A compensate for 5'NCR domain V disruptions in a cell-specific manner. *Virology* **269:**284–293.

244. **Rubinstein, S. J., T. Hammerle, E. Wimmer, and A. Dasgupta.** 1992. Infection of HeLa cells with poliovirus results in modification of a complex that binds to the rRNA promoter. *J. Virol.* **66:**3062–3068.

245. **Rueckert, R. R.** 1996. Picornaviridae: the viruses and their replication, p. 477–522. *In* B. N. Fields, D. M. Knipe, and P. M. Howley (ed.), *Fundamental Virology*, 3rd ed. Lippincott-Raven, Philadelphia, Pa.

246. **Ryan, M. D., and J. Drew.** 1994. Foot-and-mouth disease virus 2A oligopeptide mediated cleavage of an artificial polyprotein. *EMBO J.* **13:**928–933.

247. **Ryan, M. D., and M. Flint.** 1997. Virus-encoded proteinases of the picornavirus super-group. *J. Gen. Virol.* **78:**699–723.

248. **Ryan, M. D., A. M. King, and G. P. Thomas.** 1991. Cleavage of foot-and-mouth disease virus polyprotein is mediated by residues located within a 19 amino acid sequence. *J. Gen. Virol.* **72:**2727–2732.

249. **Sandoval, I. V., and L. Carrasco.** 1997. Poliovirus infection and expression of the poliovirus protein 2B provoke the disassembly of the Golgi complex, the organelle target for the antipoliovirus drug Ro-090179. *J. Virol.* **71:**4679–4693.

250. **Scheper, G. C., H. O. Voorma, and A. A. Thomas.** 1994. Binding of eukaryotic initiation factor-2 and transacting factors to the 5' untranslated region of encephalomyocarditis virus RNA. *Biochimie* **76:**801–809.

251. **Scheper, G. C., H. O. Voorma, and A. Thomas.** 1994. Base pairing with 18S ribosomal RNA in internal initiation of translation. *FEBS Lett.* **353:**271–275.

252. **Schlegel, A., T. H. Giddings, Jr., M. S. Ladinsky, and K. Kirkegaard.** 1996. Cellular origin and ultrastructure of membranes induced during poliovirus infection. *J. Virol.* **70:**6576–6588.

253. **Schwerdt, C. E., and F. L. Schaffer.** 1955. Some physical and chemical properties of purified poliomyelitis virus preparations. *Ann. N. Y. Acad. Sci.* **61:**740–750.

254. **Semler, B. L., and E. Ehrenfeld (ed.).** 1989. *Molecular Aspects of Poliovirus Infection and Detection.* American Society for Microbiology, Washington, D.C.

255. **Shaffer, D. R., E. A. Brown, and S. M. Lemon.** 1994. Large deletion mutations involving the first pyrimidine-rich tract of the 5' nontranslated RNA of human hepatitis A virus define two adjacent domains associated with distinct replication phenotypes. *J. Virol.* **68:**5568–5578.

256. **Shaffer, D. R., and S. M. Lemon.** 1995. Temperature-sensitive hepatitis A virus mutants with deletions downstream of the first pyrimidine-rich tract of the 5' nontranslated RNA are impaired in RNA synthesis. *J. Virol.* **69:**6498–6506.

257. **Shaw-Jackson, C., and T. Michiels.** 1999. Absence of internal ribosome entry site-mediated tissue specificity in the translation of a bicistronic transgene. *J. Virol.* **73:**2729–2738.

258. **Shen, Y., M. Igo, P. Yalamanchili, A. J. Berk, and A. Dasgupta.** 1996. DNA binding domain and subunit interactions of transcription factor IIIC revealed by dissection with poliovirus 3C protease. *Mol. Cell Biol.* **16:**4163–4171.

259. **Shiroki, K., T. Isoyama, S. Kuge, T. Ishii, S. Ohmi, S. Hata, K. Suzuki, Y. Takasaki, and A. Nomoto.** 1999. Intracellular redistribution of truncated La protein produced by poliovirus 3C^{pro}-mediated cleavage. *J. Virol.* **73:**2193–2200.

260. **Shiroki, K., I. Toshihiko, T. Aoki, M. Kobashi, S. Ohka, and A. Nomoto.** 1995. A new cis-acting element for RNA replication within the 5' noncoding region of poliovirus type 1 RNA. *J. Virol.* **69:**6825–6832.

261. Simoes, E. A., and P. Sarnow. 1991. An RNA hairpin at the extreme 5' end of the poliovirus RNA genome modulates viral translation in human cells. *J. Virol.* **65:** 913–921.
262. Skinner, M. A., V. Racaniello, G. Dunn, J. Cooper, P. D. Minor, and J. W. Almond. 1989. New model for the secondary structure of the 5' non-coding RNA of poliovirus is supported by biochemical and genetic data that also show that RNA secondary structure is important in neurovirulence. *J. Mol. Biol.* **207:**379–392.
263. Slobodskaya, O. R., A. P. Gmyl, S. V. Maslova, E. A. Tolskaya, E. G. Viktorova, and V. I. Agol. 1996. Poliovirus neurovirulence correlates with the presence of a cryptic AUG upstream of the initiator codon. *Virology* **221:**141–150.
264. Soloviev, V. D., T. I. Krispin, V. G. Zaslavsky, and V. I. Agol. 1968. Mechanism of resistance to enteroviruses of some primate cells in tissue culture. *J. Virol.* **2:** 553–557.
265. Sonenberg, N. 1987. Regulation of translation by poliovirus. *Adv. Virus Res.* **33:**175–204.
266. Stanway, G. 1990. Structure, function and evolution of picornaviruses. *J. Gen. Virol.* **71:**2483–2501.
267. Stanway, G., N. Kalkkinen, M. Roivainen, F. Ghazi, M. Khan, M. Smyth, O. Meurman, and T. Hyypia. 1994. Molecular and biological characteristics of echovirus 22, a representative of a new picornavirus group. *J. Virol.* **68:**8232–8238.
268. Stewart, S. R., and B. L. Semler. 1999. Pyrimidine-rich region mutations compensate for a stem-loop V lesion in the 5' noncoding region of poliovirus genomic RNA. *Virology* **264:**385–397.
269. Strebel, K., and E. Beck. 1986. A second protease of foot-and-mouth disease virus. *J. Virol.* **58:**893–899.
270. Summers, D. F., and J. V. Maizel. 1968. Evidence for large precursor proteins in poliovirus synthesis. *Proc. Natl. Acad. Sci. USA* **59:**966–971.
271. Summers, D. F., and J. V. Maizel. 1971. Determination of the gene sequence of poliovirus with pactamycin. *Proc. Natl. Acad. Sci. USA* **68:**2852–2856.
272. Summers, D. F., J. V. Maizel, and J. E. Darnell. 1965. Evidence for virus-specific noncapsid proteins in poliovirus-infected HeLa cells. *Proc. Natl. Acad. Sci. USA* **54:**505–513.
273. Svitkin, Y. V., and V. I. Agol. 1983. Translational barrier in central region of encephalomyocarditis virus genome. *Eur. J. Biochem.* **135:**145–154.
274. Svitkin, Y. V., A. Gradi, H. Imataka, S. Morino, and N. Sonenberg. 1999. Eukaryotic initiation factor 4GII (eIF4GII), but not eIF4GI, cleavage correlates with inhibition of host cell protein synthesis after human rhinovirus infection. *J. Virol.* **73:**3467–3472.
275. Svitkin, Y. V., K. Meerovitch, H. S. Lee, J. N. Dholakia, D. J. Kenan, V. I. Agol, and N. Sonenberg. 1994. Internal translation initiation on poliovirus RNA: further characterization of La function in poliovirus translation in vitro. *J. Virol.* **68:**1544–1550.
276. Taber, R., R. Rekosh, and D. Baltimore. 1971. Effect of pactamycin on synthesis of poliovirus proteins: a method for genetic mapping. *J. Virol.* **8:**395–401.
277. Takata, H., M. Obuchi, J. Yamamoto, T. Odagiri, R. P. Roos, H. Iizuka, and Y. Ohara. 1998. L* protein of the DA strain of Theiler's murine encephalomyelitis virus is important for virus growth in a murine macrophage-like cell line. *J. Virol.* **72:**4950–4955.
278. Tesar, M., S. A. Harmon, D. F. Summers, and E. Ehrenfeld. 1992. Hepatitis A virus polyprotein synthesis initiates from two alternative AUG codons. *Virology* **186:**609–618.
279. Teterina, N. L., K. Bienz, D. Egger, A. E. Gorbalenya, and E. Ehrenfeld. 1997. Induction of intracellular rearrangements by HAV proteins 2C and 2BC. *Virology* **237:** 66–77.
280. Teterina, N. L., A. E. Gorbalenya, D. Egger, K. Bienz, and E. Ehrenfeld. 1997. Poliovirus 2C proteins determinants of membrane binding and rearrangements in mammalian cells. *J. Virol.* **71:**8962–8972.
281. Thomas, A. A., R. Rijnbrand, and H. O. Voorma. 1996. Recognition of the initiation codon for protein synthesis in foot-and-mouth disease virus RNA. *J. Gen. Virol.* **77:**265–272.
282. Todd, S., J. S. Towner, D. M. Brown, and B. L. Semler. 1997. Replication-competent picornaviruses with complete genomic RNA 3' noncoding region deletions. *J. Virol.* **71:**8868–8874.
283. Tolskaya, E. A., L. I. Romanova, M. S. Kolesnikova, T. A. Ivannikova, E. A. Smirnova, N. T. Raikhlin, and V. I. Agol. 1995. Apoptosis-inducing and apoptosis-preventing functions of poliovirus. *J. Virol.* **69:**1181–1189.
284. Toyoda, H., M. J. Nicklin, M. G. Murray, C. W. Anderson, J. J. Dunn, F. W. Studier, and E. Wimmer. 1986. A second virus-encoded proteinase involved in proteolytic processing of poliovirus polyprotein. *Cell* **45:** 761–770.
285. Trono, D., R. Andino, and D. Baltimore. 1988. An RNA sequence of hundreds of nucleotides at the 5' end of poliovirus RNA is involved in allowing viral protein synthesis. *J. Virol.* **62:**2291–2299.
286. Vance, L. M., N. Moscufo, M. Chow, and B. A. Heinz. 1997. Poliovirus 2C region functions during encapsidation of viral RNA. *J. Virol.* **71:**8759–8765.
287. van Kuppeveld, F. J. M., J. G. H. Hoenderop, R. L. L. Smeets, P. H. G. Willems, H. B. Dijkman, J. M. Galama, and W. J. Melchers. 1997. Coxsackievirus protein 2B modifies endoplasmic reticulum membrane and plasma membrane permeability and facilitates virus release. *EMBO J.* **16:**3519–3532.
288. Vartapetian, A. B., A. S. Mankin, E. A. Skripkin, K. M. Chumakov, V. D. Smirnov, and A. A. Bogdanov. 1983. The primary and secondary structure of the 5'-end region of encephalomyocarditis virus RNA. A novel approach to sequencing long RNA molecules. *Gene* **26:** 189–195.
289. Ventoso, I., S. E. MacMilan, J. W. B. Hershey, and L. Carrasco. 1998. Poliovirus 2A proteinase cleaves directly the eIF-4G subunit of eIF-4G complex. *FEBS Lett.* **435:** 79–83.
290. Venuti, A., C. Di Russo, N. del Grosso, A. M. Patti, F. Ruggeri, P. R. De Stasio, M. G. Martiniello, P. Pagnotti, A. M. Degener, and M. Midulla. 1985. Isolation and molecular cloning of a fast-growing strain of human hepatitis A virus from its double-stranded replicative form. *J. Virol.* **56:**579–588.
291. Waggoner, S., and P. Sarnow. 1998. Viral ribonucleoprotein complex formation and nucleolar-cytoplasmic relocalization of nucleolin in poliovirus-infected cells. *J. Virol.* **72:**6699–6709.
292. Walter, B. L., J. H. Nguyen, E. Ehrenfeld, and B. L. Semler. 1999. Differential utilization of poly(rC) binding protein 2 in translation directed by picornavirus IRES elements. *RNA* **5:**1570–1585.
293. Wang, J., J. M. Bakkers, J. M. Galama, H. J. Bruins Slot, E. V. Pilipenko, V. I. Agol, and W. J. Melchers. 1999. Structural requirements of the higher order RNA kissing element in the enteroviral 3'UTR. *Nucleic Acids. Res.* **27:**485–490.
294. Warner, J., M. J. Madden, and J. E. Darnell. 1963. The

interaction of poliovirus RNA with *Escherichia coli* ribosomes. *Virology* **19**:393–399.
295. **Wimmer, E. (ed.).** 1994. *Cellular Receptors for Animal Viruses.* Cold Spring Harbor Laboratory Press, Cold Spring Harbor, N.Y.
296. **Wimmer, E., C. U. Hellen, and X. Cao.** 1993. Genetics of poliovirus. *Annu. Rev. Genet.* **27**:353–436.
297. **Witherell, G. W., C. S. Schultz-Witherell, and E. Wimmer.** 1995. Cis-acting elements of the encephalomyocarditis virus internal ribosomal entry site. *Virology* **214**:660–663.
298. **Xiang, W., A. Cuconati, D. Hope, K. Kirkegaard, and E. Wimmer.** 1998. Complete protein linkage map of poliovirus P3 proteins: interaction of polymerase 3Dpol with VPg and with genetic variants of 3AB. *J. Virol.* **72**:6732–6741.
299. **Xiang, W., K. Harris, L. Alexander, and E. Wimmer.** 1995. Interaction between the 5'-terminal cloverleaf and 3AB/3Cd^{pro} of poliovirus is essential for RNA replication. *J. Virol.* **69**:3658–3667.
300. **Xiang, W., A. V. Paul, and E. Wimmer.** 1997. RNA signals in entero- and rhinovirus genome replication. *Semin. Virol.* **8**:256–273.
301. **Yalamanchili, P., R. Banerjee, and A. Dasgupta.** 1997. Poliovirus-encoded protease 2APro cleaves the TATA-binding protein but does not inhibit host cell RNA polymerase II transcription in vitro. *J. Virol.* **71**:6881–6886.
302. **Yalamanchili, P., U. Datta, and A. Dasgupta.** 1997. Inhibition of host cell transcription by poliovirus: cleavage of transcription factor CREB by poliovirus-encoded protease 3Cpro. *J. Virol.* **71**:1220–1226.
303. **Yalamanchili, P., K. Weidman, and A. Dasgupta.** 1997. Cleavage of transcriptional activator Oct-1 by poliovirus encoded protease 3Cpro. *Virology* **239**:176–185.
304. **Yamasaki, K., C. C. Weihl, and R. P. Roos.** 1999. Alternative translation initiation of Theiler's murine encephalomyelitis virus. *J. Virol.* **73**:8519–8526.
305. **Yi, M., D. E. Schultz, and S. M. Lemon.** 2000. Functional significance of the interaction of hepatitis A virus RNA with glyceraldehyde 3-phosphate dehydrogenase (GAPDH): opposing effects of GAPDH and polypyrimidine tract binding protein on internal ribosome entry site function. *J. Virol.* **71**:6459–6468.
306. **Yogo, Y., and E. Wimmer.** 1972. Polyadenylic acid at the 3'-terminus of poliovirus RNA. *Proc. Natl. Acad. Sci. USA* **69**:1877–1882.
307. **Ypma-Wong, M. F., P. G. Dewalt, V. H. Johnson, J. G. Lamb, and B. L. Semler.** 1988. Protein 3CD is the major poliovirus proteinase responsible for cleavage of the P1 capsid precursor. *Virology* **166**:265–270.
308. **Ypma-Wong, M. F., D. J. Filman, J. M. Hogle, and B. L. Semler.** 1988. Structural domains of the poliovirus polyprotein are major determinants for proteolytic cleavage at Gln-Gly pairs. *J. Biol. Chem.* **263**:17846–17856.
309. **Zhang, H., S.-F. Chao, L.-H. Ping, K. Grace, B. Clarke, and S. M. Lemon.** 1995. An infectious cDNA clone of a cytopathic hepatitis A virus: genomic regions associated with rapid replication and cytopathic effect. *Virology* **212**:686–687.
310. **Zhang, S., and V. R. Racaniello.** 1997. Persistent echovirus infection of mouse cells expressing the viral receptor VLA-2. *Virology* **235**:293–301.
311. **Ziegler, E., A. M. Borman, F. G. Deliat, H. D. Liebig, D. Lugovic, K. M. Kean, T. Skern, and E. Kuechler.** 1995. Picornavirus 2A proteinase-mediated simulation of internal initiation of translation is dependent on enzymatic activity and the cleavage products of cellular proteins. *Virology* **213**:549–557.
312. **Ziegler, E., A. M. Borman, R. Kirchweger, T. Skern, and K. M. Kean.** 1995. Foot-and-mouth disease virus Lb proteinase can stimulate rhinovirus and enterovirus IRES-driven translation and cleave several proteins of cellular and viral origin. *J. Virol.* **69**:3465–3474.
313. **Zoll, J., J. M. Galama, F. J. van Kuppeveld, and W. J. Melchers.** 1996. Mengovirus leader is involved in the inhibition of host cell protein synthesis. *J. Virol.* **70**:4948–4952.
314. **Zoll, J., F. J. van Kuppeveld, J. M. Galama, and W. J. Melchers.** 1998. Genetic analysis of mengovirus protein 2A: its function in polyprotein processing and virus reproduction. *J. Gen. Virol.* **79**:17–25.

Alignments and Comparative Profiles of Picornavirus Genera

ANN C. PALMENBERG AND JEAN-YVES SGRO

13

Picornavirus sequence data have accumulated at an astonishing rate. Since the first 1,060 bases at the 3' terminus of poliovirus 1 (PV1) Mahoney genome were published in 1980 (11), the polio database alone has grown to include at least 12 complete genomes and more than 112,000 bases from >36 strains. A minimum of 150 other complete picornavirus genomes also have been sequenced, with >90 additional strains available as significant sequence fragments (>3,000 bases), in a tally that does not even begin to include several hundred thousand additional bases from a multitude of smaller segments generated in epidemiological or evolutionary studies. A rough estimate of 2,000,000 bases would not undervalue the current dataset. International sequence agencies like GenBank (www.ncbi.nlm.nih.gov/GenBank) record the published picornavirus offerings under the broad subgroup classification of "viruses." The annotated information may be searched, compared, and retrieved with standard Internet tools. But if you don't know what you're looking for, or whether a favored strain is actually on deposit in GenBank, a better place to start is the Picornavirus Sequence Database (www.iah.bbsrc.ac.uk/virus/picornaviridae), a beautifully designed web page compiled by Nick Knowles at the Institute for Animal Health, Pirbright, United Kingdom. This comprehensive site catalogues all known family members into appropriate genera and species according to the latest taxonomic designation. GenBank accession numbers, published (and unpublished) references, fragment size, and strain origin are registered for every sequence. Should you need to know, for example, whether a 327-bp fragment from the human rhinovirus HRV-72 1B gene (GenBank: Z47574) is available for comparison (9), the Picornavirus Home Page is the place to inquire. This outstanding resource, like a huge technical library, represents an invaluable research service contribution by Nick Knowles, and we are certainly indebted for his extraordinary efforts.

Nevertheless, placing books on shelves is not the same as reading them. Companion literary tools such as dictionaries or thesauruses can help make any text more informative, especially when the contents are written in a foreign language. Comparative sequence analysis, in some respects, is analogous to compiling a thesaurus for Nature's language. Although various sequence segments may appear superficially to encode similar biological meanings, it is true in Nature, as in English, that there are very few exact synonyms. That is, few "words" in either language are ever observed to exactly substitute for each other in alternative contexts without changing their logic or specific meaning. Just as the etymology of words reflects the sum of their linguistic histories, the subtle peculiarities of each sequence are indicative of unique evolutionary histories. Sequence context and content can both contribute to phenotype. Genomics is a young field, and unfortunately, when it comes to the language of life, our current interpretive skills more closely resemble gauche tourists in Paris, rather than fluent natives. Any singular ribosome still translates the delicate nuances of the basic genetic code with more precision and finesse than our best bioinformaticists. Yet we continue to compare sequences because (hubris aside) it is still one of the small number of available tools with any possibility of breaking down biological syntax into the underlying codes. Within such compilations, we vest the continual hope of teasing from shadowy precedents those common elements of circumstance and function that perhaps foretell a significant phenotypic impact. Why does *this* gene convey persistence? How does *this* internal ribosome entry site (IRES) attenuate the virus? What *specific* capsid changes might allow compromised immunity?

Since the authors' earliest feeble pairwise comparisons between the 3' untranslated regions (UTRs) of encephalomyocarditis virus (EMCV) (3) and PV1 (10), it has been clear that properly formed picornavirus alignments can have some practical use in this regard (15). Good alignments are never trivial to generate, but given that one can learn to understand and respect the principles that underlie algorithmic reconstruction of evolution, reasonable datasets can be created by judicious application of computing power and logic. Another rather trickier problem lies in the definition of a suitable presentation format for effective public data mining. In 1989, with our (then) comparative

---

Ann C. Palmenberg and Jean Yves Sgro ■ Institute for Molecular Virology, University of Wisconsin-Madison, 1525 Linden Dr., Madison, WI 53706.

sequences refined by capsid crystallographic data, we published an 11-page figure summarizing the relative orientations of 33 picornavirus P1-region sequences (16), an exercise we thought rather impressive at the time. With today's much larger alignments, that density would translate into 150 published pages, just for the current protein sequences. Obviously, the printing logistics for huge alignments are hopelessly impractical. Instead, the updated picornavirus datasets cited in this chapter have been placed on a public website (virology.wisc.edu/acp) and mirrored by the Picornavirus Home Page (above). This site also lists the strain abbreviations; gives accession numbers, sequence bibliographies, and algorithms; and provides tables of base compositions, codon frequencies, genome RNA folds (17), and other comparative picornavirus data. Reference use of this information or its future updates should cite this chapter as the published source.

HOW THE ALIGNMENTS WERE FORMED

These days anyone with a hard drive and an Internet connection can align sequences. The commonly available CLUSTAL algorithm and similar pairwise distance methods give a reasonable fit for closely related sequences or for proteins that are obvious homologues of similar length. Very nice alignments for $3C^{pro}$ and $3D^{pol}$ or within individual genera have been generated in this way (19). Genome connoisseurs, however, are always looking for new methods to tweak the data, especially in sequence regions where good fits are harder to achieve or recognize. Our previous capsid alignments were based on superimposition of virion crystal structure hydrogen-bonding maps, then extended by multiple, reiterative pairwise comparisons to include similar related sequences (16). More recently, we used those alignments as founder data for profile hidden Markov model (HMM) analyses aimed at the optimal inclusion of newer, less-related sequences (4). Profiles are position-specific scoring matrices that sum the variability for each column in an existing alignment (7), creating chained likelihood tables (a Markov model) of substitution probabilities (4). New sequences are then fit snugly against the total framework of the profile. With the HMMER program suite (Wisconsin Package Version 10.2, Genetics Computer Group, Madison, Wisc.), full-length picornavirus genome HMM-profiles (lengths of 8,000 to 9,000 bases) were calculated from the previous alignments (16). The profiles proved remarkably powerful at positioning new 5' and 3' UTRs and fitting them into the composites. Parallel polyprotein HMM-profiles (lengths of 2,500 to 3,000 amino acids) also helped ease new protein-coding sequences into logical, in-frame slots that were, by definition, consistent and optimal with regard to all other members of a given genus. Back-translation of the protein alignments and linkage with the UTR fragments gave genome-length RNA alignments that were in agreement with the best fits for the proteins and for the UTRs. The new files include (nearly) all available nonredundant sequence fragments of at least 2,000 bases in length, as listed in the Picornavirus Sequence Database (January 2001). The alignments were checked for consistency, and then refined mathematically and heuristically to (i) maximize the number of matched bases and encoded amino acids, (ii) minimize the location and frequency of indels (insertions/deletions), and (iii) emphasize the conservation of homologous features such as catalytic sites and proteolytic cleavage sites.

CURRENT PICORNAVIRUS ALIGNMENTS

The current iterations now include genome-length alignments for the seven most populous picornaviral genera (*Enterovirus, Rhinovirus, Cardiovirus, Aphthovirus, Hepatovirus, Parechovirus,* and *Teschovirus*) and extend over 173 different strains, providing formats for about 1,000,000 bases. The correlate polyprotein alignments, derived by translation of the aligned RNAs, include about 291,000 amino acids. *Kobuvirus* and *Erbovirus* data will be added when there are sufficient strains for comparison. The new datasets, clearly impractical in printed form, are Internet accessible at: virology.wisc.edu/acp. The web files are displayed as (edited) output from the GCG Wisconsin Package PRETTY program and should be downloaded with a monospace font to maintain alignment continuity. No consensus is shown, but uppercase letters highlight alignment columns where at least two-thirds of the sequences conserve an identical residue. The exact plurality required for these votes varies by alignment, as described within each file. Alternative GCG file formats (*.msf or *.rsf) may be requested by e-mail (jsgro@facstaff.wisc.edu). The website also includes RNA and protein alignments for composite picornaviral genera, covering all genome regions with common evolutionary origins (e.g., P1, 2C, 3B, 3C, and 3D).

SIMILARITY PLOTS

What, then, do the alignments teach us about synonymous regions in picornaviruses? As avowed sequence addicts, we have spent countless hours staring at alignment columns and marveling at the complex variation versus conservation in the lexicon of viral proteins. Anyone who revels in this level of detail is guaranteed to find personal enlightenment in the web files. Admittedly, however, even for the book of life, the repetitive text can become mind numbing after a while, and there is a certain truth to the adage, "One picture is worth a thousand words." In this case, we chose graphs instead of pictures, but the point is similar (or is that identical?). After many false starts with different summary methods, it was ultimately decided that only full-length polyproteins should be allowed to vote in the graph-building process. This culled many sequences from the deeper, more redundant P1 regions and kept them from overpowering the P2+P3 regions, where, invariably, there were fewer strains in each alignment. The chosen sequences (n = 3 to 33, depending upon the genus) were run through the GCG program, PLOTSIMILARITY, to capture an averaged identity score within a window (win = 20) that slid across the alignment. Window averaging smoothes the plot contours and makes it easier to identify regions with different identity profiles. Figure 1A–C shows, respectively, the relative amino acid conservation in the *Enterovirus, Rhinovirus, Aphthovirus, Hepatovirus, Parechovirus, Cardiovirus,* and *Teschovirus* polyproteins. The full-length sequences for individual species were then segregated further and independently recalculated to emphasize how they are varied among themselves, while contributing to the contours of the parental genera. All plots for all species with at least two complete members are available on the web. For brevity, only some are shown here. The number of participating sequences (n), the averaged polyprotein identity (average), and the count of alignment columns where all residues were identical (identities) are shown relative to a polyprotein map, punctuated with appropriate cleavage sites. The protein distance scales are numbered according to alignment positions in the files for each genus.

To state the obvious, conserved residues in the P2+P3 regions generally outnumber those in the P1 region for every alignment. However, the details in the distribution of conserved elements display a much more subtle and powerful pattern. Not surprisingly, and without exception, there is a 1:1 correspondence between all mapped picornavirus antigenic sites and the observed P1 troughs of limited sequence identity. In the *Rhinovirus* polyproteins, for example, the first three segments with less than 50% identity correspond exactly to the EF loop of 1B, the BC loop of 1C, and the BC loop of 1D. Better known as Nim-II, Nim-III, and Nim-IA, respectively, these are the antigenic neutralization sites on HRV14 (18, 20) and presumably other HRVs as well. The shorter Nim-IB site in the DE loop of 1D (alignment position ~720) and the COOH end of 1D are hypervariable in all rhinoviruses. The *Enterovirus* P1 troughs, as typified by poliovirus, again correspond to the Nim sites mapped on the surface of the PV1 particle (14). Also as expected, the deepest trough in the *Aphthovirus* 1D protein (position ~950) is the antigenic "FMDV-loop" between the GH strands (1). Less dominant antigenic contributions from other foot-and-mouth disease virus (FMDV) P1 segments are consistent with this profile.

Relative to these genera, the P1 regions of *Cardiovirus* and *Hepatovirus* species are almost flat lines. The EMCV and hepatitis A virus (HAV) are both represented by multiple sequences (n = 9, n = 15, respectively), but each has only one serotype. Nevertheless, the little blips within the 1B and 1D (EMCV) and at the amino acid end of 1D (HAV) indeed denote known neutralization sites (2, 5). The theiloviruses, which share less antigenic cross-reactivity than the EMCV, have deeper troughs in the same locations, presumably from the residues that contribute to this diversity. *Teschovirus* and *Parechovirus* species have not yet been mapped for epitopes, but since the graphs mirror the sequence variability in the alignments, extrapolation from the better-known viruses clearly points to several probable antigenic sites. Tracings for the human parechovirus (HPeV) P1 region plot actually superimpose quite well with many elements of the HRV plot. In contrast, the *Teschovirus* plot suggests a prominent, immunogenic FMDV loop, as well as another very reactive site in 1B.

In several of these graphs, the P1-P2 boundary marks an apparently abrupt transition in sequence conservation. To illustrate with *Teschovirus*, the data from 30 complete polyproteins, representing 11 porcine teschovirus (PTV) serotypes (21), share an average identity of 82% in the P1 region and 97% in the P2+P3 regions. The PV (83% and 96%), human enterovirus B (HEV-B) (72% and 95%), FMDV (74% and 94%), and HPeV (81% and 92%) also have abrupt transitions. Again, it is the individual sequence patterns, not the averages, that should be of interest here. Surely, immunogenic pressures are responsible for the high mutation fixation rates in the epitope-encoding regions. That is why there is local variability in the loops. But the P1 segments between these troughs, representing internal beta-sheets or helices, have, in fact, identity values quite similar to the P2+P3 region averages. That is, the infrastructure of each genome as a whole, including internal portions of the capsid region, tends to fix mutations at a uniform rate across the species lineages. On the other hand, the nonstructural regions are not uniformly equivalent either. All the plots show the central segment of protein 2C with higher than average conservation levels. The sacrosanct region spans about 150 amino acids, with 97 to 99% averaged identity, and includes the nucleoside triphosphate binding motif (Prosite #PDOC00017, [AG]-x(4)-G-K-[ST]), which probably marks the functional core of this protein. The lower than average variability here again reflects a special selective pressure that works to moderate mutation fixation, with the goal of conserving some key structure or activity that is apparently vital for all picornaviruses.

If one looks closely, each genus shows additional regions with greater or lesser genetic stability, as reflected by variability in the alignments. The FMDV 3A region and the EMCV 2A region are among the most variable in their respective species, whereas the polio, HEV-B, and PTV 3D proteins are almost invariant. These plots and the alignments that formed them record the sum of the selective pressures that honed these segments during evolution. There is nothing new about the concept of different mutational fixation rates for different regions of a genome. The concept becomes important only when we want to accurately compare genomes or use their collective histories to retrace evolution. Family history, genus phylogeny, and relationships between and among species should be followed by using the largest possible sequence fragments that are true homologues and have developed under similar selective pressures. Stated another way, long-term relationships are best fished out of the quiet end of the gene pool. Invariant regions like 2C lend themselves to comparisons outside the family. Proteins 3B, 3C, and 3D and the beta regions of P1 have obvious shared family ancestry with similar fixation rates, and their relative mutations reasonably record the history of each genus. The chaotic mutational fixation in the epitope regions, like 1D, are better suited for following short-term associations, like strain variation during outbreaks. The remaining genome regions like L, 2A, and 3A proteins and the 5' and 3' UTRs may be analogues in their functions, but they are not always genetic homologues. These regions are the best examples of loosely structured biological synonyms that can be quite useful in ordering species within genera, or strains within species, but their informational content is very sensitive to specific genome context and is rarely directly comparable.

NUCLEOTIDE PREFERENCES

If the alignments and similarity plots tabulate the thesaurus of sequence synonyms, then base composition and codon frequency data are like dictionaries of regional dialects, reflecting nucleotide preferences and codon biases that are characteristic and diagnostic of each species. The tendency for *Hepatovirus* or *Rhinovirus* species to have overabundant A+U sequences, while the *Aphthovirus* species are rich in G+C, for example, has been well documented (16). While we stirred the picornavirus sequence pot for the new alignments, it seemed opportune to revisit these parameters along the lines of the updated family taxonomy. Base composition and codon frequency data were collected for 164 strains, representing 19 of the 20 (current) picornaviral species (11). *Porcine enterovirus A* (PEV-A, 1 kb) was excluded only because there were too few bases for reliable comparison. Within the other species, several redundant strain iterations were sometimes excluded to avoid overweighting by any particular serotype. The final dataset (919 kb total) included *Bovine enterovirus* (BEV; 23 kb), *Human enterovirus A* (HEV-A; 18 kb), *Human enterovirus B* (HEV-B; 144 kb), *Human enterovirus C* (HEV-C; 16 kb), *Human*

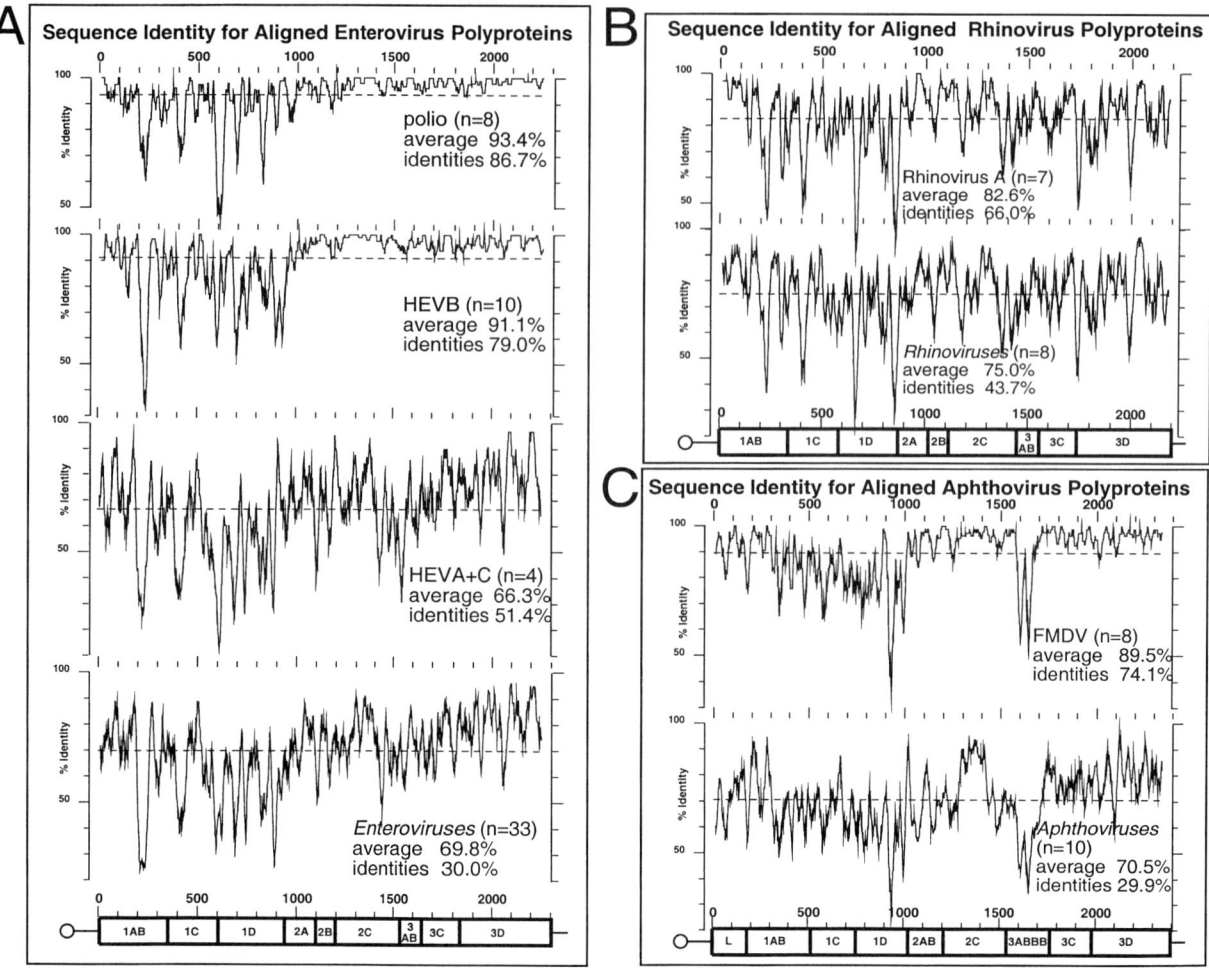

FIGURE 1 Polyprotein similarity plots. The protein alignments for picornaviral genera were culled to include only full-length sequences. The GCG program PLOTSIMILARITY calculated the average shared identity (window = 20) along the length of each alignment. The data for each genus and for separately calculated select species were plotted relative to a polyprotein map showing the cleavage site divisions and numbered according to the parental alignment columns. The dashed horizontal line and the "average" value on each plot refer to the overall identity shared among included sequences (calculated with window = 1). The "identities" value gives the percentage of alignment columns where all (n) sequences were the same. This value (occasionally) includes some locations with shared gaps, in addition to locations with identical amino acids. The Parechovirus plot is partial (1ABC only), because a full-length sequence of Ljungan virus, the type member of the LV species (GenBank: AF020521), and the only non-HPeV strain in this genus, was not available.

enterovirus D (HEV-D; 17 kb), Poliovirus (PV; 59 kb), Porcine enterovirus B (PEV-B; 7 kb), Human rhinovirus A (HRV-A; 58 kb), Human rhinovirus B (HRV-B; 10 kb), Encephalomyocarditis virus (EMCV; 77 kb), Theilovirus (ThV; 49 kb), Foot-and-mouth disease virus (FMDV; 161 kb), Equine rhinitis A virus (ERAV; 31 kb), Hepatitis A virus (HAV; 131 kb), Avian encephalomyelitis virus (AEV; 7 kb), Human parechovirus (HePV; 17 kb), Equine rhinitis B virus (ERBV; 9 kb), Porcine teschovirus (PTV; 77 kb), and Aichi virus (AiV; 8 kb). The genome base compositions [omitting 5' poly(C) tracts and 3' poly(A) tails] were very consistent within each tabulated species. The standard deviation of averaged values for any given species (e.g., %A content among all FMDV) was never greater than 2%, and more commonly, was less than 0.5%. The same was true for codon frequencies, in that the codon distribution of each sequence was closely mirrored by other members of that species. Among species, however, there was a strong skew for particular base compositions and codon frequencies (Fig. 2).

At the far end of the scale, the AiV clearly had the most anomalous composition. Although admittedly there is only one current complete sequence in this species (GenBank: AB010145), additional data from smaller 3CD-region fragments are consistent in that the C content (38%) nearly exceeds the combined purine content (19% A, 21% G) of the entire genome. Pyrimidines, therefore, make up an astonishing 62% of the AiV base count. The

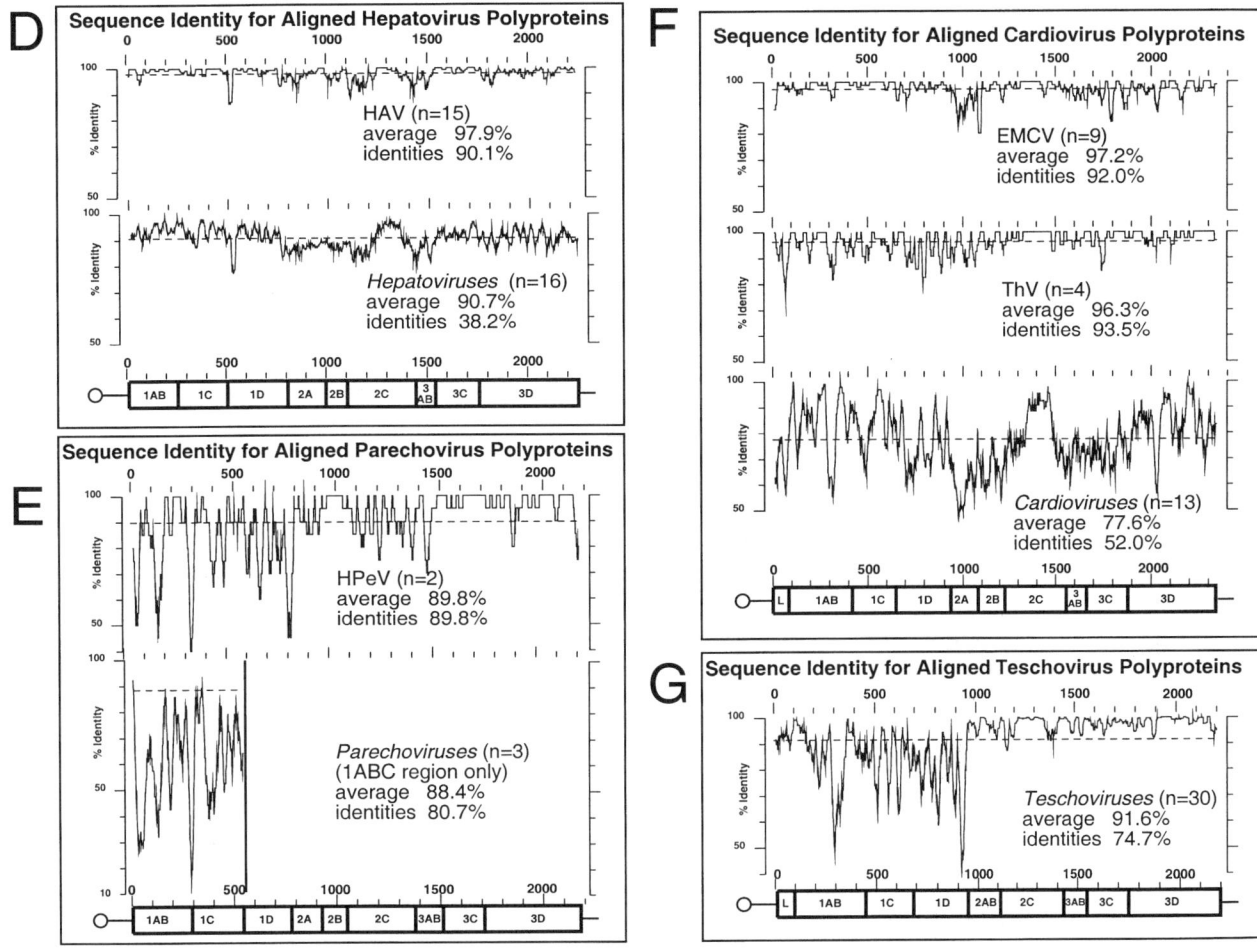

FIGURE 1 Continued

bias extends through both UTRs (A:G:C:U of 19:32:24:25%) but is most evident in the coding region, where more than half of the reading frame triplets end in C (xxA = 11%, xxG = 17%, xxC = 54%, xxU = 18%). To understand the magnitude of this extraordinary skew, it is important to remember that 5 of the 20 amino acids (Glu, Lys, Met, Gln, and Trp) representing 14% of the Aichi virus polyprotein composition cannot even be encrypted by xxC codons (e.g., Met = AUG, Lys = AAR, etc.), so the bias can only be exerted through encryption of the other 15 amino acids.

The triplet assignments in the standard genetic code are not random. The code is an evolutionary masterpiece that generally works to minimize the impact of mutational and error frequencies caused by polymerase and tRNA miscorporations. Sterically, the third codon position is the most difficult to read accurately by tRNA-mRNA pairings. Although this is the most degenerate position of the present code (perhaps originally a spacer base), more often than not, mispairings allow the same or similar amino acid to be inserted, regardless of specific nucleotide selection. The second codon position is the least error prone and probably most closely reflects the conservation of an original singlet code (4 bases, 4 amino acids), which discriminated functionality based on "inside" (hydrophobic: xCx or xUx) and "outside" (hydrophilic: xAx) amino acids.

The first position of a codon tends to signify the relative size of the encoded amino acid R-chain (small: Axx or Gxx; large: Cxx or Uxx), with a special partiality toward Gxx in eukaryotes, as a possible ribosomal proof-checking mechanism (12). Because of this codon balance, degeneracy, transitions, or errors in the first or second codon positions are likely to cause only minimum coding damage (UUA → CUA = Leu) or, at worst, permit conservative substitutions (UUA → GUA = Val). The average eukaryotic or prokaryotic protein composition tends to distribute more or less equivalently among "inside," "outside," "large," and "small" amino acids, so it is very unusual to find a significant nucleotide preference in the first two codon positions (12, 13). Among all other picornaviruses, except for AiV, this rule is generally observed, and the variance is only a few percent among other sequences in their selection of first or second codon bases (see Fig. 2). The average picornavirus ratios for Axx:Gxx:Cxx:Uxx are 30:31:19:20 (standard deviation of <4% for any base). For xAx:xGx:xCx:xUx the average ratios are 31:16:25:28 (standard deviation of <1.5% for any base). The AiV, on the other hand, has much higher than average C compositions (Cxx = 28%, xCx = 34%) at all codon bases, signifying an extraordinary selective pressure on this genome's content that carries even into the first and second codon bases as well as the third base.

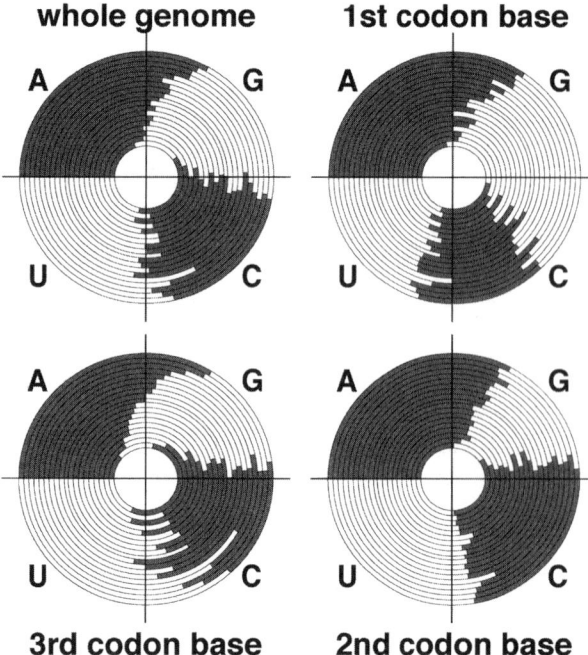

FIGURE 2 Codon and genome base compositions. Base compositions for 19 picornavirus species were summed separately, then averaged for (i) the whole genome, (ii) 1st codon base, (iii) 2nd codon base, and (iv) 3rd codon base. Each concentric ring represents an individual species, subdivided according to the averaged observed frequency (percent) of A:G:C:U. The data were sorted in ascending order by A content in the 3rd codon position, and maintain the same order in each plot: (inside ring) AiV, ThV, FMDV, ERBV, BEV, AEV, ERAV, HEV-A, EMCV, PTV, HEV-B, PV, PEV-B, HEV-C, HAV, HPeV, HEV-D, HRV-B, HRV-A (outside ring).

Other picornaviruses also have different atypical skews, though none is as dramatic as the AiV. The HAVs have high A+U content (29% and 33%) that presents as a marked preference in the third codon position (xxA = 28%, xxU = 42%, xxC = 10%) but is also influenced by an unusual underrepresentation of any codon with CG dinucleotides, such as GCG (Ala), UCG (Ser), ACG (Thr), CGX (Arg), and CCG (Pro). No codons with CG dinucleotides are used in any HAV sequence more than two to three times per reading frame, and certain codons, most notably CGG (Arg), GCG (Ala), and CCG (Pro), are excluded entirely from many genomes. *Rhinovirus* species (HRV-A and HRV-B) have similar prejudices in their preference for high A+U content, but with the ratios reversed (A = 31%, U = 29%). Again, these genomes discriminate against CGG (Arg), CCG (Pro), UCG (Ser), ACG (Thr), and GCG (Ala) codons, selecting nearly any alternative synonymous triplet at a 50- to 60-fold higher frequency than those with CG dinucleotides. The CGG (Arg), UCG (Thr), and CCG (Pro) codons are absent from most HRV sequences, and none is used more than 20 times in total among the 21,000 codons surveyed for this genus. At the other end of the scale, the FMDV has high G+C contents and favors codons ending with these bases (xxG = 27%, xxC = 37%). Consequently, the FMDV shuns a different cohort of triplets, like CUA (Leu), GUA (Val), UUA (Leu), and AUA (Ile), but is rich in CG-containing codons. Each species of *Cardiovirus, Enterovirus, Parechovirus,* and *Teschovirus* likewise can be seen to have individual characteristics that border on diagnostic, with regard to base and codon preferences. The ThV prefers U+C in the third codon position; the AEV prefers U but not C; the PV and EMCV are reasonably equivalent in their base distributions, etc.

So why should we care about these sequence tendencies? Evolution leaves its fingerprints on every page in the book of life. The clustering of base compositions and codon preferences are telling us volumes about shared lineages among viral strains, just like gene maps, IRES types, and proteolytic processing schemes are recognized predictors of familial homology. The peculiar pressures or bottlenecks that shaped one genome will have also shaped its brethren and progeny. It is hard to imagine any biological situation that would favor 54% of the codons ending in C, but in truth, even stranger skews are common in other organisms. The sequence of *Microplasma capricolum* is 25% G+C, while that of *Micrococcus leuteus* is 75% G+C (12). Originally thought to be a logical adaptation to growth temperature, most evidence now suggests that genome G+C content is more closely related to phylogeny (6) and follows whatever twisted history was survived by the parental lineage. In the prokaryotes, the presence of mutagens, suboptimal polymerase base preferences, defective repair mechanisms, or other directional mutational pressures are known to vary considerably among phylogenetic lines, and each of these pressures can contribute to a different mutational fixation rate that manifests in characteristic composition preferences (12). However bizarre the outcome, we are formed by the trials and cultures that were survived by our parents.

For eukaryotes, there is very little information about the specific pressures that might shape a given lineage. Certainly, the symmetrical methylation of CG dinucleotides has a unique structural significance in many higher DNA genomes, reducing the value and frequency of this sequence in coding regions (8). There would be no reason for a cell to support CG codons if they were not present in their own mRNAs. Moreover, unlike prokaryotes, where entire genomes usually skew as a unit, the chromosomes of vertebrates are complex mosaics of G+C-rich regions and G+C-poor regions. Eukaryotic replication occurs in multiple phases, and each phase can use different enzymes, with the G+C-rich regions generally copied before the G+C-poor regions, in every cell cycle (6). The repertoire of required tRNAs needed to translate expressed messages must therefore follow these cycles, particularly in cells with slow division times, like neurons. In short, the cumulative environment of A+U and G+C pressures can vary widely among vertebrates and tissues according to host age and cell cycle timing. We should not be surprised that our viruses adapt to these circumstances; we should only regret that we do not yet understand what these tendencies are telling us about their niches.

Comparative sequence analyses of picornaviruses are supported by NIH grant AI-17331 to A. C. Palmenberg.

REFERENCES

1. **Barnett, P. V., E. J. Ouldridge, D. J. Rowlands, F. Brown, and N. R. Parry.** 1989. Neutralizing epitopes of type O foot-and-mouth disease virus. I. Identification and characterization of three functionally independent, conformational sites. *J. Gen. Virol.* **70:**1483–1491.

2. **Boege, U., S. Onodera, D. G. Scraba, G. D. Parks, and A. C. Palmenberg.** 1991. Characterization of Mengo virus neutralization epitopes. *Virology* **181:**1–13.
3. **Drake, N. L., A. C. Palmenberg, A. Ghosh, D. R. Omilianowski, and P. Kaesberg.** 1982. Identification of the polyprotein termination site on encephalomyocarditis viral RNA. *J. Virol.* **41:**736–729.
4. **Eddy, S. R.** 1998. Profile hidden Markov models. *Bioinformatics* **14:**755–763.
5. **Emini, E. A., J. V. Hughes, D. S. Perlow, and J. Boger.** 1985. Induction of hepatitis A virus-neutralizing antibody by a virus-specific synthetic peptide. *J. Virol.* **55:**836–839.
6. **Filipski, J.** 1991. Evolution of DNA sequences. Contribution of mutational bias and selection to the origin of chromosomal compartments. *Adv. Mutagen. Res.* **2:**1–54.
7. **Gribskov, M., and S. Veretnik.** 1996. Identification of sequence patterns with profile analysis. *Methods Enzymol.* **266:**198–212.
8. **Herbert, A., and A. Rich.** 1996. Topology and formation of left-handed Z-DNA. *J. Biol. Chem.* **271:**11595–11598.
9. **Horsnell, C., R. E. Gama, P. J. Hughes, and G. Stanway.** 1995. Molecular relationships between 21 human rhinovirus serotypes. *J. Gen. Virol.* **76:**2549–2555.
10. **King, A. M. Q., F. Brown, P. Christian, T. Hovi, T. Hyypiä, N. J. Knowles, S. M. Lemon, P. D. Minor, A. C. Palmenberg, T. Skern, and G. Stanway.** 2000. Picornaviridae, p. 657–678. *In Anonymous Virus Taxonomy. Seventh Report of the International Committee for the Taxonomy of Viruses.* Academic Press, New York, N.Y.
11. **Kitamura, N., and E. Wimmer.** 1980. Sequence of 1060 3′-terminal nucleotides of poliovirus RNA as determined by a modification of the dideoxynucleotide method. *Proc. Natl. Acad. Sci. USA* **77:**3196–3200.
12. **Osawa, S.** 1995. *Evolution of the Genetic Code.* Oxford University Press, New York, N.Y.
13. **Osawa, S., T. H. Jukes, K. Watanabe, and A. Muto.** 1992. Recent evidence for evolution of the genetic code. *Microbiol. Rev.* **56:**299–264.
14. **Page, G. S., A. G. Mosser, J. M. Hogle, D. J. Filman, R. R. Rueckert, and M. Chow.** 1988. Three-dimensional structure of poliovirus serotype 1 neutralizing determinants. *J. Virol.* **62:**1781–1794.
15. **Palmenberg, A. C.** 1987. Genome organization, translation and processing in picornaviruses, p. 1–15. *In* D. J. Rolands, B. W. J. Mahy, and M. Mayo (ed.), *The Molecular Biology of Positive Strand RNA Viruses.* Academic Press, London, United Kingdom.
16. **Palmenberg, A. C.** 1989. Sequence alignments of picornaviral capsid proteins, p. 211–241. *In* B. Semler and E. Ehrenfeld (ed.), *Molecular Aspects of Picornavirus Infection and Detection.* ASM Press, Washington, D.C.
17. **Palmenberg, A. C., and J.-Y. Sgro.** 1997. Topological organization of picornaviral genomes: statistical prediction of RNA structural signals. *Semin. Virol.* **8:**231–241.
18. **Rossmann, M. G., E. Arnold, J. W. Erickson, E. A. Frankenberger, J. P. Griffith, H.-J. Hecht, J. E. Johnson, G. Kamer, M. Luo, A. G. Mosser, R. R. Rueckert, B. Sherry, and G. Vriend.** 1985. The structure of a human common cold virus (rhinovirus 14) and its functional relations to other picornaviruses. *Nature* **317:**145–153.
19. **Ryan, M. D., and M. Flint.** 1997. Virus-encoded proteinases of the picornavirus supergroup. *J. Gen. Virol.* **78:**699–723.
20. **Sherry, B., A. G. Mosser, R. J. Colonno, and R. R. Rueckert.** 1986. Use of monoclonal antibodies to identify four neutralization immunogens on a common cold picornavirus, human rhinovirus 14. *J. Virol.* **57:**246–257.
21. **Zell, R., M. Dauber, A. Krumbholz, A. Henke, E. Birch-Hirschfeld, A. Stelzner, D. Prager, and R. Wurm.** 2001. Porcine teschovirus comprise at least eleven distinct serotypes: molecular and evolutionary aspects. *J. Virol.* **75:**1620–1631.

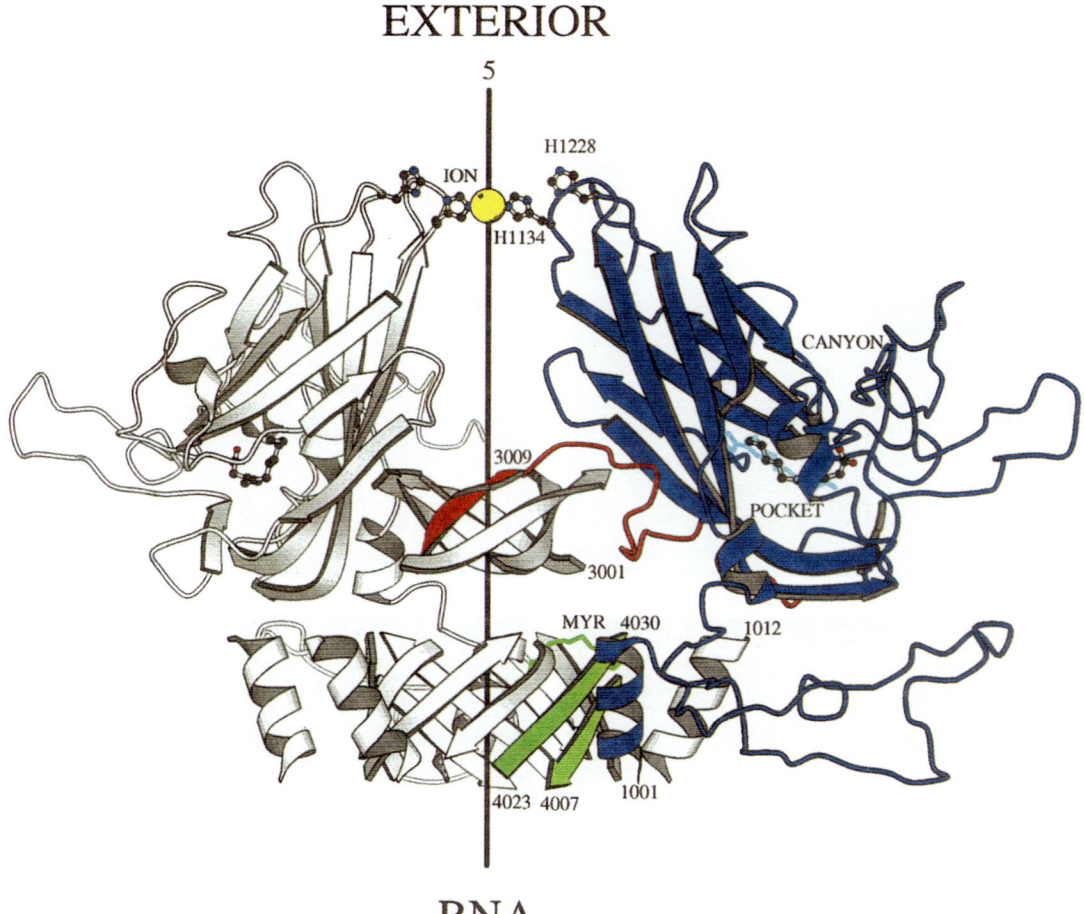

Color Plate 1 [chapter 3] A schematic diagram created using MOLSCRIPT (58) representing VP1 of HRV16, showing the binding site of the pocket factor (ball-and-stick representation) and the WIN antiviral compounds (pale blue). A cation on the fivefold axis is shown in yellow. The N termini of VP1, VP3, and VP4 interact around the fivefold axis. One copy of each of VP1 and the N termini of VP3 and VP4 are shown as blue, red, and green ribbon diagrams, respectively. The myristoylated N terminus of VP4 is labeled (MYR). Reprinted with permission from Hadfield et al. (39).

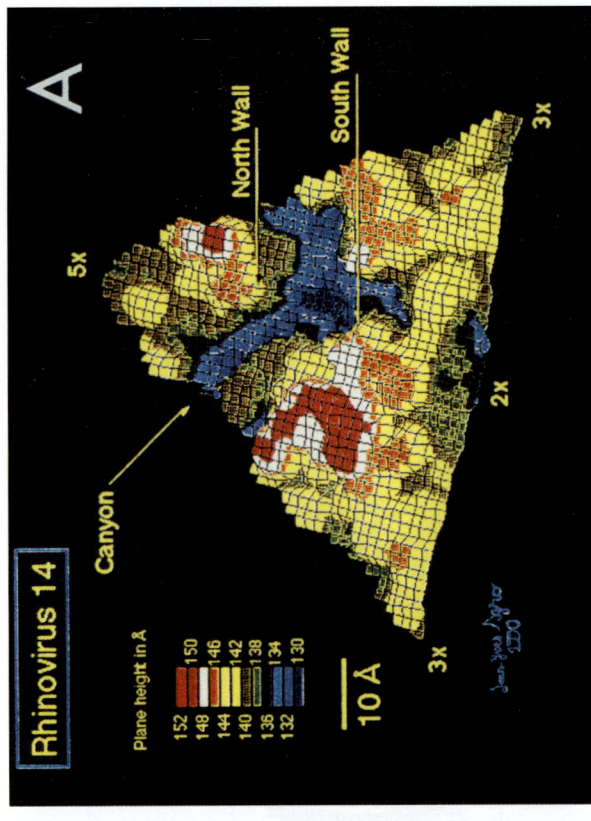
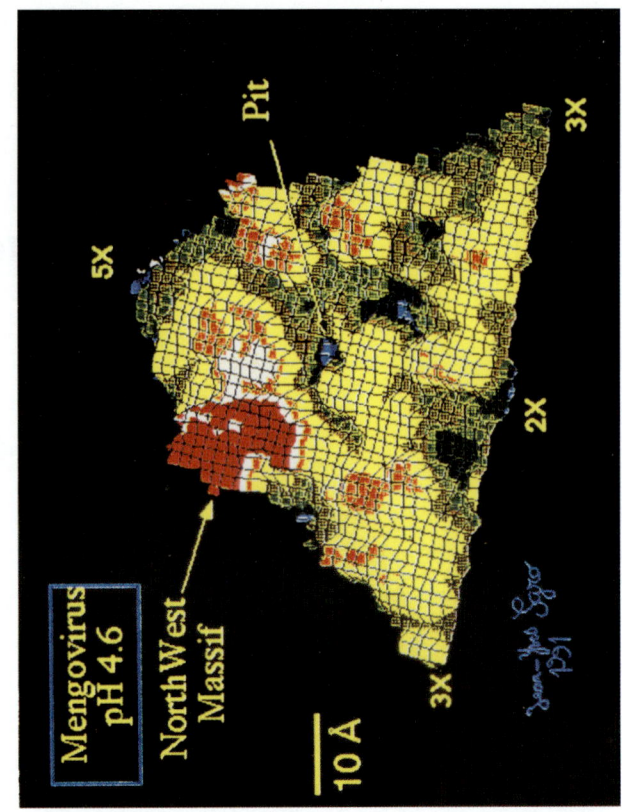
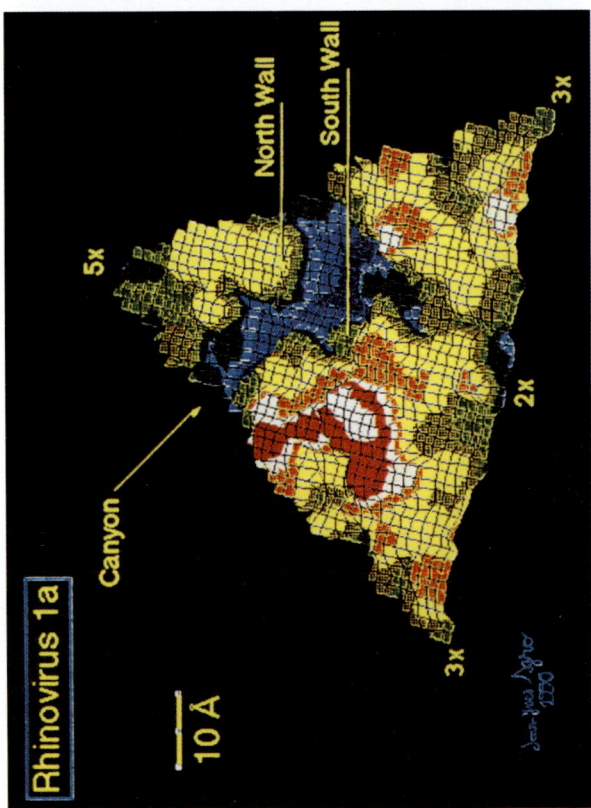
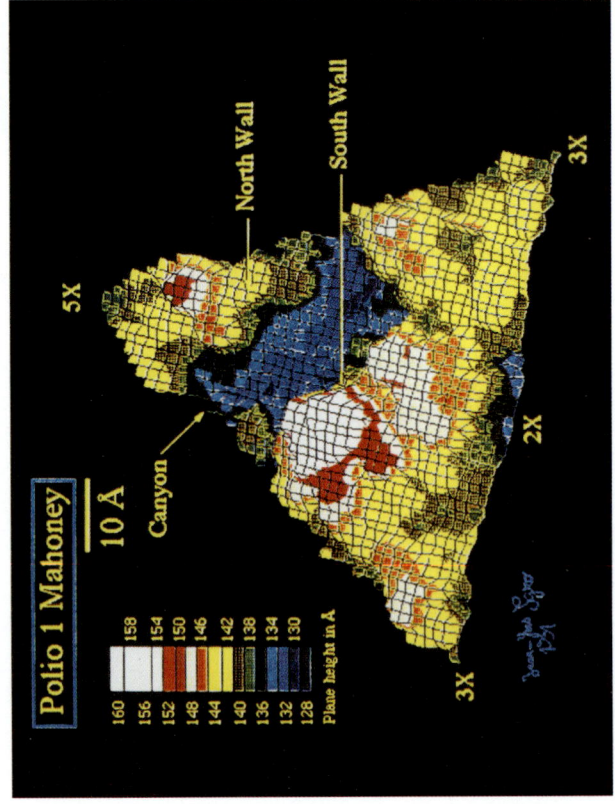

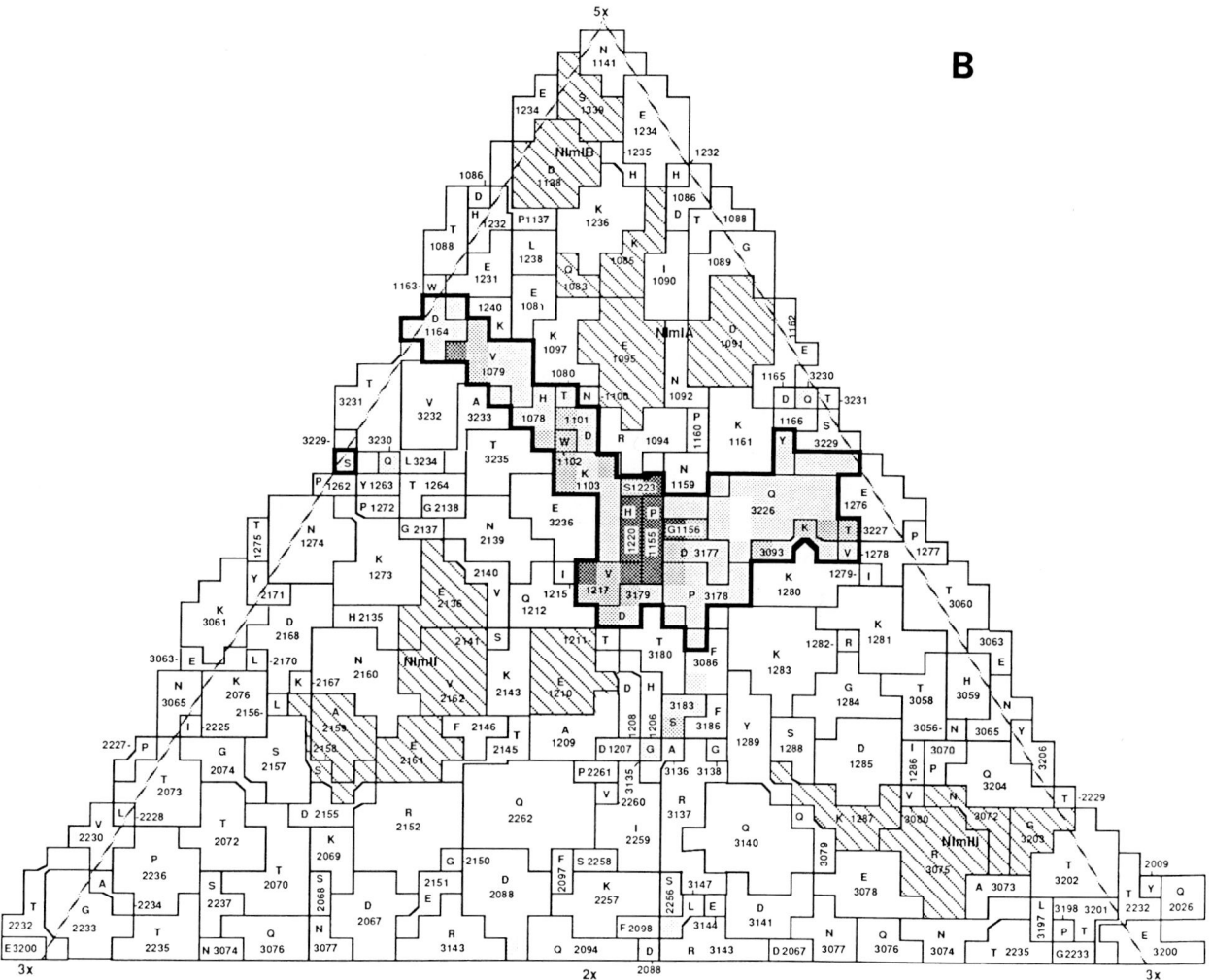

Color Plate 2 [chapter 3] Different types of representations possible with "roadmaps." The triangle represents one icosahedral asymmetric unit. The viral surface is projected onto a plane perpendicular to one icosahedral axis placed normal to the page. (A) Surface topographies of various picornaviruses: HRV1A (56), HRV14 (87), poliovirus 1 Mahoney (51), and mengovirus (74). The colors show the distance from the viral center, where blue is "low lying seas" and white is "high mountains." Images were supplied by Dr. Jean-Yves Sgro (University of Wisconsin, Madison, http://www.bocklabs.wisc.edu/topo.html). Reprinted with permission from Rotbart and Kirkegaard (90). (B) The surface of HRV14 showing the exposed areas of each amino acid in one icosahedral asymmetric unit. Residues involved in neutralizing immunogenic sites are hatched. Reprinted with permission from Rossmann and Palmenberg (89).

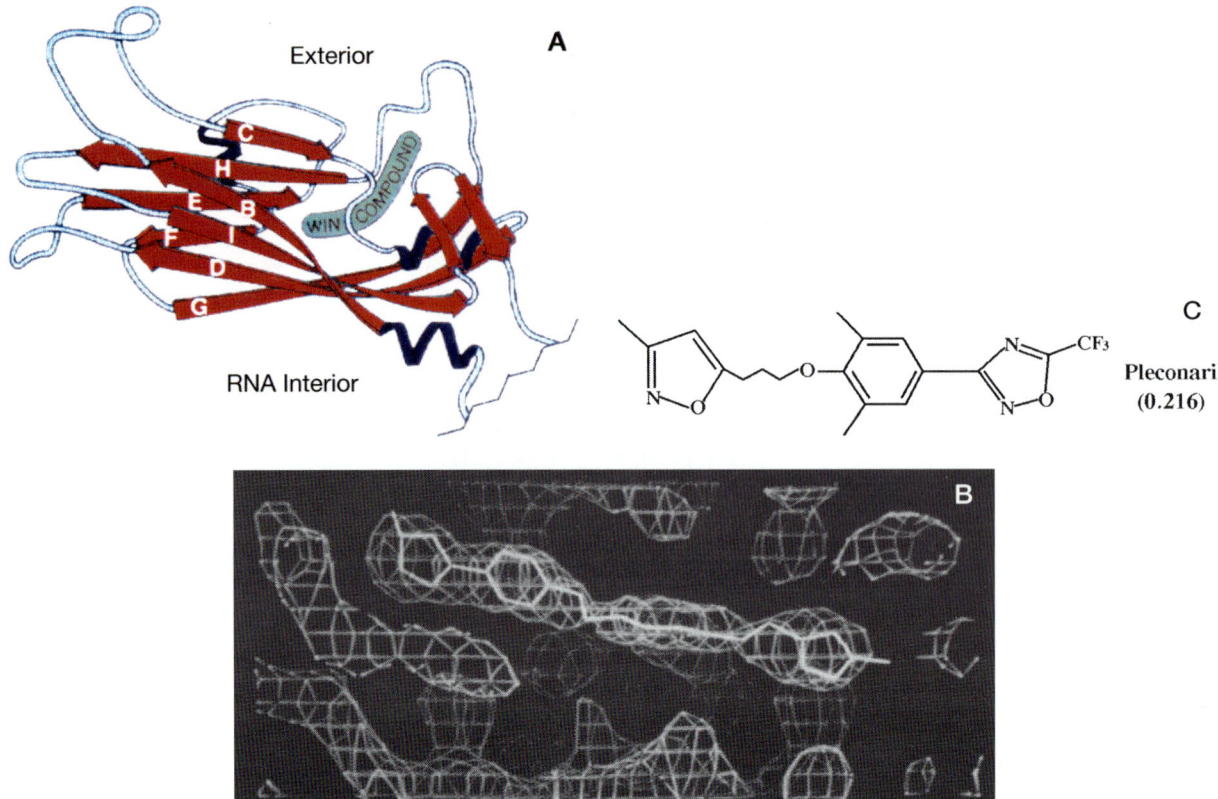

Color Plate 3 [chapter 3] Antiviral compounds bound to picornaviruses: (A) Diagrammatic representation of an antiviral compound binding within the β-barrel of VP1. (B) Electron density, at 3.0 Å resolution, of HRV14 complexed with the antiviral agent WIN 52084. This and related compounds stabilize the virus to inhibit uncoating and can also inhibit attachment. Shown is the molecular interpretation of the electron density. The compound consists of a 4-oxazaolinylphenoxy group linked to a 3-methylisoxazole group by a seven-membered aliphatic chain. The compound binds into a hydrophobic pocket in VP1 that is lined by residues that are moderately well conserved among picornaviruses. Reprinted with permission from Smith et al. (98). (C) Chemical structure of pleconaril, the compound possibly to be marketed by ViroPharma, Inc.

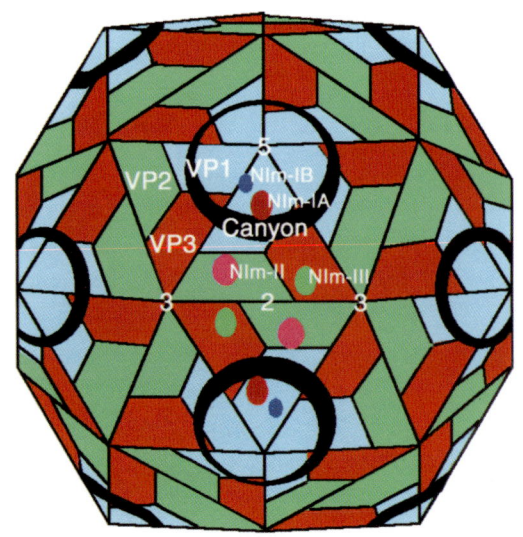

Color Plate 4 [chapter 4] Architecture of rhinovirus 14. A schematic of HRV14 is shown with the various NIm sites and canyon region labeled. VP1 to 3 are colored blue, green, and red, respectively. The four NIm sites are colored according to the scheme used in Color Plate 7A. The canyon regions are approximated by the black circles drawn around each fivefold axis.

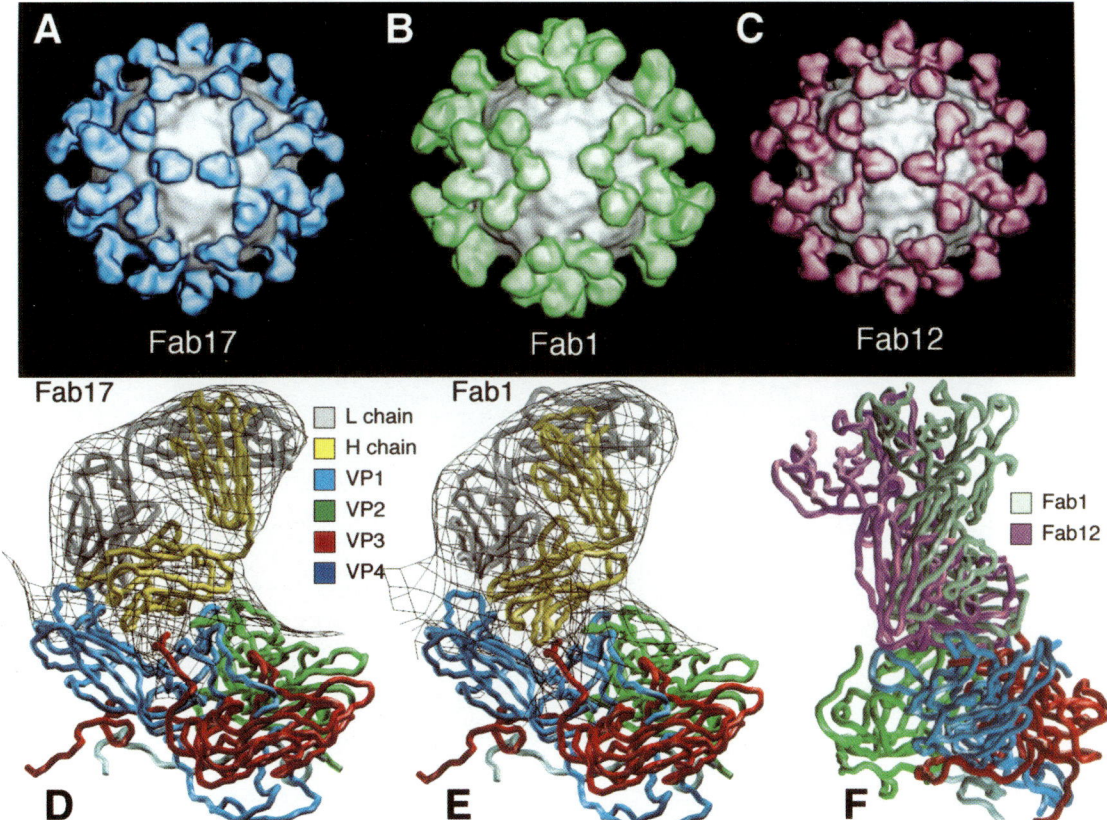

Color Plate 5 [chapter 4] Cryo-TEM analysis of HRV14 complexed with Fab17, Fab12, Fab1, and mAb17. The reconstructions of Fab17, Fab1, and Fab12 are shown in panels A to C, respectively. The virus surface is colored gray, and the antibodies are highlighted with various colors. The fitting of Fab17 and Fab1 structures into the cryo-TEM electron density is shown in panels D and E. The view here is parallel to the canyon region with the fivefold axis on the left, the twofold axis on the right, and the RNA interior on the bottom. Panel F shows an overlay of the Fab1 (green) versus Fab12 (mauve) viewed from the fivefold axis toward the twofold axis. Reprinted from the *Journal of Virology* (9) with permission from publisher.

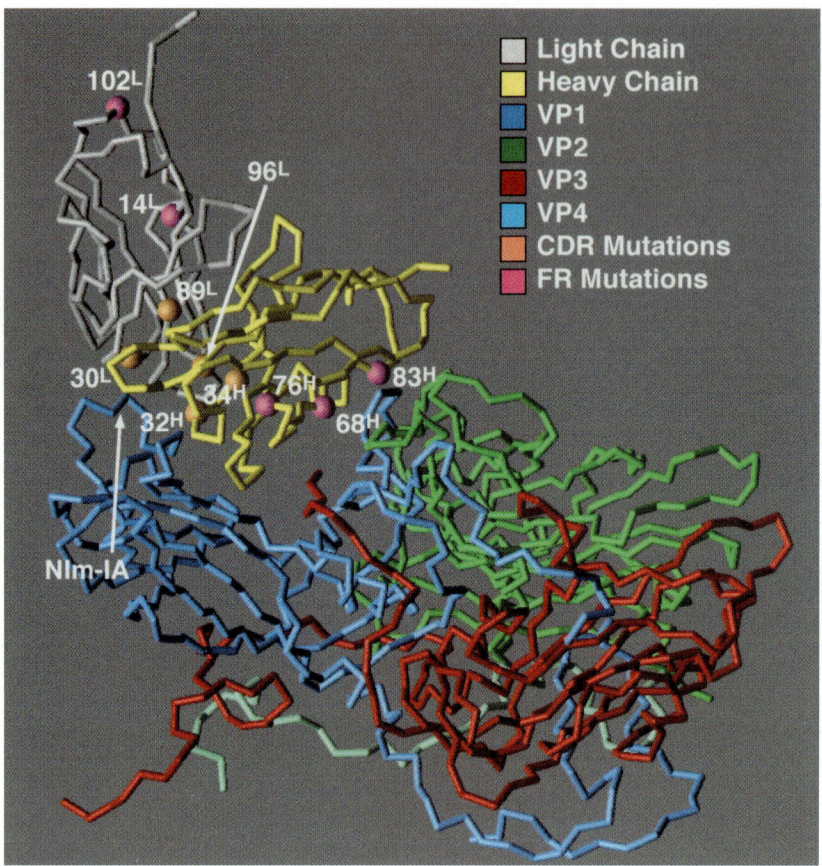

Color Plate 6 [chapter 4] Crystal structure of the Fab17-HRV14 complex. The V_H, V_L, VP1, VP2, VP3, and VP4 C-α backbones are represented by yellow, white, blue, green, red, and cyan, respectively. The differences in the Fab12 and Fab17 sequences are represented by mauve balls in the framework regions, and mutations in the CDR regions are represented by yellow balls. The view here is the same as that in Color Plate 5D and E. Note the penetration of the Fab into the canyon and the extensive contact along the south wall (the right side of the central depression). Reprinted from the *Journal of Virology* (9) with permission from publisher.

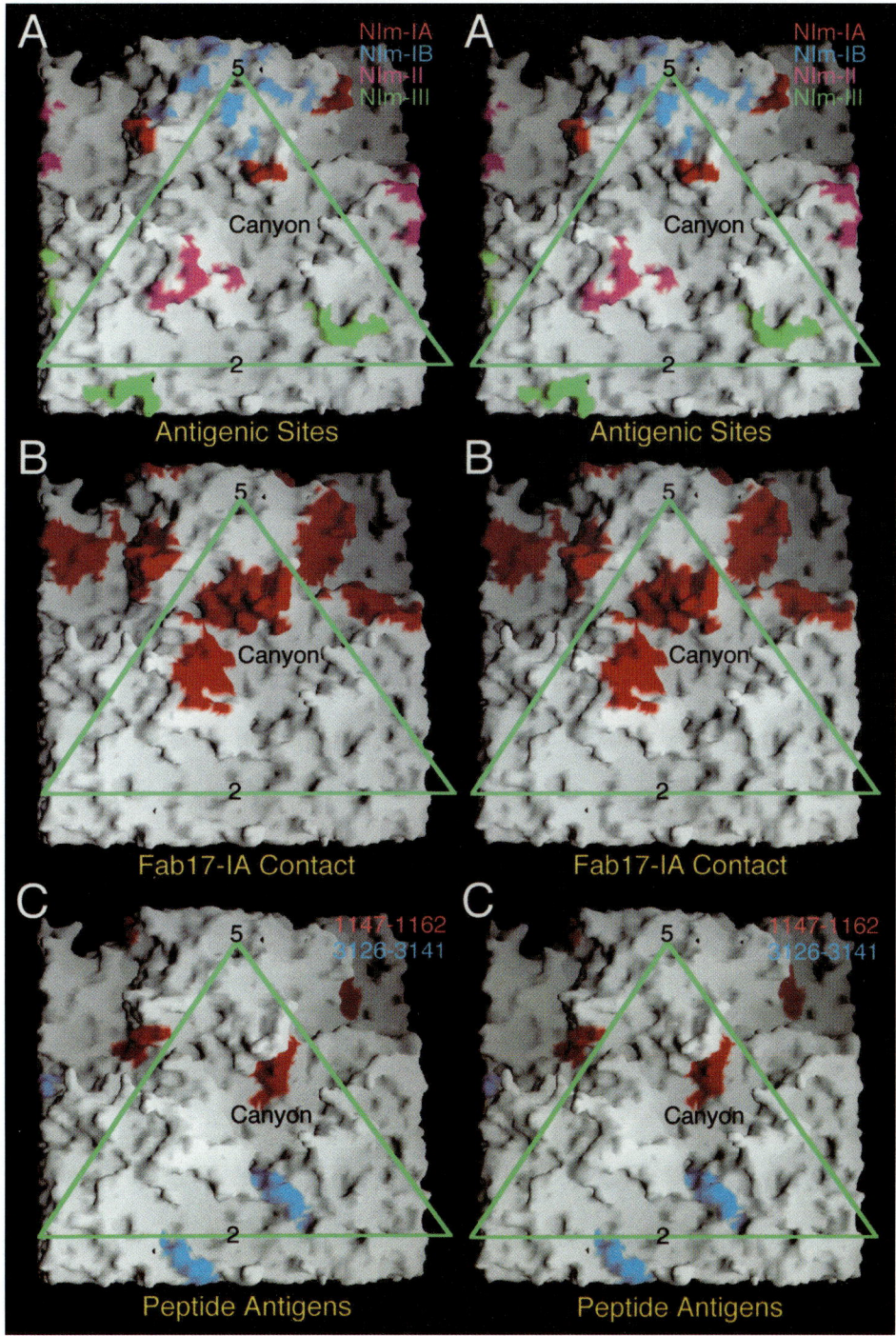

Color Plate 7 [chapter 4] Stereo images of the various locations mapped onto the surface of HRV14. In panel A the NIm sites are mapped onto a portion of the HRV14 surface. The icosahedral asymmetric unit is denoted by the green triangle and the locations of the five- and twofold axes are labeled. Panel B shows the Fab17 contact area in red. Panel C shows the surface locations of the two peptides used to elicit antibodies that exhibited cross-reactivity to several rhinovirus serotypes.

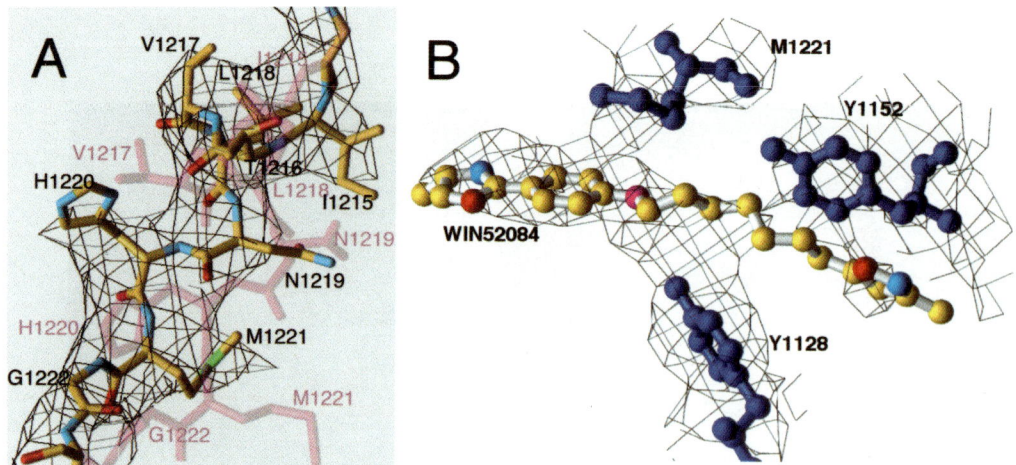

Color Plate 8 [chapter 4] Pocket factor in the HRV14-Fab17 complex. This figure shows the VP1 strand immediately above the drug pocket that moves upon binding WIN drugs (A) and the pocket factor density observed in the Fab-HRV14 crystals structure. (A) The black cage represents the electron density of this region in the Fab17-HRV14 crystal structure. The transparent mauve model is the native HRV14 structure, and the stick model (colored by atom type) is taken from the WIN-HRV14 structure. (B) The density beneath this conformational change with the WIN compound (represented by the multicolored ball and stick model) is shown as a positional reference. Some of the nearby side chains are represented by the blue ball and stick models.

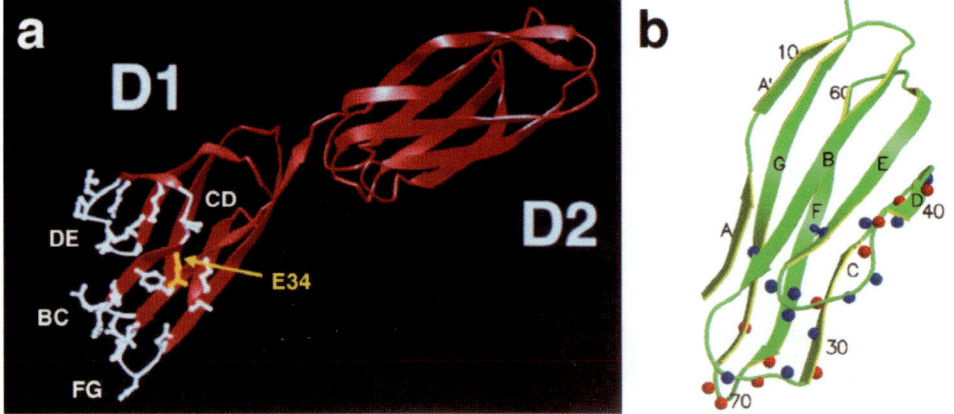

Color Plate 9 [chapter 8] (a) The ribbon diagram of ICAM-1 domains D1 and D2. The residues and loops that penetrate into the HRV canyon are colored white. Glu34, essential for LFA-1 binding, is shown in yellow. Note the elbow angle that relates the two domains. (b) Important contact residues for HRV and coxsackievirus A21 in the D1 domain. The β-strands are labeled A through G. The amino acids identified as being in the virus-receptor interface are indicated by spheres. ICAM-1 residues in contact with HRV14 and HRV16 are colored blue, while ICAM-1 residues in contact with coxsackievirus A21 are indicated in red. Modified from the *Proceedings of the National Academy of Sciences, U.S.A.* (2) with permission of the publisher.

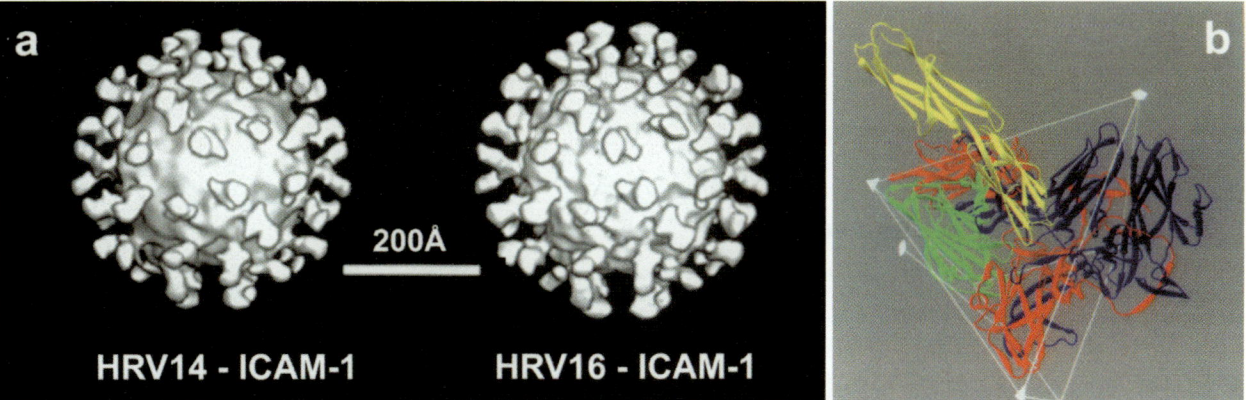

Color Plate 10 [chapter 8] (a) Cryo-EM image reconstructions of complexes between HRV14 or HRV16 and soluble D1D2 of ICAM-1 at 26 Å resolution. (b) Ribbon diagram showing the interaction of ICAM-1 (yellow) and HRV16. HRV16 proteins VP1, VP2, and VP3 are in blue, green, and red, respectively. Two symmetry-related VP1s and VP3s are shown. Some icosahedral symmetry elements and the boundary of an icosahedral asymmetric unit are shown.

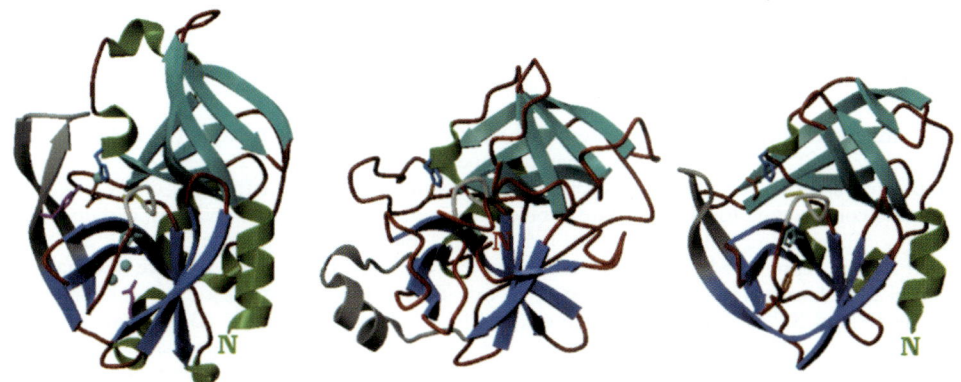

Color Plate 11 [chapter 17] Comparison of the structures of HAV 3C^{pro}, α-chymotrypsin, and PV1 3C^{pro}. Secondary structural ribbon diagrams of HAV 3C^{pro} (left), α-chymotrypsin (center), and PV1 3C^{pro} (right). The N-terminal β-barrels are represented by the cyan-colored arrows, C-terminal β-barrels by lilac arrows. The extensions in PV1 and HAV 3C^{pro} to β-strands bII1 and cII that do not form part of the β-barrels are shown in gray; the corresponding region in chymotrypsin (the "methionine loop") is also shown in gray. Helices are represented by green spiral ribbons and connecting loops by red tubes. The white segments in each of the representations denote the oxy-anion hole. The side chains of the catalytic residues (Ser, His, and Asp in α-chymotrypsin; Cys, His, and Glu in PV1-3C^{pro}; and Cys, His, H$_2$O, Asp, and Tyr in HAV 3C^{pro}) are represented in each molecule. The His161 (PV1) and His191 (HAV) of the S1 pockets of PV1 3C^{pro} and HAV 3C^{pro} that determine the cleavage specificity for P1 Gln in substrates are shown in light blue. All three molecules are represented from approximately the same vantage point.

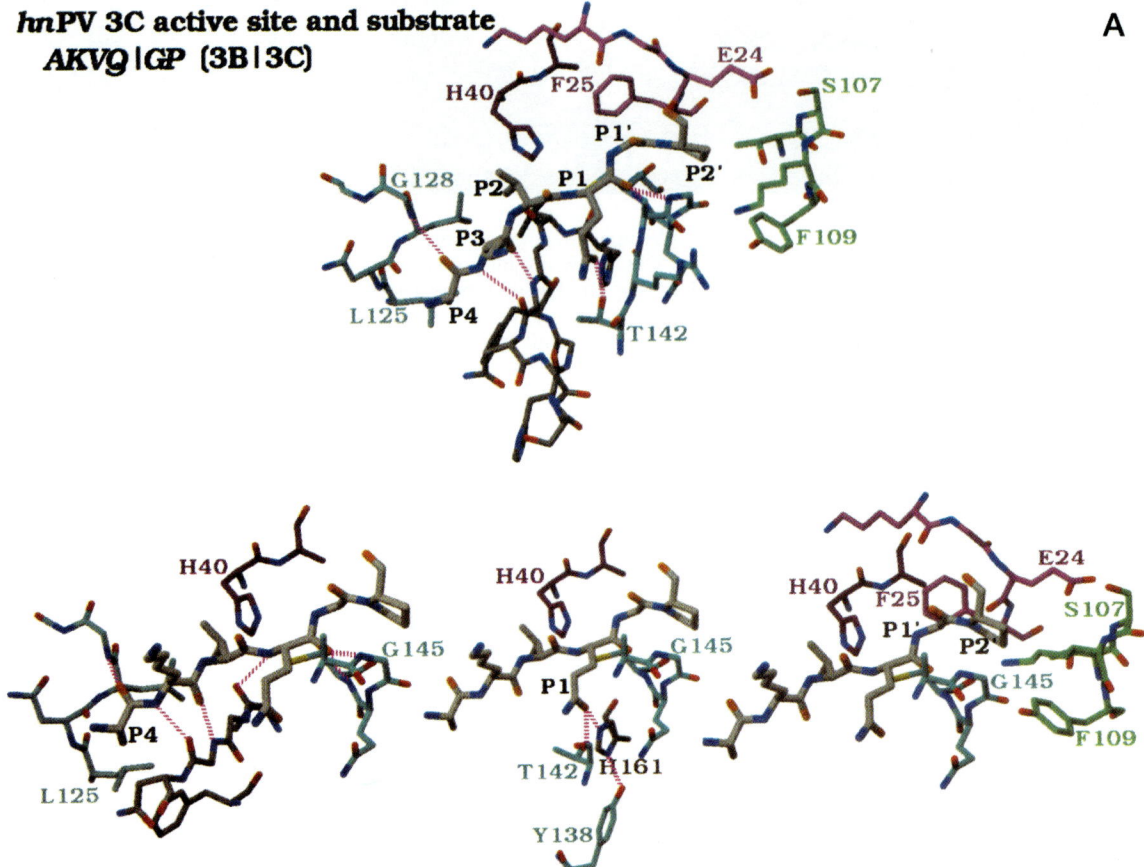

Color Plate 12 [chapter 17] Comparison of the active sites of (A) PV1 3C^{pro}, (B) HAV 3C^{pro}, and (C) HRV2 3C^{pro}. (A) A computer-generated model of residues P4 to P2' of Ala-Lys-Val-Gln-Gly-Pro (cleavage site between 3B and 3C of the polyprotein) in the active site of PV1-3C^{pro}. The atomic color coding for the substrate is blue, nitrogen; orange, oxygen; and gray, carbon. For the enzyme, color coding is blue, nitrogen; red, oxygen; the residues forming subsites S4, S2, S1, S1', and S2' are represented by different colors for the C atoms. Hydrogen bonds are designated by dashed lines between donor and acceptor atoms. Three close-ups of the subsites are shown below; S4/P4 and S2/P2 (left); S1/P1 (center); S1'/P1' and S2'/P2' (right). (B) A view of the computer-generated HAV-3C^{pro}/substrate model. The color schemes are the same as those shown in panel A. The substrate was generated from the residues of the cleavage site between VP1 and 2B of the HAV polyprotein (Leu-Phe-Ser-Gln-Ala-Lys). Hydrogen bonds are represented by dashed lines between donor and acceptor atoms. The three lower portions of the figure represent close-up views of the atomic interactions between S4/P4 and S2/P2 (left); S1/P1 (center); S1'/P1' and S2'/P2' (right). (C) A view of AG7088, a Michael addition adduct, bound in the active site of HRV2-3C^{pro} (57). The atom coloring for the inhibitor and enzyme is the same as that used in panel A. The hydrogen bonds between donor and acceptor atoms are represented by dashed lines. This inhibitor is covalently attached to the sulfur atom of Cys147.

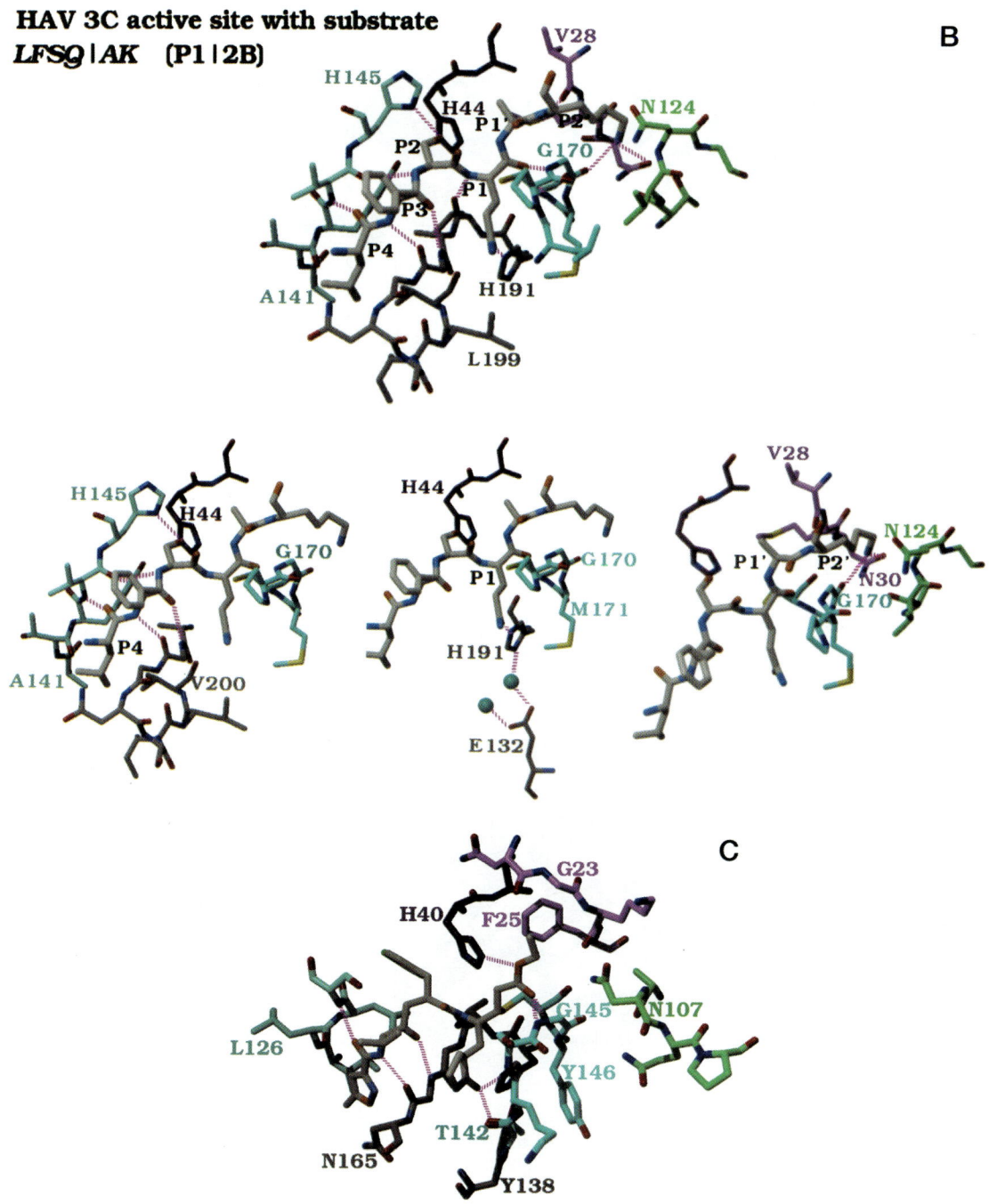

Color Plate 12 *Continued*

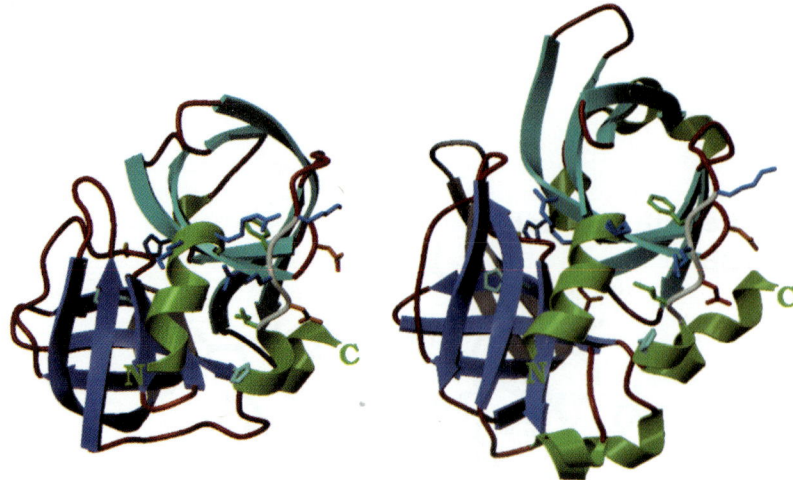

Color Plate 13 [chapter 17] RNA-binding sites on PV1-3C^{pro} (left) and on HAV-3C^{pro} (right). The segments of secondary structure are colored as in Color Plate 11. The backbone of the conserved sequence Lys-Phe-Arg-Asp-Ile is colored gray with the side chains represented (Lys and Arg, blue; Phe and Ile, green; Asp, red). The conserved segment is flanked by the two helices on the N and C termini of the molecules.

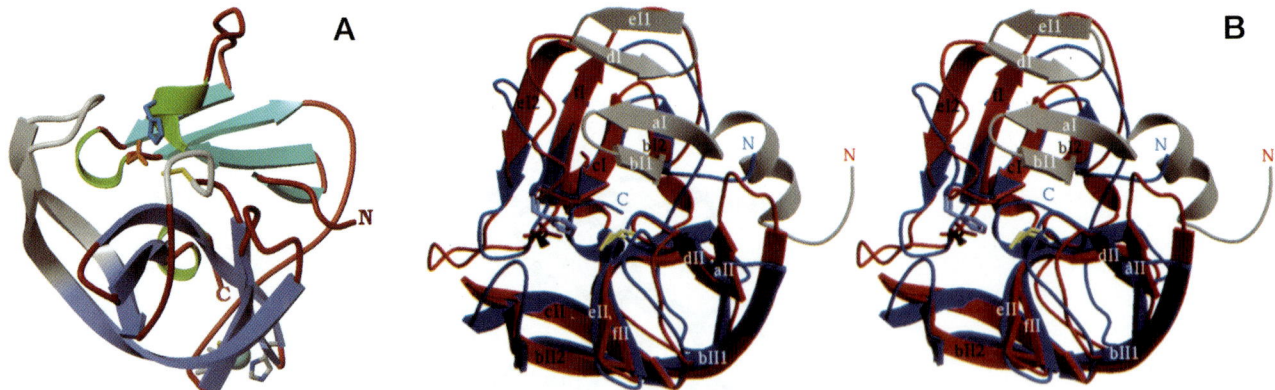

Color Plate 14 [chapter 17] The structure of HRV2 2A^{pro}. (A) A view of the HRV2-2A^{pro} showing the secondary structural units (arrows for β-strands, linking peptide segments as red tubing). The strands of the N-terminal domain are colored in cyan, those of the C-terminal domain are in lilac. The extensions to β-strands bII and cII that contain the dityrosine loop are shown in gray. Helical turns are shown as green spiral ribbons. Residues in the active site Cys106, His18, and Asp35 are represented. The Zn^{2+} binding site is also shown with the liganding residues Cys52, Cys54 and Cys112, His114 on the back side of the molecule. The Zn^{2+} is shown as a light blue sphere. The N and C termini are labeled N and C, respectively. (B) A stereodiagram showing the structural alignment of PV1-3C^{pro} (red) and HRV2-2A^{pro} (blue). The strands are labeled according to the topology of PV1 3C^{pro}. Strand labels in the N-terminal domain have the roman numeral I appended; strand labels in the C-terminal domain have the roman numeral II appended. Secondary structural elements of PV1 3C^{pro} that are missing in HRV2-2A^{pro} are colored in gray.

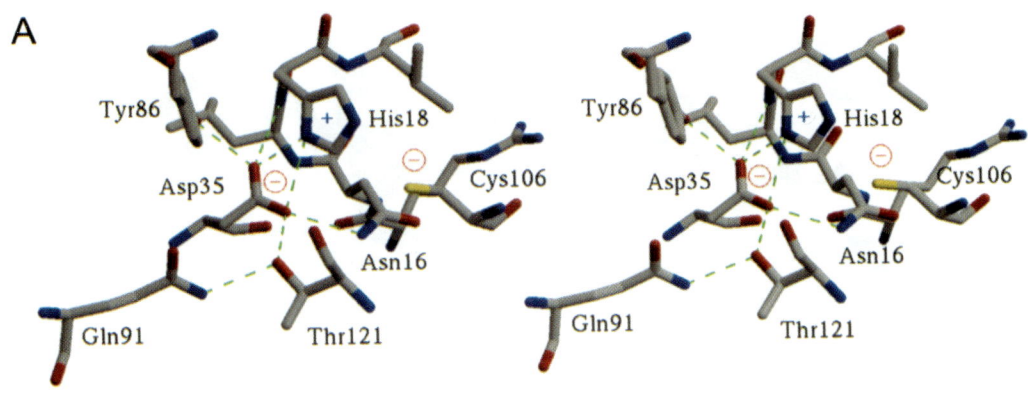

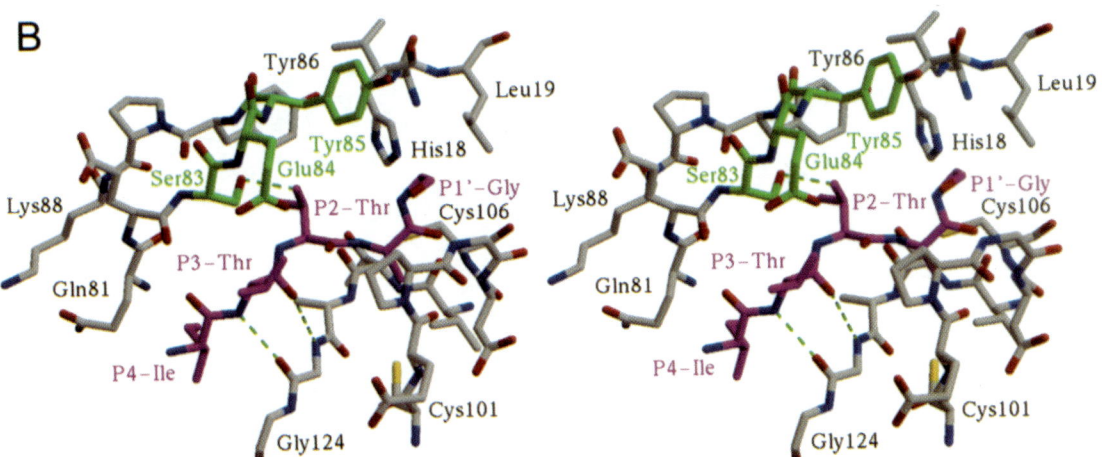

Color Plate 15 [chapter 17] The active site of HRV2 2A^pro. (A) Stereodrawing showing the region around the active site of HRV2-2A^pro. Carbon atoms are colored gray; nitrogen atoms, blue; and oxygen atoms, red. The sulfur of Cys106 is colored yellow. Probable charge status of the residues is indicated. Hydrogen bonds between donor and acceptor atoms are represented by dashed lines. (B) Stereorepresentation of a model of an oligopeptide substrate (purple) occupying subsite S4 to S1′. The pentapeptide corresponds to the sequence of the polyprotein at the junction of VP1 and 2A (-Ile-Thr-Thr-Ala-Gly-). Hydrogen bonds between the substrate and HRV2-2A^pro are represented by dashed lines. Reprinted from the *EMBO Journal* (67) with permission of the publisher.

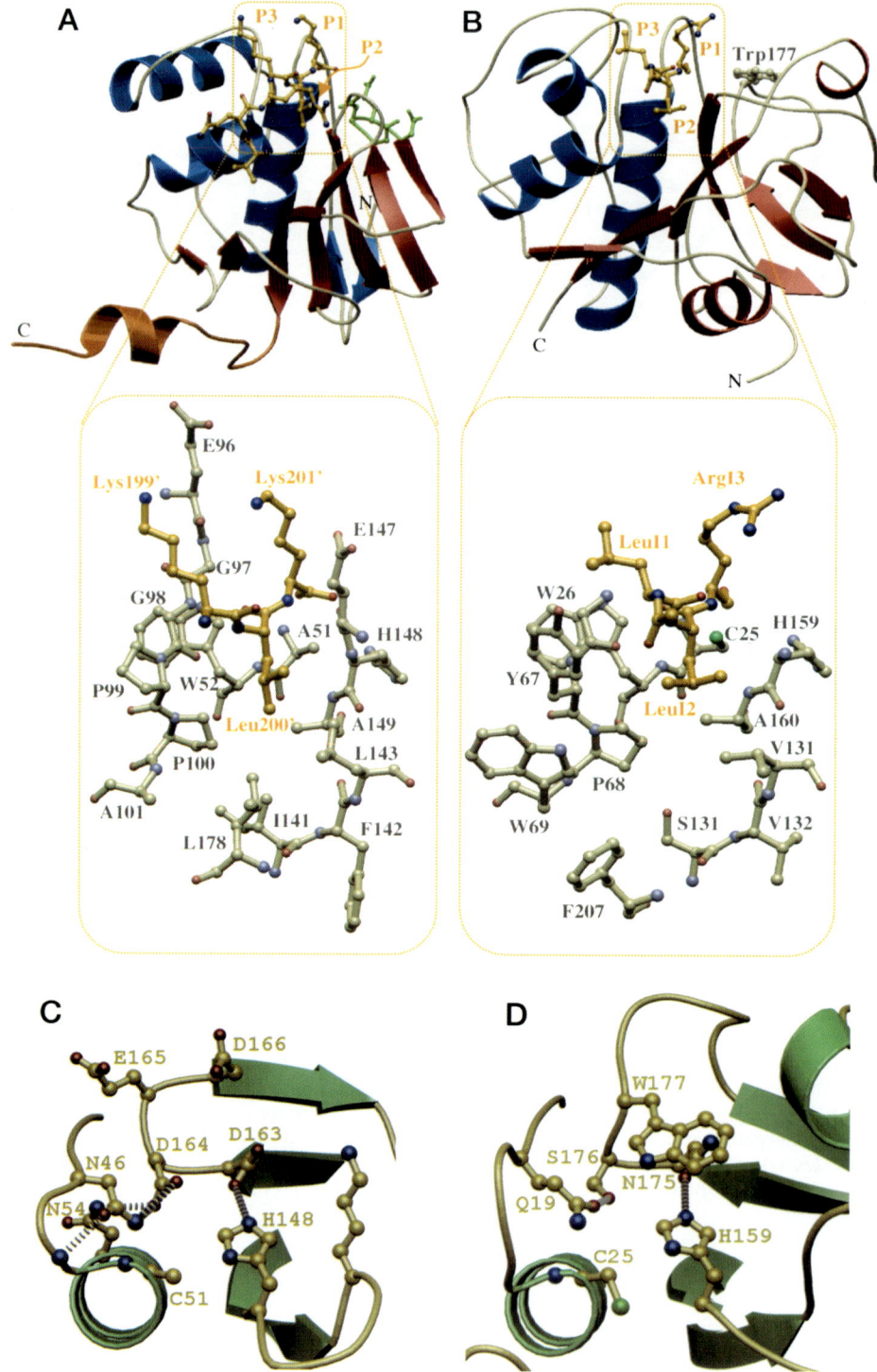

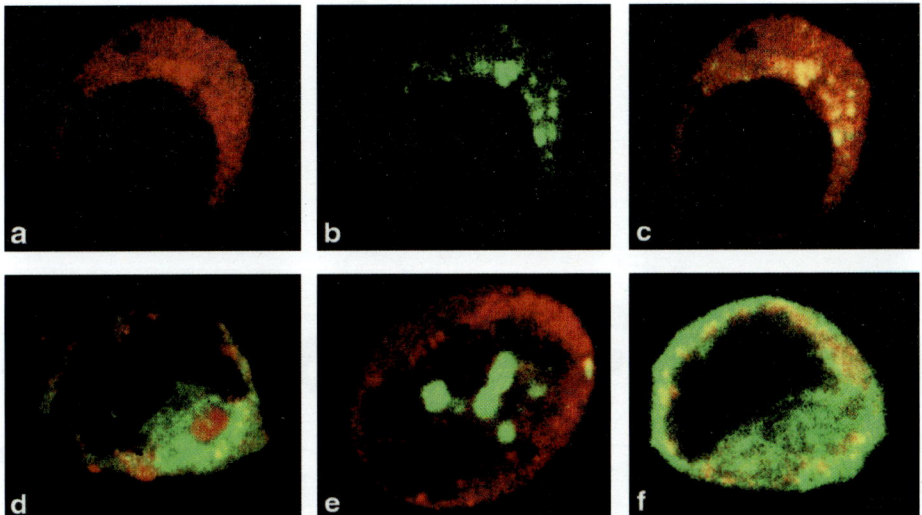

Color Plate 17 [chapter 20] Confocal laser scanning micrographs. Each image area is 19 × 22 μm. (a–c) PV-infected cell. (a) Localization of plus-strand PV RNA and (b) of minus-strand PV RNA in the same cell, visualized by fluorescent in situ hybridization. (c) Overlay of (a) and (b), plus- and minus-strand RNA colocalize in distinct structures (yellow). (d–f) Formation of the PV replication complex in *cis*. (d) Vesicles induced by protein 2BC-Flag (red) and plus-strand RNA of superinfecting PV (green). PV does not use preformed vesicles for the formation of its replication complex. (e) Transfection of a nonreplicating construct (pE5PVΔP1), coding for the entire P2 and P3 region. The induced vesicles (red) and the nonreplicating RNA (green) are found in separate structures and do not form a replication complex. (f) Transfection of a replicon, coding for the entire P2 and P3 region. The induced vesicles (green) and the replicating RNA (red) form replication complexes (yellow). (d–f) Reprinted from *Journal of Virology* (32), with permission.

Color Plate 16 [chapter 17] The structure of the FMDV L^{pro} and its comparison to papain. (A) The structure of the Lb form of the FMDV L^{pro}. View of the L^{pro} complexed to six C-terminal residues of an adjacent molecule in the unit cell. Secondary structure elements in the N-terminal domain are colored blue, those in the C-terminal domain red. The C-terminal extension is colored brown. The acidic cluster of residues Asp163, Asp164, Glu165, and Asp166 is shown in green. The dotted yellow region is expanded below to show the interactions of Lb^{pro} (gray) involved in recognizing residues Leu200′ (P2) and Lys201′ (P1) (yellow ball and stick) of an adjacent molecule. (B) The structure of papain bound to leupeptin. Standard view of papain complexed to leupeptin. Secondary structure elements in the N-terminal domain of papain are colored blue, those in the C-terminal domain red. The tryptophan residue referred to in the text is indicated. The dotted yellow region is expanded below to show the interactions of papain (gray) involved in recognizing Leu12 (P2) of leupeptin (yellow ball and stick). (C) The active site of Lb^{pro}. Arrangement of amino acid side chains around the active site of Lb^{pro}, as viewed down the central α-helix. The catalytic residues of Lb^{pro} Asn46, Cys51, His148, and Asp163 are shown. The acidic cluster (Asp163-Asp166) in the S′ binding region is also shown. The orientation of the amide group of Asn46 is maintained by a network of hydrogen-bond interactions (dotted lines) with the main-chain nitrogen of Asp49 and the side chains of Asn54 and Asp164. (D) The active site of papain. Arrangement of amino acid side chains around the active site of papain, as viewed down the central α-helix. The catalytic residues of papain Gln P-19, Cys P-25, His P-159, and Asn P-175 are shown. Hydrogen bonds are indicated. The residue Trp P-177, fully conserved in papain-like enzymes, which covers the hydrogen bond between essential catalytic residues Asn P-175 and His P-159, is also shown. The PDB coordinates used to make the drawings are 1QOL for the L^{pro} (36) and 1POP for papain complexed with leupeptin (76), respectively. Parts (C) and (D) reprinted from the *EMBO Journal* (36) with permission of the publisher. Color Plates 11 to 16 were drawn using the program MOLSCRIPT (50), with modifications by Esnouf (24) and Raster3D (61).

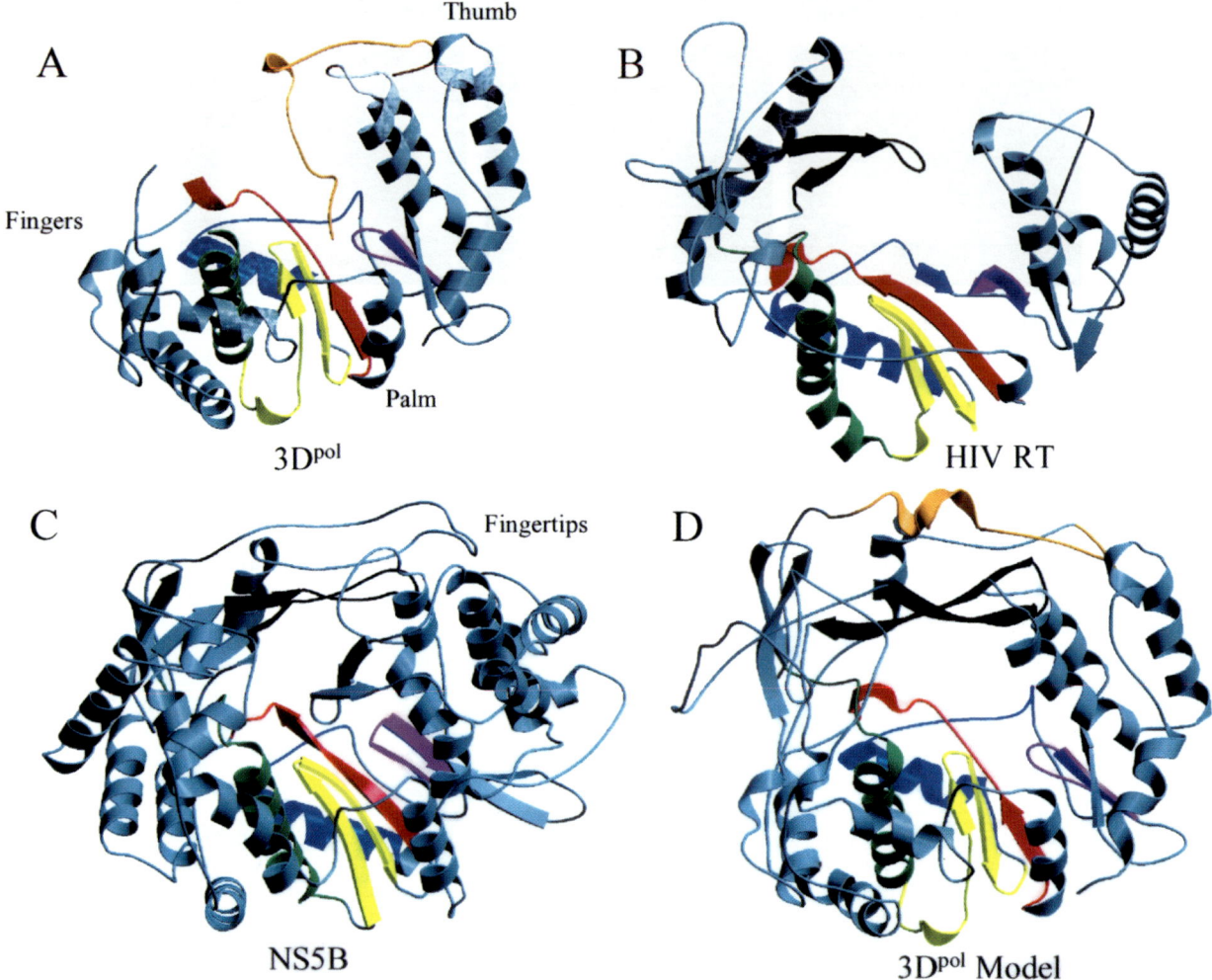

Color Plate 18 [chapter 21] Comparison of poliovirus 3D^{pol} to human immunodeficiency virus reverse transcriptase (HIV RT) and hepatitis C virus (HCV) NS5B. Crystal structure of (A) 3D^{pol} (35), (B) HCV NS5B (15, 53), and (C) HIV-1 RT (39). The molecules are colored in gray. Structural motif designations are according to Hansen et al. (35). Conserved structural motifs common to all three molecules are colored as follows: motif A, red; motif B, green; motif C, yellow; motif D, blue, motif E, purple; motif F, black. Images were rendered using MOLSCRIPT (49) and Raster3D (58). (D) Model of 3D^{pol} (complete) based upon sequence and structural homology to NS5B. Regions missing from the poliovirus crystal structure were reconstructed by superpositioning the two structures and replacing the missing regions from the 3D^{pol} structure with the corresponding region from NS5B. The amino acid side chains were changed to those of 3D^{pol} using the program O (44). Images were rendered using the program WebLab Viewer (Molecular Simulations, Inc.).

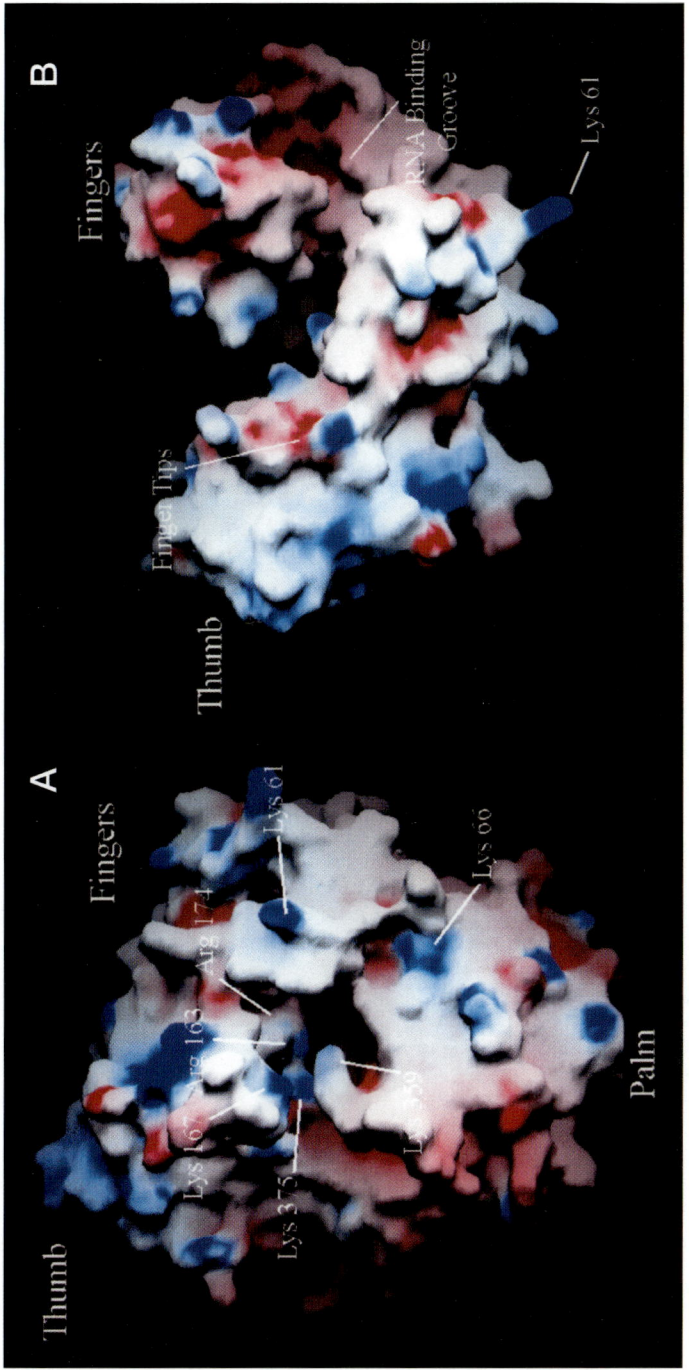

Color Plate 19 [chapter 21] Electrostatic potential diagrams of 3D^{pol}. (A) Electrostatic potential diagram of the molecular surface of 3D^{pol}. Electrostatic surface potentials were calculated for the complete 3D^{pol} model using the program GRASP (63). Regions in blue are positively charged, and those in red are negatively charged. The orientation in panel A has been rotated by 180° about the vertical axis of Color Plate 18D. The location of the fingers, palm, and thumb subdomains are noted. Basic residues lining the proposed NTP/PP$_i$ channel are labeled. Residues in these positions are predicted to make contact with nucleotides entering the active site, nucleotide in the NTP-binding site, and/or pyrophosphate. (B) Electrostatic potential diagram of the RNA-binding groove. The image is rotated by 90° about the horizontal axis of the page relative to the image shown in (A). Lys-61 has been labeled for reference. The palm subdomain is behind the molecule and cannot be seen from this view. The region in which the fingers and thumb subdomains make contact is labeled Finger Tips. The fingers subdomain is subdivided into two regions by a groove (labeled RNA Binding Groove) that may be important for nucleic acid binding based on modeling studies (Gohara and Cameron, unpublished). The RNA-binding groove is predicted to make contact with template RNA leading into the active site of the polymerase, which, in turn, may increase the stability of the enzyme on nucleic acid.

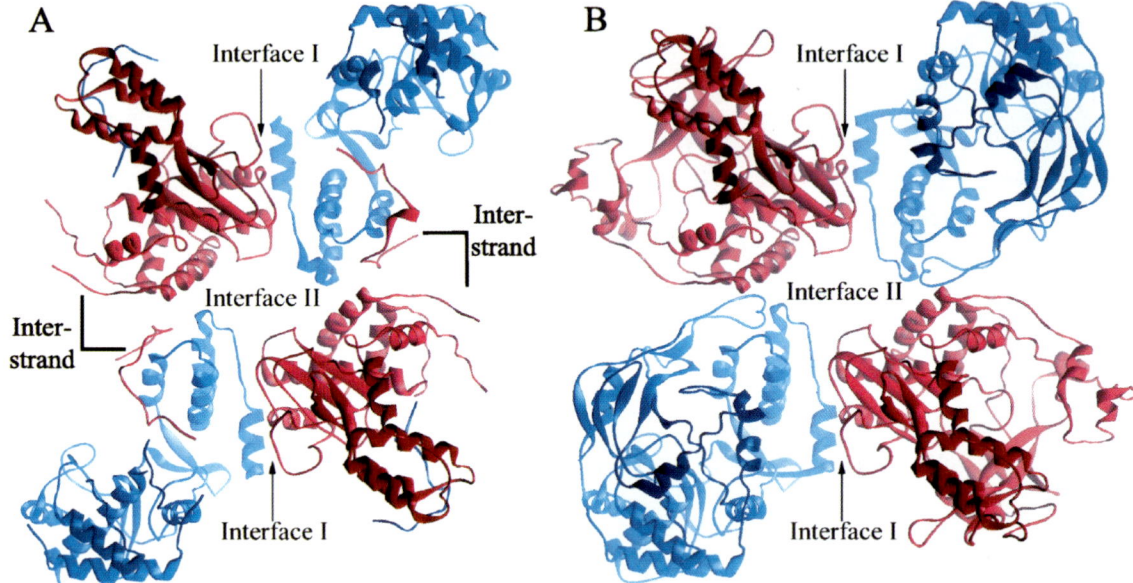

Color Plate 20 [chapter 21] Unit cell of poliovirus 3D^{pol}. (A) The unit cell of 3D^{pol} crystals based on the original structure. The unit cell is composed of two asymmetric units, each containing two molecules (one shown in red, the other shown in blue). Interfaces I and II are labeled. Interface I forms via the back of the palm of one molecule (red) and the back of the thumb of the other (blue). Interface II corresponds to the back of the fingers of one molecule (red) and the top of the thumb of the other (blue). In this image, interface II is predicted to be stabilized by intermolecular contacts of the amino terminus of one molecule (red) extending across interface II to the other (blue). (B) The unit cell of 3D^{pol} based on the complete model. Interfaces I and II form via similar interactions as those described in panel A. However, based on observations made in the NS5B structure, the amino terminus of each molecule makes intramolecular contacts with the thumb. Residues comprising interface II are the same in both panels A and B; however, the contribution of the amino terminus is different.

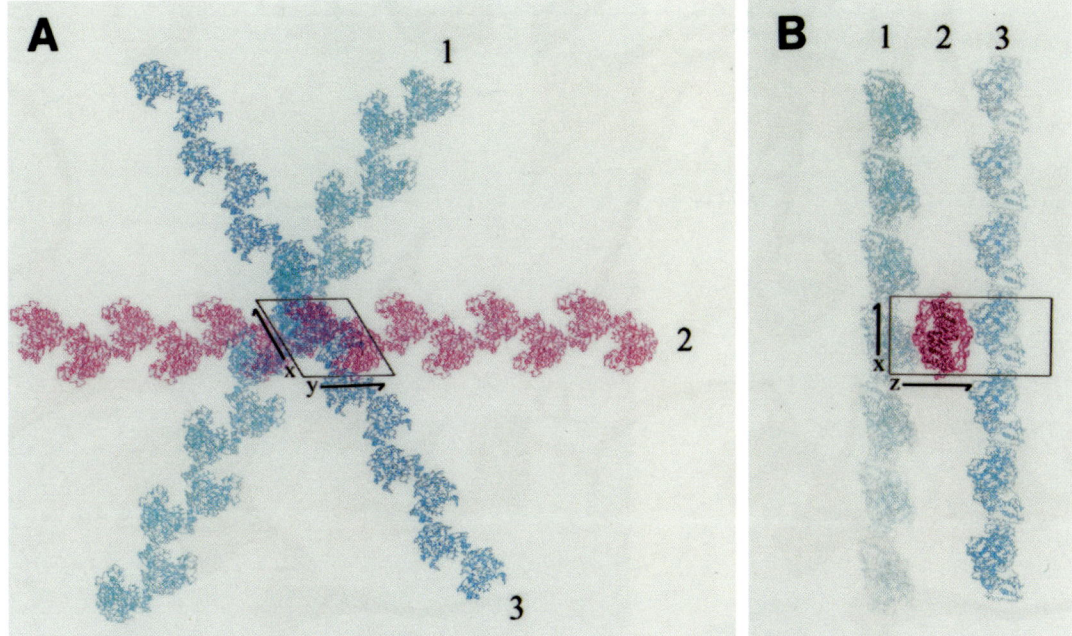

Color Plate 21 [chapter 21] Fiber formation by 3D^{pol}. Orientation of molecules involved in fiber formation occurs in a head-to-tail fashion along interface I as observed in the original crystal structure of 3D^{pol}. The unit cell is shown (black box). The two principal axes perpendicular to the view axis are labeled. (A) View down the z-axis. Each fiber shown represents a single plane (1 to 3) of fibers each stacked one on top of the other. For clarity only one fiber from each plane is shown, with the center of the plane located within the unit cell (black box). For example, the plane of the purple fiber could be constructed by translating the fiber in increments of one unit cell dimension along the x-axis in both directions. Each fiber is related to the others by rotation of 120° about the z-axis (axis perpendicular to the plane of the page) and 180° about the central axis of each fiber. (B) View down the y-axis. The image shown in panel A has been rotated by 90° about the vertical axis of the page. Planes 1 to 3 can be observed in this view. The fiber in plane 2 (purple) lies along the principal axis of this view (y-axis). In this orientation, each plane is approximately one-third the thickness of the unit cell in the z-direction. The molecules in each plane make contact with molecules in the adjacent plane via interface II.

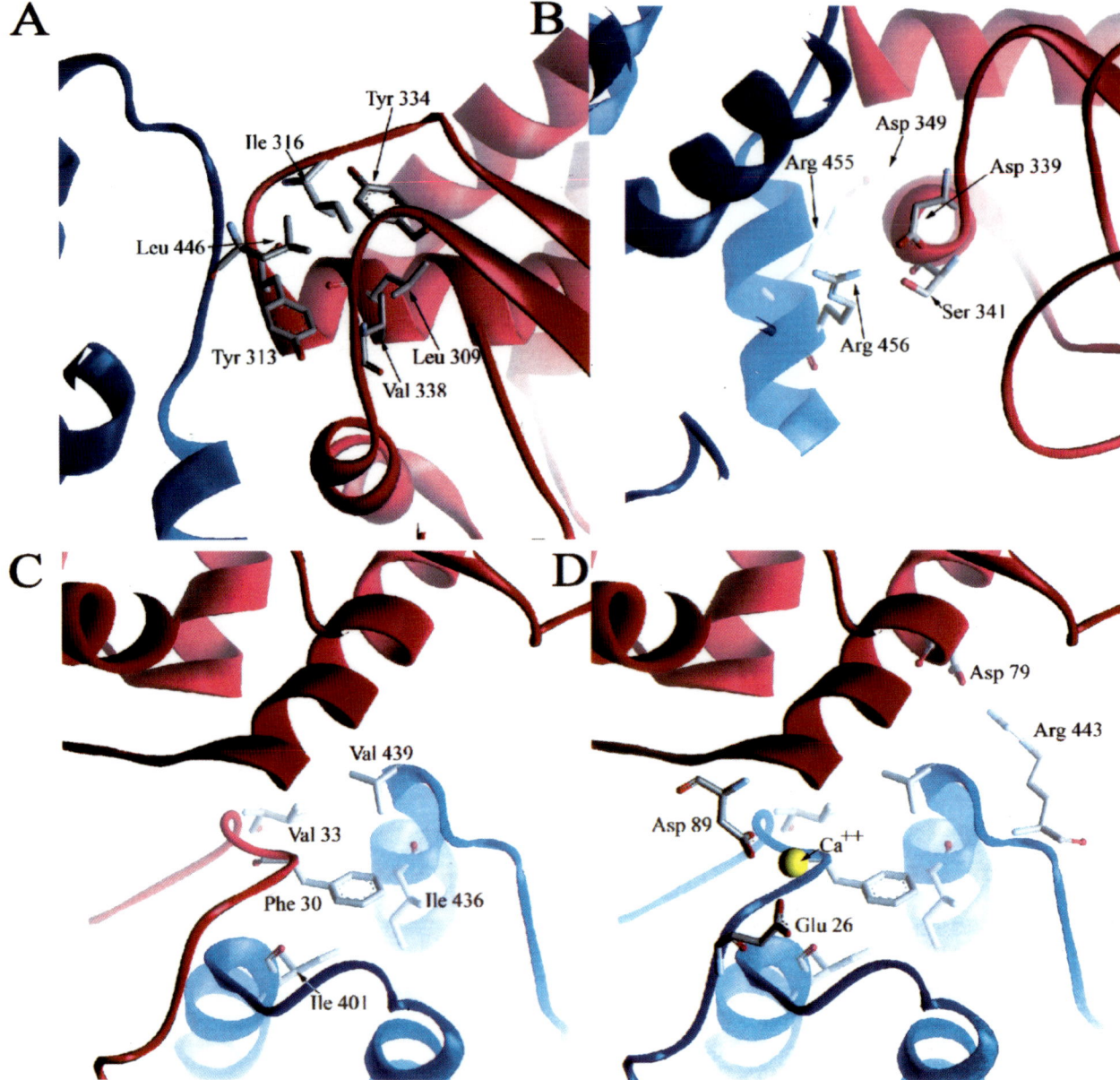

Color Plate 22 [chapter 21] Interfaces I and II. Atoms of the amino acid side chains are color coded as follows: gray, carbon; blue, nitrogen; red, oxygen. (A) Close-up view of the top of interface I. Amino acids involved in specific interactions are shown. Leu-446 on the back of the thumb of one molecule (blue) extends into a hydrophobic pocket found on the back of the palm of the other molecule (red). (B) The bottom of interface I is shown. Arg-455 hydrogen bonds to Asp-349; Arg-456 hydrogen bonds to both Asp-339 and Ser-341. The carboxyl terminus is 5 amino acids from Arg-456. (C) Interface II based on the original description by Hansen et al. (35). The amino terminus of the molecule in red extends across the junction between the two molecules and makes specific contacts with the top of the thumb of the molecule in blue. Val-33 and Phe-30 rest in a hydrophobic pocket formed by Ile-401, Ile-436, and Val-439. (D) Interface II based on the complete model for $3D^{pol}$. Amino acid side chains shown in (C) are also involved in similar interactions but have not been relabeled. The amino-terminal strand shown in red in (C) is predicted to originate from the same molecule (i.e., the blue molecule) as observed in the complete model. Additional interactions that may stabilize interface II are predicted based on both the original structure and the complete model. Asp-79 hydrogen bonds with Arg-443. Arg-443 is located on the top of the thumb in a region that consists, in part, of a basic patch. Asp-89 (red molecule) and Glu-26 (blue molecule) may be important for stabilization of interface II by serving as ligands (dashed lines) for divalent cations such as Zn^{2+} (shown here as Ca^{++} based on the original $3D^{pol}$ crystal structure).

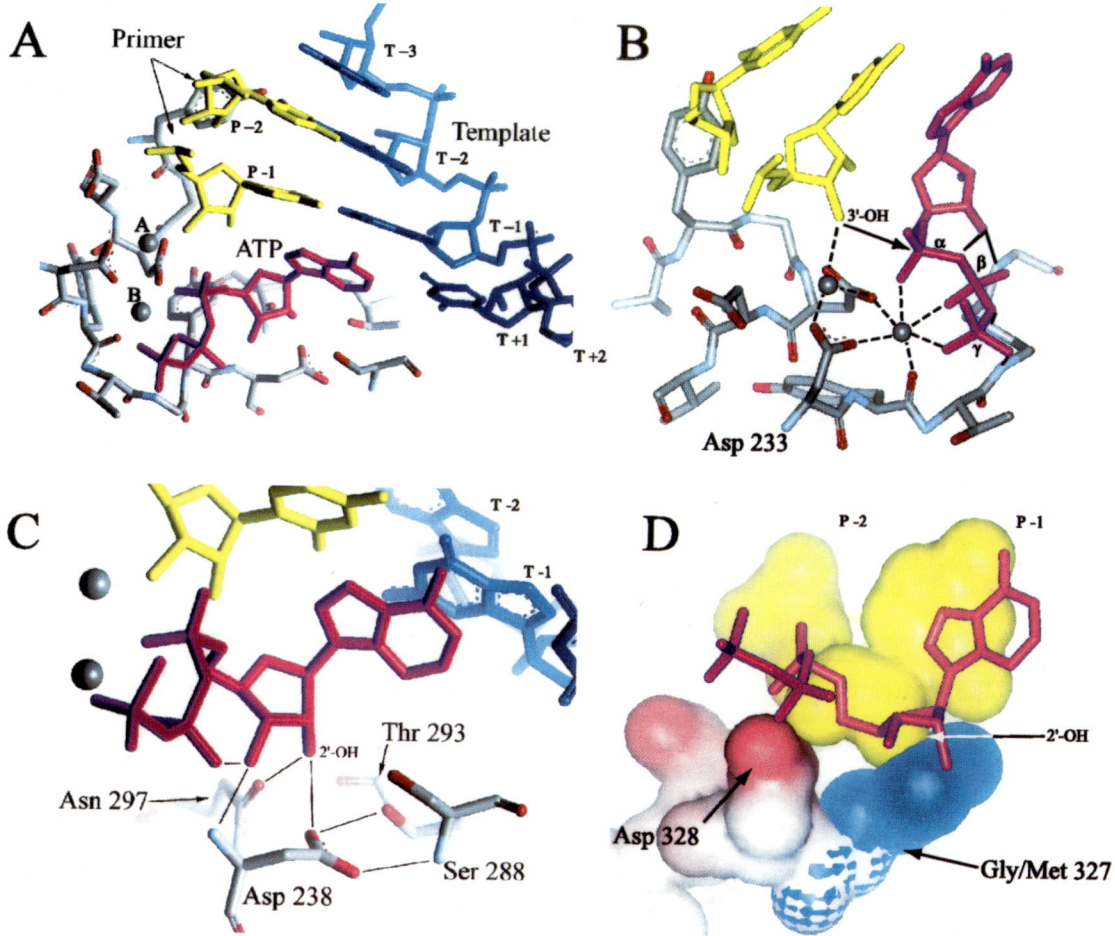

Color Plate 23 [chapter 21] Model of a 3D^{pol}-primer/template-nucleotide complex. (A) The ternary complex. Primer, template, and nucleotide are color coded as follows: primer, yellow; template, blue; nucleotide, magenta. Metal ions involved in catalysis are depicted as gray spheres. Amino acid side chains are color coded as in Color Plate 20. (B) Interaction of metal ions required for catalysis. Metal ions (labeled A and B) are coordinated by the triphosphate moiety of the incoming nucleotide (dashed lines), as well as by amino acid side chains of 3D^{pol}. Asp-233 (motif A) and Asp-328 (motif C) are strictly conserved among all nucleic acid polymerases. Asp-233, Asp-328, and the 3'-OH and oxygen atoms on the α-phosphate coordinate the metal ion at position A. The 3'-OH attacks the α-phosphorus (depicted as an arrow) of the incoming nucleotide. Metal ion B is required for stabilization of the triphosphate moiety of the incoming nucleotide and is coordinated by oxygen atoms at the α-, β-, and γ-positions of the triphosphate moiety as well as by Asp-233 and the carbonyl oxygen of Tyr-234. An oxygen on the β-phosphate hydrogen bonds to the 3'-OH as well as the backbone amide of Tyr-237. The oxygen on the γ-phosphate hydrogen bonds to the backbone amide of Gly-236. (C) Residues involved in selection of the 2'-OH are shown. Asp-238 is shown hydrogen bonding (black lines) to the 2'-OH of the incoming nucleotide as well as to Thr-293 and the backbone amide of Ser-288. Asn-297 hydrogen bonds to the 2'-OH of the incoming nucleotide as well. The 3'-OH, not labeled here for clarity, hydrogen bonds to the backbone amide of Asp-238 and an oxygen atom on the β-phosphate of the triphosphate moiety. (D) Role of the conserved glycine in the Gly-Asp-Asp motif (motif C). A surface contour of structural motif C is shown. The incoming nucleotide (magenta) and the penultimate primer nucleotide (yellow, P-2) are shown as sticks. The nucleotide on the 3' end of the primer is shown as a surface contour (yellow). The 2'-OH of the nucleotide at the 3' end of primer is labeled (arrow). Based on superpositioning with the HIV-1 ternary complex structure (32, 39), it is possible that a side chain larger than glycine (methionine in the case of HIV-1 RT, shown as a blue surface) will clash with the 2'-OH at the 3' end of primer. The presence of a glycine (as part of the Gly-Asp-Asp motif) may be required to accommodate the 2'-OH on the primer strand.

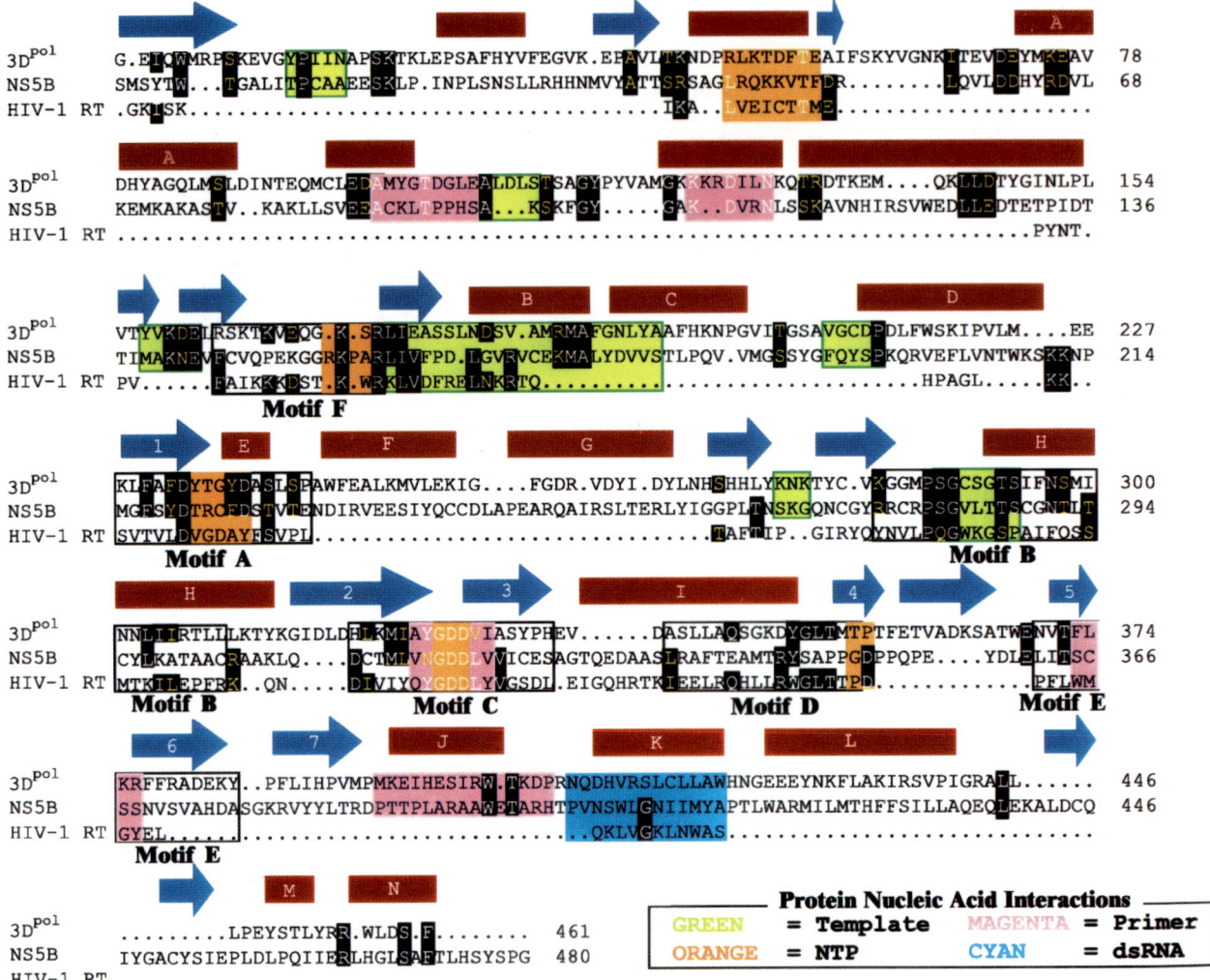

Color Plate 24 [chapter 21] Structure-based sequence alignment of 3D^{pol}, NS5B, and HIV RT. The complete sequence of 3D^{pol} is shown based on a structural alignment with NS5B and HIV-1 RT. The sequence of NS5B is shown up to residue 480. Only the sequences of structural elements of HIV-1 RT common to 3D^{pol} and NS5B are shown. Numbers at the end of lines correspond to the last amino acid in that row. For clarity, the corresponding numbers have been omitted for HIV-1 RT. Secondary structures are indicated based on those observed in the complete structure of NS5B and are shown as blue arrows (β-sheets) or red boxes (α-helices). Secondary structures are labeled according to their designation in the original 3D^{pol} structure; unlabeled boxes correspond to regions not present in the 3D^{pol} structure. Residues in white are conserved; those in yellow are conservative substitutions between the molecules. Conserved structural motifs A to F are surrounded by open black boxes. Regions predicted to make contact with nucleic acid and/or nucleotide are boxed and color coded as noted at the bottom of the figure (adapted with permission from Bressanelli et al. [15]).

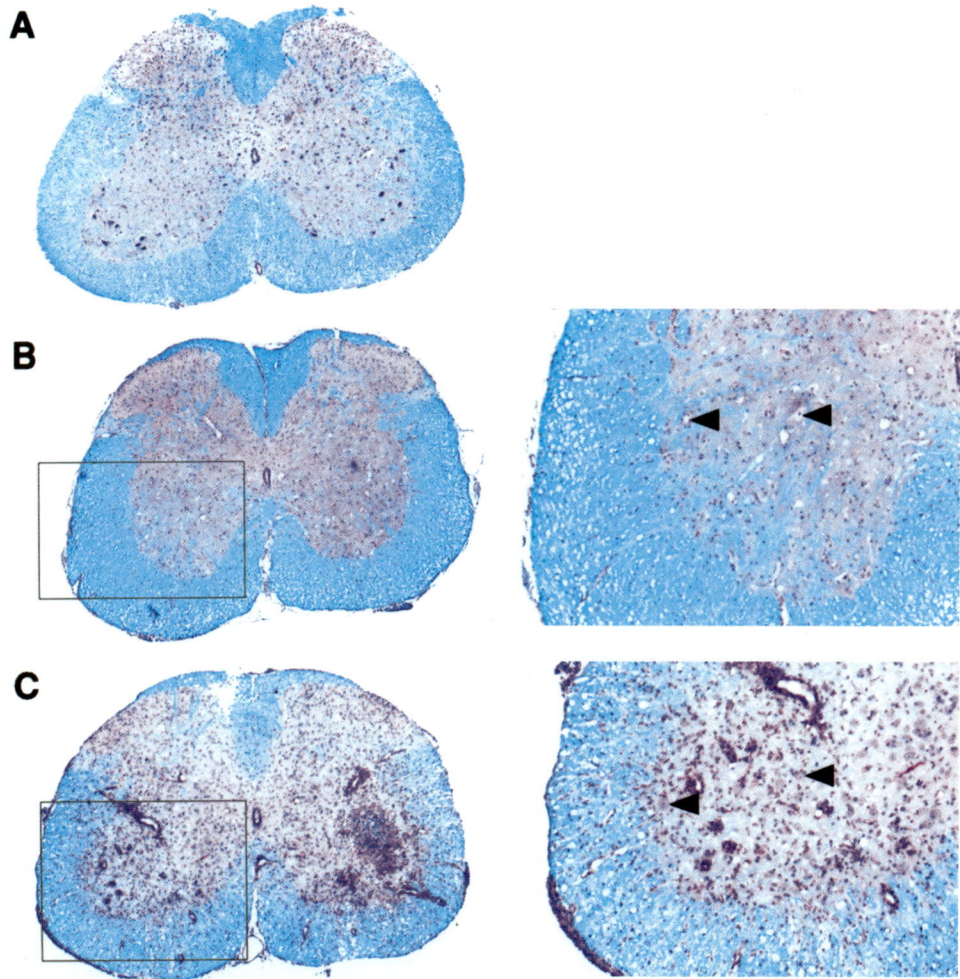

Color Plate 25 [chapter 29] Comparative neuropathology of poliovirus infection. CD155 tg mice (B) or wild-type mice (C) were infected with poliovirus by the intracerebral route. Rectangles within whole mount sections (left panels) indicate the localization of inserts shown at higher magnification (right panels). (A) Horizontal sections through the spinal cord of uninfected CD155 tg mice depict groups of large, dark-staining cells resident within the anterior horns (motor neurons). (B) Poliovirus infection selectively affects anterior horn motor neurons, which, as a result of lytic infection, are destroyed. The extraordinarily specific nature of the neuropathology of poliomyelitis can be observed at higher magnification, where the remnants of former motor neurons ("ghosts") are indicated by arrowheads. Remarkably, no other cellular compartment within the CNS shows any signs of damage. (C) Experimental infection of wild-type mice will elicit neurological symptoms only after intracerebral inoculation of poliovirus. In the absence of the human poliovirus receptor CD155, disseminated lesions affecting the entire CNS indiscriminately can be observed. Dense lymphocytic infiltrates are seen throughout the white and gray matter, and extensive tissue destruction with no discernible specificity results in the formation of a large necrotic area within the right anterior horn. The insert shown depicts intact motor neurons (arrowheads) within the spinal cord anterior horn surrounded by numerous infiltrative lesions. Luxol-fast blue, periodic acid-Schiff, hematoxylin stain; whole mount sections are shown at 4×, inserts at 12× magnification.

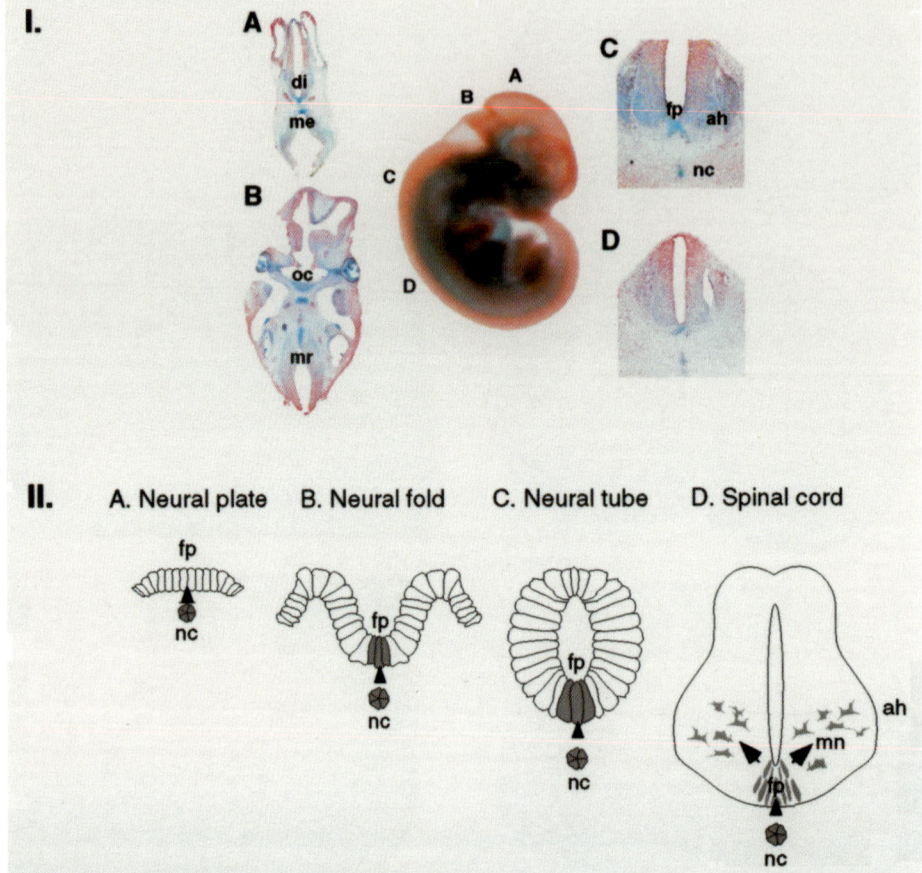

Color Plate 26 [chapter 29] (I) Activity of the CD155 promoter in the developing CNS. A–D. Transcephalic horizontal sections through mouse embryos transgenic for β-galactosidase under control of the CD155 promoter reveal cell-specific activity. The location of sections taken is indicated around the whole mount embryo in the center. CD155 promoter activity extends throughout the entire floor plate (fp) stretching from the caudal diencephalon (di; A) and the mesencephalon (me; A) into the medullary raphe (mr; B) and the spinal cord (C, D). Staining was also observed in the future optic chiasm (oc; B), the notochord (nc; C), and the spinal cord anterior horn proper (ah; C). (II) A schematic diagram of the morphogenesis of the anterior spinal cord depicts the sequence of events leading to motor neuron differentiation (A–D). Indentation of the neural plate (A) produces the neural fold (B), which, upon closure, forms the primitive neural tube (C) and spinal cord (D). The anterior commissure of the neural tube is formed by floor plate cells, which develop upon inductive signals emanating from the notochord. Floor plate cells proper are the source for inductive signals that induce motor neuron (mn) differentiation in the adjacent spinal cord anterior horn (D). The induction, differentiation, and maturation of motor neurons are critically influenced by the signaling molecule sonic hedgehog (the action of sonic hedgehog is indicated by arrows and arrowheads). X-Gal stain for β-galactosidase with eosin counterstain (32); whole mount embryo is shown at 3.2×, sections at 16× magnification.

INITIATION OF TRANSLATION

Initiation of Translation of Picornavirus RNAs: Structure and Function of the Internal Ribosome Entry Site

ELLIE EHRENFELD AND NATALYA L. TETERINA

14

TRANSLATION OF PICORNAVIRUS RNAs: HISTORICAL PERSPECTIVE

Years ago, in the pregenomics era, virologists sought to understand organisms by the tedious approach of identifying gene products rather than genes. For poliovirus (PV), the prototypic picornavirus, the analysis of virus-encoded proteins was greatly facilitated by the early observation that infection of cultured HeLa cells induced an efficient shutoff of host cell protein synthesis (see chapters 24 and 25). This allowed selective labeling of viral proteins with radioactive amino acids, which could then be visualized on sodium dodecyl sulfate-polyacrylamide gels, due to the absence of a background of labeled cellular proteins. Analyses of hundreds of such gels in several laboratories under various conditions of pulse and pulse-chase labeling led to the surprising revelation that PV RNA encoded all of its proteins from a single open reading frame that initiated translation from one initiation codon and generated a long polyprotein (~250 kDa) that underwent proteolytic processing catalyzed by active sites formed within the polyprotein sequences (see chapters 16 and 17). Although some picornavirologists went on to build productive scientific careers elucidating the details of polyprotein processing and viral protease structure and function, some of us remained puzzled by the ability of the viral RNA to direct efficient synthesis of its encoded proteins under conditions when cellular protein synthesis was inhibited. This phenomenon implied that viral protein synthesis involved a mechanism that was different in some distinct and fundamental way from that utilized by cellular mRNAs.

By the late 1970s, a skeleton of the translation mechanism utilized by the bulk of cellular mRNAs had been elucidated. The scanning model was proposed in which ribosome binding was directed by proteins bound to the m^7G cap group on the 5' ends of mRNAs, followed by translocation along the mRNA until the first AUG codon in a favorable context was encountered, resulting in initiation of translation. When the complete nucleotide sequence of the first picornavirus (PV) RNA was determined in 1981 (53, 88), it was immediately apparent that the scanning model could not be applied. The 5' end was not capped; an extremely long (742 nucleotides [nt]) and highly structured 5' untranslated region (UTR) preceded the initiating AUG codon; and numerous AUG triplets in contexts apparently favorable for initiation were present and not utilized. These observations confirmed the previous suspicions that poliovirus (and other picornaviral) mRNAs initiated translation by a unique and novel mechanism.

Early searches for RNA regions that signaled ribosome binding to viral RNAs were relatively crude: (i) Cell-free translation of encephalomyocarditis virus (EMCV) RNA after hybridization of chemically synthesized cDNA fragments to different sites in the 5' UTR showed that binding of fragments to the RNA sequence between nt 450 and the initiating AUG at nt 834 inhibited translation, whereas binding of fragments upstream of nt 450 had little or no effect on translation (95). (ii) Deletions of specific portions of the PV 5' UTR identified a region between nt 567 and 627 that appeared essential for ribosome binding and translation activity (8); other mutations throughout the region between nt 130 and 600 had measurably detrimental effects on translation (107). These findings suggested that an internal, rather than end-dependent, site on the viral RNA was capable of directing ribosome entry for initiation of translation.

More elegant proof of utilization of an internal ribosome entry site (IRES) on the viral RNA was provided by analysis of translation of bicistronic constructs engineered to encode two tandem protein sequences, separated by a viral 5' UTR (Fig. 1). Translation of the downstream cistron occurred even under conditions where the upstream cistron was prevented from being translated (44, 78), demonstrating end-independent, internal initiation. Subsequently, circular RNAs containing the EMCV IRES were constructed that bound ribosomes and directed translation of the predicted protein product (17). Taken together, these studies provided compelling evidence that ribosomes bound internally to the 5' UTR of picornavirus RNAs without the usual scanning from a capped, or uncapped, 5' terminus.

The RNA sequences that constitute an IRES extend through several hundred nucleotides and fold into complex, multidomain structures (see below). Although these

---

Ellie Ehrenfeld and Natalya L. Teterina ■ Laboratory of Infectious Diseases, National Institute of Allergy and Infectious Diseases, National Institutes of Health, Bethesda, MD 20892.

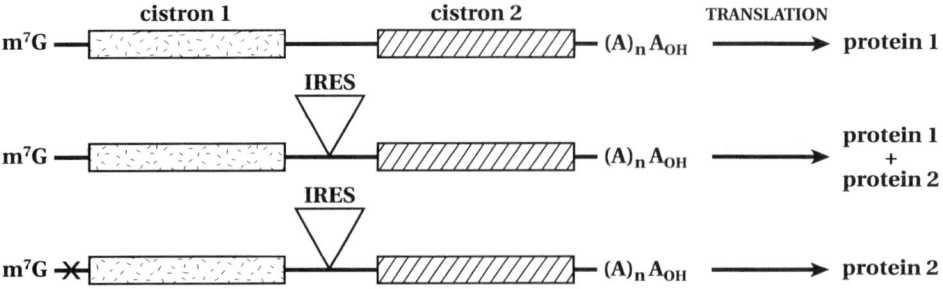

FIGURE 1 Schematic representation of bicistronic mRNAs and their translation products.

structures have not yet been visualized in three-dimensional space, they may be envisioned as forming a structural scaffold from which short, specific sequences are extended in bulges and loops fixed in space to contact proteins or other RNA segments. These proteins include both canonical translation initiation factors as well as cellular RNA binding proteins subverted to aid specific IRES utilization and thus control viral translation in different cell types (see chapter 15).

Although picornavirologists are responsible for the initial discovery of internal ribosome binding sites and for the concept of IRES function as a means of maintaining specific protein synthesis during global inhibition of cap-dependent translation, IRES elements are not unique to picornaviruses. Numerous other positive-strand RNA viruses, as well as a subset of cellular mRNAs, contain IRES elements (15, 65). The latter may allow translation of protein products under conditions such as heat shock or mitosis when the majority of protein synthesis is down-regulated, for example (18). Given the marked dissimilarities in RNA sequence and structure of these IRES elements, it appears that IRES evolution has occurred independently, multiple times, during the selection for optimal regulation of protein synthesis. For additional perspectives and for more detailed bibliographies, the reader is referred to reviews in references 24, 25, 40, 72, and 101.

STRUCTURE OF THE IRES

IRES Structures in Different Picornavirus RNAs

The IRES elements of all members of the picornavirus family are formed by approximately 450 nt within the long (600 to 1,300 nt) UTR located at the 5' ends of the RNA molecules. Although each IRES performs the same function, different picornavirus genera contain IRES elements of quite different sequence and secondary structure. On the basis of sequence comparisons and biochemical or enzymatic probing, three types of picornavirus IRES have been defined: type I in entero- and rhinoviruses; type II in cardio-, aphtho-, and parechoviruses; and type III in hepatoviruses (112). Among the three newly classified genera of picornaviruses (52), Aichi virus, representing the genus Kobuvirus, is suggested to have an IRES element most similar to type II (114); IRES elements from the Erbovirus and Teschovirus genera have not been examined. There is little sequence or secondary structure similarity among the three classes of picornavirus IRES elements, although the hepatovirus IRES appears more closely related to the type II IRES than to the type I (14). Between members of the same IRES type, sequence identity is moderate, but the predicted secondary structures are highly conserved. In accordance with the structural variance among the different IRES types, they also manifest characteristic properties of translation in vitro. For example, IRES-driven translation of cardio- and aphthovirus (type II) RNAs is accurate and efficient in rabbit reticulocyte lysates, while translation dependent on the PV or rhinovirus (type I) or hepatitis A virus (HAV) (type III) IRES is inaccurate and inefficient. Supplementation of the reticulocyte lysate with fractions from HeLa or Krebs II ascites cells improves utilization of the type I (12, 21, 82) but not the type III (31, 46) IRES.

Computer-assisted secondary structure analysis was initially applied to predict the structures of enterovirus and rhinovirus 5' UTRs (91). Several independent folding procedures all generated similar structures, composed of six stem-loop domains (I to VI). Figure 2A presents a schematic diagram of the consensus structure for the type I 5' UTR. Chemical and enzymatic probing for nucleotides involved in base pairing were generally consistent with the structure predictions (84, 98). The various models differed slightly in the folding of domain I, the central portion of domain IV, and the linker region between domains V and VI; a more recent study of the latter region by enzymatic probing of PV RNA supports the original model of Pilipenko et al. (102). In addition, phylogenetic analysis based on sequence variation found in independent virus isolates supported the existence of most of the proposed stem-loop structures by revealing extensive structure-conserving substitutions within predicted stems, a high degree of sequence conservation in predicted loops, and clustering of regions with sequence divergence in spacer regions between domains (87).

Computer predictions and phylogenetic analysis of RNA secondary structures of cardio- and aphthovirus 5' UTRs indicated that these sequences adopt a quite different pattern of stem-loop structures (23, 83). Consensus structures for cardio- and aphthovirus 5' UTRs defined 12 stem-loop domains (A–L)(Fig. 2B). The predicted structures are supported by chemical and enzymatic probing for nucleotides involved in base pairing (26, 83) and mutational analysis (45). The 5' UTR of HAV does not share

FIGURE 2 Schematic representation of the predicted stem-loop structures in the (A) poliovirus, (B) EMCV, and (C) hepatitis A virus 5' UTR of the viral RNAs.

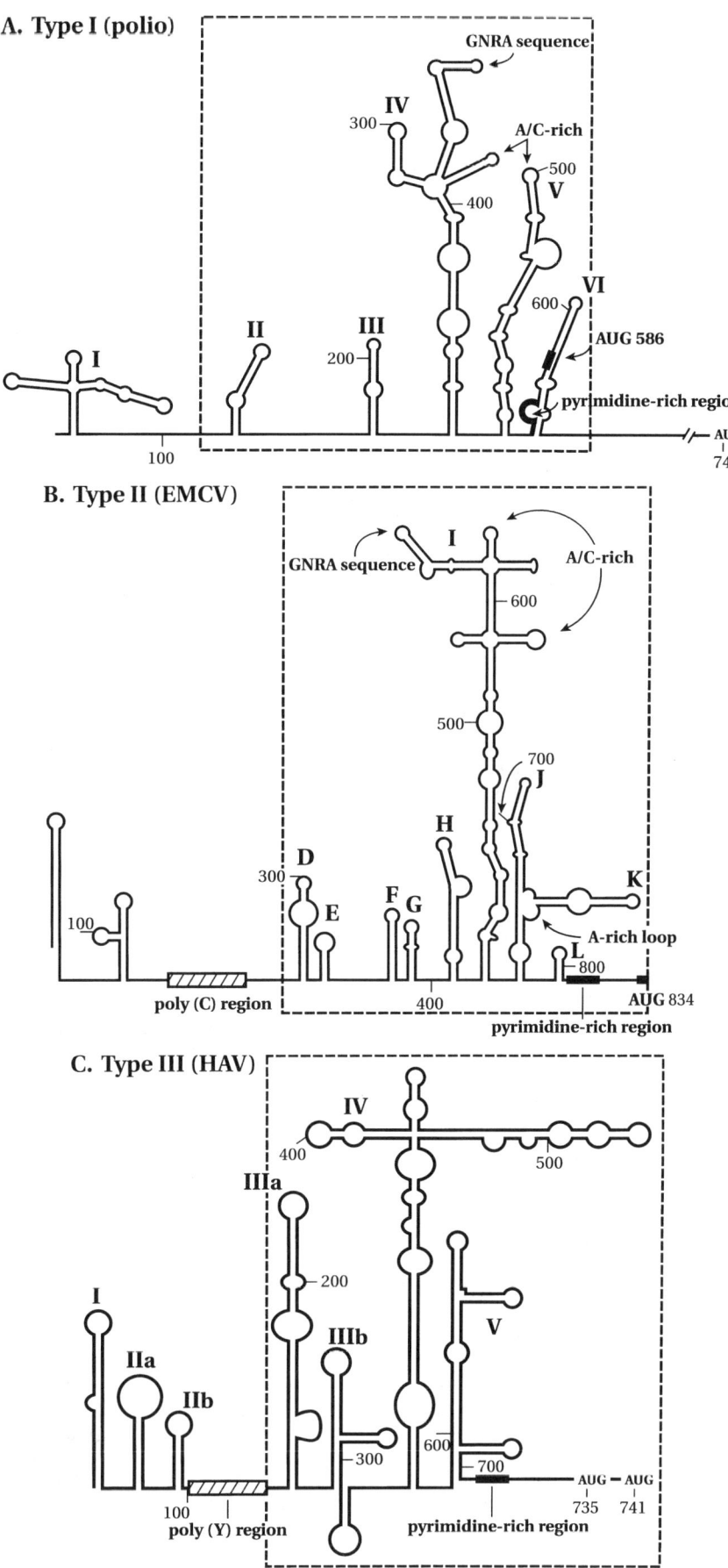

significant sequence homology with those of other picornaviruses and is considered to represent a third group of picornavirus 5′ UTRs (Fig. 2C).

Despite the marked structural differences and resulting translation properties of the three types of IRES elements in different picornaviruses, they perform the same function of directing assembly of the translation apparatus, since viable chimeric viruses can be engineered involving substitutions of one IRES type for another (3, 33, 47, 49).

Boundaries and Essential Domains of the IRES

To identify the nucleotide sequences and structures in the picornavirus 5′ UTRs that contribute to IRES function, mutations were introduced into cDNAs to generate transcripts whose translation could be evaluated in vitro or in transfected cells. In the type I IRES from PV, the 5′ boundary was placed around nt 130 and the 3′ boundary around nt 600, based on the construction of upstream and downstream deletions with little or no effect on translation efficiency in several different systems. Within these boundaries, domains II, IV, and V were essential for translation, part of domain VI could be eliminated, and deletion of the entire domain III was tolerated in a PV mutant viable in cultured cells (20, 71). Consistent with this permissible deletion, domain III is missing in all strains of bovine enterovirus (BEV) RNA. Most deletions or other mutations in the essential structures eliminated or markedly reduced IRES function, and secondary mutations that restore domain structures also restore IRES activity. The spacing between stem-loops, and possibly their three-dimensional orientation in space, may be critical. These analyses support the view that the majority of the IRES is designed to help present a few short, conserved sequences extended in loops or bulges from a highly structured scaffold that may require different amounts of stabilization in different environments. More recently, deletion analysis was used to map the IRES boundaries of coxsackievirus B3 (CVB3), another member of the enterovirus genus (61). Surprisingly, deletion of nt 1 to 529 did not affect translation levels of bicistronic constructs in vitro or in transfected cultured cells. Although the authors concluded that the CVB3 IRES is shorter than that of PV, with boundaries between nt 432 and 639, the apparently reduced requirements for upstream domains of the IRES under specific assay conditions may support the model that some IRES domains act as auxiliary structures designed to optimize accessibility of the actual ribosome entry site in a given host cell. The previously mentioned optional existence of domain III in a PV mutant and in strains of BEV may represent another example of this principle.

In the case of the EMCV 5′ UTR, which contains a type II IRES, the 5′ boundary was mapped around nt 260, at the 3′ end of the poly(C) tract. Removal of stem-loops D-H abolished translation in a bicistronic construct (43). The most critical elements for translation appear to be stem-loops I and J and single-stranded loops in the J-K domain (23, 37, 113). Mapping of the IRES in the closely related foot-and-mouth disease virus (FMDV) 5′ UTR gave similar results (6, 56, 66). Analysis of the IRES element of human parechovirus type I showed structural similarities to type II IRES elements, with a core structure consisting of domains I, J, and K; however, domains H and L, reported to be part of cardio/aphthovirus IRES elements, were apparently not required for parechovirus translation activity (70).

In all cases, the 3′ boundary of the IRES is an AUG triplet. However, the utilization of that AUG to initiate translation is a variable property, characteristic of the upstream body of the IRES (73). For example, the vast majority of ribosomes initiate translation on cardiovirus RNAs directly at the AUG at the 3′ end of the IRES, with just a few selecting the next AUG, 12 nt downstream (50, 55). For entero- and rhinoviruses, virtually no initiation occurs at the AUG at the 3′ end of the IRES; all ribosomes initiate translation approximately 150 nt downstream at the next AUG triplet (1). The aphthovirus IRES directs some initiation at its 3′ end, but the majority occurs at the next AUG further downstream (5). Hepatoviruses generally select the second of two nearly adjacent AUG triplets, at the 3′ end of the IRES (106).

Common Sequence Motifs

In addition to structural elements required to support internal initiation of translation, several sequence motifs have been conserved among all types of picornavirus IRES elements and identified as key elements in IRES function. The first is a motif described as Yn-Xm-AUG, where Yn is a pyrimidine-rich region (also called box A) (85), Xm is a spacer of 15 to 25 nt, and the AUG (box B) marks the 3′ boundary of the IRES. In the cardio-, aphtho-, and hepatoviruses (IRES types II and III), this AUG is also a translation initiation site, whereas in the entero- and rhinoviruses (IRES type I), a relatively unstructured spacer region of 30 to 150 nt separates the AUG at the end of the IRES from the AUG that starts the coding sequence (1). Both the number of pyrimidine residues in Yn and the length of Xm appear to be more important translation determinants than the precise nucleotide sequences in these motifs (45).

Some sequence motifs are found in all picornavirus IRES elements, located in single-stranded loops within the IRES structure. One is a GNRA tetraloop (where N is any nucleotide and R is a purine). The GNRA motif is located in stem-loop IV of the type I IRES, in stem-loop I in the type II IRES, and in stem-loop IV of the type III IRES (Fig. 2). In the first two cases, mutational analyses have proved the importance of this motif for IRES activity (51, 63, 93). Recent studies of tetraloop variants in the EMCV IRES implicated the 3′-terminal A residue as most crucial for IRES activity (93); however, no specific biochemical role for this motif has been identified. RNA tetraloops with GNRA consensus are often found within large RNAs with stable tertiary structures and are believed to mediate interactions between RNAs that contain the motif and other RNA or protein targets.

A second common motif is an A/C-rich sequence present in stem-loops IV and V in the type I IRES structure and in two loops of stem-loop I in type II IRES elements. Mutational studies have indicated the functional importance of these loops (63, 71), and it has been suggested that the A/C-rich loop in domain V of the PV IRES participates in the formation of a pseudoknot structure (58).

Statistical Predictions of RNA Folding

A different view of RNA folding has been applied to picornavirus genomes (75), in which it is allowed that, rather than there being a single unique minimum energy structure for large RNA molecules, there is a collection of alternative, nearly energetically equivalent configurations assumed by different molecules at any given time. Many hours of computer time were spent to algorithmically query the number of possible different pairing partners for each nucleotide in the genome, given a narrow, but arbitrary, range of energetic freedom. A pairing number (P-num) is derived for each nucleotide, representing the propensity of that base to pair with the same or alternative partners in the collection of suboptimal folds (42). Thus, bases with low P-num values exhibit strong fidelity for a specific pairing partner and those base pairs are statistically probable in all or most of the possible structures formed. It is posited that low P-num bases and their partners determine and identify biologically significant motifs, since they represent constant structures in a background of shifting configurations (41, 115).

For the picornavirus RNAs, a relatively relaxed structure is predicted, with a long, central axis of shifting base pairs, with relatively stable stems, loops, helices, and branch points extending from the central backbone. Relatively few regions contain low P-num bases; these, however, involve the 5' and 3' UTRs, including the IRES. Interestingly, the data from this approach predict that the two ends of each genome are located adjacent to each other in every molecule, although not necessarily base paired to one another.

A breathing, shifting view of structures in large RNA molecules, involving alternative pairings and re-pairings among the bases, is thermodynamically attractive and probably realistic, and may explain the need for protein binding to stabilize local structures needed for some viral functions. Support for some regions of strong inherent thermodynamic stability (low P-num bases) in the IRES comes from the observation that artificial transcripts representing individual predicted domains can compete well with long RNA molecules for specific protein binding or translation (9, 67).

HIGHER ORDER STRUCTURE

The conserved motifs in the secondary structure elements that are essential for IRES activity likely facilitate RNA-RNA or RNA-protein interactions required to maintain a higher order structure needed for proper recognition of the IRES element by the translational machinery. Models for higher ordered structures in picornavirus IRES elements have been derived by a combined approach using thermodynamic RNA folding, Monte Carlo simulation, and phylogenetic comparative analysis (59, 60). A common tertiary core structure was identified that shared a similar folded shape, in the 3' portion of all three types of picornavirus IRES elements. The core structure is formed by a region of 140 to 170 nt, depending on the genus, and includes the pyrimidine-rich region and domains that form a predicted pseudoknot. Point mutations in the pyrimidine-rich region previously shown to destroy IRES function also destroy the predicted tertiary interactions in the pseudoknot. The common structural core identified within the picornavirus IRES elements is also conserved in the 5' UTR of the divergent viruses, hepatitis C virus and pestiviruses, and thus is proposed to be a crucial element in IRES function (60).

Limitations of currently available technology for three-dimensional RNA structure analysis preclude easy experimental determination of the spatial organization of the entire IRES element. Yet, many cis-acting regulatory elements consist of complex multidomain structures whose individual domains interact with one another rather than functioning as independent units. For example, a 36-kDa protein was shown to cross-link specifically to PV IRES RNA that contained stem-loops V and VI, although no cross-linking was observed to either domain alone (36). This region comprises the conserved higher order structure predicted by Le and Maizel, described above. Genetic analyses of mutations and revertants within and between these two helical domains support the view that stem-loops V and VI interact in an essential spatial orientation to support IRES function (34, 100). Efforts to understand the structural and functional implications of such domain interactions are in preliminary phases.

It is generally accepted that long-range tertiary interactions are essential for proper folding and function of biologically active RNA. Initial attempts to study interactions between separated domains of the FMDV IRES have been reported recently (89). Pairs of the sub-IRES domain RNAs were denatured and incubated together under binding conditions, and interactions between the RNAs were observed to occur by gel mobility shift analysis. Similar studies were performed with regions of the EMCV IRES, incubated under different conditions (A. Kaminski and R. J. Jackson, personal communication). Again, specific complex formation between multiple domains was evident. Identification of specific sequences involved in these interdomain interactions, and their possible functional significance, remains to be demonstrated.

OTHER SEQUENCES AFFECTING EFFICIENCY OF IRES ACTIVITY

The picornavirus IRES elements represent relatively large complex domains composed of multiple subdomains that require correct spatial orientation and interactions to carry out IRES function. They appear to be self-contained and independent, as evidenced by their ability to be transferred en bloc to other positions, other viral genomes, or other mRNA reporter sequences, and still direct ribosome binding and initiation of translation. However, there are several indications that the efficiency of IRES utilization can be modulated by sequences outside the IRES borders.

Adjacent Sequences May Modulate Structure

A small-plaque mutant containing a 6-nt insertion after position 21, in the stable cloverleaf-like structure at the 5' terminus of PV RNA, was shown to reduce translation efficiency in infected cells by fivefold (97). Subsequently, additional mutations in the cloverleaf, as well as deletion of the entire cloverleaf, also were shown to reduce translation directed by the PV IRES (28). The 5' cloverleaf structure is clearly upstream of the 5' border of the IRES. Measurements of RNA degradation in HeLa cell extracts in vitro showed that the 5' cloverleaf plays a critical role in maintaining stability of PV RNA (4). Although degradation of mutated RNAs was not always examined as a possible cause of the reduced translation efficiency, some destabilizing mutations in the cloverleaf could be rescued from degradation by addition of an m^7G cap group to the mutant RNAs, but capping failed to restore their translation.

A biological rationale as well as a molecular mechanism has been proposed to explain the observed effects of cloverleaf mutations on IRES function (27, 28). A cellular protein, poly(C)-binding protein (PCBP), has been shown to bind two specific sites in the PV 5' NCR, both of which appear to be required for efficient translation from the PV IRES (10, 29). The mechanism by which these ribonucleoprotein complexes promote ribosome entry is not known. Translation of the viral RNA generates viral protein 3CD, which also binds to the 5' cloverleaf, forming a complex that binds PCBP even more tightly and that downregulates translation but is required for initiation of viral RNA replication (27, 76). Thus, modulation of translation activity from the PV IRES by upstream 5′-terminal sequences via protein-RNA interactions may allow viral RNA templates to be recruited for negative-strand synthesis and switch from translation to replication activity.

An opposite modulating effect of upstream 5′-terminal sequences on IRES-driven translation initiation was observed for HAV RNA translation in vitro. Deletion of the HAV 5′-terminal 138 nt, previously shown to be upstream of the IRES boundary (13), or substitution of these sequences with the terminal cloverleaf-like sequence from PV RNA, caused a fourfold enhancement of translation efficiency (32). This inhibitory effect of the HAV 5′ terminus was also observed with constructs containing the HAV 5′ NCR fused to the chloramphenicol acetyltransferase reporter gene in transfected BT7-H cells (111). A molecular explanation or rationale for these effects has not been investigated; however, the constraints of needing to accommodate the dual functions of translation and replication in adjacent regions of the viral 5′ UTR may generate inadvertent consequences for either function.

Frequent use of IRES elements to construct artificial mRNAs in a variety of eukaryotic expression vectors has produced IRES elements fused upstream of foreign RNA sequences that may be observed to influence the efficiency of the IRES-driven translation. Although of no biological significance, these observations lend credence to the view that folding patterns within the complex IRES domain are crucial for IRES activity and that sequences surrounding the IRES borders may influence the stability of neighboring sequences. These potential interactions should be borne in mind when IRES elements are engineered for expression or delivery of foreign gene products.

It should be noted that assay of IRES function in a bicistronic construct generally appears more stringent than in a monocistronic construct, perhaps due to reduced flexibility of the RNA when it is tethered upstream (23, 109).

Poly(A) Tails

Efficient translation of capped mRNAs in eukaryotic cells involves a synergistic dependence on the 5′-terminal cap structure and the 3′-terminal poly(A) tail. Stimulation by the cap group is mediated by the eIF-4 family of translation initiation factors, bound to the cap group via eIF-4E, the cap-binding protein (30). Stimulation by poly(A) is mediated via the poly(A)-binding protein (PABP) (105). The synergy in supporting translation activity between these two RNA end-binding proteins results from a physical interaction between eIF-4G, a polypeptide bound to the 5′ end via its association with eIF-4E, and PABP (38), which effectively circularizes the mRNA (110). In the case of the uncapped picornaviral RNAs, translation from all three IRES types is significantly augmented by a 3′ poly(A) tail (7, 68), suggesting that cross-talk between the IRES and the poly(A) tail occurs to modulate translation in these RNAs as well. A biochemical mechanism to explain these results has not been proposed.

HOW DOES THE IRES WORK?

Recruitment of Translation Initiation Factors and Ribosomal Subunits

During cap-dependent translation reactions, the ribosomal subunit, initiator tRNA, and all the factors and cofactors required to achieve recognition of the proper start site for protein synthesis on the mRNA are brought together via binding of the m^7G cap group at the 5′ end of the RNA to the eIF-4E subunit of eIF-4F, the cap-binding holoenzyme. The key role in organizing all of the necessary components is played by another eIF-4F subunit, eIF-4G. This large polypeptide serves as a scaffold to which many initiation factors, including one that bridges to the small ribosomal subunit, attach. (The factors and their functions in protein synthesis are described in chapter 15.) The organization of this multicomponent complex at the 5′ end of the mRNA triggers all subsequent events for carrying out synthesis of a polypeptide.

For an uncapped, IRES-containing RNA, there is no eIF-4E binding site, and thus no obvious mechanism of recruiting the key eIF-4G subunit, with all its organizational binding activities, to an appropriate site on the mRNA. Since picornavirus IRES-dependent translation requires the complete set of canonical initiation factors, except for eIF-4E (74, 77, 80, 94), the difference between cap-dependent and picornavirus IRES-dependent initiation of translation reduces to how eIF-4G is anchored to the RNA. Although little is known about the anchoring process for any of the three types of picornavirus IRES elements, a major insight into this process was gained by a series of detailed studies using toe-printing and foot-printing to show that the central portion of eIF-4G, in the presence of eIF-4A, binds directly to the J-K domain of the EMCV IRES, just upstream of the initiation site (54, 80, 81). Resolution of the molecular structure of the central portion of eIF-4G by X-ray crystallography permitted identification of a molecular surface involved in interactions with the EMCV IRES (64). The RNA structural element bound by eIF-4G consists of an oligo(A) loop and three adjacent helices at the junction of the J and K domain. More recently, direct interactions of eIF-4G with a similar structure in the aphthovirus IRES were demonstrated; importantly, point mutations that disrupted RNA binding caused severe reductions in IRES activity in vivo (62). It should be noted, however, that mutations in the EMCV IRES have been described that disrupt IRES function (113) without affecting eIF-4G binding in vitro (54), indicating that eIF-4G binding is not sufficient for translation of EMCV RNA.

The RNA structural element responsible for eIF-4G binding in cardio- and aphthoviral RNAs is conserved in the hepatovirus RNA structure as well, and may similarly account for anchoring of eIF-4G in members of this genus. No obvious equivalent structure is apparent in the type I IRES element; nevertheless a direct recruitment of eIF-4G sequences to some structural and/or sequence domain in the IRES region remains the most likely scenario for initiating the translation reaction for these viruses as well.

The critical importance of providing a mechanism for the binding of eIF-4G in order to recruit a ribosomal subunit to the mRNA was elegantly demonstrated by DeGregorio et al. (19). These authors replaced the N-terminal portion of eIF-4G with a specific RNA-binding protein, the iron response element binding protein. The chimeric protein was thus directed to the intercistronic space in a bicistronic reporter RNA, which harbored the iron response element, in HeLa cells. The eIF-4G sequence-containing protein directed translation of the downstream cistron with an efficiency approaching 15% of that driven by the hepatitis C virus IRES. Recruitment of eIF-4G to the intercistronic space via the fused specific RNA-binding protein occurred even if translation of the upstream cistron from the 5' end of the RNA was inhibited by means of a stable stem-loop structure introduced in the 5' UTR. These experiments showed that eIF-4G is sufficient to deliver a functional ribosomal subunit to the mRNA, and generated an artificial "IRES by design."

If delivery of the ribosome to the mRNA is the primary "business" of the IRES, then the business location appears to be at the 3' end of the IRES, where ribosome binding occurs. This is consistent with the prediction of a common core structural domain and the presence of conserved sequence motifs in this region. This function alone, however, cannot represent the whole story, since the borders of the IRES map well upstream of the eIF-4G binding site on the cardio- and aphthovirus RNAs, and the sizes of all the picornavirus IRES elements appear to exceed that required for an eIF-4G binding site. Additional structural domains whose sequence, integrity, and/or spatial orientation are essential for IRES function reside upstream of the proposed "business end." The function(s) provided by these additional regions of the IRES has not been elucidated. Specific binding sites for cellular factors that are or may be involved in IRES utilization have been mapped in these domains, but their biochemical roles in the translation reaction have not been identified. It is likely that the evolution of the picornavirus IRES occurred by gradual addition of domains and elements that improved its function in specific host cell environments. Thus, some additional IRES modules may have evolved to stabilize the core element directly involved in ribosome recruitment or to otherwise confer regulated, cell-specific function to the process of viral protein synthesis.

trans Action of IRES Domains

Although the concept of internal ribosome entry was developed as being mediated by *cis*-acting sequences and structures within the IRES element, several studies have demonstrated that the activities of severely defective IRES elements can be partially restored by the coexpression, in transfected cells, of the parental wild-type IRES. For example, defective forms of the EMCV IRES that contained deletions of the J domain or alterations of the conserved GNRA sequence were complemented in *trans* by coexpression of the intact EMCV IRES, but not by that of another cardiovirus, Theiler's murine encephalomyelitis virus (TMEV) or FMDV (92). Distinct, truncated regions of the EMCV IRES, insufficient to direct internal initiation alone, could also complement the defective IRES elements. IRES *trans*-complementation has been demonstrated to occur with representatives of picornaviruses containing either type I or type II IRES elements (22, 79, 103, 109). In all cases, coexpression was achieved by means of recombinant vaccinia virus expressing T7 RNA polymerase to transcribe the RNAs. Unfortunately, there have been no reports of IRES *trans*-complementation successfully performed in vitro, which likely will be required for analysis of the mechanism. However, the results are compatible with the view that IRES function is mediated by short, discrete functional motifs presented by different domains, and that different domains perform different functional activities, at least some of which may be achieved by different molecules acting in *trans*.

THE IRES AS A DETERMINANT OF VIRULENCE

The discovery of an internal ribosome binding site in picornavirus RNAs represented a major paradigm shift in our conceptual view of protein synthesis in eukaryotic cells. It had major impacts on the field of picornavirology as well as on the biochemistry of translation initiation mechanisms. After the initial publications in 1988, there occurred a flurry of activity in the early 1990s defining and characterizing the RNA sequences that form the IRES structures. A general picture emerged of a structural scaffold from which a few important sequences are presented from loops or bulges, oriented in space by extension from their stems. Ribosomal subunits attach to the mRNA at or near the AUG that marks the 3' border of the IRES, some 25 nt downstream from the start of a universal pyrimidine-rich tract.

While some laboratories are finding new interest and new approaches to structural aspects of IRES function, and additional groups are pursuing the biochemical path of identifying and characterizing the various proteins that interact with the RNA and mediate IRES function, several additional areas of research have opened as unexpected offshoots of the original IRES discovery. The first is a repeated theme connecting IRES mutations and structures with attenuation of virulence. Examples of this theme include: (i) Point mutations in stem-loop V of the PV IRES are major determinants of the attenuated phenotype of all three Sabin PV vaccine strains (69). (ii) Disruption of nucleotides in stem-loop II of the PV IRES generated viruses that retained neurovirulence in monkeys but were highly attenuated in PV-sensitive mice transgenic for the PV receptor (96). (iii) A chimeric virus in which stem-loops V and VI from the human rhinovirus IRES were substituted for the corresponding PV sequences is also highly attenuated for growth in cultured cells of neuronal origin, as well as for neurovirulence in transgenic mice or in cynomolgus monkeys inoculated intraspinally (34). (iv) Replacement of the TMEV, strain GDVII, IRES with that from FMDV produced a similarly attenuated chimeric virus (86). (v) Cardiovirulence of CVB3 and induction of myositis by CVB1 have both been mapped to sites within the IRES element (90, 108). (vi) Exchange of the PV IRES for that in CVB3 restricts the growth of the chimera in cell lines derived from a number of tissues, and attenuates the virus for heart and pancreatic disease in mice (16).

All of these phenotypic changes in virus growth patterns are presumed to result from cell- or tissue-specific differences in the quality or quantity of cellular protein factors required for interactions with IRES domains to support ribosome binding and translation initiation function. These attenuating alterations therefore represent host range mutations. For example, reconstitution of initiation complexes in vitro showed that the FMDV IRES, but not the TMEV IRES, requires a cellular protein called murine proliferation-associated protein (also designated ITAF45) that is not expressed in murine brain cells. Thus, substitution of the FMDV IRES for that of TMEV would preclude translation in the brain with a resultant loss of neurovirulence by the chimeric virus. A similar specificity has been proposed as the basis for the attenuation of Sabin PV vaccine strains, in which attenuating mutations in the IRES elements correlate with reduced translational efficiencies and restricted growth in neuronal cells but not in HeLa cells in culture (2, 57, 99, 104). Cross-linking studies have shown an impaired interaction of the Sabin 5' UTR with polypyrimidine tract-binding protein (PTB) (35), although no causal relationship between this interaction and the attenuated phenotype has been demonstrated in vivo.

Although the attribution of virulence determinants to noncoding regions of picornavirus genomes was initially surprising, mutations in the 5' UTR now constitute the largest known class of attenuated phenotypes in the picornavirus family. Virus growth in a particular tissue or cell type depends upon both the presence of cellular receptors and the presence of host factors that may be required to support the processes of translation, RNA replication, encapsidation, etc. Thus, alterations in the IRES element can regulate virus growth in a cell-specific manner to the extent that domains in the IRES require folding assistance or stabilization or catalytic functions provided by bound cellular factors.

The majority of IRES mutations studied affected translation activity in the species or cells in which they manifested an attenuated phenotype, as expected. However, in some cases, mutations clearly within the boundaries of the IRES element appear to affect either RNA replication (11, 39) or perhaps other viral functions (48, 100) as well. Given the multiple functions attributed to almost all picornaviral genes or gene products, it is perhaps to be expected that the IRES, too, will prove even more complex in function than originally predicted.

The authors thank past and present members of the laboratory for stimulating discussions and experimental data, and Dr. Ivan N. Shatsky for critical reading of the manuscript. Current work in our laboratory is supported by the National Institutes of Health.

REFERENCES

1. **Agol, V. I.** 1991. The 5'-untranslated region of picornaviral genomes. *Adv. Virus Res.* **40:**103–180.
2. **Agol, V. I., S. G. Drozdov, T. A. Ivannikova, M. S. Kolesnikova, M. B. Korolev, and E. A. Tolskaya.** 1989. Restricted growth of attenuated poliovirus strains in cultured cells of a human neuroblastoma. *J. Virol.* **63:**4034–4038.
3. **Alexander, L., H.-H. Lu, and E. Wimmer.** 1994. Poliovirus containing picornavirus type 1 and/or type 2 internal ribosomal entry site elements: genetic hybrids and the expression of a foreign gene. *Proc. Natl. Acad. Sci. USA* **91:**1406–1410.
4. **Barton, D. J., B. J. O'Donnell, and J. B. Flanegan.** 2001. 5' cloverleaf in poliovirus RNA is a cis-acting replication element required for negative-strand synthesis. *EMBO J.* **20:**1439–1448.
5. **Belsham, G. J.** 1992. Dual initiation sites of protein synthesis on foot-and-mouth disease virus RNA are selected following internal entry and scanning of ribosomes in vivo. *EMBO J.* **11:**1105–1110.
6. **Belsham, G. J., and J. K. Brangwyn.** 1990. A region of the 5' noncoding region of foot-and-mouth disease virus RNA directs efficient internal initiation of protein synthesis within cells: involvement with the role of L protease in translational control. *J. Virol.* **64:**5389–5395.
7. **Bergamini, G., T. Preiss, and M. W. Hentze.** 2000. Picornavirus IRESes and the poly(A) tail jointly promote cap-independent translation in a mammalian cell-free system. *RNA* **6:**1781–1790.
8. **Bienkowska-Szewczyk, K., and E. Ehrenfeld.** 1988. An internal 5'-noncoding region required for translation of poliovirus RNA in vitro. *J. Virol.* **62:**3068–3072.
9. **Blyn, L. B., R. Chen, B. L. Semler, and E. Ehrenfeld.** 1995. Host cell proteins binding to domain IV of the 5' noncoding region of poliovirus RNA. *J. Virol.* **69:**4381–4389.
10. **Blyn, L. B., J. S. Towner, B. L. Semler, and E. Ehrenfeld.** 1997. Requirement of poly(rC) binding protein 2 for translation of poliovirus RNA. *J. Virol.* **71:**6243–6246.
11. **Borman, A. M., F. G. Deliat, and K. M. Kean.** 1994. Sequences within the poliovirus internal ribosome entry segment control viral RNA synthesis. *EMBO J.* **13:**3149–3157.
12. **Brown, B. A., and E. Ehrenfeld.** 1979. Translation of poliovirus RNA in vitro: changes in cleavage pattern and initiation sites by ribosomal salt wash. *Virology* **97:**396–405.
13. **Brown, E. A., S. P. Day, R. W. Jansen, and S. M. Lemon.** 1991. The 5' nontranslated region of hepatitis A virus RNA: secondary structure and elements required for translation in vitro. *J. Virol.* **65:**5828–5838.
14. **Brown, E. A., A. J. Zajac, and S. M. Lemon.** 1994. In vitro characterization of an internal ribosomal entry site (IRES) present within the 5' nontranslated region of hepatitis A virus RNA: comparison with the IRES of encephalomyocarditis virus. *J. Virol.* **68:**1066–1074.
15. **Carter, M. S., K. M. Kuhn, and P. Sarnow.** 2000. Cellular internal ribosome entry site elements and the use of cDNA microarrays in their investigation, p. 615–636. *In* N. Sonenberg, J. W. B. Hershey, and M. B. Mathews (ed.), *Translational Control of Gene Expression.* Cold Spring Harbor Laboratory, Cold Spring Harbor, N.Y.
16. **Chapman, N. M., A. Ragland, J. S. Leser, K. Hofling, S. Willian, B. L. Semler, and S. Tracy.** 2000. A group B coxsackievirus/poliovirus 5' nontranslated region chimera can act as an attenuated vaccine strain in mice. *J. Virol.* **74:**4047–4056.
17. **Chen, C. Y., and P. Sarnow.** 1995. Initiation of protein synthesis by the eukaryotic translational apparatus on circular RNAs. *Science* **268:**415–417.
18. **Cornelis, S., Y. Bruynooghe, G. Denecker, S. van Huffel, S. Tinton, and R. Beyaert.** 2000. Identification and characterization of a novel cell cycle-regulated internal ribosome entry site. *Mol. Cell* **5:**597–605.
19. **De Gregorio, E., T. Preiss, and M. W. Hentze.** 1999. Translation driven by an eIF4G core domain in vivo. *EMBO J.* **18:**4865–4874.
20. **Dildine, S. L., and B. L. Semler.** 1989. The deletion of 41 proximal nucleotides reverts a poliovirus mutant containing a temperature-sensitive lesion in the 5' noncoding region of genomic RNA. *J. Virol.* **63:**847–862.
21. **Dorner, A. J., B. L. Semler, R. J. Jackson, R. Hanecak, E. Duprey, and E. Wimmer.** 1984. In vitro translation of poliovirus RNA: utilization of internal initiation sites in reticulocyte lysate. *J. Virol.* **50:**507–514.
22. **Drew, J., and G. J. Belsham.** 1994. trans Complementation by RNA of defective foot-and-mouth disease virus internal ribosome entry site elements. *J. Virol.* **68:**697–703.
23. **Duke, G. M., M. A. Hoffman, and A. C. Palmenberg.** 1992. Sequence and structural elements that contribute to efficient encephalomyocarditis virus RNA translation. *J. Virol.* **66:**1602–1609.
24. **Ehrenfeld, E.** 1996. *Initiation of Translation by Picornavirus RNAs, Translational Control.* Cold Spring Harbor Laboratory Press, Cold Spring Harbor, N.Y.
25. **Ehrenfeld, E., and B. L. Semler.** 1995. Anatomy of the poliovirus internal ribosome entry site. *Curr. Top. Microbiol. Immunol.* **203:**65–83.
26. **Evstafieva, A. G., T. Y. Ugarova, B. K. Chernov, and I. N. Shatsky.** 1991. A complex RNA sequence determines the internal initiation of encephalomyocarditis virus RNA translation. *Nucleic Acids Res.* **19:**665–671.
27. **Gamarnik, A. V., and R. Andino.** 2000. Interactions of viral protein 3CD and poly(rC) binding protein with the 5' untranslated region of the poliovirus genome. *J. Virol.* **74:**2219–2226.
28. **Gamarnik, A. V., and R. Andino.** 1998. Switch from

translation to RNA replication in positive-stranded RNA virus. *Genes Dev.* **12:**2293–2304.
29. Gamarnik, A. V., and R. Andino. 1997. Two functional complexes formed by KH domain containing proteins with the 5′ noncoding region of poliovirus RNA. *RNA* **3:**882–892.
30. Gingras, A. C., B. Raught, and N. Sonenberg. 1999. eIF4 initiation factors: effectors of mRNA recruitment to ribosomes and regulators of translation. *Annu. Rev. Biochem.* **68:**913–963.
31. Glass, M. J., and D. F. Summers. 1993. Identification of a *trans*-acting activity from liver that stimulates hepatitis A virus translation in vitro. *Virology* **193:**1047–1050.
32. Graff, J., and E. Ehrenfeld. 1998. Coding sequences enhance internal initiation of translation by hepatitis A virus RNA in vitro. *J. Virol.* **72:**3571–3577.
33. Gromeier, M., L. Alexander, and E. Wimmer. 1996. Internal ribosomal entry site substitution eliminates neurovirulence in intergeneric poliovirus recombinants. *Proc. Natl. Acad. Sci. USA* **93:**2370–2375.
34. Gromeier, M., B. Bossert, M. Arita, A. Nomoto, and E. Wimmer. 1999. Dual stem loops within the poliovirus internal ribosomal entry site control neurovirulence. *J. Virol.* **73:**958–964.
35. Gutierrez, A. L., M. Denova-Ocampo, V. R. Racaniello, and R. M. del Angel. 1997. Attenuating mutations in the poliovirus 5′ untranslated region alter its interaction with polypyrimidine tract-binding protein. *J. Virol.* **71:**3826–3833.
36. Haller, A. A., and B. L. Semler. 1995. Stem-loop structure synergy in binding cellular proteins to the 5′ noncoding region of poliovirus RNA. *Virology* **206:**923–934.
37. Hoffman, M. A., and A. C. Palmenberg. 1995. Mutational analysis of the J-K stem-loop region of the encephalomyocarditis virus IRES. *J. Virol.* **69:**4399–4406.
38. Imataka, H., A. Gradi, and N. Sonenberg. 1998. A newly identified N-terminal amino acid sequence of human eIF4G binds poly(A)-binding protein and functions in poly(A)-dependent translation. *EMBO J.* **17:**7480–7489.
39. Ishii, T., K. Shiroki, A. Iwai, and A. Nomoto. 1999. Identification of a new element for RNA replication within the internal ribosome entry site of poliovirus RNA. *J. Gen. Virol.* **80:**917–920.
40. Jackson, R. J., and A. Kaminski. 1995. Internal initiation of translation in eukaryotes: the picornavirus paradigm and beyond. *RNA* **1:**985–1000.
41. Jacobson, A. B., and M. Zuker. 1993. Structural analysis by energy dot plot of a large mRNA. *J. Mol. Biol.* **233:**261–269.
42. Jaeger, J. A., D. H. Turner, and M. Zuker. 1989. Improved predictions of secondary structures for RNA. *Proc. Natl. Acad. Sci. USA* **86:**7706–7710.
43. Jang, S. K., M. V. Davies, R. J. Kaufman, and E. Wimmer. 1989. Initiation of protein synthesis by internal entry of ribosomes into the 5′ nontranslated region of encephalomyocarditis virus RNA in vivo. *J. Virol.* **63:**1651–1660.
44. Jang, S. K., H. G. Krausslich, M. J. Nicklin, G. M. Duke, A. C. Palmenberg, and E. Wimmer. 1988. A segment of the 5′ nontranslated region of encephalomyocarditis virus RNA directs internal entry of ribosomes during in vitro translation. *J. Virol.* **62:**2636–2643.
45. Jang, S. K., and E. Wimmer. 1990. Cap-independent translation of encephalomyocarditis virus RNA: structural elements of the internal ribosomal entry site and involvement of a cellular 57-kD RNA-binding protein. *Genes Dev.* **4:**1560–1572.
46. Jia, X. Y., G. Scheper, D. Brown, W. Updike, S. Harmon, O. Richards, D. Summers, and E. Ehrenfeld. 1991. Translation of hepatitis A virus RNA in vitro: aberrant internal initiations influenced by 5′ noncoding region. *Virology* **182:**712–722.
47. Jia, X. Y., M. Tesar, D. F. Summers, and E. Ehrenfeld. 1996. Replication of hepatitis A viruses with chimeric 5′ nontranslated regions. *J. Virol.* **70:**2861–2868.
48. Johansen, L. K., and C. D. Morrow. 2000. The RNA encompassing the internal ribosome entry site in the poliovirus 5′ nontranslated region enhances the encapsidation of genomic RNA. *Virology* **273:**391–399.
49. Johnson, V. H., and B. L. Semler. 1988. Defined recombinants of poliovirus and coxsackievirus: sequence-specific deletions and functional substitutions in the 5′ noncoding regions of viral RNAs. *Virology* **162:**47–57.
50. Kaminski, A., G. J. Belsham, and R. J. Jackson. 1994. Translation of encephalomyocarditis virus RNA: parameters influencing the selection of the internal initiation site. *EMBO J.* **13:**1673–1681.
51. Kaminski, A., S. L. Hunt, C. L. Gibbs, and R. J. Jackson. 1994. Internal initiation of mRNA translation in eukaryotes. *Genet. Eng.* **16:**115–155.
52. King, A. M. Q., F. Brown, P. Christian, T. Hovi, T. Hyypiä, N. J. Knowles, S. M. Lemon, P. D. Minor, A. C. Palmenberg, T. Skern, and G. Stanway. 2000. Picornaviridae, p. 657–673. *In* M. H. V. Van Regenmortel, C. M. Fauquet, D. H. L. Bishop, C. H. Calisher, E. B. Carsten, M. K. Estes, S. M. Lemon, J. Maniloff, M. A. Mayo, D. J. McGeoch, C. R. Pringle, and R. B. Wickner (ed.), *Virus Taxonomy. Seventh Report of the International Committee for the Taxonomy of Viruses.* Academic Press, New York, N.Y.
53. Kitamura, N., B. L. Semler, P. G. Rothberg, G. R. Larsen, C. J. Adler, A. J. Dorner, E. A. Emini, R. Hanecak, J. J. Lee, S. van der Werf, C. W. Anderson, and E. Wimmer. 1981. Primary structure, gene organization and polypeptide expression of poliovirus RNA. *Nature* **291:**547–553.
54. Kolupaeva, V. G., T. V. Pestova, C. U. Hellen, and I. N. Shatsky. 1998. Translation eukaryotic initiation factor 4G recognizes a specific structural element within the internal ribosome entry site of encephalomyocarditis virus RNA. *J. Biol. Chem.* **273:**18599–18604.
55. Kong, W. P., and R. P. Roos. 1991. Alternative translation initiation site in the DA strain of Theiler's murine encephalomyelitis virus. *J. Virol.* **65:**3395–3399.
56. Kuhn, R., N. Luz, and E. Beck. 1990. Functional analysis of the internal translation initiation site of foot-and-mouth disease virus. *J. Virol.* **64:**4625–4631.
57. La Monica, N., and V. R. Racaniello. 1989. Differences in replication of attenuated and neurovirulent polioviruses in human neuroblastoma cell line SH-SY5Y. *J. Virol.* **63:**2357–2360.
58. Le, S.-Y., J.-H. Chen, N. Sonenberg, and J. V. Maizel. 1992. Conserved tertiary structure elements in the 5′ untranslated region of human enteroviruses and rhinoviruses. *Virology* **191:**858–866.
59. Le, S.-Y., and J. V. Maizel. 1998. Evolution of a common structural core in the internal ribosome entry sites of picornavirus. *Virus Genes* **16:**25–38.
60. Le, S.-Y., A. Siddiqui, and J. V. Maizel. 1996. A common structural core in the internal ribosome entry sites of picornavirus, hepatitis C virus, and pestivirus. *Virus Genes* **12:**135–147.
61. Liu, Z., C. M. Carthy, P. Cheung, L. Bohunek, J. E. Wilson, B. M. McManus, and D. Yang. 1999. Structural and functional analysis of the 5′ untranslated region of coxsackievirus B3 RNA: in vivo translational and infectivity studies of full-length mutants. *Virology* **265:**206–217.
62. Lopez de Quinto, S., and E. Martinez-Salas. 2000. Interaction of the eIF4G initiation factor with the aphthovirus

IRES is essential for internal translation initiation in vivo. *RNA* **6:**1380–1392.
63. **Lopez de Quinto, S., and E. Martinez-Salas.** 1997. Conserved structural motifs located in distal loops of aphthovirus internal ribosome entry site domain 3 are required for internal initiation of translation. *J. Virol.* **71:**4171–4175.
64. **Marcotrigiano, J., I. B. Lomakin, N. Sonenberg, T. V. Pestova, C. U. Hellen, and S. K. Burley.** 2001. A conserved HEAT domain within eIF4G directs assembly of the translation initiation machinery. *Mol. Cell* **7:**193–203.
65. **Martinez-Salas, E., R. Ramos, E. Lafuente, and S. Lopez de Quinto.** 2001. Functional interactions in internal translation initiation directed by viral and cellular IRES elements. *J. Gen. Virol.* **82:**973–984.
66. **Martinez-Salas, E., M. P. Regalado, and E. Domingo.** 1996. Identification of an essential region for internal initiation of translation in the aphthovirus internal ribosome entry site and implications for viral evolution. *J. Virol.* **70:**992–998.
67. **Meerovitch, K., Y. V. Svitkin, H. S. Lee, F. Lejbkowicz, D. J. Kenan, E. K. Chan, V. I. Agol, J. D. Keene, and N. Sonenberg.** 1993. La autoantigen enhances and corrects aberrant translation of poliovirus RNA in reticulocyte lysate. *J. Virol.* **67:**3798–3807.
68. **Michel, Y. M., D. Poncet, M. Piron, K. M. Kean, and A. Borman.** 2000. Cap-poly (A) synergy in mammalian cell-free extracts. *J. Biol. Chem.* **275:**32268–32276.
69. **Minor, P. D.** 1992. The molecular biology of poliovaccines. *J. Gen. Virol.* **73:**3065–3077.
70. **Nateri, A. S., P. J. Hughes, and G. Stanway.** 2000. In vivo and in vitro identification of structural and sequence elements of the human parechovirus 5′ untranslated region required for internal initiation. *J. Virol.* **74:**6269–6277.
71. **Nicholson, R., J. Pelletier, S.-Y. Le, and N. Sonenberg.** 1991. Structural and functional analysis of the ribosome landing pad of poliovirus type 2: *in vivo* translation studies. *J. Virol.* **65:**5886–5894.
72. **Niepmann, M.** 1999. Internal initiation of translation of picornaviruses, hepatitis C virus and pestiviruses. *Recent Res. Dev. Virol.* **1:**229–250.
73. **Ohlmann, T., and R. J. Jackson.** 1999. The properties of chimeric picornavirus IRESes show that discrimination between internal translation initiation sites is influenced by the identity of the IRES and not just the context of the AUG codon. *RNA* **5:**764–778.
74. **Ohlmann, T., M. Rau, V. M. Pain, and S. J. Morley.** 1996. The C-terminal domain of eukaryotic protein synthesis initiation factor (eIF) 4G is sufficient to support cap-independent translation in the absence of eIF4E. *EMBO J.* **15:**1371–1382.
75. **Palmenberg, A. C., and J.-Y. Sgro.** 1997. Topological organization of picornaviral genomes: statistical prediction of RNA structural signals. *Semin. Virol.* **8:**231–241.
76. **Parsley, T. B., J. S. Towner, L. B. Blyn, E. Ehrenfeld, and B. L. Semler.** 1997. Poly (rC) binding protein 2 forms a ternary complex with the 5′-terminal sequences of poliovirus RNA and the viral 3CD proteinase. *RNA* **3:**1124–1134.
77. **Pause, A., N. Methot, Y. Svitkin, W. C. Merrick, and N. Sonenberg.** 1994. Dominant negative mutants of mammalian translation initiation factor eIF-4A define a critical role for eIF-4F in cap-dependent and cap-independent initiation of translation. *EMBO J.* **13:**1205–1215.
78. **Pelletier, J., and N. Sonenberg.** 1988. Internal initiation of translation of eukaryotic mRNA directed by a sequence derived from poliovirus RNA. *Nature* **334:**320–325.
79. **Percy, N., G. J. Belsham, J. K. Brangwyn, M. Sullivan, D. M. Stone, and J. W. Almond.** 1992. Intracellular modifications induced by poliovirus reduce the requirement for structural motifs in the 5′ noncoding region of the genome involved in internal initiation of protein synthesis. *J. Virol.* **66:**1695–1701.
80. **Pestova, T. V., C. U. T. Hellen, and I. N. Shatsky.** 1996. Canonical eukaryotic initiation factors determine initiation of translation by internal ribosomal entry. *Mol. Cell. Biol.* **16:**6859–6869.
81. **Pestova, T. V., I. N. Shatsky, and C. U. T. Hellen.** 1996. Functional dissection of eukaryotic initiation factor 4F: the 4A subunit and the central domain of the 4G subunit are sufficient to mediate internal entry of 43S preinitiation complexes. *Mol. Cell. Biol.* **16:**6870–6878.
82. **Phillips, B. A., and A. Emmert.** 1986. Modulation of the expression of poliovirus proteins in reticulocyte lysates. *Virology* **148:**255–267.
83. **Pilipenko, E. V., V. M. Blinov, B. K. Chernov, T. M. Dmitrieva, and V. I. Agol.** 1989. Conservation of the secondary structure elements of the 5′-untranslated region of cardio- and aphthovirus RNAs. *Nucleic Acids Res.* **17:**5701–5711.
84. **Pilipenko, E. V., V. M. Blinov, L. I. Romanova, A. N. Sinyakov, S. V. Maslova, and V. I. Agol.** 1989. Conserved structural domains in the 5′-untranslated region of picornaviral genomes: an analysis of the segment controlling translation and neurovirulence. *Virology* **168:**201–209.
85. **Pilipenko, E. V., A. P. Gmyl, S. V. Maslova, Y. V. Svitkin, A. N. Sinyakov, and V. I. Agol.** 1992. Prokaryotic-like cis elements in the cap-independent internal initiation of translation on picornavirus RNA. *Cell* **68:**119–131.
86. **Pilipenko, E. V., T. V. Pestova, V. G. Kolupaeva, E. V. Khitrina, A. N. Poperechnaya, V. I. Agol, and C. U. Hellen.** 2000. A cell cycle-dependent protein serves as a template-specific translation initiation factor. *Genes Dev.* **14:**2028–2045.
87. **Poyry, T., L. Kinnunen, and T. Hovi.** 1992. Genetic variation in vivo and proposed functional domains of the 5′ noncoding region of poliovirus RNA. *J. Virol.* **66:**5313–5319.
88. **Racaniello, V. R., and D. Baltimore.** 1981. Cloned poliovirus complementary DNA is infectious in mammalian cells. *Science* **214:**916–919.
89. **Ramos, R., and E. Martinez-Salas.** 1999. Long-range RNA interactions between structural domains of the aphthovirus internal ribosome entry site (IRES). *RNA* **5:**1374–1383.
90. **Rinehart, J. E., R. M. Gomez, and R. P. Roos.** 1997. Molecular determinants for virulence in coxsackievirus B1 infection. *J. Virol.* **71:**3986–3991.
91. **Rivera, V. M., J. D. Welsh, and J. V. Maizel, Jr.** 1988. Comparative sequence analysis of the 5′ noncoding region of the enteroviruses and rhinoviruses. *Virology* **165:**42–50.
92. **Roberts, L. O., and G. J. Belsham.** 1997. Complementation of defective internal ribosome entry site (IRES) elements by the coexpression of fragments of the IRES. *Virology* **227:**53–62.
93. **Robertson, M. E., R. A. Seamons, and G. J. Belsham.** 1999. A selection system for functional internal ribosome entry site (IRES) elements: analysis of the requirement for a conserved GNRA tetraloop in the encephalomyocarditis virus IRES. *RNA* **5:**1167–1179.
94. **Scheper, G. C., H. O. Voorma, and A. A. Thomas.** 1992. Eukaryotic initiation factors-4E and -4F stimulate 5′ cap-dependent as well as internal initiation of protein synthesis. *J. Biol. Chem.* **267:**7269–7274.

95. Shih, D. S., I. W. Park, C. L. Evans, J. M. Jaynes, and A. C. Palmenberg. 1987. Effects of cDNA hybridization on translation of encephalomyocarditis virus RNA. *J. Virol.* **61:**2033–2037.
96. Shiroki, K., T. Ishii, T. Aoki, Y. Ota, W. X. Yang, T. Komatsu, Y. Ami, M. Arita, S. Abe, S. Hashizume, and A. Nomoto. 1997. Host range phenotype induced by mutations in the internal ribosomal entry site of poliovirus RNA. *J. Virol.* **71:**1–8.
97. Simoes, E. A., and P. Sarnow. 1991. An RNA hairpin at the extreme 5′ end of the poliovirus RNA genome modulates viral translation in human cells. *J. Virol.* **65:**913–921.
98. Skinner, M. A., V. R. Racaniello, G. Dunn, J. Cooper, P. D. Minor, and J. W. Almond. 1989. New model for the secondary structure of the 5′ non-coding RNA of poliovirus is supported by biochemical and genetic data that also show that RNA secondary structure is important in neurovirulence. *J. Mol. Biol.* **207:**379–392.
99. Slobodskaya, O. R., A. P. Gmyl, S. V. Maslova, E. A. Tolskaya, E. G. Viktorova, and V. I. Agol. 1996. Poliovirus neurovirulence correlates with the presence of a cryptic AUG upstream of the initiator codon. *Virology* **221:**141–150.
100. Stewart, S. R., and B. L. Semler. 1999. Pyrimidine-rich region mutations compensate for a stem-loop V lesion in the 5′ noncoding region of poliovirus genomic RNA. *Virology* **264:**385–397.
101. Stewart, S. R., and B. L. Semler. 1997. RNA determinants of picornavirus cap-independent translation initiation. *Semin. Virol.* **8:**242–255.
102. Stewart, S. R., and B. L. Semler. 1998. RNA structure adjacent to the attenuation determinant in the 5′-noncoding region influences poliovirus viability. *Nucleic Acids Res.* **26:**5318–5326.
103. Stone, D. M., J. W. Almond, J. K. Brangwyn, and G. J. Belsham. 1993. trans Complementation of cap-independent translation directed by poliovirus 5′ noncoding region deletion mutants; evidence for RNA-RNA interactions. *J. Virol.* **67:**6215–6223.
104. Svitkin, Y. V., T. V. Pestova, S. V. Maslova, and V. I. Agol. 1988. Point mutations modify the response of poliovirus RNA to a translation initiation factor: a comparison of neurovirulent and attenuated strains. *Virology* **166:**394–404.
105. Tarun, S. Z., and A. B. Sachs. 1995. A common function for mRNA 5′ and 3′ ends in translation initiation in yeast. *Genes Dev.* **9:**2997–3007.
106. Tesar, M., S. A. Harmon, D. F. Summers, and E. Ehrenfeld. 1992. Hepatitis A virus polyprotein synthesis initiates from two alternative AUG codons. *Virology* **186:**609–618.
107. Trono, D., R. Andino, and D. Baltimore. 1988. An RNA sequence of hundreds of nucleotides at the 5′ end of poliovirus RNA is involved in allowing viral protein synthesis. *J. Virol.* **62:**2291–2299.
108. Tu, Z., N. M. Chapman, G. Hufnagel, S. Tracy, J. R. Romero, W. H. Barry, L. Zhao, K. Currey, and B. Shapiro. 1995. The cardiovirulent phenotype of coxsackievirus B3 is determined at a single site in the genomic 5′ nontranslated region. *J. Virol.* **69:**4607–4618.
109. Van der Velden, A., A. Kaminski, R. J. Jackson, and G. J. Belsham. 1995. Defective point mutants of the encephalomyocarditis virus internal ribosome entry site can be complemented in *trans*. *Virology* **214:**82–90.
110. Wells, S. E., P. E. Hillner, R. D. Vale, and A. B. Sachs. 1998. Circularization of mRNA by eukaryotic translation initiation factors. *Mol. Cell* **2:**135–140.
111. Whetter, L. E., S. P. Day, O. Elroy-Stein, E. A. Brown, and S. M. Lemon. 1994. Low efficiency of the 5′ nontranslated region of hepatitis A virus RNA in directing cap-independent translation in permissive monkey kidney cells. *J. Virol.* **68:**5253–5263.
112. Wimmer, E., C. U. T. Hellen, and X. M. Cao. 1993. Genetics of poliovirus. *Annu. Rev. Genet.* **27:**353–436.
113. Witherell, G. W., C. S. Schultz-Witherell, and E. Wimmer. 1995. cis-Acting elements of the encephalomyocarditis virus internal ribosomal entry site. *Virology* **214:**660–663.
114. Yamashita, T., K. Sakae, H. Tsuzuki, Y. Suzuki, N. Ishikawa, N. Takeda, T. Miyamura, and S. Yamazaki. 1998. Complete nucleotide sequence and genetic organization of Aichi virus, a distinct member of the *Picornaviridae* associated with acute gastroenteritis in humans. *J. Virol.* **72:**8408–8412.
115. Zuker, M., and A. B. Jacobson. 1995. "Well-determined" regions in RNA secondary structure prediction: analysis of small subunit ribosomal RNA. *Nucleic Acids Res.* **23:**2791–2798.

Proteins Involved in the Function of Picornavirus Internal Ribosomal Entry Sites

RICHARD J. JACKSON

15

HISTORICAL PERSPECTIVE

In December 1975, Hugh Pelham, then a first-year graduate student in our group, invented the micrococcal nuclease-treated (messenger-dependent) rabbit reticulocyte lysate (56). The potential uses of the system in those days of the precloning era were much less than they are today, but we realized that one very fruitful application would be to study the expression of positive-strand RNA viral genomes: tobacco mosaic virus, tobacco rattle virus, papaya mosaic virus, cowpea mosaic virus, and encephalomyocarditis virus. The striking outcome was that the translation product patterns of all these viral RNAs, even the plant virus RNAs, generally made "sense" in relation to previously published results, and Hugh Pelham was able to exploit the lysate to add important insights into how these genomes were expressed.

However, we got a severe shock when we translated poliovirus RNA in our messenger-dependent lysate system. In contrast to every other viral RNA tested, the pattern of translation products was unrecognizable in relation to what had previously been published on the basis of infected cells, and the time course of appearance of different products could not be accommodated within a rational polyprotein processing scheme. At that time, a negative influence of inappropriate mRNA secondary structure was often invoked as the explanation for unexpected results from in vitro translation assays, but despite efforts to poison ourselves by the use of methyl mercury hydroxide pretreatment of the poliovirus RNA, we were unable to obtain an interpretable pattern of translation products by disrupting secondary structure in this way.

A critical publication at that time, certainly deserving the accolade of "citation classic" within the confines of the field, was a paper by Brown and Ehrenfeld (10), who showed for the first time in print that the translation of poliovirus RNA was inefficient and inaccurate in the rabbit reticulocyte lysate system, but accurate and efficient in HeLa cell extracts, especially if the extracts were made from virus-infected cells. Clearly, then, there was nothing about poliovirus RNA that made it inherently untranslatable: the problem lay in the translation system and not in the RNA. Subsequently, the Brown and Ehrenfeld results were confirmed by Dorner et al. (15) and by Phillips and Emmert (64), who further showed that the previously uninterpretable translation product pattern obtained when poliovirus RNA is translated in the rabbit reticulocyte lysate system was due mainly to aberrant initiation events in the 5'-proximal part of the P3 coding region (for reasons that remain entirely unexplained even to this day) and that in HeLa cell extracts (or reticulocyte lysates supplemented with HeLa cell extracts) these aberrant initiation events were suppressed, and initiation at the authentic site was enhanced, leading to a pattern of translation products close to what was expected. From that time onward, a major goal of our work, bordering almost on an obsession, was to understand how poliovirus RNA is translated correctly.

Our first reaction at that time (which predated the discovery that picornavirus RNAs are translated by internal ribosomal entry site [IRES]-dependent internal initiation) was that there might be some fundamental difference between the canonical translation initiation factors in rabbit reticulocytes as opposed to HeLa cells. With the wisdom of hindsight this was a naive premise, but, nevertheless, these thoughts led, in 1986, to the first of several annual summer visits to John Hershey's laboratory at the University of California, Davis to exploit the fact that he had a complete collection of canonical initiation factors from both HeLa cells and rabbit reticulocyte lysates in his freezer. The outcome, as would be predicted by this awesomely wise hindsight that we all have, was that supplementation of reticulocyte lysate with purified HeLa cell initiation factors did not alter the pattern of poliovirus RNA translation products significantly. Nevertheless, we did amply confirm (not that any confirmation was needed) the results of Brown and Ehrenfeld (10) that HeLa cell extracts possess at least one activity capable of achieving the desired switch in the balance of translation products; and even though the factor(s) seemed rather fragile to purification, and there were even hints of two separable factors, we were able to convince ourselves that the factor(s) did not correspond to any of the then-known canonical initiation factors present in HeLa cells.

Richard J. Jackson ■ Department of Biochemistry, University of Cambridge, Cambridge, CB2 1GA, United Kingdom.

The Discovery of IRESs in Picornavirus RNAs

The sequencing of picornavirus RNAs in the early 1980s revealed that they had rather long 5' untranslated regions (5' UTRs) of between 610 and ~1400 nucleotides [nt], depending on the particular virus species. Moreover these 5' UTRs have many AUG triplets that do not seem to be used as functional initiation codons and that are generally not highly conserved even between different isolates of the same strain of virus (67), suggesting that the great majority of these upstream AUG triplets are acquired or lost through random sequence drift, with no selective pressure either to retain or lose them. When enough sequences had been accumulated for phylogenetic comparisons to be feasible, and enough direct RNA structure probing had been done (65, 66, 73), it was clear that these 5' UTRs were highly structured. Taken together with the fact that the viral RNAs are not capped, the obvious conclusion was that they could not be translated by the scanning ribosome mechanism, which at that time was considered to be the unique and only possible mechanism of translation initiation in eukaryotes (41).

In due course, evidence for translation by direct internal ribosome entry was provided by the demonstration that the insertion of a picornavirus 5' UTR between the two cistrons of a laboratory-constructed dicistronic mRNA leads to dramatic enhancement of expression of the downstream cistron (33, 57). This discovery led directly to the concept of IRESs, cis-acting RNA elements that direct internal ribosome entry.

Coupled with the knowledge that translation of poliovirus RNA required protein factors that were largely absent from reticulocyte lysates but abundant in HeLa cells, this discovery of the unusual mode of initiation provoked the idea that there might be special dedicated translation initiation factors for IRES-dependent translation. Some of us made rather unsuccessful excursions into investigating the possibility of IRES-dependent translation in yeast, in the hope that the awesome power of yeast genetics would provide a relatively efficient and painless way of identifying such dedicated internal initiation factors. With the wisdom of hindsight, these ideas prevalent in the first half of the 1990s now seem naive and disingenuous.

Throughout the first few years following the discovery that picornavirus RNAs are translated by an IRES-dependent mechanism, the question of whether this unusual mode of initiation required the same set of canonical translation factors as is needed for the conventional scanning-dependent mechanism was largely neglected. This imbalance or oversight was eventually rectified by an important series of experiments that examined initiation complex formation on the encephalomyocarditis virus (EMCV) IRES with highly purified or recombinant initiation factors, as assayed by either sucrose density gradient centrifugation or toe-printing (60, 63). The following account discusses first the role of canonical translation initiation factors in translation dependent on picornavirus IRESs, and then goes on to discuss the involvement of other cellular proteins in IRES function.

THE ROLE OF CANONICAL INITIATION FACTORS IN INITIATION DEPENDENT ON PICORNAVIRAL IRESs

The Canonical Initiation Factors and Their Roles in Translation Initiation in General

Table 1 lists the mammalian translation initiation factors that have received general recognition but excludes other candidate factors whose role is still under debate. In brief, the normal (though not necessarily obligatory) sequence of events in initiation of translation of capped mRNAs by the conventional scanning mechanism is as follows (see reference 26 for a more detailed account). First, eIF3 binds to the 40S ribosomal subunit, followed by binding of the eIF2/Met-tRNA$_i$/GTP ternary complex. The 40S subunit, now primed for initiation, then binds to the mRNA under the influence of the eIF4 family of initiation factors, coupled to ATP hydrolysis, and with eIF1 and eIF1A playing an auxiliary but essential role (59). This is the stage at which 40S subunit scanning occurs. When the 40S subunit has engaged the correct initiation codon, presumably via base pairing between this AUG and the anticodon of the Met-tRNA$_i$ carried on the 40S subunit, the action of eIF5 and eIF5B in promoting the hydrolysis of the GTP moiety of the 40S-associated ternary complex, and the joining of the 60S ribosomal subunit, is effectively the step of commitment to initiate at that AUG codon (61). Following commitment in this way, initiation is now complete and the previously associated initiation factor proteins are thought to dissociate from the ribosome.

In this model, 40S subunits do not and cannot bind directly to the mRNA in the complete absence of initiation factors, and not even the association of eIF3 and the eIF2/Met-tRNA$_i$/GTP ternary complex with the 40S subunit is considered sufficient to facilitate small subunit binding to mRNA. Rather, it is the eIF4 family of factors that execute the "delivery" of the primed 40S subunit to the mRNA. The critical factor is the eIF4F holoenzyme complex consisting of eIF4A, an ATP-dependent RNA helicase; eIF4E, which is the only factor that binds directly to 5'-cap structures; and eIF4G, which appears to act as a scaffold (Fig. 1). In the translation of capped mRNAs by the scanning mechanism, eIF4F is thought to deliver the primed 40S subunit to the region just downstream of the cap because it is bound at the 5' end via the interaction of its eIF4E component with the cap (20). "Delivery" is a vague term deliberately chosen to hide the fact that we do not know very much about what is involved. However, some insights have come from the discovery that initiation of translation of some mRNAs does not require the complete eIF4F complex, but just the central domain of eIF4G and the associated eIF4A (Table 2).

Entero- and rhinovirus 2A and foot-and-mouth disease virus (FMDV) L proteases cleave eIF4G into an N-terminal one-third fragment, which has the eIF4E interaction site, and a C-terminal two-thirds fragment, which has the interaction site for eIF3, and both sites where eIF4A binds (20, 29, 42, 48). The resulting physical separation of the cap-binding function from the C-terminal two-thirds domain inactivates the factor for translation of capped cellular mRNAs, because the central domain of eIF4G is no longer tethered to the mRNA in the vicinity of the 5' cap. However, the translation of uncapped versions of normally capped mRNAs is actually stimulated by this cleavage of eIF4G (51, 52), or if the system is supplemented with just the central domain of eIF4G (13). Similarly, with the notable exception of the hepatitis A virus (HAV) IRES, translation dependent on picornavirus IRESs is not inhibited by cleavage of eIF4G and may even be stimulated in some circumstances (4, 6, 7, 25, 68). Thus, for uncapped mRNAs and most picornavirus IRESs, not only is eIF4E completely redundant (Table 2), but the eIF4G requirement can be fulfilled by the C-terminal two-thirds fragment or even by just the central domain (Fig. 1).

Even more striking is the case of the hepatitis C and pestivirus IRESs, which are unique (so far) among all eu-

TABLE 1 Canonical mammalian initiation factors and their roles

Factor	No. of polypeptides	Size (kDa)	Principal functions and properties
eIF1	1	12.6	Both eIF1 and 1A are needed for successful ribosome scanning to the initiation codon, and they also (especially eIF1) appear to monitor the fidelity of codon/anticodon interaction.
eIF1A	1	16.5	
eIF2	3	36.2 (α) 39.0 (β) 51.8 (γ)	Forms eIF2/Met-tRNA$_i$/GTP ternary complex, which binds to 40S ribosomal subunit in a codon-independent manner.
eIF2B	5	33.7 (α) 39.0 (β) 50.4 (γ) 57.8 (δ) 80.2 (ε)	Guanosine nucleoside exchange factor, which catalyzes exchange conversion of eIF2/GDP to eIF2/GTP. Needed for recycling of eIF2.
eIF3	10+	>600 total	Five core subunits; precise number of noncore nonstoichiometric subunits uncertain.
eIF4A(I)	1	44.4	Has RNA-dependent ATPase activity and RNA helicase activity dependent on ATP hydrolysis and eIF4B. Interacts with eIF4G at two sites. A second species, eIF4AII (46.3 kDa), is encoded by a different gene.
eIF4B	1	69.2	Precise role uncertain. Promotes RNA helicase activity of eIF4A.
eIF4E	1	25.1	Binds to 5′-cap structure. Interacts with eIF4G.
eIF4G(I)	1	171.6	Appears to fulfill a scaffold function. The central domain (see Fig. 1), in conjunction with eIF4A, appears to deliver the primed 40S subunit to the mRNA. A less abundant second species, eIF4GII (176.5 kDa), is encoded by a different gene.
eIF4F			A complex of eIF4A, 4E, and 4G (see Fig. 1).
eIF5	1	48.9	Needed for subunit joining. Promotes hydrolysis of GTP associated with eIF2.
eIF5B	1	139.0	Needed for subunit joining. Has ribosome-dependent GTPase activity.

karyotic cellular and viral RNAs in several interrelated respects: the washed 40S ribosomal subunit can bind to these RNAs at the correct site in the absence of any of the canonical initiation factors; initiation on these RNAs does not require eIF4A, 4B, 4E, or 4G or ATP hydrolysis (Table 2); nor do any of these factors appear to bind to the IRES (62). This has led to the realization that the eIF4 family of initiation factors and ATP hydrolysis are not intrinsically necessary for initiation, provided that the RNA sequence and structure are such that the small ribosomal subunit can bind directly to the mRNA at the correct site in the absence of initiation factors, as is the case with the hepatitis C virus and pestivirus IRESs, as well as all prokaryotic mRNAs. If there is no such direct binding of the small ribosomal subunit to the mRNA, as is the case with virtually all eukaryotic cellular and viral mRNAs, then, at a minimum, eIF4A and the central domain of eIF4G, in addition to ATP hydrolysis, are required to promote functional 40S subunit/mRNA interaction. In this mechanism dependent on the eIF4 family of factors and ATP hydrolysis, appropriate interaction between eIF4G and the mRNA is important to execute ribosome delivery to the correct site. This interaction can be either indirect, as happens in the translation of capped mRNAs when the eIF4G is tethered to the mRNA near its 5′ end via the binding of the associated eIF4E to the cap, or it can be achieved by direct binding of the eIF4G to the mRNA, as appears to happen with at least some picornavirus IRESs, as discussed below. A corollary is that if eIF4G could be tethered indirectly to a site in the interior of the RNA, then the prediction is that it could promote internal initiation. This has been confirmed by a clever experiment in which a synthetic IRES system was constructed consisting of an iron response element (the RNA motif that specifically binds iron regulatory protein) and a fusion protein comprising the central domain of eIF4G fused to the iron regulatory protein (14). Given that the central domain of eIF4G interacts with eIF3 (42) (Fig. 1), which itself associates tightly with the 40S ribosomal subunit (26), and since the two interactions of eIF3 (with the 40S subunit and with eIF4G) are thought to be not mutually exclusive, it is likely that there is an eIF4G/eIF3/40S subunit interaction relay, and it is this which is thought to deliver the 40S subunit to the mRNA in the vicinity of the 5′ cap.

As shown in Fig. 1, there are two sites on eIF4G to which eIF4A can bind (29). Given that the eIF4G require-

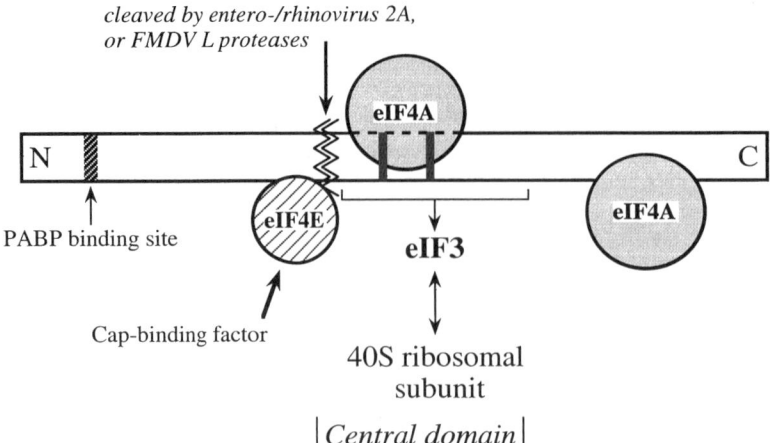

FIGURE 1 Schematic diagram of eIF4G domain structure. The eIF4G polypeptide is depicted as an open rectangle, with binding/interaction sites of PABP, eIF3, eIF4A helicase (two interaction sites), and eIF4E cap-binding factor shown (20, 48). The putative RNP-1 and RNP-2 motifs of the hypothetical RRM in the central domain are shown as vertical black bars. The indicated central domain is (so far) the minimum eIF4G fragment able to support translation initiation dependent on the EMCV IRES. The diagram is based on the more abundant and better studied eIF4G species, eIF4GI. The other minor species (eIF4GII), although only 46% homologous to eIF4GI throughout the whole protein, shows much greater homology in certain specific regions, notably in the center and toward the C terminus, suggesting that the sites of interaction with PABP, eIF3, eIF4A, and eIF4E will be in similar positions as in eIF4GI (23).

ment for initiation can be fulfilled by just the central domain in some circumstances, it must be the interaction of eIF4A with this eIF4G central domain that is important. This correlates with the fact that the equivalent of the central domain of mammalian eIF4G can be found in yeast and plant eIF4Gs, which have no counterpart of the extreme C-terminal one-third fragment of mammalian eIF4G (20, 48). Singular eIF4A and eIF4F holoenzyme complex both exhibit ATP-dependent RNA helicase activity, provided eIF4B is also present (34, 69). Unlike typical RNA and DNA helicases, this unwinding activity is claimed to be bidirectional. The eIF4F complex appeared to be about fivefold more active on a molar basis than singular eIF4A for unwinding in the $3' \rightarrow 5'$ direction, and as much as ~15-fold more active than singular eIF4A in the $5' \rightarrow 3'$ direction, provided the RNA was capped (69). These data suggest that when the cellular complement of initiation factors encounters endogenous cellular mRNAs, the pre-

TABLE 2 Characteristics of different mechanisms of initiation of translation of eukaryotic cellular and viral RNAs

	Internal initiation on:			Scanning-dependent initiation on:	
	Hepatitis C virus and pestivirus IRESs	EMCV[a] IRES	HAV IRES	Uncapped mRNA	Capped mRNA
Direct binding of washed 40S subunits in the absence of initiation factors	Yes	No	(No)[c]	No	No
Requirement for eIF4A	No	Yes	(Yes)[c]	Yes	Yes
Inhibition by dominant negative eIF4A mutants	No	Yes	Yes	Yes	Yes
Requirement for ATP hydrolysis	No	Yes[b]	(Yes)[c]	Yes	Yes
Requirement for at least part of eIF4G	No	Yes	Yes	Yes	Yes
eIF4G requirement fulfilled by central domain of eIF4G	—	Yes	(No)[c]	Yes	No
Inhibition by cleavage of eIF4G by picornavirus proteases	No	No	Yes	No	Yes
Inhibition by cap analogues (e.g., m⁷GpppG)	No	No	Yes	No	Yes
Requirement for eIF4E	No	No	Yes?	No	Yes

[a] It is thought likely that the same pattern of requirements will be shown by all picornavirus IRESs except the HAV IRES.
[b] Although initiation dependent on the EMCV IRES requires ATP hydrolysis (60, 63), significantly lower ATP concentrations are needed than for scanning-dependent initiation (30).
[c] Answers given in parentheses are considered to be the most probable outcome, but the issue has not yet been put to a direct test.

dominant outcome will be cap-dependent unwinding in the 5' → 3' direction (rather than the reverse) carried out by eIF4F complex, rather than singular eIF4A. The results leave open the possibility that unwinding in the 3' → 5' direction might occur during IRES-dependent initiation, but this remains a matter of pure speculation.

Some dominant negative mutants of eIF4A have been described, which are extremely potent inhibitors of in vitro translation (55). Translation activity can be recovered by addition of either eIF4F complex or singular eIF4A, but to effect the same degree of recovery requires sixfold more singular eIF4A than eIF4F (on a molar basis). This has led to the suggestion that the normal function of eIF4A is to recycle or treadmill through the eIF4F holoenzyme complex and that the dominant negative mutants inhibit by entering the complex but failing to exit and recycle, effectively generating a dead-end eIF4F complex (55). This in turn suggests that the principal role of eIF4A in translation initiation is as a constituent of the eIF4F complex (i.e., in association with eIF4G) and that singular eIF4A has little, if any, influence.

The central part of eIF4G may also have an RNA-binding domain of the RNP-1/RNP-2 family. This was first noted through sequence inspection of both isoforms of yeast eIF4G (22), and similar motifs can be found in eIF4G from other origins including mammals (48). However, the putative RNP-1 and RNP-2 motifs are somewhat noncanonical, and the spacing between them is atypically large. In fact, there has been no direct demonstration that it functions as an RNA-binding domain, let alone any investigation as to its specificity for particular RNA sequences.

The Role of Canonical Initiation Factors in Internal Initiation Promoted by the EMCV IRES

Of all the picornaviruses, it is the EMCV IRES that is by far the best understood, such that it has become the paradigm against which all others are compared. The cardinal features of initiation dependent on the EMCV IRES are that it is not inhibited by cleavage of eIF4G by picornavirus proteases (4, 7, 68); it is not inhibited by the 4E-BPs (eIF4E-binding proteins), which interact with eIF4E and prevent its association with eIF4G (54); and it is as sensitive to inhibition by dominant negative eIF4A mutants as is initiation by the scanning ribosome mechanism (55). Thus, eIF4E is clearly redundant, the eIF4G requirement can be satisfied by the C-terminal two-thirds or even just the central domain, and there is a strong requirement for eIF4A.

Toe-printing and sucrose gradient analyses of initiation complexes formed with highly purified initiation factors have shown that the binding of the 40S subunit to the correct initiation site on the EMCV IRES absolutely requires eIF2, 3, and 4A and either the complete native eIF4F complex (with associated eIF4A) or recombinant fragments of eIF4G, which include the central one-third domain (60, 63). Although not absolutely required, eIF4B increased the yield of complexes by about twofold. Direct binding of the central domain of eIF4G to the J-K domain of the EMCV IRES fairly close to the correct initiation site has been demonstrated by toe-printing and foot-printing (Fig. 2), and this toe-print was uninfluenced by the presence or absence of eIF4A, eIF4B, and ATP (40, 60, 63). An identical toe-print was observed when eIF4F holoenzyme complex was studied. It is not known whether the binding of eIF4G to the IRES occurs via the putative RNP-1/RNP-2 motif in the eIF4G central domain (Fig. 1). In UV-cross-linking assays with the native eIF4F holoenzymes complex and the whole EMCV IRES, all three eIF4F polypeptides, even eIF4E, were cross-linked to the IRES (63). When recombinant subdomains of eIF4G were studied using the same probe, there seemed to be cooperativity of binding (or of cross-linking) of eIF4A, eIF4B, and the central domain of eIF4G, but not the extreme C-terminal domain (63). Although the probe was the complete EMCV IRES, it seems reasonable to suppose that all three polypeptides actually bind to the J-K domain, an assumption that is supported by the fact that eIF4B in crude reticulocyte lysates can be cross-linked by UV irradiation to the J domain of the FMDV IRES in the presence of ATP (47).

The binding of the central domain of eIF4G (together with eIF4A and 4B) to the J-K domain of the EMCV IRES probably delivers the 40S subunit to the nearby initiation site via the eIF4G/eIF3/40S interaction relay. However, this cannot be sufficient to promote internal initiation; otherwise the J-K domain alone would be able to act as an efficient IRES, and the strong dependency of IRES activity on the upstream H and I domains (Fig. 2) would not be observed. At present the role of the H and I domains is unknown, but it is unlikely to be related to eIF4G binding, since fairly drastic mutations in stem-loop I have no effect on the eIF4G/J-K domain interactions. We do not know whether domains H and I bind other initiation factors or whether they are the site of ribosome-IRES interactions, but in the latter case the interactions must be rather weak, since binding of the 40S subunits to the IRES in the absence of initiation factors cannot be detected either by sucrose gradient centrifugation or by toe-printing (60).

There is compelling evidence that internal initiation on the EMCV IRES involves direct ribosome entry at the authentic initiation site (Fig. 2), with very little, if any, scanning (35, 36). Nevertheless, even when internal initiation is driven by native eIF4F holoenzyme complex with its associated eIF4A subunit, additional (singular) eIF4A is still required (60). There is also a requirement for ATP hydrolysis (60, 63), albeit lower concentrations of ATP than are needed for initiation of translation of capped mRNAs by the scanning mechanism (30). This ATP requirement can be fulfilled by dATP with reasonable efficiency (63), which correlates with the fact that dATP can support the helicase activity of singular eIF4A and of eIF4A in the eIF4F holoenzyme complex (69). The requirement for eIF4A, probably as part of the eIF4F holoenzyme complex, is further confirmed by the inhibitory effect of dominant negative eIF4A mutants (55). In fact, some old, and therefore often neglected, data imply that translation of EMCV RNA may need *more* eIF4A than does conventional scanning on globin mRNA. Partial fractionation of a cell-free system from ascites cells resulted in a greater decrease of EMCV RNA translation than globin mRNA translation. A factor that selectively restored EMCV RNA translation was purified; originally named IF$_{EMC}$, this factor subsequently turned out to be eIF4A (79).

This requirement for eIF4A and ATP hydrolysis, despite the fact that there is probably no ribosome scanning, is often thought surprising, in view of the prevailing assumption that the function of singular eIF4A is somehow associated with scanning. However, as discussed previously, the properties of dominant negative eIF4A mutants have thrown doubt on whether singular eIF4A plays a significant role in translation initiation and suggest, instead, that the main influence of eIF4A is exerted in association with

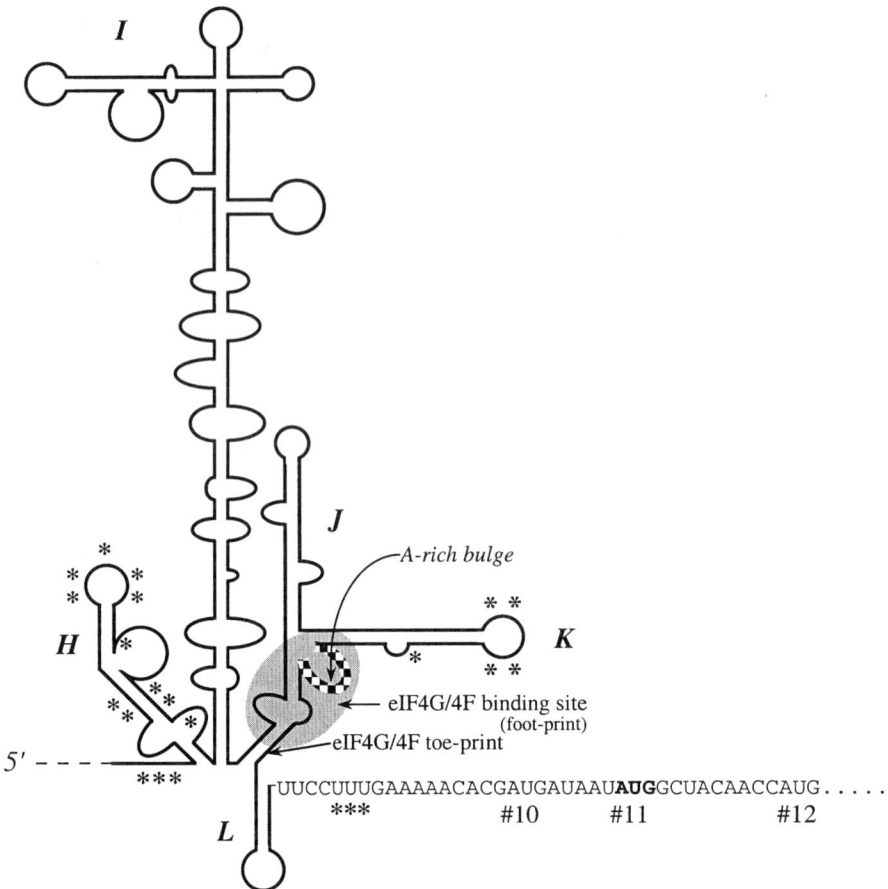

FIGURE 2 Schematic diagram of the EMCV IRES. The sequence around the authentic initiation site (AUG-11, shown in bold) is given. The various subdomains (H through L) discussed in the text are indicated. The site at which eIF4G (or eIF4F) binds as determined by foot-printing (40) is shown by stippling, and the self-consistent toe-print site (40, 60, 63) is also indicated. Asterisks denote the regions protected when PTB binds to the IRES, as determined by foot-printing/protection experiments (39). The A-rich bulge (sequence 5'-UAAAAAA-3' in EMCV strain R) is denoted by a thickened checkered line; a fortuitous expansion of this bulge by a single additional A-residue renders the activity of the IRES highly dependent on PTB (38).

eIF4G, i.e., as a subunit of eIF4F holoenzyme complex (55). It therefore seems likely that the binding of eIF4G (and associated eIF4A) to the J-K domain of the EMCV IRES not only delivers the 40S subunit to the nearby initiation site via the eIF4G/eIF3/40S subunit interaction relay, but also focuses the helicase activity of the associated eIF4A to unwind the region around the initiation site.

In scanning-dependent initiation, eIF1 and eIF1A are needed for successful scanning to the authentic initiation codon (59). In their absence, the 40S subunit stalls a short distance downstream from the cap. Delayed addition of eIF1 and eIF1A to these stalled complexes does not so much allow them to scan further from the cap, but rather it accelerates the dissociation of the stalled complexes from the mRNA. These two factors (eIF1 and eIF1A) have very little effect on the total yield of initiation complexes formed on the EMCV IRES, but they have subtle effects on which AUG codon is chosen. In the commonly used EMCV-R strain, virtually all initiation in a reticulocyte lysate translation assay is at the 11th AUG (Fig. 2), and there is almost none at AUG-10 located just 8 nt further upstream (35, 36). However, in the absence of eIF1 and eIF1A, initiation complexes form at both AUG-10 and AUG-11 in roughly equal yield (59). Addition of eIF1A slightly increases the yield of complexes at AUG-11, and eIF1 strongly decreases the yield at AUG-10, even when these additions were delayed until after complexes had formed at AUG-10. Thus these factors, especially eIF1, must destabilize complexes that have formed at AUG-10. It is not clear what features of the complex formed at AUG-10 mark it out as "incorrect" and thus target it for destabilization, but the conclusion is that both eIF1 and eIF1A are required in the initiation complex formation assay to give a pattern of relative usage of these two AUGs which accords with that observed in translation assays.

The Role of Canonical Initiation Factors in Translation Initiation Promoted by Other Picornavirus IRESs

Although we have much less direct evidence on the role of canonical initiation factors in the translation of entero-

and rhinovirus RNAs, there is no reason to believe that it is very different from the EMCV IRES paradigm. Certainly the translation of entero- and rhinovirus RNAs is not inhibited, but may even be enhanced, by cleavage of the eIF4G component of eIF4F by viral proteases (4, 6, 7, 45, 68), and is as sensitive to inhibition by dominant negative eIF4A mutants as is EMCV IRES activity. Therefore, eIF4F, or the central fragment of eIF4G, presumably binds directly to the entero- and rhinovirus IRESs. The putative binding site is not yet known and may be rather different from the binding site in the EMCV IRES (Fig. 2), which is at an A-rich bulge that has no obvious equivalent in the entero- and rhinovirus IRESs.

The HAV IRES is likely to be very different since it is inhibited by cleavage of the eIF4G component of eIF4F (3, 4, 7, 78), as well as by m^{7}GpppG cap analogue and by 4E-BP1 (I. K. Ali and R. J. Jackson, unpublished observations), which binds and sequesters eIF4E (54). These observations suggest that HAV IRES activity requires eIF4E and that the eIF4E has to be associated with eIF4G to fulfill this role. This in turn suggests the possibility that the eIF4F holoenzyme complex might bind directly, via its eIF4E subunit, to an internal site within the HAV IRES and deliver the 40S subunit to the mRNA via the eIF4G/eIF3/40S subunit interaction relay. This would be somewhat similar to what is believed to be the mechanism of translation of satellite tobacco necrosis virus RNA. This RNA is naturally uncapped, and its translation is not stimulated by capping, unless the 3' UTR is amputated or mutated, in which case translation is highly dependent on a 5' cap (75). It is known that eIF4E or the eIF4F holoenzyme complex binds to a specific stem-loop structure in the 3' UTR, and it appears that this binding somehow delivers the initiating 40S subunit to the 5'-proximal initiation site (B. M. Gazo, J. R. Gatchel, S. R. Lax, R. Ahmed, and K. S. Browning, submitted for publication).

THE ROLE OF CELLULAR RNA-BINDING PROTEINS IN PICORNAVIRUS IRES ACTIVITY

It has been known for over 20 years that poliovirus RNA translation in rabbit reticulocyte lysates is inefficient and inaccurate, especially at high RNA concentration, but can be rescued by addition of HeLa cell fractions (10, 15, 64). Subsequent publications have confirmed that this is true of other enterovirus RNAs, and is even more extreme for rhinovirus RNA (4, 5). More recent work has shown that the poliovirus IRES also functions very inefficiently in stage VI *Xenopus* oocytes, unless HeLa cell cytoplasm was co-injected or HeLa cell mRNA had been injected some time earlier (17). It has also been shown that supplementation with liver extracts, but not HeLa cell cytoplasm, stimulates the activity of the HAV IRES in reticulocyte lysate systems (21). In contrast, the cardiovirus and aphthovirus IRESs function efficiently, not only in rabbit reticulocyte lysates but also in *Xenopus* oocytes (17, 43). Thus, it is clear that the activity of at least some IRESs requires not only the supposedly ubiquitous canonical initiation factors, but also other cellular proteins that are restricted to certain tissues or cell types. This has generated considerable interest because it was thought that these tissue-specific factors might provide an explanation for the tissue tropism of the viruses, a hope that still remains largely unfulfilled.

Following the initial discovery of IRESs, the trend in the early 1990s was to try to identify these necessary additional factors by cataloguing the proteins that bind to IRESs and can be cross-linked to them by UV irradiation. However, we now know that there is no substitute for a functional assay; there are several examples of proteins that bind to an IRES apparently at a specific site, yet the binding has no effect on IRES activity (38, 77). Consequently, this discussion will ignore all the proteins (most of them still unidentified) that have been scored solely as IRES-binding proteins in UV-cross-linking assays and will focus exclusively on those that have been shown to have functional significance. To date, the proteins that meet this criterion are polypyrimidine tract-binding protein (PTB), poly(rC)-binding protein-2 (PCBP-2), unr, and, arguably, the autoantigen La.

Cellular RNA-Binding Proteins Required for Entero- and Rhinovirus IRES Activity

Given that these IRESs function inefficiently in rabbit reticulocyte lysates or *Xenopus* oocytes (4, 5, 15, 17; E. C. Brown and R. J. Jackson, unpublished observations), but efficiently in HeLa cell extracts, the usual strategy has been to try to purify and identify the HeLa cell factors that stimulate translation in the restrictive systems. The autoantigen La was the first to be discovered, although it was initially identified by virtue of the fact that it was found to bind to the region of the poliovirus IRES that represents the putative ribosome entry site. Addition of La to rabbit reticulocyte lysates was subsequently shown to give a fair stimulation of poliovirus RNA translation and to improve the accuracy of selection of the correct initiation site (46, 74). However, the concentrations of La required for this effect were significantly higher than would be present when poliovirus RNA translation in reticulocyte lysates is rescued by addition of HeLa cell extracts. Although explanations for this low specific activity of the recombinant La have been proposed, such as the possibility that the recombinant La may not be folded properly or may lack necessary post-translational modifications, the fact is that no attempt seems to have been made to test whether these explanations have any validity. Moreover, this is not a problem peculiar to recombinant La expressed in bacteria; even La purified from HeLa cells was effective only at very high concentrations (46). Thus, the current position must be that La is not a physiologically relevant stimulator (or is only of marginal relevance) of enterovirus IRES activity, but that at high concentrations it can partially mimic the physiological factors.

In uninfected cells La is considered to have a predominantly but not exclusively nuclear location (46, 50). It is true that poliovirus infection results in a redistribution of La from the nucleus to the cytoplasm (46) following removal of the extreme C terminus of La through cleavage by poliovirus 3C-protease (71). Provocative though this is, it should not be forgotten that poliovirus replicates quite well in enucleated cells (16)—indeed, very well if the progressive deterioration of enucleated cells over the time course of the infection is taken into account—and so this redistribution can only be of marginal significance for the virus life cycle.

To avoid the risk of other questionable or decidedly false positives, a strictly functional in vitro translation assay was used to purify those factors that are necessary for rhinovirus IRES activity and that are present in reticulocyte lysates at relatively low (or zero) abundance relative to HeLa cell extracts (5, 27, 28). The rhinovirus rather than poliovirus IRES was used for these assays, since it gives an even lower background of activity in the unsupplemented reticulocyte lysate, and in view of the close phylogenetic and structural relationship between the two IRESs, the expectation was that the same cellular factors would be required for both IRESs, though in fact this has turned out to be not correct. Two HeLa cell factors were isolated by this approach: when tested individually, each stimulated rhinovirus IRES activity in the reticulocyte lysate, and together their effects were at least additive and more often synergistic (27, 28). One of them was PTB, an RNA-binding protein that has been strongly implicated as a regulator of alternative splicing of pre-mRNA (76). As would be expected, therefore, PTB (also known as hnRNP I) is strongly localized in the nucleus, although there is a significant presence in the cytoplasm (19).

The other factor that stimulated HRV IRES activity was *unr* associated with a novel GH-WD repeat protein (28). *unr*, which gets its name from the fact it is encoded by a gene located just upstream of N-*ras*, is fairly ubiquitously expressed in mammalian tissues, is largely cytoplasmic, and is an essential protein, since the homozygous mouse knockout is embryonic lethal (8, 9, 31). It is a member of the cold-shock domain family of single-stranded nucleic acid-binding proteins (24), but it is unique among this family in two respects: it is the only one with as many as five cold-shock domains (Fig. 3), and all domains share a particular amino acid sequence signature not found in any other protein of the family (24, 28).

The observation that either PTB or *unr* can stimulate when added alone often causes some surprise and calls for an explanation. We believe that this is related to another peculiarity of entero- and rhinovirus IRESs: the anomalous relationship between RNA concentration and translation product yield. With most RNAs, increasing the RNA concentration results in an increase in the product yield until this yield plateaus when saturation has been attained. However, with RNAs bearing an entero- or rhinovirus IRES there is no real plateau, but instead there comes a point where a further increase in RNA concentration results in a sharp downturn in product yield. This anomalous dose response cannot be dismissed as an artifact of in vitro translation assays since it has also been noted in transfection assays, at least with the HRV IRES (7). As we have argued in detail elsewhere (27), the simplest explanation of this anomalous dose response is one that posits that IRES activity requires the simultaneous binding of two (or more) different proteins at different sites, with little or no cooperativity of binding. Under these constraints and assuming that the system contains both proteins, albeit in limiting amounts, progressively increasing the RNA concentration will reach a threshold point beyond which there will be a decrease in the absolute number, not just the relative proportion, of RNA molecules simultaneously binding both proteins. If the RNA concentration is above this critical threshold, supplementation of the system with *either* protein will elicit a stimulation, effectively by complementation.

Although both *unr* and PTB are required for efficient function of the HRV IRES, it was rather surprising (in view of the close phylogenetic relationship) to find that only PTB, and not *unr*, significantly stimulated the activity of the poliovirus IRES in rabbit reticulocyte lysate (27, 28). Addition of recombinant PTB and *unr* at realistically low concentrations stimulates HRV IRES activity as efficiently as does crude HeLa cell extract (28). However, the same is not true for the poliovirus IRES, and thus it seems likely that in addition to PTB (and also PCBP-2, which is discussed below), at least one other protein is needed for maximum poliovirus IRES activity. It will be difficult to identify this protein with the reticulocyte lysate system as a functional assay, since, unlike the HRV IRES, the poliovirus IRES works moderately efficiently in reticulocyte lysates at low RNA concentrations, and, given that these *trans*-acting factors seem to be RNA-binding proteins that act stoichiometrically with respect to RNA concentration, a sensitive assay for monitoring purification demands the use of low concentrations of mRNA. The *Xenopus* oocyte system developed by Gamarnik and Andino (17) seems a more promising approach as it is more sensitive than the reticulocyte lysate system. Efficient poliovirus IRES activity required either coinjection of HeLa cell cytoplasmic extract or previous injection of HeLa cell mRNA. Intriguingly, the HeLa cell activity behaved as a single entity of around 300 kDa, which does not correspond to any of the proteins discussed in this section.

As mentioned above, another protein identified as necessary for the activity of the entero- and rhinovirus IRESs is PCBP-2, a cytoplasmic RNA-binding protein with three KH domains. This was originally characterized as a protein that binds to stem-loop IV (1), an internal stem-loop structure in the poliovirus IRES. Because PCBPs are relatively abundant not only in HeLa cell extracts but also in rabbit reticulocyte lysates, the question of whether PCBPs are required for picornavirus IRES activity requires the use of a depletion strategy rather than the supplementation approach that was used to identify *unr*. When HeLa cell extracts were depleted of PCBPs by an affinity column procedure, they lost the capacity to support translation dependent on the poliovirus, coxsackievirus B, and rhinovirus IRESs, and addition of recombinant PCBP-2 restored the activity of these entero- and rhinovirus IRESs (2, 77). Strikingly, although PCBP-2 binds to cardio- and aphthovirus IRESs, it seems that this binding is of no functional significance, since these IRESs functioned equally well in the depleted cell-free system as in the parent extract (77).

It is particularly remarkable that only PCBP-2 but not PCBP-1 was active in restoring entero- and rhinovirus IRES activity in these assays (2). Although PCBP-1 appears to be encoded by a different gene, it differs from PCBP-2 in only 17% of residues (44), and the N-terminal region, which is believed to be the region mainly involved in RNA binding (72), shows less than 5% divergence (Fig. 3). This provocative finding suggests that we should pay more attention to investigating the relative efficiencies of the various isoforms of *unr* and PTB in supporting entero- and rhinovirus IRES activity. There are two known isoforms of *unr* (9), differing according to the inclusion or exclusion of an optionally spliced exon (Fig. 3). It was found that the smaller isoform, lacking exon 5, was the more active in supporting HRV IRES activity, although the difference was less than twofold (28). There are several variants of PTB that arise from alternative splicing of the primary transcript (53), and in addition there are PTB-like proteins, such as ROD1 (80; M. C. Wollerton and C. W. J. Smith, personal communication), which appear to be encoded by different genes. In our hands, the PTB isoforms generated by alternative splicing do not differ greatly in their ability to support rhinovirus or poliovirus IRES activity in rabbit reticulocyte lysates (Brown and Jackson, unpublished), but the PTB-like proteins encoded by different genes have yet to be tested. Although it appears that the tissue distribution of *unr*, PTB, and PCBP-2 does not provide a satisfactory explanation for the tissue tropism of var-

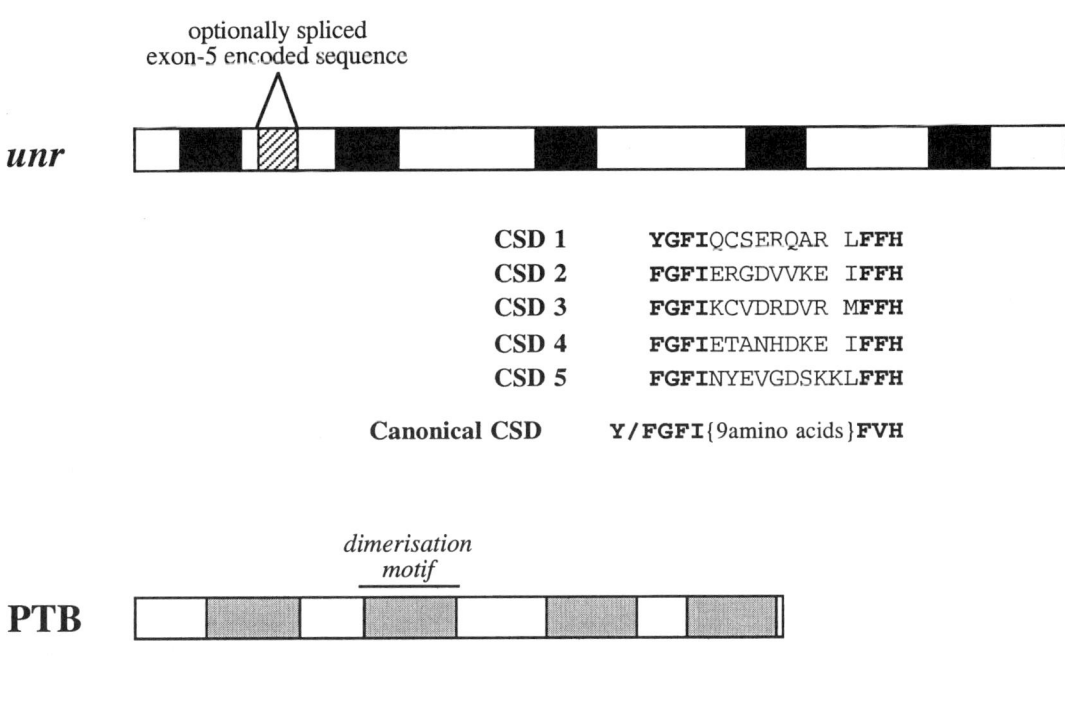

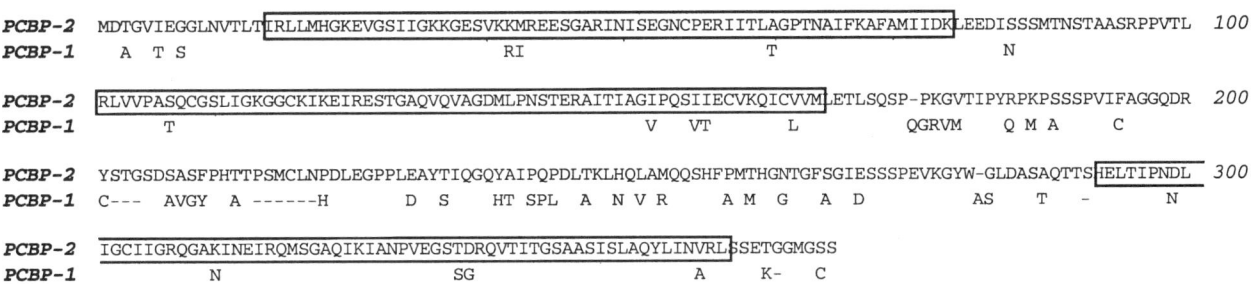

FIGURE 3 Schematic diagram of the domain structure of unr, PTB, and PCBPs. The diagrams are approximately to scale and show the five cold-shock domains (CSD) of unr in black, the four noncanonical RRMs of PTB as stippled rectangles, and the three KH-domains of PCBP-1/2 as vertically striped rectangles. The amino acid sequences of the core of each of the five CSDs of unr are given, with the amino acid residues believed to constitute the RNA-binding surface (9, 24) in bold. Note that all five CSDs of unr have the sequence FFH, which is unique to this member of the family, in contrast with the FVH motif found in all other CSD proteins (24). At the bottom is the amino acid sequence of PCBP-2, with the differences found in PCPB-1 given below. These amino acid sequences are those published by Leffers et al. (44), and the K-H domains identified by Leffers et al. are highlighted by boxed rectangles.

ious entero- and rhinoviruses, it may be that this is the wrong question to ask and what we should really be considering is the tissue distribution of different isoforms (using this term in the widest sense to include similar proteins encoded by distinct genes).

Cellular RNA-Binding Proteins and Cardio- and Aphthovirus IRES Activity

The EMCV and related cardiovirus IRESs function very efficiently not only in rabbit reticulocyte lysates but also in Xenopus oocytes (17, 43). Nevertheless, the fact that PTB has much higher affinity for the EMCV IRES than for entero- or rhinovirus IRESs, coupled with the knowledge that reticulocyte lysates contain some PTB (5), albeit at lower concentrations than HeLa cells, raised the speculation that PTB might actually play a role in the function of the EMCV IRES. This idea seemed to gain credence when it was shown that mutations in the EMCV IRES that abolished the binding of a 57-kDA protein (subsequently identified as PTB) also abolished IRES activity, while compensating mutations that restored PTB binding also restored IRES activity (32).

In a more direct test, depleting reticulocyte lysates of PTB by an affinity column approach was found to have little effect on scanning-dependent translation but resulted in a selective loss of translation dependent on the EMCV IRES, which could be restored by addition of realistically low concentrations of recombinant PTB (37). However, no evidence for PTB dependence was seen in this system with the IRES of another cardiovirus, Theiler's murine encephalomyelitis virus (TMEV). This different behavior of the EMCV and TMEV IRESs seemed counterintuitive given the close phylogenetic relationship between them (37), and given that at that time we did not know that poliovirus and rhinovirus IRESs had subtly different factor requirements. Closer study revealed that the difference was due to the fact that whereas the TMEV construct had a truly wild-type IRES and a reporter that started with viral coding sequences, the EMCV IRES that was used for this work, and also by Jang and Wimmer (32), had acquired an additional A-residue in the A-rich bulge in the J-K domain (Fig. 2) and was linked to a heterologous reporter. These differences proved to be the explanation for the differences in PTB dependence: the TMEV IRES became highly dependent on PTB if all viral coding sequences were eliminated and the A-rich bulge was enlarged by one residue, whereas the EMCV IRES became PTB independent when a wild-type IRES, without an expansion of the A-rich bulge, was linked to viral polyprotein coding sequences as reporter (38).

Depletion of PTB by a similar affinity chromatography approach reduced FMDV IRES activity to 30 to 40% of the control (49). At the time, this residual activity was said to be due to residual PTB present in the system as a result of incomplete depletion. However, a closer inspection of the data suggests that this explanation may not be valid, and certainly in a subsequent publication from the same group there was no evidence that there was any PTB associated with the subpopulation of IRESs that were being actively translated in this depleted system (70). Thus, it seems more likely that the FMDV IRES shows a partial dependence on PTB but does not absolutely require it.

What Is the Role of the Cellular RNA-Binding Proteins in IRES-Dependent Initiation?

Given the wide differences between different IRESs with respect to the requirement for these cellular *trans*-acting RNA-binding proteins, it is hard to see how any of these proteins, with the possible exception of PTB, could be performing a role similar to that of the canonical translation initiation factors as catalysts of internal initiation. It seems more likely that they act by stabilizing the appropriate three-dimensional structure of the IRES.

A particularly significant fact is that size of the A-rich bulge in the EMCV IRES and the nature of the linked reporter cistron make absolutely no difference to the binding of PTB to the IRES, or at least binding to the high-affinity site, which is stem-loop H (Fig. 2). A wild-type EMCV IRES linked to viral coding sequences and an IRES with an enlarged A-bulge linked to a heterologous reporter both bind PTB with comparable affinity, yet in the former case this binding has no influence on IRES activity and in the latter it is almost absolutely essential for such activity (38). These observations seem incompatible with the idea that PTB binding directly promotes 40S subunit entry and are much more consistent with the notion that the binding of PTB may, in special circumstances, help stabilize the appropriate three-dimensional structure of the IRES. It seems likely to be significant that PTB has four RNA recognition motifs (RRMs) in the monomer and probably exists in solution as a dimer (58), which raises the possibility that a PTB dimer could interact with the IRES at several different points, and thereby stabilize the higher-order structure. Foot-printing has indeed shown that in addition to the high-affinity site (stem-loop H), PTB interacts with several other sites (39), widely dispersed in the conventional two-dimensional representation of the secondary structure (Fig. 2). Moreover, in circumstances in which EMCV IRES activity is dependent on PTB, all four RRMs seem to be essential. The C-terminal half of PTB, with two RRMs but no dimerization motif (Fig. 3), binds equally tightly to the high-affinity site on the IRES, yet cannot support internal initiation and actually inhibits the action of full-length PTB (37), entirely consistent with the idea that it is the multipoint contact of the PTB dimer with the IRES that is critical.

Like PTB, PCBP-2 also exists as a dimer (18), and the monomeric protein has three copies of the K-H domain that is thought to be the RNA-binding surface (44). Just as the C-terminal half of PTB, which retained high-affinity binding for the EMCV IRES, inhibited the action of full-length PTB in supporting IRES activity (37), so the isolated N-terminal K-H domain of PCBP-2 is inhibitory to poliovirus RNA translation (72). As for *unr*, we do not know whether this exists as a monomer or dimer, but it has five copies of the cold-shock domain (24, 28), and mutation of any one of the five cold-shock domains abrogates the ability of *unr* to stimulate HRV IRES activity, yet does not abolish binding of the protein to the IRES (Brown and Jackson, unpublished). Thus, both PCBP-2 and *unr* also have the potential for multipoint interaction with the IRES that could help in the establishment and maintenance of the appropriate higher-order structure. Moreover, even if La may not be a physiologically relevant factor for poliovirus IRES activity, it is interesting that it, too, dimerizes, and there is evidence that this dimerization is necessary for the stimulation of poliovirus IRES activity that is observed at high La concentration (12). In conclusion, therefore, the most plausible hypothesis is that by binding at multiple points in the IRES element, PTB, PCBP-2, and *unr* serve to help in the maintenance or the attainment of the appropriate three-dimensional RNA structure.

CONCLUDING REMARKS

Given that it is 12 years since picornavirus IRESs were discovered, and over 20 years since it was first shown that correct translation of poliovirus RNA required factors that were relatively abundant in HeLa cells but largely missing from rabbit reticulocyte lysates, it sometimes seems that progress has been painfully slow. However, the past 5 years have seen a significant breakthrough in our understanding of the role of canonical initiation factors in translation dependent on the EMCV IRES, and some of the cellular RNA-binding proteins required for the activity of particular types of viral IRES have been defined. It is clear that we still have further such factors to identify for poliovirus IRES function, and it is also disappointing that the tissue distribution of the factors identified so far does not seem to provide an obvious explanation for the tissue tropism of different viruses. We are within a few years of seeing the eradication of poliovirus, largely through the widespread use of Sabin attenuated vaccine strains, yet we do not yet understand how it is that a single site mutation in the IRES of the vaccine strains restricts translation and viral replication specifically in neuronal cells, but not in HeLa cells. It would be nice if we could answer this question before such time as it becomes only of historical interest, and our students start asking us to explain what exactly is a Sabin strain and why is it significant!

I wish to thank recent and present members of my group for their numerous inputs that have helped enormously in the evolution of this chapter: Ann Kaminski, Sarah Hunt, Tuija Pöyry, Emma Brown, Iraj Ali, and Theo Ohlmann. I also thank Matt Wollerton and Chris Smith for educating me on the topic of PTB isoforms; Bert Semler for his words of wisdom on the many occasions when I have phoned him late at night (for me) for advice on obscure points of picornavirology including translation; and Karen Browning for communicating results prior to publication. Work from my own laboratory discussed in this chapter has been supported by grants from The Wellcome Trust.

REFERENCES

1. **Blyn, L. B., K. M. Swiderek, O. Richards, D. C. Stahl, B. L. Semler, and E. Ehrenfeld.** 1996. Poly(rC) binding protein 2 binds to stem-loop IV of the poliovirus RNA 5' noncoding region: identification by automated liquid chromatography-tandem mass spectrometry. *Proc. Natl. Acad. Sci. USA* **93:**11115–11120.
2. **Blyn, L. B., J. S. Towner, B. L. Semler, and E. Ehrenfeld.** 1997. Requirement of poly(rC) binding protein 2 for translation of poliovirus RNA. *J. Virol.* **71:**6243–6246.
3. **Borman, A. M., and K. M. Kean.** 1997. Intact eukaryotic initiation factor 4G is required for hepatitis A virus internal initiation of translation. *Virology* **237:**129–136.
4. **Borman, A. M., J.-L. Bailly, M. Girard, and K. M. Kean.** 1995. Picornavirus internal ribosome entry segments—comparison of translation efficiency and the requirements for optimal internal initiation of translation in vitro. *Nucleic Acids Res.* **23:**3656–3663.
5. **Borman, A. M., M. T. Howell, J. G. Patton, and R. J. Jackson.** 1993. The involvement of a spliceosome component in internal initiation of human rhinovirus RNA translation. *J. Gen. Virol.* **74:**1775–1788.
6. **Borman, A. M., R. Kirchweger, E. Ziegler, R. E. Rhoads, T. Skern, and K. M. Kean.** 1997. eIF4G and its proteolytic cleavage products: effect on initiation of protein synthesis from capped, uncapped and IRES-containing mRNAs. *RNA* **3:**186–196.
7. **Borman, A. M., P. Le Mercier, M. Girard, and K. M. Kean.** 1997. Comparison of picornaviral IRES-driven internal initiation in cultured cells of different origins. *Nucleic Acids Res.* **25:**925–932.
8. **Boussadia, O., F. Amiot, S. Cases, G. Triqueneaux, H. Jacquemin-Sablon, and F. Dautry.** 1997. Transcription of unr (upstream of N-ras) down-modulates N-ras expression in vivo. *FEBS Lett.* **420:**20–24.
9. **Boussadia, O., H. Jacquemin-Sablon, and F. Dautry.** 1993. Exon skipping in the expression of the gene immediately upstream of N-ras (unr/NRU). *Biochim. Biophys. Acta* **1172:**64–72.
10. **Brown, B. A., and E. Ehrenfeld.** 1979. Translation of poliovirus RNA in vitro: changes in cleavage pattern and initiation sites by ribosomal salt wash. *Virology* **97:**396–405.
11. [Reference deleted in proof.]
12. **Craig, A. W. B., Y. V. Svitkin, H. S. Lee, G. J. Belsham, and N. Sonenberg.** 1997. The La autoantigen contains a dimerization domain that is essential for enhancing translation. *Mol. Cell. Biol.* **17:**163–169.
13. **De Gregorio, E., T. Preiss, and M. W. Hentze.** 1998. Translational activation of uncapped mRNAs by the central part of human eIF4G is 5' end dependent. *RNA* **4:**828–836.
14. **De Gregorio, E., T. Preiss, and M. W. Hentze.** 1999. Translation driven by an eIF4G core domain in vivo. *EMBO J.* **18:**4865–4874.
15. **Dorner, A. J., B. L. Semler, R. J. Jackson, R. Hanecak, E. Duprey, and E. Wimmer.** 1984. In vitro translation of poliovirus RNA: utilization of internal initiation sites in reticulocyte lysate. *J. Virol.* **50:**507–514.
16. **Follett, E. A. C., C. R. Pringle, and T. H. Pennington.** 1975. Virus development in enucleate cells: echovirus, poliovirus, pseudorabies virus, reovirus, respiratory syncytial virus and Semliki Forest virus. *J. Gen. Virol.* **26:**183–196.
17. **Gamarnik, A. V., and R. Andino.** 1996. Replication of poliovirus in *Xenopus* oocytes requires two human factors. *EMBO J.* **15:**5988–5998.
18. **Gamarnik, A. V., and R. Andino.** 1997. Two functional complexes formed by KH domain containing proteins with the 5' noncoding region of poliovirus RNA. *RNA* **3:**882–892.
19. **Ghetti, A., S. Piñol-Roma, W. M. Michael, C. Morandi, and G. Dreyfuss.** 1992. hnRNP I, the polypyrimidine tract binding protein: distinct nuclear localization and association with hnRNPs. *Nucleic Acids Res.* **14:**3671–3678.
20. **Gingras, A. C., B. Raught, and N. Sonenberg.** 1999. eIF4 initiation factors: effectors of mRNA recruitment to ribosomes and regulators of translation. *Annu. Rev. Biochem.* **68:**913–963.
21. **Glass, M., and D. Summers.** 1993. Identification of a trans-acting activity from liver that stimulates hepatitis A virus translation in vitro. *Virology* **193:**1047–1050.
22. **Goyer, C., M. Altmann, H. S. Lee, A. Blanc, M. Deshmukh, J. L. Woolford, H. Trachsel, and N. Sonenberg.** 1993. TIF4631 and TIF4632: two yeast genes encoding the high molecular weight subunits of cap-binding protein complex (eukaryotic initiation factor 4F) contain an RNA recognition motif-like sequence and carry out an essential function. *Mol. Cell. Biol.* **13:**4860–4874.
23. **Gradi, A., H. Imataka, Y. V. Svitkin, E. Rom, B. Raught, S. Morino, and N. Sonenberg.** 1998. A novel functional human eukaryotic translation initiation factor eIF4G. *Mol. Cell. Biol.* **18:**334–342.
24. **Graumann, P. L., and M. A. Marahiel.** 1998. A superfamily of proteins that contain the cold-shock domain. *Trends Biochem. Sci.* **23:**286–290.
25. **Hambridge, S. J., and P. Sarnow.** 1992. Translational enhancement of the poliovirus 5' noncoding region mediated by virus-encoded polypeptide 2A. *Proc. Natl. Acad. Sci. USA* **89:**10272–10276.
26. **Hershey, J. W. B., and W. C. Merrick.** 2002. The pathway and mechanism of initiation of protein synthesis, p. 33–88. *In* N. Sonenberg, J. W. B. Hershey, and M. B. Mathews (ed.), *Translational Control of Gene Expression*, 2nd ed. Cold Spring Harbor Laboratory Press, Cold Spring Harbor, N.Y.
27. **Hung, S. L., and R. J. Jackson.** 1999. Polypyrimidine tract binding protein (PTB) is necessary, but not sufficient, for efficient internal initiation of translation of human rhinovirus-2 RNA. *RNA* **5:**344–359.
28. **Hunt, S. L., J. J. Hsuan, N. Totty, and R. J. Jackson.** 1999. unr, a cellular cytoplasmic RNA-binding protein with five cold-shock domains, is required for internal initiation of translation of human rhinovirus RNA. *Genes Dev.* **13:**437–448.
29. **Imataka, H., and N. Sonenberg.** 1997. Human eukaryotic translation initiation factor 4G (eIF4G) possesses two separate and independent binding sites for eIF4A. *Mol. Cell. Biol.* **17:**6940–6947.

30. Jackson, R. J. 1991. The ATP requirement for initiation of eukaryotic translation varies according to the mRNA species. *Eur. J. Biochem.* **200**:285–294.
31. Jacquemin-Sablon, H., G. Triqueneaux, S. Deschamps, M. le Maire, J. Doniger, and F. Dautry. 1994. Nucleic acid binding and intracellular localization of unr, a protein with five cold shock domains. *Nucleic Acids Res.* **22**:2643–2650.
32. Jang, S. K., and E. Wimmer. 1990. Cap-independent translation of encephalomyocarditis virus RNA–structural elements of the internal ribosomal entry site and involvement of a cellular 57-kD RNA binding protein. *Genes Dev.* **4**:1560–1572.
33. Jang, S. K., H.-G. Krausslich, M. J. H. Nicklin, G. M. Duke, A. C. Palmenberg, and E. Wimmer. 1988. A segment of the 5' nontranslated region of encephalomyocarditis virus RNA directs internal entry of ribosomes during in vitro translation. *J. Virol.* **62**:2636–2643.
34. Jaramillo, M., T. E. Dever, W. C. Merrick, and N. Sonenberg. 1991. RNA unwinding in translation: assembly of helicase complex intermediates comprising eukaryotic initiation factors eIF-4F and eIF-4B. *Mol. Cell. Biol.* **11**:5992–5997.
35. Kaminiski, A., G. J. Belsham, and R. J. Jackson. 1994. Translation of encephalomyocarditis virus RNA; parameters influencing the selection of the internal initiation site. *EMBO J.* **13**:1673–1681.
36. Kaminski, A., M. T. Howell, and R. J. Jackson. 1990. Initiation of encephalomyocarditis virus RNA translation: the authentic initiation site is not selected by a scanning mechanism. *EMBO J.* **9**:3753–3759.
37. Kaminski, A., S. L. Hunt, J. G. Patton, and R. J. Jackson. 1995. Direct evidence that polypyrimidine tract binding protein (PTB) is essential for internal initiation of encephalomyocarditis virus RNA translation. *RNA* **1**:924–938.
38. Kaminski, A., and R. J. Jackson. 1998. The polypyrimidine tract binding protein (PTB) requirement for internal initiation of translation of cardiovirus RNAs is conditional rather than absolute. *RNA* **4**:626–638.
39. Kolupaeva, V. G., C. U. T. Hellen, and I. N. Shatsky. 1996. Structural analysis of the interaction of the pyrimidine tract binding protein with the internal ribosome entry segment of encephalomyocarditis virus and foot-and-mouth disease virus. *RNA* **2**:1199–1212.
40. Kolupaeva, V. G., T. V. Pestova, C. U. T. Hellen, and I. N. Shatsky. 1998. Translation eukaryotic initiation factor 4G recognizes a specific structural element within the internal ribosome entry site of encephalomyocarditis virus RNA. *J. Biol. Chem.* **273**:18599–18604.
41. Kozak, M. 1989. The scanning model for translation: an update. *J. Cell Biol.* **108**:229–241.
42. Lamphear, B. J., R. Kirchweger, T. Skern, and R. E. Rhoads. 1995. Mapping of functional domains in eukaryotic protein synthesis initiation factor 4G (eIF4G) with picornaviral proteases. *J. Biol. Chem.* **270**:21975–21983.
43. Laskey, R. A., J. B. Gurdon, and L. V. Crawford. 1972. Translation of encephalomyocarditis viral RNA in oocytes of *Xenopus laevis*. *Proc. Natl. Acad. Sci. USA* **69**:3665–3669.
44. Leffers, H., K. Dejgaard, and J. E. Celis. 1995. Characterisation of two major cellular poly(rC)-binding human proteins each containing three K-homologous (KH) domains. *Eur. J. Biochem.* **230**:447–453.
45. Liebig, H. D., E. Ziegler, R. Yan, K. Hartmuth, H. Klump, H. Kowalski, D. Blaas, W. Sommergruber, L. Frasel, B. Lamphear, R. Rhoads, E. Kuechler, and T. Skern. 1993. Purification of 2 picornaviral 2A proteinases: interaction with eIF4γ and influence on in vitro translation. *Biochemistry* **32**:7581–7588.
46. Meerovitch, K., Y. V. Svitkin, H. S. Lee, F. Lejbkowicz, D. J. Kenan, E. K. L. Chan, V. I. Agol, J. D. Keene, and N. Sonenberg. 1993. La autoantigen enhances and corrects aberrant translation of poliovirus RNA in reticulocyte lysate. *J. Virol.* **67**:3798–3807.
47. Meyer, K., A. Petersen, M. Niepmann, and E. Beck. 1995. Interaction of eukaryotic initiation factor eIF4B with a picornavirus internal translation site. *J. Virol.* **69**:2819–2824.
48. Morley, S. J., P. S. Curtis, and V. M. Pain. 1997. eIF4G: translation's mystery factor begins to yield its secrets. *RNA* **3**:1085–1104.
49. Niepmann, M., A. Petersen, K. Meyer, and E. Beck. 1997. Functional involvement of polypyrimidine tract binding protein in translation initiation complexes with the internal ribosome entry site of foot-and-mouth-disease virus. *J. Virol.* **71**:8330–8339.
50. O'Brien, C. A., K. Margelot, and S. L. Wolin. 1993. Xenopus Ro ribonucleoproteins: members of an evolutionary conserved class of cytoplasmic ribonucleoproteins. *Proc. Natl. Acad. Sci. USA* **90**:7250–7254.
51. Ohlmann, T., M. Rau, S. J. Morley, and V. M. Pain. 1995. Proteolytic cleavage of initiation factor eIF-4γ in the reticulocyte lysate inhibits translation of capped mRNAs but enhances that of uncapped mRNAs. *Nucleic Acids Res.* **23**:334–340.
52. Ohlmann, T., M. Rau, V. M. Pain, and S. J. Morley. 1996. The C-terminal domain of eukaryotic protein synthesis initiation factor (eIF) 4G is sufficient to support cap-independent translation in the absence of eIF4E. *EMBO J.* **15**:1371–1382.
53. Patton, J. G., S. A. Mayer, P. Tempst, and B. Nadal-Ginard. 1991. Characterization and molecular cloning of polypyrimidine tract-binding protein: a component of a complex necessary for pre-mRNA splicing. *Genes Dev.* **5**:1237–1251.
54. Pause, A., G. J. Belsham, A. C. Gingras, O. Donze, T. A. Lin, J. C. Lawrence, and N. Sonenberg. 1994. Insulin dependent stimulation of protein synthesis by phosphorylation of a regulator of 5' cap function. *Nature* **371**:762–767.
55. Pause, A., N. Méthot, Y. V. Svitkin, W. C. Merrick, and N. Sonenberg. 1994. Dominant negative mutants of mammalian translation initiation factor eIF4A define a critical role for eIF4F in cap-dependent and cap-independent initiation of translation. *EMBO J.* **13**:1205–1215.
56. Pelham, H. R. B., and R. J. Jackson. 1976. An efficient mRNA-dependent translation system from rabbit reticulocyte lysates. *Eur. J. Biochem.* **67**:247–256.
57. Pelletier, J., and N. Sonenberg. 1988. Internal initiation of translation of eukaryotic mRNA directed by a sequence derived from poliovirus RNA. *Nature* **334**:320–325.
58. Pérez, I., J. G. McAfee, and J. G. Patton. 1997. Multiple RRMs contribute to RNA binding specificity and affinity for polypyrimidine tract binding protein. *Biochemistry* **36**:11881–11890.
59. Pestova, T. V., S. I. Borukhov, and C. U. T. Hellen. 1998. Eukaryotic ribosomes require initiation factors 1 and 1A to locate initiation codons. *Nature* **394**:854–859.
60. Pestova, T. V., C. U. T. Hellen, and I. N. Shatsky. 1996. Canonical eukaryotic initiation-factors determine initiation of translation by internal ribosomal entry. *Mol. Cell. Biol.* **16**:6859–6869.
61. Pestova, T. V., I. B. Lomakin, J. H. Lee, S. K. Choi, T. E. Dever, and C. U. T. Hellen. 2000. The joining of ribosomal subunits in eukaryotes requires eIF5B. *Nature* **403**:332–335.

62. Pestova, T. V., I. N. Shatsky, S. P. Fletcher, R. J. Jackson, and C. U. T. Hellen. 1998. A prokaryotic-like mode of cytoplasmic eukaryotic ribosome binding to the initiation codon during internal translation initiation of hepatitis C and classical swine fever virus RNAs. *Genes Dev.* **12:**67–83.
63. Pestova, T. V., I. N. Shatsky, and C. U. T. Hellen. 1996. Functional dissection of eukaryotic initiation-factor 4F—the 4A subunit and the central domain of the 4G subunit are sufficient to mediate internal entry of 43S preinitiation complexes. *Mol. Cell. Biol.* **16:**6870–6878.
64. Phillips, B. A., and A. Emmert. 1986. Modulation of the expression of poliovirus proteins in reticulocyte lysates. *Virology* **148:**255–267.
65. Pilipenko, E. V., V. M. Blinov, B. K. Chernov, T. M. Dmitrieva, and V. I. Agol. 1989. Conservation of the secondary structure elements in the 5′ nontranslated region of cardio- and aphthovirus RNAs. *Nucleic Acids Res.* **17:**5701–5711.
66. Pilipenko, E. V., V. M. Blinov, L. I. Romanova, A. N. Sinyakov, S. V. Maslova, and V. I. Agol. 1989. Conserved structural domains in the 5′-untranslated region of picornaviral genomes. *Virology* **168:**201–209.
67. Pöyry, T., L. Kinnunen, and T. Hovi. 1992. Genetic variation in vivo and proposed functional domains of the 5′ noncoding region of poliovirus RNA. *J. Virol.* **66:**5313–5319.
68. Roberts, L. O., R. A. Seamons, and G. J. Belsham. 1998. Recognition of picornavirus internal ribosome entry sites within cells; influence of cellular and viral proteins. *RNA* **4:**520–529.
69. Rozen, F., I. Edery, K. Meerovitch, T. E. Dever, W. C. Merrick, and N. Sonenberg. 1990. Bidirectional RNA helicase activity of eukaryotic initiation factors 4A and 4F. *Mol. Cell. Biol.* **10:**1134–1144.
70. Rust, R. C., K. Ochs, K. Meyer, E. Beck, and M. Niepmann. 1999. Interaction of eukaryotic initiation factor eIF4B with the internal ribosome entry site of foot-and-mouth disease virus is independent of the polypyrimidine tract-binding protein. *J. Virol.* **73:**6111–6113.
71. Shiroki, K., S. Isoyama, S. Kuge, T. Ishii, S. Ohmi, S. Hata, Y. Takasaki, and A. Nomoto. 1999. Intracellular redistribution of truncated La protein produced by poliovirus 3Cpro-mediated cleavage. *J. Virol.* **73:**2193–2200.
72. Silvera, D., A. V. Gamarnik, and R. Andino. 1999. The N-terminal K-homology domain of the poly(rC) binding protein is a major determinant for binding to the poliovirus 5′-untranslated region and acts as an inhibitor of viral translation. *J. Biol. Chem.* **274:**38163–38170.
73. Skinner, M. A., V. R. Racaniello, G. Dunn, J. Cooper, P. D. Minor, and J. W. Almond. 1989. New model for the secondary structure of the 5′ noncoding RNA of poliovirus is supported by biochemical and genetic data that also show that RNA secondary structure is important in neurovirulence. *J. Mol. Biol.* **207:**379–392.
74. Svitkin, Y. V., K. Meerovitch, H. S. Lee, J. N. Dholakia, D. J. Kenan, V. I. Agol, and N. Sonenberg. 1994. Internal translation initiation on poliovirus RNA: further characterization of La function in poliovirus translated in vitro. *J. Virol.* **68:**1544–1550.
75. Timmer, R. T., L. A. Benkowksi, D. Schodin, S. R. Lax, A. M. Metz, J. M. Ravel, and K. S. Browning. 1993. The 5′ and 3′ untranslated regions of satellite tobacco necrosis virus RNA affect translational efficiency and dependence on 5′ cap structure. *J. Biol. Chem.* **268:**9504–9510.
76. Valcarcel, J., and F. Gebauer. 1997. Post-transcriptional regulation: the dawn of PTB. *Curr. Biol.* **7:**R705–R708.
77. Walter, B. L., J. H. C. Nguyen, E. Ehrenfeld, and B. L. Semler. 1999. Differential utilization of poly(rC) binding protein 2 in translation directed by picornavirus IRES elements. *RNA* **5:**1570–1585.
78. Whetter, L. E., S. P. Day, O. Elroy-Stein, E. A. Brown, and S. M. Lemon. 1994. Low efficiency of the 5′ nontranslated region of hepatitis A virus RNA in directing cap-independent translation in permissive monkey kidney cells. *J. Virol.* **68:**5253–5263.
79. Wigle, D. T., and A. E. Smith. 1973. Specificity in initiation in a fractionated mammalian cell-free system. *Nat. New Biol.* **242:**136–140.
80. Yamamoto, H., K. Tsukahara, Y. Kanaoka, S. Jinno, and H. Okayama. 1999. Isolation of a mammalian homologue of a fission yeast differentiation regulator. *Mol. Cell. Biol.* **19:**3829–3841.

PROTEOLYTIC PROCESSING

Processing Determinants and Functions of Cleavage Products of Picornavirus Polyproteins

LOUIS E.-C. LEONG, CHRISTOPHER T. CORNELL, AND BERT L. SEMLER

16

Picornaviruses employ a number of unique intracellular mechanisms and novel processes during their infectious cycles resulting in their being among the most successful of viral pathogens. Successful picornavirus replication requires both cellular and viral proteins to functionally interact with each other and with RNA elements contained within the viral genome. Some of these interactions facilitate cap-independent translation initiation by internal ribosome entry (58, 98), initiation of viral-specific RNA replication on membrane vesicles within the cytoplasm to produce newly synthesized progeny RNAs (19), the processing of viral proteins from polyprotein precursors (118), and the shutoff of host protein synthesis (50). Nearly all of the virally encoded protein products necessary for these processes are found within the single, long open reading frame of the positive-stranded RNA genome of a typical picornavirus. Under normal conditions in the infected cell, the polyprotein corresponding to this complete open reading frame is never produced because virally encoded proteinases initiate polyprotein cleavage cotranslationally. Proteolytic processing mediated by these virally encoded proteinases ultimately generates numerous intermediate and mature viral polypeptides that are required for a complete infectious cycle. This mode of gene expression forgoes the synthesis and regulation of individual subgenomic mRNAs and is completely dependent on highly processive translation and accurate proteolytic processing to achieve genome replication and the subsequent production of progeny virions.

On the basis of sequence homology and virion properties (pH stability, sedimentation coefficients, and buoyant density), the picornaviruses are currently divided into six genera: aphthoviruses, cardioviruses, enteroviruses, hepatoviruses, parechoviruses, and rhinoviruses. The structural (capsid) genes reside in the P1 portion of the polyprotein, while the nonstructural gene products are found within regions of the polyprotein designated P2 and P3 (Fig. 1) (109). Exceptions to this division are found in aphthoviruses and cardioviruses, which encode leader proteins (L protein) at the amino terminus of the polyprotein. The known functions of both capsid (structural) and nonstructural protein products will be outlined in this chapter.

The processing of viral polyprotein is mediated solely by viral proteinases. In most instances, this is carried out by the 3C proteinase ($3C^{pro}$) found within the P3 region of all picornaviruses. However, there are other virally encoded proteinases that not only participate in cleavage of the viral polyprotein, but also mediate cleavage of nonviral (host) proteins. This chapter will begin with a discussion of the features of viral proteinases, continue with an outline of the functions of both precursor and mature viral polypeptides present during a picornaviral infection (summarized in Table 1), and conclude with a brief summary of nonviral substrates cleaved by viral proteinases. A detailed discussion of the structure and function of picornavirus proteinases is presented by Skern et al. in chapter 17.

VIRAL PROTEINASES

L Protein

The aphthoviruses and cardioviruses code for an L protein at the N terminus of their polyproteins. The cleavage activity of the L proteinase from foot-and-mouth disease virus (FMDV), an aphthovirus, has been well characterized. Liberated from the polyprotein via a primary cleavage event between a lysine and glycine residue at the L/P1 junction (116), amino acid alignments, protease inhibition experiments, and mutagenesis studies have identified the FMDV L proteinase as a member of the thiol protease family (46, 68, 103). Although the precise substrate specificity of the L proteinase has yet to be determined, mutagenesis studies of amino acids within the active site have revealed important aspects of substrate specificity regulation. Piccone et al. (103) mutated the active site cysteine residue to a serine residue that resulted in an L proteinase incapable of carrying out *trans* cleavages while maintaining its *cis* cleavage activity. These data suggest that a newly synthesized L proteinase, or L proteinase in the context of an L-P1 precursor polyprotein, may adopt a protein fold that specifically recognizes its in-*cis* substrate and is able to use serine as a nucleophile instead of cysteine. On the other hand, fully processed L proteinase may adopt an alternative three-

---

Louis E.-C. Leong ■ Invitrogen Corp., 1600 Faraday Ave., Carlsbad, CA 92008. *Christopher T. Cornell and Bert L. Semler* ■ Department of Microbiology and Molecular Genetics, College of Medicine, University of California, Irvine, CA 92697-4025.

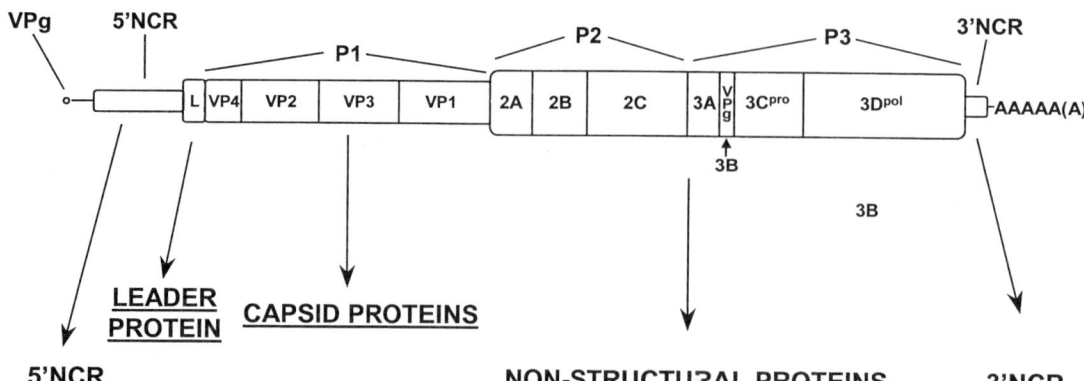

FIGURE 1 Map of proteins encoded in picornavirus genomes. Shown is a schematic of a typical picornaviral genome. The 5′ end is covalently linked to the viral protein VPg (protein 3B), and the poly(A) tail at the 3′ end is genetically coded. The polyprotein is divided into structural (P1) and nonstructural products (P2 and P3). The vertical lines represent sites along the polyprotein that are cleaved by viral proteinases; however, there are precursor proteins (e.g., 2BC, 3AB, 3CD) that have functions distinct from their mature cleavage products. Only cardioviruses and aphthoviruses encode an L protein. The viral proteinase responsible for the majority of polyprotein processing is the 3C chymotrypsin-like proteinase, and precursor polypeptides contain 3C sequences (e.g., 3CD). In addition, enteroviruses and rhinoviruses utilize the 2A proteinase to carry out the primary cleavage event between the carboxy terminus of the P1 region and the amino terminus of 2A. Cardioviruses and aphthoviruses do not contain a proteolytically active form of 2A; however, this protein is self-cleaved from the amino terminus of 2B by an undefined mechanism. The L proteinase of aphthoviruses is a cysteine-type proteinase that cleaves between its carboxy terminus and the amino terminus of VP4. The L proteinase of cardioviruses is cleaved from the polyprotein at its amino terminus by 3C. Interestingly, aphthoviruses are unique in that they encode three tandemly repeated VPgs while all other picornavirus genomes contain only one VPg.

dimensional structure required for *trans* cleavage activity that also possesses a more stringent requirement for cysteine rather than serine as an active site nucleophile. Therefore, regulation of the L proteinase substrate specificity is likely to be dependent on protein structure.

The L protein of cardioviruses has no sequence homology to the L protein of aphthoviruses and does not possess any detectable proteolytic activity. A precise function for the L protein of cardioviruses has yet to be described; however, for Theiler's murine encephalomyelitis virus (TMEV), L has been shown to be a zinc-binding protein that may have a role in host cell restricted growth (22). In addition, a TMEV protein called L*, whose amino acid sequence is out of frame with the TMEV polyprotein, has been shown to be important in virus-induced immune-mediated demyelination and essential for virus growth in cultured murine macrophage-like cells (23, 120). Unlike the *cis* cleavage of the L protein from the aphthovirus polyprotein, cleavage of the cardiovirus L protein from the P1 region is carried out by the cardiovirus 3C proteinase (94).

2A Proteinase

In contrast to the primary cleavage event in aphthoviruses that cleaves the L proteinase from the P1 region of the polyprotein, the initial processing event of the enterovirus and rhinovirus polyprotein occurs at the P1/P2 junction. Once the 2A proteinase gene product has been fully translated and can adopt a three-dimensional structure competent for proteolytic activity, it cotranslationally cleaves itself at its amino terminus to liberate the P1 polypeptide from the rest of the polyprotein. Protein crystallography studies suggest that to achieve cleavage in *cis* at its amino terminus, the mature 2A^{pro} structure would have to undergo only minor changes in the main peptide chain and torsional changes in several residues (99). The three-dimensional data also suggest that for cleavage by 2A to occur in *cis*, the requirements for substrate specificity may only be limited to having a glycine residue in the P1′ position. (Nomenclature used in this discussion of substrate specificity will be PN-P1-P1′-PN′ [112], where the scissile peptide bond is between P1 and P1′ amino acids, and N represents the amino acid position from the cleavage site.) This hypothesis is also supported by proteolytic assays (54).

The *trans* cleavage activity of 2A^{pro} is not essential for processing of the viral polyprotein. In the case of poliovirus, cleavage by the 2A proteinase occurs within the coding region of 3D^{pol} (the viral RNA-dependent RNA polymerase) to generate two products of nonessential function for

TABLE 1 Functions of picornavirus polypeptides

Protein	Functions
VP2, VP4, VP3, VP1 (capsid proteins)	Virion particle assembly Viral entry into cells
L	Host protein synthesis shutoff (aphthoviruses) Host cell-restricted viral growth (TMEV)
L*	Mediation of virally induced demyelination (TMEV)
2A	Host protein synthesis shutoff (except for aphthoviruses, cardioviruses, hepatoviruses)
2B	Alteration of membrane permeability Inhibition of cellular exocytosis Dissociation/rearrangement of endoplasmic reticulum and Golgi RNA amplification
2C	Formation of vesicles NTPase Guanidine HCl resistance
2C/2BC	RNA binding (RNA replication) Formation of vesicles
3A	Inhibition of MHC class I expression Inhibition of intracellular membrane transport
3B	Primer for RNA synthesis Covalent linkage to 5′ end of + and − strands
3AB	Membrane association of replication complexes Stimulation of 3D^{pol} Stimulation of 3CD autocleavage
3C	Viral protein processing Host protein cleavage/transcription inhibition RNA binding (RNA replication)
3CD	Viral protein processing RNA binding (RNA replication) Stimulation of VPg uridylylation
3D	VPg uridylylation RNA polymerase RNA binding

growth in cell culture, 3C′ and 3D′ (92, 128). Substrate recognition requirements for *trans* cleavage by enterovirus and rhinovirus 2A^{pro} also have shown a stringent requirement for a glycine in the P1′ position. Furthermore, peptide cleavage assays and three-dimensional analysis of poliovirus 2A^{pro} have highlighted the P2 and P4 positions of the substrate peptide as key determinants of substrate recognition, with a marked preference for isoleucine and threonine at these positions, respectively. Although 2A recognizes viral substrates, it appears that an additional critical function of the 2A proteinase of enteroviruses and rhinoviruses is the cleavage of cellular factors that are involved in cap-dependent translation. Details of these cleavages will be discussed later in this chapter.

The 2A proteinases of enteroviruses and rhinoviruses utilize a cysteine in their active sites as the nucleophilic attack group, but they differ from the L proteinase of aphthoviruses in that they do not fall into the classical definition of a cysteine proteinase. Amino acid alignments and three-dimensional protein structure studies have shown that the 2A^{pro} of enteroviruses and rhinoviruses adopts a serine protease fold similar to that of the protease chymotrypsin (12, 13, 43). Corroboration for these alignments was established by mutagenic studies of the 2A^{pro} active site amino acids (135).

The 2A proteinases of aphthoviruses and cardioviruses are not proteolytically active and the initial cleavage of these polyproteins occurs at the 2A/2B junction, before the synthesis of 3C^{pro} (48). The sequence between 2A and 2B possesses a highly conserved tetrapeptide sequence (Asn-Pro-Gly-Pro), which has been linked to an autocatalytic process that severs the tetrapeptide between the proline and glycine residue (93, 110). The exact mechanism responsible for this cleavage has yet to be elucidated, but some intriguing possibilities are reviewed by Ryan et al. in chapter 18.

3C Proteinase

Picornavirus 3C proteinases adopt a fold similar to that of the serine protease chymotrypsin (12, 13, 41, 43, 81, 86), which has been confirmed by mutagenesis studies involving 3C^{pro} (21, 49, 57, 63, 74, 76). The 3C proteinase activity carries out the majority of the proteolytic processing of the viral polyprotein. Initial studies examining the substrate recognition determinants required for processing by the 3C proteinase of poliovirus suggested that this proteinase cleaves primarily between glutamine-glycine pairs. However, only 9 of the 13 glutamine-glycine pairs present within the poliovirus polyprotein are cleaved (51, 66), suggesting 3C^{pro} substrate specificity is dictated by more than just the dipeptide sequence. It has been shown that in the case of serine proteases, the P1′ residue of the substrate does not play a significant role in substrate specificity determination. However, a requirement for a glycine at the P1′ position of many picornaviral 3C^{pro} substrates has been shown, and this requirement is thought to be due primarily to physical constraints within the substrate-binding pocket of 3C^{pro}, which allows only amino acids with small side chains to occupy the P1′ position (13, 81). Proteolytic assays with 3C^{pro} from different picornaviruses have revealed a tentative universal consensus sequence for 3C^{pro} cleavage, P4-X-X-P1-P1′, where the small amino acids glycine, alanine, and serine are preferred in the P1′ position (13, 34, 62, 79, 81, 100). Additionally, the substrate specificity pocket within 3C^{pro} contains a highly conserved histidine residue that selects primarily for glutamine in the P1 position of the substrate. This specificity for glutamine in the P1 position has been verified by proteolytic assays utilizing 3C^{pro} from different picornaviruses. The P2 and P3 positions can accept a wide number of amino acids while maintaining effective recognition by 3C^{pro} (13, 79, 81). Finally, the P4 position is an important determinant of substrate recognition and is usually a hydrophobic amino acid like alanine, valine, or isoleucine (18, 20, 27, 30, 52, 69, 91).

The evolution of picornaviruses might dictate that the P1 to PN substrate positions be identical or similar to optimize polyprotein processing and maximize the generation of mature viral proteins. However, the P1 to PN positions of the 3C^{pro} cleavage sites are not identical, even within a polyprotein derived from an individual picornavirus. It has been proposed that the variations observed in substrate determinants found at these positions may provide a mechanism for differential sensitivity to 3C^{pro} cleavage, which results in the temporal expression of mature viral proteins and their precursors. Viral protein precursors and the timely appearance of mature viral proteins are essential for viral replication. It has been demonstrated that an in vitro generated transcript of the hepatitis A virus genome bearing sequences at the 3A/3B cleavage site optimized for 3C^{pro} cleavage is unable to establish an infectious cycle (71), thereby illustrating the importance of a mechanism to delay the production of some mature viral proteins.

Further evidence supporting this notion comes from the extensively characterized 3C proteinase of poliovirus. 3CD, a precursor form of the proteinase-containing sequences of the viral RNA-dependent RNA polymerase, has been shown to possess enhanced proteolytic activity over that of the 3C proteinase by itself (95). Complete cleavage of the poliovirus P1 protein region is accomplished only by 3CD^{pro}, a process that has been shown to be dependent on a cellular polypeptide (16, 134). This cellular polypeptide may be a protein chaperone that assists in the proper folding of the P1 protein region to achieve effective processing by 3CD^{pro} (80). These and other observations led to the conclusion that substrate recognition by picornaviral proteinases is not limited to a linear amino acid sequence and is dependent on the structural presentation of the substrate.

VIRAL SUBSTRATES: STRUCTURAL POLYPEPTIDE PRODUCTS

P1 Proteins

Found within the P1 coding sequence are the capsid proteins VP4, VP2, VP3, and VP1. Initial proteolytic processing of the P1 region by the picornaviral 3C proteinase generates the capsid proteins VP0 (uncleaved VP4 and VP2), VP3, and VP1. As mentioned previously, in the case of poliovirus, the efficient cleavage of the P1 region is carried out primarily by the 3CD form of the enzyme (52, 134) and is dependent on a cellular host factor (16). Once formed, viral capsid proteins VP0, VP3, and VP1 encapsidate newly synthesized viral genomic RNA to form structures that ultimately yield infectious virus particles within the cytoplasm. The first step in this process is the formation of a protomer, consisting of VP0, VP3, and VP1. Then, five protomers come together to form a 14S pentamer (Fig. 2). In the absence of progeny RNA, 12 pentamers may assemble into an 80S procapsid structure into which a single RNA molecule is subsequently threaded, thereby forming a 150S provirion. Alternatively, the pentamers themselves may associate with newly synthesized viral RNA to form the 150S provirion structure. Independent of its pathway of production, the provirion structure is a short-lived intermediate that undergoes a final cleavage event, whereby VP0 is cleaved into VP4 and VP2 (7). This virion maturation event occurs by an undefined mechanism. Proper capsid assembly and RNA packaging are essential for virus infectivity, and cellular chaperones associate with newly synthesized virus particles and possibly contribute to virus particle assembly (80). Details surrounding the structure and assembly of capsids, as well as virion-receptor interactions, are addressed in the Virion Structure and Virus Entry sections of this volume.

In vitro synthesized viral RNAs containing large in-frame deletions within the P1 region are self-replicating in cultured cells, suggesting that the proteins required for viral RNA replication are located primarily within the P2 and P3 (nonstructural) regions of the genome (26, 61). The following section offers a comprehensive examination of the roles of these gene products during a typical picornaviral infection.

VIRAL SUBSTRATES: NONSTRUCTURAL POLYPEPTIDE PRODUCTS

P2 Proteins

A successful picornavirus infection requires the recruitment of cellular membranes to form vesicles upon which viral replication occurs. The proteins encoded within the P2 region of the picornaviral genome are thought to be required for the rearrangement of membranes within the host cell and may also play a role in the process of RNA replication. This rearrangement of cellular membranes grossly disrupts cellular functions and provides a form of compartmentalization necessary for a successful replicative cycle.

2A

Described earlier in this chapter, 2A functions primarily as a proteinase (except for the 2A proteins encoded by aphthoviruses and cardioviruses), and proteolytically active 2A protein is responsible for the primary cleavage event occurring in *cis* at its own amino terminus (between the P1 and P2 regions of the polyprotein). For poliovirus, 2A may also play a role in RNA replication (6, 77, 90). As will be described at the end of this chapter, proteolytically active 2A protein has a dramatic effect on cellular cap-dependent translation.

2B

Expression of poliovirus 2B alters intracellular membrane permeability, inhibits cellular exocytosis, and dissociates the Golgi complex (1, 10, 37, 111, 124–126). Collectively, these observations indicate that 2B contributes to the formation of replication vesicles from intracellular membranous structures during viral infection. Moreover, alterations in membrane permeability by 2B may facilitate the release of mature virions (125). In addition, 2B mutants of poliovirus have defects in RNA amplification (60).

2C and 2BC

Formation of the viral replication vesicles during virus replication has been linked to the protein 2C and its precursor 2BC. Two lines of evidence that strongly suggest this linkage are: (i) the expression of poliovirus 2BC and 2C, but not 2B, in HeLa cells leads to formation of vesicles morphologically identical to those seen during viral replication (2, 24, 117, 121); and (ii) both 2BC and 2C are associated with the viral replication vesicles themselves (14, 15).

Protein 2C has been identified as the target of guanidine-HCl, an inhibitor of viral RNA replication (104). Although the mechanism by which this occurs has not been demonstrated, it has been shown that the addition of guanidine-HCl to HeLa cellular extracts that support viral replication (85) inhibits the initiation of viral negative-strand RNA synthesis (11). A specific role for 2C in the initiation of viral negative-strand RNA synthesis has

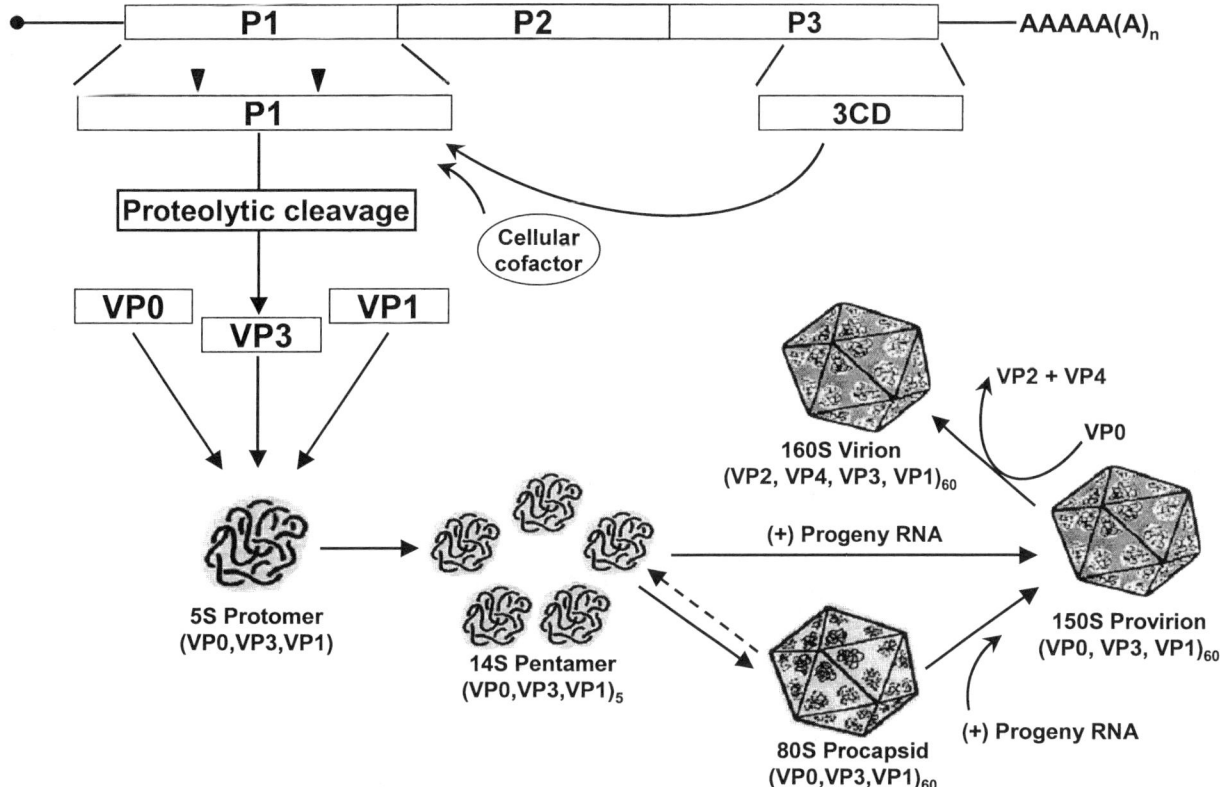

FIGURE 2 Processing of P1 capsid proteins and assembly of virion particles. 3CD carries out the cleavage of the P1 capsid precursor in a reaction that requires the activity of a cellular cofactor. This results in the formation of VP0, VP3, and VP1, which assemble into a 5S protomer. Then, five protomers assemble to form the 14S protomer. Twelve 14S protomers then either assemble around an RNA molecule or form the 80S procapsid structure into which an RNA molecule is threaded. In either case, this assembly process results in the formation of a short-lived 150S provirion. Finally, this newly formed particle undergoes a maturation event (occurring by an undefined mechanism) resulting in the cleavage of VP0 into VP2 and VP4, resulting in the production of a mature virion.

yet to be identified; however, 2C contains NTPase motifs with homology to those found in DNA helicases (42, 44, 45). While no helicase activity has been demonstrated for 2C, NTPase activities have been observed (67, 83, 84, 102). Indeed, guanidine-HCl has been shown to inhibit the NTPase activity of poliovirus protein 2C (102).

2C sequences may also play a role in the initiation of positive-strand synthesis, since 2C and 2BC have been shown to bind specific sequences in the 3' noncoding region of negative-strand viral RNA replication intermediates (8). This interaction is presumed to be mediated by two known RNA-binding motifs within 2C (108). Interestingly, the presence of the 2B domain within the 2BC precursor seems to alter the RNA sequence and structure recognition properties of the 2C protein (8, 9).

P3 Proteins

The primary function of the P3 proteins is to mediate events necessary for virus RNA replication and proteolytic processing. Like the proteins found within the P2 region of the polyprotein, P3 proteins are a set of polypeptides with diverse functions whose precursors often have different properties than their mature cleavage products.

3A and 3AB

The small hydrophobic protein 3A associates with intracellular membranes (31, 113, 122) and is also observed in its precursor form, 3AB. 3B, the genome-linked protein VPg that is covalently linked to the 5' end of both plus and minus RNA strands, is essential for virus RNA replication and may be delivered to RNA replication complexes as the precursor 3AB. Several observations support this hypothesis: (i) detergent-solubilized poliovirus 3AB stimulates 3D polymerase activity and 3CD proteolytic activity (73); (ii) detergent-solubilized poliovirus 3AB demonstrates specific and nonspecific viral RNA-binding properties (53, 130) that could target 3AB to virus RNA replication complexes; and (iii) hepatitis A viral RNAs with an optimized 3C cleavage site between 3A and 3B, which do not accumulate detectable amounts of the precursor 3AB, are deficient in viral replication (71). Although not directly demonstrating that 3B is supplied to the viral replication vesicles in the precursor form (3AB), these observations and the properties of 3AB suggest that 3AB is essential to the functions of viral replication complexes and a likely source for VPg. Additionally, 3AB may also serve to deliver the 3D RNA-dependent RNA polymerase to replication complexes, since interactions between 3AB and 3D have been demonstrated in the yeast two-hybrid assay (56, 129).

Protein 3A expression inhibits protein secretion and intracellular membrane transport in cultured cells (36, 37, 72) and has been shown to prevent the expression of major histocompatibility complex (MHC) class I molecules on the surface of the cell (32). Taken together, 3A expression could serve to inhibit cellular immunity mechanisms that rely on a properly functioning secretory pathway and could possibly assist protein 2C in the rearrangement of intracellular membranes into viral replication vesicles.

3B

The viral protein 3B, also known as VPg, is covalently linked to the 5' end of the genomic RNA (39, 75). A precise function for VPg has yet to be elucidated, but it has been shown not to be required for viral RNA infectivity in transfection experiments (88, 105, 114, 123). In vitro studies demonstrated that VPg can be uridylylated by the viral polymerase 3D at a tyrosine residue conserved among all picornaviral VPgs, and this uridylylated VPg can serve as a primer for RNA replication by the RNA-dependent RNA polymerase (97). Recently, an RNA hairpin structure required in cis for picornavirus RNA replication (termed cre, or cis-acting replication element) has been described (40, 78, 82). For poliovirus, the cre element resides within the 2C coding region and contains a conserved nucleotide motif (AAACA) that may provide a template on which uridylyl residues are covalently linked to VPg protein (107). Since VPg is found at the 5' end of both positive- and negative-strand viral RNAs (87, 101), and both negative- and positive-strand RNAs begin with uridine residues, uridylylated VPg is a likely candidate for a primer in a protein-primed mechanism of RNA synthesis initiation. The mechanism by which uridylylated VPg is translocated to the 3' poly(A) tail remains to be determined.

3C/3CD

In addition to acting as a virally encoded proteinase, 3C and 3CD also act at the level of RNA replication. 3C contains sequences that comprise an RNA-binding motif (4, 5) that has been characterized by three-dimensional studies (86) and mutagenesis experiments (3, 17, 35). For poliovirus and rhinovirus, these RNA-binding determinants within 3C have been shown to be critical for an interaction between 3C and an RNA secondary structure (known as the cloverleaf) found at the 5' end of the positive-strand RNA (3, 76). Interestingly, both poliovirus 3C and 3CD are able to form a complex at the poliovirus cloverleaf, but it is thought that 3CD is the form of 3C that forms the biologically relevant complex, binding in concert with a host protein, poly(rC)-binding protein (PCBP) (96). This complex has been shown to be required for poliovirus RNA replication and may represent a method by which the RNA-binding activity within 3C acts to deliver the poliovirus polymerase, 3D, to the replication complex. Similar to its effects on 3C proteinase activity, the presence of 3D sequences in the context of 3CD dramatically increases its ability to form the ribonucleoprotein complex (95). Some evidence exists for the presence of secondary RNA-binding determinants within the 3D portion of the 3CD polypeptide that may be critical for enhancing the RNA-binding capabilities of the molecule (C. T. Cornell and B. L. Semler, unpublished observations). Furthermore, it has been suggested that 3CD, in part, mediates a circularization of the plus-strand RNA genome by forming a protein bridge with host protein PCBP (also bound to the cloverleaf element) and poly(A)-binding protein (PABP) bound to the poly(A) tail (55). This is analogous to the circularization of cellular mRNAs that has been recently visualized and suggested as a mechanism for cellular translation initiation (127).

Data from recent studies have shown that the presence of 3CD greatly stimulates (100- to 1,000-fold) the in vitro VPg uridylylation reaction described by Wimmer and colleagues (107). The mechanism for this is unknown but may involve a direct binding of 3CD polypeptide to the cre RNA element, thereby altering its conformation and making it a more suitable template for the uridylylation reaction. Alternatively, 3CD may interact directly with the 3D polymerase to influence its VPg uridylylation activity.

3D

Protein 3D, the RNA-dependent RNA polymerase, is responsible for the synthesis of positive- and negative-strand RNAs. By itself, 3D (~52 kDa) is an effective elongating polymerase, but in vitro studies have demonstrated that polymerase activity is positively influenced by the viral protein 3AB (106). 3D-3AB interactions may facilitate localization of the polymerase to replication complexes. The 3D polymerase is also known to catalyze the VPg uridylylation reaction that is essential for RNA replication initiation (97). For encephalomyocarditis virus, the 3D polymerase has been shown to specifically recognize and bind to a region (30 nucleotides) in the 3' noncoding region immediately upstream of and including the poly(A) tail (28, 29). The picornavirus 3D RNA polymerase is an indispensable enzyme for viral replication whose biochemical properties are discussed in detail by Cameron and colleagues in chapter 21 of this volume.

CLEAVAGE OF NONVIRAL (HOST) SUBSTRATES BY VIRAL PROTEINASES

Picornavirus proteinases also carry out cleavage of host cell proteins. Since picornaviruses utilize a mechanism of translation that is cap independent, it is advantageous to the virus to inhibit nonessential cap-dependent cellular translation. In doing so, the cellular translation machinery is utilized almost exclusively for the production of viral proteins. Detailed discussions of the effects of picornavirus gene expression and replication on host cell functions are found in the Shutoff of Host Cell Translation and Transcription section of this volume.

The viral proteinase 2A of picornaviruses (except for the proteolytically inactive 2A polypeptides of aphthoviruses and cardioviruses) carries out the cleavage of eIF4G (38, 70, 115), specifically eIF4G-II (47, 119), which is an essential component of the host cap-binding complex. Cleavage of this factor occurs within the first few hours of viral infection, with total shutoff of host protein synthesis occurring at approximately 2 to 4 h postinfection. The FMDV L protein also cleaves eIF4G during an infection (33, 65), and it has been demonstrated that the carboxy-terminal cleavage fragment of eIF4G is utilized as a factor for cap-independent translation mediated by the viral internal ribosome entry site (89). It has been shown that the poliovirus 2A (131) and 3C proteinases (25) cleave TATA-binding protein, resulting in an inhibition of cellular transcription. 3C^{pro} also cleaves the cAMP-responsive element (132) and the transcriptional activator Oct-1 (133) in infected cells, which has been correlated with a reduction in cellular transcription. In addition to cleaving eIF4G and some transcription factors, enterovirus infections have also been correlated with a cleavage of PABP (59, 64), a host factor that plays a critical role in the initiation of translation on cellular mRNAs. This may also destabilize these transcripts, thereby providing an additional mechanism for the shutoff of host protein synthesis.

SUMMARY

Picornaviruses possess RNA genomes of limited coding capacity and must rely on the translation and subsequent processing of only a handful of viral gene products. The virally encoded proteinases generate both precursor and mature protein products in a timely manner so that they may carry out specific functions that are important for successful viral replication. In addition to their specificity for viral substrates, picornavirus proteinases also cleave cellular factors that dramatically affect host gene expression at the transcriptional and translational levels, further augmenting the ability of picornaviruses to very effectively complete an intracellular replication cycle and go on to infect other cells and tissues in susceptible host organisms.

REFERENCES

1. **Aldabe, R., A. Barco, and L. Carrasco.** 1996. Membrane permeabilization by poliovirus proteins 2B and 2BC. *J. Biol. Chem.* **271:**23134–23137.
2. **Aldabe, R., and L. Carrasco.** 1995. Induction of membrane proliferation by poliovirus proteins 2C and 2BC. *Biochem. Biophys. Res. Commun.* **206:**64–76.
3. **Andino, R., G. E. Rieckhof, P. L. Achacoso, and D. Baltimore.** 1993. Poliovirus RNA synthesis utilizes an RNP complex formed around the 5'-end of viral RNA. *EMBO J.* **12:**3587–3598.
4. **Andino, R., G. E. Rieckhof, and D. Baltimore.** 1990. A functional ribonucleoprotein complex forms around the 5' end of poliovirus RNA. *Cell* **63:**369–380.
5. **Andino, R., G. E. Rieckhof, D. Trono, and D. Baltimore.** 1990. Substitutions in the protease (3C^{pro}) gene of poliovirus can suppress a mutation in the 5' noncoding region. *J. Virol.* **64:**607–612.
6. **Ansardi, D. C., R. Pal-Ghosh, D. Porter, and C. D. Morrow.** 1995. Encapsidation and serial passage of a poliovirus replicon which expresses an inactive 2A proteinase. *J. Virol.* **69:**1359–1366.
7. **Arnold, E., M. Luo, G. Vriend, M. G. Rossmann, A. C. Palmenberg, G. D. Parks, M. J. Nicklin, and E. Wimmer.** 1987. Implications of the picornavirus capsid structure for polyprotein processing. *Proc. Natl. Acad. Sci. USA* **84:**21–25.
8. **Banerjee, R., A. Echeverri, and A. Dasgupta.** 1997. Poliovirus-encoded 2C polypeptide specifically binds to the 3'-terminal sequences of viral negative-strand RNA. *J. Virol.* **71:**9570–9578.
9. **Banerjee, R., W. Tsai, W. Kim, and A. Dasgupta.** 2001. Interaction of poliovirus-encoded 2C/2BC polypeptides with the 3' terminus negative-strand cloverleaf requires an intact stem-loop B. *Virology* **280:**41–51.
10. **Barco, A., and L. Carrasco.** 1998. Identification of regions of poliovirus 2BC protein that are involved in cytotoxicity. *J. Virol.* **72:**3560–3570.
11. **Barton, D. J., and J. B. Flanegan.** 1997. Synchronous replication of poliovirus RNA: initiation of negative-strand RNA synthesis requires the guanidine-inhibited activity of protein 2C. *J. Virol.* **71:**8482–8489.
12. **Bazan, J. F., and R. J. Fletterick.** 1988. Viral cysteine proteases are homologous to the trypsin-like family of serine proteases: structural and functional implications. *Proc. Natl. Acad. Sci. USA* **85:**7872–7876.
13. **Bergmann, E. M., S. C. Mosimann, M. M. Chernaia, B. A. Malcolm, and M. N. James.** 1997. The refined crystal structure of the 3C gene product from hepatitis A virus: specific proteinase activity and RNA recognition. *J. Virol.* **71:**2436–2448.
14. **Bienz, K., D. Egger, and L. Pasamontes.** 1987. Association of poliviral proteins of the P2 genomic region with the viral replication complex and virus-induced membrane synthesis as visualized by electron microscopic immunocytochemistry and autoradiography. *Virology* **160:**220–226.
15. **Bienz, K., D. Egger, Y. Rasser, and W. Bossart.** 1983. Intracellular distribution of poliovirus proteins and the induction of virus-specific cytoplasmic structures. *Virology* **131:**39–48.
16. **Blair, W. S., X. Li, and B. L. Semler.** 1993. A cellular cofactor facilitates efficient 3CD cleavage of the poliovirus P1 precursor. *J. Virol.* **67:**2336–2343.
17. **Blair, W. S., T. B. Parsley, H. P. Bogerd, J. S. Towner, B. L. Semler, and B. R. Cullen.** 1998. Utilization of a mammalian cell-based RNA binding assay to characterize the RNA binding properties of picornavirus 3C proteinases. *RNA* **4:**215–225.
18. **Blair, W. S., and B. L. Semler.** 1991. Role for the P4 amino acid residue in substrate utilization by the poliovirus 3CD proteinase. *J. Virol.* **65:**6111–6123.
19. **Bolten, R., D. Egger, R. Gosert, G. Schaub, L. Landmann, and K. Bienz.** 1998. Intracellular localization of poliovirus. *J. Virol.* **72:**8578–8585.
20. **Charini, W. A., S. Todd, G. A. Gutman, and B. L. Semler.** 1994. Transduction of a human RNA sequence by poliovirus. *J. Virol.* **68:**6547–6552.
21. **Cheah, K. C., L. E. Leong, and A. G. Porter.** 1990. Site-directed mutagenesis suggests close functional relationship between a human rhinovirus 3C cysteine protease and cellular trypsin-like serine proteases. *J. Biol. Chem.* **265:**7180–7187.
22. **Chen, H. H., W. P. Kong, and R. P. Roos.** 1995. The leader peptide of Theiler's murine encephalomyelitis virus is a zinc-binding protein. *J. Virol.* **69:**8076–8078.
23. **Chen, H. H., W. P. Kong, L. Zhang, P. L. Ward, and R. P. Roos.** 1995. A picornaviral protein synthesized out of frame with the polyprotein plays a key role in a virus-induced immune-mediated demyelinating disease. *Nat. Med.* **1:**927–931.
24. **Cho, M. W., N. Teterina, D. Egger, K. Bienz, and E. Ehrenfeld.** 1994. Membrane rearrangement and vesicle induction by recombinant poliovirus 2C and 2BC in human cells. *Virology* **202:**129–145.
25. **Clark, M. E., P. M. Lieberman, A. J. Berk, and A. Dasgupta.** 1993. Direct cleavage of human TATA-binding protein by poliovirus protease 3C in vivo and in vitro. *Mol. Cell. Biol.* **13:**1232–1237.
26. **Collis, P. S., B. J. O'Donnell, D. J. Barton, J. A. Rogers, and J. B. Flanegan.** 1992. Replication of poliovirus RNA and subgenomic RNA transcripts in transfected cells. *J. Virol.* **66:**6480–6488.
27. **Cordingley, M. G., P. L. Callahan, V. V. Sardana, V. M. Garsky, and R. J. Colonno.** 1990. Substrate requirements of human rhinovirus 3C protease for peptide cleavage in vitro. *J. Biol. Chem.* **265:**9062–9065.
28. **Cui, T., and A. G. Porter.** 1995. Localization of binding site for encephalomyocarditis virus RNA polymerase in the 3'-noncoding region of the viral RNA. *Nucleic Acids Res.* **23:**377–382.

29. Cui, T., S. Sankar, and A. G. Porter. 1993. Binding of encephalomyocarditis virus RNA polymerase to the 3′-noncoding region of the viral RNA is specific and requires the 3′-poly(A) tail. *J. Biol. Chem.* **268:**26093–26098.
30. Das, S., and A. Dasgupta. 1993. Identification of the cleavage site and determinants required for poliovirus 3C^{pro}-catalyzed cleavage of human TATA-binding transcription factor TBP. *J. Virol.* **67:**3326–3331.
31. Datta, U., and A. Dasgupta. 1994. Expression and subcellular localization of poliovirus VPg-precursor protein 3AB in eukaryotic cells: evidence for glycosylation in vitro. *J. Virol.* **68:**4468–4477.
32. Deitz, S. B., D. A. Dodd, S. Cooper, P. Parham, and K. Kirkegaard. 2000. MHC I-dependent antigen presentation is inhibited by poliovirus protein 3A. *Proc. Natl. Acad. Sci. USA* **97:**13790–13795.
33. Devaney, M. A., V. N. Vakharia, R. E. Lloyd, E. Ehrenfeld, and M. J. Grubman. 1988. Leader protein of foot-and-mouth disease virus is required for cleavage of the p220 component of the cap-binding protein complex. *J. Virol.* **62:**4407–4409.
34. Dewalt, P. G., M. A. Lawson, R. J. Colonno, and B. L. Semler. 1989. Chimeric picornavirus polyproteins demonstrate a common 3C proteinase substrate specificity. *J. Virol.* **63:**3444–3452.
35. Dewalt, P. G., and B. L. Semler. 1987. Site-directed mutagenesis of proteinase 3C results in a poliovirus deficient in synthesis of viral RNA polymerase. *J. Virol.* **61:**2162–2170.
36. Doedens, J. R., T. H. Giddings, and K. Kirkegaard. 1997. Inhibition of endoplasmic reticulum-to-Golgi traffic by poliovirus protein 3A: genetic and ultrastructural analysis. *J. Virol.* **71:**9054–9064.
37. Doedens, J. R., and K. Kirkegaard. 1995. Inhibition of cellular protein secretion by poliovirus proteins 2B and 3A. *EMBO J.* **14:**894–907.
38. Etchison, D., S. C. Milburn, I. Edery, N. Sonenberg, and J. W. Hershey. 1982. Inhibition of HeLa cell protein synthesis following poliovirus infection correlates with the proteolysis of a 220,000-dalton polypeptide associated with eucaryotic initiation factor 3 and a cap binding protein complex. *J. Biol. Chem.* **257:**14806–14810.
39. Flanegan, J. B., R. F. Pettersson, V. Ambros, N. J. Hewlett, and D. Baltimore. 1977. Covalent linkage of a protein to a defined nucleotide sequence at the 5′-terminus of virion and replicative intermediate RNAs of poliovirus. *Proc. Natl. Acad. Sci. USA* **74:**961–965.
40. Goodfellow, I., Y. Chaudhry, A. Richardson, J. Meredith, J. W. Almond, W. Barclay, and D. J. Evans. 2000. Identification of a *cis*-acting replication element within the poliovirus coding region. *J. Virol.* **74:**4590–4600.
41. Gorbalenya, A. E., V. M. Blinov, and A. P. Donchenko. 1986. Poliovirus-encoded proteinase 3C: a possible evolutionary link between cellular serine and cysteine proteinase families. *FEBS Lett.* **194:**253–257.
42. Gorbalenya, A. E., V. M. Blinov, A. P. Donchenko, and E. V. Koonin. 1989. An NTP-binding motif is the most conserved sequence in a highly diverged monophyletic group of proteins involved in positive strand RNA viral replication. *J. Mol. Evol.* **28:**256–268.
43. Gorbalenya, A. E., A. P. Donchenko, V. M. Blinov, and E. V. Koonin. 1989. Cysteine proteases of positive strand RNA viruses and chymotrypsin-like serine proteases. A distinct protein superfamily with a common structural fold. *FEBS Lett.* **243:**103–114.
44. Gorbalenya, A. E., and E. V. Koonin. 1989. Viral proteins containing the purine NTP-binding sequence pattern. *Nucleic Acids Res.* **17:**8413–8440.
45. Gorbalenya, A. E., E. V. Koonin, A. P. Donchenko, and V. M. Blinov. 1988. A conserved NTP-motif in putative helicases. *Nature* **333:**22.
46. Gorbalenya, A. E., E. V. Koonin, and M. M. Lai. 1991. Putative papain-related thiol proteases of positive-strand RNA viruses. Identification of rubi- and aphthovirus proteases and delineation of a novel conserved domain associated with proteases of rubi-, alpha-, and coronaviruses. *FEBS Lett.* **288:**201–205.
47. Gradi, A., Y. V. Svitkin, H. Imataka, and N. Sonenberg. 1998. Proteolysis of human eukaryotic translation initiation factor eIF4GII, but not eIF4GI, coincides with the shutoff of host protein synthesis after poliovirus infection. *Proc. Natl. Acad. Sci. USA* **95:**11089–11094.
48. Grubman, M. J., and B. Baxt. 1982. Translation of foot-and-mouth disease virion RNA and processing of the primary cleavage products in a rabbit reticulocyte lysate. *Virology* **116:**19–30.
49. Grubman, M. J., M. Zellner, G. Bablanian, P. W. Mason, and M. E. Piccone. 1995. Identification of the active-site residues of the 3C proteinase of foot-and-mouth disease virus. *Virology* **213:**581–589.
50. Haller, A. H., and B. L. Semler. 1995. Translation and host cell shut off, p. 113–133. *In* H. A. Rotbart (ed.), *Human Enterovirus Infections.* ASM Press, Washington, D.C.
51. Hanecak, R., B. L. Semler, C. W. Anderson, and E. Wimmer. 1982. Proteolytic processing of poliovirus polypeptides: antibodies to polypeptide P3-7c inhibit cleavage at glutamine-glycine pairs. *Proc. Natl. Acad. Sci. USA* **79:**3973–3977.
52. Harris, K. S., S. R. Reddigari, M. J. Nicklin, T. Hammerle, and E. Wimmer. 1992. Purification and characterization of poliovirus polypeptide 3CD, a proteinase and a precursor for RNA polymerase. *J. Virol.* **66:**7481–7489.
53. Harris, K. S., W. Xiang, L. Alexander, W. S. Lane, A. V. Paul, and E. Wimmer. 1994. Interaction of poliovirus polypeptide 3CD^{pro} with the 5′ and 3′ termini of the poliovirus genome. Identification of viral and cellular cofactors needed for efficient binding. *J. Biol. Chem.* **269:**27004–27014.
54. Hellen, C. U., C. K. Lee, and E. Wimmer. 1992. Determinants of substrate recognition by poliovirus 2A proteinase. *J. Virol.* **66:**3330–3338.
55. Herold, J., and R. Andino. 2001. Poliovirus RNA replication requires genome circularization through a protein-protein bridge. *Mol. Cell* **7:**581–591.
56. Hope, D. A., S. E. Diamond, and K. Kirkegaard. 1997. Genetic dissection of interaction between poliovirus 3D polymerase and viral protein 3AB. *J. Virol.* **71:**9490–9498.
57. Ivanoff, L. A., T. Towatari, J. Ray, B. D. Korant, and S. R. Petteway, Jr. 1986. Expression and site-specific mutagenesis of the poliovirus 3C protease in *Escherichia coli.* *Proc. Natl. Acad. Sci. USA* **83:**5392–5396.
58. Jang, S. K., H. G. Krausslich, M. J. Nicklin, G. M. Duke, A. C. Palmenberg, and E. Wimmer. 1988. A segment of the 5′ nontranslated region of encephalomyocarditis virus RNA directs internal entry of ribosomes during in vitro translation. *J. Virol.* **62:**2636–2643.
59. Joachims, M., P. C. Van Breugel, and R. E. Lloyd. 1999. Cleavage of poly(A)-binding protein by enterovirus proteases concurrent with inhibition of translation in vitro. *J. Virol.* **73:**718–727.
60. Johnson, K. L., and P. Sarnow. 1991. Three poliovirus 2B mutants exhibit noncomplementable defects in viral RNA amplification and display dosage-dependent dominance over wild-type poliovirus. *J. Virol.* **65:**4341–4349.
61. Kaplan, G., and V. R. Racaniello. 1988. Construction and characterization of poliovirus subgenomic replicons. *J. Virol.* **62:**1687–1696.

62. **Kean, K. M., N. Teterina, and M. Girard.** 1990. Cleavage specificity of the poliovirus 3C protease is not restricted to Gln-Gly at the 3C/3D junction. *J. Gen. Virol.* **71**(Pt. 11):2553–2563.
63. **Kean, K. M., N. L. Teterina, D. Marc, and M. Girard.** 1991. Analysis of putative active site residues of the poliovirus 3C protease. *Virology* **181**:609–619.
64. **Kerekatte, V., B. D. Keiper, C. Badorff, A. Cai, K. U. Knowlton, and R. E. Rhoads.** 1999. Cleavage of poly(A)-binding protein by coxsackievirus 2A protease in vitro and in vivo: another mechanism for host protein synthesis shutoff? *J. Virol.* **73**:709–717.
65. **Kirchweger, R., E. Ziegler, B. J. Lamphear, D. Waters, H. D. Liebig, W. Sommergruber, F. Sobrino, C. Hohenadl, D. Blaas, and R. E. Rhoads.** 1994. Foot-and-mouth disease virus leader proteinase: purification of the Lb form and determination of its cleavage site on eIF-4 gamma. *J. Virol.* **68**:5677–5684.
66. **Kitamura, N., B. L. Semler, P. G. Rothberg, G. R. Larsen, C. J. Adler, A. J. Dorner, E. A. Emini, R. Hanecak, J. J. Lee, S. van der Werf, C. W. Anderson, and E. Wimmer.** 1981. Primary structure, gene organization and polypeptide expression of poliovirus RNA. *Nature* **291**:547–553.
67. **Klein, M., H. J. Eggers, and B. Nelsen-Salz.** 1999. Echovirus 9 strain barty non-structural protein 2C has NTPase activity. *Virus Res.* **65**:155–160.
68. **Kleina, L. G., and M. J. Grubman.** 1992. Antiviral effects of a thiol protease inhibitor on foot-and-mouth disease virus. *J. Virol.* **66**:7168–7175.
69. **Kong, J. S., S. Venkatraman, K. Furness, S. Nimkar, T. A. Shepherd, Q. M. Wang, J. Aube, and R. P. Hanzlik.** 1998. Synthesis and evaluation of peptidyl Michael acceptors that inactivate human rhinovirus 3C protease and inhibit virus replication. *J. Med. Chem.* **41**:2579–2587.
70. **Krausslich, H. G., M. J. Nicklin, H. Toyoda, D. Etchison, and E. Wimmer.** 1987. Poliovirus proteinase 2A induces cleavage of eucaryotic initiation factor 4F polypeptide p220. *J. Virol.* **61**:2711–2718.
71. **Kusov, Y., and V. Gauss-Muller.** 1999. Improving proteolytic cleavage at the 3A/3B site of the hepatitis A virus polyprotein impairs processing and particle formation, and the impairment can be complemented in *trans* by 3AB and 3ABC. *J. Virol.* **73**:9867–9878.
72. **Lama, J., and L. Carrasco.** 1992. Expression of poliovirus nonstructural proteins in *Escherichia coli* cells. Modification of membrane permeability induced by 2B and 3A. *J. Biol. Chem.* **267**:15932–15937.
73. **Lama, J., A. V. Paul, K. S. Harris, and E. Wimmer.** 1994. Properties of purified recombinant poliovirus protein 3AB as substrate for viral proteinases and as co-factor for RNA polymerase 3D^{pol}. *J. Biol. Chem.* **269**:66–70.
74. **Lawson, M. A., and B. L. Semler.** 1991. Poliovirus thiol proteinase 3C can utilize a serine nucleophile within the putative catalytic triad. *Proc. Natl. Acad. Sci. USA* **88**:9919–9923.
75. **Lee, Y. F., A. Nomoto, B. M. Detjen, and E. Wimmer.** 1977. A protein covalently linked to poliovirus genome RNA. *Proc. Natl. Acad. Sci. USA* **74**:59–63.
76. **Leong, L. E., P. A. Walker, and A. G. Porter.** 1993. Human rhinovirus-14 protease 3C (3C^{pro}) binds specifically to the 5′-noncoding region of the viral RNA. Evidence that 3C^{pro} has different domains for the RNA binding and proteolytic activities. *J. Biol. Chem.* **268**:25735–25739.
77. **Li, X., H. H. Lu, S. Mueller, and E. Wimmer.** 2001. The C-terminal residues of poliovirus proteinase 2A(pro) are critical for viral RNA replication but not for cis- or trans-proteolytic cleavage. *J. Gen. Virol.* **82**:397–408.
78. **Lobert, P. E., N. Escriou, J. Ruelle, and T. Michiels.** 1999. A coding RNA sequence acts as a replication signal in cardioviruses. *Proc. Natl. Acad. Sci. USA* **96**:11560–11565.
79. **Long, A. C., D. C. Orr, J. M. Cameron, B. M. Dunn, and J. Kay.** 1989. A consensus sequence for substrate hydrolysis by rhinovirus 3C proteinase. *FEBS Lett.* **258**:75–78.
80. **Macejak, D. G., and P. Sarnow.** 1992. Association of heat shock protein 70 with enterovirus capsid precursor P1 in infected human cells. *J. Virol.* **66**:1520–1527.
81. **Matthews, D. A., W. W. Smith, R. A. Ferre, B. Condon, G. Budahazi, W. Sisson, J. E. Villafranca, C. A. Janson, H. E. McElroy, and C. L. Gribskov.** 1994. Structure of human rhinovirus 3C protease reveals a trypsin-like polypeptide fold, RNA-binding site, and means for cleaving precursor polyprotein. *Cell* **77**:761–771.
82. **McKnight, K. L., and S. M. Lemon.** 1998. The rhinovirus type 14 genome contains an internally located RNA structure that is required for viral replication. *RNA* **4**:1569–1584.
83. **Mirzayan, C., and E. Wimmer.** 1992. Genetic analysis of an NTP-binding motif in poliovirus polypeptide 2C. *Virology* **189**:547–555.
84. **Mirzayan, C., and E. Wimmer.** 1994. Biochemical studies on poliovirus polypeptide 2C: evidence for ATPase activity. *Virology* **199**:176–187.
85. **Molla, A., A. V. Paul, and E. Wimmer.** 1991. Cell-free, de novo synthesis of poliovirus. *Science* **254**:1647–1651.
86. **Mosimann, S. C., M. M. Cherney, S. Sia, S. Plotch, and M. N. James.** 1997. Refined X-ray crystallographic structure of the poliovirus 3C gene product. *J. Mol. Biol.* **273**:1032–1047.
87. **Nomoto, A., B. Detjen, R. Pozzatti, and E. Wimmer.** 1977. The location of the polio genome protein in viral RNAs and its implication for RNA synthesis. *Nature* **268**:208–213.
88. **Nomoto, A., N. Kitamura, F. Golini, and E. Wimmer.** 1977. The 5′-terminal structures of poliovirion RNA and poliovirus mRNA differ only in the genome-linked protein VPg. *Proc. Natl. Acad. Sci. USA* **74**:5345–5349.
89. **Ohlmann, T., M. Rau, V. M. Pain, and S. J. Morley.** 1996. The C-terminal domain of eukaryotic protein synthesis initiation factor (eIF) 4G is sufficient to support cap-independent translation in the absence of eIF4E. *EMBO J.* **15**:1371–1382.
90. **Pal-Ghosh, R., and C. D. Morrow.** 1993. A poliovirus minireplicon containing an inactive 2A proteinase is expressed in vaccinia virus-infected cells. *J. Virol.* **67**:4621–4629.
91. **Pallai, P. V., F. Burkhardt, M. Skoog, K. Schreiner, P. Bax, K. A. Cohen, G. Hansen, D. E. Palladino, K. S. Harris, and M. J. Nicklin.** 1989. Cleavage of synthetic peptides by purified poliovirus 3C proteinase. *J. Biol. Chem.* **264**:9738–9741.
92. **Pallansch, M. A., O. M. Kew, B. L. Semler, D. R. Omilianowski, C. W. Anderson, E. Wimmer, and R. R. Rueckert.** 1984. Protein processing map of poliovirus. *J. Virol.* **49**:873–880.
93. **Palmenberg, A. C.** 1990. Proteolytic processing of picornaviral polyprotein. *Annu. Rev. Microbiol.* **44**:603–623.
94. **Parks, G. D., G. M. Duke, and A. C. Palmenberg.** 1986. Encephalomyocarditis virus 3C protease: efficient cell-free expression from clones which link viral 5′ noncoding sequences to the P3 region. *J. Virol.* **60**:376–384.
95. **Parsley, T. B., C. T. Cornell, and B. L. Semler.** 1999. Modulation of the RNA binding and protein processing activities of poliovirus polypeptide 3CD by the viral RNA polymerase domain. *J. Biol. Chem.* **274**:12867–12876.

96. Parsley, T. B., J. S. Towner, L. B. Blyn, E. Ehrenfeld, and B. L. Semler. 1997. Poly (rC) binding protein 2 forms a ternary complex with the 5′-terminal sequences of poliovirus RNA and the viral 3CD proteinase. *RNA* **3:**1124–1134.
97. Paul, A. V., J. H. van Boom, D. Filippov, and E. Wimmer. 1998. Protein-primed RNA synthesis by purified poliovirus RNA polymerase. *Nature* **393:**280–284.
98. Pelletier, J., and N. Sonenberg. 1988. Internal initiation of translation of eukaryotic mRNA directed by a sequence derived from poliovirus RNA. *Nature* **334:**320–325.
99. Petersen, J. F., M. M. Cherney, H. D. Liebig, T. Skern, E. Kuechler, and M. N. James. 1999. The structure of the 2A proteinase from a common cold virus: a proteinase responsible for the shut-off of host-cell protein synthesis. *EMBO J.* **18:**5463–5475.
100. Petithory, J. R., F. R. Masiarz, J. F. Kirsch, D. V. Santi, and B. A. Malcolm. 1991. A rapid method for determination of endoproteinase substrate specificity: specificity of the 3C proteinase from hepatitis A virus. *Proc. Natl. Acad. Sci. USA* **88:**11510–11514.
101. Pettersson, R. F., V. Ambros, and D. Baltimore. 1978. Identification of a protein linked to nascent poliovirus RNA and to the polyuridylic acid of negative-strand RNA. *J. Virol.* **27:**357–365.
102. Pfister, T., and E. Wimmer. 1999. Characterization of the nucleoside triphosphatase activity of poliovirus protein 2C reveals a mechanism by which guanidine inhibits poliovirus replication. *J. Biol. Chem.* **274:**6992–7001.
103. Piccone, M. E., M. Zellner, T. F. Kumosinski, P. W. Mason, and M. J. Grubman. 1995. Identification of the active-site residues of the L proteinase of foot-and-mouth disease virus. *J. Virol.* **69:**4950–4956.
104. Pincus, S. E., D. C. Diamond, E. A. Emini, and E. Wimmer. 1986. Guanidine-selected mutants of poliovirus: mapping of point mutations to polypeptide 2C. *J. Virol.* **57:**638–646.
105. Racaniello, V. R., and D. Baltimore. 1981. Cloned poliovirus complementary DNA is infectious in mammalian cells. *Science* **214:**916–919.
106. Richards, O. C., and E. Ehrenfeld. 1998. Effects of poliovirus 3AB protein on 3D polymerase-catalyzed reaction. *J. Biol. Chem.* **273:**12832–12840.
107. Rieder, E., A. V. Paul, D. W. Kim, J. H. van Boom, and E. Wimmer. 2000. Genetic and biochemical studies of poliovirus cis-acting replication element cre in relation to VPg uridylylation. *J. Virol.* **74:**10371–10380.
108. Rodriguez, P. L., and L. Carrasco. 1995. Poliovirus protein 2C contains two regions involved in RNA binding activity. *J. Biol. Chem.* **270:**10105–10112.
109. Rueckert, R. R., and E. Wimmer. 1984. Systematic nomenclature of picornavirus proteins. *J. Virol.* **50:**957–959.
110. Ryan, M. D., A. M. King, and G. P. Thomas. 1991. Cleavage of foot-and-mouth disease virus polyprotein is mediated by residues located within a 19 amino acid sequence. *J. Gen. Virol.* **72:**2727–2732.
111. Sandoval, I. V., and L. Carrasco. 1997. Poliovirus infection and expression of the poliovirus protein 2B provoke the disassembly of the Golgi complex, the organelle target for the antipoliovirus drug Ro-090179. *J. Virol.* **71:**4679–4693.
112. Schechter, I., and A. Berger. 1967. On the size of the active site in proteases. I. Papain. *Biochem. Biophys. Res. Commun.* **27:**157–162.
113. Semler, B. L., C. W. Anderson, R. Hanecak, L. F. Dorner, and E. Wimmer. 1982. A membrane-associated precursor to poliovirus VPg identified by immunoprecipitation with antibodies directed against a synthetic heptapeptide. *Cell* **28:**405–412.
114. Semler, B. L., A. J. Dorner, and E. Wimmer. 1984. Production of infectious poliovirus from cloned cDNA is dramatically increased by SV40 transcription and replication signals. *Nucleic Acids Res.* **12:**5123–5141.
115. Sommergruber, W., H. Ahorn, H. Klump, J. Seipelt, A. Zoephel, F. Fessl, E. Krystek, D. Blaas, E. Kuechler, H. D. Liebig, et al. 1994. 2A proteinases of coxsackie- and rhinovirus cleave peptides derived from eIF-4G via a common recognition motif. *Virology* **198:**741–745.
116. Strebel, K., and E. Beck. 1986. A second protease of foot-and-mouth disease virus. *J. Virol.* **58:**893–899.
117. Suhy, D. A., T. H. Giddings, Jr., and K. Kirkegaard. 2000. Remodeling the endoplasmic reticulum by poliovirus infection and by individual viral proteins: an autophagy-like origin for virus-induced vesicles. *J. Virol.* **74:**8953–8965.
118. Summers, D. F., and J. V. J. Maizel. 1968. Evidence for large precursor proteins in poliovirus synthesis. *Proc. Natl. Acad. Sci. USA* **59:**966–971.
119. Svitkin, Y. V., A. Gradi, H. Imataka, S. Morino, and N. Sonenberg. 1999. Eukaryotic initiation factor 4GII (eIF4GII), but not eIF4GI, cleavage correlates with inhibition of host cell protein synthesis after human rhinovirus infection. *J. Virol.* **73:**3467–3472.
120. Takata, H., M. Obuchi, J. Yamamoto, T. Odagiri, R. P. Roos, H. Iizuka, and Y. Ohara. 1998. L* protein of the DA strain of Theiler's murine encephalomyelitis virus is important for virus growth in a murine macrophage-like cell line. *J. Virol.* **72:**4950–4955.
121. Teterina, N. L., K. Bienz, D. Egger, A. E. Gorbalenya, and E. Ehrenfeld. 1997. Induction of intracellular membrane rearrangements by HAV proteins 2C and 2BC. *Virology* **237:**66–77.
122. Towner, J. S., T. V. Ho, and B. L. Semler. 1996. Determinants of membrane association for poliovirus protein 3AB. *J. Biol. Chem.* **271:**26810–26818.
123. van der Werf, S., J. Bradley, E. Wimmer, F. W. Studier, and J. J. Dunn. 1986. Synthesis of infectious poliovirus RNA by purified T7 RNA polymerase. *Proc. Natl. Acad. Sci. USA* **83:**2330–2334.
124. van Kuppeveld, F. J., J. M. Galama, J. Zoll, and W. J. Melchers. 1995. Genetic analysis of a hydrophobic domain of coxsackie B3 virus protein 2B: a moderate degree of hydrophobicity is required for a cis-acting function in viral RNA synthesis. *J. Virol.* **69:**7782–7790.
125. van Kuppeveld, F. J., J. G. Hoenderop, R. L. Smeets, P. H. Willems, H. B. Dijkman, J. M. Galama, and W. J. Melchers. 1997. Coxsackievirus protein 2B modifies endoplasmic reticulum membrane and plasma membrane permeability and facilitates virus release. *EMBO J.* **16:**3519–3532.
126. van Kuppeveld, F. J., W. J. Melchers, K. Kirkegaard, and J. R. Doedens. 1997. Structure-function analysis of coxsackie B3 virus protein 2B. *Virology* **227:**111–118.
127. Wells, S. E., P. E. Hillner, R. D. Vale, and A. B. Sachs. 1998. Circularization of mRNA by eukaryotic translation initiation factors. *Mol. Cell* **2:**135–140.
128. Wimmer, E., C. U. Hellen, and X. Cao. 1993. Genetics of poliovirus. *Annu. Rev. Genet.* **27:**353–436.
129. Xiang, W., A. Cuconati, D. Hope, K. Kirkegaard, and E. Wimmer. 1998. Complete protein linkage map of poliovirus P3 proteins: interaction of polymerase 3D^{pol} with VPg and with genetic variants of 3AB. *J. Virol.* **72:**6732–6741.
130. Xiang, W., A. Cuconati, A. V. Paul, X. Cao, and E. Wimmer. 1995. Molecular dissection of the multifunc-

tional poliovirus RNA-binding protein 3AB. *RNA* **1:** 892–904.
131. **Yalamanchili, P., R. Banerjee, and A. Dasgupta.** 1997. Poliovirus-encoded protease 2A^{pro} cleaves the TATA-binding protein but does not inhibit host cell RNA polymerase II transcription in vitro. *J. Virol.* **71:**6881–6886.
132. **Yalamanchili, P., U. Datta, and A. Dasgupta.** 1997. Inhibition of host cell transcription by poliovirus: cleavage of transcription factor CREB by poliovirus-encoded protease 3C^{pro}. *J. Virol.* **71:**1220–1226.
133. **Yalamanchili, P., K. Weidman, and A. Dasgupta.** 1997. Cleavage of transcriptional activator Oct-1 by poliovirus encoded protease 3C^{pro}. *Virology* **239:**176–185.
134. **Ypma-Wong, M. F., P. G. Dewalt, V. H. Johnson, J. G. Lamb, and B. L. Semler.** 1988. Protein 3CD is the major poliovirus proteinase responsible for cleavage of the P1 capsid precursor. *Virology* **166:**265–270.
135. **Yu, S. F., and R. E. Lloyd.** 1991. Identification of essential amino acid residues in the functional activity of poliovirus 2A protease. *Virology* **182:**615–625.

Structure and Function of Picornavirus Proteinases

TIM SKERN, BERNHARD HAMPÖLZ, ALBA GUARNÉ, IGNACIO FITA,
ERNST BERGMANN, JENS PETERSEN, AND MICHAEL N. G. JAMES

17

The information in the picornavirus plus-strand RNA genome is encoded in a single open reading frame. The protein synthesis machinery of the infected cell generates a single polypeptide, designated the viral polyprotein, from this open reading frame. The success of viral replication depends absolutely on the activity of proteinases encoded within the polyprotein to process it into the mature viral proteins. Furthermore, viral proteinases enhance the replication of their respective viruses by cleaving specific cellular proteins, thereby modulating the metabolism of the host.

The three-dimensional structures of three types of picornaviral proteinases have now been solved by X-ray crystallography (1, 36, 58, 67). This chapter summarizes the implications of these structures on the proteolytic mechanisms, the substrate specificities, and the functions of the proteinases in infected cells.

THE PICORNAVIRAL POLYPROTEIN

The picornaviral polyproteins can be divided into three regions, designated P1, P2, and P3 (Fig. 1) (71). These correspond to the N-terminal capsid protein precursor (P1, containing the four capsid proteins 1A–1D), the middle of the polyprotein containing three of the nonstructural proteins (P2, the three proteins 2A–2C), and the most C-terminal segment of the polyprotein containing four nonstructural proteins (P3, proteins 3A–3D). In the cardio- and aphthoviruses, a protein known as the leader (L) protein precedes P1 (Fig. 1). The patterns of proteolytic processing in six genera of picornaviruses will now be summarized briefly.

Primary Cleavages on the Polyprotein

The hepato- and parechoviruses encode only a single proteolytic enzyme and are therefore proteolytically the simplest of the picornaviruses (Fig. 1). In these viruses, $3C^{pro}$ carries out both primary cleavage events, with the initial cleavage occurring between the P2 proteins 2A and 2B (56) and the second between 2C and 3A. In contrast, other genera encode a 2A protein with proteolytic activity that is responsible for carrying out the cleavage that separates the capsid precursor P1 from the precursor of the nonstructural proteins, P2–P3. In rhino- and enteroviruses, the 2A ($2A^{pro}$) proteins are cysteine proteinases having a chymotrypsin-like fold (7, 31). They cleave their respective polyproteins between the C terminus of VP1 and their own N terminus. In contrast, the 2A proteins of cardio- and aphthoviruses perform the primary cleavage between the C terminus of 2A and the N terminus of 2B (Fig. 1), thereby generating a P1-2A precursor (63, 73). In addition, they bear no sequence similarity to the 2A proteins of rhino- and enteroviruses nor to any other proteinases. However, the cardio- and aphthovirus 2A proteins are, despite the differences in length, related to each other. Thus, of the 19 amino acids that comprise the 2A protein of aphthoviruses (73), 5 of the 7 most C-terminal residue amino acids are identical to those found at the C terminus of the 140-amino-acid cardiovirus 2A protein (23). The mechanism of action of the cardio- and aphthovirus 2A proteins remains unclear; it is discussed by Ryan et al. in chapter 18.

Processing in the cardio- and aphthoviruses has a further unusual feature, brought about by the presence of the leader protein. In the aphthoviruses, the leader protein is a papain-like cysteine proteinase (L^{pro}) which cleaves between its own C terminus and the N terminus of VP4 (Fig. 1) (80). In cardioviruses, however, the leader protein possesses no proteolytic activity, and cleavage between its C terminus and the N terminus of VP4 is mediated by $3C^{pro}$ in a secondary cleavage. The function of the leader protein in cardioviruses is unclear.

Secondary Cleavages on the Viral Polyprotein

As can be seen in the polyprotein processing maps for poliovirus (PV) and foot-and-mouth disease virus (FMDV)

Tim Skern and Bernhard Hampölz ■ Institute of Medical Biochemistry, Vienna Bio Center, University of Vienna, Dr. Bohr-Gasse 9/3, A-1030 Vienna, Austria. *Alba Guarné and Ignacio Fita* ■ Centre d'Investigació i Desenvolupament (CSIC), Jordi Girona Salgado 18-26, E-08034 Barcelona, Spain. *Ernst Bergmann and Michael N. G. James* ■ CIHR Group in Protein Structure and Function, Department of Biochemistry, University of Alberta, Edmonton, Alberta T6G 2H7, Canada. *Jens Petersen* ■ Astra Zeneca, R & D Molndal, S-431 83 Molndal, Sweden.

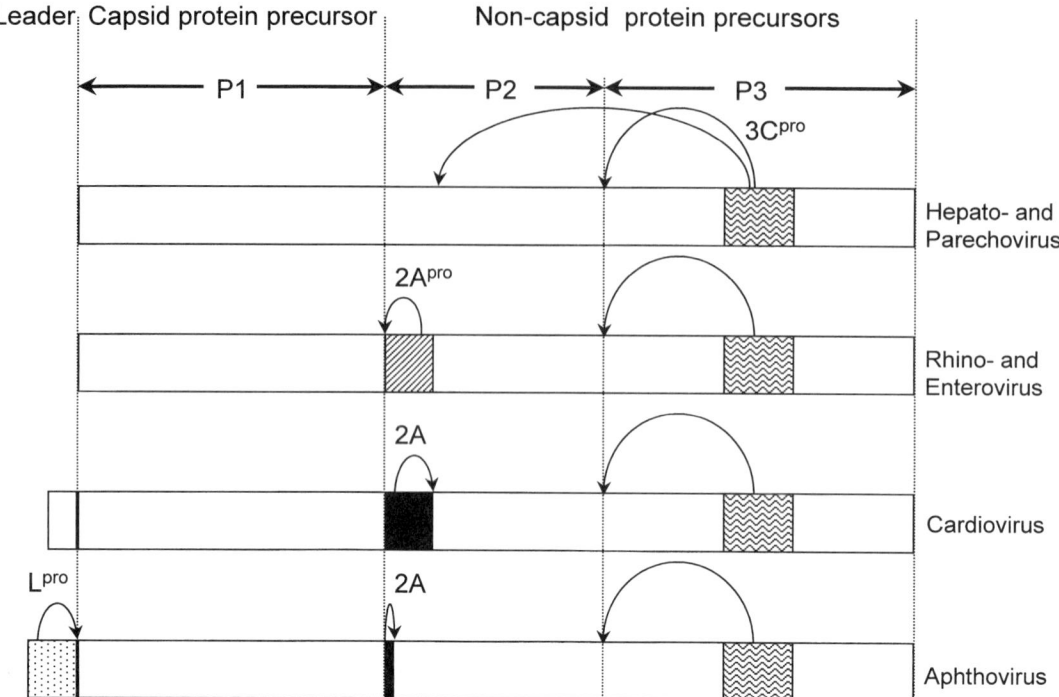

FIGURE 1 Proteolytic processing in picornaviruses. Variations in primary cleavage events among six picornavirus genera. The polyproteins of the indicated viruses are shown schematically as open boxes. Primary cleavages are indicated. The different shadings of the 2A protein reflect the differences in mechanism and size in this protein. The 2A protein of hepato- and parechoviruses has not been shown to possess proteolytic activity.

shown in Fig. 2A and 2B, respectively, the $3C^{pro}$ performs the majority of the secondary processing steps on the polyprotein. In PV, but not in other picornaviruses, two cleavages are carried out by the precursor of $3C^{pro}$, $3CD^{pro}$ (Fig. 2A). These are between the capsid proteins VP0 and VP3 and between VP3 and VP1 (44, 89). This function of 3CD has not yet been demonstrated for other picornaviruses. The reason for this requirement in poliovirus, but not in other picornaviruses, is not clear.

Another secondary cleavage peculiar to poliovirus and certain human rhinovirus (HRV) serotypes is a cleavage by the $2A^{pro}$ in the protein 3CD to give the alternate products 3C' and 3D' (38, 59). The biological relevance of this cleavage is, however, not clear, as elimination of the cleavage site (sequence Gln-Gly) in poliovirus by site-directed mutagenesis does not affect replication of the virus (see reference 52 and references therein).

The final cleavage to take place is that between the capsid proteins VP4 and VP2. The precursor of these proteins, VP0, is assembled into the new viral particles. During maturation of the viral particles, an as yet unknown proteolytic activity carries out the cleavage of VP0. As the cleaved bond appears to be protected against proteolysis from external agents since it is in the assembled capsid, efforts have been directed to defining a catalytic activity consisting of amino acids from the capsid and parts of the RNA molecule. Thus, serine 10 of VP2 in HRV14 was proposed to be the nucleophile carrying out catalysis (5). However, as replacement of the serine 10 with alanine did not disrupt cleavage, this theory was discarded. Recently, Curry et al. (20) proposed that a conserved histidine in VP2, together with the RNA, could be the proteolytic agent for the maturation cleavage. This hypothesis remains to be proven.

Cleavages of Cellular Proteins during Viral Replication

During the replication of a picornavirus, the physiology and ultrastructure of the infected cells are drastically modified. Thus, cellular RNA and protein synthesis as well as protein trafficking are inhibited. Furthermore, the cell's ultrastructure undergoes dramatic changes that are visible in the light microscope and are known as the cytopathic effect (70). In addition, a large-scale vesicularization takes place. Although the molecular mechanisms bringing about these effects are not fully understood, picornaviral proteinases have been shown to cleave a number of cellular proteins (summarized in Table 1). Many of these cleavages have been implicated in the events leading to the modulations of cellular physiology described above.

The most intensely investigated cleavage of a cellular protein is that of eukaryotic initiation factor (eIF) 4GI and its recently described homologue, eIF4GII. Cleavage of these proteins is carried out by the $2A^{pro}$ of entero- and rhinoviruses and the L^{pro} of FMDV (22, 34, 54, 81). Although the sites of cleavage on eIF4GI by these two proteinases lie seven amino acids apart (Gly_{634}*Arg for the L^{pro} and Arg_{641}*Gly for the $2A^{pro}$) (47, 51) (numbering according to reference 40), in each case the cleavage leads to the inability of the host cell to initiate protein synthesis on its own capped mRNA. This phenomenon is known as the host-cell protein shutoff. Viral protein synthesis is unaffected as viral protein translation initiates internally at a site on the viral mRNA known as the internal ribosome

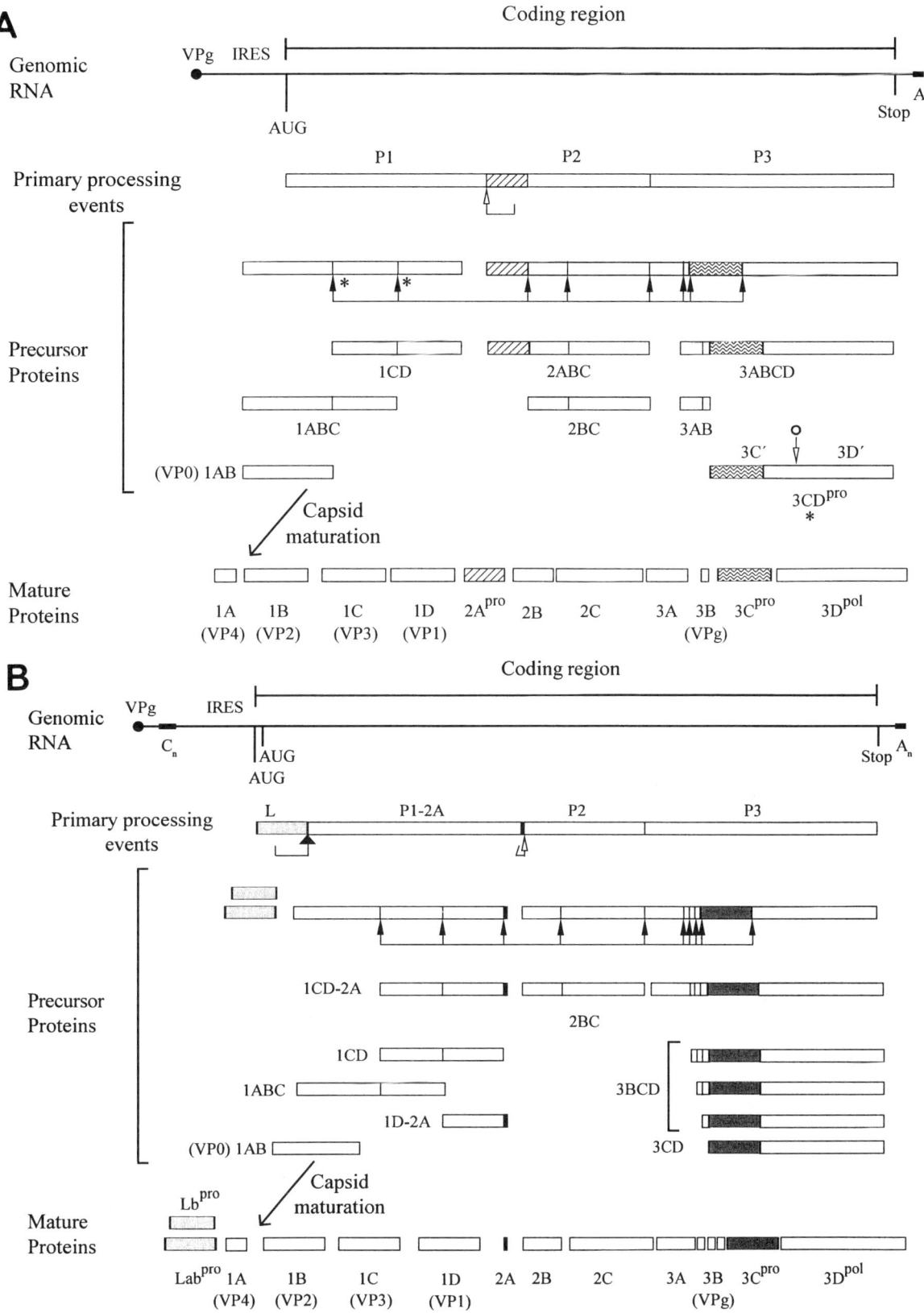

FIGURE 2 (A) Proteolytic processing map of poliovirus. The RNA genome of the virus is shown at the top as a black line. The positions of the IRES, the initiating AUG and stop codons, and the poly(A) tail are indicated. The polyprotein is indicated as an open box. Positions of the proteinases and their cleavage sites are indicated. 2A^{pro} cleavages are indicated by an open arrow, 3C^{pro} cleavages by a closed arrow. An open circle indicates the secondary 2A^{pro} cleavage; an asterisk indicates cleavages carried out by 3CD^{pro}. (B) Proteolytic processing map of FMDV. The cleavages are keyed as in (A) except that the fat closed arrow depicts the site of L^{pro} processing. No cleavage sites for 3CD^{pro} have been determined. Adapted from reference 8.

TABLE 1 Cellular proteins cleaved by picornaviral proteinases

Protein cleaved	Effect	Picornavirus	Proteinase	Reference
Eukaryotic initiation factor 4GI (eIF4GI)	Reduction in host cell translation (host-cell shutoff)	HRV, PV, CV, FMDV	$2A^{pro}$ L^{pro} $3C^{pro}$	54 22 9
Eukaryotic initiation factor 4GII (eIF4GII)		PV, RV	$2A^{pro}$	34 81
Eukaryotic initiation factor 4A (eIF4A)		FMDV	$3C^{pro}$	9
Poly(A)-binding protein	Reduction in host cell translation or viral replication?	CV, PV	$2A^{pro}$	45 43
Transcription factor IIIC	Reduction in host transcription	PV	$3C^{pro}$	18
TATA-binding protein	Reduction in host transcription	PV	$3C^{pro}$	19 87
TATA-binding protein	Reduction in host transcription	PV	$2A^{pro}$	85
CREB (cyclic AMP-responsive element binding protein)	Inhibition of CREB-activated transcription	PV	$3C^{pro}$	86
Transcriptional activator Oct-1	Inhibition of transcriptional activation	PV	$3C^{pro}$	88
Dystrophin	Modulation of cell ultrastructure?	CV	$2A^{pro}$	6
Microtubule-associated protein-4	Modulation of cell ultrastructure?	PV	$3C^{pro}$	42
Cytokeratin 8	Modulation of cell ultrastructure?	HRV, CV	$2A^{pro}$	77
Histone H3	?	FMDV	$3C^{pro}$	25 82

entry site (IRES). Whether the enzymes cleave eIF4G directly or indirectly in a mechanism involving the activation of a cellular proteinase is still a matter of debate (see references 16, 17, 29 and references therein). This issue is discussed in more detail in chapters 24 and 26.

eIF4GI and eIF4A, an ATP-dependent RNA helicase, have recently been shown to be substrates for the $3C^{pro}$ during FMDV infection (9). These cleavages occur late in infection; indeed, the $3C^{pro}$-induced cleavage of eIF4GI is only observed in viruses deleted in L^{pro}. Thus, the significance of these cleavages is not clear at present.

Two groups have independently identified a further protein of the translation machinery, poly(A)-binding protein (PABP), as a target of polio- and coxsackievirus (CV) $2A^{pro}$ (43, 45). This protein binds to the poly(A) tail of mRNAs as well as to the N-terminal domain of eIF4G. It thus appears to play a role in the initiation of protein synthesis despite its recognition of the part of the mRNA 3′ to the termination codon. However, as the cleavage of PABP occurs significantly later than that of eIF4G, it is unclear whether PABP inactivation is connected to the shutoff of host-cell protein synthesis. Instead, it seems possible that the cleavage is required to prevent PABP bound to the poly(A) tail of the picornaviral RNA from being incorporated into the maturing viral capsid.

The shutoff of all three classes of host-cell transcription in cells infected by picornaviruses has also been investigated (18, 19, 21, 26, 69). Davies et al. (21) reported that the transient expression of the PV $2A^{pro}$ reduced host-cell RNA synthesis by 20-fold. Further progress in understanding this effect has, however, not been made. Only one protein belonging to the transcriptional machinery of a mammalian cell has been shown to be cleaved by an entero- or rhinoviral $2A^{pro}$, namely, the TATA-binding protein (TBP) by the $2A^{pro}$ of poliovirus (85). However, this cleavage does not seem to be detrimental to the function of TBP and thus cannot be responsible for the observed shutoff of host cell transcription by $2A^{pro}$. It has been suggested that the effect on host-cell transcription is an indirect consequence of the $2A^{pro}$-mediated shutoff of host-cell protein synthesis (85).

In contrast, the presence of PV $3C^{pro}$ could inhibit Pol-II-mediated transcription in vivo and in vitro (19, 87). Once again, cleavage of TBP was observed; however, in this case, the function of the transcription factor was abrogated (19, 87). Subsequent work (86, 88) showed that the Oct-1 binding protein and the transcription factor CREB are substrates for poliovirus $3C^{pro}$, implying that poliovirus also inhibits transcription via these more specific routes (Table 1). Cleavage of a specific factor involved in Pol-III-mediated transcription, transcription factor IIIC (TFIIIC), has also been observed (18). It is not clear whether the proteins of the transcriptional machinery cleaved by the poliovirus $3C^{pro}$ are general targets for the $3C^{pro}$ of other picornaviruses.

Last, with regard to transcription, the cleavage of histone H3 has been observed by FMDV $3C^{pro}$ and was reported to inhibit cellular transcription. However, the mechanism and significance of this observation are not clear (25, 82).

Three proteins cleaved in infected cells have been identified that may be involved in leading to the ultrastructural changes observed in the infected cell. These are microtubule-associated protein-4, a target of $3C^{pro}$ (42); dystrophin, a target of coxsackievirus B3 $2A^{pro}$ (6); and cytokeratin 8, a target of both HRV2 and CVB4 $2A^{pro}$ (77). It has been speculated that the cleavage of dystrophin in cardiac smooth muscle may represent a link between coxsackieviral infection and cardiac insufficiency (6). The cleavage of cytokeratin 8 may cause disruption of the microtubular network and so facilitate cell lysis and virus release. Given the extensive and massive structural changes that take place in infected cells, it seems highly likely that other cellular protein targets for picornaviral proteinases will be found in the future.

STRUCTURES OF PICORNAVIRAL PROTEINASES

The crystal structures of several picornaviral proteinases have been published recently (Table 2). This chapter will discuss these structures in terms of their mechanisms of action and specificities and how the proteinases have evolved to be able to carry out their specific roles in the replication of the respective viruses.

The 3C^{pro}

Background

The picornaviral 3C^{pro} proteins were classified by inhibitor studies as belonging to the cysteine proteinase family (30, 66). Mutational analyses, amino acid sequence comparisons, and three-dimensional modeling all implied, however, that the proteins probably possessed a protein fold similar to that found in serine proteinases such as chymotrypsin (4, 7, 31, 32, 41). The three-dimensional structures of the 3C^{pro} from hepatitis A virus (HAV), HRV14, HRV2, and PV1 provided final proof of this relationship (1, 14, 57, 58, 62). In addition, the three-dimensional structures also revealed the basis of substrate specificity in these enzymes. For example, as can be seen in Table 3, the 3C^{pro} from PV1 and HAV are specific for Gln at *P1*. However, the preferences at *P4* and *P2* and in the *P'* region differ significantly. Examination of the three-dimensional structures of these enzymes showed that these specificities are a consequence of the divergent geometries of the substrate-binding sites. The nomenclature of cleavage sites is that of Berger and Schechter (10), in which the residue at the C terminus generated by cleavage of the peptide bond is designated *P1*, preceded by the *P2* residue, etc., and the residue at the newly generated N terminus is designated *P1'*, etc. Sites on the proteinase that bind specifically to various parts of the substrate are designated *S1* and *S1'*, etc. For the purpose of this chapter, this nomenclature is written in italics to distinguish between the nomenclature used to describe the parts of the picornaviral polyprotein.

The Structures of the PV1 and HAV 3C^{pro} and Comparison with Chymotrypsin

The overall folds of the 3C^{pro} from PV1 and HAV are clearly similar to that of chymotrypsin (Color Plate 11, following p. 156). Chymotrypsin, the prototypic serine proteinase, consists of two antiparallel β-barrels, with six β-strands (labeled a to f) in each barrel. The active site and substrate-binding site of chymotrypsin lie on the surface of the molecule close to the junction of the two barrels. Chymotrypsin has an activation domain that involves parts of the N-terminal domain and some residues of the C-terminal domain. This activation domain undergoes a large conformational change when the precursor chymotrypsinogen is converted to chymotrypsin by a single trypsin cleavage at Arg15-Ile16 of chymotrypsinogen. The two domains of chymotrypsin are "lashed" together by interactions at the N terminus of the N domain with the β-barrel of the C domain and by interactions of the C-terminal helix of the C domain with the β-barrel of the N domain. Similar interactions are also seen in the 3C^{pro} of PV1, HRV2, HRV14, and HAV.

It is likely that the conversion of the precursor of the 3C^{pro} to the active form of the enzyme also involves large conformational changes. The polypeptide forming the junction between 3B and 3C likely lies in the substrate binding groove of 3C and is cleaved by 3C when it is fully folded. The N-terminal residues of 3C then fold into the α-helix that is a unique feature of the 3C^{pro} enzymes. This conformational change removes the residues occupying the *S'* subsites of the 3C^{pro} thereby creating an a substrate-accessible open active site on the enzyme. In addition, the N-terminal helix interacts with residues of the C-terminal β-barrel and the C-terminal helix of 3C^{pro} interacts with the parts of the N-terminal β-barrel. Thus, a major difference between the picornaviral 3C^{pro} and the chymotrypsin family of serine proteinases is the presence of α-helices at both the N and C termini of the 3C^{pro} enzymes whereas chymotrypsin has an α-helix only at the C terminus of the molecule.

Structural Superposition and Sequence Alignments

Now that the three-dimensional structures of several 3C^{pro} are known at relatively high resolution, it is possible to carry out a structurally based sequence alignment (Table 4 and Fig. 3) to evaluate the percent identity of the amino acid positions of the 3C^{pro} relative to the serine proteinase family. Such an alignment among the 3C enzymes also helps in the evaluation of the subsite specificities of the several enzymes from the different picornaviral genera.

The enteroviral 3C^{pro} (PV1) and rhinoviral 3C^{pro} (HRV2) are the most similar in 3D fold (root mean squared [rms] difference of 0.71 Å for 173 common Cα atom pairs) (Table 4) and in sequence (43% identical). The 3C proteinases from these two genera are most similar in size as well (182 and 183 amino acid residues). HAV 3C^{pro} is

TABLE 2 Published structures of picornaviral proteinases

Proteinase	Cellular homologue	Virus	Number of amino acids	Catalytic triad	Modification[a]	Reference
3C^{pro}	Chymotrypsin	HAV	219	C172, H44, Y143	C24S, C172A	1
						14
		HRV14	182	C146, H40, E71		58
		PV1	183	C147, H40, E71		62
		HRV2	182	C147, H40, E71		57
2A^{pro}	*Streptomyces griseus* proteinase B	HRV2	142	C106, H18, D35		67
Lb^{pro}	Papain	FMDV O$_{1k}$	173	C51, H148, D163	C51A	35, 36

[a] The structure is that of the native protein unless otherwise stated.

TABLE 3 The sequences of the cleavage sites of the 3C^{pro} of HAV and PV1

Protein junction	HAV^a	PV1^b
VP2/VP3	LSTQ*MMRN	PRLQ*GLPV
VP3/VP1	VTTQ*VGDD	ALAQ*GLGQ
VP1/2A	LSTE*SMMS	
2A/2B	**LFSQ*AKIS**	AMEQ*GITN
2B/2C	LRTQ*SFSN	VIKQ*GDSW
2C/3A	LWSQ*GIDD	ALFQ*GPLQ
3A/3B	**IPAE*GVYH**	**AGHQ*GAYT**
3B/3C	VESQ*STLE	AKVQ*GPGF
3C/3D	IESQ*RIMK	TQSQ*GEIP
	P P'	P P'
	4 21	4 1 12
Specificity	LXSQ*XX	AXXQ*GP
	I TE	T L
	V A	V I
		P D
		A
		E

^{a}Reference 11.
^{b}Reference 48.

much larger (219 residues) and has significantly reduced similarity to PV1 3C^{pro} and to HRV2 3C^{pro} in these comparisons. The rms differences are 1.37 Å and 1.31 Å for 135 and 134 common C$^\alpha$ atoms, respectively. The sequence identities relative to HAV 3C^{pro} are also reduced by more than half as well (16.9% and 20.2% for PV1 3C^{pro} and HRV2 3C^{pro}, respectively). Figure 3 shows that there are only a few regions having conserved sequences among the three molecules. In addition to the segments that support the two active site residues (Hydrophobe)$_4$-Pro-Ser/Thr-His-Ala and Gly-Xaa-Cys-Gly-Gly-(Hydrophobe)$_2$, there are three other regions of conserved amino acid sequence and 3D structure. One region (Leu-Gly-Val-Xaa-Asp) is the second strand of the N-terminal β-barrel (bI1). A second region of conserved sequence and structure is the RNA-binding segment in the polypeptide that links the two β-barrels together (Lys-Phe-Arg-Asp-Ile). These five residues are conserved in the entero-, rhino-, and hepatoviruses but not in the cardio-, aphtho-, or parechoviruses. The final highly conserved segment surrounds the S1 pocket specificity determinant (Hydrophobe)$_2$-Gly-(Hydrophobe)-His-Val/Ile-Ala/Gly-Gly. This region is conserved in all six genera and defines the specificity for glutamine as the P1 residue for 3C^{pro} cleavage on the polypeptide.

The final column in Table 4 lists a pairwise comparison of the three viral 3C^{pro} to the bacterial serine proteinase *Streptomyces griseus* protease B (SGPB). This enzyme was selected for the comparison because it is approximately the same size (185 residues) as PV1 3C^{pro} and HRV2 3C^{pro} (183 and 182 residues, respectively). It is, however, somewhat smaller than HAV 3C^{pro} (219 residues). The increased values for the rms d values (range, 1.42 Å to 1.52 Å) and the decreased number of C$^\alpha$ atoms that make up the rms differences (range, 91 to 101) show the much larger evolutionary distance between the bacterial serine proteinases and the viral 3C^{pro} enzymes. The last row of the lower triangular matrix shows that the sequence identities of the viral 3C^{pro} with the bacterial SGPB ranges from 6.5 to 11.9%, the lowest in the table. The two most extensive regions of sequence and structural identity between the 3C^{pro} and the serine proteinases are in the region of the active site nucleophile (3C^{pro}, Gly-Gln-Cys-Gly-Gly; SGPB, Gly-Asp-Ser-Gly-Gly) and the region of the S1 specificity pocket (3C^{pro}, Val-Ile-Gly-Met-His-Val-Gly-Gly; SGPB, Ala-Ile-Gly-Leu-Thr-Ser-Gly-Gly). It is truly remarkable that this very low sequence identity correctly identified the 3C^{pro} fold as closely related to the chymotrypsin serine proteinase family (7, 31, 32).

Active Sites

In chymotrypsin there are three side chains associated with the catalytic hydrolysis of suitable substrates by the active site: the nucleophilic serine 195, the general acid/base histidine 57, and the aspartic acid 102 that is usually associated with orienting His57 properly for the proton transfer reactions (Color Plate 11). In addition to these residues, there is the oxyanion hole, an electrophilic feature provided by two main-chain hydrogen bonds that stabilizes the negative charge developing on the carbonyl oxygen of the peptide substrate during catalysis. These features are also present in the 3C^{pro} although some of the roles are played by different residue types.

Examination of the structures of PV1 and HAV 3C^{pro} reveals a similar orientation of the main chains as observed in the serine proteinases. The catalytic nucleophile, however, is a cysteine residue in the 3C^{pro} enzymes. The role of the general acid/base proton transporter is played by histidine and there is a similarly folded polypeptide that provides the oxyanion binding site. The orienting role of Asp102 in the serine proteinases is provided by a glutamic acid side-chain carboxylate in the enteroviral and rhinoviral 3C^{pro}. However, HAV 3C^{pro}, in spite of having an aspartate 84 that could fulfill this role, has no negatively charged group within hydrogen-bonding distance to the imidazole ring of the general acid/base histidine 44. The

TABLE 4 Pairwise structural comparisons among 3C proteinases and SGPB^a

	PV1 3C	HRV2 3C	HAV 3C	SGPB
PV1 3C	—	0.71 Å (173)	1.37 Å (135)	1.42 Å (101)
HRV2 3C	43.2%	—	1.31 Å (134)	1.47 Å (92)
HAV 3C	16.9%	20.2%	—	1.52 Å (91)
SGPB	10.4%	6.5%	11.9%	—

^{a}The upper triangular matrix gives the root main square differences for common C$^\alpha$ atoms (Å). The PDB accession codes for the coordinate data sets used here are: PV1 3C molecule B, available from M. James; HRV2 3C, 1CQQ; HAV 3C molecule A, 1HAV; SGPB, 3SGB. The numbers in parentheses refer to the number of pairs of C$^\alpha$ atoms in each superposition. The lower part of the matrix contains the percentages of identical residues in the overlapped pairs. The superpositions were done using Swiss PDB Viewer (http://www.expasy.ch/spdbv/) (37).

```
HAV-3C    1     STLEI-AGL  VRK-NLVQFG  VGEKNGSVRW  VMNALGVKDD  WLLVPSHAYK
PV1-3C    1     GPGFDY-AVA MAKRNIVTAT  TSK------G  EFTMLGVHDN  VAILPTHASP
HRV-3C    1     GPEEEFGMSL -IKHNSCVIT  TEN------G  KFTGLGVYDR  FVVVPTHADP
                   .           * *                 *** *       ..*.**

HAV-3C    48    FEKDYEMMEF YFNRGGTYY-  SISAGNVVIQ  SLDV---GFQ  DVVLMKVPTI
PV1-3C    44    G------ESI VID----GKE  VEI---LDAK  ALEDAAGTNL  EITIITLKRN
HRV-3C    44    G------KEI QVDG-----I  TTK--VIDSY  DLYNKNGIKL  EITVLKLDRN
                   .           .         .           *         .....  .

HAV-3C    94    PKFRDITQHF IKKGDVPRAL  NRLATLVTTV  N-GTPMLISE  GPLKMEEKAT
PV1-3C    81    EKFRDIRPHI PTQIT----E  TNDGVLIVNT  SKYPNMYVPV  GAVTEQGYLN
HRV-3C    81    EKFRDIRRYI PNNED----D  YPNCNLALLA  NQPEPTIINV  GDVVSYGNIL
                 *****  .              *                  ..  *  .

HAV-3C    143   YVHKKNDGTT VDLTVDQAWR  GKGEGLPGMC  GGALVSSNQS  IQNAILGIHV
PV1-3C    127   AG-------- -GAQTARTLM  YNFPTAAGQC  GGVITCT---  --GKVIGMHV
HRV-3C    127   LSG------- --NQTARMLK  YSYPTKSGYC  GGVLYK----  -IGQVLGIHV
                              .          .* * **.               ...*.**

HAV-3C    193   AGGNSILVAK LVTQEMFQNI  DKKIESQ
PV1-3C    163   GGNGSHGFAA ALKRSYFTQS  Q
HRV-3C    163   GGNGRDGFSA MLLRSYFTDV  Q
                 .*    .  .  . *
```

FIGURE 3 Structural alignments of the 3C proteinases from HAV, PV1, and HRV2. Asterisks under the residue symbols of the sequence for HRV 3C indicate identical residues in all three proteins. Dots indicate that highly similar residues are in the same positions in all three proteins. The alignments are based on the structural superpositions done in Table 4.

side chain of Asp84 points away from His44 and is involved in an ion pair interaction with the side chain of Lys202. The side chain of Tyr143 in HAV 3C^{pro} points toward the catalytic histidine residue but is not directly hydrogen bonded to it. Bergmann et al. (14) have proposed that the deprotonated phenolate side chain of Tyr143 could assist in orienting the catalytic imidazolium electrostatically. In support of this idea, the site-directed mutation of Tyr143 to phenylalanine reduces the catalytic rate by a factor of 20 (B. Malcolm, unpublished data). More work needs to be done to fully evaluate the catalytic mechanism of the 3C^{pro} enzymes.

Substrate Binding by Picornaviral 3C^{pro}

The X-ray structures of PV1 3C^{pro} and HAV 3C^{pro} have been superimposed by least-squares methods (see previous section) onto the crystallographically determined structure of the complex of OMTKY3 bound to SGPB. This gave a good model for the substrate binding to the viral 3C^{pro} once the side chains of P4 to P2' in OMTKY3 were exchanged to those of the best cleavage sites of the 3C^{pro}. PV1 3C^{pro} had the 3B/3C cleavage sequence Ala-Lys-Val-Gln-Gly-Pro inserted (Color Plate 12A, following p. 156) and the sequence Leu-Phe-Ser-Gln-Ala-Lys was inserted for the HAV 3C^{pro} (Color Plate 12B). More detailed views of the substrate-binding pockets for residues P4, P1, P1', and P2' are also shown in these figures. The inhibitor developed for HRV2 3C^{pro} by Agouron Pharmaceuticals (57) also emphasizes the binding sites S4 to S1' for that enzyme (Color Plate 12C). On the one hand, these several views illustrate the differences in substrate specificity of the PV1 3C^{pro} and the HAV 3C at P4 and at P1'. On the other hand, they show that in spite of having the same glutamine specificity at P1, the arrangement and nature of the residues in PV1 3C^{pro} and in HAV 3C^{pro} that confer this P1 specificity are different.

Recognition of the P1 Residue

Both HAV 3C^{pro} and PV1 3C^{pro} show an almost absolute specificity for glutamine at the P1 position. In both cases, the primary determinant of this specificity is an uncharged histidine residue (His191 in HAV and His161 in PV1) in the S1 pocket. However, the residues that orient the histidine and maintain it in the uncharged form are different in the two enzymes. In HAV, this role is performed by the buried side chain of Glu132; in PV1, the orientation is performed by Tyr138 and Thr142 (14, 62).

In PV1 3C^{pro} the p-OH group of Tyr138 donates a hydrogen bond to the $N^{\delta 1}$ atom of His161. Therefore, the $N^{\epsilon 2}$ atom of His161 will be protonated to ensure the neutrality of His161. The proton on $N^{\epsilon 2}$ of His161 is thus donated to the carbonyl oxygen of the glutamine side chain in the P1 position of a substrate. Also contributing to this recognition of the glutamine P1 residue is Thr142, which donates a proton from its γOH group to the carbonyl oxygen of the P1 glutamine (Color Plate 12A). This hydrogen-bonding scheme is also observed in the structure of HRV2 3C^{pro} complexed to the Agouron inhibitor AG7088 that has a cyclized analogue of glutamine as the P1 residue (57).

The S1 pocket of HAV 3C^{pro} has a neutral His191 that is protonated on $N^{\epsilon 2}$ to provide recognition for the carbonyl oxygen of a P1 glutamine. The side chain of Glu132 is buried in the hydrophobic interior of the C-terminal domain of HAV 3C^{pro}. It is surrounded by Leu and Ala residues. In such cases the pKa of the carboxylate of glutamic residues is elevated to ~9.5 from the normal value of 4.5 in aqueous buffer (68). There are two buried water molecules associated with the carboxylate of Glu132 and one mediates H bonding from Glu132 to His191 $N^{\delta 1}$. This hydrogen bonding environment of His191 ensures a neutral side chain with a hydrogen bond donor function for hydrogen bond recognition of the P1 glutamine carbonyl oxygen.

Recognition of the P4 Residue

The HAV 3C^{pro} has a preference for large hydrophobic P4 residues, which is explained by a large open S4 pocket lined by Ala141, Val200, and C$^\beta$ of Tyr143. In contrast, the PV enzyme has a much smaller P4 pocket, filled mostly by the side chain of Leu125 and Phe170. Thus, only residues containing small hydrophobic residues (i.e., Ala) can be accommodated in the P4 position of a substrate. HRV2 3C^{pro} has a similar small S4 pocket with similar hydrophobic residues filling it (Ile125, Phe170).

Recognition of the P2 Residue

Examination of Table 3 shows that HAV 3C^{pro} has a strong preference for Ser or Thr residues in P2, whereas the S2 binding site in PV1 3C^{pro} seems to allow almost any side chain but with a mild preference for large hydrophobes. In HAV 3C^{pro} the Ser or Thr side chains of P2 residues either donate or receive a hydrogen bond from the imidazole side chain of His145 (Color Plate 12B). The S2 binding pocket is much larger in the entero- and rhinoviral 3C^{pro} enzymes.

Recognition of the P1' and P2' Residues

The PV1 3C^{pro} enzyme has an absolute requirement for glycine at P1' and a noticeable preference for proline or hydrophobic residues at P2'. In contrast, the HAV 3C^{pro} does not seem to have a strong amino acid preference at these positions. These differences can be explained by the variations in the position of β-strand bI1 in the N-terminal β-barrel (nomenclature from reference 14). In PV1, this strand lies adjacent to the active site and, together with Phe25, prevents any residues with side chains larger than that of glycine from being accommodated at the P1' site. The presence of Gly at P1' and the frequent occupancy of P2' by Pro suggest that the substrate is turned out of the active site and away from β-strand bI1. In the HAV enzyme, in contrast, β-strand bI1 is further away from the active site, allowing sufficient space for the accommodation of larger, charged residues such as lysine at P2'. The S2' pocket in HAV 3C^{pro} has been visualized in the structure of the complex with iodoacetylvalylphenylalanine-NH2 (13). HAV 3C^{pro} accommodates a P2' NH hydrogen bonding to the carbonyl of Val28. In addition, there is a large pocket on the surface of HAV 3C^{pro} that will accommodate large P2' side chains such as the phenylalanine in this inhibitor (Color Plate 12B).

The RNA Binding Site of 3C^{pro}

The 5' and 3' noncoding regions of the genomes of picornaviruses have signals that are required for RNA replication and the initiation of protein synthesis. The 5'-terminal ~100 nucleotides of entero-, rhino-, and hepatoviruses begin with a predicted cloverleaf that is required for viral replication but does not have a binding site for the RNA-dependent RNA polymerase (3D^{pol}). Rather, this cloverleaf has been shown to interact with either the 3C^{pro} or its precursor 3CD^{pol} (3, 53); binding of the cloverleaf to the precursor is about 10-fold stronger (2). Subsequent autocatalysis of 3CD^{pro} would generate the mature 3D^{pol} at the correct site for the initiation of RNA synthesis.

3C^{pro} and 3CD^{pro} bind to a single stem-loop in this cloverleaf (27 nucleotides) as part of a ternary complex of which the Poly(rC)-binding protein is the third member (27, 65). The stem-loop has two GUAC self-complementary sequences in each of stem I and stem II, a U-rich 3 × 3 internal bubble, and a 3-nucleotide hairpin loop (UAU). The 14-residue stem-loop has recently had its solution structure determined by nuclear magnetic resonance (39).

The region on 3C^{pro} that has the RNA recognition site is on the opposite side of the proteinase to the active proteolytic site (Color Plate 13, following p. 156). The RNA-binding site comprises one face each of the N- and C-terminal helices as well as that part of the polypeptide chain that links the N- and C-terminal β-barrels of 3C^{pro}. The amino acid sequence of the residues involved in RNA binding is Lys-Phe-Arg-Asp-Ile; this sequence of five amino acids is conserved among most of the entero-, rhino-, and hepatoviruses, implying that RNA binding has nearly as tight evolutionary constraints as does the proteolytic activity (12, 14, 58). A complete understanding of the molecular interactions involved in binding a specific RNA cloverleaf structure awaits the determination of the structure of the protein-RNA complex.

Structure of 2A^{pro}

Background

Toyoda et al. (83) showed that the 2A protein of poliovirus was a proteinase capable of cleaving between the C terminus of VP1 and its own N terminus. Subsequent work also identified the corresponding proteins of rhino- and coxsackieviruses as proteinases. As in the case of 3C^{pro}, inhibitor studies showed that 2A^{pro} was a cysteine proteinase (49) and modeling studies predicted that the protein possessed a chymotrypsin-like fold, albeit more closely related to the smaller serine proteinases, such as SGPB and α-lytic proteinase (7). There are several differences between the 2A^{pro} and 3C^{pro}. First, the 2A^{pro} only cleaves the viral polyprotein at its own N terminus but not at its own C terminus (3C^{pro} performs this cleavage) (see Fig. 2B). Second, the third residue of the catalytic triad in all 2A^{pro} so far examined is Asp. Third, the determinants of substrate specificity are different. 2A^{pro} can accept a wide variety of amino acids as the P1 residue, whereas the 3C^{pro} has, as described above, an almost absolute requirement for Gln at P1. Instead, the determinants of substrate specificity for 2A^{pro} lie at positions P4, P2, P1', and P2'. This is clearly illustrated by comparison of the two sequenced cleavage sites of HRV2 2A^{pro}, IleIleThrThrAla*GlyProSerAsp on the viral polyprotein and LeuSerThrArg*GlyProProArg on eIF4GI (51).

The Structure of HRV2 2A^{pro} and Comparison to SGPB and PV1 3C^{pro}

Recently, the three-dimensional structure of HRV2 2A^{pro} has been determined (67). Comparisons with the structures of SGPB and the several 3C^{pro} illuminate the molecular basis of some of the differences in cleavage specificity.

The overall fold of HRV2 2A^{pro} is shown in Color Plate 14A (following p. 156). Like SGPB and the 3C proteinases, HRV2 2A^{pro} comprises two subdomains, built up by β-strands as found in chymotrypsin. However, the N-terminal subdomain of HRV2 2A^{pro} has only four β-strands and thus differs from SGPB and all other proteinases with a chymotrypsin-like fold that have eight β-strands. Nevertheless, the positions and orientations of the active site residues, His18, Asp35, and Cys106, are very similar to those of the active site residues of SGPB, His57, Asp102, and Ser195 (Color Plate 14A).

Another unusual feature of the HRV2 2A^{pro} molecule is the presence of a zinc ion, coordinated at the beginning of the second subdomain on the opposite face of the molecule to the active site by three cysteine residues (Cys52, Cys54, and Cys112) and one histidine residue (His114) (79, 84). Inhibitor studies (78), coupled with the distance (20 Å) of the zinc ion to the active site, indicate that the zinc ion is not involved in catalysis. Instead, it seems more likely that the zinc ion maintains the structural integrity of the protein, compensating in some way for the four missing β-strands of the N-terminal domain. Pertinently, perhaps, certain chymotrypsin-like proteinases such as elastase have a disulfide bridge (Cys136 to Cys201) at the same spatial position as the zinc ion in HRV2 2A^{pro}. As disulfide bridges do not normally form inside the cell, given the reducing environment, the HRV2 2A^{pro} may have evolved the zinc-binding site to achieve the equivalent stability donated by the disulfide bridge in elastase. The presence of a similar, but not identical, zinc coordination site in the chymotrypsin-like serine proteinase of hepatitis C virus strengthens this idea (46, 55).

Structural Comparison to 3C^{pro} Enzymes

The superimposition of the structures of HRV2 2A^{pro} and PV1 3C^{pro} highlights the difference in architecture of the N-terminal subdomains (Color Plate 14B). The structural superposition of HRV2 2A^{pro} with PV1 3C^{pro} results in an rms d of 1.57 Å for 93 common C$^\alpha$ atom pairs. Figure 4 shows the structurally based sequence alignment of these two enzymes. The parts of the N-terminal domain of PV1 3C^{pro} that are not present in HRV2 2A^{pro} are the N-terminal α-helix and β-strands aI, bI1, dI, and eI1 (Color Plate 14B). The C-terminal domain of HRV2 2A is very similar to that of PV1 3C^{pro}. There is a six-residue insertion in HRV2 2A^{pro} over that of PV1 3C^{pro} in a β-hairpin between β-strands bII2 and cII (Color Plate 14A and B) that has been dubbed the "dityrosine loop." Overall, the sequence identity between PV1 3C^{pro} and HRV2 2A^{pro} is 18.3%. The majority of the identical residues are in the C-terminal domain (Fig. 4). There is no zinc-binding site in 3C^{pro}.

Active Site of HRV2 2A^{pro}

There is extensive hydrogen bonding in the active site of HRV2 2A^{pro} (Color Plate 15A, following p. 156). Much of the hydrogen bonding involves Asp35, the carboxylate of which is almost certainly negatively charged as it is the recipient of six potential H-bonds, three to each oxygen atom. The negative change charge on Asp35 would have a strong stabilizing effect on a positively charged imidazolium ring of His18. Therefore, the simplest view of the 2A^{pro} active site is a negatively charged thiolate nucleophile (Cys106) with a positively charged general acid/base histidine residue (His18), as found in papain-like enzymes. Use of aklylating agents supports this view; however, the ion-pair formed does differ from that in papain, as its presence is confined to the same, unusually narrow pH range in which the enzyme is catalytically competent (75). Thus, the hydrolytic mechanism is closely related to that of the 3C^{pro} enzymes involving a covalently attached thioester that results from the breakdown of the tetrahedral intermediate by departure of the protonated leaving group.

Substrate Specificity in HRV2 2A^{pro}

The X-ray structure of SGPB complexed to the turkey ovomucoid variant Ala[18] (OMTKY3) was superposed onto the X-ray structure of HRV2 2A^{pro} to evaluate the substrate specificities for HRV2 2A^{pro}. It was noted that the β-hairpin 82-89 (the dityrosine loop) made several contacts that were too close to the P4 to P2' segment of the OMTKY3-Ala[18] variant. In particular, the side chain of Tyr85 had to be rotated to relieve some of these contacts. The final model for the probable binding mode of an hexapeptide substrate (P4 to P2') is shown in Color Plate 15B.

P1 Residue Interactions

There is little enzyme recognition of the side chain of the P1 residue (78). Substrates with P1 residues such as Thr, Leu, Phe, and Tyr had comparable cleavage efficiency to Ala. Positively charged P1 residues were cleaved quite well, but negatively charged residues (Asp and Glu) were not cleaved at all. Cys101 fills out the S1 pocket in HRV2 2A^{pro} and the pocket is relatively flat. This is likely the major reason for the relatively weak discrimination among side chains in peptide substrates. The discrimination against the negatively charged side chains of Asp and Glu in P1 is due likely to the presence of the negatively charged side chains of Glu98, Glu102, and Asp125 surrounding the S1 pocket.

P2 Residue Interactions

There is quite a pronounced preference for a Thr side chain in the P2 position of substrates. This preference may arise from the potential hydrogen-bonding interaction of the O$^\gamma$ atom of the Thr in P2 with a Ser at position 83 in the dityrosine flap. Little or no cleavage occurs when valine is in the P2 position of an equivalent substrate.

P4 Residue Interactions

There is a strong preference for a P4 hydrophobe such as Leu or Ile. The S4 binding results from a long and narrow but quite hydrophobic pocket that should favor Leu or Ile. The S4 hydrophobic pocket is made up in part by Ile80, Ile96, Ala122, and Ala129.

```
PV1-3C    3    GFDYAVAMAK  RNIVTATTSK  GEFTMLGVHD  NVAILPTHAS  PGESIVIDGK
HRV2-2A.  1                        G  PSDMYVHVGN  -LIYRNLHLF  NSEM------
                                  .*   .      *    .*

PV1-3C    53   EVEILDAKAL  EDAAGTNLEI  TIITLKRNEK  FADIRPHIPT  QITETNDGVL
HRV2-2A.  25   ---HESILVS  -----YSSDL  IIYRT---NT  VGD--DYIPS  C-DCTQ-ATY
                  . ..               . .    *    .  *   **.    *   .

PV1-3C    103  IVNTSKYPNM  YVPVGAVTEQ  GYLNAGG---  ---AQTARTL  MYNFPTAAGQ
HRV2-2A.  60   YCKH---KNR  YFPI-TVTSH  DWYEIQESEY  YPKHIQYNLL  IGEGPCEPGD
                  .        *  * *..**    .              *. .  .*.

PV1-3C    147  CGGVITCTGK  VIGMHVGGNG  SHGFAAALK-  -RSYFTQSQ
HRV2-2A.  106  CGGKLLCKHG  VIGIVTAGGD  NHVAFIDLRH  FHCAEEQ
               ***.^       ***. *   .   *.  .       *
```

FIGURE 4 Sequence alignment based on the structures of PV1 3C^{pro} and HRV2 2A^{pro}.

P1' and P2' Residue Interactions

The most important residues for the substrate specificity of HRV2 2A^{pro} seem to be Gly at position P1' and Pro at position P2'. The most restricting residues that limit the P1' residue to Gly are His18 and Leu19. Tyr85 may also interfere with a side chain at P1', but until a structure of a complex with a suitable inhibitor is determined, this latter point is speculative. At present it is not clear why Pro is almost exclusively the P2' residue.

Structure of L^{pro}

Background

The L^{pro}, the first protein on the polyprotein of FMDV, was identified as a proteinase in 1986 (80). As translation initiation occurs at one of two AUG codons 84 nucleotides apart, L^{pro} can exist in one of two forms, designated Lab^{pro} and Lb^{pro} (74). Both forms show the same enzymatic properties (60). The two known functions of the L^{pro} are to cleave itself from the growing polyprotein by cleavage at its own C terminus and to cleave the eIF4G homologues, thus preventing the host cell from translating its own capped mRNA. The amino acid sequences at the two known cleavage sites have been determined. These are ArgLysLeuLys*GlyAlaGlyGln at the junction of the C terminus of L^{pro} and VP4 on the polyprotein (64) and AlaAsnLeuGly*ArgThrThrLeu on eIF4GI (47). Inhibitor studies, mutational analysis, and amino acid alignments all implied that the L^{pro} was a cysteine proteinase with a mechanism and overall fold similar to papain, a proteinase from the papaya plant. Papain serves as a prototype for the CA clan of cysteine proteinases (15, 33, 72). However, the low overall identity of the L^{pro} to papain, the unusual difference in amino acid sequence of the cleavage sites, and the ability of the enzyme to process itself at its own C terminus showed clearly that the prototypic papain-like fold has been strongly modified in order to achieve the dual cleavage specificity.

Structure of the L^{pro} and Comparison with Papain

The structure of the Lb form of the FMDV L^{pro} has been determined by X-ray crystallography (35, 36). The protein was expressed in bacteria as the inactive mutant C51A in which the nucleophilic cysteine was replaced by alanine (47, 90). The overall fold of the L^{pro} is compared to that of papain in Color Plate 16A and 16B, following p. 156. The rms difference is 1.49 Å for 65 common C$^\alpha$ atoms in the two molecules. Both proteinases comprise two domains, an α-helical domain and a β-sheet domain; these are referred to as the left and right domains, respectively, based on their position in the standard view of papain used in Color Plate 16. The major differences are the lack of any prominent surface loops in the Lb^{pro} and the presence of a C-terminal extension in Lb^{pro}.

The active site of the molecule lies at the interface of the two domains. Both papain and the FMDV L^{pro} possess a catalytic dyad comprising a cysteine (A51 in L^{pro} and P-C25 in papain) present at the top of the central helix (Color Plate 16C and 16D) and a histidine (H148 in L^{pro} and P-H159 in papain) located adjacent to the nucleophilic cysteine. In papain, the imidazole group of this histidine residue is oriented by Asn175 whereas in the L^{pro}, Asp163 carries out this role.

Substrate Binding to FMDV L^{pro}

As stated above, the FMDV L^{pro} recognizes at least two different substrates, one on the viral polyprotein and one on the host protein eIF4GI. Thus, the FMDV L^{pro} appears to have two different specificities. How, therefore, does FMDV L^{pro} recognize and bind a substrate? Comparison of the cleavage sites shows that a hydrophobic bulky residue, a leucine, is present at the P2 position in both cleavage sites. This preference is common to many members of the papain family. However, the residues at the other positions (P3, P1, and P1') vary; in fact, these residues change their charge from one substrate, the viral polyprotein, to the other, the cellular protein eIF4G. What is the molecular architecture of L^{pro} requiring the presence of a leucine residue at P2 while allowing the presence of positively charged amino acids at either P1 and P1'? Insight into these questions was obtained from the L^{pro} crystal structure (36), in which the L^{pro} molecules were packed such that the C-terminal residues of one molecule were found in the substrate-binding site of an adjacent one. This structure represents, in fact, the complex of the L^{pro} with the P side of its primary substrate and allowed the molecular interactions occurring in the recognition of substrate by L^{pro} to be examined in detail.

The substrate interacts with L^{pro} in an extended antiparallel β-sheet configuration forming hydrogen bonds to the main chain of residue Gly98 (Color Plate 16A). The most important interactions in the L^{pro} substrate-binding groove are clearly with the P2 leucine residue. Comparison with the P2 binding pocket of papain in complex with the peptide inhibitor leupeptin reveals that the S2 pockets of the two enzymes are topologically very similar, forming a deep hydrophobic cavity. The cavity is formed in the L^{pro} by the side chains of residues L178, I141, L143, A149, P99, P100, and A101 as well as main-chain interactions from F142, H148, A149, and W52 (Color Plate 16A). Thus, the FMDV L^{pro} appears to have evolved a similar P2 binding pocket to anchor the substrate by a hydrophobic residue as in papain, but has also developed a higher level of specificity by creating additional and sophisticated binding pockets for residues in positions P1 and P1'.

Recognition of the P1 Residue

As the side chain of the P2 leucine residue is pointing down into the S2 pocket, the adjacent P1 and P3 residues point upward and away from the enzyme. For the polyprotein substrate, the P1 lysine residue establishes weak ionic interactions with the carboxyl groups of Glu96 and Glu147 that help to stabilize the charge whereas the aliphatic parts of their side chains provide a hydrophobic environment for the side chain of the lysine. Thus, only lysine or a similar residue such as arginine can be well accommodated at P1. The side chains of most other amino acids will clash either sterically or ionically with the residues of this narrow S1 slot. Glycine, lacking a side chain, will not interfere with the residues building the S1 slot; however, it will contribute little to the binding energy. In fact, the presence of glycine at P1 in substrates of papain is unusual; it is not clear why the glycine can be accepted at this position in the L^{pro}.

Recognition of the P1' Residue

Let us now turn to interactions at the P1' site. Here, no direct structural information on an enzyme substrate complex is available. Nevertheless, comparison of S' regions of the L^{pro} structure with those of papain reveals the greatest differences between the enzymes and indicates how the arginine present at P1' in the eIF4GI cleavage site could be accommodated. In papain, the S1' site is built up by residues P-Glu142, P-Ala136, and P-Ala137 and lies to the right of the active site residues shown in Color Plate 16D. These residues are not present in the L^{pro}. In contrast, we propose that S1' interactions in the L^{pro} involve the region containing four negatively charged residues (Asp163, Asp164, Glu165, and Asp166) (Color Plate 16C). This area is not available in papain as it is protected from the environment by Trp177 (Color Plate 16B and 16D).

Asp164 could quite easily accommodate positively charged residues at position P1', such as the arginine residue found in the eIF4GI cleavage site. Nevertheless, the presence of the acidic cluster does not require that a substrate has to have basic residues at the P' site, as is the case in the cleavage sequence of the polyprotein, which has glycine and alanine residues in this region.

In summary, the FMDV L^{pro} has evolved to recognize two specific substrates at two different cleavage sites by providing a deep hydrophobic pocket to interact specifically with residues such as leucine at the P2 site, and subsequently modulating the interaction through subtle requirements at the P1 or P1' sites. Would it not have been easier for the FMDV L^{pro} to have evolved to recognize a unique cleavage site? This would mean cleaving between L and VP4 at a site containing a P1 Gly and a P1' Arg, as found in the cleavage site of eIF4GI, or cleaving the eIF4GI between a P1 Lys and a P1' Gly, as found in the polyprotein cleavage site. The first possibility cannot be an option as the N-terminal region of VP4 contains the recognition signal for myristoylation (GlyAlaGlyXSer); any attempt of the virus to introduce basic residues would lead to an inability to myristoylate VP4 and hence a defect in viral replication. The second option does not seem possible either, as the sequence LeuLys*Gly cannot be found in a position that would allow proteolysis to separate the eIF4GI binding domains for eIF4E and eIF4A.

CONCLUDING REMARKS

The examination of the 3D structures of 3C^{pro}, 2A^{pro}, and L^{pro} has significantly furthered our understanding of the mode of actions of these proteins. Certain general features can now be noted. First, all the proteinases so far examined have evolved a device to prevent product inhibition following self-processing. In the 3C^{pro} and L^{pro}, a short α-helix is formed at the newly generated N terminus and C terminus, respectively, preventing the chain from reaching back and blocking the active site. In contrast, in HRV2 2A^{pro} at least, ionic interactions involving the newly generated N terminus keep the active site free of the processed terminus. A second general feature is that the active sites and catalytic mechanisms of the picornaviral proteinases are significantly different from the prototypes to which they are related.

Nevertheless, crucial aspects remain unclear. Why is the active site nucleophile of 3C^{pro} and 2A^{pro} cysteine and not serine? Is it the requirement for the imidazolium-thiolate ion pair? Or is it simply the presence of the sulfur atom, which prevents collapse of the oxyanion hole, as has been proposed (14)? How does the structure of the 3C^{pro} part of 3CD differ from the mature protein? How do both structures bind to the RNA hairpin loop? Are the ideas of how L^{pro} and 2A^{pro} interact with eIF4GI correct? Is the C terminus of L^{pro} involved in the recognition and cleavage of eIF4G, as has been recently suggested (28)?

The answers to these questions await the determination of suitable structures, especially those involving proteinase-inhibitor or proteinase-RNA complexes.

REFERENCES

1. **Allaire, M., M. M. Chernaia, B. A. Malcolm, and M. N. G. James.** 1994. Picornaviral 3C cysteine proteinases have a fold similar to chymotrypsin-like serine proteinases. *Nature* **369:**72–76.
2. **Andino, R., G. E. Rieckhof, P. L. Achacoso, and D. Baltimore.** 1993. Poliovirus RNA synthesis utilizes an RNP complex formed around the 5'-end of viral RNA. *EMBO J.* **12:**3587–3598.
3. **Andino, R., G. E. Rieckhof, and D. Baltimore.** 1990. A functional ribonucleoprotein complex forms around the 5' end of poliovirus RNA. *Cell* **63:**369–380.
4. **Argos, P., G. Kamer, M. J. H. Nickelin, and E. Wimmer.** 1984. Similarity in gene organisation and homology between proteins of animal picornaviruses and a plant comovirus suggest a common ancestry of these virus families. *Nucleic Acids Res.* **12:**7251–7267.
5. **Arnold, E., M. Luo, G. Vriend, M. G. Rossmann, A. C. Palmenberg, G. D. Parks, M. J. Nicklin, and E. Wimmer.** 1987. Implications of the picornavirus capsid structure for polyprotein processing. *Proc. Natl. Acad. Sci. USA* **84:**21–25.
6. **Badorff, C., G. H. Lee, B. J. Lamphear, M. E. Martone, K. P. Campbell, R. E. Rhoads, and K. U. Knowlton.** 1999. Enteroviral protease 2A cleaves dystrophin: evidence of cytoskeletal disruption in an acquired cardiomyopathy. *Nat. Med.* **5:**320–326.
7. **Bazan, J. F., and R. J. Fletterick.** 1988. Viral cysteine proteases are homologous to the trypsin-like family of serine proteases: structural and functional implications. *Proc. Natl. Acad. Sci USA* **85:**7872–7876.
8. **Belsham, G. J.** 1993. Distinctive features of foot-and-mouth disease virus, a member of the picornavirus family; aspects of virus protein synthesis, protein processing and structure. *Prog. Biophys. Mol. Biol.* **60:**241–260.
9. **Belsham, G. J., G. M. McInerney, and N. Ross Smith.** 2000. Foot-and-mouth disease virus 3C protease induces cleavage of translation initiation factors eIF4A and eIF4G within infected cells. *J. Virol.* **74:**272–280.
10. **Berger, A., and I. Schechter.** 1970. Mapping the active site of papain with the aid of peptide substrates and inhibitors. *Philos. Trans. R. Soc. London Ser. B* **257:**249–264.
11. **Bergmann, E. M.** 1998. Hepatitis A virus picornain 3C, p. 713–715. *In* A. Barrett, N. Rawlings, and J. F. Woessner (ed.), *Handbook of Proteolytic Enzymes.* Academic Press, London, United Kingdom.
12. **Bergmann, E. M., and M. N. G. James.** 1999. Proteolytic enzymes of the viruses of the family picornaviridae, p. 139–163. *In* B. Dunn (ed.), *Proteinases of Infectious Agents.* Academic Press, San Diego, Calif.
13. **Bergmann, E. M., and M. N. G. James.** 2000. The 3C proteinases of picornaviruses and other positive-sense, single-stranded viruses, p. 117–143. *In* K. von der Helm and B. Korant (ed.), *Handbook of Experimental Pharmacology*, vol. XXVIII. *Proteases as Targets for Therapy.* Springer Verlag, Heidelberg, Germany.
14. **Bergmann, E. M., S. C. Mosimann, M. M. Chernaia, B. A. Malcolm, and M. N. G. James.** 1997. The refined crystal structure of the 3C gene product from hepatitis A virus: specific proteinase activity and RNA recognition. *J. Virol.* **71:**2436–2448.
15. **Berti, P. J., and A. C. Storer.** 1995. Alignment/phylogeny of the papain superfamily of cysteine proteases. *J. Mol. Biol.* **246:**273–283.
16. **Bovee, M. L., B. J. Lamphear, R. E. Rhoads, and R. E. Lloyd.** 1998. Direct cleavage of eIF4G by poliovirus 2A protease is inefficient in vitro. *Virology* **245:**241–249.

17. **Bovee, M. L., W. E. Marissen, M. Zamora, and R. E. Lloyd.** 1998. The predominant eIF4G-specific cleavage activity in poliovirus-infected HeLa cells is distinct from 2A protease. *Virology* **245:**229–240.
18. **Clark, M. E., T. Hammerle, E. Wimmer, and A. Dasgupta.** 1991. Poliovirus proteinase-3C converts an active form of transcription factor-IIIC to an inactive form—a mechanism for inhibition of host cell polymerase-III transcription by poliovirus. *EMBO J.* **10:**2941–2947.
19. **Clark, M. E., P. M. Lieberman, A. J. Berk, and A. Dasgupta.** 1993. Direct cleavage of human TATA-binding protein by poliovirus protease 3C *in vivo* and *in vitro*. *Mol. Cell. Biol.* **13:**1232–1237.
20. **Curry, S., E. Fry, W. Blakemore, R. Abu-Ghazaleh, T. Jackson, A. King, S. Lea, J. Newman, and D. Stuart.** 1997. Dissecting the roles of VP0 cleavage and RNA packaging in picornavirus capsid stabilization: the structure of empty capsids of foot-and-mouth disease virus. *J. Virol.* **71:**9743–9752.
21. **Davies, M. V., J. Pelletier, K. Meerovitch, N. Sonenberg, and R. J. Kaufman.** 1991. The effect of poliovirus proteinase 2A^{pro} expression on cellular metabolism—inhibition of DNA replication, RNA polymerase-II transcription, and translation. *J. Biol. Chem.* **266:**14714–14720.
22. **Devaney, M. A., V. N. Vakharia, R. E. Lloyd, E. Ehrenfeld, and M. J. Grubman.** 1988. Leader protein of foot-and-mouth disease virus is required for cleavage of the p220 component of the cap-binding protein complex. *J. Virol.* **62:**4407–4409.
23. **Dougherty, W. G., and B. L. Semler.** 1993. Expression of virus-encoded proteinases—functional and structural similarities with cellular enzymes. *Microbiol. Rev.* **57:**781–822.
24. **Esnouf, R.** 1997. An extensively modified version of Molscript that includes greatly enhanced colouring capacities. *J. Mol. Graphics* **15:**133–138.
25. **Falk, M. M., P. R. Grigera, I. E. Bergmann, A. Zibert, G. Multhaup, and E. Beck.** 1990. Foot-and-mouth disease virus protease-3C induces specific proteolytic cleavage of host cell histone-H3. *J. Virol.* **64:**748–756.
26. **Fradkin, L. G., S. K. Yoshinaga, A. J. Berk, and A. Dasgupta.** 1987. Inhibition of host cell RNA polymerase III-mediated transcription by poliovirus: inactivation of specific transcription factors. *Mol. Cell. Biol.* **7:**3880–3887.
27. **Gamarnik, A. V., and R. Andino.** 1997. Two functional complexes formed by KH domain containing proteins with the 5′ noncoding region of poliovirus RNA. *RNA* **3:**882–892.
28. **Glaser, W., R. Cencic, and T. Skern.** 2001. Foot-and-mouth disease leader proteinase: involvement of C-terminal residues in self-processing and cleavage of eIF4GI. *J. Biol. Chem.* **276:**35473–35481.
29. **Glaser, W., and T. Skern.** 2000. Extremely efficient cleavage of eIF4G by picornaviral proteinases L and 2A *in vitro*. *FEBS Lett.* **480:**151–155.
30. **Gorbalenya, A. E., and Y. V. Svitkin.** 1983. Protease of encephalomyocarditis virus: purification and role of the SH groups in processing of the structural proteins precursor. *Biochemistry (USSR)* **48:**385–395.
31. **Gorbalenya, A. E., V. M. Blinov, and A. P. Donchenko.** 1986. Poliovirus-encoded proteinase 3C: a possible evolutionary link between cellular serine and cysteine proteinase families. *FEBS Lett.* **194:**253–257.
32. **Gorbalenya, A. E., A. P. Donchenko, V. M. Blinov, and E. V. Koonin.** 1989. Cysteine proteases of positive strand RNA viruses and chymotrypsin-like serine proteases. A distinct protein superfamily with a common structural fold. *FEBS Lett.* **243:**103–114.
33. **Gorbalenya, A. E., E. V. Koonin, and M. M. Lai.** 1991. Putative papain-related thiol proteases of positive-strand RNA viruses. Identification of rubi- and aphthovirus proteases and delineation of a novel conserved domain associated with proteases of rubi-, alpha-, and coronaviruses. *FEBS Lett.* **288:**201–205.
34. **Gradi, A., Y. V. Svitkin, H. Imataka, and N. Sonenberg.** 1998. Proteolysis of human eukaryotic translation initiation factor eIF4GII, but not eIF4GI, coincides with the shutoff of host protein synthesis after poliovirus infection. *Proc. Natl. Acad. Sci. USA* **95:**11089–11094.
35. **Guarné, A., B. Hampoelz, W. Glaser, X. Carpena, J. Tormo, I. Fita, and T. Skern.** 2000. Structural and biochemical features distinguish the foot-and-mouth disease virus leader proteinase from other papain-like enzymes. *J. Mol. Biol.* **302:**1227–1240.
36. **Guarné, A., J. Tormo, K. Kirchweger, D. Pfistermueller, I. Fita, and T. Skern.** 1998. Structure of the foot-and-mouth disease virus leader protease: a papain-like fold adapted for self-processing and eIF4G recognition. *EMBO J.* **17:**7469–7479.
37. **Guex, N., and M. C. Peitsch.** 1997. SWISS-MODEL and the Swiss-PDBViewer: an environment for comparative protein modeling. *Electrophoresis* **18:**2714–2723.
38. **Hanecak, R., B. L. Semler, C. W. Anderson, and E. Wimmer.** 1982. Proteolytic processing of poliovirus polypeptides: antibodies to polypeptide P3-7c inhibit cleavage at glutamine-glycine pairs. *Proc. Natl. Acad. Sci. USA* **79:**3973–3977.
39. **Huang, H., A. Alexandrov, X. Chen, I. T. Barnes, H. Zhang, K. Dutta, and S. M. Pascal.** 2001. Structure of an RNA hairpin from HRV-14. *Biochemistry* **40:**8055–8064.
40. **Imataka, H., A. Gradi, and N. Sonenberg.** 1998. A newly identified N-terminal amino acid sequence of human eIF4G binds poly(A)-binding protein and functions in poly(A)-dependent translation. *EMBO J.* **17:**7480–7489.
41. **Ivanoff, L. A., T. Towatari, J. Ray, B. D. Korant, and S. R. Petteway, Jr.** 1986. Expression and site-specific mutagenesis of the poliovirus 3C protease in *Escherichia coli*. *Proc. Natl. Acad. Sci. USA* **83:**5392–5396.
42. **Joachims, M., K. S. Harris, and D. Etchison.** 1995. Poliovirus protease 3C mediates cleavage of microtubule-associated protein 4. *Virology* **211:**451–461.
43. **Joachims, M., P. C. Van Breugel, and R. E. Lloyd.** 1999. Cleavage of poly(A)-binding protein by enterovirus proteases concurrent with inhibition of translation in vitro. *J. Virol.* **73:**718–727.
44. **Jore, J., B. De Geus, R. J. Jackson, P. H. Pouwels, and B. E. Enger-Valk.** 1988. Poliovirus protein 3CD is the active protease for processing of the precursor protein P1 *in vitro*. *J. Gen. Virol.* **69:**1627–1636.
45. **Kerekatte, V., B. D. Keiper, C. Badorff, A. Cai, K. U. Knowlton, and R. E. Rhoads.** 1999. Cleavage of poly(A)-binding protein by coxsackievirus 2A protease in vitro and in vivo: another mechanism for host protein synthesis shutoff? *J. Virol.* **73:**709–717.
46. **Kim, J. L., K. A. Morgenstern, C. Lin, T. Fox, M. D. Dwyer, J. A. Landro, S. P. Chambers, W. Markland, C. A. Lepre, E. T. O'Malley, S. L. Harbeson, C. M. Rice, M. A. Murcko, P. R. Caron, and J. A. Thomson.** 1996. Crystal structure of the hepatitis C virus NS3 protease domain complexed with a synthetic NS4A cofactor peptide. *Cell* **87:**343–355.
47. **Kirchweger, R., E. Ziegler, B. J. Lamphear, D. Waters, H. D. Liebig, W. Sommergruber, F. Sobrino, C. Hohenadl, D. Blaas, R. E. Rhoads, and T. Skern.** 1994. Foot-and-mouth disease virus leader proteinase: purifica-

tion of the Lb form and determination of its cleavage site on eIF-4 gamma. *J. Virol.* **68:**5677–5684.
48. **Kitamura, N., B. L. Semler, P. G. Rothberg, G. R. Larsen, C. J. Adler, A. J. Dorner, E. A. Emini, R. Hanecak, J. J. Lee, S. van der Werf, C. W. Anderson, and E. Wimmer.** 1981. Primary structure, gene organization and polypeptide expression of poliovirus RNA. *Nature* **291:**547–553.
49. **Koenig, H., and B. Rosenwirth.** 1988. Purification and partial characterization of poliovirus protease 2A by means of a functional assay. *J. Virol.* **62:**1243–1250.
50. **Kraulis, P. J.** 1991. MOLSCRIPT: a program to produce both detailed and schematic plots of protein structures. *J. Appl. Crystallogr.* **24:**946–950.
51. **Lamphear, B. J., R. Yan, F. Yang, D. Waters, H. D. Liebig, H. Klump, E. Kuechler, T. Skern, and R. E. Rhoads.** 1993. Mapping the cleavage site in protein synthesis initiation factor eIF-4 gamma of the 2A proteases from human coxsackievirus and rhinovirus. *J. Biol. Chem.* **268:**19200–19203.
52. **Lee, C.-K., and E. Wimmer.** 1988. Proteolytic processing of poliovirus polyprotein: elimination of 2A^{pro} mediated alternative cleavage of polypeptide 3CD by in vitro mutagenesis. *Virology* **166:**405–414.
53. **Leong, L. E. C., P. A. Walker, and A. G. Porter.** 1993. Human rhinovirus-14 protease-3C (3C^{pro}) binds specifically to the 5′-noncoding region of the viral RNA—evidence that 3C^{pro} has different domains for the RNA binding and proteolytic activities. *J. Biol. Chem.* **268:**25735–25739.
54. **Lloyd, R. E., M. J. Grubman, and E. Ehrenfeld.** 1988. Relationship of p220 cleavage during picornavirus infection to 2A proteinase sequencing. *J. Virol.* **62:**4216–4223.
55. **Love, R. A., H. E. Parge, J. A. Wickersham, Z. Hostomsky, N. Habuka, E. W. Moomaw, T. Adachi, and Z. Hostomska.** 1996. The crystal structure of hepatitis C virus NS3 proteinase reveals a trypsin-like fold and a structural zinc binding site. *Cell* **87:**331–342.
56. **Martin, A., N. Escriou, S. F. Chao, M. Girard, S. M. Lemon, and C. Wychowski.** 1995. Identification and site-directed mutagenesis of the primary (2A/2B) cleavage site of the hepatitis A virus polyprotein: functional impact on the infectivity of HAV RNA transcripts. *Virology* **213:**213–222.
57. **Matthews, D. A., P. S. Dragovich, S. E. Webber, S. A. Fuhrman, A. K. Patick, L. S. Zalman, T. F. Hendrickson, R. A. Love, T. J. Prins, J. T. Marakovits, R. Zhou, J. Tikhe, C. E. Ford, J. W. Meador, R. A. Ferre, E. L. Brown, S. L. Binford, M. A. Brothers, D. M. DeLisle, and S. T. Worland.** 1999. Structure-assisted design of mechanism-based irreversible inhibitors of human rhinovirus 3C protease with potent antiviral activity against multiple rhinovirus serotypes. *Proc. Natl. Acad. Sci. USA* **96:**11000–11007.
58. **Matthews, D. A., W. W. Smith, R. A. Ferre, B. Condon, G. Budahazi, W. Sisson, J. E. Villafranca, C. A. Janson, H. E. McElroy, C. L. Gribskov, and S. Worland.** 1994. Structure of human rhinovirus 3C protease reveals a trypsin-like polypeptide fold, RNA-binding site, and means for cleaving precursor polyprotein. *Cell* **77:**761–771.
59. **McLean, C., T. J. Matthews, and R. R. Rueckert.** 1976. Evidence of ambiguous processing and selective degradation in the noncapsid proteins of rhinovirus 1A. *J. Virol.* **19:**903–914.
60. **Medina, M., E. Domingo, J. K. Brangwyn, and G. J. Belsham.** 1993. The 2 species of the foot-and-mouth disease virus leader protein, expressed individually, exhibit the same activities. *Virology* **194:**355–359.
61. **Merrit, E., and M. Murphy.** 1994. Raster3D version 2.0. A program for photorealistic molecular graphics. *Acta Crystallogr.* **D50:**869–873.
62. **Mosimann, S. C., M. M. Cherney, S. Sia, S. Plotch, and M. N. G. James.** 1997. Refined X-ray crystallographic structure of the poliovirus 3C gene product. *J. Mol. Biol.* **273:**1032–1047.
63. **Palmenberg, A. C.** 1990. Proteolytic processing of picornaviral polyprotein. *Annu. Rev. Microbiol.* **44:**603–623.
64. **Palmenberg, A. C.** 1989. Sequence alignments of picornaviral capsid proteins, p. 211–241. *In* B. L. Semler and E. Ehrenfeld (ed.), *Molecular Aspects of Picornavirus Infection and Detection.* American Society for Microbiology, Washington, D.C.
65. **Parsley, T. B., J. S. Towner, L. B. Blyn, E. Ehrenfeld, and B. L. Semler.** 1997. Poly (rC) binding protein 2 forms a ternary complex with the 5′-terminal sequences of poliovirus RNA and the viral 3CD proteinase. *RNA* **3:**1124–1134.
66. **Pelham, H. R. B.** 1978. Translation of encephalomyocarditis virus RNA *in vitro* yields an active proteolytic processing enzyme. *Eur. J. Biochem.* **85:**457–462.
67. **Petersen, J. F., M. M. Cherney, H. D. Liebig, T. Skern, E. Kuechler, and M. N. James.** 1999. The structure of the 2A proteinase from a common cold virus: a proteinase responsible for the shut-off of host-cell protein synthesis. *EMBO J.* **18:**5463–5475.
68. **Qasim, M. A., M. R. Ranjbar, R. Wynn, S. Anderson, and M. Laskowski.** 1995. Ionizable P1 residues in serine proteinase inhibitors undergo large pKa shifts on complex formation. *J. Biol. Chem.* **270:**27419–27422.
69. **Rubinstein, S. J., and A. Dasgupta.** 1989. Inhibition of rRNA synthesis by poliovirus-specific inactivation of transcription factors. *J. Virol.* **63:**4689–4696.
70. **Rueckert, R.** 1996. The picornaviruses, p. 609–654. *In* B. Fields, D. Knipe, and P. Howley (ed.), *Fields Virology,* vol. 1. Lippincott-Raven, Philadelphia, Pa.
71. **Rueckert, R. R., and E. Wimmer.** 1984. Systematic nomenclature of picornavirus proteins. *J. Virol.* **50:**957–959.
72. **Ryan, M., and M. Flint.** 1997. Virus-encoded proteinases of the picornavirus super-group. *J. Gen. Virol.* **78:**699–723.
73. **Ryan, M. D., A. M. Q. King, and G. P. Thomas.** 1991. Cleavage of foot-and-mouth disease virus polyprotein is mediated by residues located within a 19 amino acid sequence. *J. Gen. Virol.* **72:**2727–2732.
74. **Sangar, D. V., S. E. Newton, D. J. Rowlands, and B. E. Clarke.** 1987. All foot and mouth disease virus serotypes initiate protein synthesis at two separate AUGs. *Nucleic Acids Res.* **15:**3305–3315.
75. **Sarkany, Z., T. Skern, and L. Polgar.** 2000. Characterization of the active site thiol group of rhinovirus 2A proteinase. *FEBS Lett.* **481:**289–292.
76. **Schroeder, E., C. Phillips, E. Garman, K. Harlos, and C. Crawford.** 1993. X-ray crystallographic structure of a papain leupeptin complex. *FEBS Lett.* **315:**38–42.
77. **Seipelt, J., H. D. Liebig, W. Sommergruber, C. Gerner, and E. Kuechler.** 2000. 2A proteinase of human rhinovirus cleaves cytokeratin 8 in infected HeLa cells. *J. Biol. Chem.* **275:**20084–20089.
78. **Sommergruber, W., H. Ahorn, A. Zophel, I. Maurer-Fogy, F. Fessl, G. Schnorrenberg, H. D. Liebig, D. Blaas, E. Kuechler, and T. Skern.** 1992. Cleavage specificity on synthetic peptide substrates of human rhinovirus-2 proteinase-2A. *J. Biol. Chem.* **267:**22639–22644.
79. **Sommergruber, W., G. Casari, F. Fessl, J. Seipelt, and T. Skern.** 1994. The 2A proteinase of human rhinovirus is a zinc containing enzyme. *Virology* **204:**815–818.
80. **Strebel, K., and E. Beck.** 1986. A second protease of foot-and mouth disease virus. *J. Virol.* **58:**893–899.

81. **Svitkin, Y. V., A. Gradi, H. Imataka, S. Morino, and N. Sonenberg.** 1999. Eukaryotic initiation factor 4GII (eIF4GII), but not eIF4GI, cleavage correlates with inhibition of host cell protein synthesis after human rhinovirus infection. *J. Virol.* **73:**3467–3472.
82. **Tesar, M., and O. Marquardt.** 1990. Foot-and-mouth disease virus protease 3C inhibits cellular transcription and mediates cleavage of histone H3. *Virology* **174:**364–374.
83. **Toyoda, H., M. J. H. Nicklin, M. G. Murray, C. W. Anderson, J. J. Dunn, F. W. Studier, and E. Wimmer.** 1986. A second virus-encoded proteinase involved in proteolytic processing of poliovirus polyprotein. *Cell* **45:**761–770.
84. **Voss, T., R. Meyer, and W. Sommergruber.** 1995. Spectroscopic characterization of rhinoviral protease 2A: Zn is essential for the structural integrity. *Protein Sci.* **4:**2526–2531.
85. **Yalamanchili, P., R. Banerjee, and A. Dasgupta.** 1997. Poliovirus-encoded protease $2A^{pro}$ cleaves the TATA-binding protein but does not inhibit host cell RNA polymerase II transcription in vitro. *J. Virol.* **71:**6881–6886.
86. **Yalamanchili, P., U. Datta, and A. Dasgupta.** 1997. Inhibition of host cell transcription by poliovirus: cleavage of transcription factor CREB by poliovirus-encoded protease $3C^{pro}$. *J. Virol.* **71:**1220–1226.
87. **Yalamanchili, P., K. Harris, E. Wimmer, and A. Dasgupta.** 1996. Inhibition of basal transcription by poliovirus: a virus-encoded protease ($3C^{pro}$) inhibits formation of TBP-TATA box complex *in vitro*. *J. Virol.* **70:**2922–2929.
88. **Yalamanchili, P., K. Weidman, and A. Dasgupta.** 1997. Cleavage of transcriptional activator Oct-1 by poliovirus encoded protease $3C^{pro}$. *Virology* **239:**176–185.
89. **Ypma-Wong, M. F., P. G. Dewalt, V. H. Johnson, J. G. Lamb, and B. L. Semler.** 1988. Protein 3CD is the major poliovirus proteinase responsible for cleavage of the P1 capsid precursor. *Virology* **166:**265–270.
90. **Ziegler, E., A. M. Borman, F. G. Deliat, H. D. Liebig, D. Jugovic, K. M. Kean, T. Skern, and E. Kuechler.** 1995. Picornavirus 2A proteinase-mediated stimulation of internal initiation of translation is dependent on enzymatic activity and the cleavage products of cellular proteins. *Virology* **213:**549–557.

The Aphtho- and Cardiovirus "Primary" 2A/2B Polyprotein "Cleavage"

MARTIN D. RYAN, GARRY LUKE, LORRAINE E. HUGHES,
VANESSA M. COWTON, EDWIN TEN DAM, XUEJUN LI,
MICHELLE L. L. DONNELLY, AMIT MEHROTRA, AND DAVID GANI

18

SEQUENCES INVOLVED IN THE PRIMARY 2A/2B CLEAVAGE

Early work on poliovirus polyprotein processing revealed the existence of two proteinases within the polyprotein and that the primary cleavage, which served to separate the capsid protein region of the polyprotein (P1) from the replicative protein polyprotein domain (P2), was mediated by the 2A proteinase ($2A^{pro}$) cleaving at its own N terminus (Fig. 1A) (44). In the case of the aphtho- and cardioviruses, however, the primary cleavage in this region of the polyprotein was known to be different, occurring at the C terminus of 2A (Fig. 1A) (11, 24, 31). In the aphtho- and cardioviruses, therefore, this primary cleavage results in the 2A protein remaining as a C-terminal extension of P1 until it is cleaved from P1 during secondary processing (33). Precursor forms spanning the 2A/2B junction are not observed in aphtho- or cardiovirus polyprotein processing. Comparison of the sequences of the 2A regions of different picornaviruses showed that the entero- and rhinoviruses possessed highly similar 2A proteinases. While the cardiovirus 2A proteins (between 142 and 157 amino acids [aa]) were of a size similar to that of entero- and rhinovirus $2A^{pro}$, no sequence similarity was apparent. Indeed, the 2A region of aphthoviruses was thought to be only 16 aa in length. The extremely short aphthovirus 2A region did, however, show sequence similarity with the C-terminal region of the longer cardiovirus 2A proteins (Fig. 1B).

Experiments analyzing the endogenous processing properties of recombinant aphthovirus (foot-and-mouth disease virus [FMDV]) polyproteins in which either the upstream- or downstream contexts of 2A were deleted showed that the 2A oligopeptide region did not function as part of a larger precursor form. Deletion of sequences immediately upstream did have an effect in that "cleavage" became "highly efficient" (~90%) rather than complete. Deletions downstream of 2A (although maintaining the N-terminal proline residue of protein 2B) did not appear to affect cleavage (34). These studies indicated that the cleavage activity could be a property of the 2A oligopeptidic region alone. Consistent with this notion, studies on the endogenous processing properties of domains of the cardiovirus Theiler's murine encephalomyelitis virus (TMEV) polyprotein localized the 2A/2B cleavage activity within the 2AB region (2). The 2A/2B cleavage activity of the cardiovirus encephalomyocarditis virus (EMCV) was mapped to the C-terminal third of 2A plus the N-terminal half of 2B (14). In this study the importance of the conservation of the sequence at the cleavage site, and the cleavage site itself (-NPG ⇓ P-), was confirmed. Deletions within the TMEV 2A protein, although leaving the C-terminal region intact, resulted in genomes that were competent, although impaired, in RNA replication and showed reduced virus titers (22, 49). Interestingly, the TMEV 2A protein could not substitute for mengovirus 2A protein (49).

These observations were extended by analyzing the self-processing properties of artificial polyprotein systems. Polyproteins comprised two reporter proteins (chloramphenicol acetyltransferase [CAT]; β-glucuronidase [GUS]) flanking 2A (together with the N-terminal proline residue of protein 2B) forming [CAT2AGUS] were encoded by a single open reading frame (ORF) (35). Translation reactions in vitro were programmed with transcripts derived from either the control construct pCATGUS (encoding CAT and GUS in a single ORF) or pCAT2AGUS. The translation profiles showed that the FMDV 2A region mediated a cleavage at its own C terminus, as in native FMDV processing, and that this cleavage occurred with high efficiency, but not to completion (~90%) (Fig. 2A)—as was observed in the recombinant FMDV polyproteins in which sequences N terminal of 2A were deleted. A nested set of deletions extending from the N terminus into the FMDV 2A sequence showed that cleavage occurred with only 13 aa remaining, but not 11 aa (Fig. 2B). Furthermore, a precursor-product relationship was shown not to exist between uncleaved [CAT2AGUS] and the GUS and [CAT2A] cleavage products. Following the arrest of protein

---

Martin D. Ryan, Garry Luke, Lorraine E. Hughes, Vanessa M. Cowton, Edwin ten Dam, and Xuejun Li ■ Centre for Biomolecular Sciences, School of Biology, University of St. Andrews, Biomolecular Sciences Building, North Haugh, St. Andrews, Fife KY16 9ST, Scotland. *Michelle L. L. Donnelly* ■ Marie Curie Research Institute, The Chart, Oxted, Surrey RH8 0TL, United Kingdom. *Amit Mehrotra and David Gani* ■ The School of Chemistry, The University of Birmingham, Edgbaston, Birmingham B15 2TT, United Kingdom.

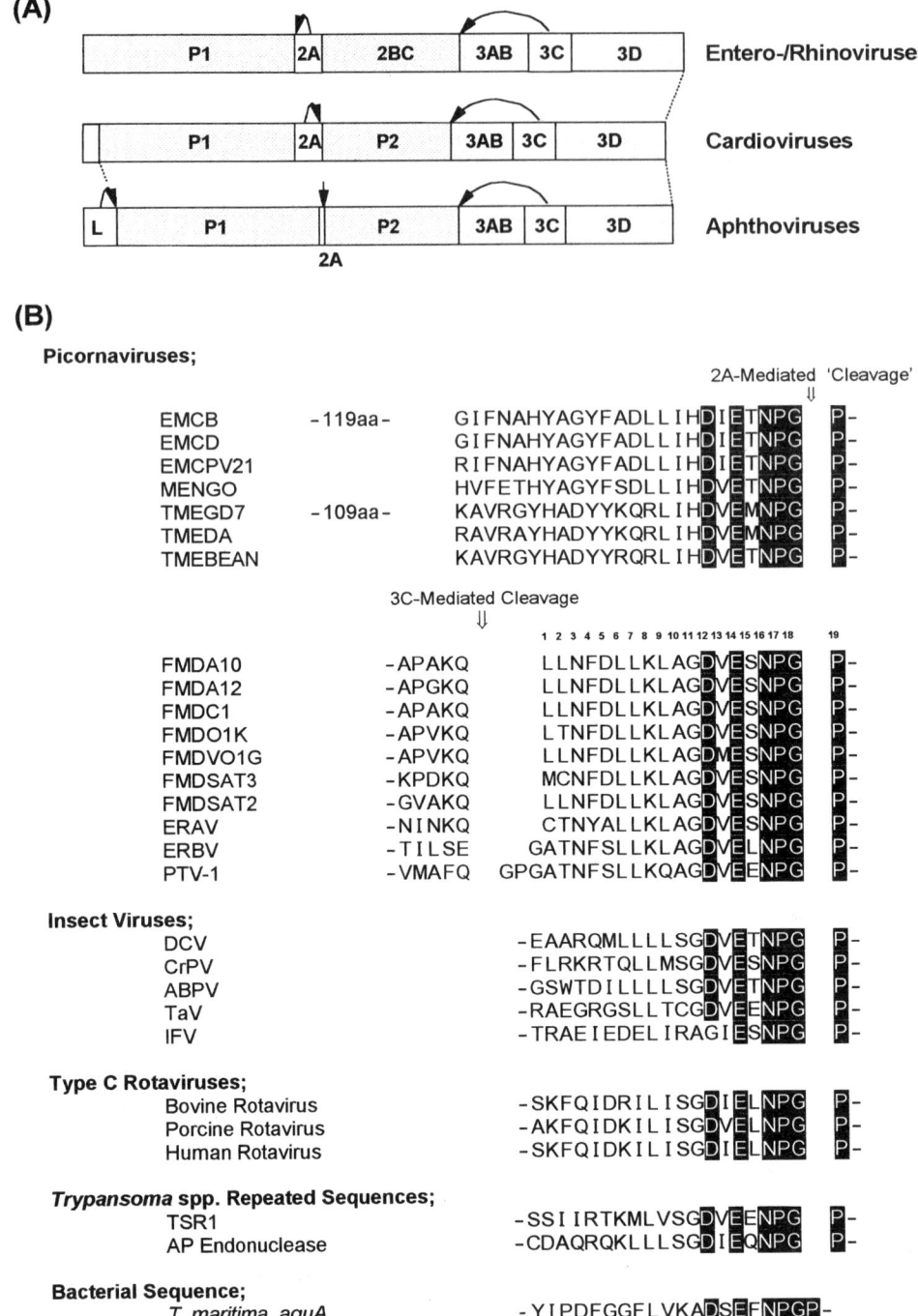

FIGURE 1 Picornavirus polyproteins. (A) The polyprotein organizations of entero-, rhino-, cardio-, and aphthoviruses are shown together (boxed areas) with the sites of primary polyprotein cleavage. (B) The sequences of the C-terminal region of cardioviruses and the 2A region of aphthoviruses are shown together with 2A-like sequences from other virus and cellular sequences.

synthesis, the [CAT2AGUS] translation product was stable and did not subsequently cleave into [CAT2A] and GUS. Cleavage occurred, therefore, cotranslationally, but not posttranslationally. With such artificial reporter polyprotein systems the 2A/2B cleavage activity of both EMCV and TMEV was subsequently mapped to the C-terminal 18 aa of their 2A proteins (together with the N-terminal proline of 2B)—these cardiovirus sequences being as efficient as the FMDV 2A in mediating cleavage. In addition, the influence on cleavage activity of the upstream sequences proximal to FMDV 2A was more finely mapped to within the C-terminal 5 aa of protein 1D (5). Restoration of this 5-aa sequence increased the cleavage activity to >99% (Fig. 2B) (5, 6). Interestingly, expression of these artificial

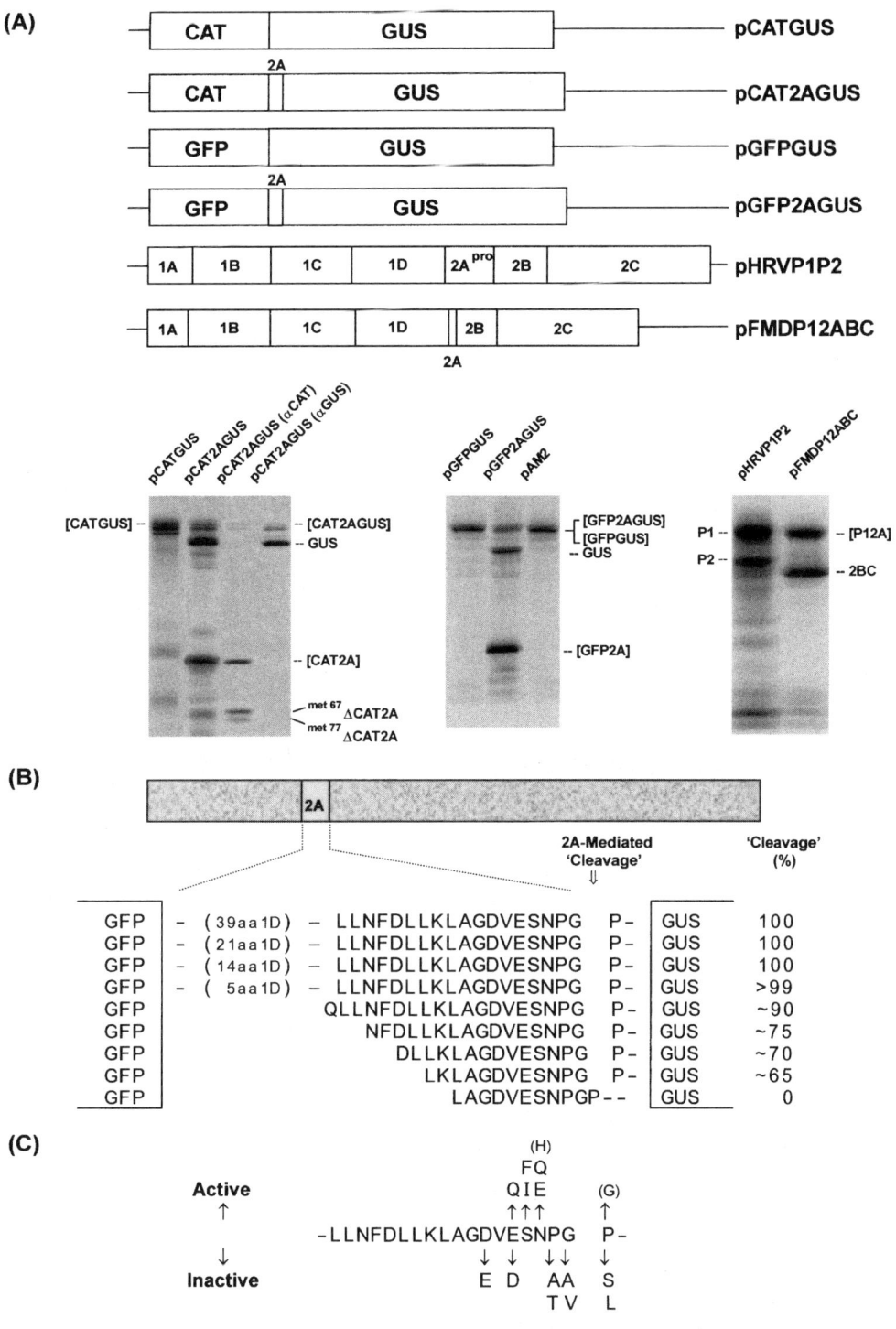

FIGURE 2 Translational analyses. Artificial reporter polyproteins (boxed areas) used to program in vitro translation systems are shown together with translation profiles obtained from rabbit reticulocyte lysates. (A) The FMDV region was either N-terminally extended by the incorporation of FMDV 1D sequences or by stepwise deletion. (B) Cleavage activities (%) are shown. (C) Site-directed mutants of FMDV 2A were constructed and the cleavage activities analyzed with in vitro translation systems.

polyproteins in a prokaryotic system did not reveal any cleavage activity. The presence of a 3C proteinase cleavage site conserved among FMDVs (also present in the same position in newly sequenced related viruses) led us to propose that FMDV 2A is 18 rather than 16 aa long (Fig. 1B).

We found significant levels of internal initiation occurred within CAT using these in vitro translation systems, which compromised our quantitative analyses (see below). Internal initiation sites within CAT were identified by N-terminal deletion and immunoprecipitation studies (Fig. 2A). We now use green fluorescent protein (GFP), rather than CAT, in our artificial polyprotein cleavage assay systems. Translation profiles obtained from [GFP2AGUS] constructs show very little internal initiation (Fig. 2A). Data obtained with this system are entirely consistent with the [CAT2AGUS] polyprotein, but translation profiles may be quantified much more accurately.

To determine whether the RNA sequence of this region, rather than the peptide sequence which it encoded, was responsible for cleavage, we engineered a construct (pAM2) that contained the FMDV 2A sequence in a [GFP2AGUS] construct, although out of frame (+2 frame) with respect to the GFP and GUS sequences. Translation profiles obtained from this construct showed no cleavage activity (Fig. 2A). Our conclusions from these data were that (i) the cleavage activity per se was a function of the aphthovirus 18-aa 2A peptide sequence, (ii) the C-terminal 18 aa of the cardiovirus 2A protein is functionally equivalent, (iii) proximal upstream sequences were influential in but not critical for this activity, and (iv) cleavage did not occur in *Escherichia coli*.

MUTAGENETIC ANALYSES OF 2A-MEDIATED CLEAVAGE

For purposes of this discussion, the numbering scheme shown in Fig. 1B is used. Inspection of picornavirus (and nonpicornavirus, see below) 2A sequences shows that only the -DxExNPG ⇓ P- motif is conserved in nature. Sequences immediately upstream of this motif that were shown to be either critical or very important for the activity are, however, not conserved. In a study in which this motif was subjected to site-directed mutagenesis, Hahn and Palmenberg found mutation of the (completely) conserved residues of this motif to either abrogate or very severely affect activity (14). The single exception to this was an E14D mutant in which partial activity was observed. We have performed site-directed mutagenesis on the FMDV 2A sequence, and our data are summarized in Fig. 2C. We find that, at variance with the EMCV mutagenesis, the FMDV E14D mutant is not active, although the E14Q mutant showed partial activity. Residue S15 shows natural sequence variation (Fig. 1B), and mutant forms not found in nature (S15F, S15I) are partially active. Residue N16 can be mutated while retaining partial cleavage activity, but mutation of both P17 and G18 abrogates activity. Interestingly, P19 (the N-terminal residue of protein 2B) shows very slight activity when mutated to glycine, but not to serine or leucine (6).

While we have shown that the sequences immediately upstream of the conserved -DxExNPGP- motif are critical for activity, inspection of the available sequences in this region reveals that there are a number of different "solutions" that nature has adopted in different groups of picornaviruses and other viruses described below. Mutants of the conserved motif uniformly show either substantially lower or no cleavage activity.

"2A-LIKE" SEQUENCES

Probing the databases for sequences containing this conserved motif shows the presence of 2A-like sequences in other virus polyproteins (Fig. 1B). We have tested these 2A-like sequences (as indicated in Fig. 1) by insertion of the 2A-like sequences into our [GFP-GUS] reporter system (6). Not surprisingly, the picornavirus 2A sequences from the equine rhinoviruses types A and B and PTV-1 are active.

Insect Viruses

In the case of the insect viruses Drosophila C virus (DCV; accession no. AF014388), cricket paralysis virus (CrPV; accession no. AF218039), acute bee paralysis virus (ABPV; accession no. AF150629), and *Thosea asigna* virus (TaV; accession no. AF062037), their 2A-like sequences, when inserted between GFP and GUS, showed high cleavage activity. In the case when cleavage was >99%, uncleaved [GFP'2A'GUS] material was only barely detectable. In the case of infectious flacherie virus (IFV; accession no. AB000906), however, the 2A-like sequence was only partially active in our assay system (~50%). It can be seen that the -DxExNPGP- motif is not conserved but differs from the consensus by D12G (Fig. 1B).

In the case of IFV, we propose that the 2A-like sequence functions as it does in picornaviruses—to bring about a primary cleavage between polyprotein domains comprising the capsid proteins and those comprising the replicative proteins (Fig. 3A). In the case of DCV, CrPV, and ABPV, however, the 2A-like sequence occurs toward the beginning of ORF1 (replicative proteins; Fig. 3A), whereas in TaV, the 2A-like sequence is present within the capsid protein precursor. In this case the activity of the 2A-like sequence has been demonstrated by N-terminal sequencing of the capsid protein cleavage products (29).

Type C Rotaviruses

The 2A-like sequence is present in human, bovine, and porcine type C rotavirus nonstructural protein 34 (NS34; gene 6; accession no. AJ132203, L12390, and M69115, respectively). Analysis of these 2A-like sequences in our [GFP'2A'GUS] system showed much lower cleavage activity than that observed for other 2A-like sequences (6). Interestingly, the type C rotavirus NS34 protein may be aligned with the NS3 protein of type A rotaviruses but has an additional double-stranded RNA binding domain at its C terminus. Inspection of alignments of this domain with other dsRNA binding domains shows this domain to start immediately downstream of the 2A-like sequence (Fig. 3B).

Trypanosoma Repeated Sequences

2A-like sequences are present within repeated sequences in *Trypanosoma cruzi* (accession no. X83098) and *Trypanosoma brucei* (accession no. X05710 and S28721). Surprisingly, these 2A-like sequences are in different types of insertion element. Ribosomal insertion mobile elements (RIMEs) insert themselves into trypanosome rDNA genes. These elements, in turn, are themselves disrupted by insertions. In the case of *T. cruzi* a RIME may contain the insertion of a non-long terminal repeat (LTR) retrotransposon (L1Tc) (19). This element has three main ORFs: ORF1 (L1Tca) has significant similarity to the human AP endonuclease protein, ORF2 has significant similarity to retrotranscriptase-related sequences from non-LTR retrotransposons, and ORF3 encodes a gag-like protein (Fig. 3C). The 2A-like sequence is present in the N-terminal portion of the AP endonuclease-like sequence (L1Tca) and, interestingly, the similarity with other AP endonuclease protein family members starts immediately after the 2A-like sequence (Fig. 3C).

In *T. brucei*, however, the RIME is disrupted by the insertion of a different type of element with a single, long ORF encoding a reverse transcriptase-like protein (Fig. 3C) (19). The 2A-like sequence is formed by the juxtaposition of two ORFs during transposition: the N-terminal portion being derived from the RIME sequence and the C-terminal portion being derived from the reverse transcriptase-like protein (Fig. 3C). We have inserted these 2A-like sequences into our [GFP'2A'GUS] system and found both to be active (6). We propose, therefore, that in both cases the 2A-like sequence serves to generate either the "mature" AP endonuclease-like protein (*T. cruzi*) or "mature" reverse transcriptase-like protein (*T. brucei*) by cleaving these proteins from their fusion partners.

Cellular Sequences

Probing the databases for the presence of the conserved -DxExNPGP- motif reveals (to date) only one further occurrence. This motif is present within the thermophilic eubacterium *Thermatoga maritima augA* gene product α-glucuronidase (accession no. P96105). Insertion of this 2A-like sequence (Fig. 1B) into our reporter system shows, however, this 2A-like sequence to be inactive (6). This observation is consistent with our previous analyses of the N-terminally truncated forms of 2A: the -DxExNPGP- motif alone is not sufficient to confer self-cleavage but requires an appropriate upstream context.

STRUCTURE OF 2A

We have used a range of secondary structural prediction algorithms on 2A and 2A-like sequences. The consensus that emerges is that of a helical structure followed by a tight turn (-NPG-). The prediction of an α-helical structure was supported by dynamic molecular modeling performed upon the FMDV 2A sequence (36). In this structural model residues D5, K8, D12, and N16 align along one side of the proposed α-helical segment, an arrangement that remained stable in dynamic simulations. Two salt bridges, D5 and K8 (in an $i, i + 3$ arrangement) and K8 and D12 ($i, i + 4$), and a hydrogen bonding interaction between D12 and N16 ($i, i + 4$) could serve to stabilize this structure.

MECHANISM OF CLEAVAGE ACTIVITY

In our first report of 2A-mediated cleavage of an artificial polyprotein system we put forward three hypotheses to explain these data: (i) that FMDV served as a substrate for a host-cell proteinase, (ii) that 2A represented a novel type of proteolytic element, or (iii) that 2A in some way interfered in peptide bond formation (35).

The "Substrate" Hypothesis

In this model 2A represents a substrate for a cellular proteinase that would need to be both very efficient and very tightly coupled to translation, since cleavage occurs cotranslationally, but not posttranslationally (35). At present there are no reports of such a ribosome-associated proteinase. 2A has been used for many biotechnological purposes and, as such, a wide range of recombinant self-processing systems have been expressed in a wide range of cell types, including mammalian, insect, plant, and fungal (3, 4, 10, 15, 18, 20, 25, 28, 38–40, 42, 45, 46). Such a proteinase would, therefore, need both to be present in this range of cell types and to have conserved its substrate specificity. Our site-directed mutagenesis data (only part of which is presented here) do not resolve this issue since the different mutant forms could represent, for example, substrates with different binding affinities for the hypothetical cellular proteinase. It should be noted here, however, that some point mutants we have constructed (which show no cleavage) are over 10 residues N terminal of the cleavage site. Similarly, it could be argued that our observations regarding the influence of the upstream sequences reflect their role in protein folding vis-à-vis the "presentation" of the site of cleavage to this hypothetical proteinase.

The "Proteinase" Hypothesis

Perhaps dispensing with the protein "architecture" required by a proteinase to recognize a substrate in *trans*, to cleave a peptide bond, then regenerate the nucleophile, could enable such a short sequence to function as a single-turnover *cis*-acting proteolytic element. In considering a novel *cis*-acting proteolytic activity for 2A, the presence of conserved potential nucleophiles (D, E, S/T) within the canonical motif was of great interest. Indeed, asparagine residues are known to mediate peptide bond cleavage via a mechanism similar to the β-aspartyl shift (reviewed in reference 48). Here our site-directed mutagenesis data are more informative. Mutation of D12 either abrogates cleavage (D12H, see reference 14; D12E, Fig. 2C) or very severely affects it (D12N, see reference 14). The IFV 2A-like sequence is active and has a glycine residue in this position (Fig. 1B). The E14Q mutation retains (reduced) activity (Fig. 2C). These two "candidate" nucleophilic residues do not appear, therefore, to function in the manner of an acidic proteinase. Although serine or threonine (both nucleophiles in proteinases) are present in all aphthoviruses and many cardioviruses, natural sequence variation in this position (Fig. 1B) precludes S15/T15 functioning in the manner of a serine or threonine proteinase. Mutation of N16 and retention of activity exclude peptide bond cleavage via a mechanism similar to the β-aspartyl shift. On the basis of the site-directed mutagenesis and natural sequence variation data sets, a proteolytic mechanism seems improbable.

The "Translational" Hypothesis

Analysis of the in vitro translation profiles obtained from both [CAT2AGUS] and [GFP2AGUS] showed a common, remarkable feature. Proteins were radiolabeled with ^{35}S-methionine and the distribution of radioactivity in the accumulated products was quantified by phosphorimaging (normalized for methionine contents). The upstream translation product (either [CAT2A] or [GFP2A]) was present in a molar excess over the downstream translation product, GUS. This effect varied between rabbit reticulocyte lysates, where ratios were commonly 5:1, and wheat germ extracts, where ratios were commonly 15:1. Interestingly, extension of the N-terminal FMDV protein 2B residues present immediately downstream of 2A in our reporter polyproteins (from just -P- to -PFFF-) increased the observed imbalance dramatically (data not shown).

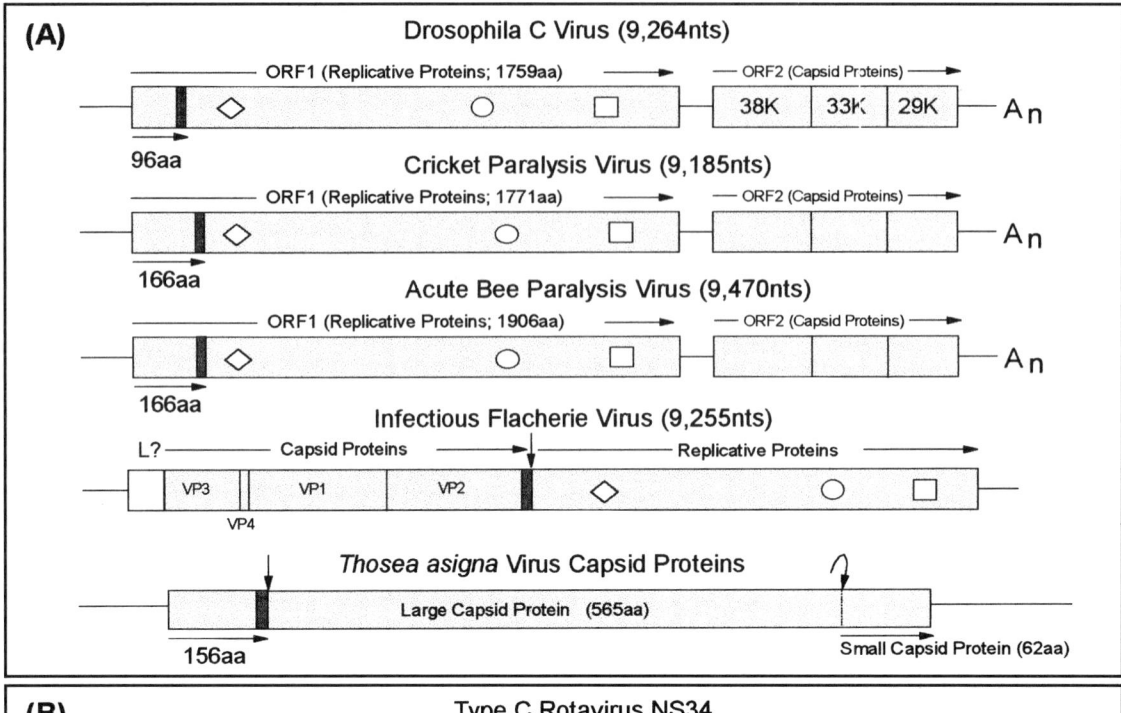
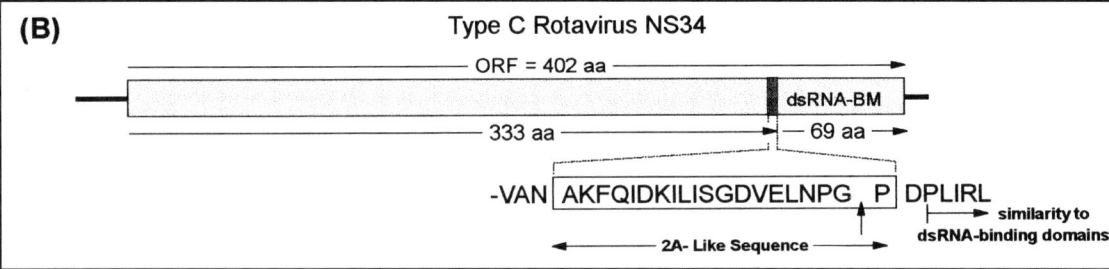
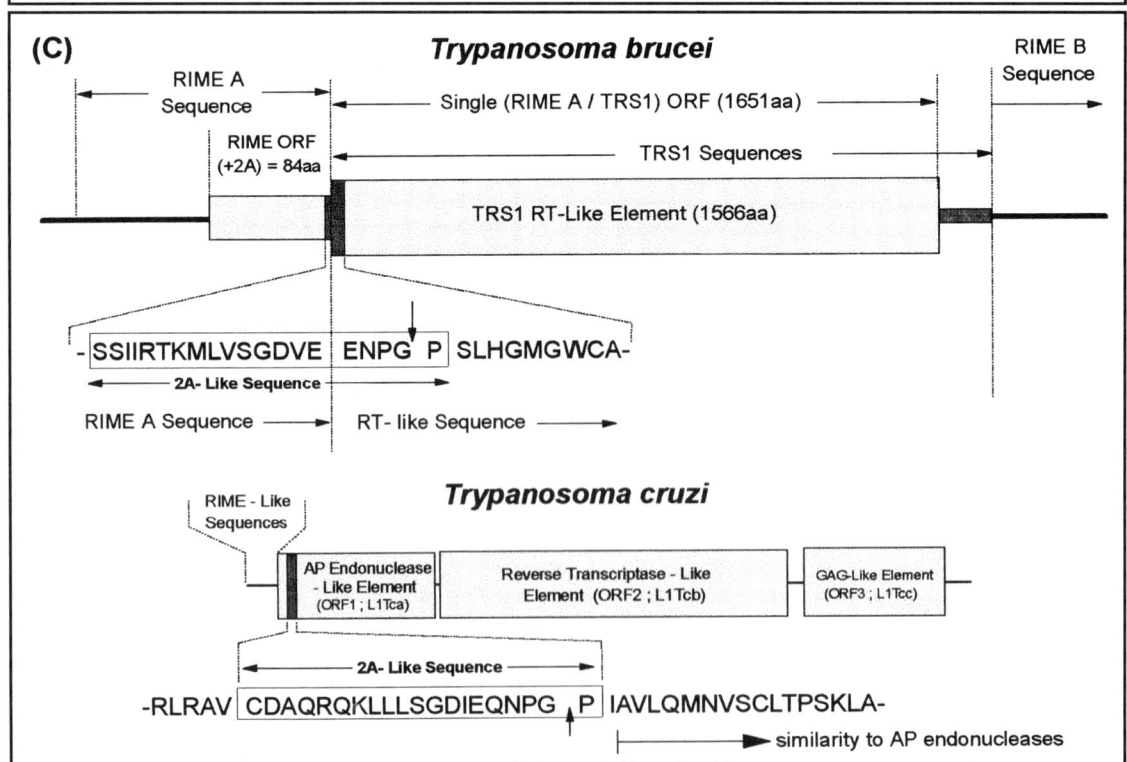

The products we are measuring are those that have accumulated: a function of both protein synthesis and degradation. Protein degradation studies showed this explanation could not account for our observed product imbalances (7). An alternative explanation for this product imbalance could be that significant premature termination of transcription or translation was occurring, at random, in these coupled systems. This would give rise to a polar effect resulting in a greater level of synthesis of sequences N terminal to the polyprotein system. In our system this effect coupled with cleavage at a specific site could explain this imbalance. To address this question two types of approaches were adopted: first, to reverse the gene order—to place the (longer) GUS sequence upstream of GFP by making a [GUS2AGFP] polyprotein. Second, a control construct encoding polyprotein encoding the [P1P2] from human rhinovirus 14 (HRV14) was made—in this case P1 and P2 are cleaved by a known, characterized proteinase, 2A^{pro}. Analyses of the [GUS2AGFP] construct showed molar excess of the [GUS2A] cleavage product over GFP, whereas analysis of the HRV14 [P1P2] construct showed the *proteolytic* cleavage products P1 and P2 to be present in ratios of between 1.3 and 1.2 to 1 (Fig. 2A) (7). This showed that our translation systems were able to synthesize long ORFs (HRV14 [P1P2] is some 55% longer than [GFP2AGUS]) and observe ratios of ~1:1 when this should be the case. Interestingly, translation of a construct (pFMDP12ABC) encoding the [P12A2BC] region of the FMDV polyprotein, in which 2A is in its entirely native protein context, showed the cleavage products [P12A] and [2BC] also to be present in ratios of between 1.2 and 1.1 to 1 (Fig. 2A) (7).

From this work we concluded that the molar excess of the translation product N terminal of 2A over that C-terminal of 2A was a product of inserting the 2A sequence into our artificial polyprotein systems: its functioning in a suboptimal polyprotein context. This is supported by the data whereby sequences immediately N terminal of 2A affect its activity. These effects have, however, given us a new insight into the mechanism of 2A-mediated cleavage.

A TRANSLATIONAL MODEL OF 2A CLEAVAGE ACTIVITY

Given that the substrate and proteinase hypotheses are improbable, taken together with our observations on the imbalance of the translation products, how can cleavage be explained? We have proposed a mechanism whereby two specific translation products may be obtained from a single ORF by modification of the elongation stage of translation. In our model the upstream translation product ([P12A], aphthoviruses; [L-P1-2A], cardioviruses; [GFP2A], artificial systems) is released from the translation complex by the cleavage of the ester linkage between the nascent peptide and the tRNA to which it is attached (7, 36).

The scheme we have proposed is shown in Fig. 4. The individual steps are outlined here and discussed below. Step (i): The peptide bond between P17 and G18 is synthesized; deacylated tRNA^{gly} is present in the P site and (2A)peptidyl-tRNA is present in the A site of the ribosome. Step (ii): Following translocation, the 2A-peptidyl-tRNA is translocated to the P site, the deacylated tRNA^{gly} is translocated to the E site, and deacylated tRNA^{asn} exits the complex. An interaction between the putative helical portion of 2A and the exit pore of the eukaryotic ribosome serves to fix the orientation of the base of the helix within the peptidyl-transferase center of the ribosome. The tight turn (-NPG-) repositions the peptide-tRNA ester linkage away from a conformation that would (normally) lead to peptide bond formation. Step (iii): Prolyl-tRNA enters the A site. The normal nucleophilic attack performed by prolyl-tRNA upon the electrophilic center (the glycyl carbonyl carbon atom) is inhibited due to the reorientation of this center—peptide bond formation is inhibited. Step (iv): The 2A-peptidyl-tRNA^{gly} ester bond is hydrolyzed. Step (v): The nascent polypeptide is released from the translation complex—cleavage. The P site is now occupied by deacylated tRNA^{gly}, the A site being occupied by prolyl-tRNA. Step (vi): Deacylated tRNA^{pro} exits the complex, deacylated tRNA^{gly} is translocated from the P to E site, prolyl-tRNA is translocated from the A to P site, and the next aminoacyl-tRNA enters the A site to continue translation—synthesizing a discrete downstream translation product.

This proposed translational model of 2A cleavage activity is novel and represents yet another method whereby viruses modify the host cell's translation process for their own purposes. Such modifications include leaky scanning, reinitiation, suppression of termination, ribosomal frameshifting, internal ribosome entry, and ribosomal "hopping." Indeed, it has emerged that many of these strategies used by viruses to control protein biogenesis are, in fact, also used by cells themselves. Here various aspects of our model will be discussed in light of our data and observations others have made on the process of translation.

2A:Ribosome Interactions

An early observation was that the 2A protein of EMCV was associated with ribosomes prepared from EMCV-infected Krebs-II cell extracts (21). Presumably the components that comprise the exit pore of ribosomes have evolved to minimize any potential interactions with nascent polypeptides. An increasing body of literature now shows, however, that certain peptide sequences may interact with this ribosome structure and in doing so can bring about a "pause" in the elongation cycle and, indeed, inhibit peptidyl-transferase activity (12, 16, 32). During the translation of bacteriophage T4 *gene 60* a ribosomal "hop" occurs from codon 47 to a matched "landing" codon 50 nucleotides downstream (47). Of specific relevance to our model is the finding that a requirement for this translational bypass is a 16-aa *cis*-acting sequence (residues 17 to 30) in the nascent chain, probably acting in the exit channel of the ribosome (47). This type of translational control

FIGURE 3 2A-like sequences. (A) Insect virus polyproteins are shown together with the location of the 2A-like sequence (shaded rectangle), picornavirus protein 2C-like domain (open circles), proteinase domain (open squares), and polymerase domains (open diamonds). (B) The position of the type C rotavirus 2A-like sequence (shaded rectangle) is shown. (C) The sequence and position of the 2A-like sequences from *Trypanosoma* spp. repeated sequences are shown (shaded rectangle).

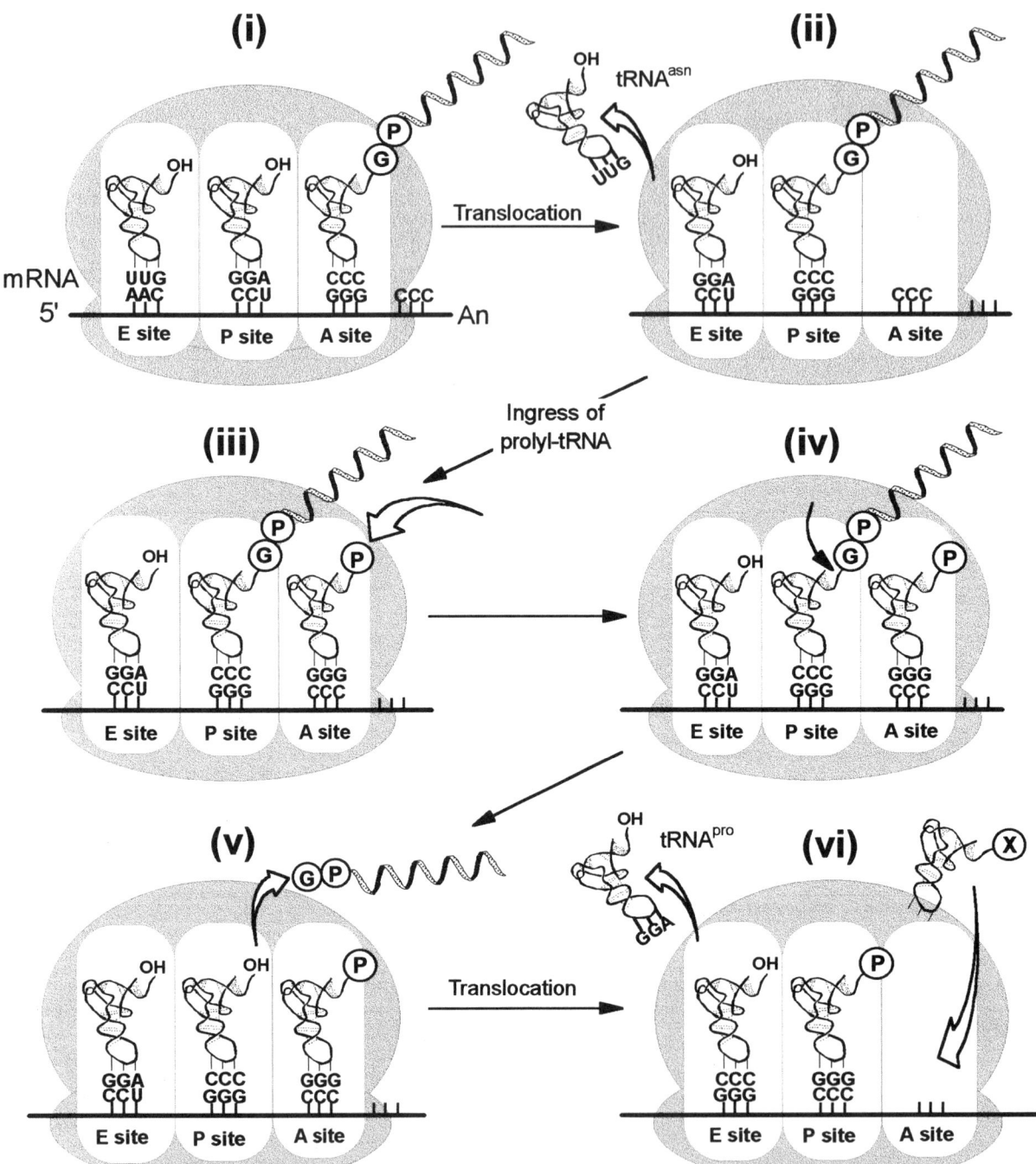

FIGURE 4 Translational model of 2A-mediated "cleavage." Step (i): The synthesis of the 2A peptide sequence is completed with the 2A-peptidyl-tRNA complex in the ribosomal A site. Step (ii): This complex is translocated from the A to P site by eEF2. Step (iii): Prolyl-tRNA is bound to the A site. Step (iv): Cleavage of the peptide-tRNA ester linkage occurs. Step (v): The nascent peptide is released from the ribosome. Step (vi): Prolyl-tRNA is translocated from the A to P site, the next aminoacyl-tRNA is bound to the A site, and translation of the downstream product continues.

has also been implicated in the expression of cellular genes (reviewed in references 8 and 9).

The structural model of 2A we have developed is one of a helix with a tight turn at its C terminus. In this model the helical portion of 2A would, at a specific stage in the elongation/translocation cycle, interact with the exit pore of the ribosome. This would result in 2A adopting a specific, fixed orientation and it conferring a strong spatial constraint upon the tight turn at the base of the helix, reorienting the peptide-tRNA ester linkage away from its normal conformers. The length of the proposed helical portion of the 2A sequence is some 27 Å, which could be entirely accommodated within the exit tunnel of the ribosome, some 100 Å long (1).

Inhibition of Peptidyl-Transferase Activity

During peptide bond formation the peptidyl-tRNA electrophilic center (P site) must occupy a space within the peptidyl-transferase site, which is accessible by the nucleophilic center of the aminoacyl-tRNA (A site). Our site-directed mutagenetic data show that if this incoming nucleophile is prolyl-tRNA, then cleavage occurs extremely efficiently; if the nucleophile is glycyl-tRNA, then cleavage occurs extremely inefficiently; and if the nucleophile is any other aminoacyl-tRNA, then cleavage does not occur at all. It is known that prolyl-tRNA is the poorest nucleophile of all the possible aminoacyl-tRNAs for two reasons: first, that the nitrogen is a secondary amine but, perhaps more important, that this secondary amino group is sterically hindered due to its location in a five-membered pryolidone ring structure. When analogues of the antibiotic puromycin were tested for inhibition of translation, the poorest analogue was that containing proline (23). Furthermore, 3′-O-prolyl adenosine was found to be the worst 3′-O-aminoacyl adenosine substrate for peptidyl-transferase activity (37). Interestingly, in both studies glycine proved to be the next poorest nucleophile—consistent with our site-directed mutagenesis data.

Recent analyses of the function of the putative catalytic bases within the peptidyl-transferase center has led to the proposal that transpeptidation is promoted not through chemical catalysis but simply by the proper positioning of the substrates (27)—the essence of our model is that this precise positioning is subverted by the nascent 2A sequence, thereby inhibiting transpeptidation.

Cleavage of the 2A Peptidyl-tRNA Ester Linkage

Given that peptide bond formation between G18 and P19 is inhibited by either or both of the mechanisms described above, how could this ester bond be cleaved? Presumably the intrinsic rate of ester bond cleavage is not sufficient to account for the observed rapid rate of cotranslational cleavage, since (i) peptidyl-tRNA hydrolase is required to "scavenge" peptidyl-tRNAs arising from abortive termination, and (ii) a system has evolved in bacteria (tmRNA) to rescue "stalled" translation complexes where truncation of the mRNA has occurred. This implies that the peptidyl-tRNA ester linkage within the cytoplasm or within such a translational complex is relatively stable under physiological conditions. We have proposed a mechanism in which the ester moiety is activated as an electrophile precisely in the same manner as in peptidyl transfer but that the nucleophile is an activated water molecule. Magnesium ions are known to be required for peptidyl-transferase activity, and we have suggested that a Mg^{2+} ion can bind at the base of the 2A helix axis (36), positioning the Mg^{2+} ion in the negatively charged field of the helix dipole, together with a coordinated water molecule, perfectly for attack on the peptidyl-tRNA ester carbonyl group.

Synthesis of Full-Length [GFP2AGUS] Translation Products

One notable difference between 2A activity in its native polyprotein context and in our artificial polyprotein systems is that 10% of the translation products are full length. When these constructs were modified by the addition of just 5 aa of the native polyprotein upstream context of 2A, the amount of uncleaved translation product was much reduced (5, 7). The FMDV 2A is suboptimal in heterologous protein contexts and requires sequences from the C terminus of FMDV capsid protein 1D for complete cleavage. If the function of the helical portion of 2A is to interact with the exit pore of the ribosome, thereby "fixing" the reverse turn at its base, then the 18-aa 2A sequence, by itself, is too short to accomplish this completely. The increased conformational space of the carbonyl carbon would permit the prolyl-tRNA to access this electrophilic center and form a peptide bond. Increasing the length by 5 aa could, however, have the effect of increasing the binding to the ribosomal exit pore and restricting the conformational freedom of the carbonyl carbon. Consistent with this notion is the observation that N-terminal truncation of 2A sequence resulted in increased peptide bond formation (35). The lack of conservation immediately upstream of the conserved -DxExNPG P- motif suggests that there are a (limited) number of ways in which 2As can interact with the ribosomal exit pore to achieve the correct orientation of the reverse-turn-ester linkage within the peptidyl-transferase center.

Synthesis of the Discrete Downstream Translation Product

Following cleavage of the ester bond, a deacylated tRNA is present in the P site and a prolyl- (rather than peptidyl-) tRNA occupies the A site—a situation analogous, but not identical, to normal peptide bond synthesis. Translocation of the prolyl-tRNA into the P site would permit ingress of the next aminoacyl-tRNA and synthesis of the downstream translation product to occur. Were the A site to be unoccupied at this stage, we suggest termination of translation might well occur. The kinetics of the hydrolysis of the ester bond would need to be such that it be slower than the combined rate of (i) the translocation of (2A)peptidyl-tRNA from the A to P site plus (ii) the overall process of binding prolyl-tRNA into the A site.

The Imbalance in Synthesis—Cleavage in the Ribosomal A Site?

Immediately after the addition of G18 to the growing nascent chain the (2A)peptidyl-tRNA complex is present within the A site of the ribosome. One can envisage that were this complex to reside in the A site for relatively prolonged periods, then cleavage could occur in this site. This would result in deacylated tRNAs being present in both P and A sites—directly analogous to termination of translation. This would, therefore, result in the synthesis of the upstream translation product alone. It was shown that during the course of a picornavirus infection, perhaps not surprisingly, the rate of ribosome processivity decreases (13, 30, 41), although the rate-limiting steps are not known. Interestingly, translation studies on cardiovirus RNA using Krebs-2 cell-free extracts showed a "translational barrier" in the central region of the genome that could be overcome by the addition of eEF2 (43).

The Imbalance in Synthesis—Cleavage in the Ribosomal P Site?

Cleavage of the ester bond while the peptidyl-tRNA complex was in the P site could occur in two states: the A site occupied by prolyl-tRNA or the A site being unoccupied. If the A site were unoccupied, then, presumably, this situation mimics that which occurs in the termination of translation and the ribosome subunits would dissociate. Were cleavage of the ester bond to occur while the A site was occupied by prolyl-tRNA (Fig. 4, step v), then the closest analogous situation that would occur during normal translation is that of dipeptidyl-tRNA in the P site during the early stages of protein synthesis. Translation complexes with short nascent peptides are less stable than those with longer peptides (17), an effect exacerbated by hydrophobic residues (26).

In summary, we and others have shown the aphtho- and cardiovirus 2A/2B cleavage is mediated by an oligopeptidic region, representing either the whole (aphthoviruses) or part (cardioviruses) of the 2A region. We provide evidence that this method of protein biogenesis is not confined to the picornaviruses, but is used by other RNA viruses and virus-like mobile genetic elements. We have, however, analyzed only the 2A-like tracts that corresponded to the 18-aa region of FMDV. The figures given for the cleavage activities may very well, therefore, not represent the true activities of these sequences in their native protein contexts, but be the product of the (suboptimal) lengths of the 2A-like sequences we analyzed. The mechanism that is consistent with all of our translational and site-directed mutagenetic data is one of modification of the host-cell translational process at a specific site within the polyprotein. In our model of cleavage, 2A acts as a *cis*-acting hydrolase element (not an enzyme sensu stricto), rather than a proteinase, and we propose the term "chysel" to refer to its intriguing activity.

We gratefully acknowledge the Biotechnology and Biological Sciences Research Council and The Wellcome Trust for supporting this work.

REFERENCES

1. **Ban, N., P. Nissen, J. Hansen, M. Capel, P. B. Moore, and T. A. Steitz.** 1999. Placement of protein and RNA structures into a 5Å-resolution map of the 50S ribosomal subunit. *Nature* **400**:841–847.
2. **Batson, S., and K. Rundell.** 1991. Proteolysis at the 2A/2B junction in Theiler's murine encephalomyelitis virus. *Virology* **181**:764–767.
3. **Chaplin, P. J., E. B. Camon, B. Villarreal-Ramos, M. Flint, M. D. Ryan, and R. A. Collins.** 1999. Production of interleukin-12 as a self-processing polypeptide. *J. Interferon Cytokine Res.* **19**:235–241.
4. **de Felipe, P., V. Martín, M. L. Cortés, M. D. Ryan, and M. Izquierdo.** 1999. Use of the 2A sequence from foot-and-mouth disease virus in the generation of retroviral vectors for gene therapy. *Gene Ther.* **6**:198–208.
5. **Donnelly, M. L. L., D. Gani, M. Flint, S. Monoghan, and M. D. Ryan.** 1997. The cleavage activity of aphtho- and cardiovirus 2A proteins. *J. Gen. Virol.* **78**:13–21.
6. **Donnelly, M. L. L., L. E. Hughes, G. Luke, X. Li, H. Mendoza, E. ten Dam, D. Gani, and M. D. Ryan.** 2001. The 'cleavage' activities of FMDV 2A site-directed mutants and naturally-occurring '2A-like' sequences. *J. Gen. Virol.* **82**:1027–1041.
7. **Donnelly, M. L. L., G. Luke, A. Mehrotra, X. Li, L. E. Hughes, D. Gani, and M. D. Ryan.** 2001. Analysis of the aphtovirus 2A/2B polyprotein 'cleavage' mechanism indicates not a proteolytic reaction, but a novel translational effect: a putative ribosomal 'skip'. *J. Gen. Virol.* **82**:1013–1025.
8. **Farabaugh, P. J.** 1996. Programmed translational frameshifting. *Microbiol. Rev.* **60**:103–134.
9. **Gesteland, R. F., and J. F. Atkins.** 1996. Recoding: dynamic reprogramming of translation. *Annu. Rev. Biochem.* **65**:741–768.
10. **Gopinath, K., J. Wellink, C. Porta, K. M. Taylor, G. P. Lomonossoff, and A. van Kammen.** 2000. Engineering cowpea mosaic virus RNA-2 into a vector to express heterologous proteins in plants. *Virology* **267**:159–173.
11. **Grubman, M. J., and B. Baxt.** 1982. Translation of foot-and-mouth disease virion RNA and processing of the primary cleavage products in a rabbit reticulocyte lysate. *Virology* **116**:19–30.
12. **Gu, Z., R. Harrod, E. J. Rogers, and P. S. Lovett.** 1994. Anti-peptidyl transferase leader peptides of attenuation-regulated chloramphenicol-resistance genes. *Proc. Natl. Acad. Sci. USA* **91**:5612–5616.
13. **Hackett, P. B., E. Egberts, and P. Traub.** 1978. Translation of ascites and mengovirus RNA in fractionated cell free systems from uninfected and mengovirus-infected Ehrlich-ascites-tumor cells. *Eur. J. Biochem.* **83**:341–352.
14. **Hahn, H., and A. C. Palmenberg.** 1996. Mutational analysis of the encephalomyocarditis virus primary cleavage. *J. Virol.* **70**:6870–6875.
15. **Halpin, C., S. E. Cooke, A. Barakate, A. El Amrani, and M. D. Ryan.** 1999. Self-processing polyproteins—a system for co-ordinate expression of multiple proteins in transgenic plants. *Plant J.* **17**:453–459.
16. **Harrod, R., and P. S. Lovett.** 1995. Peptide inhibitors of peptidyltransferase alter the conformation of domains IV and V of large subunit rRNA: a model for nascent peptide control of translation. *Proc. Natl. Acad. Sci. USA* **92**:8650–8654.
17. **Karimi, R., M. Y. Pavlov, V. Heurgue-Hamard, R. H. Buckingham, and M. Ehrenberg.** 1998. Initiation factors IF1 and IF2 synergistically remove peptidyl-tRNAs with short polypeptides from the P-site of translating *Escherichia coli* ribosomes. *J. Mol. Biol.* **281**:241–252.
18. **Kokuho, T., S. Watanabe, Y. Yokomizo, and S. Inumaru.** 1999. Production of biologically active, heterodimeric porcine interleukin-12 using a monocistronic baculoviral expression system. *Jap. Vet. Immunol. Immunopathol.* **72**:289–302.
19. **Martin, F., C. Maranon, M. Olivares, C. Alonso, and M. C. Lopez.** 1995. Characterization of a non-long terminal repeat retrotransposon cDNA (L1Tc) from *Trypanosoma cruzi*: homology of the first ORF with the ape family of DNA repair enzymes. *J. Mol. Biol.* **247**:49–59.
20. **Mattion, N. M., E. C. Harnish, J. C. Crowley, and P. A. Reilly.** 1996. Foot-and-mouth disease virus 2A protease mediates cleavage in attenuated Sabin 3 poliovirus vectors engineered for delivery of foreign antigens. *J. Virol.* **70**:8124–8127.
21. **Medvedkina, O. A., I. V. Scarlat, N. O. Kalinina, and V. I. Agol.** 1974. Virus-specific proteins associated with ribosomes of Krebs-II cells infected with encephalomyocarditis virus. *FEBS Lett.* **39**:4–8.
22. **Michiels, T., V. DeJong, R. Rodrigus, and C. Shaw-Jackson.** 1997. Protein 2A is not required for Theiler's virus replication. *J. Virol.* **71**:9549–9556.

23. **Nathans, D., and A. Niedle.** 1963. Structural requirements for puromycin inhibition of protein synthesis. *Nature* **197**:1076–1077.
24. **Palmenberg, A. C., G. D. Parks, D. J. Hall, R. H. Ingraham, T. W. Seng, and P. V. Pallai.** 1992. Proteolytic processing of the cardioviral P2 region: primary 2A/2B cleavage in clone-derived precursors. *Virology* **190**:754–762.
25. **Percy, N., W. S. Barclay, A. Garcia-Sastre, and P. Palese.** 1994. Expression of a foreign protein by influenza A virus. *J. Virol.* **68**:4486–4492.
26. **Picking, W. D., O. W. Odom, T. Tsalkova, I. Serdyuk, and B. Hardesty.** 1991. The conformation of nascent polylysine and polyphenylalanine peptides on ribosomes. *J. Biol. Chem.* **266**:1534–1542.
27. **Polacek, N., M. Gaynor, A. Yassin, and A. S. Mankin.** 2001. Ribosomal peptidyl transferase can withstand mutations at the putative catalytic nucleotide. *Nature* **411**:498–501.
28. **Precious, B., D. F. Young, A. Bermingham, R. Fearns, M. D. Ryan, and R. E. Randall.** 1995. Inducible expression of the P, V, and NP genes of the paramyxovirus simian virus 5 in cell lines and an examination of the NP-P and NP-V interactions. *J. Virol.* **69**:8001–8010.
29. **Pringle, F. M., K. H. J. Gordon, T. N. Hanzlik, J. Kalmakoff, P. D. Scotti, and V. K. Ward.** 1999. A novel capsid expression strategy for *Thosea asigna* virus (*Tetraviridae*). *J. Gen. Virol.* **80**:1855–1863.
30. **Ramabhadran, T. V., and R. E. Thatch.** 1981. Translational elongation rate changes in encephalomyocarditis virus-infected and interferon-treated cells. *J. Virol.* **39**:573–583.
31. **Robertson, B. H., M. J. Grubman, G. N. Weddell, D. M. Moore, J. D. Welsh, T. Fischer, D. J. Dowbenko, D. G. Yansura, B. Small, and D. G. Kleid.** 1985. Nucleotide and amino acid sequence coding for polypeptides of foot-and-mouth disease virus type A12. *J. Virol.* **54**:651–660.
32. **Rogers, E. J., and P. S. Lovett.** 1994. The *cis*-effect of a nascent peptide on its translating ribosome: influence of the cat-86 leader pentapeptide on translation at leader codon 6. *Mol. Microbiol.* **12**:181–186.
33. **Ryan, M. D., G. J. Belsham, and A. M. Q. King.** 1989. Specificity of substrate-enzyme interactions in foot-and-mouth disease virus polyprotein processing. *Virology* **173**:35–45.
34. **Ryan, M. D., A. M. Q. King, and G. P. Thomas.** 1991. Cleavage of foot-and-mouth disease virus polyprotein is mediated by residues located within a 19 amino acid sequence. *J. Gen. Virol.* **72**:2727–2732.
35. **Ryan, M. D., and J. Drew.** 1994. Foot-and-mouth disease virus 2A oligopeptide mediated cleavage of an artificial polyprotein. *EMBO J.* **13**:928–933.
36. **Ryan, M. D., M. L. L. Donnelly, A. Lewis, A. P. Mehrotra, J. Wilkie, and D. Gani.** 1999. A model for non-stoichiometric, co-translational protein scission in eukaryotic ribosomes. *Bioorganic Chem.* **27**:55–79.
37. **Rychlik, I., J. Cerna, S. Chladek, P. Pulkrabek, and J. Zemlicka.** 1970. Substrate specificity of ribosomal peptidyl transferase. *Eur. J. Biochem.* **16**:136–142.
38. **Schmidt, M., and A. Rethwilm.** 1995. Replicating foamy virus-based vectors directing high-level expression of foreign genes. *Virology* **210**:167–178.
39. **Smerdou, C., and P. Liljestrom.** 1999. Two-helper RNA system for production of recombinant Semliki Forest virus particles. *J. Virol.* **73**:1092–1098.
40. **Smolenska, L., L. M. Roberts, D. Learmonth, A. J. Porter, W. J. Harris, T. M. A. Wilson, and S. S. Cruz.** 1998. Production of a functional single chain antibody attached to the surface of a plant virus. *FEBS Lett.* **441**:379–382.
41. **Summers, D. F., J. V. Maizel, and J. E. Darnell.** 1967. Decrease in size and synthetic activity of poliovirus polysomes late in the infectious cycle. *Virology* **31**:427–435.
42. **Suzuki, N., L. M. Geletka, and D. L. Nuss.** 2000. Essential and dispensable virus-encoded replication elements revealed by efforts to develop hypoviruses as gene expression vectors. *J. Virol.* **74**:7568–7577.
43. **Svitkin, Y. V., and V. I. Agol.** 1983. Translational barrier in central region of encephalomyocarditis virus genome. *Eur. J. Biochem.* **133**:145–154.
44. **Toyoda, H., M. J. H. Nicklin, M. G. Murray, C. W. Anderson, J. J. Dunn, F. W. Studier, and E. Wimmer.** 1986. A second virus-encoded proteinase involved in proteolytic processing of poliovirus polyprotein. *Cell* **45**:761–770.
45. **van der Ryst, E., T. Nakasone, A. Habel, A. Venet, E. Gomard, R. Altmeyer, M. Girard, and A. M. Borman.** 1998. Study of the immunogenicity of different recombinant mengo viruses expressing HIV1 and SIV epitopes. *Res. Virol.* **149**:5–20.
46. **Varnavski, A. N., and A. A. Khromykh.** 1999. Noncytopathic flavivirus replicon RNA-based system for expression and delivery of heterologous genes. *Virology* **255**:366–375.
47. **Weiss, R., W. Huang, and D. Dunn.** 1990. A nascent peptide is required for ribosomal bypass of the coding gap in bacteriophage T4 gene 60. *Cell* **62**:117–126.
48. **Wright, H. T.** 1991. Nonenzymatic deamidation of asparaginyl and glutaminyl residues in proteins. *Crit. Rev. Biochem. Mol. Biol.* **26**:1–52.
49. **Zoll, J., F. J. M. van Kuppeveld, J. M. D. Galama, and W. J. G. Melchers.** 1998. Genetic analysis of mengovirus protein 2A: its function in polyprotein processing and in virus production. *J. Gen. Virol.* **79**:17–25.

VIRAL RNA REPLICATION

Possible Unifying Mechanism of Picornavirus Genome Replication

ANIKO V. PAUL

19

Picornaviruses, like other RNA viruses, are unique in their ability to synthesize RNA on an RNA template. To achieve this task they induce the synthesis of a special RNA-dependent RNA polymerase. Since viral RNAs are linear molecules, these enzymes have to employ special methods to initiate replication while retaining the integrity of the 5' end of their genomes. Picornaviral RNA polymerases face an additional problem because the viral RNAs contain two different types of termini. The 5' end of the plus-strand RNA contains heteropolymeric sequences and the terminal UMP is covalently liked to a tyrosine residue in a small protein, called VPg (Fig. 1) (4, 68, 117). On the other hand, the 3' end of the RNA is terminated with a genetically encoded poly(A) tail (31, 146), where minus-strand RNA synthesis must begin. The nonspecific poly(A) sequences, however, cannot provide specificity to the RNA polymerase during the initiation of RNA synthesis. As we will see later, the picornaviral RNA polymerases devised ingenious ways to overcome these problems.

It is generally accepted that picornaviral RNA replication proceeds via the following pathway:

+strand RNA → −strand RNA synthesis → RF →
+strand RNA synthesis → RI → +strand RNA

where RF (replicative form) is double-stranded RNA and RI (replicative intermediate) is partially double and partially single-stranded (141).

In this review an attempt will be made to summarize all the pertinent experimental evidence that is currently available and to propose a unified model for picornavirus RNA replication. These data are derived from three types of experiments. In the simplest type, purified enzymes are used to study biochemical reactions in vitro. The second in complexity are those studies that use crude replication complexes isolated either from infected cells or from coupled translation/replication reactions of viral RNA. Finally, the most difficult method involves studying reactions in the infected cell itself. Since most of the available information is derived from studies of poliovirus, a member of the *Enterovirus* genus and the prototype of *Picornaviridae* (118; G. Stanway, F. Brown, P. D. Christian, H. Tapani, T. Hyypia, A. M. Q. King, N. J. Knowles, S. M. Lemon, P. D. Minor, M. A. Pallansch, A. C. Palmenberg, and T. Skern, Abstr. XI Meet. Eur. Study Group Mol. Biol. Picornaviruses, abstr. A07, 2000), the models will be based primarily on this system. Whenever important differences with other picornaviruses exist, e.g., members of the genus *Rhinovirus* (human rhinoviruses [HRV]), *Hepatovirus* (hepatitis A virus [HAV]), *Cardiovirus* (encephalomyocarditis virus [EMCV]), *Aphthovirus* (foot-and-mouth disease virus [FMDV]), or others, they will be discussed separately. It should be emphasized that since very little is known about the details of the process, the models are highly speculative and will surely change in the future. Specifically, I will (i) summarize the viral and cellular factors required for RNA replication, (ii) discuss the coupling of RNA translation and replication, (iii) describe the products of RNA synthesis, (iii) propose a unified model of picornaviral minus- and plus-strand RNA synthesis, and (iv) compare protein-primed RNA and DNA synthesis. Because of the limited scope of this article, previous models (130), no longer under consideration, will not be discussed.

VIRAL AND CELLULAR FACTORS REQUIRED FOR RNA REPLICATION

Viral Proteins

Both biochemical and genetic studies have shown that all of the nonstructural proteins (Fig. 1) (60) are involved in poliovirus RNA replication (reviewed in reference 141). Due to the small size of the virus, the genetic information encoded in the viral genome is utilized in the form of both mature and precursor polypeptides (118). The functions of the polypeptides encoded by the P2 domain are the least understood, but they are known to have a strong influence on the biochemical and structural changes that are induced in the host cell following virus infection. The proteins of the P3 domain are those that are most directly involved in the process of RNA synthesis.

Aniko V. Paul ■ Department of Molecular Genetics and Microbiology, State University of New York at Stony Brook, Stony Brook, NY 11790.

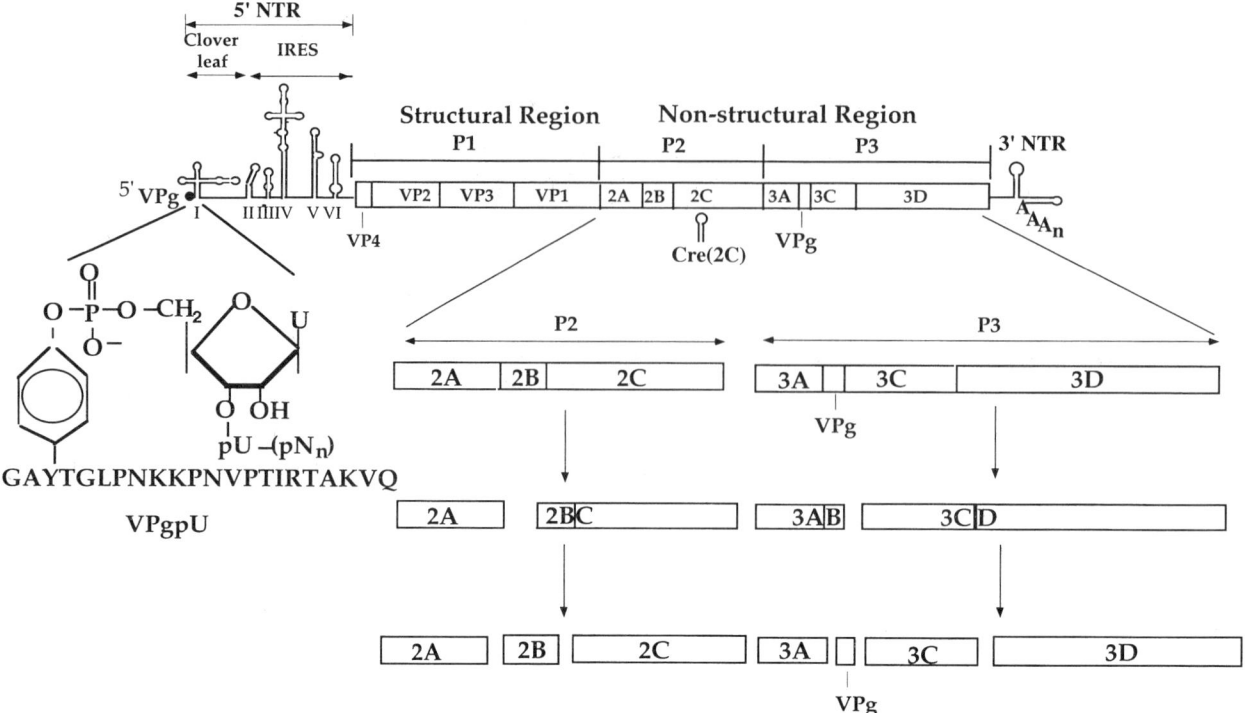

FIGURE 1 Structure of poliovirus genomic RNA and processing of the polyprotein. The single-stranded RNA of poliovirus is shown with the terminal protein VPg at its 5' end and the 3' NTR with the poly(A) tail at its 3' end. The 5' NTR consists of the cloverleaf and the large IRES element. The location of the cre(2C) hairpin in the coding region of 2C is indicated. The attachment site of the 5'-terminal UMP to the tyrosine of VPg is shown enlarged. The polyprotein contains structural (P1) and nonstructural (P2, P3) domains. Processing of the P2 and P3 precursors of the polyprotein by 3C^{pro}/3CD^{pro} is shown enlarged, with vertical lines indicating the proteinase cleavage sites.

Proteins of the P2 Domain

The members of this group of polypeptides are 2A^{pro}, 2B, 2BC, and 2C^{ATPase}. Protein 2A^{pro} is encoded by all picornaviruses but differs widely in size and function among its members (54, 118). Only the 2A polypeptides of entero- and rhinoviruses are bona fide proteinases (designated 2A^{pro}) whose primary function is to cleave the polyprotein in cis between domains P1/P2 (reviewed in reference 48). In addition, 2A^{pro} is involved in the inhibition of host cell protein synthesis (reviewed in reference 123). The 2A polypeptides of HAV and EMCV have no proteolytic activity and that of FMDV is only 16 residues long (118). Whereas mutations in the coding region of poliovirus 2A^{pro} have been shown to cause partial or full inhibition of viral replication (71, 84, 137, 147), no such function has been found to be associated with the 2A protein of HAV (46) and of Theiler's virus (82). Although 2A^{pro} of poliovirus is definitely involved in some step(s) of viral RNA synthesis (71), the mechanism by which the protein participates in genome replication remains obscure.

Very little is known about the function of the picornaviral protein 2B. Expression of 2B in mammalian cells has been associated with a block of secretory transport (30), disassembly of the Golgi complex (120), permeabilization of the plasma membrane (2), and induction of membrane proliferation (3) and rearrangements (129). Similarly, the expression of 2BC induces membrane proliferation (3) and rearrangements (21, 129) in the host cell leading to the formation of vesicles to which the replication complexes are attached (15, 21, 129). Through yeast two-hybrid analysis, poliovirus proteins 2B, 2BC, and 2C were found to interact with each other in all combinations except for 2C/2C (24). Genetic analysis of 2B/2B interaction has shown this protein to be important for RNA replication (24).

Protein 2C^{ATPase} is a very complex protein that is highly conserved among picornaviruses (43) and is abundant in viral replication complexes (14, 15). The 2C^{ATPase} of poliovirus contains an N-terminal amphipathic helix (97), a membrane-binding region (32), two RNA-binding domains (112), and a zinc-binding cysteine-rich motif (102). The protein is known to have an ATPase activity (103, 111), which is inhibited by low concentration of guanidine hydrochloride (103), a potent inhibitor of picornavirus RNA replication in vivo (23). Although the protein contains domains conserved among a superfamily of helicases (42, 43), no helicase activity has yet been found to be associated with it (103). Genetic analyses have implicated this protein in a variety of functions during viral replication such as virus uncoating (70), host cell membrane rearrangement (21, 129), RNA replication (reviewed in reference 141), and encapsidation (136a). The biochemical mechanisms by which 2C^{ATPase} engages in these processes is not known. Recently, in an in vitro translation/replication system, which produces viable poliovirus (85), 2C^{ATPase} was found to be required just prior to or during initiation of minus-strand RNA synthesis (12).

Proteins of the P3 Domain

During translation of poliovirus RNA the P3 precursor is generated from the polyprotein by a fast cleavage event at the amino terminus of the 3A-coding region. The P3 polypeptide then undergoes rapid processing to yield two important, relatively stable and multifunctional precursors, 3AB and 3CD^{pro} (Fig. 1, Table 1) (reviewed in reference 48). This is followed by partial processing of the precursors to their final cleavage products 3A, 3B, 3C^{pro}, and 3D^{pol} (Table 1). Some of these proteins interact with each other to form homo- or heterodimers or even oligomerize (45, 95, 142).

Despite its small size (12 kDa), the small basic protein 3AB appears to have multiple functions, which can be assayed in vitro (Table 1) (49, 67, 96, 106, 143, 144). By itself 3AB is a nonspecific RNA-binding protein (49, 96, 143) but when complexed with 3CD^{pro} it specifically binds both to the 5′ cloverleaf and the 3′ nontranslated region (NTR) (49, 143, 144). The possible roles of these RNA-protein interactions will be discussed later. The C-terminal domain of 3A contains a stretch of hydrophobic amino acids, which are believed to provide it with a site of attachment to the membranes during replication (40, 124, 133). Although the glycosylation of 3A in translation extracts has been observed (28), such modification does not appear to be essential for the growth of poliovirus (29). Enviroxime, an inhibitor of rhino- and poliovirus RNA replication, was shown to interact with 3A and to preferentially inhibit plus-strand RNA synthesis (50).

The picornaviral VPg is 20 to 24 amino acids in length and contains a fully conserved and essential tyrosine at position 3, the attachment site to the RNA (43, 62, 118, 145). FMDV encodes three VPgs in tandem (35), whereas the other picornaviruses encode only one (43). Interestingly, when two tandem VPgs are engineered into poliovirus, the resulting virus is quasi-infectious and retains only the N-terminal peptide while the second is deleted (19). The replacement of PV1 VPg with that of HRV14 VPg, but not with that of HRV2 VPg, results in a viable poliovirus (A. V. Paul, J. Peters, and E. Wimmer, submitted). In vitro PV1 and HRV2 VPgs can be uridylylated by their cognate RNA polymerases on either poly(A) or viral RNA templates (39a, 39b, 99, 100, 109).

Protein 3CD^{pro} is the precursor of both proteinase 3C^{pro} and the RNA polymerase 3D^{pol}. Its primary function is the processing of all cleavage sites in the entero- and rhinovirus polyprotein with the exception of VP4/VP2 and P1/P2. Cleavages occur most often at glutamine/glycine cleavage sites (reviewed in reference 48). In addition, 3CD^{pro} has multiple functions as an RNA-binding protein (5, 6, 49, 94, 99, 109, 144). The RNA-binding domain is located in the 3C^{pro} polypeptide, but this activity appears to be modulated by parts of the 3D^{pol} protein (93). As discussed above, when complexed with 3AB, 3CD^{pro} interacts specifically with the 5′ cloverleaf and the 3′ NTR (49, 144). This polypeptide also binds the 5′ cloverleaf when complexed with the cellular protein poly(rC)-binding protein (PCBP2) (38, 94). In addition, 3CD^{pro} of PV1 and HRV2 interact with their cognate cis-acting RNA element [cre(2C) and cre(2A), respectively] along with 3D^{pol} and VPg during the reaction in which VPg is uridylylated in vitro (39b, 99, 109).

The RNA polymerases of poliovirus and HRV2 are dependent in vitro on an RNA template (34, 39a, 39b) and on a primer, either RNA, DNA, or VPg (34, 39a, 39b, 99, 100). The primary activities of the enzymes are the elongation of an oligonucleotide primer that is annealed to a template (Table 1) (34, 39a) and the covalent attachment of UMP to the hydroxyl group of tyrosine in VPg (39b, 99, 100). The poliovirus enzyme has the ability to unwind a double-stranded RNA during transcription (20) and to switch templates (7). It also catalyzes other types of reactions in vitro, such as reverse transcription and RNA chain initiation, but these occur only with low efficiencies and under special reaction conditions (8). Although PV1 3D^{pol} is a soluble protein, a fraction of it is associated with membranous replication complexes in infected cells (14). This association is believed to be mediated by protein-protein interactions involving membrane-bound 3AB (52). A partial structure of poliovirus 3D^{pol} has recently been solved and was found to have the structure typical for polymerases with finger, palm, and thumb domains (45). Both in vitro (45, 95) and in vivo (142) studies suggest that this protein assembles into oligomers, a form that appears to favor both the elongation and RNA-binding activity of the polymerase (95).

The processing of the P3 domain of other picornaviral polyproteins, such as that of EMCV (A. G. Aminev and A. C. Palmenberg, Abstr. XI Meet. Eur. Study Group Mol. Biol. Picornaviruses, abstr. D06, 2000) or HAV (64), is different from that of poliovirus in that 3ABC is also a stable intermediate and appears to be important for viral RNA replication (64). The binding of HAV 3ABC to the 5′ and 3′ NTRs of the HAV genome is specific and much stronger than the binding of either 3AB or 3C^{pro} (64, 65). In contrast to poliovirus, the 3C^{pro} polypeptides of HAV (63) and of HRV14 (69) appear to possess a specific RNA-binding activity toward their 5′ NTRs.

Cellular Proteins

During the past few years there has been increasing evidence that RNA viruses use cellular factors for the transcription and replication of their genomes, although normal eukaryotic cells do not possess a machinery to support RNA-dependent RNA synthesis. Indeed, these factors have cellular functions that are entirely different from RNA synthesis. They either modify proteins, such as kinases, or are components of the cell's normal RNA processing or translation machineries (reviewed in reference 66). The putative host factors involved in picornavirus RNA replication are listed in Table 2. The earliest reported host factors in poliovirus RNA replication were a protein kinase and a uridylyl transferase, but these are no longer under consideration (145). More recently, on the basis of the in vitro translation/replication system (85), Barton et al. suggested that one or more cellular factors are required for poliovirus minus-strand RNA synthesis (11). Gamarnik and Andino have observed that both poliovirus RNA translation and replication in *Xenopus* oocytes require cellular factors (36). The existence of important host factors for poliovirus and CBV3 RNA replication has also been predicted from mammalian host range phenotypes (148). The identity of these factors has not yet been determined.

In other studies the cellular polypeptide Sam68 was found to interact with poliovirus 3D^{pol} in the yeast two-hybrid system (75). Waggoner and Sarnow reported an interaction of the poliovirus 3′ NTR sequences with the human protein nucleolin, which relocalizes in the cytoplasm

TABLE 1 Properties and functions of proteins encoded by the P3 domain of the poliovirus polyprotein

Protein	Properties and functions	References
3A	Required for RNA replication	40, 50, 52, 143
	Membrane associated	40, 133
	Inhibits host protein secretion	29
	Substrate for glycosylation	28
	Interacts with 3AB	142
	Dimerizes	142
3B	Required for RNA replication	62, 141, and references therein
	Covalently linked to plus- and minus-strand RNA	89
	Substrate for uridylylation	100
	Weakly stimulates $3D^{pol}$ activity in vitro	96
	Weakly stimulates $3CD^{pro}$ autoprocessing	83
	Interacts with $3D^{pol}$ or $3CD^{pro}$	142
$3C^{pro}$	Processes viral proteins	48 and references therein
	Cleaves host proteins	27, 113
	Weakly binds to 5' cloverleaf with 3AB	49
$3D^{pol}$	Required for RNA replication	141 and references therein
	Uridylylates VPg	99, 100
	Elongates RNA chains	34
	Unwinds double-stranded RNA during polymerization	20
	Binds to RNA	95
	Has terminal adenylyltransferase activity	88
	Can switch templates	7
	Interacts with cellular protein Sam68	75
	Interacts with $3CD^{pro}$, 3B, 3AB	142
	Dimerizes	45, 95
3AB	Required for RNA replication	40, 133, 143
	Associated with membranes	40, 133
	Binds to RNA (nonspecific)	96, 143
	Binds to 5' cloverleaf with $3CD^{pro}$	49, 143
	Binds to 3' NTR with $3CD^{pro}$ or $3D^{pol}$	49
	Substrate for glycosylation	28
	Stimulates $3D^{pol}$ activity in vitro	67, 96, 106, 107
	Stimulates $3CD^{pro}$ autoprocessing in vitro	83
	Interacts with $3D^{pol}$, $3CD^{pro}$	52, 83, 142
	Oligomerizes	142
$3CD^{pro}$	Required for RNA replication	5, 6, 109, 141, 144
	Processes viral proteins	48 and references therein
	Processes cellular protein	114
	Binds to 5' cloverleaf with 3AB	49, 144
	Binds to 5' cloverleaf with PCBP2	38, 94
	Interacts strongly with 3B, 3AB	83, 142
	Interacts weakly with $3D^{pol}$, $3CD^{pro}$	142
	Binds to 3' NTR with 3AB	49
	Binds to PV1 cre(2C)	109

during poliovirus infection (138). Again, the role of these interactions remains unknown.

The other host factors listed in Table 2 have been identified through their interaction with cis-acting elements in picornaviral genomes. It is important to point out that not all of these RNA-protein interactions are necessarily relevant to picornavirus RNA replication. The only one of these factors characterized thus far is PCBP2, which specifically interacts with two domains of the poliovirus 5' NTR, the cloverleaf structure and stem-loop IV of the internal ribosome entry site (IRES) (17, 38, 94). A report by Herold and Andino has indicated that human poly(A)-binding protein (PABP), a potential new host factor in RNA replication, is able to interact in vitro with PCBP2, poliovirus $3CD^{pro}$, and the 3' NTR-poly(A) (51a). The binding of PABP to the poly(A) tail might explain the

TABLE 2 Viral and cellular proteins binding to picornaviral cis-replicating RNA elements[a]

Virus	+Cloverleaf	−Cloverleaf	3′ NTR-poly(A)	cre(2C)
Poliovirus:				
PV1(M)				
Viral proteins	3AB/3CD^{pro} [49, 143, 144]	2C [9]	3AB/3CD^{pro} [49]	3CD^{pro} [109]
Cellular proteins	PCBP2 (with 3CD^{pro}) [5, 38, 94]	p36, p38 kDa [114]	p34, p36 [131]	p50 [109]
	ΔEF1-α (with 3CD^{pro}) [49]		Nucleolin [138]	
	PABP (with 3CD^{pro}) [51a]		PABP [51a]	
PV3				
Cellular proteins			p34–36, p60, p70 kDa [79]	
HRV14				
Viral protein	3C^{pro} [69]			
Cellular proteins			p34–36 kDa [131]	
			p34–36, p60, p70 kDa [79]	
CB4				
Cellular proteins			p34–36, p60, p70 kDa [79]	
EMCV				
Viral protein			3D^{pol} [25, 26]	

Virus	+ 5′ nt 1–148	3′ NTR-poly(A)
HAV		
Viral proteins	3AB, 3ABC, 3C^{pro} [63, 64]	3AB, 3ABC [64]
Cellular proteins		p38, p45, p57, p84, p110 kDa [64, 65]

[a] Brackets indicate references.

presence of RF molecules in the infected cell with protruding poly(A) tails (51). A possible role of PABP in minus-strand RNA synthesis will be described later.

The cis-acting RNA Elements

Purified poliovirus RNA polymerase 3D^{pol} can copy any RNA in the presence of a primer in a soluble in vitro system. However, in the infected cell 3D^{pol} replicates exclusively poliovirus RNA. Therefore, it was predicted that the viral RNA must express specific signals for the recognition of the replication proteins in order to achieve specificity in vivo. Most studies have concentrated on the 3′ and 5′ terminal structures in picornaviral RNAs, which were considered to possess all of the cis-acting signals required by the replication proteins to initiate transcription (reviewed in references 1 and 145). These termini were designated as origins of replication at the left and right ends of the RNA, oriR and oriL, respectively (105). Only recently has the importance of internal sequences in the coding region of the polyprotein become clear.

The 5′ Cloverleaf (oriL)

All picornaviruses contain 5′-terminal nucleotide sequences that form complex structures typical for entero- and rhinoviruses, on one hand, and cardio-, aphtho-, and hepatoviruses on the other (5, 6, 110, 145). In all of these structures the 5′-phosphate of the terminal UMP is covalently linked to the hydroxyl group of a tyrosine in VPg (Fig. 1) (4, 43, 68, 117). In entero- and rhinoviruses the 5′-terminal structure resembles a cloverleaf, also referred to as domain I (Fig. 2A) (110), while the corresponding elements of other picornaviruses have less-defined structures.

The first evidence that the cloverleaf is involved in RNA replication was provided by Andino et al. (5, 6). These authors have shown the formation of a specific RNA-protein (RNP) complex consisting of viral protein 3CD^{pro}, a cellular protein p36, and the cloverleaf of poliovirus RNA. This cellular protein was subsequently identified by Blyn et al. as PCBP2, and its splice variant, PCBP1 (17). Mutational analysis of the cloverleaf revealed that 3CD^{pro} interacts with stem-loop d (5, 38, 94, 144) while PCBP2 binds to stem-loop b (5, 38, 94). The binding of this protein complex to the cloverleaf was predicted to be required both for plus- and minus-strand RNA synthesis (6, 38, 51a) and possibly also for regulating the switch from translation to replication (37).

Proteins 3AB and 3CD^{pro}, which interact with each other both in vitro (83) and in vivo (142), also form a specific RNP complex with the 5′ cloverleaf of poliovirus. Numerous genetic and biochemical experiments have shown that the 3AB/3CD^{pro}/cloverleaf RNP has an essential role in poliovirus RNA replication. First, a genetic link between 3AB's function and cloverleaf-RNP formation was established using 3AB mutants (144). Second, both RNP formation and replication phenotypes covaried with mutations in the cloverleaf (49, 144). Protein 3AB, just as PCBP2, makes contact with stem-loop b of the cloverleaf (49). Whether the PCBP2-cloverleaf and the 3AB-cloverleaf interactions with 3CD^{pro} are important at the same or different stages of RNA replication is not yet known.

Similar studies by Leong et al. and Walker et al. demonstrated the interaction of HRV14 3C^{pro} both with the HRV14 and PV1 cloverleaf structures in stem-loop d (69, 139). In contrast to HRV14 3C^{pro}, the 3C^{pro} of PV1 is es-

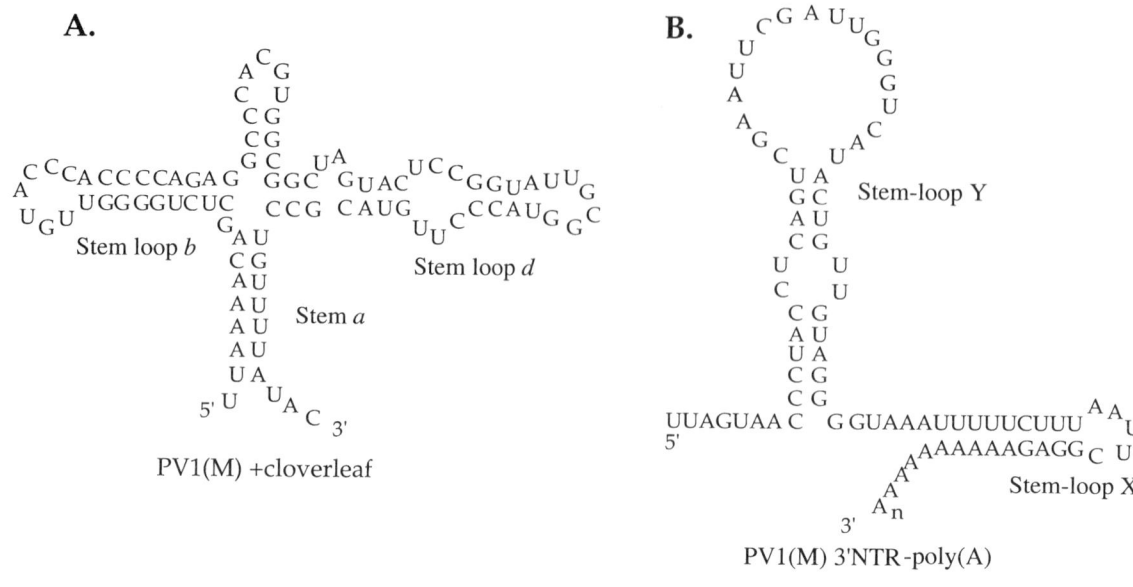

FIGURE 2 Predicted secondary structures of picornaviral *cis*-replicating elements. (A) The PV1(M) 5′ cloverleaf. (B) The PV1(M) 3′ NTR-poly(A). (C) The PV1(M) *cre*(2C), HRV14 *cre*(VP1), and HRV2 *cre*(2A) RNAs. The conserved sequences in the loops are shown with bold letters. Also shown (boxed in) is the conserved sequence in all the known internal *cis*-replicating elements of picornaviral RNAs. See Note Added in Proof.

sentially inactive in the interaction with the cloverleaf (49), and PV1 3CD^pro recognizes only the PV1 and not the HRV14 cloverleaf (144).

The 3' NTR-Poly(A) (oriR)

Mutational analysis of the heteropolymeric sequences in the 3' NTR of entero- and rhinoviruses indicated that this region is important for RNA replication. Pilipenko et al. proposed that the picornaviral 3' NTRs have highly ordered structures that can be grouped into three types: a single stem-loop in rhinoviruses (X), a two-stem-loop structure in polioviruses (X, Y) (Fig. 2B), and a three-stem-loop structure in coxsackieviruses and echoviruses (X, Y, Z) (104). For poliovirus, CBV3, and HRV14 the predicted structures were verified by enzymatic and chemical analysis (78, 104).

Two different models have been proposed for the structure of the poliovirus 3' NTR. The first is a pseudoknot formed by domain Y and upstream sequences (56). The second is an interaction between stem-loops X and Y resulting in a "kissing" interaction (78, 105). Mutational analyses of poliovirus and CBV3 3' NTR mutants strongly favor the latter model over the pseudoknot (78). This conclusion is based on studies of mutants with weakened "kissing" interactions that resulted in defective RNA replication while mutations in the proposed pseudoknot showed little or no effect on viral growth.

On the basis of these findings, Pilipenko et al. proposed that the 3' NTR and the poly(A) tail form the origin of replication, oriR, for minus-strand RNA synthesis (105). This was followed by the unexpected discovery that the 3' NTR of poliovirus can be exchanged with that of HRV14 or CBV4 and the resulting viruses have nearly normal growth properties (115). Even more surprising was the finding that the 3' NTRs of poliovirus (132) or HRV14 are dispensable (81, 132). Deletion of the poliovirus 3' NTR resulted in viruses impaired in replication, but revertants could be isolated that contained mutations scattered over the entire genome (D. M. Brown and B. L. Semler, Abstr. XI Meet. Eur. Study Group Mol. Biol. Picornaviruses, abstr. G10, 2000).

Numerous studies have attempted to find specific binding of cellular or viral proteins to picornaviral 3' NTRs (Table 2). Among the viral proteins PV1 3AB/3CD^pro were found to bind to the PV1 3' NTR (49), EMCV 3D^pol to the EMCV 3' NTR (25, 26), and HAV 3AB and 3ABC to the HAV 3' NTR (64, 65). Cellular protein nucleolin has shown high affinity toward the PV1 3' NTR (138). Todd et al. reported the binding of two unidentified cellular proteins (p34, p36) to the PV1 and HRV14 3' NTRs (131). Mutations in the 3' NTR that resulted in reduced binding also interfered with viral growth. Mellits et al. reported the binding of the same factor(s) not only to the 3' NTR of PV3 and HRV14 but also of CBV4 (79). Interestingly, the binding of a cellular protein p38 to the 3'-terminal sequences of HAV was found to be optimal only when the RNA probes contained some C-terminal sequences of 3D^pol, in addition to the 3' NTR and the poly(A) sequences (65).

The poly(A) tail of picornaviruses is variable; it is the shortest in cardioviruses (35 nucleotides [nt]) and longest in aphthoviruses (100 nt) (118). That of poliovirus is about 90 nt long (146) and it is known to be genetically encoded, that is, it is transcribed from poly(U) in the minus strands (31). Spector and Baltimore have reported that a poliovirus with a poly(A) tail of less than 20 nt retains only 5% of the wild-type infectivity (126). Sarnow observed that the minimum length of the poly(A) tail on poliovirus RNA transcripts is 12 nt (121). Similar conclusions were reached by Herold and Andino, who showed that poliovirus minus-strand synthesis depends on a poly(A) tail of at least 12 nt (51a). This is exactly the same length necessary for the human PABP to interact with the 3' NTR-poly(A) in vitro (51a).

Internal cis-Acting Element (oriI)

The first cis-acting element in the coding sequences of a picornavirus RNA was discovered by McKnight and Lemon (76, 77). This RNA segment consists of a hairpin structure in the coding sequence of the capsid protein VP1 of HRV14. A similar cis-acting element was recently described by Goodfellow et al. in the coding sequence of poliovirus protein 2C [cre(2C)] (41). Although the PV1 and HRV14 cis-replicating elements (Fig. 2C) differ in sequence and structure, they have similar functions in vivo. Both elements are required in the context of the plus strand and are position independent in function, and disruption of both results in the failure to synthesize minus strands (41, 77). These similarities suggested not only that they have the same role in replication but also that other picornaviruses might contain similar elements. This was proven to be the case when a cis-acting internal RNA hairpin was identified in the coding sequence of VP2 in the *Cardiovirus* genus of TMEV and mengovirus (72). The TMEV element could be functionally exchanged with that of mengovirus but not with that of poliovirus or HRV14 (72). We have recently discovered a similar cis-replicating element in the coding sequence of 2A^pro of HRV2, a member of the *Rhinovirus* genus (Fig. 2C) (39b).

As will be shown later, the cre(2C) element of poliovirus or the cre(2A) of HRV2 have at least two possible roles. First, they offer a site of recognition and binding for 3CD^pro prior to the in vitro uridylylation of VPg by 3D^pol (39b, 99, 109). Second, they serve as a specific template in vitro for the protein priming reaction (39b, 99, 109). Therefore, the PV1 cre(2C) or the HRV2 cre(2A) hairpins might be designated as oriI, the internal origin (or origin of initiation) of minus- and/or plus-strand RNA synthesis.

The Cloverleaf at the 3' End of Minus-Strand RNA

The sequence complementary to the plus-strand cloverleaf also forms a similar structure. Although mutational analysis of this structure suggested that it is not important for RNA replication (6), the specific binding of proteins to this structure has been reported. Roehl and Semler (114) and Roehl et al. (113) found two cellular proteins (p36 and p38) that specifically bound to the poliovirus minus-strand cloverleaf at about 3 to 4 h after infection. It was shown that p38, a product of processing by 3C^pro/3CD^pro, bound to the nucleotides 5 to 10 region (plus-strand numbers) of PV1 minus-strand RNA (113). Deletion of these sequences, which reduced the binding of the protein, also rendered this RNA noninfectious in transfection experiments (113). Banerjee et al. have reported a specific binding of poliovirus protein 2C to the minus-strand cloverleaf (9). This interaction was shown to require the sequence of UGUUU in stem *a* of the minus-strand cloverleaf in the form of a double-stranded structure (9). It should be noted that the 2C polypeptide analyzed by Banerjee et al. (9) was a renatured product isolated originally from an insoluble fraction after expression in *Escherichia coli*. Pfister and

Wimmer have observed that such renatured 2C protein lacks ATPase activity (unpublished results). In contrast, a soluble fusion protein isolated also after expression in *E. coli* that exhibited strong ATPase activity failed to bind to the minus-strand cloverleaf structure (T. Pfister and E. Wimmer, unpublished results).

The IRES

The primary function of the IRES is undoubtedly to promote the translation of the picornaviral genome (57, 58, 101, 141). However, certain mutations in this structure appear to also influence RNA replication. The first such report by Borman et al. (18) described a 3-nt deletion in domain V of the polio IRES in a dicistronic poliovirus that contained the EMCV IRES between P1 and P2. This virus exhibited a phenotype in RNA replication (18). Recently, a deletion mutant in stem-loop II of the poliovirus IRES was shown to be defective both in translation and in RNA replication (55). How these mutations affect RNA replication is not yet known. This is particularly mysterious in view of the fact that the poliovirus IRES can be functionally replaced not only by the IRESs of picornaviruses such as EMCV, HRV2, and HRV14 but also by that of HCV, an RNA element that shows no apparent similarity to picornaviral IRESs (43, 141). Whether the function of the IRES is required directly during RNA synthesis or for the switch between translation and replication is not yet known.

Membranous Structures

Picornavirus RNA replication takes place in the cytoplasm of the host cell and can also occur in enucleated cells (87). Electron microscopic studies of poliovirus-infected cells revealed that most of the cytoplasmic space of the infected cell is occupied by membranous vesicles, which exhibit a rosette-like structure with the replication complex in its center (15). Vesicle induction is determined by the $2C^{ATPase}$ moiety of viral protein 2BC while the 2B domain of the precursor controls the morphology of the vesicles. These structures are derived mostly from membranes of the endoplasmic reticulum and the Golgi complex and are associated with viral proteins 2B, 2BC, and $2C^{ATPase}$ (15, 129). Protein 3AB also interacts with the membranes through the hydrophobic domain of its 3A moiety (40, 133). It is generally assumed that 3AB, through its binding to $3D^{pol}$ and $3CD^{pro}$, recruits these proteins to the replication complex, which by themselves are unable to associate with membranes (52, 142). Membranous vesicles isolated from infected cells have been shown to contain not only single-stranded RNA but also double-stranded intermediates, the RF and RI (16).

Although much information is available about the structure and protein components of vesicles in infected cells, the role of membranes in RNA replication is still not clear. It has been suggested that membranes act as a scaffold for the assembly of the replication complex or to protect the viral RNA from degradation by cellular enzymes. Alternatively, they serve to concentrate the viral proteins at the site of RNA synthesis or to physically separate the viral RNA template from other cellular mRNAs. Interestingly, recent studies suggest that the formation of the poliovirus replication complex requires coupled viral translation, vesicle production, and viral RNA synthesis (33). These and other questions about the structure and function of membranous structures in picornaviral infection will be addressed in more detail in chapter 20.

COUPLING BETWEEN VIRAL RNA TRANSLATION AND REPLICATION

Early studies with defective interfering particles (DI) have suggested that in picornaviruses translation and replication are coupled (reviewed in references 1 and 43). This hypothesis was supported by the findings of Novak and Kirkegaard, who studied the growth of replication-incompetent mutants by complementation in *trans* (91). They demonstrated that replication of poliovirus genomes whose translation was terminated from $2A^{pro}$ into the $3D^{pol}$ coding sequences could not be rescued in *trans*. A requirement to translate in *cis* could be attributed to a requirement for the *cis*-delivery of nascent proteins to the site of RNA synthesis, most likely during the first round of translation early in infection (43, 91). Alternatively, the passage of ribosomes through this region is required, altering the secondary structure of the RNA segment (91). Why there is a coupling of translation and replication is not yet understood, but it appears to be a common characteristic of plus-strand RNA viruses. This phenomenon has also been observed, for example, with cowpea mosaic virus (*Comovirus*) (136), tobacco etch virus (*Potyvirus*) (73), and mouse hepatitis virus (*Coronavirus*) (28a).

PRODUCTS OF RNA SYNTHESIS IN VITRO AND IN VIVO

RNA Synthesis In Vivo

During the first 3 h of infection the accumulation of viral RNA in the cell is exponential, followed by a 1-h linear phase during which about 80% of the total RNA is produced (reviewed in reference 108). When RNA synthesis reaches a maximum, about 2,000 to 3,000 molecules/cell/min are produced and it takes less than a minute for the synthesis of a full-length RNA. Three different species of viral RNA, all VPg-linked, can be found in the infected cell. The first species that can be detected following virus infection is the multistranded structure of the RI. About 90% of the total RI molecules contain genome-length minus strands and a varying number of complementary strands of varying length. The structures are partially double stranded. The major species of RNA in the infected cell is single-stranded RNA of plus-strand polarity that is identical to virion RNA. Viral double-stranded RNA, the RF, is fully double stranded. It is continuously formed during the infection at a relatively low rate. All minus strands are associated with RI or RF and no free minus strands are detectable in vivo. It is generally accepted that the RF is an intermediate of replication rather than an artifact of the isolation procedure (1, 141). In addition to high-molecular-weight RNAs, VPgpUpU can also be detected in the infected cells (22).

A novel system was developed by Gamarnik and Andino to study poliovirus replication in *Xenopus* oocytes (36). Microinjection of poliovirus RNA in oocytes results in a complete cycle of replication and production of infectious particles. Two cytoplasmic HeLa cell proteins (or protein complexes) are required for poliovirus replication, one for translation, the other for replication (36). *Xenopus* oocytes are also able to support the replication of mengovirus but without the need for any additional cellular extract (39). In contrast, the replication of HRV14 in this system depends on the presence of a cellular factor that is required for translation (39).

RNA Synthesis In Vitro

With Purified Proteins

When poliovirus RNA is incubated in vitro with purified $3D^{pol}$ and an oligo(U) primer, full-length negative strands can be synthesized (10). This "elongation" reaction proceeds efficiently on poly(A) (34) or any 3' polyadenylated template with no specificity for poliovirus templates. Poly(A) also serves as template for the uridylylation of VPg in vitro in reactions catalyzed by purified PV1(M) or HRV2 $3D^{pol}$ (39a, 99, 100):

$$VPg + 3D^{pol} + poly(A) + UTP + Mn^{2+}(Mg^{2+}) \rightarrow$$
$$VPgpU \rightarrow VPgpUpU \rightarrow VPg\text{-}poly(U)$$

The final product is VPg-linked poly(U), the 5' end of minus-strand RNA (89). Interestingly, when full-length poliovirus or HRV2 RNAs are used as templates in this in vitro assay instead of poly(A), the primary templates for the synthesis of VPgpUpU are the cre(2C) (41) and cre(2A) RNA (39b) hairpins, respectively (39b, 99, 100). The reactions are strongly stimulated by the addition of $3CD^{pro}$ (39b, 99, 100):

$$VPg + 3D^{pol} + cre\ RNA + 3CD^{pro} + UTP$$
$$+ Mg^{2+}(Mn^{2+}) \rightarrow VPgpU \rightarrow VPgpUpU$$

The elongation of the precursors into minus strands is inefficient (39b, 99, 100).

With Crude Replication Complexes

Crude replication complexes (CRCs) isolated from poliovirus-infected cells are active in viral RNA synthesis in vitro, and they contain all three species of viral-specific RNAs as well as viral and cellular proteins (127, 128, 135). In the presence of nucleoside triphosphates VPg is uridylylated to VPgpU and VPgpUpU, which can be chased into VPg-UUAAAACAG, the first nine nucleotides of plus-strand RNA, and into full-length plus strands (127, 128). A similar complex from HeLa cells infected with the Sabin type 1 strain of poliovirus, which is temperature sensitive (ts) for replication, is defective in the synthesis of VPgpU and VPgpUpU at the restrictive temperature, but elongation is unaffected (135). Recently the ts synthesis of the precursors was shown to be due to a Tyr73His change in the RNA polymerase protein of the Sabin type 1 strain of poliovirus (98).

Treatment of CRCs with detergent (NP40) abolishes the synthesis of VPgpUpU but has no effect on the elongation of RNA chains, suggesting that initiation is dependent on the integrity of membranous structures (128, 135). This observation contrasts with the ability of $3D^{pol}$ to uridylylate VPg in the in vitro system that lacks membranes (39a, 39b, 99, 100, 109). One possible explanation of these conflicting data is that detergent treatment does not interfere with VPg uridylylation per se, but rather with the processing of 3AB or of a larger precursor of VPg, which normally occurs in a membrane-bound form (67). Alternatively, the CRC assures high concentration of reaction partners in tightly sequestered complexes. Treatment with detergent dilutes the reaction partners below minimal concentration, an effect particularly relevant to $3D^{pol}$ (1, 95).

Translation and Replication in HeLa Cell-Free Extracts

A novel cell-free system was developed by Molla et al. in which both viral protein synthesis and RNA replication take place, resulting in the de novo synthesis of infectious poliovirus that is indistinguishable from that isolated from tissue culture (85). When poliovirus RNA is incubated in a cell-free extract of HeLa cells under the appropriate ionic conditions, the viral RNA is translated into the polyprotein, which is subsequently cleaved to yield all the viral proteins. These proteins carry out replication of the RNA, which is then encapsidated. This system has been applied by several groups to study poliovirus replication (11, 12, 51, 134). Barton et al. have shown that replication complexes isolated from such reactions contained replicative intermediate RNA and VPg-linked genome-length plus-strand RNA in large excess over minus-strand RNA (11). The initiation of minus-strand synthesis was found to require the guanidine-inhibited activity of protein $2C^{ATPase}$ and one or more soluble factors (11, 12). Since the in vitro reaction in which VPg is uridylylated on the cre(2C) template does not require either $2C^{ATPase}$ or host factors, it is possible that the function of these proteins is required prior to that step. For example, these proteins might be required at some stage of vesicle synthesis or assembly of replication complexes.

PROPOSED MODEL OF PICORNAVIRUS RNA REPLICATION

After entry of the picornavirus into the host cell, the viral RNA is used as template first for translation and then for minus-strand RNA synthesis. It is generally assumed that translation has to be terminated prior to minus-strand synthesis since the ribosomes and the RNA polymerase would otherwise have to travel on the same template but in opposite directions. Using an in vitro translation reaction of a poliovirus replicon RNA and purified $3D^{pol}$, Gamarnik and Andino have observed that the polymerase is unable to replicate the input RNA template while it is undergoing translation (37). They proposed that the switch from translation to minus-strand RNA synthesis is achieved when a critical concentration of $3CD^{pro}$ accumulates in the infected cell. Then the binding of $3CD^{pro}$ to the cloverleaf would repress viral translation by sequestering PCBP2, a host RNA-binding protein essential for poliovirus IRES function, an event that would promote minus-strand RNA synthesis. An unanswered question about this model is why the large amount of $3CD^{pro}$ in the infected cell at the peak of RNA replication is not causing a premature inhibition of the continuing translation of the viral RNA (1, 145). Recently Barton et al. (13) have reported similar experiments with the in vitro translation/replication system of poliovirus (85) and have also come to the conclusion that translating ribosomes inhibit negative-strand RNA synthesis.

Herold and Andino recently proposed a model in which the poliovirus genome circularizes prior to or during minus-strand RNA synthesis by way of an interaction of the cellular PABP with the poly(A) tail on the one hand and PCBP2/$3CD^{pro}$/5' cloverleaf on the other (51a). This model is based on an observation that PABP appears to physically interact with $3CD^{pro}$, PCBP2, and the poly(A) tail both in vitro and in vivo. Formation of the large RNP complex, presumably accompanying the circularization of the genome, was found to be required for minus-strand RNA synthesis (51a). Another potential function of the PABP-poly(A) interaction could be to prevent nonspecific uridylylation on the poly(A) tail sequences, an activity that is intrinsic to the polymerase protein (100).

Figure 3 shows the proposed model of minus-strand RNA synthesis on a circularized genome (51a). It is important to point out that it is not clear at what stage of the overall process circularization of the genome might occur or what its function might be. At least in vitro the initiation reaction itself does not require a circularized RNA and the primary template for VPg uridylylation by either the PV1(M) or HRV2 polymerase is not the poly(A) tail but the *cre*(2C) or *cre*(2A) RNAs, respectively (39b, 99).

Model of Minus-Strand RNA Synthesis

Recognition and Selection of the Viral RNA Template

Prior to the initiation of minus-strand RNA synthesis, the RNA polymerase has to recognize its own viral RNA in a pool of cellular mRNAs and then select it as the only template for transcription. As we will show below, at least one step in the recognition of the poliovirus template RNA might occur at the internal RNA hairpin [*cre*(2C)] and require the presence of 3CD^{pro} (99, 109).

Initiation of Minus-Strand Synthesis

It was more than 20 years ago when it was discovered that in poliovirus-infected cells both plus and minus strands were VPg-linked (89). Subsequently the presence of VPgpUpU was discovered in poliovirus-infected cells (22) and the synthesis of VPg-linked precursors was also observed in CRCs (127, 128, 135). These findings led to a model for the initiation of RNA synthesis in which VPg serves as the primer for the RNA polymerase (140). This model was supported by the observation that the poliovirus RNA polymerase is strictly primer dependent (34).

Only recently has it been shown directly in an in vitro reaction that 3D^{pol} of PV1(M) and HRV2 catalyzes the uridylylation of VPg on a poly(A) template yielding VPgpU and VPgpUpU, which can be elongated into VPg-linked poly(U) (39a, 100), the 5' end of minus strands (89). Although these results suggested that in vivo initiation might occur on the poly(A) tail, they could not explain the specificity of the process. The function of the poly(A) tail in the initiation reaction was further challenged when it was discovered that the uridylylation of VPg on full-length poliovirus RNA, but not on a poly(A) template, was strongly stimulated by purified 3CD^{pro} (99). Furthermore, deletion of either the poly(A) tail or the entire 3' NTR-poly(A) from full-length poliovirus RNAs had very little effect on the ability of these transcripts to serve as templates for the protein-priming reaction (99). These observations were surprising for two reasons. They showed not only that the poly(A) tail was not the primary template in full-length viral RNA but also that the 3' NTR was not the site recognized by the uridylylation complex formed by 3D^{pol}, 3CD^{pro}, VPg, and UTP.

A subsequent in vitro analysis of the *cis*-acting RNA elements of poliovirus and HRV2 has revealed that they serve as templates for the synthesis of VPgpU and VPgpUpU, in a reaction dependent on the RNA-binding

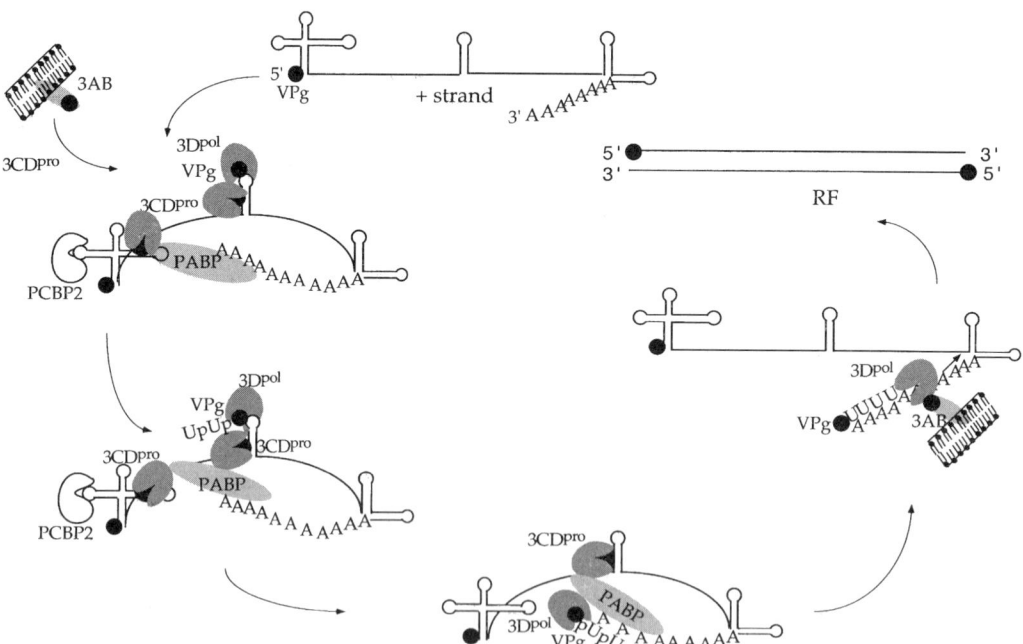

FIGURE 3 Proposed model of picornaviral minus-strand RNA synthesis. An RNP complex formed around the 5' cloverleaf interacts with the PABP bound to the 3' NTR-poly(A) resulting in a circularized genome (51a). Proteinase 3CD^{pro} cleaves membrane-bound 3AB to yield VPg and 3A. 3D^{pol}, 3CD^{pro}, and VPg form a complex with the *cre* RNA hairpin. The polymerase synthesizes VPgpU and VPgpUpU using the A$_1$A$_2$ACA sequence in the loop as template, and the complex is transferred to the 3' end of the poly(A) tail. The VPg-linked precursors then serve as primer for 3D^{pol} during the elongation step, a reaction possibly stimulated by membrane-bound 3AB.

activity of 3CD^pro (39b, 99, 109) (Fig. 3 and 4). All the known picornaviral internal *cis*-acting elements, the *cre*(2C) of PV1 (41), the *cre*(VP1) of HRV14 (76, 77), the *cre*(VP2) loop of TMEV and mengovirus (72), and the *cre*(2A) of HRV2 (39b), contain a conserved sequence of 5 nt (AAACA) either in the loop or in a bulge of the hairpin structure (Fig. 2C) (99). In addition, they are required for minus-strand synthesis (41, 77). Interestingly, the first two As in the conserved sequence of PV1(M) and HRV2 *cre* RNAs were found to be essential for the synthesis of VPgpU and of VPgpUpU, for RNA replication in vivo, and for viral viability (39b, 109). Both the PV1 *cre*(2C) and the HRV2 *cre*(2A) RNAs could be functionally exchanged in the VPg-uridylylation assay with the VP1 stem-loop of HRV14 (99), suggesting that other picornaviral internal *cre* RNAs also have the same function. It should be noted that in B-cluster enteroviruses the predicted conserved motif is AAAUG, assuming that the corresponding RNA segment in the 2C-coding region constitutes the *cis*-replicating element (41, 109).

One might ask why is it preferable for a picornavirus to use an internal site, rather than the poly(A) tail, for a template during the protein priming reaction. A simple answer to this question might be that such a process, which uses the specificity of both viral sequences and of 3CD^pro, reduces or eliminates the chance that the polymerase will use the wrong template for transcription. It is interesting to note that such a model could also account for the near absence of "negative" RI molecules in infected cells. Initiation at the internal site could not continue concurrently with minus-strand RNA synthesis. It will be interesting to see whether the replication of a number of VPg-linked plant viral RNAs that lack poly(A) tails (*Sobemovirus, Luteovirus, Enamovirus, Barnavirus*) (125) is also initiated at an internal *oriI* or at the 3' end of the plus strand.

Since VPg is always linked to an UMP in picornaviral RNAs (4, 117), one would expect that the RNA polymerase possesses strict specificity toward UTP in the nucleotidylylation reaction it catalyzes. In addition, based on the polarity of the A_1A_2ACA sequence, A_2 would be expected to serve as template nucleotide for VPgpU synthesis. Surprisingly, both expectations turned out to be incorrect. Poliovirus 3D^pol is able to covalently link GMP, CMP, or AMP to VPg on mutant templates containing C, G, or U in the first position of the A_1A_2ACA sequence, respectively, but not (<10%) when the templates contain the same nucleotides in the second position (109; A. V. Paul, E. Rieder, and E. Wimmer, submitted). The nucleotidylylated proteins can not be elongated to VPgpNpU (N is G, C, or A). These characteristics of PV1(M) 3D^pol, which are shared by HRV2 3D^pol (39b), are consistent with a "slide-back" model (reviewed in reference 119) for the synthesis of VPgpUpU. According to this model, A_1 of the A_1A_2ACA sequence of PV *cre*(2C) RNA is the template nucleotide for the linkage of UMP to VPg by 3D^pol (Fig. 4; see Fig. 6A). This is followed by the slide-back of VPgpU to hydrogen bond with A_2. The second UMP is then added again by 3D^pol on the A_1 template nucleotide.

The question of which precursor polypeptide supplies VPg for the uridylylation reaction is still unresolved. It has

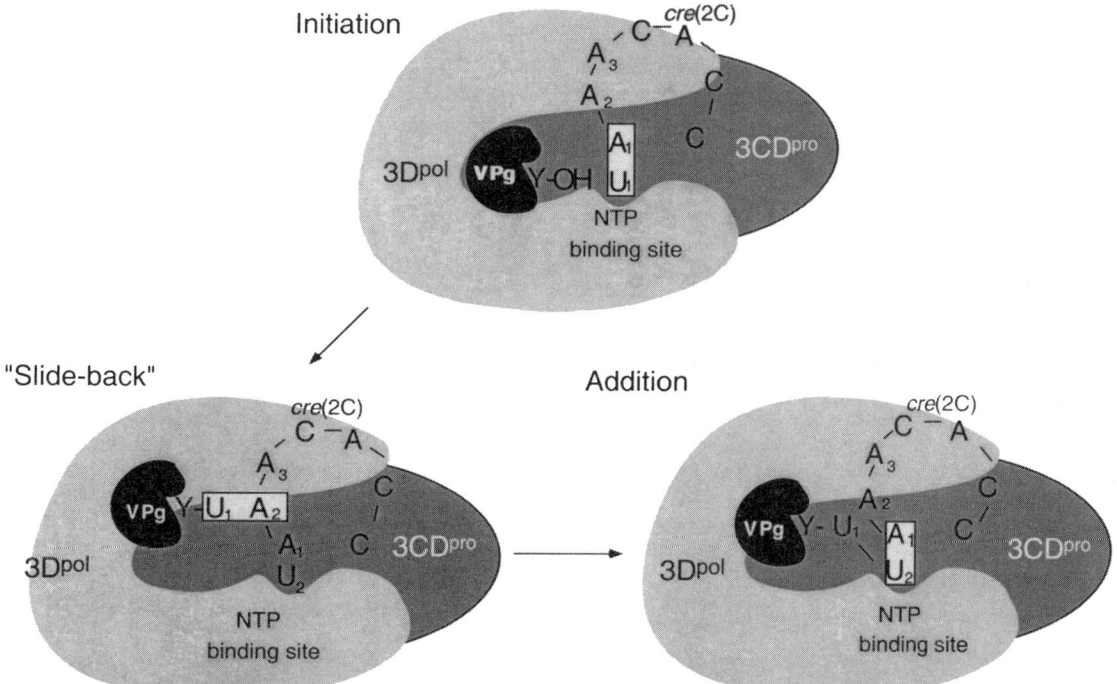

FIGURE 4 Slide-back model of VPgpUpU synthesis by PV1(M) 3D^pol. Proteins 3D^pol, 3CD^pro, and VPg form a complex with the PV1(M) *cre*(2C) RNA hairpin. Using A_1 in the A_1A_2ACA sequence of the loop as template, the complementary nucleotide is selected and 3D^pol catalyzes the formation of a phosphodiester bond between UMP and the hydroxyl group of tyrosine in VPg. VPgpU then slides back and hydrogen bonds with A_2 and the second UMP is added on the A_1 template nucleotide.

been generally accepted that membrane-bound 3AB serves this function following its cleavage by 3CD^{pro} to 3A and VPg (1, 40, 108, 133). However, recent studies by Towner et al. suggest that in vivo a larger P3-derived polypeptide such as 3ABC or 3BCD might be the true precursor (134). These authors observed that a mutation in 3AB, causing a severe replication defect, could be efficiently complemented in vivo in *trans* by providing a P3 precursor but not the mature 3AB polypeptide. Another unanswered question concerns the identity of the protein that is uridylylated in vivo. Although VPg is a good substrate for uridylylation in vitro, for optimal activity it is required at 50-fold higher concentration than the polymerase protein (39a, 39b, 99, 100). This suggests the possibility that in vivo a precursor of VPg, with higher affinity to either the RNA or the polymerase than the VPg peptide itself, might be the true substrate for the reaction. At least in the case of cardioviruses this possibility is supported by the observation that during viral infection both VPg and large precursors (3ABC, 2C3AB) can be labeled with ^{32}P (Aminev and Palmenberg, Abstr. XI Meet. Eur. Study Group Mol. Biol. Picornaviruses, 2000, abstr. no. D06). These large precursors are relatively stable intermediates of polyprotein processing during the replication of cardioviruses, unlike in the case of enteroviruses (Aminev and Palmenberg, Abstr. XI Meet. Eur. Study Group Mol. Biol. Picornaviruses, 2000, abstr. no. D06). It should also be noted that uridylylated 3AB or 3ABC or P3 polypeptides have not been found in poliovirus-infected cells (E. Wimmer, unpublished observations).

Translocation of Precursors to the 3′ End of the Plus Strand

It is reasonable to assume that the precursors would be released from the *ori*I RNA and translocated to the 3′ end of the plus strand prior to elongation into minus strands. Unfortunately, nothing is known about this process, and one can only speculate about how this might occur. Whether PABP or PABP/3CD^{pro} (51a) is involved in positioning the poly(A) tail near the *cre*(2C), as depicted on the model (Fig. 3), is not yet known. It is likely that 3CD^{pro} is involved in binding the 3D^{pol}-VPg complex to the template during the protein-priming reaction since neither 3D^{pol} nor VPg has a high affinity to this RNA structure (109). The interaction of 3D^{pol} and VPg with each other and with 3CD^{pro} has been previously demonstrated (142). Therefore, one might expect that either 3CD^{pro} has to be autoprocessed to release the other proteins or that 3D^{pol} would have to undergo a conformational change so that together with VPgpUpU it can be released from the 3CD^{pro}/*cre*(2C) complex and transferred to the 3′ end of the poly(A) tail. The 3′ NTR might provide a specific binding site for 3D^{pol} and/or 3CD^{pro} so that VPgpUpU can be delivered exclusively to the viral poly(A) tail. Whether a direct physical interaction occurs between the 3′ NTR-poly(A) tail and the *cre*(2C) hairpin during this stage of replication remains to be determined. In this context it is interesting to point out that an interaction between an internal *cis*-acting RNA element and the 3′ NTR of a potyvirus RNA genome has been previously reported. Tobacco etch virus, a member of the picornavirus superfamily, contains a *cis*-acting RNA element in its genome, which forms a series of hairpin structures involving RNA both from the coding sequences of its coat protein (CP) and the 3′ NTR (44, 73). Interestingly, this internal *cis*-acting element in the CP domain has a strong similarity to that of the picornaviruses in that it contains an essential stretch of AAACA sequence in a bulge of one of the hairpins. Whether this sequence has anything to do with a protein-priming reaction during potyvirus replication is not yet known.

Elongation of VPgpUpU into Minus-Strand RNA

It is a general characteristic of in vitro protein-primed nucleic acid synthesis that nucleotidylylated precursors are in excess over elongated species of viral DNAs or RNAs (53, 100, 119). Although elongation of poliovirus VPgpUpU into VPg-linked poly(U) on a poly(A) template occurs quite readily in vitro (100), no efficient elongation into minus strands has yet been achieved when the precursors are produced on the *cre*(2C) hairpin of the polioviral RNA template (99). Therefore, it is likely that the problem is with the transfer of the precursors to the poly(A) tail rather than with the elongation step itself. There are at least two possible explanations why the translocation/elongation is inefficient in the in vitro reaction. The simplest is that in addition to 3D^{pol}, 3CD^{pro}, and VPg other viral or cellular factors are required. Second is that only those RNA molecules that have been translated are able to function in these processes. This possibility is supported by the finding that a mutation in the *cre*(2C) RNA can not be complemented in *trans* (109).

The elongation step most likely involves a structural change of the enzyme. The affinity of the polymerase for its template is expected to be relatively high during the protein-priming step but subsequently low so that it can move along its template during the elongation of the primer. The structural change in the polymerase might, for example, involve a dissociation of oligomers (45, 95) into monomers. Both the RNA-binding (95) and uridylylating activity of 3D^{pol} (39a, 39b, 99, 100) are known to be enhanced under conditions that favor oligomerization.

Of all the poliovirus proteins, only 3AB has been shown to have a stimulatory effect on the elongation reaction by 3D^{pol}. In vitro 3AB stimulates RNA synthesis by 3D^{pol} when an oligonucleotide primer is used on a poly(A) or an RNA template (67, 96, 106, 107). The stimulatory effect is only seen when the enzyme concentration is low (96) and it appears to be due to a stabilization of some primer-template complexes (107). Whether 3AB stimulates the elongation of VPg-linked oligonucleotides during minus-strand RNA synthesis in vivo remains to be determined. Another unresolved question concerns the identity of the enzyme that is responsible for the unwinding of the highly structured regions in picornaviral RNAs, such as the 3′ NTR, the *ori*I hairpin, or the 5′ NTR, during minus-strand synthesis. Cho et al. have provided one possible answer by showing that in vitro 3D^{pol} itself has an unwinding activity while in the process of elongation (20).

Plus-Strand RNA Synthesis

In poliovirus-infected cells, the overall ratio of plus to minus strands is about 50:1, suggesting that each minus strand serves as template for the synthesis of many plus strands (92). This is in agreement with the finding that only the RF and the RI contain minus strands while free minus strands are never observed. Interestingly, the existence of circular forms of RF in EMCV-infected cells has been demonstrated, but their role in replication is not known (116). It is generally accepted that the RF is a true intermediate in the replication process rather than an isolation artifact (1, 141). Figure 5 illustrates the proposed model of picornaviral plus-strand RNA synthesis starting from the double-stranded RF.

Initiation of Plus-Strand Synthesis

It is reasonable to assume that the first step in the initiation reaction is again the uridylylation of VPg. Since there is a large excess of plus-strand RNA over minus-strand RNA in infected cells, it is conceivable that the *cre*(2C) would produce an excess of VPgpUpU waiting to be used for initiation of plus-strand RNA also. This scenario is appealing since it does not require the presence of two mechanisms for VPgpUpU synthesis. However, since the 5' and 3' ends of the picornaviral genome are very different, two different mechanisms might exist for the synthesis of the VPg-linked precursors. It is possible that a distinct uridylylation reaction takes place on a 3'-terminal segment of the minus strand (Fig. 5). This is supported by the observation that the integrity of the 5'-terminal plus-strand sequences is important both for plus-strand and for minus-strand RNA synthesis (5, 6, 37). Although most RNA templates, except the mRNA (90) in the infected cell, are VPg-linked (89), the function, if any, of the genome-linked VPg in plus-strand RNA synthesis is not yet known. There is no need to postulate a distant internal site as template for uridylylation, since, unlike the poly(A) tail, the minus-strand cloverleaf contains virus-specific sequences. The use of such an internal site would also require an extensive unwinding of the RF prior to plus-strand synthesis.

The two 3'-terminal As of the minus-strand cloverleaf are potential templates for the synthesis of VPgpU and VPgpUpU (Fig. 5). These same two As (Us at the 5' end of plus strand), however, can be deleted from poliovirus (47) and CBV3 RNAs (61), but not from HAV RNA (47). Upon transfection into mammalian cells, poliovirus and CVB3 progeny have regained the two terminal Us. These results could be interpreted to mean that the precursors are made in a template-independent reaction. This, however, is unlikely since in vitro $3D^{pol}$ is unable to catalyze uridylylation of VPg in the absence of a template (100). Alternatively, the two terminal As could be regenerated by polyadenylation of the 3' end of the minus strand, an activity intrinsic to $3D^{pol}$ in vitro (88). Finally, uridylylation might occur at another site in the cloverleaf followed by translocation to the 3' end of the minus strand, deriving specificity only from RNA/protein interactions rather than from sequence complementarity of precursor and template. For example, a potential site for template is two adjacent As in a well-conserved AAACA sequence in stem *a* of the minus-strand cloverleaf, whose integrity is required for viral viability (6). These same nucleotides form the complement of the UGUUU sequence predicted by Banerjee et al. to be required for 2C binding (9). The use of either the two terminal As or the site in stem *a* would require only minimal unwinding of the cloverleaf prior to the protein-priming reaction.

How the end of the double-stranded structure in the RF would become destabilized or unwound is not yet known. Protein $2C^{ATPase}$, which has a conserved helicase motif and ATPase activity (Fig. 5) (42, 103, 111), was initially predicted to carry out this reaction. However, no helicase activity has yet been found to be associated with this protein (103). Alternatively, the destabilizing may be achieved not

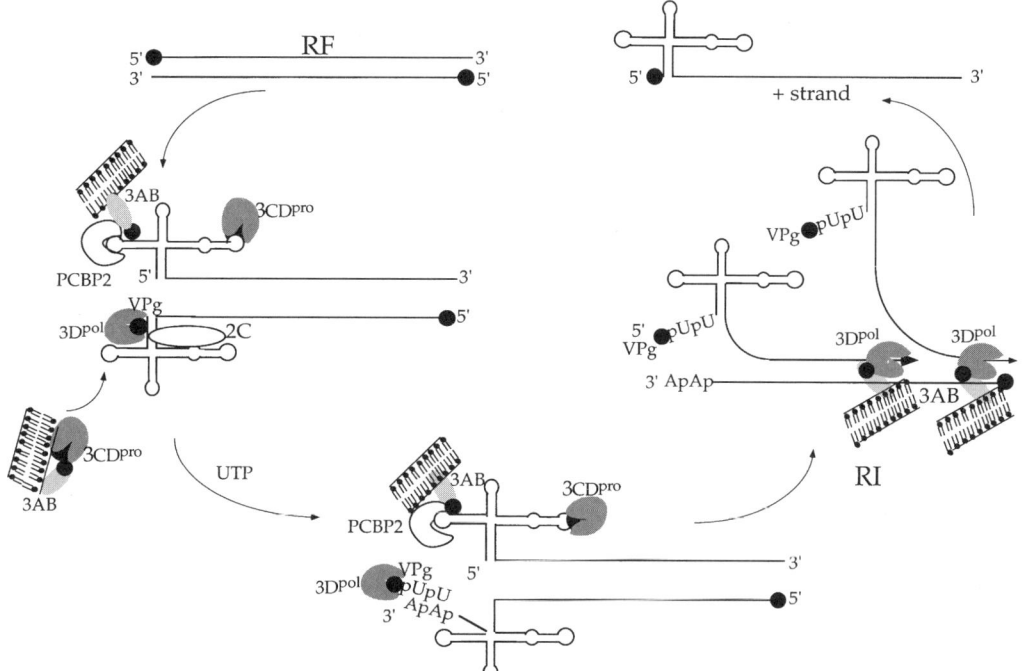

FIGURE 5 Proposed model of picornaviral plus-strand RNA synthesis. The end of the RF is unwound by the binding of PCBP2/3CD^{pro} and 3AB/3CD^{pro} to the plus strand and of 2C to the minus strand of the 5' cloverleaf. 3CD^{pro} catalyzes the cleavage of membrane-bound 3AB to 3A and VPg, and 3CD^{pro} undergoes autoprocessing. The polymerase synthesizes VPgpUpU using the 3'-terminal two As of the minus strand as template. The precursors are elongated into plus strands by the polymerase, possibly using the stimulatory activity of membrane-bound 3AB.

A.

	Picornavirus 3D^{pol}	Phage Φ29 DP
Template	5' A A A C A 3'	5' T A C T T T 3'
Protein-priming	5' A A A C A 3' U p-VPg	5' T A C T T T 3' A p-TP
"Slide-back"	5' A A A C A 3' U p-VPg	5' T A C T T T 3' A p-TP
Elongation (addition)	5' A A A C A 3' U U p-VPg	5' T A C T T T 3' A A p-TP

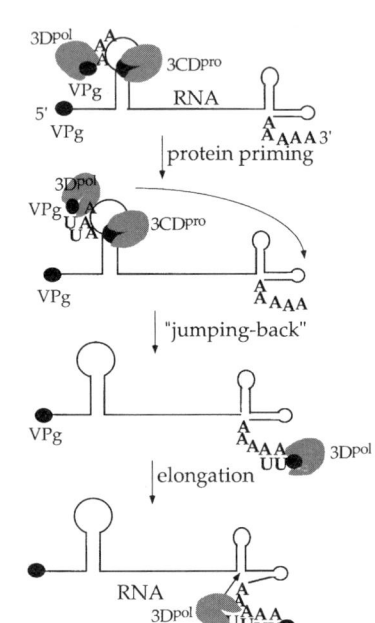

B. Picornavirus minus strand RNA

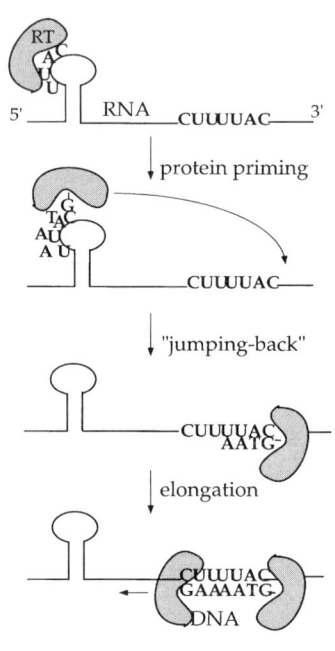

Hepatitis B virus cDNA

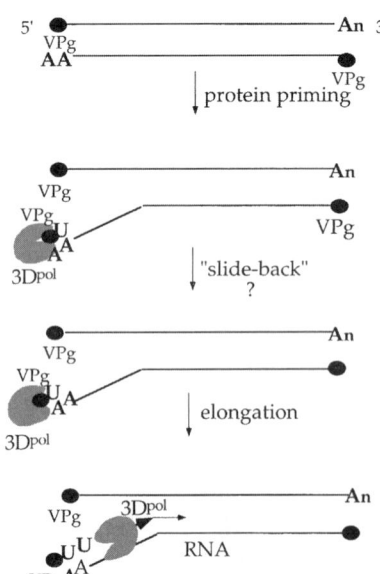

C. Picornavirus plus strand RNA

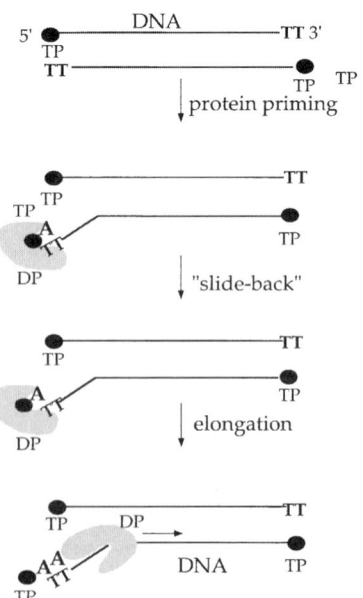

Phage Φ29 DNA

with a helicase but rather with proteins binding near the end of the RF, thereby separating the strands and stabilizing the structures of both the plus- and minus-strand cloverleaf structures (1, 5, 145). This possibility was suggested by the finding that the integrity of the plus-strand cloverleaf is required for plus-strand RNA synthesis (5). In addition, it has been shown that 3CD^{pro} binds to the plus-strand cloverleaf when complexed either with 3AB (49, 144) or PCBP2 (38, 94) while 2C and an unidentified cellular protein p38 bind to the minus-strand structure (9, 113, 114). It is interesting to note that DNA polymerases (adenovirus and phages Φ29 or PRD1), which use their double-stranded DNA genome as the template for protein priming, also do not use a helicase but rather helix-destabilizing proteins to unwind the end of their DNAs (119 and references therein).

It has also been suggested that a cellular helicase might assist in unwinding the RF since a double-stranded picornavirus RNA is infectious (86). Interestingly, the RF is noninfectious in enucleated cells although these cells can normally replicate single-stranded RNA (87). These observations might be interpreted to mean that the function of a nuclear protein is involved in the unwinding of the RF (1).

The exact source of the 3D^{pol} and VPg molecules used in the protein-priming step is not yet known. One possibility is that these proteins are produced following proteolytic cleavage of the 3CD^{pro} and 3AB molecules, which previously bound as a complex to the plus-strand cloverleaf (5, 49, 144). Alternatively, additional 3CD^{pro} and 3AB molecules are recruited for this purpose (Fig. 5). In either case, in vitro studies have shown that 3AB stimulates the autoprocessing of 3CD^{pro} to yield 3D^{pol} and 3C^{pro} (83) and 3CD^{pro} cleaves membrane-bound 3AB to 3A and VPg (67). That either 3AB or a 3AB-containing polypeptide is the precursor of VPg is supported by two lines of evidence. First, mutations engineered into the hydrophobic and membrane-binding domain of 3A cause defects in plus-strand RNA synthesis (40). Second, enviroxime, an antiviral compound that inhibits the replication of rhinoviruses and enteroviruses, and targets the 3A protein, specifically inhibits both initiation and elongation of plus-strand RNA in infected cells (50).

Elongation of VPgpUpU into Plus-Strand RNA

Elongation in vitro of an oligonucleotide primer on a minus-strand RNA template into full-length plus-strand RNA has not yet been observed. Similarly, there is nothing known about the steps involved in the elongation of VPgpUpU into plus-strand RNA. If the VPg-linked precursors were made at a distant location, then a translocation from that distant site to the 3' end would also be required prior to elongation.

It could be hypothesized that initiation of minus-strand synthesis on plus strands can only occur once, that is, if double-stranded RNA is not a substrate for minus-strand synthesis. On the other hand, protein priming near the end of the genome would permit multiple initiations before completion of a plus strand resulting in a RI molecule that is mainly double stranded (Fig. 5). This would lead to the observed excess of plus strands over minus strands during genome replication.

COMPARISON OF PROTEIN-PRIMED RNA AND DNA REPLICATION

Several stages in the process of picornaviral RNA replication are remarkably similar to protein-primed DNA synthesis by the DNA polymerases of adenovirus, bacteriophages Φ29, PRD1, and Cp-1 (59, 74, 80, 119), or the reverse transcriptase (RT) of hepatitis B virus (HBV) (53, 122). During initiation of picornaviral minus-strand RNA synthesis the slide-back mechanism for the synthesis of VPgpUpU (Fig. 3) is to a large extent the same as that used by the DNA polymerase of phage Φ29 for the deoxyadenylylation of its terminal protein (TP) (Fig. 6A). Poliovirus 3D^{pol} uses A_1 of the 5'-A_1A_2ACA-3' sequence in cre(2C) (109; A. V. Paul, E. Rieder, and E. Wimmer, submitted) while phage Φ29 DNA polymerase uses T_1 of the 5'-TACTT$_1$T$_2$-3' sequence (80, 119) as the template for the attachment of the first nucleotide to the terminal protein. There is a slide-back (3' → 5') of the nucleotidylylated proteins to the adjacent positions (VPgpU to A_2 and TPdA to T_2) followed by the addition of the second nucleotide using again position 1 (A_1 and T_1, respectively) as the template. One difference between the two systems is that while 3D^{pol} uses the internal cre RNA as template for the nucleotidylylation reaction, the DNA polymerases use sequences at the 3' end of their partially opened double-stranded DNAs. As a consequence of the difference between the location of the template nucleotides, elongation of VPgpUpU on the cre hairpin is aborted, but the elongation of TP-dAdA on the DNA template continues. It is generally assumed that the functions of the slide-back (or jump-back) mechanism used by the bacteriophage DNA polymerases are to regenerate the 5' end of their linear DNA strands and to enhance the specificity of the reaction (59, 74, 80, 119). One might speculate that the slide-back mechanism is used by 3D^{pol} to overcome the problem created by the enzyme's lack of strict nucleotide

FIGURE 6 Comparison of protein-primed RNA and DNA synthesis. (A) Initiation of picornaviral minus-strand RNA synthesis and phage Φ29 DNA synthesis. The slide-back mechanism is used by the picornaviral RNA polymerase and by phage Φ29 DNA polymerase (80) for the synthesis of the dinucleotidylylated protein precursors. Details of the mechanism are described in the text. (B) Picornaviral minus-strand RNA synthesis and HBV cDNA synthesis. Both viral polymerases use an internal RNA hairpin as the template for the protein-priming reaction and the nucleotidylylated proteins are translocated to the 3' end of the plus strand where they are elongated into the complementary strands (53, 99, 122). (C) Picornaviral plus-strand RNA synthesis and phage Φ29 DNA synthesis (80). The end of the double-stranded template is first unwound by the binding of proteins to the plus and minus strands. The viral polymerases use the 3' end of their RNA/DNA strand as template for the nucleotidylylation reaction. The precursors are elongated into complementary RNA/DNA strands. RT, reverse transcriptase; DP, DNA polymerase; TP, terminal protein.

specificity in the nucleotidylylation reaction. Without a proofreading activity 3D^{pol} would not be able to remove the incorrect nucleotide from VPgpN (N is A or C or G). The slide-back step, however, would ensure that a mutant VPgpN is not elongated since N would not hydrogen bond with A$_2$.

The overall process of picornaviral minus-strand RNA synthesis might resemble protein-primed cDNA synthesis by the reverse transcriptase of HBV (Fig. 6B) (53, 122). Both of these viruses use an internal RNA hairpin as template for the nucleotidylylation of a viral protein (VPg for PV1 and RT for HBV) and for synthesis of a short oligonucleotide (UU for PV1, GTAA for HBV) attached to the hydroxyl group of a tyrosine. The second step in cDNA synthesis, and possibly also in RNA synthesis, involves the translocation of the nucleotidylylated proteins to or near the 3' end of the plus strand. This is followed by the elongation of the protein-linked primer into minus strands by the polymerase. The mechanism of transfer and what provides the specificity of this process are not yet known. Clearly, the short homology between the donor and acceptor sites is not sufficient to specify the site of translocation. For HBV RT it has been shown that sequences far upstream of the attachment site are necessary for either the transfer or elongation reaction (122). Both viral polymerases recruit additional proteins(s) for optimal protein priming and polymer synthesis. Poliovirus 3D^{pol} uses 3CD^{pro} (99, 109) and HBV RT requires a chaperone complex of cellular proteins (53, 122).

The proposed model of picornaviral plus-strand RNA synthesis might resemble protein-primed DNA synthesis catalyzed by the polymerases of adenovirus or bacteriophages Φ29, PRD1, and Cp-1 (Fig. 6C) (59, 74, 80, 119). These processes commence on a partially opened double-stranded structure and the polymerases use sequences near the 3' end of their DNA/RNA strands as templates for the nucleotidylylation reaction. As mentioned above, the DNA polymerases use a slide-back or jump-back mechanism during the initiation of protein-primed DNA synthesis (Fig. 6A). In comparison, picornaviral plus-strand RNA synthesis might be initiated by the uridylylation of VPg by 3D^{pol} on the two 3' terminal As of the minus strand in the partially opened RF. Whether the slide-back mechanism is used for the initiation of picornaviral plus-strand RNA synthesis remains to be determined.

CONCLUDING REMARKS

Progress in the field of picornavirus RNA replication during the past 35 years has been slow, and the work has proved to be exceedingly difficult. Recently a great deal of information has accumulated on the subject of viral factors required for replication. In addition, there has been progress in understanding the specificity of the viral template and the protein-priming reaction used for the initiation of minus-strand RNA synthesis. In the introduction I have mentioned that picornaviruses appear to have developed ingenious ways to overcome the problems caused by the peculiar nature of their plus-stranded linear genomes. By utilizing an internal RNA hairpin for the synthesis of the primer for minus-strand RNA synthesis, the RNA polymerase might solve the problem caused by the presence of the nonspecific poly(A) sequences at the 3' end of its genome. In view of this, it can be understood why the enzyme would select a protein rather than an oligonucleotide primer for minus-strand RNA synthesis. VPg with only two nucleotides attached to it, and in a complex with 3D^{pol} (and/or other proteins), could be easily removed from the internal location and transferred to the 3' end of the poly(A) tail.

Among the many unanswered questions remain the role of host factors, what provides specificity to the transfer of the VPg-linked precursors to the poly(A) tail, and where the synthesis of plus strands is initiated. If it is indeed true that translation, replication, and vesicle formation are all coupled in vivo, then reconstitution of an in vitro replication system from purified protein components will be very difficult. It is likely that from now on more of the information will be derived from complex and in vivo-like systems such as the unique cell-free translation/replication system. It is hoped that in the future the combination of knowledge gained from all the genetic and biochemical approaches will lead to further insights into the mechanism of picornaviral RNA replication.

I thank E. Wimmer for a critical reading of this manuscript.

NOTED ADDED IN PROOF

Recently, evidence has been presented that *cre*(2C)-dependent uridylylation is required for synthesis of poliovirus positive-strand but not negative-strand RNA (K. E. Murray, T. R. Lyons, A. W. Roberts, and D. J. Barton; B. J. Morasco, L. S. Silvestri, and J. B. Flanegan; XII Meet. Eur. Study Group Mol. Biol. Picornaviruses, March 2002). At the same meeting, another group (Y. Yang, R. Rijnbrand, E. Wimmer, A. Paul, A. Martin, and S. Lemon) presented evidence that the sequence required for HRV14 *cre* function is GXXXAAAXXXXXA and not the AAACA sequence indicated in Fig. 2C of this chapter. Our recent studies indicate that the same motif is also required for poliovirus *cre*(2C) function (J. Yin, A. Paul, and E. Wimmer, in preparation).

REFERENCES

1. **Agol, V. I., A. V. Paul, and E. Wimmer.** 1999. Paradoxes of the replication of picornaviral genomes. *Virus Res.* **62:**129–147.
2. **Aldabe, R., A. Barco, and L. Carrasco.** 1996. Membrane permeabilization by poliovirus proteins 2B and 2BC. *J. Biol. Chem.* **271:**23134–23137.
3. **Aldabe, R., and L. Carrasco.** 1995. Induction of membrane proliferation by poliovirus protein 2C and 2BC. *Biochem. Biophys. Res. Commun.* **206:**64–76.
4. **Ambros, V., and D. Baltimore.** 1978. Protein is linked to the 5' end of poliovirus RNA by a phosphodiester linkage to tyrosine. *J. Biol. Chem.* **253:**5263–5266.
5. **Andino, R., G. E. Rieckhof, P. L. Achacoso, and D. Baltimore.** 1993. Poliovirus RNA synthesis utilizes an RNP complex formed around the 5' end of viral RNA. *EMBO J.* **12:**3587–3598.
6. **Andino, R., G. E. Rieckhof, and D. Baltimore.** 1990. A functional ribonucleoprotein complex forms around the 5' end of poliovirus RNA. *Cell* **63:**369–380.
7. **Arnold, J. J., and C. E. Cameron.** 1999. Poliovirus RNA-dependent RNA polymerase (3D^{pol}) is sufficient for template switching in vitro. *J. Biol. Chem.* **274:**2706–2716.
8. **Arnold, J. J., S. K. B. Ghosh, and C. E. Cameron.** 1999. Poliovirus RNA-dependent RNA polymerase (3D^{pol}). Divalent cation modulation of primer, template, and nucleotide selection. *J. Biol. Chem.* **274:**37060–37069.
9. **Banerjee, R., A. Echeverri, and A. Dasgupta.** 1997. Poliovirus-encoded 2C polypeptide specifically binds to the 3'-terminal sequences of viral negative-strand RNA. *J. Virol.* **71:**9570–9578.

10. Baron, M. H., and D. Baltimore. 1982. In vitro copying of viral positive strand RNA by poliovirus replicase. Characterization of the reaction and its products. *J. Biol. Chem.* **257:**12359–12366.
11. Barton, D. J., E. P. Black, and J. B. Flanegan. 1995. Complete replication of poliovirus in vitro: preinitiation RNA replication complexes require soluble cellular factors for the synthesis of VPg-linked RNA. *J. Virol.* **69:**5516–5527.
12. Barton, D. J., and J. B. Flanegan. 1997. Synchronous replication of poliovirus RNA: initiation of negative-strand RNA synthesis requires the guanidine-inhibited activity of protein 2C. *J. Virol.* **71:**8482–8489.
13. Barton, D. J., B. J. Morasco, and J. B. Flanegan. 1999. Translating ribosomes inhibit poliovirus negative-strand RNA synthesis. *J. Virol.* **73:**10104–10112.
14. Bienz, K., D. Egger, Y. Rasser, and W. Bossart. 1983. Intracellular distribution of poliovirus proteins and the induction of virus-specific cytoplasmic structures. *Virology* **131:**39–48.
15. Bienz, K., D. Egger, M. Troxler, and L. Pasamontes. 1990. Structural organization of poliovirus RNA replication is mediated by viral proteins of the P2 genomic region. *J. Virol.* **64:**1156–1163.
16. Bienz, K., D. Egger, T. Pfister, and M. Troxler. 1992. Structural and functional characterization of the poliovirus replication complex. *J. Virol.* **66:**2740–2747.
17. Blyn, L. B., K. M. Swiderek, O. Richards, D. C. Stahl, B. L. Semler, and E. Ehrenfeld. 1996. Poly(rC) binding protein 2 binds to stem-loop IV of the poliovirus RNA 5' noncoding region: identification by automated liquid chromatography-tandem mass spectrometry. *Proc. Natl. Acad. Sci. USA* **93:**11115–11120.
18. Borman, A. M., F. G. Deliat, and K. M. Kean. 1994. Sequences within the poliovirus internal ribosome entry segment control viral RNA synthesis. *EMBO J.* **13:**3149–3157.
19. Cao, X., R. J. Kuhn, and E. Wimmer. 1993. Replication of poliovirus RNA containing two VPg coding sequences leads to a specific deletion event. *J. Virol.* **67:**5572–5578.
20. Cho, M. W., O. C. Richards, T. M. Dmitrieva, V. Agol, and E. Ehrenfeld. 1993. RNA duplex unwinding activity of poliovirus RNA-dependent RNA polymerase 3D^{pol}. *J. Virol.* **67:**3010–3018.
21. Cho, M. W., N. Teterina, D. Egger, K. Bienz, and E. Ehrenfeld. 1994. Membrane rearrangement and vesicle induction by recombinant poliovirus 2C and 2BC in human cells. *Virology* **202:**129–145.
22. Crawford, N. M., and D. Baltimore. 1983. Genome-linked protein VPg of poliovirus is present as free VPg and VPgpUpU in poliovirus-infected cells. *Proc. Natl. Acad. Sci. USA* **80:**7452–7455.
23. Crowther, D., and J. L. Melnick. 1961. Studies on the inhibitory action of guanidine on poliovirus multiplication in cell cultures. *Virology* **15:**65–74.
24. Cuconati, A., W. Xiang, F. Lahser, T. Pfister, and E. Wimmer. 1998. A protein linkage map of the P2 nonstructural proteins of poliovirus. *J. Virol.* **72:**1297–1307.
25. Cui, T., and A. G. Porter. 1995. Localization of binding site for encephalomyocarditis virus RNA polymerase in the 3'-noncoding region of the viral RNA. *Nucleic Acids Res.* **23:**377–382.
26. Cui, T., S. Sankar, and A. G. Porter. 1993. Binding of encephalomyocarditis virus RNA polymerase to the 3'-noncoding region of the viral RNA is specific and requires the 3'-poly(A) tail. *J. Biol. Chem.* **268:**26093–26098.
27. Das, S., and A. Dasgupta. 1993. Identification of the cleavage site and determinants required for poliovirus 3C^{pro}-catalyzed cleavage of human TATA-binding transcription factor TBP. *J. Virol.* **67:**3326–3331.
28. Datta, U., and A. Dasgupta. 1994. Expression and subcellular localization of poliovirus VPg-precursor protein 3AB in eukaryotic cells: evidence for glycosylation in vitro. *J. Virol.* **68:**4468–4477.
28a. De Groot, R. J., R. G. Van Der Most, and W. J. M. Spaan. 1992. The fitness of defective interfering murine coronavirus DI-a and its derivatives is decreased by nonsense and frameshift mutations. *J. Virol.* **66:**5898–5905.
29. Doedens, J. R., T. H. Giddings, Jr., and K. Kirkegaard. 1997. Inhibition of endoplasmic reticulum-to-Golgi traffic by poliovirus protein 3A: genetic and ultrasound analysis. *J. Virol.* **71:**9054–9064.
30. Doedens, J. R., and K. Kirkegaard. 1995. Inhibition of cellular protein secretion by poliovirus proteins 2B and 2BC. *EMBO J.* **14:**894–907.
31. Dorsch-Haesler, K., Y. Yogo, and E. Wimmer. 1975. Evidence from in vitro RNA synthesis that poly(A) of the poliovirus genome is genetically encoded. *J. Virol.* **16:**1512–1517.
32. Echeverri, A. C., and A. Dasgupta. 1995. Amino terminal regions of poliovirus 2C protein mediate membrane binding. *Virology* **208:**540–553.
33. Egger, D., N. Teterina, E. Ehrenfeld, and K. Bienz. 2000. Formation of the poliovirus replication complex requires coupled viral translation, vesicle production, and viral RNA synthesis. *J. Virol.* **74:**6570–6580.
34. Flanegan, J. B., and D. Baltimore. 1977. Poliovirus-specific primer-dependent RNA polymerase able to copy poly(A). 1977. *Proc. Natl. Acad. Sci. USA* **74:**3677–3680.
35. Forss, S., and H. Schaller. 1982. A tandem repeat gene in a picornavirus. *Nucleic Acids Res.* **10:**6441–6450.
36. Gamarnick, A. V., and R. Andino. 1996. Replication of poliovirus in Xenopus oocytes requires two human factors. *EMBO J.* **15:**5988–5998.
37. Gamarnik, A. V., and R. Andino. 1998. Switch from translation to RNA replication in a positive-stranded RNA virus. *Genes Dev.* **12:**2293–2304.
38. Gamarnik, A. V., and R. Andino. 2000. Interactions of viral protein 3CD and poly(rC) binding protein with the 5' untranslated region of the poliovirus genome. *J. Virol.* **74:**2219–2226.
39. Gamarnik, A. V., N. Boddeker, and R. Andino. 2000. Translation and replication of human rhinovirus type 14 and mengovirus in Xenopus oocytes. *J. Virol.* **74:**11983–11987.
39a. Gerber, K., E. Wimmer, and A. V. Paul. 2001. Biochemical and genetic studies of the initiation of human rhinovirus 2 RNA replication: purification and enzymatic analysis of the RNA-dependent RNA polymerase 3D^{pol}. *J. Virol.* **75:**10969–10978.
39b. Gerber, K., E. Wimmer, and A. V. Paul. 2001. Biochemical and genetic studies of the initiation of human rhinovirus 2 RNA replication: identification of a *cis*-replicating element in the coding sequence of 2A^{pro}. *J. Virol.* **75:**10979–10990.
40. Giachetti, C., S. S. Hwang, and B. L. Semler. 1992. Cis-acting lesions targeted to the hydrophobic domain of a poliovirus membrane protein involved in RNA replication. *J. Virol.* **66:**6045–6057.
41. Goodfellow, I., Y. Chaudhry, A. Richardson, J. Meredith, J. W. Almond, W. Barclay, and D. J. Evans. 2000. Identification of a *cis*-acting replication element within the poliovirus coding region. *J. Virol.* **74:**4590–4600.
42. Gorbalenya, A. E., E. V. Koonin, and Y. I. Wolf. 1990. A new superfamily of putative NTP-binding domains encoded by genomes of small DNA and RNA viruses. *FEBS Lett.* **262:**145–148.
43. Gromeier, M., E. Wimmer, and A. E. Gorbalenya. 1999. Genetics, pathogenesis and evolution of picornaviruses, p. 287–343. *In* E. Domingo, R. Webster, and J. Holland (ed.), *Origin and Evolution of Viruses.* Academic Press, San Diego, Calif.
44. Haldeman-Cahill, R., J.-A. Daros, and J. C. Carrington. 1998. Secondary structures in the capsid coding sequence

and 3' nontranslated region involved in amplification of the tobacco etch virus genome. *J. Virol.* **72:**4072–4079.
45. **Hansen, J. L., A. M. Long, and S. C. Schultz.** 1997. Structure of the RNA-dependent RNA polymerase of poliovirus. *Structure* **5:**1109–1122.
46. **Harmon, S. A., S. U. Emerson, Y. K. Huang, D. F. Summers, and E. Ehrenfeld.** 1995. Hepatitis A viruses with deletions in the 2A gene are infectious in cultured cells and marmosets. *J. Virol.* **69:**5576–5581.
47. **Harmon, S. A., O. C. Richards, D. F. Summers, and E. Ehrenfeld.** 1991. The 5'-terminal nucleotides of hepatitis A virus RNA, but not poliovirus RNA, are required for infectivity. *J. Virol.* **65:**2757–2760.
48. **Harris, K. S., C. U. T. Hellen, and E. Wimmer.** 1990. Proteolytic processing in the replication of picornaviruses. *Semin. Virol.* **1:**323–333.
49. **Harris, K. S., W. Xiang, L. Alexander, W. S. Lane, A. V. Paul, and E. Wimmer.** 1994. Interaction of poliovirus polypeptide 3CD[pro] with the 5' and 3' termini of the poliovirus genome. *J. Biol. Chem.* **269:**27004–27014.
50. **Heinz, B. A., and L. M. Vance.** 1995. The antiviral compound enviroxime targets the 3A coding region of rhinovirus and poliovirus. *J. Virol.* **69:**4189–4197.
51. **Herold, J., and R. Andino.** 2000. Poliovirus requires a precise 5' end for efficient positive-strand RNA synthesis. *J. Virol.* **74:**6394–6400.
51a. **Herold, J., and R. Andino.** 2001. Poliovirus RNA replication requires genome circularization through a protein-protein bridge. *Mol. Cell* **7:**581–591.
52. **Hope, D. A., S. E. Diamond, and K. Kirkegaard.** 1997. Genetic dissection of interaction between poliovirus 3D polymerase and viral protein 3AB. *J. Virol.* **71:**9490–9498.
53. **Hu, J., and C. Seeger.** 1997. RNA signals that control DNA replication in hepadnaviruses. *Semin. Virol.* **8:**205–211.
54. **Hughes, P. J., and G. Stanway.** 2000. The 2A proteins of three diverse picornaviruses are related to each other and to the H-rev 107 family of proteins involved in the control of cell proliferation. *J. Gen. Virol.* **81:**201–207.
55. **Ishii, T., K. Shiroki, A. Iwai, and A. Nomoto.** 1999. Identification of a new element for RNA replication within the internal ribosome entry site of poliovirus RNA. *J. Gen. Virol.* **80:**917–920.
56. **Jacobson, S. J., D. A. M. Konings, and P. Sarnow.** 1993. Biochemical and genetic evidence for a pseudoknot structure at the 3' terminus of the poliovirus RNA genome and its role in viral RNA amplification. *J. Virol.* **67:**2961–2971.
57. **Jang, S. K., H. G. Krausslich, M. J. H. Nicklin, G. M. Duke, A. C. Palmenberg, and E. Wimmer.** 1988. A segment of the nontranslated region of encephalomyocarditis virus RNA directs internal entry of ribosomes during in vitro translation. *J. Virol.* **62:**2636–2643.
58. **Jang, S. K., M. V. Davies, R. J. Kaufman, and E. Wimmer.** 1989. Initiation of protein synthesis by internal entry of ribosomes into the 5' nontranslated region of encephalomyocarditis virus RNA in vivo. *J. Virol.* **63:**1651–1660.
59. **King, A. J., and P. C. van der Vliet.** 1994. A precursor terminal protein-trinucleotide intermediate during initiation of adenovirus DNA replication: regeneration of molecular ends in vitro by a jumping back mechanism. *EMBO J.* **13:**5786–5792.
60. **Kitamura, N., B. L. Semler, P. G. Rothberg, G. R. Larsen, C. J. Adler, A. J. Dorner, E. A. Emini, R. Hanecak, J. J. Lee, S. van der Werf, C. W. Anderson, and E. Wimmer.** 1981. Primary structure, gene organization, polypeptide expression of poliovirus RNA. *Nature* **291:**547–553.
61. **Klump, W. M., I. Bergmann, B. C. Muller, D. Ameis, and R. Kandolf.** 1990. Complete nucleotide sequence of infectious coxsackievirus B3 cDNA: two initial 5' uridine residues are regained during plus strand synthesis. *J. Virol.* **64:**1573–1583.
62. **Kuhn, R. J., H. Tada, M. F. Ypma-Wong, B. L. Semler, and E. Wimmer.** 1988. Mutational analysis of the genome-linked protein VPg of poliovirus. *J. Virol.* **62:**4207–4215.
63. **Kusov, Y. Y., and V. Gauss-Muller.** 1997. In vitro RNA binding of the hepatitis A virus proteinase 3C(HAV 3C[pro]) to secondary structure elements within the 5' terminus of the HAV genome. *RNA* **3:**291–302.
64. **Kusov, Y. Y., G. Morace, C. Probst, and V. Gauss-Muller.** 1997. Interaction of hepatitis A virus (HAV) precursor proteins 3AB and 3ABC with the 5' and 3' termini of the HAV RNA. *Virus Res.* **51:**151–157.
65. **Kusov, Y., M. Weitz, G. Dollenmeier, and V. Gauss-Muller.** 1996. RNA-protein interactions at the 3' end of the hepatitis A virus RNA. *J. Virol.* **70:**1890–1897.
66. **Lai, M. C.** 1998. Cellular factors in the transcription and replication of viral RNA genomes: a parallel to DNA-dependent transcription. *Virology* **244:**1–12.
67. **Lama, J., A. V. Paul, K. S. Harris, and E. Wimmer.** 1994. Properties of purified recombinant poliovirus protein 3AB as substrate for viral proteinases and as co-factor for RNA polymerase 3D[pol]. *J. Biol. Chem.* **269:**66–70.
68. **Lee, Y. F., A. Nomoto, B. M. Detjen, and E. Wimmer.** 1977. A protein covalently linked to poliovirus genome RNA. *Proc. Natl. Acad. Sci. USA* **74:**59–63.
69. **Leong, L. E.-C., P. A. Walker, and A. G. Porter.** 1993. Human rhinovirus-14 protease 3C (3C[pro]) binds specifically to the 5' noncoding region of the viral RNA. *J. Biol. Chem.* **268:**25735–25739.
70. **Li, J. P., and D. Baltimore.** 1990. An intragenic revertant of poliovirus 2C mutant has an uncoating defect. *J. Virol.* **64:**1102–1107.
71. **Li, X., H. H. Lu, S. Muller, and E. Wimmer.** 2001. The C-terminal residues of poliovirus proteinase 2A[pro] are critical for viral RNA replication but not for cis- and trans-proteolytic cleavage. *J. Gen. Virol.* **82:**397–408.
72. **Lobert, P.-E., N. Escriou, J. Ruelle, and T. Michiels.** 1999. A coding RNA sequence acts as a replication signal in cardioviruses. *Proc. Natl. Acad. Sci. USA* **96:**11560–11565.
73. **Mahajan, S., V. V. Dolja, and J. C. Carrington.** 1996. Roles of the sequence encoding tobacco etch virus capsid protein in genome amplification: requirements for the translation process and a cis-active element. *J. Virol.* **70:**4370–4379.
74. **Martin, A. C., L. Blanco, P. Garcia, M. Salas, and J. Mendez.** 1996. In vitro protein-primed initiation of pneumococcal phage Cp-1 DNA replication occurs at the third 3' nucleotide of the linear template: a stepwise sliding-back mechanism. *J. Mol. Biol.* **260:**369–377.
75. **McBride, A. E., A. Schlegel, and K. Kirkegaard.** 1996. Human protein Sam68 relocalization and interaction with poliovirus RNA polymerase in infected cells. *Proc. Natl. Acad. Sci. USA* **93:**2296–2301.
76. **McKnight, K. L., and S. L. Lemon.** 1996. Capsid coding sequence is required for efficient replication of human rhinovirus 14 RNA. *J. Virol.* **70:**1941–1952.
77. **McKnight, K. L., and S. M. Lemon.** 1998. The rhinovirus type 14 genome contains an internally located RNA structure that is required for viral replication. *RNA* **4:**1569–1584.
78. **Melchers, W. J. G., J. G. J. Hoenderop, H. J. Bruins Slot, C. W. A. Pleij, E. V. Pilipenko, V. I. Agol, and J. M. D. Galama.** 1997. Kissing of the two predominant hairpin loops in the coxsackie B virus 3' untranslated region is the essential structural feature of the origin of replication required for negative-strand RNA synthesis. *J. Virol.* **71:**686–696.
79. **Mellits, K. H., J. M. Meredith, J. B. Rohll, D. J. Evans, and J. W. Almond.** 1998. Binding of a cellular factor to

the 3' untranslated region of the RNA genomes of entero- and rhinoviruses plays a role in virus replication. *J. Gen. Virol.* **79:**1715–1723.
80. Mendez, J., L. Blanco, J. A. Esteban, A. Bernad, and M. Salas. 1992. Initiation of Φ29 DNA replication occurs at the second 3' nucleotide of the linear template: a sliding back mechanism for protein-primed DNA replication. *Proc. Natl. Acad. Sci. USA* **89:**9579–9583.
81. **Meredith, J. M., J. B. Rohll, J. W. Almond, and D. J. Evans.** 1999. Similar interactions of the poliovirus and rhinovirus 3D polymerases with the 3' untranslated region of rhinovirus 14. *J. Virol.* **73:**9952–9958.
82. **Michiels, T., V. Dejong, R. Rodrigus, and C. Shaw-Jackson.** 1997. Protein 2A is not required for Theiler's virus replication. *J. Virol.* **71:**9549–9556.
83. **Molla, A., K. S. Harris, A. V. Paul, S. H. Shin, J. Mugavero, and E. Wimmer.** 1994. Stimulation of poliovirus proteinase 3C^{pro}-related proteolysis by the genome-linked VPg and its precursor 3AB. *J. Biol. Chem.* **269:**27015–27020.
84. **Molla, A., A. V. Paul, M. Schmid, S. K. Jang, and E. Wimmer.** 1993. Studies on dicistronic polioviruses implicate viral proteinase 2A^{pro} in RNA replication. *Virology* **196:**739–747.
85. **Molla, A., A. V. Paul, and E. Wimmer.** 1991. Cell-free *de novo* synthesis of poliovirus. *Science* **254:**1647–1651.
86. **Montagnier, L., and F. K. Sanders.** 1963. Replicative form of encephalomyocarditis virus ribonucleic acid. *Nature* **199:**664.
87. **Morgan-Detjen, B., J. Lucas, and E. Wimmer.** 1978. Poliovirus single-stranded RNA and double-stranded RNA: differential infectivity in enucleate cells. *J. Virol.* **27:**582–586.
88. **Neufeld, K. L., J. M. Galarza, O. C. Richards, D. F. Summers, and E. Ehrenfeld.** 1994. Identification of terminal adenylyl transferase activity of the poliovirus polymerase 3D^{pol}. *J. Virol.* **68:**5811–5818.
89. **Nomoto, A., B. Detjen, R. Pozzatti, and E. Wimmer.** 1977. The location of the polio genome protein in viral RNAs and its implication for RNA synthesis. *Nature* **268:**208–213.
90. **Nomoto, A., N. Kitamura, F. Golini, and E. Wimmer.** 1977. The 5'-terminal structures of poliovirion RNA and poliovirus mRNA differ only in the genome-linked protein VPg. *Proc. Natl. Acad. Sci. USA* **74:**5345–5349.
91. **Novak, J. E., and K. Kirkegaard.** 1994. Coupling between genome translation and replication in an RNA virus. *Genes Dev.* **8:**1726–1737.
92. **Novak, J. E., and K. Kirkegaard.** 1991. Improved method for detecting poliovirus negative strands used to demonstrate specificity of positive-strand encapsidation and the ratio of positive to negative strands in infected cells. *J. Virol.* **65:**3384–3387.
93. **Parsley, T. B., C. T. Cornell, and B. L. Semler.** 1999. Modulation of the RNA binding and protein processing activities of poliovirus polypeptide 3CD by the viral RNA polymerase domain. *J. Biol. Chem.* **274:**12867–12876.
94. **Parsley, T. B., J. S. Towner, L. B. Blyn, E. Ehrenfeld, and B. L. Semler.** 1997. Poly(rC) binding protein 2 forms a ternary complex with the 5'-terminal sequences of poliovirus RNA and the viral 3CD proteinase. *RNA* **3:**1124–1134.
95. **Pata, J. D., S. C. Schultz, and K. Kirkegaard.** 1995. Functional oligomerization of poliovirus RNA-dependent RNA polymerase. *RNA* **1:**466–477.
96. **Paul, A. V., X. Cao, K. S. Harris, J. Lama, and E. Wimmer.** 1994. Studies with poliovirus polymerase 3D^{pol}. Stimulation of poly(U) synthesis in vitro by purified poliovirus protein 3AB. *J. Biol. Chem.* **269:**29173–29181.
97. **Paul, A. V., A. Molla, and E. Wimmer.** 1994. Studies of a putative amphipathic helix in the N-terminus of poliovirus protein 2C. *Virology* **199:**188–199.
98. **Paul, A. V., J. Mugavero, J. Yin, S. Hobson, S. Schultz, J. H. van Boom, and E. Wimmer.** 2000. Studies on the attenuation phenotype of polio vaccines: poliovirus RNA polymerase derived from Sabin type 1 sequence is temperature sensitive in the uridylylation of VPg. *Virology* **272:**72–84.
99. **Paul, A. V., E. Rieder, D. W. Kim, J. H. van Boom, and E. Wimmer.** 2000. Identification of an RNA hairpin in poliovirus RNA that serves as the primary template in the in vitro uridylylation of VPg. *J. Virol.* **74:**10359–10370.
100. **Paul, A. V., J. H. van Boom, D. Fillipov, and E. Wimmer.** 1998. Protein-primed RNA synthesis by purified poliovirus RNA polymerase. *Nature* **393:**280–284.
101. **Pelletier, J., and N. Sonenberg.** 1988. Internal initiation of translation of eukaryotic mRNA directed by a sequence derived from poliovirus RNA. *Nature* **334:**320–325.
102. **Pfister, T., K. W. Jones, and E. Wimmer.** 2000. A cysteine-rich motif in poliovirus protein 2C^{ATPase} is involved in RNA replication and binds zinc in vitro. *J. Virol.* **74:**334–343.
103. **Pfister, T., and E. Wimmer.** 1999. Characterization of the nucleoside triphosphatase activity of poliovirus protein 2C reveals a mechanism by which guanidine inhibits poliovirus replication. *J. Biol. Chem.* **274:**6992–7001.
104. **Pilipenko, E. V., S. V. Maslova, A. N. Sinyakov, and V. I. Agol.** 1992. Towards identification of *cis*-acting elements involved in the replication of enterovirus and rhinovirus RNAs: a proposal for the existence of tRNA-like terminal structures. *Nucleic Acids Res.* **20:**1739–1745.
105. **Pilipenko, E. V., K. V. Poperechny, S. V. Maslova, W. J. G. Melchers, H. J. Slot, and V. I. Agol.** 1996. Cis-element, *oriR*, involved in the initiation of (−) strand poliovirus RNA: a quasi-globular multi-domain RNA structure maintained by tertiary ("kissing") interactions. *EMBO J.* **15:**5428–5436.
106. **Plotch, S. J., and O. Palant.** 1995. Poliovirus protein 3AB forms a complex with and stimulates the activity of the viral RNA polymerase, 3D^{pol}. *J. Virol.* **69:**7169–7179.
107. **Richards, O. C., and E. Ehrenfeld.** 1998. Effects of poliovirus 3AB protein on 3D polymerase-catalyzed reaction. *J. Biol. Chem.* **273:**12832–12840.
108. **Richards, O. C., and E. Ehrenfeld.** 1990. Poliovirus RNA replication. *Curr. Top. Microbiol. Immunol.* **161:**90–119.
109. **Rieder, E., A. V. Paul, D. W. Kim, J. H. van Boom, and E. Wimmer.** 2000. Genetic and biochemical studies of poliovirus *cis*-acting replication element *cre* in relation to VPg uridylylation. *J. Virol.* **74:**10371–10380.
110. **Rivera, V. M., J. D. Welsh, and J. V. Maizel.** 1988. Comparative sequence analysis of the 5' noncoding region of the enteroviruses and rhinoviruses. *Virology* **165:**42–50.
111. **Rodriguez, P. L., and L. Carrasco.** 1993. Poliovirus protein 2C has ATP-ase and GTP-ase activities. *J. Biol. Chem.* **268:**8105–8110.
112. **Rodriguez, P. L., and L. Carrasco.** 1995. Poliovirus 2C contains two regions involved in RNA binding activity. *J. Biol. Chem.* **270:**10105–10112.
113. **Roehl, H. H., T. B. Parsley, T. V. Ho, and B. L. Semler.** 1997. Processing of a cellular polypetide by 3CD proteinase is required for poliovirus ribonucleoprotein complex formation. *J. Virol.* **71:**578–585.
114. **Roehl, H. H., and B. L. Semler.** 1995. Poliovirus infection enhances the formation of two ribonucleoprotein complexes at the 3' end of viral negative-strand RNA. *J. Virol.* **69:**2954–2961.
115. **Rohll, J. B., D. H. Moon, D. J. Evans, and J. W. Almond.** 1995. The 3' untranslated region of picornavirus

RNA: features required for efficient genome replication. *J. Virol.* **69**:7835–7844.
116. Romanova, L. I., and V. I. Agol. 1979. Interconversion of linear and circular forms of double-stranded RNA of encephalomyocarditis virus. *J. Virol.* **93**:574–577.
117. Rothberg, P. G., T. J. R. Harris, A. Nomoto, and E. Wimmer. 1978. O^4-(5'-uridylyl)tyrosine is the bond between the genome-linked protein and the RNA of poliovirus. *Proc. Natl. Acad. Sci. USA* **75**:4868–4872.
118. Rueckert, R. R. 1996. Picornaviridae: the viruses and their replication, p. 609–654. *In* B. N. Fields, D. M. Knipe, and P. M. Howley (ed.), *Fields Virology*, 3rd ed. Lippincott-Raven Publishers, Philadelphia, Pa..
119. Salas, M., J. T. Miller, J. Leis, and M. L. DePamphilis. 1996. Mechanism for priming DNA synthesis, p. 131–176. *In* M. L. DePamphilis (ed.), *DNA Replication in Eukaryotic Cells*. Cold Spring Harbor Laboratory Press, Cold Spring Harbor, N.Y.
120. Sandoval, I. V., and L. Carrasco. 1997. Poliovirus infection and expression of the poliovirus protein 2B provoke the disassembly of the Golgi complex, the organelle target for the antipoliovirus drug Ro-090179. *J. Virol.* **71**:4679–4693.
121. Sarnow, P. 1989. Role of 3'-end sequences in infectivity of poliovirus transcripts made in vitro. *J. Virol.* **63**:467–470.
122. Seeger, C., and W. S. Mason. 1996. Replication of the hepatitis virus genome, p. 815–831. *In* M. L. DePamphilis (ed.), *DNA Replication in Eukaryotic Cells*. Cold Spring Harbor Laboratory Press, Cold Spring Harbor, N.Y.
123. Seipelt, J., A. Guarne, E. Bergmann, M. James, W. Sommergruber, I. Fita, and T. Skern. 1999. The structures of picornaviral proteinases. *Virus Res.* **62**:159–168.
124. Semler, B. L., C. W. Anderson, R. Hanecak, L. F. Dorner, and E. Wimmer. 1982. A membrane-associated precursor to poliovirus VPg identified by immunoprecipitation with antibodies directed against a synthetic heptapeptide. *Cell* **28**:405–412.
125. Shaw, J. G. 1996. Plant viruses, p. 499–532. *In* B. N. Fields, D. M. Knipe, and P. M. Howley (ed.), *Fields Virology*, 3rd ed. Lippincott-Raven Publishers, Philadelphia, Pa.
126. Spector, D. H., and D. Baltimore. 1974. Requirement of 3'-terminal poly(adenylic acid) for the infectivity of poliovirus RNA. *Proc. Natl. Acad. Sci. USA* **71**:2983–2987.
127. Takeda, N., R. J. Kuhn, C. F. Yang, T. Takegami, and E. Wimmer. 1986. Initiation of poliovirus plus-strand RNA synthesis in a membrane complex of infected HeLa cells. *J. Virol.* **60**:43–53.
128. Takegami, T., R. J. Kuhn, C. W. Anderson, and E. Wimmer. 1983. Membrane-dependent uridylylation of the genome-linked protein VPg of poliovirus. *Proc. Natl. Acad. Sci. USA* **80**:7447–7451.
129. Teterina, N. L., K. Bienz, D. Egger, A. E. Gorbalenya, and E. Ehrenfeld. 1997. Induction of intracellular membrane rearrangements by HAV proteins 2C and 2BC. *Virology* **237**:66–77.
130. Tobin, G. J., D. C. Young, and J. B. Flanegan. 1989. Self-catalyzed linkage of poliovirus terminal protein VPg to poliovirus RNA. *Cell* **59**:511–519.
131. Todd, S., J. H. C. Nguyen, and B. L. Semler. 1995. RNA-protein interactions directed by the 3' end of human rhinovirus genomic RNA. *J. Virol.* **69**:3605–3614.
132. Todd, S., J. S. Towner, D. M. Brown, and B. L. Semler. 1997. Replication-competent picornaviruses with complete genomic RNA 3' noncoding region deletions. *J. Virol.* **71**:8868–8874.
133. Towner, J. S., T. V. Ho, and B. L. Semler. 1996. Determinants of membrane association for poliovirus protein 3AB. *J. Biol. Chem.* **271**:26810–26818.
134. Towner, J. S., M. M. Mazanet, and B. L. Semler. 1998. Rescue of defective poliovirus RNA replication by 3AB-containing precursor polyproteins. *J. Virol.* **72**:7191–7200.
135. Toyoda, H., C. F. Yang, N. Takeda, A. Nomoto, and E. Wimmer. 1987. Analysis of RNA synthesis of type 1 poliovirus by using an in vitro molecular genetic approach. *J. Virol.* **61**:2816–2822.
136. Van Bokhoven, H., O. L. Gall, D. Kasteel, J. Verver, J. Wellink, and A. V. Kammen. 1993. Cis- and trans-acting elements in cowpea mosaic virus RNA replication. *Virology* **195**:377–386.
136a.Vance, L. M., N. Moscufo, M. Chow, and B. A. Heinz. 1997. Poliovirus 2C region functions during encapsidation of viral RNA. *J. Virol.* **71**:8759–8765.
137. Ventoso, I., A. Barco, and L. Carrasco. 1998. Mutational analysis of poliovirus 2A^{pro}. Distinct inhibitory functions of 2A^{pro} on translation and transcription. *J. Biol. Chem.* **273**:27960–27967.
138. Waggoner, S., and P. Sarnow. 1998. Viral ribonucleoprotein complex formation and nucleolar-cytoplasmic relocalization of nucleolin in poliovirus-infected cells. *J. Virol.* **72**:6699–6709.
139. Walker, P. A., L. E.-C. Leong, and A. G. Porter. 1995. Sequence and structural determinants of the interaction between the 5'-noncoding region of picornavirus RNA and rhinovirus protease 3C. *J. Biol Chem.* **270**:14510–14516.
140. Wimmer, E. 1982. Genome-linked proteins of viruses. *Cell* **28**:199–201.
141. Wimmer, E., C. U. T. Hellen, and X. Cao. 1993. Genetics of poliovirus. *Annu. Rev. Genet.* **27**:353–436.
142. Xiang, W., A. Cuconati, D. Hope, K. Kirkegaard, and E. Wimmer. 1998. Complete protein linkage map of poliovirus P3 proteins: interaction of polymerase 3D^{pol} with VPg and with genetic variants of 3AB. *J. Virol.* **72**:6732–6741.
143. Xiang, W., A. Cuconati, A. V. Paul, X. Cao, and E. Wimmer. 1995. Molecular dissection of the multifunctional poliovirus RNA-binding protein 3AB. *RNA* **1**:892–904.
144. Xiang, W., K. S. Harris, L. Alexander, and E. Wimmer. 1995. Interaction between the 5'-terminal cloverleaf and 3AB/3CD^{pro} of poliovirus is essential for RNA replication. *J. Virol.* **69**:3658–3667.
145. Xiang, W., A. V. Paul, and E. Wimmer. 1997. RNA signals in entero- and rhinovirus genome replication. *Semin. Virol.* **8**:256–273.
146. Yogo, Y., and E. Wimmer. 1972. Polyadenylic acid at the 3'-terminus of poliovirus RNA. *Proc. Natl. Acad. Sci. USA* **69**:1877–1882.
147. Yu, S. F., P. Benton, M. Bovee, J. Sessions, and R. E. Lloyd. 1995. Defective RNA replication by poliovirus mutants deficient in 2A protease cleavage activity. *J. Virol.* **69**:247–252.
148. Zell, R., K. Klingel, M. Sauter, U. Fortmuller, and R. Kandolf. 1995. Coxsackieviral proteins functionally recognize the polioviral cloverleaf structure of the 5' NTR of a chimeric enterovirus RNA: influence of species-specific host cell factors in virus growth. *Virus Res.* **39**:87–103.

Role of Cellular Structures in Viral RNA Replication

DENISE EGGER, RAINER GOSERT, AND KURT BIENZ

20

VIRUS REPLICATION AND VIRUS-INDUCED HOST CELL DESTRUCTION ARE COUPLED

During their replication cycles many viruses extensively affect host cell morphology. Pathologists diagnosed viral diseases on the basis of morphological characteristics of the diseased tissue long before the nature and biology of viruses were known. The take-off of modern experimental virology was the observation by Enders (33) that in cultured cells poliovirus (PV) induces morphological alterations, termed cytopathic effect (CPE). Subsequently, CPE could be used as an easy marker for virus replication in cell cultures.

Picornaviruses, with the possible exception of hepatitis A virus (HAV), induce cell alterations that culminate ultimately in cell death. The cell-killing property is the reason for the pathogenicity of these viruses, since the extent of cell destruction in an infected organ determines the severity of the symptoms in the organism. Picornavirus-induced cell alterations and cell destruction are directly coupled to viral replication (16). This was also demonstrated in coxsackievirus-infected muscles of mice where viral RNA replication located to the foci of gradual destruction of the contractile material (11, 53, 54). That cell destruction, and hence virulence, is coupled to virus replication implies that pathogenicity of a virus cannot be diminished, e.g., for production of attenuated vaccine or for gene transfer purposes, without reducing viability of the virus. In fact, oral PV vaccine strains consist of PV mutants with highly restricted growth in neural tissue (44, 45). In permissive cells, however, PV Sabin vaccine strains are as virulent, i.e., cell killing, as wild-type PV (unpublished data).

Recently, it was found that apoptosis can also lead to picornavirus-related cell death (1). The mechanisms of CPE and apoptosis are different. CPE consists of nuclear alterations and, essentially, in a restructuring of cellular membranes that are involved in or even necessary for efficient viral replication. Apoptosis is a cellular suicide program and may be triggered by many different stimuli, including viral infections (72), against which it is thought to be a defense mechanism (56). In PV- or Theiler's virus-infected cell cultures, apoptosis occurs under restricted viral growth conditions (1, 50, 81), whereas in HAV-infected cell cultures, apoptosis seems the prevalent mechanism of cell death (20, 43). In picornavirus-infected organs of humans or animals, cells can be found showing characteristics of either CPE or apoptosis (40, 71, 84). It is an open discussion whether the clinical outcome of an infection depends on the balance between apoptosis and viral replication-mediated cell killing (2).

VIRAL RNA REPLICATION REQUIRES ALTERED CELLULAR MEMBRANES

Structural Features of the Infected Cell

In a PV-infected cell culture, CPE observed by low-power light microscopy (LM) is characterized by cell rounding and nuclear condensation, followed by shrinkage and detachment of the cells from their support. Cytoplasmic alterations, which have been described in the LM as "cytoplasmic eosinophilic paranuclear mass" (70) (Fig. 1b), consist at the ultrastructural level of a great number of membranous vesicles (Fig. 1a). They are densely packed, so that the outer lipid layers of two adjacent vesicular membranes seem to be fused into a single membrane of three lipid layers (28). The presence of cytoplasmic material and virions within some of the vesicles points to an autophagic process (28). Investigations on cryofixed vesicles confirmed the presence of autophagic vacuoles (74, 75a). Early in infection, few if any autophagic vacuoles seem to be present (12, 13, 19). As the infection progresses, the amount of vesicles in the cytoplasm increases, seemingly at the expense of the rER, which finally disappears almost completely (13, 15).

Virus-induced vesicles are characteristic of infections by PV, coxsackievirus, foot-and-mouth disease virus, and Theiler's virus (11, 15, 18, 28, 36, 74, 88) as well as for rhino- and mengovirus (unpublished data). Only HAV was found to induce vesicle-like membrane alterations of somewhat different morphology. They consist of tightly associated oblong vesicles forming an interwoven membranous structure, which was thus termed a tubular-vesicular network (43).

Denise Egger, Rainer Gosert, and Kurt Bienz ■ Institute for Medical Microbiology, University of Basel, CH-4003 Basel, Switzerland.

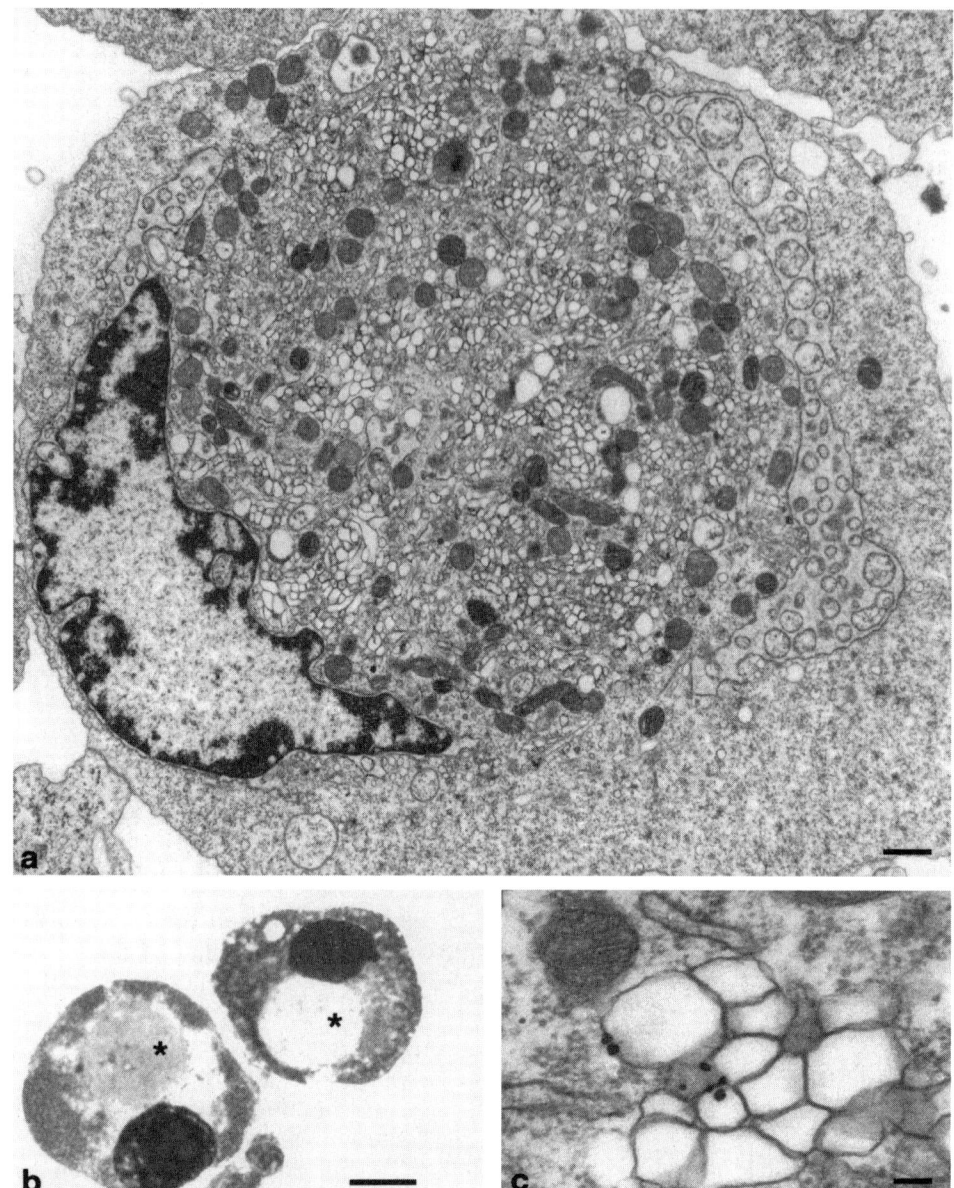

FIGURE 1 Morphology of and viral RNA synthesis in PV-infected HEp-2 cells. (a) Electron microscopic picture shows a large field of polioviral vesicles. Bar, 1 μm. (b) Giemsa-stained cells in the LM, the large cytoplasmic eosinophilic inclusion (*) corresponds to the vesiculated area in Fig. 1a. Bar, 10 μm. (c) High-resolution autoradiograph, silver grains indicate incorporation of ^{3}H-uridin into viral RNA on the surface of PV vesicles. Bar, 100 nm.

Intracellular Site of Viral RNA Synthesis

Biochemical and morphological analyses of PV-, coxsackievirus-, and HAV-infected cells showed that viral RNA synthesis is connected to the virus-induced vesicles described above (11, 16, 21, 22, 34, 39, 62, 77; R. Gosert, D. Egger, and K. Bienz, submitted for publication). However, the exact biochemical mechanism of the membrane involvement in RNA transcription is still unclear. High-resolution autoradiography pictures suggested that PV RNA synthesis proceeds on the outer surface of the vesicles (12) (Fig. 1c). Since up to a 100-fold higher amount of plus- than minus-strand RNA is synthesized in the infected cell (5, 19, 39, 64), the autoradiography findings, which cannot discriminate between plus- and minus-strand RNA, reflect predominantly plus-strand RNA synthesis.

Plus- and minus-strand PV RNA syntheses proceed in parallel throughout the replication cycle (19, 64). It was suggested that membranes may be involved in the initiation step of minus-strand RNA synthesis by providing membrane-bound precursor(s) of VPg (83), found to be the primer of plus- as well as minus-strand RNA synthesis (46, 67, 76). By fluorescent in situ hybridization, minus-strand RNA was always found to colocalize to plus-strand RNA (19) (Color Plate 17a–c, following p. 156). Additional rather large amounts of plus-strand RNA, apparently not associated with minus strands, could be observed. By combined in situ localization of viral RNA and membrane-bound viral proteins, both RNA species were always found associated with the vesicular membranes. The authors concluded from their data that plus-strand RNA is copied into minus strand within plus- and minus-strand-RNA-containing membranous structures, from where the resulting double-stranded replicative form (RF) would be released and transformed into a still vesicle-bound, plus-strand-producing replicative intermediate (RI) (19).

Nonstructural viral proteins associated with the membranes of the picornavirus-induced vesicles include the P2 proteins 2B, 2C and its precursor 2BC, and the P3 protein 3A and its precursors. The P2 proteins have been shown by electron microscopic immunocytochemistry to be exclusively associated with the vesicles, so that they can be used as markers for these membranes (12, 13, 43, 74). The P2 proteins seem to interact with membranes via their amphipathic helices (8, 29, 30, 55, 65, 78, 85) and/or hydrophobic domains (87), whereas protein 3A(B) has characteristics of an intrinsic membrane protein (25, 82).

With the possible exception of 2A, the P2 and P3 proteins are directly or indirectly involved in the replication of the viral genome. 3D^{pol}, an RNA-dependent RNA polymerase (7, 35) with unwinding activity (23), and the uridylylated form of VPg (3B), the primer of RNA synthesis (63, 67), are directly involved in the RNA polymerization process. In addition to polymerase, primer, and protease functions, P3 proteins have been reported to form a membrane-bound complex for initiation of viral RNA synthesis and to interact with each other for the proteolytic maturation of 3D^{pol} and with cellular protein to inhibit translation as a prerequisite for viral minus-strand RNA synthesis (see "Formation and Biological Significance of the Viral Replication Complex" below) (37, 38, 46, 60, 83, 91). The P2 proteins are involved in the structural alteration of the host cell membranes necessary for RNA replication (see "Formation of PV Vesicles" below). However, they seem to exert different additional functions. Guanidine HCl, an inhibitor of viral RNA synthesis, has its target in the protein 2C sequence (69). The guanidine-sensitive functions include inhibition of the ATPase activity of 2C (68), 2C-mediated attachment of the replication complex to the vesicular membranes (17), and initiation of minus-strand RNA synthesis (10). Protein 2B was reported to change the permeability of cellular membranes (3, 47, 49, 85, 86).

Viral RNA Synthesis in Subcellular Fractions

Membrane-containing fractions from uninfected cells can act as coupled translation/transcription systems and, if programmed with viral RNA, will support de novo PV production (9, 61). Subcellular vesicle-containing fractions isolated from PV-infected cells are active in viral RNA synthesis in vitro. Analysis of such fractions revealed important details of structure and function of the vesicles and their relation to viral replication steps and viral molecules. The isolated vesicles have the propensity to associate in characteristic arrangements, termed rosettes (13, 14, 17) (Fig. 2). These higher-order structures encompass the site of viral RNA replication, i.e., the replication complex. They contain genome-length RNA, RI, and RF (14) and initiate plus-strand synthesis in vitro to produce mature genome-length progeny RNA in the RI (31).

A very tight configuration of the rosette precludes the entry of hybridization probes. Therefore, attempts to obtain more information on the spatial arrangement of the different RNA species within the rosette were unsuccessful (14).

Rosettes can be dissociated into single vesicles, which are still capable of initiating plus-strand RNA synthesis. Individual vesicles exhibit longer or shorter membranous tubules and carry RI with protruding, i.e., RNase-sensitive, 5′ ends of nascent plus-strand RNA. The minus-strand-

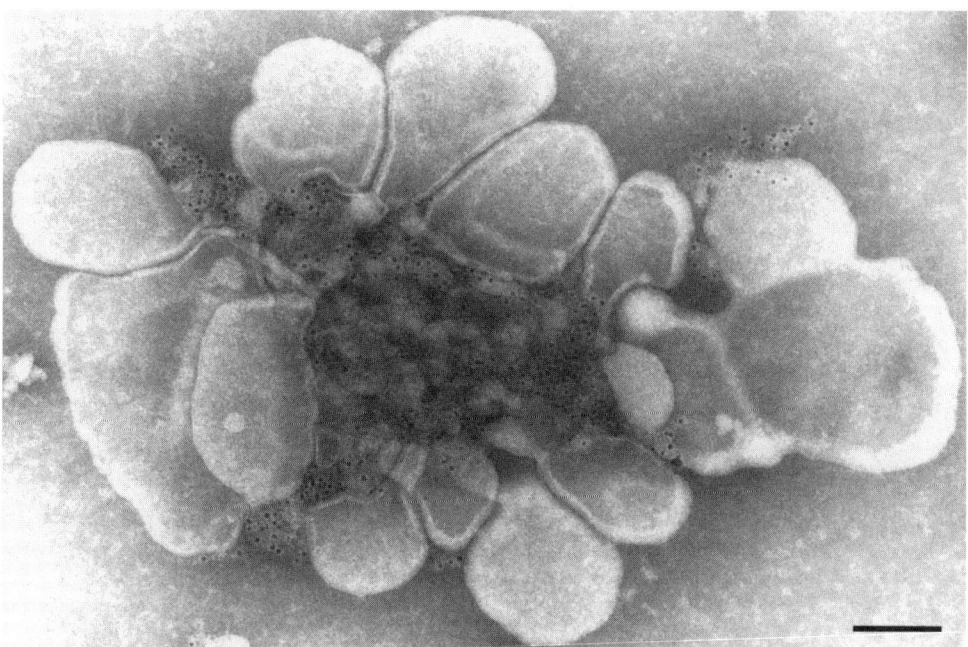

FIGURE 2 An isolated, native replication complex appears as a rosette-like structure. Tubules of the vesicles point toward the center of the rosette. Immunogold labeling for PV proteins 2B and 2C and precursors. Bar, 100 nm.

containing core of the RI is protected from exogenously added RNase, possibly by being covered with proteins of the viral replication complex. Interestingly, individual vesicles can reform intact rosettes (31).

Vesicular membranes have been found to be necessary for initiation of plus-strand RNA synthesis (31). The functional advantage of a rosette over a single vesicle might be a high local concentration of components needed for RNA synthesis and the enhanced chance for the replicating RNA to undergo a subsequent initiation event on a vesicular membrane.

FORMATION OF PV VESICLES

An induction role for the P2 protein 2BC in vesicle formation was suggested by experiments in which the cleavage of the viral polyprotein was inhibited (15). Expression of individual viral proteins in HeLa cells also pointed to the viral protein 2BC as the protein responsible for triggering the vesicle formation process (4, 24, 30, 78), possibly assisted by protein 3A (75a). By expressing different domains of this protein, it was found that the N-terminal part of 2C (amino acids 1 to 274) alone was sufficient to produce vesicles. This domain of 2C contains an amphipathic helix, which confers membrane association to the polypeptide (29, 30, 78), and an NTP-binding motif (42, 59, 79) with ATPase activity (68). An involvement of this ATPase activity in membrane rearrangement is a matter of discussion (68).

It has been debated extensively whether membrane structures originally engaged in retrograde membrane transport, and thus being Golgi-derived, or whether membranes of the anterograde transport, which starts at the ER, represent the origin of the polioviral vesicles. Arguments that vesicular structures belonging to the retrograde pathway contribute to the PV vesicle population include the observation that ARF1, the GTPase of the COPI complex of the retrograde vesicular transport (reviewed in reference 89), was found to be necessary for virus reproduction in a cell-free system (27). Experiments using a flavonoid, a retrograde transport inhibitor, were interpreted to mean that the Golgi would be a primary target of PV, particularly of the protein 2B (73).

Results from experiments with brefeldin A (BFA), which inhibits PV replication, yielded distinct interpretations and thus could not completely clarify the issue of whether vesicles consist of Golgi- or ER-derived membranes (48, 57). Likewise, isolated vesicles immunoprecipitated with antibodies against viral protein 2C were found to contain marker proteins of the ER but also of Golgi and lysosomes (74).

An involvement of the anterograde vesicular traffic was inferred from morphological and immunocytochemical investigations suggesting that the vesicles bud from the ER (12, 75a) and that Golgi membranes are recruited secondarily and only after the formation of ER-derived PV vesicles is well under way (19).

Recent experiments in our laboratory visualized the vesicle budding process at the ER and demonstrated that the formation of vesicles is part of the anterograde transport. The anterograde membrane flow in the uninfected cell starts by binding of the GTPase Sar1 to the ER and, subsequently, of the coat protein complex II proteins (COPII: sec23/24p and sec13/31p) (reviewed in references 75 and 89). Using antibodies against COPII components, we have shown that budding of the PV vesicles from the ER is a COPII-mediated cellular process, whereby viral proteins seem to determine the site of vesicle formation (72a).

FORMATION AND BIOLOGICAL SIGNIFICANCE OF THE VIRAL REPLICATION COMPLEX

Replication of viral RNA proceeds in a highly ordered, rosette-like replication complex, consisting of replicating viral RNA, viral and cellular proteins, and tubulated vesicles. Recent experiments indicated that the formation of a functional replication complex is a *cis*-acting process coupling viral translation, vesicle budding, and viral RNA synthesis (32).

The mechanisms governing the formation of a functional replication complex were investigated by expressing the viral membrane-binding protein 2BC or the entire set of P2 and P3 proteins that induce vesicles similar to those found during PV infection (24, 77a). It was tested whether preformed vesicles were able to contribute in *trans* to replication complexes formed by a superinfecting PV. Rather unexpectedly, PV uses neither preformed vesicles nor otherwise altered ER membranes for its own replication complex formation, suggesting that vesicles can only be used in RNA replication if they have been formed and provided with the relevant proteins translated from the same RNA that will be replicated in the corresponding replication complex (32). This view is supported by the findings that viral RNA has first to be translated in order to be replicated (64), that all components of the replication complex have to be delivered to the replication complex directly following translation (26, 83), and finally that PV replication occurs only after uninterrupted translation of the P2-P3 coding sequences (66).

Formation of replication complexes also requires active viral RNA replication. Precluding RNA-dependent RNA synthesis inhibits the association of viral RNA and vesicles into a replication complex (Color Plate 17d–f), regardless of whether viral RNA synthesis is suppressed by mutations in the RNA or protein 3D, or by a chemical inhibitor (guanidine HCl) (32, 77a).

Formation of the replication complex in *cis*, as well as its apparent impermeability for constituents of higher molecular weight (14, 76), largely precludes an exchange of viral and cellular molecules between a replication complex and the remainder of the cell or another replication complex. This might explain why there is limited complementation of nonstructural protein functions in *trans* (51, 80, 90) and why the recently described *cis*-acting replication element, present on the plus-strand RNA and required for initiation of RNA synthesis, needs to be provided in *cis* (41). In contrast, other virus families, such as the *Flaviviridae*, exhibit an open replication complex allowing for complementation in *trans* (52).

For PV RNA replication, translation of an individual RNA molecule has to be down-regulated to allow for transcription. The proposed mechanism for this switch consists of an enhanced 3CD-mediated binding of the cellular poly(rC)-binding protein to the 5′-cloverleaf structure of plus-strand viral RNA (37, 38). It is not clear whether sequestration of this regulatory process in the compartment of the replication complex contributes to the proper local concentration of the molecules involved.

Membrane-associated replication complexes are commonly found in cells infected with plus-strand RNA viruses. Although different RNA viruses use and transform diverse cellular membrane compartments for building up a replication complex, these viruses have in common that their RNA replication depends on the presence of membranes. DNA replication, in contrast, proceeds without the support of membranous structures. During DNA replication, topoisomerases cut one strand of the dsDNA repeatedly and thus allow for unwinding of comparably short DNA fragments. In contrast, the viral RF RNA, which is built up as an intermediate in RNA replication, has to unwind in its full length during transcription. With the length of 2.7 µm for the 7.5 kb of PV RNA (58), considerable steric problems must be overcome during the unwinding process. Conceivably, membranes may serve as a scaffold to prevent tangling and back-hybridization of replicating RNA, thus allowing for the observed fast RNA synthesis of less than a minute's duration for a full-length RNA strand of PV (6).

REFERENCES

1. **Agol, V. I., G. A. Belov, K. Bienz, D. Egger, M. S. Kolesnikova, N. T. Raikhlin, L. I. Romanova, E. A. Smirnova, and E. A. Tolskaya.** 1998. Two types of death of poliovirus-infected cells: caspase involvement in the apoptosis but not cytopathic effect. *Virology* **252:**343–353.
2. **Agol, V. I., G. A. Belov, K. Bienz, D. Egger, M. S. Kolesnikova, L. I. Romanova, L. V. Sladkova, and E. A. Tolskaya.** 2000. Competing death programs in poliovirus-infected cells: commitment switch in the middle of the infectious cycle. *J. Virol.* **74:**5534–5541.
3. **Aldabe, R., A. Barco, and L. Carrasco.** 1996. Membrane permeabilization by poliovirus proteins 2B and 2BC. *J. Biol. Chem.* **271:**23134–23137.
4. **Aldabe, R., and L. Carrasco.** 1995. Induction of membrane proliferation by poliovirus proteins 2C and 2BC. *Biochem. Biophys. Res. Commun.* **206:**64–76.
5. **Andino, R., G. E. Rieckhof, and D. Baltimore.** 1990. A functional ribonucleoprotein complex forms around the 5' end of poliovirus RNA. *Cell* **63:**369–380.
6. **Baltimore, D.** 1969. The replication of picornavirus, p. 101–176. In H. B. Levy (ed.), *The Biochemistry of Viruses*. Marcel Dekker, New York, N.Y.
7. **Baltimore, D., R. Franklin, H. J. Eggers, and I. Tamm.** 1963. Poliovirus-induced RNA polymerase and the effects of virus-specific inhibitors on its production. *Proc. Natl. Acad. Sci. USA* **49:**843–849.
8. **Barco, A., and L. Carrasco.** 1995. A human virus protein, poliovirus protein 2BC, induces membrane proliferation and blocks the exocytic pathway in the yeast *Saccharomyces cerevisiae*. *EMBO J.* **14:**3349–3364.
9. **Barton, D. J., E. P. Black, and J. B. Flanegan.** 1995. Complete replication of poliovirus in vitro: preinitiation RNA replication complexes require soluble cellular factors for the synthesis of VPg-linked RNA. *J. Virol.* **69:**5516–5527.
10. **Barton, D. J., and J. B. Flanegan.** 1997. Synchronous replication of poliovirus RNA: initiation of negative-strand RNA synthesis requires the guanidine-inhibited activity of protein 2C. *J. Virol.* **71:**8482–8489.
11. **Bienz, K., D. Egger, G. Bienz-Isler, and H. Loeffler.** 1972. Light and electron microscopic autoradiography of coxsackievirus A 1 infected muscles: viral RNA synthesis and inhibition of host cell RNA synthesis. *Arch. Gesamte. Virusforsch.* **39:**35–47.
12. **Bienz, K., D. Egger, and L. Pasamontes.** 1987. Association of polioviral proteins of the P2 genomic region with the viral replication complex and virus-induced membrane synthesis as visualized by electron microscopic immunocytochemistry and autoradiography. *Virology* **160:**220–226.
13. **Bienz, K., D. Egger, and T. Pfister.** 1994. Characteristics of the poliovirus replication complex. *Arch. Virol. Suppl.* **9:**147–157.
14. **Bienz, K., D. Egger, T. Pfister, and M. Troxler.** 1992. Structural and functional characterization of the poliovirus replication complex. *J. Virol.* **66:**2740–2747.
15. **Bienz, K., D. Egger, Y. Rasser, and W. Bossart.** 1983. Intracellular distribution of poliovirus proteins and the induction of virus-specific cytoplasmic structures. *Virology* **131:**39–48.
16. **Bienz, K., D. Egger, Y. Rasser, and W. Bossart.** 1980. Kinetics and location of poliovirus macromolecular synthesis in correlation to virus-induced cytopathology. *Virology* **100:**390–399.
17. **Bienz, K., D. Egger, M. Troxler, and L. Pasamontes.** 1990. Structural organization of poliovirus RNA replication is mediated by viral proteins of the P2 genomic region. *J. Virol.* **64:**1156–1163.
18. **Bienz, K., D. Egger, and D. A. Wolff.** 1973. Virus replication, cytopathology, and lysosomal enzyme response of mitotic and interphase Hep-2 cells infected with poliovirus. *J. Virol.* **11:**565–574.
19. **Bolten, R., D. Egger, R. Gosert, G. Schaub, L. Landmann, and K. Bienz.** 1998. Intracellular localization of poliovirus plus- and minus-strand RNA visualized by strand-specific fluorescent in situ hybridization. *J. Virol.* **72:**8578–8585.
20. **Brack, K., W. Frings, A. Dotzauer, and A. Vallbracht.** 1998. A cytopathogenic, apoptosis-inducing variant of hepatitis A virus. *J. Virol.* **72:**3370–3376.
21. **Butterworth, B. E., E. J. Shimshick, and F. Y. Yin.** 1976. Association of polioviral RNA polymerase complex with phospholipid membranes. *J. Virol.* **19:**457–466.
22. **Caliguiri, L. A., and I. Tamm.** 1970. The role of cytoplasmic membranes in poliovirus biosynthesis. *Virology* **42:**100–111.
23. **Cho, M. W., O. C. Richards, T. M. Dmitrieva, V. Agol, and E. Ehrenfeld.** 1993. RNA duplex unwinding activity of poliovirus RNA-dependent RNA polymerase 3Dpol. *J. Virol.* **67:**3010–3018.
24. **Cho, M. W., N. Teterina, D. Egger, K. Bienz, and E. Ehrenfeld.** 1994. Membrane rearrangement and vesicle induction by recombinant poliovirus 2C and 2BC in human cells. *Virology* **202:**129–145.
25. **Ciervo, A., F. Beneduce, and G. Morace.** 1998. Polypeptide 3AB of hepatitis A virus is a transmembrane protein. *Biochem. Biophys. Res. Commun.* **249:**266–274.
26. **Collis, P. S., B. J. O'Donnell, D. J. Barton, J. A. Rogers, and J. B. Flanegan.** 1992. Replication of poliovirus RNA and subgenomic RNA transcripts in transfected cells. *J. Virol.* **66:**6480–6488.
27. **Cuconati, A., A. Molla, and E. Wimmer.** 1998. Brefeldin A inhibits cell-free, de novo synthesis of poliovirus. *J. Virol.* **72:**6456–6464.
28. **Dales, S., H. J. Eggers, I. Tamm, and G. E. Palade.** 1965. Electron microscopic study of the formation of poliovirus. *Virology* **26:**379–389.
29. **Echeverri, A., R. Banerjee, and A. Dasgupta.** 1998. Amino-terminal region of poliovirus 2C protein is sufficient for membrane binding. *Virus Res.* **54:**217–223.
30. **Echeverri, A. C., and A. Dasgupta.** 1995. Amino terminal regions of poliovirus 2C protein mediate membrane binding. *Virology* **208:**540–553.
31. **Egger, D., L. Pasamontes, R. Bolten, V. Boyko, and K. Bienz.** 1996. Reversible dissociation of the poliovirus replication complex: functions and interactions of its components in viral RNA synthesis. *J. Virol.* **70:**8675–8683.

32. **Egger, D., N. Teterina, E. Ehrenfeld, and K. Bienz.** 2000. Formation of the poliovirus replication complex requires coupled viral translation, vesicle production, and viral RNA synthesis. *J. Virol.* **74:**6570–6580.
33. **Enders, J. F.** 1955. Developments in tissue culture, p. 221–223. In *Poliomyelitis: Papers and Discussions Presented at the Third International Poliomyelitis Conference.* Lippincott, Philadelphia, Pa.
34. **Etchison, D., and E. Ehrenfeld.** 1981. Comparison of replication complexes synthesizing poliovirus RNA. *Virology* **111:**33–46.
35. **Flanegan, J., and D. Baltimore.** 1977. Poliovirus-specific primer dependent RNA polymerase able to copy poly(A). *Proc. Natl. Acad. Sci. USA* **74:**3677–3680.
36. **Frankel, G., Y. Lorch, P. Karlik, and A. Friedmann.** 1987. Fractionation of Theiler's virus-infected BHK21 cell homogenates: isolation of virus-induced membranes. *Virology* **158:**452–455.
37. **Gamarnik, A. V., and R. Andino.** 2000. Interactions of viral protein 3CD and poly(RC) binding protein with the 5′ untranslated region of the poliovirus genome. *J. Virol.* **74:**2219–2226.
38. **Gamarnik, A. V., and R. Andino.** 1998. Switch from translation to RNA replication in a positive-stranded RNA virus. *Genes Dev.* **12:**2293–2304.
39. **Giachetti, C., and B. L. Semler.** 1991. Roles of a viral membrane polypeptide in strand-specific initiation of poliovirus RNA synthesis. *J. Virol.* **65:**2647–2654.
40. **Girard, S., T. Couderc, J. Destombes, D. Thiesson, F. Delpeyroux, and B. Blondel.** 1999. Poliovirus induces apoptosis in the mouse central nervous system. *J. Virol.* **73:**6066–6072.
41. **Goodfellow, I., Y. Chaudhry, A. Richardson, J. Meredith, J. W. Almond, W. Barclay, and D. J. Evans.** 2000. Identification of a *cis*-acting replication element within the poliovirus coding region. *J. Virol.* **74:**4590–4600.
42. **Gorbalenya, A. E., E. V. Koonin, and Y. I. Wolf.** 1990. A new superfamily of putative NTP-binding domains encoded by genomes of small DNA and RNA viruses. *FEBS Lett.* **262:**145–148.
43. **Gosert, R., D. Egger, and K. Bienz.** 2000. A cytopathic and a cell culture adapted hepatitis-A virus strain differ in cell killing but not in intracellular membrane rearrangements. *Virology* **266:**157–169.
44. **Gromeier, M., B. Bossert, M. Arita, A. Nomoto, and E. Wimmer.** 1999. Dual stem loops within the poliovirus internal ribosomal entry site control neurovirulence. *J. Virol.* **73:**958–964.
45. **Gromeier, M., S. Mueller, D. Solecki, B. Bossert, G. Bernhardt, and E. Wimmer.** 1997. Determinants of poliovirus neurovirulence. *J. Neurovirol.* **3:**S35–S38.
46. **Harris, K. S., W. Xiang, L. Alexander, W. S. Lane, A. V. Paul, and E. Wimmer.** 1994. Interaction of poliovirus polypeptide 3CDpro with the 5′ and 3′ termini of the poliovirus genome. Identification of viral and cellular cofactors needed for efficient binding. *J. Biol. Chem.* **269:**27004–27014.
47. **Irurzun, A., J. Arroyo, A. Alvarez, and L. Carrasco.** 1995. Enhanced intracellular calcium concentration during poliovirus infection. *J. Virol.* **69:**5142–5146.
48. **Irurzun, A., L. Perez, and L. Carrasco.** 1992. Involvement of membrane traffic in the replication of poliovirus genomes: effects of brefeldin A. *Virology* **191:**166–175.
49. **Jecht, M., C. Probst, and V. GaussMuller.** 1998. Membrane permeability induced by hepatitis A virus proteins 2B and 2BC and proteolytic processing of HAV 2BC. *Virology* **252:**218–227.
50. **Jelachich, M. L., and H. L. Lipton.** 1996. Theiler's murine encephalomyelitis virus kills restrictive but not permissive cells by apoptosis. *J. Virol.* **70:**6856–6861.
51. **Johnson, K. L., and P. Sarnow.** 1991. Three poliovirus 2B mutants exhibit noncomplementable defects in viral RNA amplification and display dosage-dependent dominance over wild-type poliovirus. *J. Virol.* **65:**4341–4349.
52. **Khromykh, A. A., P. L. Sedlak, and E. G. Westaway.** 2000. *cis*- and *trans*-acting elements in flavivirus RNA replication. *J. Virol.* **74:**3253–3263.
53. **Klingel, K., C. Hohenadl, A. Canu, M. Albrecht, M. Seemann, G. Mall, and R. Kandolf.** 1992. Ongoing enterovirus-induced myocarditis is associated with persistent heart muscle infection: quantitative analysis of virus replication, tissue damage, and inflammation. *Proc. Natl. Acad. Sci. USA* **89:**314–318.
54. **Klingel, K., P. Rieger, G. Mall, H. C. Selinka, M. Huber, and R. Kandolf.** 1998. Visualization of enteroviral replication in myocardial tissue by ultrastructural in situ hybridization: identification of target cells and cytopathic effects. *Lab. Invest.* **78:**1227–1237.
55. **Kusov, Y. Y., C. Probst, M. Jecht, P. D. Jost, and V. GaussMuller.** 1998. Membrane association and RNA binding of recombinant hepatitis A virus protein 2C. *Arch. Virol.* **143:**931–944.
56. **LeGrand, E. K.** 2000. Implications of early apoptosis of infected cells as an important host defense. *Med. Hypotheses.* **54:**591–596.
57. **Maynell, L. A., K. Kirkegaard, and M. W. Klymkowsky.** 1992. Inhibition of poliovirus RNA synthesis of brefeldin A. *J. Virol.* **66:**1985–1994.
58. **Meyer, J., R. E. Lundquist, and J. V. Maizel, Jr.** 1978. Structural studies of the RNA component of the poliovirus replication complex. II. Characterization by electron microscopy and autoradiography. *Virology* **85:**445–455.
59. **Mirzayan, C., and E. Wimmer.** 1992. Genetic analysis of an NTP-binding motif in poliovirus polypeptide 2C. *Virology* **189:**547–555.
60. **Molla, A., K. S. Harris, A. V. Paul, S. H. Shin, J. Mugavero, and E. Wimmer.** 1994. Stimulation of poliovirus proteinase 3Cpro-related proteolysis by the genome-linked protein VPg and its precursor 3AB. *J. Biol. Chem.* **269:**27015–27020.
61. **Molla, A., A. V. Paul, and E. Wimmer.** 1991. Cell-free, de novo synthesis of poliovirus. *Science* **254:**1647–1651.
62. **Mosser, A. G., L. A. Caliguiri, and I. Tamm.** 1972. Incorporation of lipid precursors into cytoplasmic membranes of poliovirus-infected HeLa cells. *Virology* **47:**39–47.
63. **Nomoto, A., B. Detjen, R. Pozzatti, and E. Wimmer.** 1977. The location of the polio genome protein in viral RNAs and its implication for RNA synthesis. *Nature* **268:**208–213.
64. **Novak, J. E., and K. Kirkegaard.** 1994. Coupling between genome translation and replication in an RNA virus. *Genes Dev.* **8:**1726–1737.
65. **Paul, A. V., A. Molla, and E. Wimmer.** 1994. Studies of a putative amphipathic helix in the N-terminus of poliovirus protein 2C. *Virology* **199:**188–199.
66. **Paul, A. V., J. Mugavero, A. Molla, and E. Wimmer.** 1998. Internal ribosomal entry site scanning of the poliovirus polyprotein: implications for proteolytic processing. *Virology* **250:**241–253.
67. **Paul, A. V., J. H. vanBoom, D. Filippov, and E. Wimmer.** 1998. Protein-primed RNA synthesis by purified poliovirus RNA polymerase. *Nature* **393:**280–284.
68. **Pfister, T., and E. Wimmer.** 1999. Characterization of the nucleoside triphosphatase activity of poliovirus protein 2C reveals a mechanism by which guanidine inhibits poliovirus replication. *J. Biol. Chem.* **274:**6992–7001.

69. Pincus, S. E., D. C. Diamond, E. A. Emini, and E. Wimmer. 1986. Guanidine-selected mutants of poliovirus: mapping of point mutations to polypeptide 2C. *J. Virol.* **57:**638–646.
70. Reissig, M., D. W. Howes, and J. L. Melnick. 1956. Sequence of morphological changes in epithelial cell cultures infected with poliovirus. *J. Exp. Med.* **104:**289–304.
71. Roivainen, M., S. Rasilainen, P. Ylipaasto, R. Nissinen, J. Ustinov, L. Bouwens, D. L. Eizirik, T. Hovi, and T. Otonkoski. 2000. Mechanisms of coxsackievirus-induced damage to human pancreatic beta-cells. *J. Clin. Endocrinol. Metab.* **85:**432–440.
72. Roulston, A., R. C. Marcellus, and P. E. Branton. 1999. Viruses and apoptosis. *Annu. Rev. Microbiol.* **53:**577–628.
72a. Rust, R. C., L. Landmann, R. Gosert, B. L. Tang, W. J. Hong, H. P. Hauri, D. Egger, and K. Bienz. 2001. Cellular COPII proteins are involved in production of the vesicles that form the poliovirus replication complex. *J. Virol.* **75:**9808–9818.
73. Sandoval, I. V., and L. Carrasco. 1997. Poliovirus infection and expression of the poliovirus protein 2B provoke the disassembly of the Golgi complex, the organelle target for the antipoliovirus drug Ro-090179. *J. Virol.* **71:**4679–4693.
74. Schlegel, A., T. H. Giddings, Jr., M. S. Ladinsky, and K. Kirkegaard. 1996. Cellular origin and ultrastructure of membranes induced during poliovirus infection. *J. Virol.* **70:**6576–6588.
75. Springer, S., A. Spang, and R. Schekman. 1999. A primer on vesicle budding. *Cell* **97:**145–148.
75a. Suhy, D. A., T. H. Giddings, and K. Kierkegaard. 2000. Remodeling the endoplasmic reticulum by poliovirus infection and by individual viral proteins: an autophagy-like origin for virus-induced vesicles. *J. Virol.* **74:**8953–8965.
76. Takeda, N., R. J. Kuhn, C. F. Yang, T. Takegami, and E. Wimmer. 1986. Initiation of poliovirus plus-strand RNA synthesis in a membrane complex of infected HeLa cells. *J. Virol.* **60:**43–53.
77. Takegami, T., R. J. Kuhn, C. W. Anderson, and E. Wimmer. 1983. Membrane-dependent uridylylation of the genome-linked protein VPg of poliovirus. *Proc. Natl. Acad. Sci. USA* **80:**7447–7451.
77a. Teterina, N. L., D. Egger, K. Bienz, D. M. Brown, B. L. Semler, and E. Ehrenfeld. 2001. Requirements for assembly of poliovirus replication complexes and negative-strand RNA synthesis. *J. Virol.* **75:**3841–3850.
78. Teterina, N. L., A. E. Gorbalenya, D. Egger, K. Bienz, and E. Ehrenfeld. 1997. Poliovirus 2C protein determinants of membrane binding and rearrangements in mammalian cells. *J. Virol.* **71:**8962–8972.
79. Teterina, N. L., K. M. Kean, A. E. Gorbalenya, V. I. Agol, and M. Girard. 1992. Analysis of the functional significance of amino acid residues in the putative NTP-binding pattern of the poliovirus 2C protein. *J. Gen. Virol.* **73:**1977–1986.
80. Teterina, N. L., W. D. Zhou, M. W. Cho, and E. Ehrenfeld. 1995. Inefficient complementation activity of poliovirus 2C and 3D proteins for rescue of lethal mutations. *J. Virol.* **69:**4245–4254.
81. Tolskaya, E. A., L. I. Romanova, M. S. Kolesnikova, T. A. Ivannikova, E. A. Smirnova, N. T. Raikhlin, and V. I. Agol. 1995. Apoptosis-inducing and apoptosis-preventing functions of poliovirus. *J. Virol.* **69:**1181–1189.
82. Towner, J. S., T. V. Ho, and B. L. Semler. 1996. Determinants of membrane association for poliovirus protein 3AB. *J. Biol. Chem.* **271:**26810–26818.
83. Towner, J. S., M. M. Mazanet, and B. L. Semler. 1998. Rescue of defective poliovirus RNA replication by 3AB-containing precursor polyproteins. *J. Virol.* **72:**7191–7200.
84. Tsunoda, I., C. I. Kurtz, and R. S. Fujinami. 1997. Apoptosis in acute and chronic central nervous system disease induced by Theiler's murine encephalomyelitis virus. *Virology* **228:**388–393.
85. van Kuppeveld, F. J., J. M. Galama, J. Zoll, P. J. van den Hurk, and W. J. Melchers. 1996. Coxsackie B3 virus protein 2B contains cationic amphipathic helix that is required for viral RNA replication. *J. Virol.* **70:**3876–3886.
86. van Kuppeveld, F. J., W. J. Melchers, K. Kirkegaard, and J. R. Doedens. 1997. Structure-function analysis of coxsackie B3 virus protein 2B. *Virology* **227:**111–118.
87. van Kuppeveld, F. J., P. J. J. C. vandenHurk, W. vanderVlient, J. M. D. Galama, and W. J. G. Melchers. 1997. Chimeric coxsackie B3 virus genomes that express hybrid coxsackievirus-poliovirus 2B proteins: functional dissection of structural domains involved in RNA replication. *J. Gen. Virol.* **78:**1833–1840.
88. Weber, S., H. Granzow, F. Weiland, and O. Marquardt. 1996. Intracellular membrane proliferation in *E. coli* induced by foot-and-mouth disease virus 3A gene products. *Virus Genes* **12:**5–14.
89. Wieland, F., and C. Harter. 1999. Mechanisms of vesicle formation: insights from the COP system. *Curr. Opin. Cell Biol.* **11:**440–446.
90. Wimmer, E., C. U. T. Hellen, and X. Cao. 1993. Genetics of poliovirus. *Annu. Rev. Genet.* **27:**353–436.
91. Xiang, W., K. S. Harris, L. Alexander, and E. Wimmer. 1995. Interaction between the 5'-terminal cloverleaf and 3AB/3CDpro of poliovirus is essential for RNA replication. *J. Virol.* **69:**3658–3667.

Molecular Biology of Picornaviruses
Editors, B. L. Semler and E. Wimmer
©2002 ASM Press, Washington, DC 20036-2904

Poliovirus RNA-Dependent RNA Polymerase (3D^{pol}): Structure, Function, and Mechanism

CRAIG E. CAMERON, DAVID W. GOHARA, AND JAMIE J. ARNOLD

21

Replication of the poliovirus genome has been studied for many decades by using a variety of molecular, genetic, biochemical, and structural approaches (1, 71, 83, 98, 99). These studies have uncovered most, if not all, of the virus-encoded proteins and RNA sequences/structures required for genome replication. The polyprotein produced by translation of viral RNA can be divided into three regions: P1, P2, and P3. P1 encodes viral structural proteins; P2 and P3 encode viral nonstructural proteins. Interestingly, all of the nonstructural proteins of the virus are thought to be involved in the genome replication process. For example, proteins encoded by the P2 region of the genome are important for converting the host cell cytoplasm into an environment conducive for efficient production of genomes (2, 3, 20, 22, 25, 28, 84, 85, 88, 90). Proteins encoded by the P3 region of the genome, however, are thought to participate more directly in the genome replication process (4, 5, 101, and references therein). The fourth and final protein domain of the P3 region of the viral polyprotein is the RNA-dependent RNA polymerase (RdRP), 3D^{pol}, the core component of the replication machinery.

Since the initial report of RdRP activity in poliovirus-infected cells (29), many laboratories have worked to understand this enzyme. These studies have led to the overexpression of 3D^{pol} in *Escherichia coli* (33, 59, 61, 62, 73, 80, 82), biochemical and biological analysis of 3D^{pol} and derivatives of 3D^{pol} produced by using site-directed mutagenesis (6–8, 11, 12, 16, 19, 21, 23, 24, 30, 32, 36, 40, 41, 54, 60, 67–70, 72, 76–79, 93–96), solution of the crystal structure of 3D^{pol} (35), and construction of a structural model for 3D^{pol} in complex with substrates: primer/template and nucleotide (32).

Given the vast literature that has accumulated over the years with 3D^{pol} as the primary focus, it is impossible to provide a comprehensive review of this information here. Therefore, in this chapter, we will focus primarily on studies performed over the past 4 years that have permitted a more detailed appreciation of the structure, function, and mechanism of this prototypic RdRP.

STRUCTURE OF 3D^{pol}: RELATIONSHIP TO OTHER POLYMERASES

One of the most important contributions to our understanding of 3D^{pol} function was the solution of the crystal structure of 3D^{pol} by Schultz and colleagues in 1997 (35). This structure provided the first glimpse into the architecture of an RdRP. Given the existence of structures for the other three classes of nucleic acid polymerase (26, 39, 47, 66, 86), structural information for 3D^{pol} also filled in a gap that existed for many years.

A ribbon diagram of 3D^{pol} is shown in Color Plate 18A, following p. 156. The overall topology of 3D^{pol} is very similar to that of the other classes of nucleic acid polymerase. This enzyme can be compared to a cupped right hand with "fingers," "palm," and "thumb" subdomains. The fingers and thumb subdomains are likely involved in nucleic acid binding; the palm subdomain is likely involved in nucleic acid and nucleotide binding along with catalysis. While both the palm and thumb subdomains provided clear electron density for model construction, a substantial portion of the fingers subdomain (amino acids 38 to 66, 98 to 180, and 270 to 290) was disordered and is absent from the model. The location of this missing region of the fingers subdomain can be approximated by comparison of the 3D^{pol} structure to that of reverse transcriptase (RT) from human immunodeficiency virus (HIV) shown in Color Plate 18B.

The palm subdomain of 3D^{pol} is composed of five conserved motifs, designated motifs A to E (see Color Plate 18A). As discussed in greater detail below, these conserved regions of the palm subdomain are involved in nucleotide binding (motifs A and B) (9, 13, 14, 18, 31, 32, 74), phosphoryl transfer (motif C) (10, 40, 41, 92, 93, 97), structural integrity of the palm subdomain (motif D) (17), and nucleic acid binding (motif E) (38, 42, 75). In addition, a sixth conserved structural motif (motif F) was identified based on modeling of the 3D^{pol} ternary complex (32) and evaluation of the hepatitis C virus (HCV) polymerase structure (15, 53). This motif is located in the fingers sub-

---

Craig E. Cameron, David W. Gohara, and Jamie J. Arnold ■ Department of Biochemistry and Molecular Biology, Pennsylvania State University, University Park, PA 16802.

domain and is likely involved in binding to the triphosphate moiety of the nucleotide substrate. Similar functions can be ascribed to motifs A–F of HIV RT (Color Plate 18B) (39) and the RdRP from HCV, NS5B (Color Plate 18C) (53).

Amino-terminal to the fingers subdomain is a region of $3D^{pol}$ predicted to be unique to the RdRP compared to other classes of nucleic acid polymerase. This region corresponds to amino acids 1 to 97 of $3D^{pol}$. Residues 1 to 11 and 38 to 66 are disordered. Residues 12 to 37 form a strand that may comprise part of the thumb subdomain, and residues 67 to 97 form a helix that is located beneath the fingers subdomain. Based on the Schultz structure, it was not possible to determine how the strand and helix are connected. In fact, it was proposed that the amino-terminal strand might originate from a different $3D^{pol}$ molecule and constitute an oligomerization domain. However, an alternative hypothesis can be put forward based on the crystal structure of HCV NS5B (53).

As indicated in Color Plate 18C, HCV NS5B has a completely encircled active site owing to extensive interactions between the unique amino-terminal region of this enzyme (termed the fingertips in Color Plate 18C) and the thumb subdomains. By using sequence and structural homology between $3D^{pol}$ and NS5B, it is possible to construct a complete model of $3D^{pol}$, including the missing portion of the fingers subdomain and the amino-terminal region (Color Plate 18D). This model of $3D^{pol}$ suggests that this enzyme may also have a completely encircled active site as a result of interactions between the fingertips and the thumb subdomains. It should be noted that to build the complete model of $3D^{pol}$, the 12 to 37 strand shown in the Schultz structure as a part of the thumb subdomain had to be repositioned. These residues are colored orange in the models shown in Color Plate 18A and 18D.

The possible existence of an interaction between the fingertips and the thumb subdomains of $3D^{pol}$ has interesting functional implications. For example, as a result of these putative interactions, a channel is formed that may facilitate entry of nucleotides into or exit of pyrophosphate from the catalytic center (Color Plate 19A, following p. 156). That negatively charged molecules like nucleotides and pyrophosphate would be attracted to this channel is supported by the fact that the entrance to the channel is decorated by an array of conserved lysines and arginines. Interestingly, one of these residues, Lys-61, has been implicated in the affinity of $3D^{pol}$ for nucleotides (76, 77, 79).

The proposed interaction between the fingertips and thumb subdomains also contributes to formation of a long groove on the surface of the enzyme sufficient to accommodate 10 nucleotides of RNA (Color Plate 19B). This value is in agreement with that determined biochemically (12). The nucleic acid-binding site of this enzyme should be much less dynamic than those polymerases that lack the fingertips-thumb interaction. The lack of conformational flexibility between the fingers and thumb subdomains should permit a more stable association of $3D^{pol}$ with nucleic acid if dissociation of the polymerase-nucleic acid complex is driven by movement (intrinsic dynamics) of the fingers and/or thumb subdomains. In agreement with this hypothesis is the finding that the half-life of a $3D^{pol}$-primer/template complex is 0.3 to 2 h at 37°C (7), a value 1,000-fold more stable than that of a comparable HIV RT-primer/template complex (45).

OLIGOMERIZATION OF $3D^{pol}$

The preceding discussion highlights the similarity of $3D^{pol}$ with other classes of nucleic acid polymerase. While features unique to $3D^{pol}$ may exist, for example, the so-called fingertips, this subdomain likely exists in all RdRPs based on the two RdRP structures available to date. In contrast, two potential interaction/oligomerization domains were also observed in the crystal structure of $3D^{pol}$. These interaction surfaces have no structural homologues in any other polymerases for which structural information is available, including the RdRP from HCV. The two interaction domains have been termed interfaces I and II (Color Plate 20A, following p. 156) (35).

Based on the crystal structure, both interfaces are predicted to have extensive interaction surfaces. Interface I is formed from the back of the palm of one subunit interacting with the back of the thumb of a second subunit and buries 1,480 Å^2 of solvent-accessible surface area (35). Interface II is formed from interactions between the residues 12 to 37 of one subunit interacting with the thumb of a second subunit. This interaction of the 12 to 37 strand would be stabilized by interaction of the back of the fingers of one subunit (helix composed of residues 67 to 97 of the amino-terminal region) with the top of the thumb of a second subunit. As discussed above, our modeling studies based on the structure of HCV NS5B would change the intermolecular interaction between the 12 to 37 strand and the thumb (Color Plate 20A) to an intramolecular interaction (Color Plate 20B). However, the remaining intermolecular interactions at interface II would remain intact, and none of the interactions at interface I would be affected by the presence of the fingertips. The head-to-tail interaction of polymerase molecules via interface I produces fibers that extend indefinitely (Color Plate 21A, following p. 156). Each molecule of the fiber is rotated 180° and translated 44 Å relative to the adjacent molecule. Fiber-fiber interactions will occur via interface II (Color Plate 21B).

Interface I can be divided into two regions based on the location of residues important for interface stability on the back of the thumb. The first region is located at the top of the thumb (Color Plate 22A, following p. 156). A single residue at the top of the thumb (Leu-446) inserts into a hydrophobic pocket on the back of the palm of the second subunit. This hydrophobic pocket is formed by Leu-309, Tyr-313, Ile-316, Tyr-334, and Val-338. The second region is located at the bottom of the thumb (Color Plate 22B). Arginines 455 and 456 of the thumb hydrogen bond to aspartic acids 349 and 339, respectively, of the palm. In addition, Arg-456 may also interact with Ser-341.

Interface II can be divided into two regions based on the requirement for the interaction to be intermolecular in nature. For example, the interaction between the 12 to 37 strand and the thumb can arise either by means of an intermolecular interaction or an intramolecular interaction (Color Plate 22C and 22D). In contrast, the interaction between the 67 to 97 helix and top of the thumb can only occur by means of an intermolecular interaction (Color Plate 22D). We will refer to the former region of interface II as II-A and the latter region of interface II as II-B. Formation of interface II-A is driven by insertion of the side chain of Phe-30 into a hydrophobic pocket composed of Val-33, Ile-401, Ile-436, and Val-439 (Color Plate 22C). Formation of interface II-B involves coordination of a divalent cation (Ca^{2+} in Color Plate 22D) by Glu-26 from one subunit and Asp-89 from the second subunit. In addition, hydrogen bonding between Asp-79 from one subunit and Arg-443 from the second subunit should also stabilize interface II-B (Color Plate 22D).

Does interface II-A arise from an inter- or intramolecular interaction? Cross-linking experiments performed by the Schultz laboratory have shown that intermolecular interactions can, in fact, occur at interface II (37). Therefore, the model presented in Color Plate 18D is clearly speculative. However, recent structural data for the RdRP from rabbit hemorrhagic disease virus show intramolecular interactions at interface II-A (K. Ng and M. N. James, personal communication). This enzyme belongs to the same supergroup as poliovirus polymerase and shares significant homology with this enzyme (48, 100).

The ability to define the oligomerization domains in such great detail permits us to ask whether these domains are present in all picornavirus polymerases. If all picornavirus polymerases interact via similar interfaces, then it is reasonable to expect that residues critical to the stability of the interface will be conserved in all enzymes or change in a manner consistent with retention of polymerase-polymerase interactions. The result of such an analysis is presented in Table 1. Interface I should form in all picornavirus polymerases. All of the residues comprising this interaction surface are conserved or change in a manner that should not disrupt this interface. Interaction between the 12 to 37 strand and the thumb, interface II-A, should also occur in all picornavirus polymerases. However, interaction between the bottom of the fingers and the top of the thumb, interface II-B, may not occur in all picornavirus polymerases. For example, neither Glu-26 nor Asp-79, ligands to the divalent cation critical for the intermolecular interaction, is conserved (Table 1).

Is there a biological role for polymerase oligomerization? Given the extensive nature of the interactions comprising interface I and the apparent conservation of this particular interface within the family of picornavirus polymerases, it seems reasonable to conclude that this interface has some biological function. In support of this conclusion, Diamond and Kirkegaard have shown that changing arginines 455 and 456, residues critical to the integrity of interface I, to alanine renders the virus inviable (24). The initial explanation for this phenotype was based on the observation that $3D^{pol}$ shows strong cooperativity in binding nucleic acid, and with some RNA templates (for example, Fig. 1A), complete coating of the RNA is essential for utilization of the RNA by $3D^{pol}$ (67). Therefore, destabilization of interface I would be predicted to diminish directly RNA binding and indirectly polymerase activity. A direct role for interface I in cooperative binding of $3D^{pol}$ to RNA has recently been established by biochemical characterization of $3D^{pol}$ derivatives containing mutations at positions 455, 456, or other positions (37). Biochemical and biological analyses of poliovirus derivatives with changes at position 446 (top of thumb) and 342 (back of palm) provide additional support for the architecture of interface I shown in Color Plate 22A and 22B and a requirement for this interface in virus multiplication (37). Finally, mutations found in $3D^{pol}$-coding sequence of the Sabin poliovirus type 1 may confer temperature sensitivity to this mutant virus by altering the efficiency of interface I formation and/or the stability of this interface (69).

Our laboratory has also performed studies to probe the function of interface I. Biological studies using a poliovirus replicon have shown that mutations similar to those discussed above that disrupt interface I preclude RNA synthesis in vivo. Biochemical analysis of the corresponding $3D^{pol}$ derivatives in vitro failed to show defects in protein stability, binding to synthetic RNA primer/templates, or polymerase activity (S. K. Ghosh, H. B. Pathak, S. Sharma, J. Graci, and C. E. Cameron, unpublished results). Interface I mutants also retain the capacity to uridylylate VPg when the reaction is templated by the recently discovered cis-acting replication element (cre) (34, 70). However, the efficiency of this reaction cannot be stimulated by 3CD when interface I mutants are employed. These data suggest that an interaction between 3D and 3CD may exist that is mediated by interactions with interface I. It is worth noting that the Wimmer laboratory has demonstrated an interaction between 3D and 3CD by using the yeast two-hybrid system (101). This 3D-3CD interaction may be required for efficient uridylylation of VPg, an obligatory step for synthesis of progeny viral genomes. It must be stressed that this interpretation is currently only speculation. The development of a coherent model to explain the function of interface I will be an important contribution to our understanding of not only $3D^{pol}$ structure-function relationships but also mechanisms controlling initiation of viral RNA synthesis.

Interface II-A clearly also has an important role in poliovirus polymerase function and consequently in virus multiplication as mutations that are predicted to disrupt this interface inactivate polymerase activity (37). Two models have been presented for interface II-A formation based on the nature of the interaction—that is, inter- or intramolecular. At this time, we would like to propose the possibility that both types of interaction occur in vivo, thereby expanding the functional capabilities of $3D^{pol}$. For example, intermolecular interactions would permit association of $3D^{pol}$ fibers (Color Plate 21B) and enable formation of a $3D^{pol}$ lattice that might act as a scaffold for RNA replication and/or other processes essential for virus multiplication. Intramolecular interactions would permit a stable association of polymerase with nascent RNA and/or template as discussed above. A more rigorous analysis of this interface in vitro and in vivo is necessary to understand better the structure and function of this interface.

MODEL OF A $3D^{pol}$-PRIMER/TEMPLATE-NUCLEOTIDE COMPLEX

To gain additional insight into the structural basis for $3D^{pol}$ function, we constructed a model for a ternary complex of $3D^{pol}$ (32) based on structural information available for HIV RT (39). In Color Plate 23A, following p. 156, the central core of the polymerase active site, primarily the palm subdomain, is shown with bound primer/template, incoming nucleotide (ATP), and two magnesium ions. By using this ternary complex model, we have identified structural features of this enzyme required for phosphoryl transfer, coupling of correct nucleotide binding to catalytic efficiency and ribonucleotide specificity.

Two divalent cations are required for polymerase-catalyzed phosphoryl transfer reactions (87). This requirement for divalent cations has been demonstrated biochemically for $3D^{pol}$ (8, 29, 41). The ability to model two magnesium ions in the $3D^{pol}$ ternary complex supports the

TABLE 1 Conservation of residues among structural features of poliovirus 3D[pol]

Residue	Conservation[a]	Interaction[b]
Interface I[c]		
Leu-309	Hydrophobic (Leu, Ile, Val)	Leu-446
Tyr-313	Strictly conserved	Leu-446
Ile-316	Hydrophobic (Ile, Val, Phe)	Leu-446
Tyr-334	Hydrophobic (Tyr, Phe, Thr)	Leu-446
Val-338	Hydrophobic (Val, Leu, Ile)	Leu-446
Asp-339	Highly conserved (Asp 90%, Gln)	Arg-456
Ser-341	Charged (Ser, Glu, Asp, Asn, Gln)	Arg-456
Asp-349	Charged (Asp, Lys, Ser, Glu)	Arg-455
Leu-446	Hydrophobic (Leu, Ile, Val, Ala)	Leu-309, Tyr-313, Ile-316, Tyr-334, Val-338
Arg-455	Conserved (Arg, His)	Asp-349
Arg-456	Charged (Arg, Lys, Asp, Glu)	Asp-339, Ser-341
Interface II		
Glu-26	Charged (Glu, Arg, Lys, His, Gln)	Metal ion
Phe-30	Hydrophobic (Phe, Tyr, Ala)	Ile-401, Ile-436, Val-439
His-31	Highly conserved (His 90%, Arg, Tyr)	Met-86
Val-33	Highly conserved (Val 80%, Ile)	Phe-30, Val-439
Asp-79	Charged (Asp, Glu, Lys)	Arg-443
Asp-89	Partly conserved (Asp 50%, Phe 30%, Gly 20%)	Metal ion
Ile-401	Hydrophobic (Ile, Val, Leu)	Phe-30, Ile-436
Ile-436	Hydrophobic (Ile, Phe, Val)	Phe-30, Ile-401
Val-439	Highly conserved (Val 80%, Leu, Cys)	Phe-30, Val-33
Arg-443	Charged (Arg, Lys)	Asp-79
Fingers (NTP)		
Lys-159	Strictly conserved	Contacts with incoming nucleotide
Arg-163	Strictly conserved	α-Phosphate of bound NTP
Lys-167	Strictly conserved	Contacts with incoming nucleotide
Lys-172	Strictly conserved	γ-Phosphate of bound NTP
Arg-174	Strictly conserved	α-Phosphate of bound NTP
Palm/thumb[e]		
Lys-359	Highly conserved (Lys 95%, Ala 5%)	Contacts with incoming nucleotide
Lys-375[d]	Strictly conserved	Primer backbone: P−1, P−2
Arg-376	Strictly conserved	Primer backbone: P−2, P−3
RNA binding groove[e]		
Ser-115	Highly conserved (Ser 90%, Ala 10%)	Nucleotide base: T+3
Arg-136	Partly conserved (Arg 40%, Lys 40%, Asn, Gly, Ala)	RNA backbone: T+4
Lys-143	Charged (Glu, Lys, Arg)	RNA backbone: T+4, T+5
Asp-146	Partly conserved (Asp 60%, Asn 30%, Lys 10%)	Nucleotide base: T+5
Tyr-157	Hydrophobic (Tyr, Phe, Cys)	Sugar stacking: T+3
Lys-278	Charged (Lys, Arg, Asn, Glu, Ser)	Nucleotide base: T+3
dsRNA[e]		
Lys-395	Highly conserved (Lys 80%, [Glu, Asp, Asn] 15%, Val 5%)	Primer/template duplex: P−3/T−3
Glu-399	Partly conserved (Glu 70%, Ser 10%, Ala 20%)	Primer/template duplex: P−3/T−3
Arg-408	Charged ([Arg, Lys, Ser] 90%, Ala, Gly)	Primer/template duplex: P−4/T−4, P−5/T−5
Gln-411	Highly conserved (Gln 90%, Glu, Lys, Ser)	Primer/template duplex: T−7
Asp-412	Highly conserved (Asp 70%, Glu 30%)	Primer/template duplex: P−6/T−6, T−7
Arg-415	Partly conserved (Arg 50%, Glu, Met, Thr, Leu, Ile)	Primer/template duplex: T−6
Ser-416	Highly conserved (Ser 80%, Asn 20%)	Primer/template duplex: P−4

[a] Conservation was determined based on sequence alignment of the RNA-dependent RNA polymerases from foot-and-mouth disease virus, encephalomyocarditis virus, mengovirus, hepatitis A virus, poliovirus, echovirus, coxsackie A virus, coxsackie B virus, and human rhinovirus (A. C. Palmenberg, http://www.bocklabs.wisc.edu/acp; A. C. Palmenberg, personal communication).
[b] Interactions were determined using the program "CONTACT" from the CCP4 suite of programs. Interatomic distance cutoffs were set between 2.8 and 3.3 Å.
[c] Residues in boldfaced type are from the same side of either interface I or II (i.e., blue molecule in Color Plates 20 and 22).
[d] Residues that are underlined have been mutated. The mutations and phenotypes are listed in Table 2.
[e] Interactions are based on a comparison of the 3D[pol] ternary complex model with HIV-1 RT.

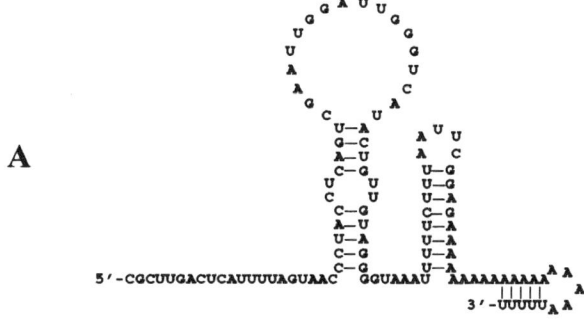

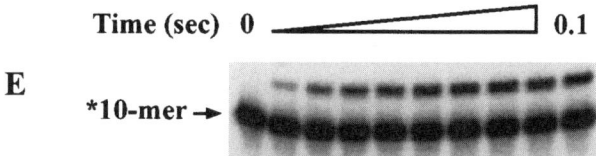

FIGURE 1 Substrates employed to study poliovirus polymerase in vitro. (A) Hairpin substrate (67). (B) Homopolymeric primer/template substrate (dT$_{15}$/rA$_{30}$) (6). (C) Heteropolymeric primer/template substrate (8). (D) sym/sub (7). (E) 3D^{pol}-catalyzed incorporation of AMP into sym/sub (7).

hypothesis that the chemical mechanism of the RdRP will be similar to the DNA polymerases. The magnesium ions have been designated A and B. Metal A is coordinated by the 3'-OH of primer, Asp-233 of motif A, and Asp-328 of motif C (Color Plate 23B). Asp-328 is a part of the Gly-Asp^{328}-Asp RdRP signature (48). The primary function of metal A is to activate the 3'-OH nucleophile by lowering the pK$_a$ of this moiety. In addition, metal A may serve to stabilize negative charge that forms during the reaction. Metal B is also coordinated by Asp-233 and Asp-328 (Color Plate 23B). However, this metal also has extensive interactions with oxygens of the triphosphate moiety of the incoming nucleotide (Color Plate 23B). The interaction between metal B and the triphosphate likely stabilizes the triphosphate in a conformation competent for catalysis.

The appropriate conformation of the triphosphate moiety of the incoming nucleotide is essential for efficient phosphodiester bond formation. The simplest explanation for this requirement is that an optimal distance exists between the 3'-OH of primer and the alpha phosphorus of the incoming nucleotide for attack of the phosphorus by the activated hydroxyl. Increasing the distance between the alpha phosphorus and hydroxyl should decrease the rate of phosphoryl transfer (52). Therefore, the enzyme has evolved several mechanisms to ensure the proper orientation of the triphosphate. In addition to the divalent cations, residues in motif F (Lys-159, Arg-163, Lys-167, Lys-172, and Arg-174) (see Table 1) interact with and stabilize the triphosphate moiety of the incoming nucleotide. This motif is also found in RT but is not found in other classes of nucleic acid polymerase (Color Plate 24, following p. 156) (32, 39, 53).

Interestingly, the position of the triphosphate is also linked to the presence of the correct sugar configuration—that is, the presence of hydroxyls at both the 2' and 3' positions of the nucleotide. As indicated in Color Plate 23B, motif A, in particular Asp-233, participates in the stabilization of metal B in the active site. This metal also interacts with the triphosphate of the incoming nucleotide. Motif A forms a β-turn-α structure with Asp-233 residing in the β-strand (Color Plate 23B). The position of this strand is modulated by the position of the carboxy-terminal α-helix. One residue critical for determining the position of this α-helix is Asp-238 (Color Plate 23C). Asp-238 is located in the ribose-binding pocket and either directly or indirectly interacts with the 2′-OH of the ribonucleotide (D. W. Gohara and C. E. Cameron, unpublished results). In the absence of a 2′-OH, the orientation of the Asp-238 side chain will change, causing movement of Asp-233, which, in turn, will decrease catalytic efficiency owing to the increased mobility of the triphosphate moiety of the incoming nucleotide.

The position of the Asp-238 side chain is also dependent on the presence of the 3′-OH. The amide nitrogen of the Asp-238 residue hydrogen bonds to the 3′-OH of the incoming nucleotide. This interaction limits the dynamics of this residue and the corresponding side chain. Removing the 3′-OH of the incoming nucleotide would, therefore, decrease catalytic efficiency in a manner similar to that described above for the 2′-OH by increasing the mobility of the triphosphate. The absence of a 3′-OH on the incoming nucleotide may also increase the mobility of the triphosphate as a result of loss of the hydrogen bond between the 3′-OH and the oxygen of the beta phosphorus of the nucleotide (Color Plate 23C) (Gohara and Cameron, unpublished). A mechanism linking the presence of the correct base to a catalytically competent orientation of the triphosphate likely serves to minimize incorporation of nucleotides with an incorrect base and may involve interactions within the ribose-binding pocket.

Additional mechanisms exist to ensure selection for binding of ribonucleotides (rNTPs) instead of 2′-deoxyribonucleotides (2′-dNTPs). For example, Asn-297, a residue located in motif B that is conserved in all animal virus RdRPs, is in a position that permits hydrogen bonding of its side chain to the 2′-OH. Changing this residue to alanine produces a 3D^{pol} derivative that is essentially incapable of distinguishing between ATP and 2′-dATP (Gohara and Cameron, unpublished). The wild-type enzyme incorporates ATP 200-fold more efficiently than 2′-dATP (7, 32; J. J. Arnold and C. E. Cameron, unpublished results; Gohara and Cameron, unpublished). Apparently, this level of selection is sufficient to preclude incorporation of 2′-dNMPs into the poliovirus genome, perhaps a reflection of the low cytosolic availability of 2′-dNTPs. In prokaryotes, however, the selectivity may need to be greater than 200 and a unique, more stringent mechanism for rNTP selection may exist. Consistent with this possibility is the finding that the constellation of residues predicted to occupy the ribose-binding pocket in bacteriophage Qβ replicase is different from that shown in Color Plate 23C for 3D^{pol}. In particular, Asp-238, Asn-297, and Ser-288 have been changed to Ser, Glu, and Met, respectively, in Qβ replicase (48). It will be interesting to determine whether incorporation of these changes into 3D^{pol} supports catalytic activity and modulates the stringency of rNTP/2′-dNTP selection.

Nucleotide specificity of most nucleic acid polymerases can be modulated by the divalent cation employed in the reaction; this observation holds for 3D^{pol} (8; Gohara and Cameron, unpublished). In the presence of Mn^{2+}, rNTPs are utilized by 3D^{pol} only sixfold better than 2′-dNTPs (Arnold and Cameron, unpublished; Gohara and Cameron, unpublished). This apparent dependence of nucleotide specificity on the nature of the divalent cation employed may reflect the ability of the divalent cation to preorganize the substrate for catalysis. One fundamental difference between the interaction of various divalent cations with the triphosphate moiety of nucleotides is the affinity of the interaction (55). This difference in affinity is usually manifested by changes in the kinetics of dissociation of the metal from the metal-nucleotide complex (55). In particular, Mg^{2+} binds less tightly to the triphosphate of the nucleotide than Mn^{2+}. As a result, retention of Mg^{2+} in the active site long enough for catalysis to occur requires the appropriate positioning of all ligands. As discussed above, the position of several of the ligands to the Mg^{2+} can be modulated by the presence or absence of interactions at sites remote from the catalytic center, such as the ribose-binding pocket. In contrast, Mn^{2+} dissociates very slowly from the metal-nucleotide complex and, therefore, may not require the full complement of interactions in the ribose-binding pocket to support a catalytically active conformation of the triphosphate.

Although the use of Mn^{2+} as the divalent cation in polymerization reactions permits a few nucleotides with the incorrect sugar configuration or base to be incorporated, processive incorporation of these same incorrect nucleotides is not observed (9). The inability to incorporate processively 2′-dNTPs may be a reflection of restrictions imposed by motif C of 3D^{pol} on the nature of the 3′ end of primer required for catalysis to occur. The signature Gly-Asp-Asp motif of RdRPs is located at the top of the motif C loop. The presence of Gly-327 permits the ultimate nucleotide of primer to be held in position for catalysis as long as this nucleotide contains a 2′-OH (Color Plate 23D). Therefore, once a 2′-dNMP is incorporated into primer, the efficiency of the subsequent incorporation should be decreased owing to the inappropriate position of the 3′-OH. Consistent with this hypothesis is the fact that polymerases that use DNA primers more efficiently than RNA primers, HIV RT for example, have a larger residue at this position. In the case of HIV RT, the structurally analogous residue is a methionine. The presence of such a large residue should not only facilitate binding to a primer with a 2′-dNMP located at the ultimate position but also antagonize binding to a primer with an rNMP at this position (Color Plate 23D) (91; Gohara and Cameron, unpublished). Interestingly, changing Gly-327 to Ala in 3D^{pol} increases the efficiency of nucleotide incorporation after incorporation of a 2′-dNMP (Gohara and Cameron, unpublished).

The primary limitation of the existing structural model is that the exact position of amino acid side chains is not known with accuracy. This limitation does not pose a problem with interpretation in the catalytic center or nucleotide-binding pocket given the limited number of side-chain conformations and the extensive use of hydrogen bonding at these sites. However, information regarding the precise interactions of 3D^{pol} with nucleic acid is more difficult to acquire. To circumvent this problem, we have constructed a sequence alignment between 3D^{pol}, HCV NS5B, and HIV RT that has been constrained in part by structural information (Color Plate 24).

This alignment has proved to be useful in making predictions regarding the regions of 3D^{pol} that interact with the nucleic acid backbone, base pairs within the primer/template duplex, and the bases of the template (Table 1). Interactions with the backbone should be important for stability of the 3D^{pol}-nucleic acid complex. Interactions with the base pairs of the duplex may be important for "proofreading" of incorporated nucleotides. Interactions with the template may facilitate local unwinding of any

RNA structure that may impede processive replication of the genome (19). Support for the functional significance of the residues listed in Table 1 derives from the fact that these residues are highly conserved in the RdRPs of all picornavirus family members (Table 1). In addition, several of the residues located in these functional domains have been altered by site-directed mutagenesis and shown to produce virus that is either temperature sensitive for growth or inviable (Table 2).

FUNCTIONAL ANALYSIS OF 3D^{pol}

Until recently, mechanistic evaluation of the polymerase catalytic cycle has not been possible. This gap persisted for so long because of the absence of nucleic acid substrates that permit polymerase activity to be monitored by using end-labeled primers. Traditional polymerase assays for 3D^{pol} employed homopolymeric primer/templates (for example, Fig. 1B). Evidence for polymerase activity is obtained readily by using [α-^{32}P]-UTP; however, very few primers are actually extended in reactions employing this type of substrate (6). The ability to incorporate many nucleotides in these reactions reflects the ability of 3D^{pol} to employ a template-switching mechanism to incorporate nucleotides with these substrates (6). Complexes composed of 3D^{pol} and nascent RNA can move from one template in the reaction to another. By using a 30-nucleotide (nt) homopolymeric RNA template, products greater than 300 nt can be produced (6). Given the added complexity associated with the use of homopolymeric primer/templates, this class

TABLE 2 Mutations introduced in poliovirus 3D^{pol}

Location	Mutation[a]	Phenotype In vivo	Phenotype In vitro	Interactions	Conservation[b]	Reference(s)
Fingers	A29C		D	Interface II	Low conservation	37
	F30A		D	Fingertips	Conserved (65%)	37
	K51A/D53A	TS		Fingertips	Conserved charge	24
	E55A/E56A	TS		Nucleic acid	Conserved charge	24
	E98A/D99A	TS		Nucleic acid	Conserved charge negative	24
	D105A/E108A	SP		Nucleic acid	Conserved charge	24
	K125A/K126A/K127A	D		Nucleic acid	Highly conserved basic	24
	R136A/D137A	TS		Nucleic acid	Highly conserved negative	24
	G149-I-I150[c]	D	D	Nucleic acid	–	16
	I256-L-G257	TS	R	Surface	–	16
	K276L	TS		Nucleic acid	Partly conserved	76, 78, 79
Palm	**K61L**	D	D	Nucleotide	Strictly conserved	76, 78, 79
	D71A/E72A	D			Conserved charge negative	24
	D79A/H80	TS			His conserved (70%)	24
Motif A	E226A/E227A	SP		Nucleic acid	Low conservation	24
	D238A	D	D	Nucleotide (2'-OH)	Highly conserved (98%)	32[d]
	L241-I-S242	D	D	Perturb motif A	–	16
Motif B	C290-S-S291	D	D	Perturb motif B	–	16
	T293A		R	Nucleotide (2'-OH)	Strictly conserved	32[d]
	N297A/D	D/TS	R	Nucleotide (2'-OH)	Strictly conserved	32[d]
Motif C	G327A/V/M		R/R/D	Primer (2'-OH)	Strictly conserved	32[d]
	D328E/H/N/Q		D	Metal ion	Strictly conserved	41
	D329E/N		D	Metal ion	Strictly conserved	41
Motif D	T353-T-M354	SP		Hydrophobic core	–	16
Motif E	K375A/R376A	D		Primer grip	Highly conserved basic	24
	L342A	TS	R	Interface I	Partly conserved (60%)	37
	D349R	WT	R	Interface I	Partly conserved (40%)	37
Thumb	**D381A/E382A/K383A**	D		Stability (H-bond)	Highly conserved negative	24
	K395A/E396A	D		dsRNA	Lys conserved (70%)	24
	H398A/E399A	D		dsRNA	Glu conserved (70%)	24
	K405A/D406A	D		dsRNA	Highly conserved (85%)	24
	D412A/H413A	D		dsRNA	Highly conserved basic	24
	N424D/H/Y	(SP/TS)	TS/TS/WT/TS	Stability	Conserved basic (80%)	16
	E426A/E427A/E428A	TS		Stability	Conserved charge	24
	L446A		R	Interface I	Partly conserved (40%)	37
	R455A/R456A	D		Interface I	Highly conserved	24

[a] Residues on the surface are in boldfaced type.
[b] See footnote a, Table 1.
[c] Inserted residues are indicated as capitalized letters flanked by residues amino- and carboxy-terminal to the insertion.
[d] Gohara and Cameron, unpublished.

of substrate does not provide significant insight into the catalytic mechanism and does not provide precise information regarding the effects of mutations in $3D^{pol}$-coding sequence on function.

Primer/template substrates similar to those employed to study DNA polymerases and reverse transcriptases (Fig. 1C) have also been employed to study $3D^{pol}$ activity (8). Again, very few productive complexes assemble—that is, complexes with the active site of $3D^{pol}$ located over the 3′ end of primer (8). In fact, with these more traditional primer/templates it appears that as much as 70% of the enzyme partitions in a conformation in which the 3′ end of template is located in the $3D^{pol}$ active site (8). Binding of $3D^{pol}$ in the "incorrect" orientation on these substrates appears to be driven by the enzyme's preference for a 5′ overhang in the primer strand. This preference makes sense both biochemically and biologically. For example, the ability of $3D^{pol}$ to move between templates while retaining nascent RNA suggests that a greater number of interactions may occur between $3D^{pol}$ and nascent RNA than between $3D^{pol}$ and template. Moreover, recombination between poliovirus genomes is known to occur frequently in vivo, and a template-switching mechanism is employed during this process (27, 43, 46, 89).

In spite of the fact that $3D^{pol}$ utilizes a 5′ overhang to direct binding in vitro, this enzyme retains the capacity to bind primer/templates in multiple orientations. Therefore, it seemed plausible that by using a symmetrical primer/template (Fig. 1D), stoichiometric assembly of substrates might be realized. This hypothesis proved to be correct (7). The symmetrical substrate shown in Fig. 1D is referred to as sym/sub.

The initial binding of $3D^{pol}$ to sym/sub is slow. Nevertheless, the resulting $3D^{pol}$-sym/sub complex isomerizes to form an extraordinarily stable complex ($t_{1/2} \sim 30$ min to 2 h) that appears to contain a single polymerase monomer (7). Incorporation of single (Fig. 1E) and multiple nucleotides can be evaluated by using this substrate, and this reaction is fast (7). Under saturating conditions of nucleotide, incorporation of a single nucleotide will take only 10 to 40 msec (7). Together, these data predict that a single polymerase monomer should be sufficient to replicate an entire genome in under 2 min, a biologically reasonable time scale (83), without dissociating from nascent RNA. Additional support for the biological relevance of $3D^{pol}$-sym/sub complexes is that analysis of $3D^{pol}$ derivatives with sym/sub predicts biological phenotypes more accurately than other assays, for example, the poly(rU) polymerase assay (32).

The ability to construct $3D^{pol}$ derivatives, evaluate their elongation rates in vitro, and determine the consequence of these changes in vivo has provided additional support for the possibility that genome replication is coupled kinetically to processes upstream (translation) (64) and downstream (packaging) (65). Decreasing the elongation rate of $3D^{pol}$ by 2.5-fold relative to wild-type enzyme produces virus that is temperature sensitive for growth; a fivefold reduction produces inviable virus (32). If only a fivefold decrease in elongation rate is necessary to kill the virus population, then development of antivirals targeting the viral RdRP may be easier than previously imagined.

The availability of sym/sub has facilitated elucidation of the kinetic mechanism for single nucleotide incorporation catalyzed by $3D^{pol}$ (Arnold and Cameron, unpublished). Presentation of the details of this mechanism is beyond the scope of this review; however, the mechanism is fully consistent with structural information, especially regarding the mechanism for rNTP/dNTP selection and correct/incorrect rNTP selection.

As implied in the discussion above, binding of nucleotides is a two-step process. The first step recognizes the triphosphate and the second step organizes the triphosphate for catalysis in a manner that depends on the correct sugar configuration and the correct base. Consistent with this model is the finding that most nucleotides, rNTPs and dNTPs (correct and incorrect), are bound by the enzyme equivalently (Table 3). Specificity shows up primarily in the efficiency of incorporation, a reflection of how well and how long the triphosphate is positioned for attack by the 3′-OH of primer. This conclusion appears to be valid regardless of sequence context (Table 3). It is also worth noting that selection for the correct nucleotide ranges from 5,000 (incorrect pyrimidine-purine pair) to 500,000 (incorrect pyrimidine-pyrimidine pair) during the incorporation step (Table 3 and unpublished results). These data are consistent with the observation that transitions are more prevalent in the poliovirus genome than transversions (21). Finally, $3D^{pol}$ will incorporate nucleotide analogues in vitro, such as the RNA virus mutagen, ribavirin (RTP in Table 3), and 2-aminopurine (2APTP in Table 3). The ability to assay quantitatively the incorporation of nucleotide analogues may assist in development of antiviral nucleotides specific for the viral RdRP.

The preceding discussion has emphasized studies of the $3D^{pol}$-catalyzed elongation reaction. Initiation of poliovirus RNA synthesis requires the 22-amino-acid primer, $3B^{VPg}$. An understanding of the mechanism of peptide-primed initiation of RNA synthesis by $3D^{pol}$ has been pioneered by Paul and Wimmer using poly(rA) or oligo(rA) templates (68). The products of this reaction are VPg-pU, VPg-pUpU, and VPg-poly(U). The solution conditions required for this reaction are quite similar to those required for the elongation reaction. However, Mn^{2+} is the preferred divalent cation, and a concentration of $3B^{VPg}$ in the μM range is required.

The use of poly(rA) as a template for this reaction assumed, quite reasonably, that initiation occurred at the 3′ end of poliovirus RNA. While poliovirus RNA also serves as a template for uridylylation of VPg, this reaction does not require the poly(A) tail of the genome (70). This observation led to the identification of the centrally located *cre* as the template for uridylylation (70). *cre*-templated uridylylation is equivalently efficient in both Mg^{2+} and Mn^{2+} and is stimulated 30-fold by $3CD^{pro}$ (70). *cre* is a 61-nt stem-loop located in the 2C-coding region of poliovirus RNA; functionally equivalent structures likely exist in all picornaviruses (34, 57, 81). Biochemical and genetic data suggest that the upper half of this structure is important for uridylylation activity, with residues in the loop serving as the template (81). The RNA-binding activity of the 3C domain of $3CD^{pro}$ is required for its stimulatory properties (70). To date, only the components have been identified for this reaction. It is likely that the future will provide an understanding of the stoichiometry and mechanism for assembly of this initiation complex, along with mechanisms to transfer the product to the 3′ end of poliovirus RNA.

INSIGHT INTO THE POLIOVIRUS REPLICATION COMPLEX

It is clear that the availability of structural information for $3D^{pol}$ has shed light on our understanding of $3D^{pol}$ function,

TABLE 3 Kinetic and thermodynamic constants for $3D^{pol}$ catalyzed nucleotide incorporation

Substrates		Kinetic parameters	
Nucleic acid	Nucleotide	K_d μM	k_{pol} s^{-1}
sym/sub-U			
GCA**U**CCCGGG	ATP[a]	133.5 ± 18.1	86.7 ± 3.7
GGGCCC**U**ACG	2'-dATP[a]	284.3 ± 59.1	0.80 ± 0.06
	3'-dATP[b]	317.5 ± 51.7	1.40 ± 0.09
	2APTP[b]	85.3 ± 23.4	1.95 ± 0.17
	ATPαS[b]	88.8 ± 23.5	20.6 ± 1.6
	GTP[c]	310.0 ± 29.6	0.013 ± 0.001
	RTP[c,d]	496 ± 21	0.014 ± 0.001
	ITP[c]	189 ± 22	0.034 ± 0.002
sym/sub-C			
GAU**C**CCGGG	RTP[c]	430 ± 79	0.019 ± 0.002
GGGCCC**C**UAG	GTP[c]	3.8 ± 0.7	56.7 ± 2.8
	ITP[e]	6.9 ± 0.8	23.3 ± 0.7
sym/sub-A			
GCU**A**CCCGGG	UTP[b]	97.5 ± 2.0	266 ± 2
GGGCCC**A**UCG			
sym/sub-G			
CAU**G**CCCGGG	CTP[c]	19.2 ± 3.2	157 ± 8
GGGCCC**G**UAC			
sym/sub-I			
CAU**I**CCCGGG	CTP[e]	177 ± 33	116 ± 9
GGGCCC**I**UAC	UTP[e]	1120 ± 123	0.036 ± 0.002
sym/sub-R[d]			
CAU**R**CCCGGG	CTP[c]	493 ± 41	8.5 ± 0.3
GGGCCC**R**UAC	UTP[c]	551 ± 127	7.6 ± 0.6
sym/sub-UA			
GC**A**UCCCGGGA	UTP[b]	407.1 ± 42.9	318.1 ± 18.2
AGGGCCCU**A**CG			

[a] Values taken from reference 32.
[b] Values taken from Arnold and Cameron, unpublished.
[c] Values taken from reference 21.
[d] R, ribavirin, which is 1-β-D-ribofuranosyl-1,2,4-triazole-3-carboxamide.
[e] Values taken from D. Maag and C. E. Cameron, unpublished results.

especially our understanding of the catalytic mechanism, substrate recognition, and the union of these two processes. However, in vivo, $3D^{pol}$ does not act alone. This enzyme is the central component of the replication machinery, but it must interact with other viral and/or cellular proteins to arrive at the right place at the right time for initiation of genome replication. It is quite clear that viral factors, for example, 3AB and $3CD^{pro}$, can modulate various activities of $3D^{pol}$ in vitro (50, 51, 72). As discussed above, the oligomerization domain(s) may be critical for aspects of replication complex assembly. However, other sites for protein-protein interactions may exist on the surface of $3D^{pol}$.

To date, alanine-scanning, biological screening, and site-directed mutagenesis have revealed only a few $3D^{pol}$ residues necessary for interaction with other poliovirus proteins or cellular proteins. Most of the characterized mutations in $3D^{pol}$-coding sequence that are located on the surface of the enzyme are implicated in binding nucleic acid or stabilizing protein structure (Table 2). The exceptions are Asp-71, Glu-72, Asp-79, and His-80 (Table 2). These residues were targeted in the clustered charged-to-alanine mutagenesis study of $3D^{pol}$ performed by the Kirkegaard laboratory and shown to be critical for virus multiplication (24). These residues are located on the back of the palm subdomain, and there is no obvious structural explanation for the observed biological phenotype. It is possible that these residues are involved in protein-protein interactions critical for assembly of the replication complex. Thus, alanine-scanning mutagenesis of solvent-accessible residues in general may prove useful in the identification of other $3D^{pol}$-interacting surfaces.

One additional approach that has been used to address the question, what constitutes the replication complex, is the yeast two-hybrid system (22, 101). This analysis has demonstrated the interaction of $3D^{pol}$ with most of the stable P3-derived proteins; the one exception is with the 3C protease (101). In addition, this system has been exploited to delineate interaction surfaces on $3D^{pol}$; the $3D^{pol}$-3AB interaction has been mapped onto $3D^{pol}$ and is located near motif E (Val-391) (38). The yeast two-hybrid system has also been an important tool for the identification of a cellular protein that interacts with $3D^{pol}$, Sam68 (Src-associated in mitosis, 68 kDa) (56). During poliovirus infection, Sam68 relocalizes from the nucleus to the cytoplasm and coimmunoprecipitation data place Sam68 within replication complexes. Localization of the Sam68-binding site on $3D^{pol}$ has not been reported. By employing modifications of the yeast two-hybrid system, for example, the reverse two-hybrid system, it may be possible to uncover quite efficiently all of the 3D^{pol} interaction surfaces with single-amino-acid-level resolution.

FUTURE DIRECTIONS

In this chapter, we have shown that over the past few years a remarkable amount of information has become available that has increased our understanding of the structure, function, and mechanism of 3D^{pol}. In fact, in most respects, our understanding of 3D^{pol} is now equivalent to that of other classes of nucleic acid polymerase. Clearly, much work remains to be completed. A few additional structures will have a significant impact on our understanding of the structure-function relationships of 3D^{pol}. For example, a complete structure of 3D^{pol} is needed to solve the mystery surrounding interface II. A structure of 3D^{pol} in complex with substrates is needed to define the path of the nucleic acid through the enzyme, thus providing a structural basis for the increased affinity for nascent RNA relative to template. Given the many interactions between 3D^{pol} and other viral nonstructural proteins and cellular proteins, a more quantitative analysis of these interactions may shed light on replicase composition, stoichiometry, and assembly, thus facilitating reconstitution of genome replication in vitro from purified components. Finally, while a variety of assays exist now that permit elucidation of the biochemical and biophysical properties of 3D^{pol}, it is important to begin to interrogate more rigorously the biological relevance of these properties.

REFERENCES

1. **Agol, V. I., A. V. Paul, and E. Wimmer.** 1999. Paradoxes of the replication of picornaviral genomes. *Virus Res.* **62:** 129–147.
2. **Aldabe, R., A. Barco, and L. Carrasco.** 1996. Membrane permeabilization by poliovirus proteins 2B and 2BC. *J. Biol. Chem.* **271:**23134–23137.
3. **Aldabe, R., and L. Carrasco.** 1995. Induction of membrane proliferation by poliovirus proteins 2C and 2BC. *Biochem. Biophys. Res. Commun.* **206:**64–76.
4. **Andino, R., G. E. Rieckhof, P. L. Achacoso, and D. Baltimore.** 1993. Poliovirus RNA synthesis utilizes an RNP complex formed around the 5′-end of viral RNA. *EMBO J.* **12:**3587–3598.
5. **Andino, R., G. E. Rieckhof, and D. Baltimore.** 1990. A functional ribonucleoprotein complex forms around the 5′ end of poliovirus RNA. *Cell* **63:**369–380.
6. **Arnold, J. J., and C. E. Cameron.** 1999. Poliovirus RNA-dependent RNA polymerase (3Dpol) is sufficient for template switching in vitro. *J. Biol. Chem.* **274:**2706–2716.
7. **Arnold, J. J., and C. E. Cameron.** 2000. Poliovirus RNA-dependent RNA polymerase (3D(pol)). Assembly of stable, elongation-competent complexes by using a symmetrical primer-template substrate (sym/sub). *J. Biol. Chem.* **275:**5329–5336.
8. **Arnold, J. J., S. K. Ghosh, and C. E. Cameron.** 1999. Poliovirus RNA-dependent RNA polymerase (3D(pol)). Divalent cation modulation of primer, template, and nucleotide selection. *J. Biol. Chem.* **274:**37060–37069.
9. **Astatke, M., K. Ng, N. D. Grindley, and C. M. Joyce.** 1998. A single side chain prevents *Escherichia coli* DNA polymerase I (Klenow fragment) from incorporating ribonucleotides. *Proc. Natl. Acad. Sci. USA* **95:**3402–3407.
10. **Bakhanashvili, M., O. Avidan, and A. Hizi.** 1996. Mutational studies of human immunodeficiency virus type 1 reverse transcriptase: the involvement of residues 183 and 184 in the fidelity of DNA synthesis. *FEBS Lett.* **391:** 257–262.
11. **Barton, D. J., B. J. Morasco, and J. B. Flanegan.** 1996. Assays for poliovirus polymerase, 3D(pol), and authentic RNA replication in HeLa S10 extracts. *Methods Enzymol.* **275:**35–57.
12. **Beckman, M. T., and K. Kirkegaard.** 1998. Site size of cooperative single-stranded RNA binding by poliovirus RNA-dependent RNA polymerase. *J. Biol. Chem.* **273:** 6724–6730.
13. **Bonnin, A., J. M. Lazaro, L. Blanco, and M. Salas.** 1999. A single tyrosine prevents insertion of ribonucleotides in the eukaryotic-type phi29 DNA polymerase. *J. Mol. Biol.* **290:**241–251.
14. **Boyer, P. L., S. G. Sarafianos, E. Arnold, and S. H. Hughes.** 2000. Analysis of mutations at positions 115 and 116 in the dNTP binding site of HIV-1 reverse transcriptase. *Proc. Natl. Acad. Sci. USA* **97:**3056–3061.
15. **Bressanelli, S., L. Tomei, A. Roussel, I. Incitti, R. L. Vitale, M. Mathieu, R. De Francesco, and F. A. Rey.** 1999. Crystal structure of the RNA-dependent RNA polymerase of hepatitis C virus. *Proc. Natl. Acad. Sci. USA* **96:**13034–13039.
16. **Burns, C. C., M. A. Lawson, B. L. Semler, and E. Ehrenfeld.** 1989. Effects of mutations in poliovirus 3Dpol on RNA polymerase activity and on polyprotein cleavage. *J. Virol.* **63:**4866–4874.
17. **Canard, B., K. Chowdhury, R. Sarfati, S. Doublie, and C. C. Richardson.** 1999. The motif D loop of human immunodeficiency virus type 1 reverse transcriptase is critical for nucleoside 5′-triphosphate selectivity. *J. Biol. Chem.* **274:**35768–35776.
18. **Cases-Gonzalez, C. E., M. Gutierrez-Rivas, and L. Menendez-Arias.** 2000. Coupling ribose selection to fidelity of DNA synthesis. The role of Tyr-115 of human immunodeficiency virus type 1 reverse transcriptase *J. Biol. Chem.* **275:**19759–19767.
19. **Cho, M. W., O. C. Richards, T. M. Dmitrieva, V. Agol, and E. Ehrenfeld.** 1993. RNA duplex unwinding activity of poliovirus RNA-dependent RNA polymerase 3Dpol. *J. Virol.* **67:**3010–3018.
20. **Cho, M. W., N. Teterina, D. Egger, K. Bienz, and E. Ehrenfeld.** 1994. Membrane rearrangement and vesicle induction by recombinant poliovirus 2C and 2BC in human cells. *Virology* **202:**129–145.
21. **Crotty, S., D. Maag, J. J. Arnold, W. Zhong, J. Y. Lau, Z. Hong, R. Andino, and C. E. Cameron.** 2000. The broad-spectrum antiviral ribonucleoside ribavirin is an RNA virus mutagen. *Nat. Med.* **6:**1375–1379.
22. **Cuconati, A., W. Xiang, F. Lahser, T. Pfister, and E. Wimmer.** 1998. A protein linkage map of the P2 nonstructural proteins of poliovirus. *J. Virol.* **72:**1297–1307.
23. **Dasgupta, A., M. H. Baron, and D. Baltimore.** 1979. Poliovirus replicase: a soluble enzyme able to initiate copying of poliovirus RNA. *Proc. Natl. Acad. Sci. USA* **76:**2679–2683.
24. **Diamond, S. E., and K. Kirkegaard.** 1994. Clustered charged-to-alanine mutagenesis of poliovirus RNA-dependent RNA polymerase yields multiple temperature-sensitive mutants defective in RNA synthesis. *J. Virol.* **68:** 863–876.
25. **Doedens, J. R., and K. Kirkegaard.** 1995. Inhibition of cellular protein secretion by poliovirus proteins 2B and 3A. *EMBO J.* **14:**894–907.
26. **Doublie, S., S. Tabor, A. M. Long, C. C. Richardson, and T. Ellenberger.** 1998. Crystal structure of a bacteriophage T7 DNA replication complex at 2.2 A resolution. *Nature* **391:**251–258.

27. Duggal, R., A. Cuconati, M. Gromeier, and E. Wimmer. 1997. Genetic recombination of poliovirus in a cell-free system. *Proc. Natl. Acad. Sci. USA* **94:**13786–13791.
28. Egger, D., N. Teterina, E. Ehrenfeld, and K. Bienz. 2000. Formation of the poliovirus replication complex requires coupled viral translation, vesicle production, and viral RNA synthesis. *J. Virol.* **74:**6570–6580.
29. Flanegan, J. B., and D. Baltimore. 1977. Poliovirus-specific primer-dependent RNA polymerase able to copy poly(A). *Proc. Natl. Acad. Sci. USA* **74:**3677–3680.
30. Flanegan, J. B., and D. Baltimore. 1979. Poliovirus polyuridylic acid polymerase and RNA replicase have the same viral polypeptide. *J. Virol.* **29:**352–360.
31. Gao, G., M. Orlova, M. M. Georgiadis, W. A. Hendrickson, and S. P. Goff. 1997. Conferring RNA polymerase activity to a DNA polymerase: a single residue in reverse transcriptase controls substrate selection. *Proc. Natl. Acad. Sci. USA* **94:**407–411.
32. Gohara, D. W., S. Crotty, J. J. Arnold, J. D. Yoder, R. Andino, and C. E. Cameron. 2000. Poliovirus RNA-dependent RNA polymerase (3Dpol): structural, biochemical, and biological analysis of conserved structural motifs A and B. *J. Biol. Chem.* **275:**25523–25532.
33. Gohara, D. W., C. S. Ha, S. Kumar, B. Ghosh, J. J. Arnold, T. J. Wisniewski, and C. E. Cameron. 1999. Production of "authentic" poliovirus RNA-dependent RNA polymerase (3D(pol)) by ubiquitin-protease-mediated cleavage in *Escherichia coli*. *Protein Expr. Purif.* **17:**128–138.
34. Goodfellow, I., Y. Chaudhry, A. Richardson, J. Meredith, J. W. Almond, W. Barclay, and D. J. Evans. 2000. Identification of a *cis*-acting replication element within the poliovirus coding region. *J. Virol.* **74:**4590–4600.
35. Hansen, J. L., A. M. Long, and S. C. Schultz. 1997. Structure of the RNA-dependent RNA polymerase of poliovirus. *Structure* **5:**1109–1122.
36. Hey, T. D., O. C. Richards, and E. Ehrenfeld. 1986. Synthesis of plus- and minus-strand RNA from poliovirion RNA template in vitro. *J. Virol.* **58:**790–796.
37. Hobson, S. D., E. S. Rosenblum, O. C. Richards, K. Richmond, K. Kirkegaard, and S. C. Schultz. 2001. Oligomeric structures of poliovirus polymerase are important for function. *EMBO J.* **20:**1153–1163.
38. Hope, D. A., S. E. Diamond, and K. Kirkegaard. 1997. Genetic dissection of interaction between poliovirus 3D polymerase and viral protein 3AB. *J. Virol.* **71:**9490–9498.
39. Huang, H., R. Chopra, G. L. Verdine, and S. C. Harrison. 1998. Structure of a covalently trapped catalytic complex of HIV-1 reverse transcriptase: implications for drug resistance. *Science* **282:**1669–1675.
40. Jablonski, S. A., and C. D. Morrow. 1993. Enzymatic activity of poliovirus RNA polymerases with mutations at the tyrosine residue of the conserved YGDD motif: isolation and characterization of polioviruses containing RNA polymerases with FGDD and MGDD sequences. *J. Virol.* **67:**373–381.
41. Jablonski, S. A., and C. D. Morrow. 1995. Mutation of the aspartic acid residues of the GDD sequence motif of poliovirus RNA-dependent RNA polymerase results in enzymes with altered metal ion requirements for activity. *J. Virol.* **69:**1532–1539.
42. Jacques, P. S., B. M. Wohrl, M. Ottmann, J. L. Darlix, and S. F. Le Grice. 1994. Mutating the "primer grip" of p66 HIV-1 reverse transcriptase implicates tryptophan-229 in template-primer utilization *J. Biol. Chem.* **269:**26472–26478.
43. Jarvis, T. C., and K. Kirkegaard. 1992. Poliovirus RNA recombination: mechanistic studies in the absence of selection. *EMBO J.* **11:**3135–3145.
44. Jones, T. A., J. Y. Zou, S. W. Cowan, and Kjeldgaard. 1991. Improved methods for binding protein models in electron density maps and the location of errors in these models. *Acta Crystallogr. A* **47:**110–119.
45. Kati, W. M., K. A. Johnson, L. F. Jerva, and K. S. Anderson. 1992. Mechanism and fidelity of HIV reverse transcriptase *J. Biol. Chem.* **267:**25988–25997.
46. Kirkegaard, K., and D. Baltimore. 1986. The mechanism of RNA recombination in poliovirus. *Cell* **47:**433–443.
47. Kohlstaedt, L. A., J. Wang, J. M. Friedman, P. A. Rice, and T. A. Steitz. 1992. Crystal structure at 3.5 A resolution of HIV-1 reverse transcriptase complexed with an inhibitor. *Science* **256:**1783–1790.
48. Koonin, E. V. 1991. The phylogeny of RNA-dependent RNA polymerases of positive-strand RNA viruses. *J. Gen. Virol.* **72:**2197–2206.
49. Kraulis, P. J. 1991. MOLSCRIPT: a program to produce both detailed and schematic plots of protein structures. *J. Appl. Crystallogr.* **24:**946–950.
50. Lama, J., A. V. Paul, K. S. Harris, and E. Wimmer. 1994. Properties of purified recombinant poliovirus protein 3aB as substrate for viral proteinases and as co-factor for RNA polymerase 3Dpol. *J. Biol. Chem.* **269:**66–70.
51. Lama, J., M. A. Sanz, and P. L. Rodriguez. 1995. A role for 3AB protein in poliovirus genome replication. *J. Biol. Chem.* **270:**14430–14438.
52. Lawson, S. L., W. W. Wakarchuk, and S. G. Withers. 1996. Effects of both shortening and lengthening the active site nucleophile of *Bacillus circulans* xylanase on catalytic activity. *Biochemistry* **35:**10110–10118.
53. Lesburg, C. A., M. B. Cable, E. Ferrari, Z. Hong, A. F. Mannarino, and P. C. Weber. 1999. Crystal structure of the RNA-dependent RNA polymerase from hepatitis C virus reveals a fully encircled active site. *Nat. Struct. Biol.* **6:**937–943.
54. Lubinski, J. M., L. J. Ransone, and A. Dasgupta. 1987. Primer-dependent synthesis of covalently linked dimeric RNA molecules by poliovirus replicase. *J. Virol.* **61:**2997–3003.
55. Martin, R. B. 1990. *In* H. Sigel and A. Sigel (ed.), *Metal Ions in Biological Systems*, vol. 26. Dekker, New York, N.Y.
56. McBride, A. E., A. Schlegel, and K. Kirkegaard. 1996. Human protein Sam68 relocalization and interaction with poliovirus RNA polymerase in infected cells. *Proc. Natl. Acad. Sci. USA* **93:**2296–2301.
57. McKnight, K. L., and S. M. Lemon. 1998. The rhinovirus type 14 genome contains an internally located RNA structure that is required for viral replication. *RNA* **4:**1569–1584.
58. Merritt, E. J., and M. E. P. Meurphy. 1997. Raster3D version 2.0—a program for photorealistic molecular graphics. *Acta Crystallogr. D* **50:**869–873.
59. Morrow, C. D., B. Warren, and M. R. Lentz. 1987. Expression of enzymatically active poliovirus RNA-dependent RNA polymerase in *Escherichia coli*. *Proc. Natl. Acad. Sci. USA* **84:**6050–6054.
60. Neufeld, K. L., J. M. Galarza, O. C. Richards, D. F. Summers, and E. Ehrenfeld. 1994. Identification of terminal adenylyl transferase activity of the poliovirus polymerase 3Dpol. *J. Virol.* **68:**5811–5818.
61. Neufeld, K. L., O. C. Richards, and E. Ehrenfeld. 1991. Expression and characterization of poliovirus proteins 3BVPg, 3Cpro, and 3Dpol in recombinant baculovirus-infected *Spodoptera frugiperda* cells. *Virus Res.* **19:**173–188.
62. Neufeld, K. L., O. C. Richards, and E. Ehrenfeld. 1991. Purification, characterization, and comparison of poliovirus RNA polymerase from native and recombinant sources. *J. Biol. Chem.* **266:**24212–24219.

63. Nicholls, A., K. Sharp, and B. Honig. 1991. Protein folding and association: insights from the interfacial and thermodynamic properties of hydrocarbons. *Proteins* **11:**281–296.
64. Novak, J. E., and K. Kirkegaard. 1994. Coupling between genome translation and replication in an RNA virus. *Genes Dev.* **8:**1726–1737.
65. Nugent, C. I., K. L. Johnson, P. Sarnow, and K. Kirkegaard. 1999. Functional coupling between replication and packaging of poliovirus replicon RNA. *J. Virol.* **73:**427–435.
66. Ollis, D. L., C. Kline, and T. A. Steitz. 1985. Domain of *E. coli* DNA polymerase I showing sequence homology to T7 DNA polymerase. *Nature* **313:**818–819.
67. Pata, J. D., S. C. Schultz, and K. Kirkegaard. 1995. Functional oligomerization of poliovirus RNA-dependent RNA polymerase. *RNA* **1:**466–477.
68. Paul, A. V., J. H. van Boom, D. Filippov, and E. Wimmer. 1998. Protein-primed RNA synthesis by purified poliovirus RNA polymerase. *Nature* **393:**280–284.
69. Paul, A. V., J. Mugavero, J. Yin, S. Hobson, S. Schultz, J. H. van Boom, and E. Wimmer. 2000. Studies on the attenuation phenotype of polio vaccines: poliovirus RNA polymerase derived from Sabin type 1 sequence is temperature sensitive in the uridylylation of VPg. *Virology* **272:**72–84.
70. Paul, A. V., E. Rieder, D. W. Kim, J. H. van Boom, and E. Wimmer. 2000. Identification of an RNA hairpin in poliovirus RNA that serves as the primary template in the in vitro uridylylation of VPg. *J. Virol.* **74:**10359–10370.
71. Pilipenko, E. V., S. V. Maslova, A. N. Sinyakov, and V. I. Agol. 1992. Towards identification of *cis*-acting elements involved in the replication of enterovirus and rhinovirus RNAs: a proposal for the existence of tRNA-like terminal structures. *Nucleic Acids Res.* **20:**1739–1745.
72. Plotch, S. J., and O. Palant. 1995. Poliovirus protein 3AB forms a complex with and stimulates the activity of the viral RNA polymerase, 3Dpol. *J. Virol.* **69:**7169–7179.
73. Plotch, S. J., O. Palant, and Y. Gluzman. 1989. Purification and properties of poliovirus RNA polymerase expressed in *Escherichia coli*. *J. Virol.* **63:**216–225.
74. Polesky, A. H., M. E. Dahlberg, S. J. Benkovic, N. D. Grindley, and C. M. Joyce. 1992. Side chains involved in catalysis of the polymerase reaction of DNA polymerase I from *Escherichia coli*. *J. Biol. Chem.* **267:**8417–8428.
75. Powell, M. D., M. Ghosh, P. S. Jacques, K. J. Howard, S. F. Le Grice, and J. G. Levin. 1997. Alanine-scanning mutations in the "primer grip" of p66 HIV-1 reverse transcriptase result in selective loss of RNA priming activity. *J. Biol. Chem.* **272:**13262–13269.
76. Richards, O. C., S. Baker, and E. Ehrenfeld. 1996. Mutation of lysine residues in the nucleotide binding segments of the poliovirus RNA-dependent RNA polymerase. *J. Virol.* **70:**8564–8570.
77. Richards, O. C., and E. Ehrenfeld. 1997. One of two NTP binding sites in poliovirus RNA polymerase required for RNA replication. *J. Biol. Chem.* **272:**23261–23264.
78. Richards, O. C., and E. Ehrenfeld. 1998. Effects of poliovirus 3AB protein on 3D polymerase-catalyzed reaction. *J. Biol. Chem.* **273:**12832–12840.
79. Richards, O. C., J. L. Hansen, S. Schultz, and E. Ehrenfeld. 1995. Identification of nucleotide binding sites in the poliovirus RNA polymerase. *Biochemistry* **34:**6288–6295.
80. Richards, O. C., L. A. Ivanoff, K. Bienkowska-Szewczyk, B. Butt, S. R. Petteway, M. A. Rothstein, and E. Ehrenfeld. 1987. Formation of poliovirus RNA polymerase 3D in *Escherichia coli* by cleavage of fusion proteins expressed from cloned viral cDNA. *Virology* **161:**348–356.
81. Rieder, E., A. V. Paul, D. W. Kim, J. H. van Boom, and E. Wimmer. 2000. Genetic and biochemical studies of poliovirus *cis*-acting replication element *cre* in relation to VPg uridylylation. *J. Virol.* **74:**10371–10380.
82. Rothstein, M. A., O. C. Richards, C. Amin, and E. Ehrenfeld. 1988. Enzymatic activity of poliovirus RNA polymerase synthesized in *Escherichia coli* from viral cDNA. *Virology* **164:**301–308.
83. Rueckert, R. R. 1996. *Picornaviridae: The Viruses and Their Replication*, 3rd ed., vol. 1. Lippincott-Raven Publishers, Philadelphia, Pa.
84. Sandoval, I. V., and L. Carrasco. 1997. Poliovirus infection and expression of the poliovirus protein 2B provoke the disassembly of the Golgi complex, the organelle target for the antipoliovirus drug Ro-090179. *J. Virol.* **71:**4679–4693.
85. Schlegel, A., T. H. Giddings, M. S. Ladinsky, and K. Kirkegaard. 1996. Cellular origin and ultrastructure of membranes induced during poliovirus infection. *J. Virol.* **70:**6576–6588.
86. Sousa, R., Y. J. Chung, J. P. Rose, and B. C. Wang. 1993. Crystal structure of bacteriophage T7 RNA polymerase at 3.3 A resolution. *Nature* **364:**593–599.
87. Steitz, T. A., and J. A. Steitz. 1993. A general two-metal-ion mechanism for catalytic RNA. *Proc. Natl. Acad. Sci. USA* **90:**6498–6502.
88. Suhy, D. A., T. H. Giddings, and K. Kirkegaard. 2000. Remodeling the endoplasmic reticulum by poliovirus infection and by individual viral proteins: an autophagy-like origin for virus-induced vesicles. *J. Virol.* **74:**8953–8965.
89. Tang, R. S., D. J. Barton, J. B. Flanegan, and K. Kirkegaard. 1997. Poliovirus RNA recombination in cell-free extracts. *RNA* **3:**624–633.
90. Teterina, N. L., A. E. Gorbalenya, D. Egger, K. Bienz, and E. Ehrenfeld. 1997. Poliovirus 2C protein determinants of membrane binding and rearrangements in mammalian cells. *J. Virol.* **71:**8962–8972.
91. Thrall, S. H., R. Krebs, B. M. Wohrl, L. Cellai, R. S. Goody, and T. Restle. 1998. Pre-steady-state kinetic characterization of RNA-primed initiation of transcription by HIV-1 reverse transcriptase and analysis of the transition to a processive DNA-primed polymerization mode. *Biochemistry* **37:**13349–13358.
92. Wakefield, J. K., S. A. Jablonski, and C. D. Morrow. 1992. In vitro enzymatic activity of human immunodeficiency virus type 1 reverse transcriptase mutants in the highly conserved YMDD amino acid motif correlates with the infectious potential of the proviral genome. *J. Virol.* **66:**6806–6812.
93. Walker, D. E., D. McPherson, S. A. Jablonski, S. McPherson, and C. D. Morrow. 1995. An aspartic acid at amino acid 108 is required to rescue infectious virus after transfection of a poliovirus cDNA containing a CGDD but not SGDD amino acid motif in 3Dpol. *J. Virol.* **69:**8173–8177.
94. Ward, C. D., and J. B. Flanegan. 1992. Determination of the poliovirus RNA polymerase error frequency at eight sites in the viral genome. *J. Virol.* **66:**3784–3793.
95. Ward, C. D., M. A. Stokes, and J. B. Flanegan. 1988. Direct measurement of the poliovirus RNA polymerase error frequency in vitro. *J. Virol.* **62:**558–562.
96. Wells, V. R., S. J. Plotch, and J. J. DeStefano. 2001. Determination of the mutation rate of poliovirus RNA-dependent RNA polymerase. *Virus Res.* **74:**119–132.
97. Wilson, J. E., A. Aulabaugh, B. Caligan, S. McPherson, J. K. Wakefield, S. Jablonski, C. D. Morrow, J. E.

Reardon, and P. A. Furman. 1996. Human immunodeficiency virus type-1 reverse transcriptase. Contribution of Met-184 to binding of nucleoside 5′-triphosphate. *J. Biol. Chem.* **271:**13656–13662.
98. **Wimmer, E., C. U. Hellen, and X. Cao.** 1993. Genetics of poliovirus. *Annu. Rev. Genet.* **27:**353–436.
99. **Wimmer, E., and A. Nomoto.** 1993. Molecular biology and cell-free synthesis of poliovirus. *Biologicals* **21:**349–356.
100. **Wirblich, C., H. J. Thiel, and G. Meyers.** 1996. Genetic map of the calicivirus rabbit hemorrhagic disease virus as deduced from in vitro translation studies. *J. Virol.* **70:**7974–7983.
101. **Xiang, W., A. Cuconati, D. Hope, K. Kirkegaard, and E. Wimmer.** 1998. Complete protein linkage map of poliovirus P3 proteins: interaction of polymerase 3Dpol with VPg and with genetic variants of 3AB. *J. Virol.* **72:**6732–6741.

Picornavirus Genetics: an Overview

VADIM I. AGOL

22

The term "picornavirus genetics" is used in a variety of meanings. The aim of this chapter is to overview the mechanisms underlying the stability and especially the variability of the picornavirus phenotype and genotype. Also, the principles of genetic analysis of viral functions and of manipulations with the viral genome will be briefly considered. More detailed discussions of these problems and additional references may be found in other chapters of this book as well as in excellent informative reviews, old (46, 127) and more recent (60, 61, 98, 242).

Genetics is dealing with genes. In the case of picornaviruses, the very notion of "gene" is ambiguous. If we accept, with appropriate specifications, the one-gene-one-polypeptide definition, we will then have to define what is a single polypeptide in the viruses in which a variety of "mature" proteins are generated by limited proteolysis of a polyprotein, the product of a single open reading frame. No consensus solution of this semantic issue is currently available (for a discussion, see reference 242). For the sake of simplicity, we will consider a gene as a unit encoding a terminal ("mature") functional product of the polyprotein cleavage.

MILESTONES IN PICORNAVIRUS GENETICS

Studies on phenotypic variability of picornaviruses had begun long before tools for genomic studies became available. Perhaps the first evidence for antigenic and host range variations in picornaviruses was obtained with foot-and-mouth disease virus as early as in the 1920s (27). Later on, variants of poliovirus capable of infecting mice rather than only primates were described (12, 73). Antigenic variability of poliovirus (existence of three serotypes) (22, 30), changes of its host range (139, 140), and virulence (129, 204) became obvious. The discovery of the ability of poliovirus to grow in cultured cells (80) made potentially possible a great variety of genetic experiments. A key step forward was the introduction of the plaque technique for quantitation and cloning of picornaviruses (69). All these seminal discoveries were made before the genetic material of a picornavirus had been identified as RNA in 1955 (44, 211).

Mutagenesis of poliovirus in vivo (by growing it in the presence of proflavine) and in vitro (by chemical treatment of the virus and its RNA) was accomplished soon thereafter (24, 70). Meanwhile, a variety of in vitro phenotypic markers, notably, thermosensitivity of reproduction and resistance to inhibitors, have been described (reviewed in references 88 and 213). Realization of genetic heterogeneity of any, even clonal, population of picornaviruses (as well as other viruses) was a major contribution to picornavirus genetics (59, 62, 221).

By studying the inheritance of phenotypic markers in the progeny of mixed infections (two-factor crosses), genetic recombination between poliovirus variants was demonstrated early in the 1960s (104, 137). Soon thereafter the first linkage maps of poliovirus temperature-sensitive (*ts*) mutations were generated (45). Biochemical proof of the recombination (i.e., evidence that genomic segments and/or proteins of a recombinant had indeed been derived from different parents) came nearly two decades later (123, 200). Meanwhile, the existence of another type of genomic rearrangement, deletions, in defective interfering (DI) poliovirus genomes was documented (41, 42).

Complementation between guanidine-sensitive and guanidine-dependent poliovirus mutants was independently described in 1964 by several groups (6, 48, 239). On the other hand, interference between poliovirus mutants under certain conditions has also been demonstrated (47, 158).

The establishment of the primary structure of poliovirus RNA (126, 189) followed by sequencing of other picornavirus genomes gave an indispensible tool for the direct characterization of genetic variability, whereas demonstration of the infectivity of poliovirus cDNA (190) paved the path for a variety of interventions in the structure of the viral genome. It will not be an exaggeration to state that the whole modern picornavirus genetics stemmed from these two breakthrough achievements made in 1981.

New, not yet fully explored possibilities are opened with the demonstration of cell-free picornavirus (poliovirus) reproduction (165).

Vadim I. Agol ■ M. P. Chumakov Institute of Poliomyelitis & Viral Encephalitides, Russian Academy of Medical Sciences, Moscow Region 142782; and M. V. Lomonosov Moscow State University, Moscow 119899, Russia.

VARIABILITY OF THE PHENOTYPE

Properties of picornaviruses grown under standard conditions are generally fairly stable. On the other hand, variability of the phenotypic properties of these viruses is also a widespread phenomenon. This variability either can be generated experimentally, e.g., by changing conditions for the virus growth or introduction of mutations, or result from mostly undefined events during viral evolution.

Fitness Variability

Fitness reflects the relative ability to produce stable infectious progeny in a given environment (61). With such a broad definition, the majority of phenotypically expressed mutations affect viral fitness in one manner or another. Fitness may be evaluated by comparing viral variants with respect to their progeny yields under certain conditions or by assaying their competitive potential upon mixed infection.

The comparative viral yields are usually estimated in single-cycle experiments or, semiquantitatively, by plaque sizes (in the latter case, one should be aware, however, that the components of the overlay, e.g., agar sulfated polysaccharides, may selectively affect reproduction of certain viral variants). Viral variants may generate equal harvest under some conditions but not under the others. Poliovirus mutants with an altered ability to grow at low (66; see also reference 63) or especially high (148) temperatures (cold-sensitive and thermosensitive, respectively) are classical examples of picornavirus phenotype variability (relevant early studies reviewed in reference 46). Mutants unable to grow under certain restrictive conditions are referred to as conditionally lethal.

For comparative fitness assays, the mixtures of viral variants (one of them being a reference virus with the assigned fitness value of 1) are subjected to multiple consecutive passages, and the changes in relative proportions of each component are assayed in the course of their cocultivation (151; reviewed in reference 60). Although the interpretation of such experiments may sometimes not be straightforward (for example, the relative fitness may depend on the multiplicity of infection; cf. 214), even subtle differences in fitness could be revealed in many cases by this approach. However, the possibility of genetic alterations in the assayed viruses upon their cultivation should be taken into account.

Resistance to Inhibitors

The easy appearance of drug-resistant picornavirus variants is a great benefit for genetic studies but creates formidable problems for the development of antiviral therapeutics.

A variety of synthetic hydrophobic compounds inhibit uncoating of some picornaviruses, e.g., rhinoviruses and enteroviruses, through interaction with the capsid. However, mutants resistant to, or dependent on the presence of, these drugs can readily be selected (8, 74, 103, 166). The resistance may be due to a decreased capacity of the virions to bind the inhibitor or to their enhanced ability to productively react with cellular receptors in the presence of the bound drug (100, 216).

Guanidine HCl, in millimolar concentrations, was among the first discovered inhibitors of intracellular reproduction of enteroviruses (195). However, guanidine-resistant (g^r) and guanidine-dependent (g^d) mutants readily accumulate upon virus growth in the presence of the drug (146, 160). The same is true of the similarly acting inhibitor 2-(α-hydroxybenzyl)-benzimidazole (75). Numerous other examples of picornavirus drug resistance are known.

Host Range Variability

Not only do different picornaviruses vary in their host range, but also such variation may be observed for a given virus. Most poliovirus strains are infectious exclusively for primates or primate-derived cells. Nevertheless, some strains of this virus belonging to serotype 2 were demonstrated to be neurovirulent for mice (12). Selection of mice-pathogenic variants from type 1 and type 3 poliovirus populations (115, 139, 140; see also reference 49) was among the first demonstrations of picornavirus potential to change its host range. The virus could also be adapted to grow in chicken embryos (197).

In some cases, the host range change appears to require adaptation to a new cellular receptor. Certain mutations of the human poliovirus receptor inactivate its ability to mediate entry of the viral genome into the cell. Poliovirus variants able to overcome this barrier can be selected (43, 241). The already mentioned acquisition by poliovirus mutants of pathogenicity for mice may be caused by their ability to interact with a noncognate (murine) receptor protein (115). Normally, foot-and-mouth disease virus (FMDV) enters host cells through interaction of an Arg-Gly-Asp (RGD) motif on its VP1 capsid protein with cellular integrins (111, 171). However, viral mutants lacking the RGD motif can be selected (153). They are able to infect cells (even possessing no relevant integrin and therefore normally nonsusceptible to FMDV) by using other noncognate receptors (15).

Not only viral entry but also intracellular steps of picornavirus reproduction may be restricted in a host-specific manner. A specific requirement of the FMDV internal ribosome entry site (IRES) for a cell-cycle-dependent host protein may contribute to inability of this virus to grow in nondividing cells (181). Efficiency of mengovirus reproduction in mice and murine cells but not in HeLa cells highly depends on the length of the 5′ UTR poly(C) tract (68, 150). Some alterations of the replicative cis-acting element oriL (so-called cloverleaf) of coxsackievirus B3 may result in host range changes (244). Mutations in the regions of hepatitis A virus (HAV) RNA that are involved in its replication and translation (e.g., 5′ UTR and P2-coding region) also specifically affect viral growth in certain host cells (52, 77, 95).

Antigenic Variability

Antigenic changes may occur in picornaviruses relatively rapidly, for example, even upon a short-term infection of individual hosts with either the Sabin-vaccine (162) or wild-type (wt) (107, 124) polioviruses. Not surprisingly, polioviruses isolated during an outbreak are heterogeneous with respect to antigenic properties (108). The same is true also of other picornaviruses. The antigenic changes obviously reflect selective pressure of the immune system.

An efficient tool for experimentally studying antigenic variation became available with the advent of the monoclonal antibodies technique. Numerous escape mutants (i.e., mutants selected in the presence of, and resistant to, an antibody) of poliovirus (78, 163), human rhinovirus (217), FMDV (25, 224), and other picornaviruses (23, 223) have been selected and characterized. On the other hand, antigenic changes may occur "spontaneously," that is, without selection, for example, in in vitro cultivated virus (57, 215).

Variability of Pathogenicity

The pathogenic potential of picornaviruses may vary in two respects: (i) viral variants may be more or less virulent, in the sense that different doses of a virus are required to inflict similar clinical signs (at the extreme, even the highest possible dose may fail to produce any signs); and (ii) the variants may cause different clinical patterns.

Attenuated (less virulent) variants of poliovirus (9, 96, 109, 129, 204, 220), FMDV (33, 56, 155), cardioviruses (68, 179), HAV (26, 119, 188), and other picornaviruses have been selected or engineered. In some cases, such attenuated variants are used as live vaccines, the best known example being the Sabin strains of poliovirus (205). From the practical viewpoint, it is important that such attenuated variants retain, at least to a significant degree, their capacity to grow in standard cell cultures.

With enteroviruses, it is a common situation that a given virus may cause different diseases, whereas the same set of symptoms can be inflicted by different viruses (159). Strains of coxsackievirus B3 differ from one another in their cardiovirulence, whereas strains of coxsackievirus B4 vary in their ability to induce diabetes (33, 71). An impressive example of the capacity of a picornavirus to cause different diseases is Theiler's murine encephalomyelitis virus (TMEV): some strains of this virus inflict acute fatal encephalomyelitis, whereas others are causative agents of a chronic demyelinating disease (112, 145). The potential of a given TMEV strain to trigger a specific clinical pattern can be additionally changed as a result of a single (or a few) point mutation(s) (183).

The examples presented illustrate only a small part of a very broad range of phenotypic variations of picornaviruses. They give, however, a general idea about the amount of work ahead, if one of the ultimate goals of picornavirus genetics is to uncover the molecular nature of viral behavior.

VARIABILITY OF THE GENOME

Point Mutations

Picornavirus RNA replication is not fully faithful. Miscorporation of nucleotides is a common phenomenon upon RNA synthesis by viral RNA polymerases. There are at least two general mechanisms resulting in mistakes of copying. The enzyme may make an error in selecting a noncomplementary nucleotide for insertion into the nascent strand. Another possibility may consist in a kind of "stuttering," a property shared to a certain extent by all of the RNA polymerases and responsible, for example, for the polyadenylation or cotranscriptional "editing" in negative-strand RNA viruses (51). The enzyme, together with the 3' end of the nascent strand, may make one or more steps backward and then continue faithful elongation. The probability of such backward movement depends on the nucleotide sequence in the contact region of the template and nascent strands as well as on their context.

The picornavirus RNA polymerase, like analogous enzymes of other RNA viruses, lacks the ability to remove the erroneously incorporated nucleotide (the proofreading activity), characteristic of many DNA polymerases. This explains why the rate of nucleotide misincorporation is rather high. For poliovirus, the mutation frequencies in vitro (238) and in vivo (53, 54, 237) were roughly estimated to lie between 10^{-3} and 10^{-5} substitutions per site per replication, with transitions occurring much more frequently than transversions (131). These estimates suggest that the synthesis of each copy of a full-length RNA genome is accompanied, on average, by a mutation (64). Hence, the progeny of even a single viral RNA molecule is not a homogeneous "clone" but rather a highly heterogeneous population of related genomes bearing mutations at various sites. Such populations were dubbed "quasispecies" (reviewed in references 61 and 62). In fact, the mutation rate is so high that it nearly approaches the level that would result in extinction of a population ("the error catastrophe"). Therefore, chemical mutagenes are able to increase the mutation rate only to a relatively moderate extent (105, 219); further increase in this rate may simply kill viruses (49a).

Although the majority of possible mutations are phenotypically neutral (121), many others are expected to diminish or abolish the replicative capacity of the RNA, e.g., because of the damage to its essential replicative cis-elements, inactivation of replicative viral proteins, or just interference with translation due to generation of the stop codons (as is known, translation is strictly coupled to replication; cf. 172). Some mutations may be detrimental to genome encapsidation. Thus, although it is not very unlikely that all theoretically possible single and even double mutations are generated during reproduction of a large enough viral population, in reality the progeny is markedly less heterogeneous.

It is unclear to what extent the error rates of RNA polymerases of different picornaviruses differ from one another. We are aware of no mutator type mutations (i.e., changing the mutation rate) of the picornavirus RNA polymerases. It may be supposed that the existing level of fidelity of the viral RNA polymerases maintains an optimal balance between genome stability and variability.

Genome Rearrangements

Types of Rearrangements

Genome rearrangements may be caused by intermolecular or intramolecular events. Recombination is a typical manifestation of the former, whereas both intermolecular and intramolecular reactions may lead to deletions or insertion (including duplications) of the genetic material. Recombination can readily be registered upon mixed infection with different variants of a virus, but it also likely occurs between sibling molecules in a singly infected cell. Deletions/insertions compatible with virus viability are detected in the coding and noncoding RNA segments of different picornaviruses (18, 38, 83, 94, 169, 234) although they are observed less frequently compared to point mutations. Nonviable, helper-dependent picornavirus particles containing RNA molecules with extended deletions, so-called DI genomes, may be present in laboratory viral stocks and their abundance is markedly enhanced upon serial high multiplicity-of-infection (MOI) passages (41, 42). The dependence on MOI suggests that intermolecular interactions are likely involved in the generation of the deletions, although intramolecular rearrangement cannot be excluded either. The DI deletions vary in size but are confined to the capsid protein-coding region and do not change the reading frame (134).

A special case of genomic rearrangements is represented by changes in the length of internal homopolymeric regions, i.e., poly(C) (84, 102, 194) and poly(A) (82). The simplest explanation of these changes is "stuttering" of the viral RNA polymerase (see above).

Mechanisms of Rearrangements

Replicative Rearrangements. Genomic rearrangements may arise by two different mechanisms, replicative or nonreplicative (Fig. 1). Until recently, only the replicative mechanism (also referred to as template switching or copy choice) was considered feasible with regard to the recombination between genomes of RNA viruses, in general, and picornaviruses, in particular (2, 45, 113, 242). One of the strongest, though obviously indirect, pieces of evidence for the existence of template switching is preciseness of recombination in many systems. Two questions are central to template switching: (i) Why does the polymerase stop elongation on, and dissociate from, the original template? and (ii) how is the anchoring site selected?

A given level of processivity is an inherent property of any RNA polymerase, and the picornavirus enzymes also may jump from one template to another (13). In principle, the processivity can be modulated by interactions of the catalytic subunit of the enzyme with yet to be defined ligands as well as by the local structure of the template and nascent strands. It was suggested, for example, that secondary structure elements (199) and A-U-rich regions (122) may facilitate the dissociation of picornavirus elongating complexes and the detachment of the enzyme together with the 3' end of the nascent strand from the template. It seems likely that any errors due to either the "true" misincorporation or stuttering may result in pausing and hence in an enhanced probability of dissociation (178). If so, such dissociation may be regarded as a kind of proofreading mechanism instrumental in discarding erroneously copied genomes.

Although the crossover sites may be widely distributed along the genome, their location does not appear to be entirely random (230), consistent with the significance of the local structure of the parting and/or anchoring sites. The reported dependence of the distributions of crossovers upon temperature (67) could also be explained by changes in the strength of the local template/nascent strand or RNA/enzyme interactions affecting either dissociation or reassociation of the elongation complex. On the other hand, nonrandom distribution of the crossover sites may be due in part also to low fitness (or even lethal phenotype) of certain combinations of genome segments derived from heterologous partners. This factor perhaps explains a relatively low abundance of natural picornavirus recombinants with crossovers within the capsid protein-coding region.

Poliovirus recombination was suggested to occur predominantly during minus-strand RNA synthesis (125). Although the interpretation of relevant experiments has been challenged (39), the preponderance of recombination events during the minus-strand synthesis seems logical in view of markedly higher abundance, in the infected cell, of free single-stranded RNA molecules of positive polarity, which could provide a pool of potential acceptor templates.

The dissociated 3' terminus of the nascent strand, possibly complexed to the RNA polymerase, may land onto a precisely homologous site of another template molecule. In this case, recombination is called homologous and precise. It seems plausible that identity of parting and anchoring sites is a major factor ensuring the preciseness of the landing. In line with this notion is the fact that the frequency of recombination between different poliovirus serotypes is markedly lower than between the variants of the same serotype (231). The structures of the crossover sites indicate that strictly identical sequences in the parting and anchoring sites can be rather short (only a few nucleotides) or even absent (125, 199, 230). Thus, parting and anchoring sites should perhaps be similar but not necessarily identical.

An apparently limited length of identical or even similar sequences in parting/anchoring sites poses a problem of how, during homologous recombination, the proper anchoring oligonucleotide could be selected among a great number of related sites likely present throughout the entire genome. One of the possible solutions to this problem may consist in the assumption that the actual length of the heteroduplex between the parting and anchoring sites is significantly larger than usually assumed, although the pairing should not necessarily be complete. It could also be imagined that secondary structure elements assist in bring-

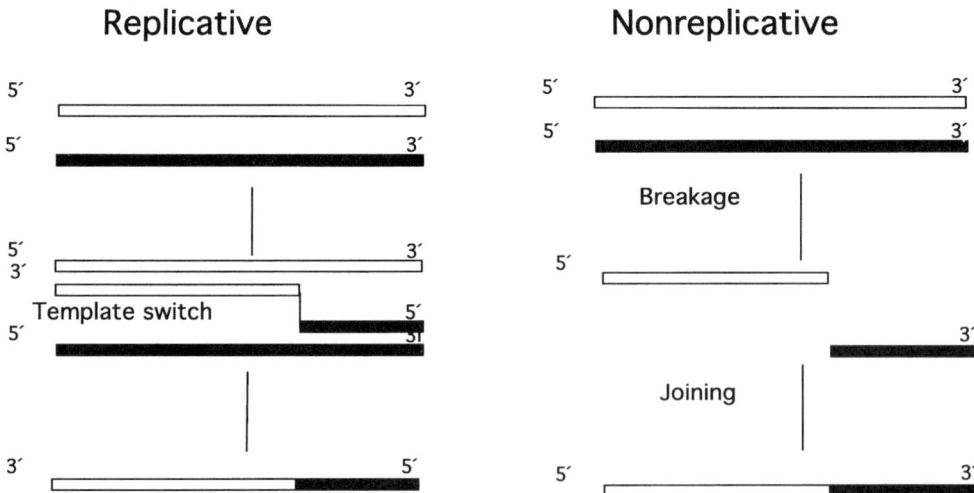

FIGURE 1 Two modes of recombination between RNA genomes. In the replicative mode, the synthesis of a nascent strand is started on one parental RNA molecule and is completed on another, due to template switching. Alternatively, fragments of different parental RNA molecules may be covalently joined in a nonreplicative reaction.

ing homologous sites of two templates to close proximity (Fig. 2) (199, 230), but experimental evidence supporting this hypothesis is difficult to produce. Predominance of homologous, as opposed to nonhomologous, recombinants among the progeny of mixed infection could well be due to the negative selection of incorrect genomes. Nevertheless, generation of homologous recombinants under nonselective conditions was also reported (114).

Obviously, template switching mechanistically similar to that occurring during recombination can also generate deletions and insertions, if the nascent strand jumps between

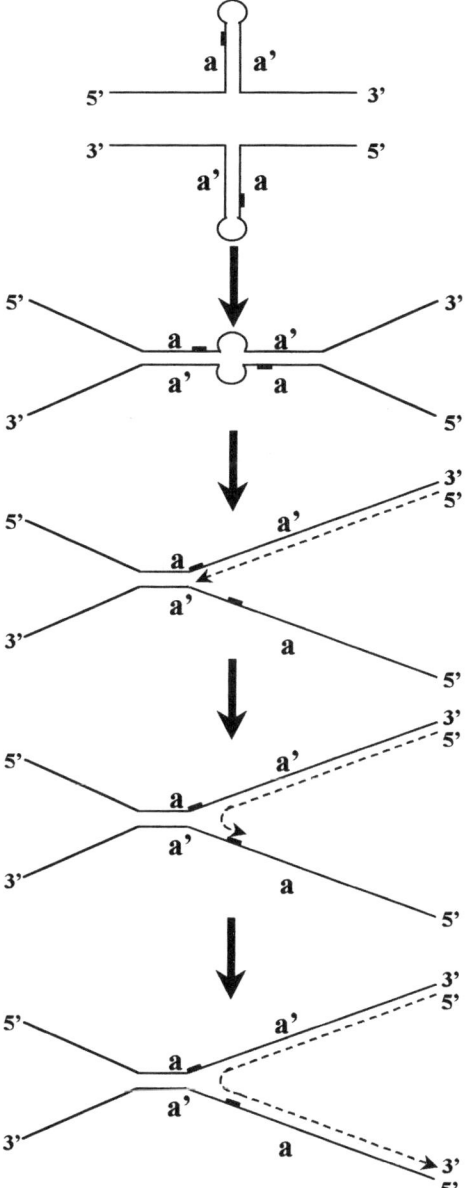

FIGURE 2 A model showing how heteroduplex formation may facilitate finding the proper anchoring site upon precise replicative recombination. Two homologous RNA molecules may form a heteroduplex through interaction between identical secondary structure elements. As a result, the to-be parting and anchoring sites on these molecules are brought in close proximity.

structurally identical (or similar) direct repeats located at different loci of the same or different templates (199). It may be hypothesized that, when the deletions are short (cf. 178), the new anchoring site may possibly be reached by the polymerase sliding, together with the 3' end of the nascent strand, along the template.

There is a class of genomic rearrangements, e.g., among deletions in picornavirus DI genomes, in which the to-be-joined termini of the RNA segments do not appear to contain repeated sequences. In other words, the parting and anchoring sites in these cases exhibit no obvious signs of similarity. To explain the origin of such rearrangements in the framework of the template switch mechanism, a model involving guiding RNA sequences was proposed. The guide may pair with the ends of the recombining partners and thus bring them in close proximity to one another (134). In principle, other parts of the viral genome or even cellular RNA may serve as guiding molecules, but the experimental support of such mechanism is still lacking.

Nonreplicative Rearrangements. Template switching is not the only possible way for generating nonhomologous rearrangements of viral RNAs. A nonreplicative mechanism could well operate in such cases (40, 91). Two key steps of this mechanism are represented by the cleavage of the recombining partners and joining of the fragments thereby generated. These two reactions could theoretically be accomplished either in a concerted fashion or in succession.

There are different hypothetical possibilities for the generation of recombining partners: cleavages by cellular RNases or self-cleaving cryptic ribozymes and premature termination of nascent strands (90). At least one of the variants of the joining reaction requires 3'-phosphate and 5'-OH groups (90). Such structures of the ligated termini suggest that some cellular enzyme should perhaps be involved but its nature is yet to be determined. For example, RNA 3'-terminal phosphate cyclase (86) may in principle convert the terminal 3'-phosphate into cyclic 2',3'-phosphate, which may subsequently be ligated to the 5'-OH group with (192) or without (135) involvement of additional enzymes.

Nonreplicative rearrangements are expected to be predominantly nonhomologous. It cannot be excluded that some of the known insertions of foreign RNA sequences (e.g., derived from ribosomal RNA) (37; A. P. Gmyl, unpublished) into the coding part of the viral genome may be generated nonreplicatively.

Biological Significance of Rearrangements

Viral RNA rearrangements of any kind (recombination, deletions, insertions) may contribute to genome plasticity and evolution. On the other hand, recombination may serve quite the opposite function of maintaining the stability of the genome. As discussed above, the progeny of a single viral genome may harbor a variety of different mutations, including adverse ones. Recombination between such altered RNA molecules may result in the regeneration of the parental-type genome. When host-to-host transfers are accomplished by relatively small doses of virus and the trend to fitness decline is expected (see below), such a rescue mechanism may be particularly important (3).

Genome Plasticity

Any function of the picornaviral genome can perhaps be accomplished by numerous different combinations of nucleotide sequences and, in the case of viral proteins, amino acid sequences. As natural and engineered variability of viral genomes hints, the degeneracy should be enormous and the existing viruses appear to use only a minute subset of the sequence space, which can ensure a specific phenotype. This fact creates a significant potential for evolution and plasticity of the viral genome. Genome plasticity refers to two distinct but related phenomena: (i) retention of viability (with or without phenotypic changes) after genomic changes, and (ii) spontaneous restoration of lost or damaged functions by acquisition of alternative genome structures.

The ease with which g^s and g^d poliovirus mutants could be selected upon virus cultivation in the presence of guanidine (146, 160) was one of the first illuminating illustrations of the propensity of the viral genome to adapt to unfavorable conditions. Remarkably, similar alterations of the sensitivity to guanidine may be caused by different nucleotide changes (14, 184, 232).

In 1985, viable, though phenotypically altered, poliovirus mutants were generated by insertion of a triplet into the polyprotein reading frame (21). Then, viable mutants with deletions or insertions both in the 3' untranslated and 5' untranslated regions (3' UTR and 5' UTR, respectively) (133, 209) were engineered. It became obvious that a genome function damaged by introduced mutations could often be restored by the acquisition of suppressor mutations (pseudoreversions through second-site mutations). Thus, replicative defects caused by short deletions in the poliovirus 5' UTR could be phenotypically cured by additional rather extended deletions occurring spontaneously upon cultivation of the debilitated mutants (58, 180). The engineered defects may be functionally so severe that no parental type genomes could be detected in the progeny; instead, each viable offspring contains a modified (pseudoreversion type) RNA. Such genomes are referred to as quasi-infectious (93). Regaining of fitness after a given detrimental mutation may occur by markedly different genomic changes (82, 91, 132, 180).

A striking example of picornavirus genome plasticity is provided by experiments with modifications of the picornavirus 3' UTR. In enteroviruses, this part of viral RNA is represented by a complex multidomain quasi-globular structure maintained by kissing interactions between loops of its two helical elements (157, 164, 182, 236). Mutations destroying the kissing interaction or changing mutual orientation of its helical elements (156) resulted in a significant loss of fitness, as judged by the acquisition of ts, quasi-infectious, or lethal phenotypes, associated with a severe suppression of viral RNA replication. It is believed that this complex structure, called oriR, is involved in the initiation of negative-strand RNA synthesis. However, the replacement of enterovirus oriR by structurally unrelated 3' UTR of human rhinovirus 14 (198) or its partial and even complete deletion (228, 229) resulted in a viable virus. The replicative potential of such viruses may be associated, at least in part, with adaptive compensating mutations in the viral RNA polymerase (161; cf. also discussion of this issue in reference 5).

Certain mutations in the replicative and translational control elements of the poliovirus 5' UTR can be compensated by second-site mutations in the noncapsid proteins 3C and 2A, respectively (10, 202).

The ability of FMDV to compensate for mutational alterations in the RGD motif of VP1 (normally used for entry into susceptible cells) by switching to alternative cellular receptors (15, 153) is an illustration of another type of plasticity.

Genome Evolution

There are a number of fundamental questions pertinent to the evolution of picornaviruses that cannot presently be answered. We do not know from where the putative common picornavirus precursor came and how it evolved to the existing variety of picornaviruses. On the other hand, studies on diverse evolutionary aspects are a "hot spot" of current picornavirus research.

Isolates of a wild-type virus separated geographically or temporarily from one another usually exhibit more or less marked differences in their nucleotide and amino acid sequences. The estimated rate of the natural evolution of poliovirus is 1 to 2% nucleotides per year (120). The potential to generate mutations of different sorts (nucleotide substitutions and rearrangements) is inherent in the replicative mechanism of picornaviruses. The evolution consists in consecutive fixation of a minute portion of these mutations. In addition, more or less extended rearrangements of the viral genome, such as deletions (18, 38, 83, 94, 169), duplications (177), insertions, and recombinations (see below) occur, though apparently much more rarely.

Some of the rules governing mutation fixation are obvious. Genomic changes that increase and decrease viral fitness are expected to be preferentially selected for and against, respectively. However, the majority of accumulated mutations appear to be phenotypically neutral or nearly so (85, 121, 206). This is true of not only the so-called silent (synonymous) mutations (e.g., most of the nucleotide substitutions at the third codon positions), which do not change the primary structure of the encoded protein, but also of many nonsynonymous replacements. "RNA viruses change far more than they adapt" (206).

Fixation of neutral mutations is largely due to sampling, upon transmission of a virus, of relatively small portions from heterogeneous quasispecies populations. Such a mechanism ensures fixation of mutations nearly regardless of their adaptive value (except of course the lethal ones). A neutral or debilitating substitution can also be fixed as a "passenger" accompanying a selective advantageous mutation. Obviously, the probability of fixation of neutral and detrimental mutations should dramatically depend on the size of the viral population involved in the infection of the subsequent host system. The smaller is the population, the higher is the chance. Evolution based on random sampling is expected to result in either maintenance of viral fitness at a more or less constant level (due to the preponderance of neutral mutations among the total possible substitutions) or even fitness decrease (due to the fact that phenotypically adverse mutations are more common than favorable ones). The latter phenomenon is known as "Muller's ratchet." On the other hand, the trend toward loss of fitness may be interrupted by stochastic appearance of fitness-increasing mutations. The above notions have found clear-cut support in experiments with plaque-to-plaque (bottlenecking) versus large-culture passages of FMDV and other RNA viruses (60, 61, 65, 81). There is ground to believe that random sampling is a major contributing factor to the natural evolution of poliovirus both in human organisms and in human populations (3, 85).

Assuming an approximately constant frequency of replicative errors made by the RNA polymerase of a given virus, the rate of accumulation of neutral mutations should depend largely on the number of cycles of viral reproduction per time unit. Therefore, on the average, it is expected to be roughly constant through time. In other words, the evolving viral genomes behave as molecular clocks (76, 92, 206). This fact was used for the estimation of the time of divergence (the "age") of picornaviral populations (cf. 85, 110, 226, 245). The reliability of these clocks may not, however, be very high, especially if nucleotide (rather than amino acid) substitutions are analyzed during relatively short and relatively long periods of time. The former situation may be associated with significant contributions of positive or negative selection, whereas the problem with the latter is that the degree of divergence tends to be leveled off with time (in particular, due to back mutations). The analysis of amino acid substitutions has another drawback, a much slower rate of fixation.

It should also be kept in mind that viruses are generally evolving not as isolated populations. Competition (214) and recombination (2) between populations may significantly alter the natural history of a virus.

Although the mechanisms of picornavirus speciation are yet to be determined, there is a good deal of knowledge, based on comparative analysis of amino acid and nucleotide sequences, of relatedness between different picornavirus genera and species ("evolutionary" or "phylogenetic" trees) (cf. 98, 154, 222). Hypothetical models of the evolution of picornaviruses can be derived from these data (98). When similar analysis is used for characterization of different isolates of a given species, valuable information about the geographical distribution of picornavirus variants (143, 152, 168, 193) and routes of their spread (187, 218) can be obtained.

VIRAL INTERACTIONS

A cell may be infected by more than a single virus. Different viral genomes may interact with one another, resulting in generation of recombinant progeny. On the other hand, proteins encoded by different viruses may help, or interfere with, reproduction of each other, directly or indirectly, e.g., by altering intracellular conditions. Moreover, essentially similar interactions occur between sibling genomes or their products even in a singly infected cell.

Complementation

Complementation in viruses refers to the capacity of rescuing the function of a gene product of one virus by a product encoded by a similar gene of another virus. The two complementing genomes may be deficient in products of different genes, and being expressed within the same cell, they may supply the respective missing functions to each other. Complementation may also be unilateral, when a deficient function of a virus is restored, for example, by a wild-type helper. The restoration may also be due to interactions between proteins encoded by the same genes of two partners carrying different deteriorating mutations each. This phenomenon is explained by the ability of differently damaged oligomeric proteins to form, in certain cases, a functionally competent tertiary structure.

In picornaviruses, however, there are several features that seriously complicate the problem (242). One such feature is the strategy of genome expression by making viral proteins via stepwise cleavage of the viral polyprotein. The function of intermediate cleavage products of the polyprotein may differ from those of its constituent "mature" components.

There is ample evidence that capsid proteins can be provided in *trans*. Phenotypic mixing (generation of mosaic capsids composed of proteins originating from parents belonging to different serotypes) and genome masking (encapsidation of the RNA into a capsid provided by the helper virus of a different serotype) are long known phenomena (48, 138, 240). The same capacity is clearly illustrated also by the existence of viral particles composed of DI RNA and capsid of a helper virus (41, 134). With noncapsid proteins, however, the situation is much more complicated.

A good example of a well-complementable protein is 2A polypeptide of enteroviruses (20). This is not necessarily true of 2A of other picornaviruses (it should be noted that very few complementation studies have been carried out in picornaviruses other than enteroviruses). For example, the relevant region of the FMDV polyprotein is involved in the polyprotein self-cleavage (203) and hence is expected to be required in *cis*.

On the other hand, at least certain lesions of poliovirus 2B cannot be rescued in *trans* (20, 116, 227). The explanation of this fact is not obvious but is perhaps somehow related to the fact that 2B (as such or as a component of the 2BC precursor) seems to serve not (or not only) as a direct participant of the replicative reactions but rather is involved in the rearrangement of intracellular membranes in the infected cells, thereby creating an appropriate environment for replication. At least some of these alterations appear irreversible and irreparable.

With other nonstructural proteins, the situation is not so straightforward: their lesions were reported to be and not to be complementable. Unilateral and mutual rescue of poliovirus mutants with altered sensitivity to guanidine was the first example of complementation between picornaviruses (6, 48, 239). Because g^s and g^d mutations map to 2C (184, 232), these observations indicate that 2C lesions can be rescued in *trans*. Similarly, relatively efficient *trans*-rescue of engineered poliovirus 2C mutants was reported (141, 142). Just the opposite conclusion, however, was derived from experiments with some other engineered 2C mutations (227). Certain 3A mutations appear to be complementable (20), whereas others are not (89). Also, different 3D lesions exhibited poor (20, 227) and relatively efficient (7, 36) capacity to be rescued in *trans*.

Explanations for such an apparent inconsistency could be different. Most, if not all, picornavirus proteins are polyfunctional. Just as an example, 3D polymerase is involved in VPg uridylylation (176) and initiation of RNA strand and its elongation; it has to interact with some other viral nonstructural proteins (243), with itself (175), and possibly with some host proteins; it should also be able to recognize appropriate terminal and internal *cis*-acting RNA replicative elements, etc. One may assume that some of these properties can be complemented, while others cannot. Furthermore, functions and properties of a "mature" viral protein may differ from the properties of this protein when it is a part of a less processed precursor. Thus, a mutation in poliovirus 3A can be restored in *trans* by 3ABCD but not by 3AB (233). Another possibility may be related to the presence of replicative *cis*-acting signals within the coding region (93). Mutational inactivation of such signals should likely bring about noncomplementable defects.

A special mode of complementation, dubbed intragenomic, was observed with an engineered poliovirus in which a deficient function of mutated VPg moiety of 3AB was partially rescued by another functional 3AB gene in the same genome but controlled by a separate IRES (32).

Existence of complementation at the RNA (rather than protein) level was also suggested on the basis of experiments in which impaired function of mutated picornavirus IRES was partially restored by coexpression of homologous intact IRES or of its fragments (196, 225).

New possibilities for complementation analysis are opened with the development of cell-free systems for picornavirus reproduction (67).

The biological significance of complementation between picornaviruses under natural conditions is unknown, but since mixed infections of human beings (and perhaps animals) with different enteroviruses are not uncommon, complementation between coexisting agents seems possible.

Interference

Picornaviruses may interfere with each other. The viruses may compete for host cell receptors (50) or interference may occur at the intracellular level. Different mechanisms may be responsible for the latter phenomenon. One may involve viral proteins forming functional oligomers: inclusion of structurally different subunits provided by the coinfecting partner into such oligomers may result in functional inactivation of the entire structure (negative dominance). Another possibility is related to the old idea about the limiting number of active sites capable of ensuring viral reproduction. One may envision, for example, that intracellular membranes altered by one virus cannot be utilized for the replication of its partner. Some recent findings concerning the effect of poliovirus proteins on the rearrangement of the intracellular membrane network (72) are in line with such an assumption. However, discrimination between different mechanisms upon the analysis of a given case of interference is a difficult task.

It is likely that a kind of interference takes place even between the sibling molecules. Such interference may limit the viral yield per infected cell. This mode of viral self-control is yet to be explored.

Recombination

The mechanisms of recombination between picornaviruses have already been considered (in "Genome Rearrangements" above). Here, it is appropriate just to mention that this type of viral interaction is not a purely laboratory phenomenon but occurs not infrequently in nature. For example, children receiving trivalent Sabin poliovirus vaccine regularly excrete intertypic recombinants (31). Intertypic recombinants between Sabin strains or between Sabin and *wt* strains are found relatively often among viruses isolated from cases of so-called vaccine-associated poliomyelitis (38a, 87, 99, 119a, 144). Natural intertypic recombinants of other picornaviruses are also described (28, 130, 207). Interspecies recombination appears to make a significant contribution to the evolution of picornaviruses (106, 208).

GENETIC ANALYSIS

Mutational Analysis

There are two general approaches to linking specific phenotypic traits to specific genes or their parts: (i) identification of mutations associated with a distinct phenotype, and (ii) observation of phenotypic effects of engineered mutations in specific genes. Mutational analysis is a highly powerful tool but a few cautionary remarks seem appropriate.

Mapping a mutation(s) responsible for a given viral phenotype may require sequencing of the entire genome, if it is not firmly established that the phenotype is associated solely with a specific genomic fragment. To guarantee correctness of the assignment, the putative mutation(s) should be reintroduced into the viral RNA followed by assaying the phenotype of the engineered virus. Since many phenotypic traits are quantitative rather than qualitative, on the one hand, and altered phenotypes are often associated with multiple mutations, on the other hand, accurate mapping may turn out rather difficult.

The second approach, exploration of a viral gene function(s) by introducing site-directed mutations, may be associated with other complications. The mutations may interfere with such general processes as translation, polyprotein processing, or RNA replication, thereby affecting functions of nontarget genes as well. In some cases, the engineered mutations may affect only one of several functions of a multifunctional gene. Moreover, the affected function may be important or even essential under certain conditions (e.g., in the infected animal) but completely dispensable under others (e.g., in tissue culture cells).

The power of genetic analysis can often be markedly enhanced when introduction of a debilitating mutation is followed by selecting and studying revertants with completely or partially restored functional properties. The genomes of some of such revertants may really return to their parental structure, but in other cases restoration of the phenotype may be due to second-site mutations. Such pseudoreversions may provide very useful information about the structure-function relationship of the genomic region affected by the mutation (58, 180, 182) as well as about interactions between different genes or *cis*-elements (10, 161).

Complementation Analysis

At an early step of picornavirus research, it seemed reasonable to exploit classical complementation analysis to estimate the number of viral genes. Attempts were undertaken to define separate "complementation groups" by grouping mutants unable to complement each other but able to complement reproduction of mutants belonging to other groups (46). However, these attempts produced no clear-cut results for the reasons discussed in the section "Complementation." After the genomes of several picornaviruses had been sequenced, there was no longer any need to count viral genes by this sort of analysis.

On the other hand, the ability or inability to rescue in *trans* an impaired function by the relevant viral protein may provide valuable information about possible molecular mechanisms involved (36, 89, 116, 232, 233).

Recombinational Analysis

Like complementation, recombination was among the first approaches to characterize the structure of the picornavirus genome. Two-factor and three-factor crosses were used to generate genetic (linkage) maps showing the relative positions of different *ts* mutations with specific phenotypes (46). The assignment of the guanidine target to nonstructural proteins, and specifically to 2C (79, 210, 231), and first approximate mapping of poliovirus attenuation mutants (4) were done by crossing appropriate picornaviruses. Soon thereafter, however, a more powerful and versatile technique of recombination analysis based on cDNA technology was introduced (128, 136). Variants of this technique are now in common use.

REPLICONS, CHIMERAS, AND VECTORS

With the advent of cDNA technology it became possible to generate different kinds of artificial picornavirus genomes useful for elucidating some fundamental problems or serving applied purposes.

One type of such constructs is represented by replicons, i.e., portions of the viral genome able to replicate either autonomously or assisted by a helper but unable by themselves to generate infectious particles. In fact, natural replicons, DI genomes ("Genome Rearrangements" section), have been known for a long while. Similar replicons with deletions in the capsid-encoding regions of the genome (sometimes partially replaced by marker foreign genes) can readily be engineered (16, 101, 118). They are used, for example, in attempts to define essential cis-elements for replication and packaging and to explore other important features of viral replication (cf. 174, 186).

Designing chimeras between different picornaviruses is another approach to solve some fundamental and applied problems. Exchange of a portion of poliovirus 5′ UTR for appropriate regions of coxsackievirus B3 results in viable viruses sometimes exhibiting a ts phenotype (117, 212). Replacing poliovirus IRES by the corresponding element of rhinovirus leads to a severe loss of monkey virulence without a significant impairment of virus growth in standard cell lines (96). A similar effect can be obtained by exchanging the coxsackievirus B3 5′ UTR for the homologous region of the poliovirus genome (34). This approach may be used for the design of attenuated viral variants, and it also points to IRES involvement in determining viral host range. Shuffling IRES domains between different picornaviruses permits also a more precise mapping of cis-elements responsible for these effects (97, 181).

Other variants of engineered chimerical viruses contain polyproteins composed of segments derived from different picornaviruses (17, 55, 147, 235). Such constructs proved to be useful for studying specificity of viral protein/RNA and protein/protein interactions.

Picornavirus genomes have also been modified to encode antigenic determinants of other RNA and DNA viruses with the prospect of using them either as vaccines or diagnostic or research tools (e.g., 11, 29, 185). For similar purposes, appropriate determinants of nonviral genes are also being inserted into picornavirus genomes (e.g., 149, 173, 201). On the other hand, picornavirus IRESs are widely used in different vectors to ensure efficient translation of target proteins (e.g., 1, 170, 191). An important point of concern with chimeras design is their genetic stability (167).

CONCLUDING REMARKS

As with other biological systems, the picornavirus genome has evolved a mechanism for maintaining a balance between variability and stability. In general terms, these mechanisms are understandable, if not to say obvious. Variability is undoubtedly due to error-prone picornaviral RNA polymerases, which in addition exhibit limited processivity (ensuring template-switch recombination). Another potential contribution to genome variability may come from the propensity of RNA molecules to recombine in a nonreplicative mode. In view of the robustness of the viral genome (the capacity to perform a specific function by a very great number of more or less diverse protein and RNA structures), these mechanisms often produce viable variants. The main reason for genome stability is evidently a strong selective pressure.

On the other hand, the current understanding of the mechanisms of picornavirus genome variability and stability is rather superficial and limited. It not only lacks predictive power (although admittedly the direction of further evolution is unpredictable in principle) but also fails to explain the evolutionary history of the viral family in terms other than similarity and divergence between viral species or genera. Gaining deeper insights into these fundamental problems is a challenging and feasible goal for forthcoming research.

Current work in the author's laboratory is supported by grants from INTAS, Russian Foundation for Basic Research, and National Multiple Sclerosis Society (United States).

REFERENCES

1. **Adam, M. A., N. Ramesh, A. D. Miller, and W. R. Osborne.** 1991. Internal initiation of translation in retroviral vectors carrying picornavirus 5′ nontranslated regions. *J. Virol.* **65:**4985–4990.
2. **Agol, V. I.** 1997. Recombination and other genomic rearrangements in picornaviruses. *Semin. Virol.* **8:**1–9.
3. **Agol, V. I., G. A. Belov, E. A. Cherkasova, E. V. Gavrilin, M. S. Kolesnikova, L. I. Romanova, and E. A. Tolskaya.** 2001. Some problems of molecular biology of poliovirus infection relevant to pathogenesis and viral spread. *Dev. Biol.* (Basel) **105:**43–50.
4. **Agol, V. I., V. P. Grachev, S. G. Drozdov, M. S. Kolesnikova, V. G. Kozlov, N. M. Ralph, L. I. Romanova, E. A. Tolskaya, A. V. Tyufanov, and E. G. Viktorova.** 1984. Construction and properties of intertypic poliovirus recombinants: first approximation mapping of the major determinants of neurovirulence. *Virology* **136:**41–55.
5. **Agol, V. I., A. V. Paul, and E. Wimmer.** 1999. Paradoxes of the replication of picornaviral genomes. *Virus Res.* **62:**129–147.
6. **Agol, V. I., and G. A. Shirman.** 1964. Interaction of guanidine-sensitive and guanidine-dependent variants of poliovirus in mixedly infected cells. *Biochem. Biophys. Res. Commun.* **17:**28–33.
7. **Agut, H., K. M. Kean, O Fichot, J. Morasco, J. B. Flanegan, and M. Girard.** 1989. A point mutation in the poliovirus polymerase gene determines a complementable temperature-sensitive defect of RNA replication. *Virology* **168:**302–311.
8. **Ahmad, A. L., A. B. Dowsett, and D. A. Tyrrell.** 1987. Studies of rhinovirus resistant to an antiviral chalcone. *Antiviral Res.* **8:**27–39.
9. **Almond, J. W., D. Stone, K. Burke, M. A. Skinner, A. J. Macadam, D. Wood, M. Ferguson, and P. D. Minor.** 1993. Approaches to the construction of new candidate poliovirus type 3 vaccine strains. *Dev. Biol. Stand.* **78:**161–169.
10. **Andino, R., G. E. Rieckhof, D. Trono, and D. Baltimore.** 1990. Substitutions in the protease (3Cpro) gene of poliovirus can suppress a mutation in the 5′ noncoding region. *J. Virol.* **64:**607–612.
11. **Andino, R., D. Silvera, S. D. Suggett, P. L. Achacoso, C. J. Miller, D. Baltimore, and M. B. Feinberg.** 1994.

Engineering poliovirus as a vaccine vector for the expression of diverse antigens. *Science* **265**:1448–1451.

12. **Armstrong, C.** 1939. Successful transfer of the Lansing strain of poliomyelitis virus from the cotton rat to the white mouse. *Public Health Rep.* **54**:2302–2305.
13. **Arnold, J. J., and C. E. Cameron.** 1999. Poliovirus RNA-dependent RNA polymerase (3Dpol) is sufficient for template switching in vitro. *J. Biol. Chem.* **274**:2706–2716.
14. **Baltera, R. F., Jr., and D. R. Tershak.** 1989. Guanidine-resistant mutants of poliovirus have distinct mutations in peptide 2C. *J. Virol.* **63**:4441–4444.
15. **Baranowski, E., C. M. Ruiz-Jarabo, N. Sevilla, D. Andreu, E. Beck, and E. Domingo.** 2000. Cell recognition by foot-and-mouth disease virus that lacks the RGD integrin-binding motif: flexibility in aphthovirus receptor usage. *J. Virol.* **74**:1641–1647.
16. **Barclay, W., Q. Li, G. Hutchison, D. Moon, A. Richardson, N. Percy, J. W. Almond, and D. J. Evans.** 1998. Encapsidation studies of poliovirus subgenomic replicons. *J. Gen. Virol.* **79**:1725–1734.
17. **Bell, Y. C., B. L. Semler, and E. Ehrenfeld.** 1999. Requirements for RNA replication of a poliovirus replicon by coxsackievirus B3 RNA polymerase. *J. Virol.* **73**:9413–9421.
18. **Beneduce, F., G. Pisani, M. Divizia, A. Pana, and G. Morace.** 1995. Complete nucleotide sequence of a cytopathic hepatitis A virus strain isolated in Italy. *Virus Res.* **36**:299–309.
19. **Bergstrom, C. T., P. McElhany, and L. A. Real.** 1999. Transmission bottlenecks as determinants of virulence in rapidly evolving pathogens. *Proc. Natl. Acad. Sci. USA* **96**:5095–5100.
20. **Bernstein, H. D., P. Sarnow, and D. Baltimore.** 1986. Genetic complementation among poliovirus mutants derived from an infectious cDNA clone. *J. Virol.* **60**:1040–1049.
21. **Bernstein, H. D., N. Sonenberg, and D. Baltimore.** 1985. Poliovirus mutant that does not selectively inhibit host cell protein synthesis. *Mol. Cell. Biol.* **5**:2913–2923.
22. **Bodian, D., L. M. Morgan, and H. A. Howe.** 1949. Differentiation of types of poliomyelitis virus. III. The grouping of fourteen strains into three basic immunological types. *Am. J. Hyg.* **49**:234–245.
23. **Boege, U., D. Kobasa, S. Onodera, G. D. Parks, A. C. Palmenberg, and D. G. Scraba.** 1991. Characterization of mengo virus neutralization epitopes. *Virology* **181**:1–13.
24. **Boeyé, A.** 1959. Induction of mutation in poliovirus by nitrous acid. *Virology* **9**:691–700.
25. **Bolwell, C., B. E. Clarke, N. R. Parry, E. J. Ouldridge, F. Brown, and D. J. Rowlands.** 1989. Epitope mapping of foot-and-mouth disease virus with neutralizing monoclonal antibodies. *J. Gen. Virol.* **70**:59–68.
26. **Bradley, D. W., C. A. Schable, K. A. McCaustland, E. H. Cook, B. L. Murphy, H. A. Fields, J. W. Ebert, C. Wheeler, and J. E. Maynard.** 1984. Hepatitis A virus: growth characteristics of in vivo and in vitro propagated wild and attenuated virus strains. *J. Med. Virol.* **14**:373–386.
27. **Brooksby, J. B.** 1958. The virus of foot-and-mouth disease. *Adv. Virus Res.* **5**:1–37.
28. **Bunch, T., E. Rieder, and P. Mason.** 1994. Sequence of the S fragment of foot-and-mouth disease virus type A12. *Virus Genes* **8**:173–175.
29. **Burke, K. L., D. J. Evans, O. Jenkins, J. Meredith, E. D. D'Souza, and J. W. Almond.** 1989. A cassette vector for the construction of antigen chimaeras of poliovirus. *J. Gen. Virol.* **70**:2475–2479.
30. **Burnet, F. M., and J. Macnamara.** 1931. Immunological differences between strains of poliomyelitis virus. *Br. J. Exp. Pathol.* **12**:57–61 (quoted in reference 73).
31. **Cammack, N., A. Phillips, G. Dunn, V. Patel, and P. D. Minor.** 1988. Intertypic genomic rearrangements of poliovirus strains in vaccinees. *Virology* **167**:507–514.
32. **Cao, X., and E. Wimmer.** 1995. Intragenomic complementation of a 3AB mutant in dicistronic polioviruses. *Virology* **209**:315–326.
33. **Cao, X. M., I. E. Bergmann, and E. Beck.** 1991. Comparison of the 5' and 3' untranslated genomic regions of virulent and attenuated foot-and-mouth disease viruses (strains O1 Campos and C3 Resende). *J. Gen. Virol.* **72**:2821–2825.
34. **Chapman, N. M., A. Ragland, J. S. Leser, K. Hofling, S. Willian, B. L. Semler, and S. Tracy.** 2000. A group B coxsackievirus/poliovirus 5' nontranslated region chimera can act as an attenuated vaccine strain in mice. *J. Virol.* **74**:4047–4056.
35. **Chapman, N. M., A. I. Ramsingh, and S. Tracy.** 1997. Genetics of coxsackievirus virulence. *Curr. Top. Microbiol.* **223**:227–258.
36. **Charini, W. A., C. C. Burns, E. Ehrenfeld, and B. L. Semler.** 1991. trans rescue of a mutant poliovirus RNA polymerase function. *J. Virol.* **65**:2655–2665.
37. **Charini, W. A., S. Todd, G. A. Gutman, and B. L. Semler.** 1994. Transduction of a human RNA sequence by poliovirus. *J. Virol.* **68**:6547–6552.
38. **Charpentier, N., M. Davila, E. Domingo, and C. Escarmis.** 1996. Long-term, large-population passage of aphthovirus can generate and amplify defective noninterfering particles deleted in the leader protease gene. *Virology* **223**:10–18.
38a. **Cherkasova, E. A., E. A. Korotkova, M. L. Yakovenko, O. E. Ivanova, T. P. Eremeeva, K. M. Chumakov, and V. I. Agol.** 2002. Long-term circulation of vaccine-derived poliovirus that causes paralytic disease. *J. Virol.* **76**:6791–6799.
39. **Chetverin, A. B.** 1999. The puzzle of RNA recombination. *FEBS Lett.* **460**:1–5.
40. **Chetverin, A. B., H. V. Chetverina, A. A. Demidenko, and V. I. Ugarov.** 1997. Nonhomologous RNA recombination in a cell-free system: evidence for a transesterification mechanism guided by secondary structure. *Cell* **88**:503–513.
41. **Cole, C. N., and D. Baltimore.** 1973. Defective interfering particles of poliovirus. II. Nature of the defect. *J. Mol. Biol.* **76**:325–343.
42. **Cole, C. N., D. Smoler, E. Wimmer, and D. Baltimore.** 1971. Defective interfering particles of poliovirus. I. Isolation and physical properties. *J. Virol.* **7**:478–485.
43. **Colston, E. M., and V. R. Racaniello.** 1995. Poliovirus variants selected on mutant receptor-expressing cells identify capsid residues that expand receptor recognition. *J. Virol.* **69**:4823–4829.
44. **Colter, J. S., H. H. Bird, A. W. Moyer, and R. A. Brown.** 1957. Infectivity of ribonucleic acid isolated from virus infected tissues. *Virology* **4**:522–532.
45. **Cooper, P. D.** 1968. A genetic map of poliovirus temperature-sensitive mutants. *Virology* **35**:584–596.
46. **Cooper, P. D.** 1977. Genetics of picornaviruses. *Comp. Virol.* **9**:133–207.
47. **Cords, C. E., and J. J. Holland.** 1964. Interference between enteroviruses and conditions affecting its reversal. *Virology* **22**:226–234.
48. **Cords, C. E., and J. J. Holland.** 1964. Replication of poliovirus RNA induced by heterologous virus. *Proc. Natl. Acad. Sci. USA* **51**:1080–1082.
49. **Couderc, T., J. Hogle, H. Le Blay, F. Horaud, and B. Blondel.** 1993. Molecular characterization of mouse-virulent poliovirus type I Mahoney mutants: involvement of residues of polypeptides VP1 and VP2 located on the

inner surface of the capsid protein shell. *J. Virol.* **67:** 3808–3817.

49a. Crotty, S., C. E. Cameron, and R. Andino. 2001. RNA virus error catastrophe: direct molecular test by using ribavirin. *Proc. Natl. Acad. Sci. USA* **98:**6895–6900.

50. **Crowell, R. L., and B. J. Landau.** 1983. Receptors in the initiation of picornavirus infection. *Comp. Virol.* **18:** 1–43.

51. **Curran, J., and D. Kolakofsky.** 1999. Replication of paramyxoviruses. *Adv. Virus Res.* **54:**403–422.

52. **Day, S. P., P. Murphy, E. A. Brown, and S. M. Lemon.** 1992. Mutations within the 5' nontranslated region of hepatitis A virus RNA which enhance replication in BS-C-1 cells. *J. Virol.* **66:**6533–6540.

53. **de la Torre, J. C., C. Giachetti, B. L. Semler, and J. J. Holland.** 1992. High frequency of single-base transitions and extreme frequency of precise multiple-base reversion mutations in poliovirus. *Proc. Natl. Acad. Sci. USA* **89:** 2531–2535.

54. **de la Torre, J. C., E. Wimmer, and J. J. Holland.** 1990. Very high frequency of reversion to guanidine resistance in clonal pools of guanidine-dependent type 1 poliovirus. *J. Virol.* **64:**664–671.

55. **Dewalt, P. G., M. A. Lawson, R. J. Colonno, and B. L. Semler.** 1989. Chimeric picornavirus polyproteins demonstrate a common 3C proteinase substrate specificity. *J. Virol.* **63:**3444–3452.

56. **Diez, J., M. Hofner, E. Domingo, and A. I. Donaldson.** 1990. Foot-and-mouth disease virus strains isolated from persistently infected cell cultures are attenuated for mice and cattle. *Virus Res.* **18:**3–7.

57. **Diez, J., M. G. Mateu, and E. Domingo.** 1989. Selection of antigenic variants of foot-and-mouth disease virus in the absence of antibodies, as revealed by an in situ assay. *J. Gen. Virol.* **70:**3281–3289.

58. **Dildine, S. L., and B. L. Semler.** 1989. The deletion of 41 proximal nucleotides reverts a poliovirus mutant containing a temperature-sensitive lesion in the 5' noncoding region of genomic RNA. *J. Virol.* **63:**847–862.

59. **Domingo, E., M. Davila, and J. Ortin.** 1980. Nucleotide sequence heterogeneity of the RNA from a natural population of foot-and-mouth-disease virus. *Gene* **11:**333–346.

60. **Domingo, E., C. Escarmís, L. Menéndez-Arias, and J. J. Holland.** 1999. Viral quasi-species and fitness variations, p. 141–161. *In* E. Domingo, R. G. Webster, and J. J. Holland (ed.), *Origin and Evolution of Viruses*. Academic Press, San Diego, Calif.

61. **Domingo, E., and J. J. Holland.** 1997. RNA virus mutations and fitness for survival. *Annu. Rev. Microbiol.* **51:** 151–178.

62. **Domingo, E., E. Martinez-Salas, F. Sobrino, J. C. de la Torre, A. Portela, J. Ortin, C. Lopez-Galindez, P. Perez-Brena, N. Villanueva, R. Najera, S. VandePol, D. Steinhauer, N. De Polo, and J. J. Holland.** 1985. The quasi-species (extremely heterogeneous) nature of viral RNA genome populations: biological relevance—a review. *Gene* **40:**1–8.

63. **Dove, A. W., and V. R. Racaniello.** 1997. Cold-adapted poliovirus mutants bypass a postentry replication block. *J. Virol.* **71:**4728–4735.

64. **Drake, J. W., and J. J. Holland.** 1999. Mutation rates among RNA viruses. *Proc. Natl. Acad. Sci. USA* **96:** 13910–13913.

65. **Duarte, E., D. Clarke, A. Moya, E. Domingo, and J. Holland.** 1992. Rapid fitness losses in mammalian RNA virus clones due to Muller's ratchet. *Proc. Natl. Acad. Sci. USA* **89:**6015–6019.

66. **Dubes, G. R., and M. Chapin.** 1956. Cold-adapted genetic variants of polioviruses. *Science* **124:**586–588.

67. **Duggal, R., and E. Wimmer.** 1999. Genetic recombination of poliovirus in vitro and in vivo: temperature-dependent alteration of crossover sites. *Virology* **258:**30–41.

68. **Duke, G. M., J. E. Osorio, and A. C. Palmenberg.** 1990. Attenuation of mengo virus through genetic engineering of the 5' noncoding poly(C) tract. *Nature* **343:**474–476.

69. **Dulbecco, R., and M. Vogt.** 1954. Plaque formation and isolation of pure lines with polioviruses. *J. Exp. Med.* **99:** 167–182.

70. **Dulbecco, R., and M. Vogt.** 1958. Studies on the induction of mutations in poliovirus by proflavine. *Virology* **5:** 236–243.

71. **Dunn, J. J., N. M. Chapman, S. Tracy, and J. R. Romero.** 2000. Genomic determinants of cardiovirulence in coxsackievirus B3 clinical isolates: localization to the 5' nontranslated region. *J. Virol.* **74:**4787–4794.

72. **Egger, D., N. Teterina, E. Ehrenfeld, and K. Bienz.** 2000. Formation of the poliovirus replication complex requires coupled viral translation, vesicle production, and viral RNA synthesis. *J. Virol.* **74:**6570–6580.

73. **Eggers, H. J.** 1999. Milestones in early poliomyelitis research (1840 to 1949). *J. Virol.* **73:**4533–4535.

74. **Eggers, H. J., and B. Rosenwirth.** 1988. Isolation and characterization of an arildone-resistant poliovirus 2 mutant with an altered capsid protein VP1. *Antiviral Res.* **9:** 23–35.

75. **Eggers, H. J., and I. Tamm.** 1962. On the mechanism of selective inhibition of enterovirus multiplication by 2-(α-hydroxybenzyl)-benzimidazole. *Virology* **18:**426–438.

76. **Elena, S. F., F. Gonzalez-Candelas, and A. Moya.** 1992. Does the VP1 gene of foot-and-mouth disease virus behave as a molecular clock? *J. Mol. Evol.* **35:**223–229.

77. **Emerson, S. U., Y. K. Huang, C. McRill, M. Lewis, and R. H. Purcell.** 1992. Mutations in both the 2B and 2C genes of hepatitis A virus are involved in adaption to growth in cell culture. *J. Virol.* **66:**650–654.

78. **Emini, E. A., B. A. Jameson, A. J. Lewis, G. R. Larsen, and E. Wimmer.** 1982. Poliovirus neutralization epitopes: analysis and localization with neutralizing monoclonal antibodies. *J. Virol.* **43:**997–1005.

79. **Emini, E. A., J. Leibowitz, D. C. Diamond, J. Bonin, and E. Wimmer.** 1984. Recombinants of Mahoney and Sabin strain poliovirus type 1: analysis of in vitro phenotypic markers and evidence that resistance to guanidine maps in the nonstructural proteins. *Virology* **137:**74–85.

80. **Enders, J. F., T. H. Weller, and F. C. Robbins.** 1949. Cultivation of the Lansing strain of poliomyelitis virus in cultures of various human embryonic tissues. *Science* **109:** 85–87.

81. **Escarmis, C., M. Davila, N. Charpentier, A. Bracho, A. Moya, and E. Domingo.** 1996. Genetic lesions associated with Muller's ratchet in an RNA virus. *J. Mol. Biol.* **264:** 255–267.

82. **Escarmis, C., M. Davila, and E. Domingo.** 1999. Multiple molecular pathways for fitness recovery of an RNA virus debilitated by operation of Muller's ratchet. *J. Mol. Biol.* **285:**495–505.

83. **Escarmis, C., J. Dopazo, M. Davila, E. L. Palma, and E. Domingo.** 1995. Large deletions in the 5'-untranslated region of foot-and-mouth disease virus of serotype C. *Virus Res.* **35:**155–167.

84. **Escarmis, C., M. Toja, M. Medina, and E. Domingo.** 1992. Modifications of the 5' untranslated region of foot-and-mouth disease virus after prolonged persistence in cell culture. *Virus Res.* **26:**113–125.

85. **Gavrilin, G. V., E. A. Cherkasova, G. Yu. Lipskaya, O. M. Kew, and V. I. Agol.** 2000. Evolution of circulating wild poliovirus and of vaccine-derived poliovirus in an

immunodeficient patient: a unifying model. *J. Virol.* **74:** 7381–7390.
86. **Genschik, P., E. Billy, M. Swianiewicz, and W. Filipowicz.** 1997. The human RNA 3'-terminal phosphate cyclase is a member of a new family of proteins conserved in Eucarya, Bacteria and Archaea. *EMBO J.* **16:**2955–2967.
87. **Georgescu, M. M., F. Delpeyroux, M. Tardy-Panit, J. Balanant, M. Combiescu, A. A. Combiescu, S. Guillot, and R. Crainic.** 1994. High diversity of poliovirus strains isolated from the central nervous system from patients with vaccine-associated paralytic poliomyelitis. *J. Virol.* **68:**8089–8101.
88. **Ghendon, Y. Z.** 1972. Conditional-lethal mutants of animal viruses. *Prog. Med. Virol.* **14:**68–90.
89. **Giachetti, C., S. S. Hwang, and B. L. Semler.** 1992. cis-acting lesions targeted to the hydrophobic domain of a poliovirus membrane protein involved in RNA replication. *J. Virol.* **66:**6045–6057.
90. **Gmyl, A. P., E. V. Belousov, S. V. Maslova, E. V. Khitrina, A. B. Chetverin, and V. I. Agol.** 1999. Nonreplicative RNA recombination in poliovirus. *J. Virol.* **73:** 8958–8965.
91. **Gmyl, A. P., E. V. Pilipenko, S. V. Maslova, G. A. Belov, and V. I. Agol.** 1993. Functional and genetic plasticities of the poliovirus genome: quasi-infectious RNAs modified in the 5'-untranslated region yield a variety of pseudorevertants. *J. Virol.* **67:**6309–6316.
92. **Gojobori, T., E. N. Moriyama, and M. Kimura.** 1990. Molecular clock of viral evolution, and the neutral theory. *Proc. Natl. Acad. Sci. USA* **87:**10015–10018.
93. **Goodfellow, I., Y. Chaudhry, A. Richardson, J. Meredith, J. W. Almond, W. Barclay, and D. J. Evans.** 2000. Identification of a cis-acting replication element within the poliovirus coding region. *J. Virol.* **74:**4590–4600.
94. **Graff, J., C. Kasang, A. Normann, M. Pfisterer-Hunt, S. M. Feinstone, and B. Flehmig.** 1994. Mutational events in consecutive passages of hepatitis A virus strain GBM during cell culture adaptation. *Virology* **204:**60–68.
95. **Graff, J., A. Normann, and B. Flehmig.** 1997. Influence of the 5' noncoding region of hepatitis A virus strain GBM on its growth in different cell lines. *J. Gen. Virol.* **78:**1841–1849.
96. **Gromeier, M., L. Alexander, and E. Wimmer.** 1996. Internal ribosomal entry site substitution eliminates neurovirulence in inter-generic poliovirus recombinants. *Proc. Natl. Acad. Sci. USA* **93:**2370–2375.
97. **Gromeier, M., B. Bossert, M. Arita, A. Nomoto, and E. Wimmer.** 1999. Dual stem loops within the poliovirus internal ribosomal entry site control neurovirulence. *J. Virol.* **73:**958–964.
98. **Gromeier, M., E. Wimmer, and A. E. Gorbalenya.** 1999. Genetics, pathogenesis and evolution of picornaviruses, p. 287–343. *In* E. Domingo, R. G. Webster, and J. J. Holland (ed.), *Origin and Evolution of Viruses.* Academic Press, San Diego, Calif.
99. **Guillot, S., V. Caro, N. Cuervo, E. Korotkova, M. Combiescu, A. Persu, A. Aubert-Combiescu, F. Delpeyroux, and R. Crainic.** 2000. Natural genetic exchanges between vaccine and wild poliovirus strains in humans. *J. Virol.* **74:**8434–8443.
100. **Hadfield, A. T., M. A. Oliveira, K. H. Kim, I. Minor, M. J. Kremer, B. A. Heinz, D. Shepard, D. C. Pevear, R. R. Rueckert, and M. G. Rossmann.** 1995. Structural studies on human rhinovirus 14 drug-resistant compensation mutants. *J. Mol. Biol.* **253:**61–73.
101. **Hagino-Yamagishi, K., and A. Nomoto.** 1989. In vitro construction of poliovirus defective interfering particles. *J. Virol.* **63:**5386–5392.
102. **Harris, T. J., and F. Brown.** 1977. Biochemical analysis of a virulent and an avirulent strain of foot-and-mouth disease virus. *J. Gen. Virol.* **34:**87–105.
103. **Heinz, B. A., R. R. Rueckert, D. A. Shepard, F. J. Dutko, M. A. McKinlay, M. Fancher, M. G. Rossmann, J. Badger, and T. J. Smith.** 1989. Genetic and molecular analyses of spontaneous mutants of human rhinovirus 14 that are resistant to an antiviral compound. *J. Virol.* **63:**2476–2485.
104. **Hirst, G. K.** 1962. Genetic recombination with Newcastle disease virus, polioviruses and influenza. *Cold Spring Harbor Symp. Quant. Biol.* **27:**303–308.
105. **Holland, J. J., E. Domingo, J. C. de la Torre, and D. A. Steinhauer.** 1990. Mutation frequencies at defined single codon sites in vesicular stomatitis virus and poliovirus can be increased only slightly by chemical mutagenesis. *J. Virol.* **64:**3960–3962.
106. **Hughes, P. J., C. North, P. D. Minor, and G. Stanway.** 1989. The complete nucleotide sequence of coxsackievirus A21. *J. Gen. Virol.* **70:**2943–2952.
107. **Huovilainen, A., T. Hovi, L. Kinnunen, K. Takkinen, M. Ferguson, and P. Minor.** 1987. Evolution of poliovirus during an outbreak: sequential type 3 poliovirus isolates from several persons show shifts of neutralization determinants. *J. Gen. Virol.* **68:**1373–1378.
108. **Huovilainen, A., L. Kinnunen, M. Ferguson, and T. Hovi.** 1988. Antigenic variation among 173 strains of type 3 poliovirus isolated in Finland during the 1984 to 1985 outbreak. *J. Gen. Virol.* **69:**1941–1848.
109. **Iizuka, N., M. Kohara, K. Hagino-Yamagishi, S. Abe, T. Komatsu, K. Tago, M. Arita, and A. Nomoto.** 1989. Construction of less neurovirulent polioviruses by introducing deletions into the 5' noncoding sequence of the genome. *J. Virol.* **63:**5354–5363.
110. **Ishiko, H., N. Takeda, K. Miyamura, N. Kato, M. Tanimura, K. H. Lin, M. Yin-Murphy, J. S. Tam, G. F. Mu, and S. Yamazaki.** 1992. Phylogenetic analysis of a coxsackievirus A24 variant: the most recent worldwide pandemic was caused by progenies of a virus prevalent around 1981. *Virology* **187:**748–759.
111. **Jackson, T., D. Sheppard, M. Denyer, W. Blakemore, and A. M. King.** 2000. The epithelial integrin alphavbeta6 is a receptor for foot-and-mouth disease virus. *J. Virol.* **74:**4949–4956.
112. **Jakob, J., and R. P. Roos.** 1996. Molecular determinants of Theiler's murine encephalomyelitis-induced disease. *J. Neurovirol.* **2:**70–77.
113. **Jarvis, T. C., and K. Kirkegaard.** 1991. The polymerase in its labyrinth: mechanisms and implications of RNA recombination. *Trends Genet.* **7:**186–191.
114. **Jarvis, T. C., and K. Kirkegaard.** 1992. Poliovirus RNA recombination: mechanistic studies in the absence of selection. *EMBO J.* **11:**3135–3145.
115. **Jia, Q., S. Ohka, K. Iwasaki, K. Tohyama, and A. Nomoto.** 1999. Isolation and molecular characterization of a poliovirus type 1 mutant that replicates in the spinal cords of mice. *J. Virol.* **73:**6041–6047.
116. **Johnson, K. L., and P. Sarnow.** 1991. Three poliovirus 2B mutants exhibit noncomplementable defects in viral RNA amplification and display dosage-dependent dominance over wild-type poliovirus. *J. Virol.* **65:**4341–4349.
117. **Johnson, V. H., and B. L. Semler.** 1988. Defined recombinants of poliovirus and coxsackievirus: sequence-specific deletions and functional substitutions in the 5'-noncoding regions of viral RNAs. *Virology* **162:**47–57.
118. **Kaplan, G., and V. R. Racaniello.** 1988. Construction and characterization of poliovirus subgenomic replicons. *J. Virol.* **62:**1687–1696.

119. Karron, R. A., R. Daemer, J. Ticehurst, E. D'Hondt, H. Popper, K. Mihalik, J. Philips, S. Feinstone, and R. H. Purcell. 1988. Studies of prototype live hepatitis A virus vaccines in primate models. *J. Infect. Dis.* **157:** 338–345.
119a. Kew, O., V. Morris-Glasgow, M. Landaverde, C. Burns, J. Shaw, Z. Garib, J. Andre, E. Blackman, C. J. Freeman, J. Jorba, R. Sutter, G. Tambinia, L. Venczel, C. Perdreira, F. Laender, H. Shimizu, T. Yoneyama, T. Miyamura, H. van der Avoort, M. S. Oberste, D. Kilpatrick, S. Cochi, M. Pallansch, and C. de Quadros. 2002. Outbreak of poliomyelitis in Hispaniola associated with circulating type 1 vaccine-derived poliovirus. *Science* **296:**356–359.
120. Kew, O. M., M. N. Mulders, G. Y. Lipskaya, E. E. da Silva, and M. A. Pallansch. 1995. Molecular epidemiology of poliovirus. *Semin. Virol.* **6:**401–414.
121. Kimura, M. 1983. *The Neutral Theory of Molecular Evolution.* Cambridge University Press, Cambridge, United Kingdom.
122. King, A. M. 1988. Preferred sites of recombination in poliovirus RNA: an analysis of 40 intertypic cross-over sequences. *Nucleic Acids Res.* **16:**11705–11723.
123. King, A. M., D. McCahon, W. R. Slade, and J. W. Newman. 1982. Recombination in RNA. *Cell* **29:**921–928.
124. Kinnunen, L., A. Huovilainen, T. Poyry, and T. Hovi. 1990. Rapid molecular evolution of wild type 3 poliovirus during infection in individual hosts. *J. Gen. Virol.* **71:**317–324.
125. Kirkegaard, K., and D. Baltimore. 1986. The mechanism of RNA recombination in poliovirus. *Cell* **47:**433–443.
126. Kitamura, N., B. L. Semler, P. G. Rothberg, G. R. Larsen, C. J. Adler, A. J. Dorner, E. A. Emini, R. Hanecak, J. J. Lee, S. Werf, C. W. Anderson, and E. Wimmer. 1981. Primary structure, gene organization and polypeptide expression of poliovirus RNA. *Nature* **291:**547–553.
127. Koch, F., and G. Koch. 1985. *The Molecular Biology of Poliovirus.* Springer-Verlag, Vienna, Austria.
128. Kohara, M., T. Omata, A. Kameda, B. L. Semler, H. Itoh, E. Wimmer, and A. Nomoto. 1985. In vitro phenotypic markers of a poliovirus recombinant constructed from infectious cDNA clones of the neurovirulent Mahoney strain and the attenuated Sabin 1 strain. *J. Virol.* **53:**786–792.
129. Koprowski, H., G. A. Jarvis, and T. W. Norton. 1952. Immune responses in human volunteers upon oral administration of a rodent-adapted strain of poliomyelitis virus. *Am. J. Hyg.* **55:**108–126.
130. Krebs, O., and O. Marquardt. 1992. Identification and characterization of foot-and-mouth disease virus O1 Burgwedel/1987 as an intertypic recombinant. *J. Gen. Virol.* **73:**613–619.
131. Kuge, S., N. Kawamura, and A. Nomoto. 1989. Strong inclination toward transition mutation in nucleotide substitutions by poliovirus replicase. *J. Mol. Biol.* **207:** 175–182.
132. Kuge, S., N. Kawamura, and A. Nomoto. 1989. Genetic variation occurring on the genome of an in vitro insertion mutant of poliovirus type 1. *J. Virol.* **63:**1069–1075.
133. Kuge, S., and A. Nomoto. 1987. Construction of viable deletion and insertion mutants of the Sabin strain of type 1 poliovirus: function of the 5′ noncoding sequence in viral replication. *J. Virol.* **61:**1478–1487.
134. Kuge, S., I. Saito, and A. Nomoto. 1986. Primary structure of poliovirus defective-interfering particle genomes and possible generation mechanisms of the particles. *J. Mol. Biol.* **192:**473–487.
135. Lafontaine, D., D. Beaudry, P. Marquis, and J. P. Perreault. 1995. Intra- and intermolecular nonenzymatic ligations occur within transcripts derived from the peach latent mosaic viroid. *Virology* **212:**705–709.
136. La Monica, N., C. Meriam, and V. R. Racaniello. 1986. Mapping of sequences required for mouse neurovirulence of poliovirus type 2 Lansing. *J. Virol.* **57:**515–525.
137. Ledinko, N. 1963. Genetic recombination with poliovirus type 1. Studies of crosses between a normal horse serum-resistant mutant and several guanidine-resistant mutants of the same strain. *Virology* **20:**107–119.
138. Ledinko, N., and G. K. Hirst. 1961. Mixed infection of HeLa cells with polioviruses types 1 and 2. *Virology* **14:** 107–119.
139. Li, C. P., and K. Habel. 1951. Adaptation of Leon strain of poliomyelitis virus to mice. *Proc. Soc. Exp. Biol. Med.* **78:**233–238.
140. Li, C. P., and M. Schaeffer. 1953. Adaptation of type 1 poliomyelitis virus to mice. *Proc. Soc. Exp. Biol. Med.* **82:**477–481.
141. Li, J. P., and D. Baltimore. 1988. Isolation of poliovirus 2C mutants defective in viral RNA synthesis. *J. Virol.* **62:**4016–4021.
142. Li, J. P., and D. Baltimore. 1990. An intragenic revertant of a poliovirus 2C mutant has an uncoating defect. *J Virol.* **64:**1102–1107.
143. Lipskaya, G. Y., E. A. Chervonskaya, G. I. Belova, S. V. Maslova, T. N. Kutateladze, S. G. Drozdov, M. Mulders, M. A. Pallansch, O. M. Kew, and V. I. Agol. 1995. Geographical genotypes (geotypes) of poliovirus case isolates from the former Soviet Union: relatedness to other known poliovirus genotypes. *J. Gen. Virol.* **76:** 1687–1699.
144. Lipskaya, G. Y., A. R. Muzychenko, O. K. Kutitova, S. V. Maslova, M. Equestre, S. G. Drozdov, R. Perez Bercoff, and V. I. Agol. 1991. Frequent isolation of intertypic poliovirus recombinants with serotype 2 specificity from vaccine-associated polio cases. *J. Med. Virol.* **35:** 290–296.
145. Lipton, H. L., and M. L. Jelachich. 1997. Molecular pathogenesis of Theiler's murine encephalomyelitis virus-induced demyelinating disease in mice. *Intervirology* **40:** 143–152.
146. Loddo, B., W. Ferrari, A. Spaneda, and G. Brotzu. 1962. In vitro guanidine-resistance and guanidine-dependence of poliovirus. *Experientia* **18:**518–519.
147. Lu, H. H., X. Li, A. Cuconati, and E. Wimmer. 1995. Analysis of picornavirus 2A(pro) proteins: separation of proteinase from translation and replication functions. *J. Virol.* **69:**7445–7452.
148. Lwoff, A. Factors influencing evolution of viral disease at the cellular level and in the organism. *Bacteriol. Rev.* **23:**109–124.
149. Mandl, S., L. J. Sigal, K. L. Rock, and R. Andino. 1998. Poliovirus vaccine vectors elicit antigen-specific cytotoxic T cells and protect mice against lethal challenge with malignant melanoma cells expressing a model antigen. *Proc. Natl. Acad. Sci. USA* **95:**8216–8221.
150. Martin, L. R., Z. C. Neal, M. S. McBride, and A. C. Palmenberg. 2000. Mengovirus and encephalomyocarditis virus poly(C) tract lengths can affect virus growth in murine cell culture. *J. Virol.* **74:**3074–3081.
151. Martinez, M. A., C. Carrillo, F. Gonzalez-Candelas, A. Moya, E. Domingo, and F. Sobrino. 1991. Fitness alteration of foot-and-mouth disease virus mutants: measurement of adaptability of viral quasispecies. *J. Virol.* **65:** 3954–3957.

152. **Martinez, M. A., J. Dopazo, J. Hernandez, M. G. Mateu, F. Sobrino, E. Domingo, and N. J. Knowles.** 1992. Evolution of the capsid protein genes of foot-and-mouth disease virus: antigenic variation without accumulation of amino acid substitutions over six decades. *J. Virol.* **66:** 3557–3565.
153. **Martinez, M. A., N. Verdaguer, M. G. Mateu, and E. Domingo.** 1997. Evolution subverting essentiality: dispensability of the cell attachment Arg-Gly-Asp motif in multiply passaged foot-and-mouth disease virus. *Proc. Natl. Acad. Sci. USA* **94:**6798–6802.
154. **Marvil, P., N. J. Knowles, A. P. Mockett, P. Britton, T. D. Brown, and D. Cavanagh.** 1999. Avian encephalomyelitis virus is a picornavirus and is most closely related to hepatitis A virus. *J. Gen. Virol.* **80:**653–662.
155. **Mason, P. W., M. E. Piccone, T. S. Mckenna, J. Chinsangaram, and M. J. Grubman.** 1997. Evaluation of a live-attenuated foot-and-mouth disease virus as a vaccine candidate. *Virology* **227:**96–102.
156. **Melchers, W. J., J. M. Bakkers, H. J. Bruins Slot, J. M. Galama, V. I. Agol, and E. V. Pilipenko.** 2000. Cross-talk between orientation-dependent recognition determinants of a complex control RNA element, the enterovirus oriR. *RNA* **6:**976–987.
157. **Melchers, W. J. G., H. Heenderop, H. J. Bruins Slot, C. Pleij, E. V. Pilipenko, V. I. Agol, and J. Galama.** 1997. Kissing of the two predominant hairpin loops in the coxsackie B virus 3′UTR in the origin of replication required for (−) strand RNA synthesis. *J. Virol.* **71:**686–696.
158. **Melnick, J. L.** 1953. Poliomyelitis. *Adv. Virus Res.* **1:** 229–275.
159. **Melnick, J. L.** 1996. Enteroviruses: polioviruses, coxsackieviruses, echoviruses, and newer enteroviruses, p. 655–712. *In* B. N. Fields, D. M. Knipe, and P. M. Howley (ed.), *Fields Virology*, 3rd ed. Lippincott-Raven, Philadelphia, Pa.
160. **Melnick, J. L., D. Crowther, and J. Barrera-Oro.** 1961. Rapid development of drug resistant mutants of poliovirus. *Science* **134:**557.
161. **Meredith, J. M., J. B. Rohll, J. W. Almond, and D. J. Evans.** 1999. Similar interactions of the poliovirus and rhinovirus 3D polymerases with the 3′ untranslated region of rhinovirus 14. *J. Virol.* **73:**9952–9958.
162. **Minor, P. D., A. M. John, M. Ferguson, and J. P. Icenogle.** 1986. Antigenic and molecular evolution of the vaccine strain of type 3 poliovirus during the period of excretion by a primary vaccinee. *J. Gen. Virol.* **67:** 693–706.
163. **Minor, P. D., G. C. Schild, J. Bootman, D. M. Evans, M. Ferguson, P. Reeve, M. Spitz, G. Stanway, A. J. Cann, R. Hauptmann, L. D. Clarke, R. C. Mountford, and J. W. Almond.** 1983. Location and primary structure of a major antigenic site for poliovirus neutralization. *Nature* **301:**674–679.
164. **Mirmomeni, M. H., P. J. Hughes, and G. Stanway.** 1997. An RNA structure in the 3′ untranslated region of enteroviruses is necessary for efficient replication. *J. Virol.* **71:**2363–2370.
165. **Molla, A., A. V. Paul, and E. Wimmer.** 1991. Cell-free, de novo synthesis of poliovirus. *Science* **254:**1647–1651.
166. **Mosser, A. G., and R. R. Rueckert.** 1993. WIN 51711-dependent mutants of poliovirus type 3: evidence that virions decay after release from cells unless drug is present. *J. Virol.* **67:**1246–1254.
167. **Mueller, S., and E. Wimmer.** 1998. Expression of foreign proteins by poliovirus polyprotein fusion: analysis of genetic stability reveals deletions and formation of cardioviruslike open reading frames. *J. Virol.* **72:**20–31.
168. **Mulders, M. N., G. Y. Lipskaya, H. G. A. M. van der Avoort, M. P. G. Koopmans, O. M. Kew, and A. M. van Loon.** 1995. Molecular epidemiology of wild poliovirus type 1 in Europe, the Middle East and the Indian subcontinent. *J. Infect. Dis.* **171:**1399–1405.
169. **Mulders, M. N., J. H. Reimerink, M. Stenvik, I. Alaeddinoglu, H. G. van der Avoort, T. Hovi, and M. P. Koopmans.** 1999. A Sabin vaccine-derived field isolate of poliovirus type 1 displaying aberrant phenotypic and genetic features, including a deletion in antigenic site 1. *J. Gen. Virol.* **80:**907–916.
170. **Murakami, M., H. Watanabe, Y. Niikura, T. Kameda, K. Saitoh, M. Yamamoto, Y. Yokouchi, A. Kuroiwa, K. Mizumoto, and H. Iba.** 1997. High-level expression of exogenous genes by replication-component retrovirus vectors with an internal ribosomal entry site. *Gene* **202:** 23–29.
171. **Neff, S., D. Sa-Carvalho, E. Rieder, P. W. Mason, S. D. Blystone, E. J. Brown, and B. Baxt.** 1998. Foot-and-mouth disease virus virulent for cattle utilizes the integrin alpha(v)beta3 as its receptor. *J. Virol.* **72:**3587–3594.
172. **Novak, J. E., and K. Kirkegaard.** 1994. Coupling between genome translation and replication in an RNA virus. *Genes Dev.* **8:**1726–1737.
173. **Novak, M. J., L. E. Smythies, S. A. McPherson, P. D. Smith, and C. D. Morrow.** 1999. Poliovirus replicons encoding the B subunit of Helicobacter pylori urease elicit a Th1 associated immune response. *Vaccine* **17:** 2384–2391.
174. **Nugent, C. I., K. L. Johnson, P. Sarnow, and K. Kirkegaard.** 1999. Functional coupling between replication and packaging of poliovirus replicon RNA. *J. Virol.* **73:**427–435.
175. **Pata, J. D., S. C. Schultz, and K. Kirkegaard.** 1995. Functional oligomerization of poliovirus RNA-dependent RNA polymerase. *RNA* **1:**466–477.
176. **Paul, A. V., J. H. van Boom, D. Filippov, and E. Wimmer.** 1998. Protein-primed RNA synthesis by purified poliovirus RNA polymerase. *Nature* **393:**280–284.
177. **Pilipenko, E. V., V. M. Blinov, and V. I. Agol.** 1990. Gross rearrangements within the 5′-untranslated region of the picornaviral genomes. *Nucleic Acids Res.* **18:** 3371–3375.
178. **Pilipenko, E. V., A. P. Gmyl, and V. I. Agol.** 1995. A model for rearrangements in RNA genomes. *Nucleic Acids Res.* **23:**1870–1875.
179. **Pilipenko, E. V., A. P. Gmyl, S. V. Maslova, E. V. Khitrina, and V. I. Agol.** 1995. Attenuation of Theiler's murine encephalomyelitis virus by modifications of the oligopyrimidine/AUG tandem, a host-dependent translational cis-element. *J. Virol.* **69:**864–870.
180. **Pilipenko, E. V., A. P. Gmyl, S. V. Maslova, Y. V. Svitkin, A. N. Sinyakov, and V. I. Agol.** 1992. A prokaryotic-like cis-element in the cap-independent internal initiation of translation on picornavirus RNA. *Cell* **68:**119–131.
181. **Pilipenko, E. V., T. V. Pestova, V. G. Kolupaeva, E. V. Khitrina, A. N. Poperechnaya, V. I. Agol, and C. U. Hellen.** 2000. A cell cycle-dependent protein serves as a template-specific translation initiation factor. *Genes Dev.* **14:**2028–2045.
182. **Pilipenko, E. V., K. V. Poperechny, S. V. Maslova, W. J. G. Melchers, H. J. Bruins Slot, and V. I. Agol.** 1996. Cis-element, oriR, involved in the initiation of (−) strand poliovirus RNA: a quasi-globular multidomain RNA structure maintained by tertiary ("kissing") interaction. *EMBO J.* **19:**5428–5436.
183. **Pilipenko, E. V., E. G. Viktorova, E. V. Khitrina, S. V. Maslova, N. Jarousse, M. Brahic, and V. I. Agol.** 1999.

Distinct attenuation phenotypes caused by mutations in the translational starting window of Theiler's murine encephalomyelitis virus. *J. Virol.* **73:**3190–3196.
184. **Pincus, S. E., H. Rohl, and E. Wimmer.** 1987. Guanidine-dependent mutants of poliovirus: identification of three classes with different growth requirements. *Virology* **157:**83–88.
185. **Porter, D. C., D. C. Ansardi, and C. D. Morrow.** 1995. Encapsidation of poliovirus replicons encoding the complete human immunodeficiency virus type 1 gag gene by using a complementation system which provides the P1 capsid protein in trans. *J. Virol.* **69:**1548–1555.
186. **Porter, D. C., D. C. Ansardi, J. Wang, S. McPherson, Z. Moldoveanu, and C. D. Morrow.** 1998. Demonstration of the specificity of poliovirus encapsidation using a novel replicon which encodes enzymatically active firefly luciferase. *Virology* **243:**1–11.
187. **Poyry, T., L. Kinnunen, J. Kapsenberg, O. Kew, and T. Hovi.** 1990. Type 3 poliovirus/Finland/1984 is genetically related to common Mediterranean strains. *J. Gen. Virol.* **71:**2535–2541.
188. **Provost, P. J., P. A. Conti, P. A. Giesa, F. S. Banker, E. B. Buynak, W. J. McAleer, and M. R. Hilleman.** 1983. Studies in chimpanzees of live, attenuated hepatitis A vaccine candidates. *Proc. Soc. Exp. Biol. Med.* **172:**357–363.
189. **Racaniello, V. R., and D. Baltimore.** 1981. Molecular cloning of poliovirus cDNA and determination of the complete nucleotide sequence of the viral genome. *Proc. Natl. Acad. Sci. USA* **78:**4887–4891.
190. **Racaniello, V. R., and D. Baltimore.** 1981. Cloned poliovirus complementary DNA is infectious in mammalian cells. *Science* **214:**916–919.
191. **Ramesh, N., S. T. Kim, M. Q. Wei, M. Khalighi, and W. R. Osborne.** 1996. High-titer bicistronic retroviral vectors employing foot-and-mouth disease virus internal ribosome entry site. *Nucleic Acids Res.* **24:**2697–2700.
192. **Reid, C. E., and D. W. Lazinski.** 2000. A host-specific function is required for ligation of a wide variety of ribozyme-processed RNAs. *Proc. Natl. Acad. Sci. USA* **97:**424–429.
193. **Rico-Hesse, R., M. A. Pallansch, B. K. Nottay, and O. M. Kew.** 1987. Geographic distribution of wild poliovirus type 1 genotypes. *Virology* **160:**311–322.
194. **Rieder, E., T. Bunch, F. Brown, and P. W. Mason.** 1993. Genetically engineered foot-and-mouth disease viruses with poly(C) tracts of two nucleotides are virulent in mice. *J. Virol.* **67:**5139–5345.
195. **Rightsel, W. A., J. R. Dice, R. J. McAlpine, E. A. Timm, I. W. McLean, G. J. Dixon, and F. M. Schabel.** 1961. Antiviral effect of guanidine. *Science* **134:**558–559.
196. **Roberts, L. O., and G. J. Belsham.** 1997. Complementation of defective picornavirus internal ribosome entry site (IRES) elements by the coexpression of fragments of the IRES. *Virology* **227:**53–62.
197. **Roca-Garcia, M., A. W. Moyer, and H. R. Cox.** 1953. Poliomyelitis. 2. Propagation of MEF-1 strain of poliomyelitis virus in developing chick embryo by yolk sac inoculation. *Proc. Soc. Exp. Biol. Med.* **81:**519–525.
198. **Rohll, J. B., D. H. Moon, D. J. Evans, and J. W. Almond.** 1995. The 3′ untranslated region of picornavirus RNA: features required for efficient genome replication. *J. Virol.* **69:**7835–7844.
199. **Romanova, L. I., V. M. Blinov, E. A. Tolskaya, E. G. Viktorova, M. S. Kolesnikova, E. A. Guseva, and V. I. Agol.** 1986. The primary structure of crossover regions of intertypic poliovirus recombinants: a model of recombination between RNA genomes. *Virology* **155:**202–213.

200. **Romanova, L. I., E. A. Tolskaya, M. S. Kolesnikova, and V. I. Agol.** 1980. Biochemical evidence for intertypic genetic recombination of polioviruses. *FEBS Lett.* **1:**109–112.
201. **Rose, C., W. Andrews, M. Ferguson, J. McKeating, J. Almond, and D. Evans.** 1994. The construction and characterization of poliovirus antigen chimeras presenting defined regions of the human T lymphocyte marker CD4. *J. Gen. Virol.* **75:**969–977.
202. **Rowe, A., G. L. Ferguson, P. D. Minor, and A. J. Macadam.** 2000. Coding changes in the poliovirus protease 2A compensate for 5′NCR domain V disruptions in a cell-specific manner. *Virology* **269:**284–293.
203. **Ryan, M. D., and M. Flint.** 1997. Virus-encoded proteinases of the picornavirus supergroup. *J. Gen. Virol.* **78:**699–723.
204. **Sabin, A. B.** 1955. Behavior of chimpanzee-avirulent poliomyelitis viruses in experimentally infected human volunteers. *Am. J. Med. Sci.* **230:**1–8.
205. **Sabin, A. B.** 1985. Oral poliovirus vaccine: history of its development and use, and current challenge to eliminate poliomyelitis from the world. *J. Infect. Dis.* **151:**420–436.
206. **Sala, M., and S. Wain-Hobson.** 1999. Drift and conservatism in RNA virus evolution: are they adapting or merely changing? p. 115–140. *In* E. Domingo, R. G. Webster, and J. J. Holland (ed.), *Origin and Evolution of Viruses*. Academic Press, San Diego, Calif.
207. **Santti, J., H. Harvala, L. Kinnunen, and T. Hyypia.** 2000. Molecular epidemiology and evolution of coxsackievirus A9. *J. Gen. Virol.* **81:**1361–1372.
208. **Santti, J., T. Hyypia, L. Kinnunen, and M. Salminen.** 1999. Evidence of recombination among enteroviruses. *J. Virol.* **7:**8741–8749.
209. **Sarnow, P., H. D. Bernstein, and D. Baltimore.** 1986. A poliovirus temperature-sensitive RNA synthesis mutant located in a noncoding region of the genome. *Proc. Natl. Acad. Sci. USA* **83:**571–575.
210. **Saunders, K., A. M. King, D. McCahon, J. W. Newman, W. R. Slade, and S. Forss.** 1985. Recombination and oligonucleotide analysis of guanidine-resistant foot-and-mouth disease virus mutants. *J. Virol.* **56:**921–929.
211. **Schwerdt, C. E., and F. L. Schaffer.** 1955. Some physical and chemical properties of purified poliomyelitis virus preparations. *Ann. N. Y. Acad. Sci.* **61:**740–750.
212. **Semler, B. L., V. H. Johnson, and S. Tracy.** 1986. A chimeric plasmid from cDNA clones of poliovirus and coxsackievirus produces a recombinant virus that is temperature-sensitive. *Proc. Natl. Acad. Sci. USA* **83:**1777–1781.
213. **Sergiescu, D., F. Horodniceanu, and A. Aubert-Combiescu.** 1972. The use of inhibitors in the study of picornavirus genetics. *Prog. Med. Virol.* **14:**123–199.
214. **Sevilla, N., C. M. Ruiz-Jarabo, G. Gomez-Mariano, E. Baranowski, and E. Domingo.** 1998. An RNA virus can adapt to the multiplicity of infection. *J. Gen. Virol.* **79:**2971–2980.
215. **Sevilla, N., N. Verdaguer, and E. Domingo.** 1996. Antigenically profound amino acid substitutions occur during large population passages of foot-and-mouth disease virus. *Virology* **225:**400–405.
216. **Shepard, D. A., B. A. Heinz, and R. R. Rueckert.** 1993. WIN 52035-2 inhibits both attachment and eclipse of human rhinovirus 14. *J. Virol.* **67:**2245–2254.
217. **Sherry, B., and R. Rueckert.** 1985. Evidence for at least two dominant neutralization antigens on human rhinovirus 14. *J. Virol.* **53:**137–143.
218. **Shulman, L. M., R. Handsher, C. F. Yang, S. J. Yang, J. Manor, A. Vonsover, Z. Grossman, M. Pallansch, E.

Mendelson, and O. M. Kew. 2000. Resolution of the pathways of poliovirus type 1 transmission during an outbreak. *J. Clin. Microbiol.* **38:**945–952.
219. Sierra, S., M. Dávila, P. R. Lowenstein, and E. Domingo. 2000. Response of foot-and-mouth disease virus to increased mutagenesis: influence of viral load and fitness in loss of infectivity. *J. Virol.* **74:**8316–8323.
220. Slobodskaya, O. R., A. P. Gmyl, S. V. Maslova, E. A. Tolskaya, E. G. Viktorova, and V. I. Agol. 1996. Poliovirus neurovirulence correlates with the presence of a cryptic AUG upstream of the initiator codon. *Virology* **221:**141–150.
221. Sobrino, F., M. Davila, J. Ortin, and E. Domingo. 1983. Multiple genetic variants arise in the course of replication of foot-and-mouth disease virus in cell culture. *Virology* **128:**310–318.
222. Stanway, G., and T. Hyypia. 1999. Parechoviruses. *J. Virol.* **73:**5249–5254.
223. Stapleton, J. T., and S. M. Lemon. 1987. Neutralization escape mutants define a dominant immunogenic neutralization site on hepatitis A virus. *J. Virol.* **61:**491–498.
224. Stave, J. W., J. L. Card, D. O. Morgan, and V. N. Vakharia. 1988. Neutralization sites of type O1 foot-and-mouth disease virus defined by monoclonal antibodies and neutralization-escape virus variants. *Virology* **62:**21–29.
225. Stone, D. M., J. W. Almond, J. K. Brangwyn, and G. J. Belsham. 1993. trans complementation of cap-independent translation directed by poliovirus 5' noncoding region deletion mutants: evidence for RNA-RNA interactions. *J. Virol.* **67:**6215–6223.
226. Takeda, N., M. Tanimura, and K. Miyamura. 1994. Molecular evolution of the major capsid protein VP1 of enterovirus 70. *J. Virol.* **68:**854–862.
227. Teterina, N. L., W. D. Zhou, M. W. Cho, and E. Ehrenfeld. 1995. Inefficient complementation activity of poliovirus 2C and 3D proteins for rescue of lethal mutations. *J. Virol.* **69:**4245–4254.
228. Todd, S., and B. L. Semler. 1996. Structure-infectivity analysis of the human rhinovirus genomic RNA 3' noncoding region. *Nucleic Acids Res.* **24:**2133–2142.
229. Todd, S., J. S. Towner, D. M. Brown, and B. L. Semler. 1997. Replication-competent picornaviruses with complete genomic RNA 3' noncoding region deletions. *J. Virol.* **71:**8868–8874.
230. Tolskaya, E. A., L. I. Romanova, V. M. Blinov, E. G. Viktorova, A. N. Sinyakov, M. S. Kolesnikova, and V. I. Agol. 1987. Studies on the recombination between RNA genomes of poliovirus: the primary struture and nonrandom distribution of crossover regions in the genomes of intertypic poliovirus recombinants. *Virology* **161:**54–62.
231. Tolskaya, E. A., L. I. Romanova, M. S. Kolesnikova, and V. I. Agol. 1983. Intertypic recombination in poliovirus: genetic and biochemical studies. *Virology* **124:**121–132.
232. Tolskaya, E. A., L. I. Romanova, M. S. Kolesnikova, A. P. Gmyl, A. E. Gorbalenya, and V. I. Agol. 1994. Genetic studies on the NTP-binding pattern containing 2C protein of poliovirus: possible mechanism of guanidine effect on 2C function and evidence for importance of 2C oligomerization. *J. Mol. Biol.* **236:**1310–1323.
233. Towner, J. S., M. M. Mazanet, and B. L. Semler. 1998. Rescue of defective poliovirus RNA replication by 3AB-containing precursor polyproteins. *J. Virol.* **72:**7191–7200.
234. Toyoda, H., M. Kohara, Y. Kataoka, T. Suganuma, T. Omata, N. Imura, and A. Nomoto. 1984. Complete nucleotide sequences of all three poliovirus serotype genomes. Implication for genetic relationship, gene function and antigenic determinants. *J. Mol. Biol.* **174:**561–585.
235. van Kuppeveld, F. J., P. J. van den Hurk, W. van der Vliet, J. M. Galama, and W. J. Melchers. 1997. Chimeric coxsackie B3 virus genomes that express hybrid coxsackievirus-poliovirus 2B proteins: functional dissection of structural domains involved in RNA replication. *J. Gen. Virol.* **78:**1833–1840.
236. Wang, J., J. M. Bakkers, J. M. Galama, H. J. Bruins Slot, E. V. Pilipenko, V. I. Agol, and W. J. Melchers. 1999. Structural requirements of the higher order RNA kissing element in the enteroviral 3'UTR. *Nucleic Acids Res.* **27:**485–449.
237. Ward, C. D., and J. B. Flanegan. 1992. Determination of the poliovirus RNA polymerase error frequency at eight sites in the viral genome. *J. Virol.* **66:**3784–3793.
238. Ward, C. D., M. A. Stokes, and J. B. Flanegan. 1988. Direct measurement of the poliovirus RNA polymerase error frequency in vitro. *J. Virol.* **62:**558–562.
239. Wecker, E., and G. Lederhilger. 1964. Curtailment of the latent period by double infection with polioviruses. *Proc. Natl. Acad. Sci. USA* **52:**246–251.
240. Wecker, E., and G. Lederhilger. 1964. Genomic masking produced by double infection of HeLa cells with heterotypic polioviruses. *Proc. Natl. Acad. Sci. USA* **52:**705–709.
241. Wien, M. W., S. Curry, D. J. Filman, and J. M. Hogle. 1997. Structural studies of poliovirus mutants that overcome receptor defects. *Nat. Struct. Biol.* **4:**666–674.
242. Wimmer, E., C. U. Hellen, and X. Cao. 1993. Genetics of poliovirus. *Annu. Rev. Genet.* **27:**353–436.
243. Xiang, W., A. Cuconati, D. Hope, K. Kirkegaard, and E. Wimmer. 1998. Complete protein linkage map of poliovirus P3 proteins: interaction of polymerase 3Dpol with VPg and with genetic variants of 3AB. *J. Virol.* **72:**6732–6741.
244. Zell, R., K. Klingel, M. Sauter, U. Fortmuller, and R. Kandolf. 1995. Coxsackieviral proteins functionally recognize the polioviral cloverleaf structure of the 5'-NTR of a chimeric enterovirus RNA: influence of species-specific host cell factors on virus growth. *Virus Res.* **39:**87–103.
245. Zhang, G., D. T. Haydon, N. J. Knowles, and J. W. McCauley. 1999. Molecular evolution of swine vesicular disease virus. *J. Gen. Virol.* **80:**639–651.

Error Frequencies of Picornavirus RNA Polymerases: Evolutionary Implications for Virus Populations

ESTEBAN DOMINGO, ERIC BARANOWSKI, CRISTINA ESCARMÍS,
FRANCISCO SOBRINO, AND JOHN J. HOLLAND

23

INTRODUCTION: OVERVIEW OF RNA VIRUS EVOLUTION

Evolution, or change in genetic composition of a population with time, is the result of a number of sequential steps involving a complex interplay between intrinsic modifications of the genetic makeup of the organisms and environmental influences. Viruses are no exception. The main steps that have been identified in the evolution of RNA viruses, starting with a single infectious genome of any virus group, are (i) genetic variation, notably very high mutation rates (and in some cases also high recombination rates) during RNA genome replication which soon leads to complex mutant distributions termed viral quasispecies (57–59); (ii) competitive rating among components of the mutant spectra of quasispecies replicating at the same site in a defined environment; and (iii) positive selection, random sampling events, and genetic drift acting on heterogeneous viral populations, which leads to genetic diversification of viral populations in space and time. Diversification can occur (and it often occurs) in a single infected individual, since multiple cells, tissues, and organs offer a mosaic of different environments suitable for the selective growth of different variants generated during replication. A number of overviews of animal and plant RNA virus evolution have been published in recent years. The reader can find relevant information in references 42, 45, 50, 77, 92, 133, and 134.

In this chapter, we first examine key features of the three main stages in virus evolution with examples drawn from several virus groups, and then we review specific results with picornaviruses, as well as implications of high mutation rates and quasispecies dynamics for this important and diverse group of pathogens.

ERROR-PRONE RNA SYNTHESIS

Mutation rates, or number of misincorporations per nucleotide copied, for RNA viruses are generally in the range of 10^{-3} to 10^{-5} substitutions per nucleotide copied, as evidenced by measurements employing biochemical and genetic procedures with several viruses (11, 48, 53), including viruses regarded as monotypic antigenically such as measles virus (166). Mutation frequencies, or numbers of mutations per nucleotide found in viral populations (when comparing consensus sequences of independent isolates or individual genomes from one isolate), are also high, although in this case the range of values is expanded to cover 10^{-2} to 10^{-5} substitutions per nucleotide. As examples, the mutation frequencies in the polymerase (3D) gene among cocirculating foot-and-mouth disease virus isolates from the same outbreak were in the range of 7.0×10^{-4} to 2.8×10^{-3} substitutions per nucleotide (193). Within a human immunodeficiency virus (HIV)-infected individual, mutation frequencies in *pol* of HIV-1 quasispecies can reach 1.1×10^{-2} substitutions per nucleotide (139). Obviously, this broad range of values is influenced by selective forces as well as by distance (number of replication rounds) from a clonal origin of the virus under analysis. In long-lasting, chronic viral infections such as those with HIV-1, its simian counterpart simian immunodeficiency virus, or human hepatitis C virus, diversity among components of the mutant spectra develops in a readily apparent way, and results obtained with these viruses have lent increasing support to the direct influence of a quasispecies dynamics in viral pathogenesis and adaptability in vivo (45, 66, 69, 70, 74, 94).

Generally elevated mutation frequencies have been also observed with other RNA genetic elements, including retroelements and DNA genomes, which use RNA copies as replication intermediates, such as the hepadnaviruses, notably human hepatitis B virus. These mutation rates and frequencies are about a millionfold larger than those estimated for cellular DNA replication (51, 52), although increased cell mutation rates and frequencies (hypermutation) are occasionally seen, such as during generation of immunoglobulin gene diversity, in some types of cancer

---

Esteban Domingo, Eric Baranowski, and Cristina Escarmís ■ Centro de Biología Molecular "Severo Ochoa," Universidad Autónoma de Madrid, Cantoblanco, 28049 Madrid, Spain. *Francisco Sobrino* ■ Centro de Biología Molecular "Severo Ochoa," and CISA-INIA, 28130 Valdeolmos, Madrid, Spain. *John J. Holland* ■ Department of Biology and Center for Molecular Genetics, University of California, San Diego, La Jolla, CA 92093-0116.

cells, and in some populations of bacteria, among other examples (as a review of the common features in the dynamics of genetic change in viruses and cells, including prokaryotic and eukaryotic pathogens, see reference 45).

Studies with bacterial and animal DNA polymerases, and retroviral reverse transcriptases, suggest that high mutation rates of RNA viruses are influenced decisively by the absence of proofreading-repair activities and can be also modulated by the structure of the enzyme domains involved in polynucleotide synthesis. In many cellular DNA polymerases, a proofreading activity is associated with a 3' to 5' exonuclease, which is present as a distinct structural domain in the enzymes (19, 81, 177, 183). No such domain has been detected in the three-dimensional structures of viral RNA-dependent RNA polymerases or reverse transcriptases (84, 177). Alignment of 3D polymerase proteins of different picornavirus genera (120, 208; N. J. Knowles and A. Palmenberg, www.iah.bbsrc.ac.uk/virus/picornaviridae/sequencedatabase/alignments/alignmts.hts) suggests that no domain that could be assigned to a proofreading-repair exonucleolytic activity is encoded within the picornaviral polymerase gene. The absence of proofreading-repair activity is also supported by in vitro fidelity measurements carried out with viral nucleic acid polymerases under a variety of experimental conditions and using different fidelity assays (6, 23, 181, 197). However, it cannot be excluded that some cellular proteins could be associated at times with viral polymerases, resulting in modulation of error levels. As an example, mutation rates for HIV may be influenced by the regulatory viral protein Vpr (114, 115).

Recent studies with reverse transcriptase (RT) of HIV suggest that copying fidelity of viral replicases may also be influenced by amino acid replacements in the enzyme. Some replacements around the active site of RT may enhance copying fidelity (195) while other replacements may decrease fidelity (121). Variations of up to 100-fold in copying accuracy have been documented, although such figures may be influenced by the assays used for the measurements. Some mutants of RT display an increased ability to remove chain-terminating nucleoside analogues (3'-azido-3'-deoxythymidine [zidovudine]) from the growing chain by pyrophosphorolysis (4) or by ribonucleotide-dependent phosphorolysis (123, 127). It has also been suggested that attack by pyrophosphate could contribute to error correction by the poliovirus polymerase (6). Evidence of effects of amino acid replacements on picornaviral replicase accuracy is still lacking, although they are likely to occur in view of shared structural and functional features among the nucleic acid polymerases examined to date (6, 19, 79, 84, 177, 183).

The Inevitable Generation of Mutant Swarms: The Quasispecies

With average mutation rates approximating 10^{-4} substitutions per nucleotide copied, an RNA genome of about 10^4 residues will incorporate an average of one mutation each time one genomic molecule is synthesized. Since every productively infected cell produces 1 to 10^6 progeny genomes, viral replication must unavoidably lead to the continuous synthesis of variant genomes within cells, tissues, and organs of an infected host. Many experiments with viruses replicating in cell culture and in vivo have documented that negative selection maintains at low frequencies those mutants with defects in replication, and many of these may be eliminated from subsequent generations of virus production, depending on relative fitness levels (47, 48). In spite of mutant filtering by negative selection, clones of RNA viruses rapidly evolve into complex mutant distributions (or mutant swarms), the viral quasispecies (42, 49, 57–59, 91, 94). Virologists have adapted a generalized quasispecies concept to describe dynamic distributions of nonidentical but closely related mutant and recombinant viral genomes subjected to a continuous process of genetic variation, competition, and selection (42, 145). Genomes of RNA viruses (and possibly also of some DNA viruses) (see reference 45) cannot be described as a defined unique structure, but as a weighted average of a large number of different individual sequences (49).

Since the original theoretical quasispecies concept proposed by Eigen and his colleagues (57–59) involved steady-state, equilibrium distributions with an infinite number of genomes, some alternative term akin to quasispecies could be considered to refer to virus populations. However, invention of another term would have been unwarranted given the pioneering theoretical developments of Eigen and associates and the obvious conceptual relevance of their initial theoretical work to the observations with RNA viruses. Also, the possible alternative term "polymorphism" employed in classical population genetics is not adequate since it does not convey the capacity for exploration of sequence space, which is paramount to viral genome adaptability. With the levels of heterogeneity and viral load often seen in infected individuals, RNA virus populations include potentially all possible single mutants and decreasing amounts of multiple mutants (20, 45, 49, 59). Furthermore, the term polymorphism excluded (at least in its original formulations) unique and rare alleles that are genuine components of viral quasispecies (further discussion of the appropriateness of the term "quasispecies" is provided in reference 45 and references therein). The key issue in viral quasispecies is not whether mutant distributions are in equilibrium or not, but whether they offer a dynamic and adaptive-prone ensemble of nonidentical genomes. Recent evidence verifies that they do. Generation of complex mutant swarms to the point that invalidates the concept of the wild type as a defined genomic sequence appears increasingly to be a general adaptive strategy of pathogenic RNA viruses, some DNA viruses, and some types of cell populations (review in reference 45).

Levels of adaptation are reflected in relative fitness values, which can be quantitated by growth-competition experiments in cell culture or in vivo (26, 93; review in reference 47). The population dynamics of virus multiplication has a direct influence on the evolution of fitness values: large population passages in a defined environment generally tend to produce virus populations with increased fitness values (64, 141, 143, 144, 198) while limitations in the number of infectious viruses transferred (inefficient infection or introduction of population bottlenecks) generally lead to populations with low fitness, at times near viral extinction (28, 31, 45, 47, 48, 54, 55, 60, 63, 205, 206). However, it must be stressed that fitness gains or losses depend on both the initial fitness of the viral quasispecies and the size of the population bottleneck introduced. As shown with vesicular stomatitis virus (142), the higher the initial fitness of a virus the less severe must the bottleneck be to avoid fitness loss (review in reference 47). The very clear and dramatic effects of population size and dynamics on viral fitness constitute additional evidence of high mutation rates, of selective ranking of components of mutant spectra, and of the non-neutral character of many subsets of mutations occurring in viral quasispecies. RNA viruses are changing continuously and grasping opportunities for adaptation, sometimes gradually, sometimes suddenly.

Long-Term Evolution

Generation of quasispecies swarms in vivo is the first step in the process of genetic diversification of viruses in nature, operating in complex, mutual, intimate interaction with their hosts (102). Viral quasispecies, as observed experimentally, are the result of a complex interplay between intrinsic (mutant generation) and extrinsic (environmental changes and stochastic events) influences acting on replicating ensembles. Random sampling of one or a limited number of viral genomes can occur within hosts through migration of free virions or infected cells. It is probably frequent also in some types of host-to-host transmission such as aerosol spread of respiratory viruses. In any newly infected individual host, recurrent complex evolutionary cycles of mutant generation, competition, selection, migration, bottlenecks, etc., may modify transiently organized mutant distributions (9, 14, 16, 17, 22, 26–32, 42–49, 54–57, 59, 60, 63, 64, 66, 69, 70, 74, 75, 82, 91–96, 101, 117–119, 126, 141, 143, 144, 150, 160, 162, 198, 205, 206).

Estimates from phylogenetic analyses suggest that RNA viruses evolve (i.e., fix mutations in their consensus sequences) at rates that are frequently in the range of 10^{-2} to 10^{-4} substitutions per nucleotide per year (reviews in references 45 and 48). These values can exceed by one million-fold those estimated for functional cellular genes. Evolutionary rates for viruses are obviously average values encompassing periods of even faster evolution during active viral replication under selective pressures, and periods of stasis (very slow evolution) due to limited replication or replication near population equilibrium (without modification of the consensus sequence) (2, 199). Thus, the dual possibility of population equilibrium or disequilibrium, uniquely manifested by a quasispecies population structure and dynamics, permits virus stability or change, as needed. Since a steady accumulation of mutations over long time periods is rarely observed, genetic distances between viruses cannot be used reliably to infer times of divergence (45).

In many positive-strand RNA viruses, including picornaviruses, RNA recombination is frequent and it may have a decisive influence on virus evolution (100a, 103, 106, 138). Likewise, genome segment reassortment plays an important role in diversification of viruses with a segmented genome (199). The picture of RNA virus population structure and evolution outlined in previous paragraphs is fully manifested in its many facets when picornaviruses are examined at the population level.

Error Frequencies during Replication of Picornaviruses: Response to Drugs and Antibodies

Picornaviruses have the rare and experimentally useful property that they can become dependent on some inhibitory drugs for replication. This remarkable paradox has been exploited from early times to estimate rates of transitions between drug-sensitive, drug-resistant, and drug-dependent picornavirus mutants. In one of the very early studies with guanidine hydrochloride, Melnick and colleagues (126) documented the rapid development of drug-resistant poliovirus in cell culture and in monkeys, stating that "the phenomenon of drug resistance poses yet another problem in the search for a satisfactory viral chemotherapeutic agent." This sentence anticipated by more than 40 years the dramatic consequences of HIV resistance to antiviral agents and the general problem of microbial evolution toward pathogens that are increasingly refractory to inhibitory treatments. Eggers and Tamm in 1965 pioneered studies with coxsackievirus A9 and the drug 2(-α-hydroxybenzyl)-benzimidazole (HBB), an inhibitor of virus replication; a frequency of the order of "10^{-4} mutations per replication" was estimated for the transition between HBB dependence and HBB independence (56). Mutants with varying degrees of resistance to HBB arose and were selected in the course of passage of sensitive virus in the presence of the drug. Eggers and Tamm proposed that similar events could underlie selection of guanidine-resistant poliovirus mutants upon passage of sensitive poliovirus in the presence of guanidine (108).

Guanidine resistance maps in protein 2C (3, 152, 165). The drug inhibits the ATPase activity of 2C (151). The frequency of guanidine-resistant revertants in six clonal pools of guanidine-dependent mutants of poliovirus type 1 was $(6.5 \pm 6.3) \times 10^{-4}$. From this value, and since all amino acid replacements occurred at a single position, the minimal corrected base substitution frequency per nucleotide in the relevant codon was estimated to be $(2.1 \pm 1.9) \times 10^{-4}$ (39).

A number of hydrophobic compounds (arildone, chalcone, pirodavir, 4′, 6′-dichloroflavan, and the WIN series) accommodate into a hydrophobic pocket located at the base of the canyon around the fivefold axes of the enterovirus and rhinovirus capsid (176). These compounds probably displace the natural lipidic pocket factor, and by so doing they inhibit uncoating (and in some cases attachment to cells) (71) and may protect the viruses against inactivation by heat and acid or alkaline pH (reviewed in references 135, 159, and 174). Drug-resistant and drug-dependent mutants are isolated with high frequencies both in cell culture and in vivo (reviewed in references 43, 135, 174, and 187). Human rhinovirus 14 mutants showing low-level resistance to the WIN compound 52084 (methyl derivative of disoxaril, 5-[7-[4-(4,5 dihydro-2-oxazolyl)phenoxy]heptyl]-3-methyl-isoxazole) occurred at frequencies of 1×10^{-3} to 4×10^{-4}, while the frequency of high-level resistant mutants was 10-fold lower (87). The frequency of rhinovirus 9 mutants resistant to the chalcone R0-09-0410 was 1×10^{-5} (1); resistant rhinovirus mutants were also selected in vivo (35). There are probably many routes to drug resistance (136, 174), including amino acid replacements in the wall of the pocket preventing accommodation of the drug into the pocket (termed "exclusion" mutants), and replacements elsewhere in the capsid that affect viral uncoating (83, 87, 135). Resistant mutants display decreased affinity for the drug or increased affinity for the receptor, and often show low fitness values relative to their parental counterparts (reviewed in reference 135).

Another series of loci for which we have an instrument for quantifying mutants are antigenic sites, and the tools are neutralizing antibodies and cytotoxic T cells, although the latter have not been much used in the case of picornaviruses, perhaps because of evidence that protection against picornaviral diseases is mainly associated with the humoral branch of the immune response (132, 188). In an early analysis of clinical isolates of coxsackievirus B4 mutants, changes at one or more epitopes were detected at frequencies exceeding 10^{-2} (153). In the absence of immunological pressure, using plaque-purified coxsackievirus B4 in cell culture, changes at one or more epitopes were found at frequencies greater than 10^{-2} (154). Monoclonal antibody-resistant (MAR) mutants of poliovirus type 3 were found at frequencies of 10^{-3} to 10^{-5} in several viral clones and vaccine strains (61, 130, 131). A similar range can be estimated for foot-and-mouth disease virus (FMDV) from the data of Xie et al. (202) and in infected swine (27). MAR mutant frequencies are not related to the number of serotypes described for a given picornavirus genus: for the monotypic mengovirus and the extremely diverse (more than 100 serotypes) rhinovirus, MAR mutant frequencies were 3×10^{-3} to 5×10^{-5} (21) and 10^{-4} to 10^{-5} (172), respectively. For hepatitis A virus, a value of 3×10^{-3} was reported (179).

MAR mutant frequencies vary for different epitopes, probably reflecting distinct constraints to variation, as well as constraints to the type and numbers of amino acid residues that can provide anchor points with different affinity for the antibody. This appears to be the case in some discontinuous, complex epitopes of FMDV, with MAR frequencies ranging from 10^{-5} to 10^{-7} (107, 125). Moreover, frequencies can be greatly underestimated by phenotypic masking of mutant genomes assembled into wild-type envelopes or capsids (27, 95, 189) or by lower fitness of MAR mutants relative to their parental wild types (47, 80, 118). Because of these several effects, MAR mutant frequencies cannot be directly related to mutation rates.

Picornavirus variants displaying different degrees of resistance to polyclonal antisera raised in animals can also be selected. For several viruses, antigenic variants can become dominant even in the absence of, or diminished amounts of, selecting antibodies (reviewed in reference 46; see recent observations with picornaviruses replicating in immunodeficient hosts in references 9, 17, 101, and 117). However, in the case of FMDV the types of amino acid substitutions found in antigenic variants selected by antibodies were distinct from the substitutions found in such variants arising in the absence of antibodies (22, 41). Minimal genetic change can lead to a significant antigenic modification: an epitope involved in neutralization of an FMDV antigenic subtype was generated as a result of a single amino acid replacement in the capsid of another FMDV subtype (88). One particular human rhinovirus type yielded antigenic variants much more readily than other types, to the point at which some selected mutants no longer belonged to the original antigenic group (148). Although the basis for antigenic variation and diversification among picornaviral genera remains a mystery, the results with human rhinovirus suggest the possibility that particular isolates with a dominant and structurally flexible antigenic site may act as sources of additional variants (88, 148).

This brief account of mutation frequencies with regard to drug- and antibody-binding domains underscores the large fractions of many types of mutants that must populate mutant spectra, their characterization being limited by the availability of selective agents and tests for quantification. Myriad mutants provide the raw material for picornavirus adaptability in manners still to be discovered since we are aware of only a minute portion of the selective constraints that confront viruses as they complete successive life cycles in infected hosts.

Biochemical Measurements of Error Rates and Frequencies in Picornaviruses

The high mutation frequencies observed during replication of viruses in cell culture and in host organisms have been paralleled by observations of low fidelity of viral polymerases in cell-free systems and in purified form. Well-documented examples in virology are the studies over recent decades with Qβ replicase (20) and retroviral RTs (7, 13, 128).

Studies with picornaviral RNA-dependent RNA polymerases (replicases) face limitations derived from the difficulties in obtaining purified enzymes capable of sustaining multiple rounds of template-dependent copying. Pioneer work with encephalomyocarditis virus and poliovirus RNA-dependent RNA polymerases (34, 67, 68, 149, 164; reviewed in reference 82) has led to enzyme (3D) preparations that show template-dependent and primer-dependent activity that can be stimulated by other poliovirus-coded proteins (5, 82). Ward et al. (197) used homopolymeric templates to quantitate error rates in the range of 7×10^{-4} to 5.4×10^{-3} misincorporations per nucleotide copied, using poly(A), poly(C), and poly(I) as templates, and equimolar amounts of complementary (correct) and noncomplementary (incorrect) nucleotide substrates. An eightfold increase in the elongation rate, brought about by an increase in the magnesium ion concentration in the reaction mixture, resulted in a fivefold increase in error frequency (197). Other in vitro fidelity assays on heteropolymeric templates yielded values around 4×10^{-4} substitutions per nucleotide (199a).

A different biochemical approach to the determination of error frequencies developed by Steinhauer and Holland (182) involves the measurement of the proportion of RNase T1-resistant molecules at a defined site of a viral genome occupied by a guanosine (G) and surrounded by non-G residues. (RNase T1 cleaves specifically at G residues on single-stranded RNA.) Resistant genomes were shown to include U, C, or A at the site under study, thus providing a direct measurement of error frequency at the G site (180, 182). Ward and Flanegan (196) adapted this procedure to poliovirus and determined error frequencies in the range of 3.2×10^{-3} to 5.0×10^{-3} (with a mean value of $[4.1 \pm 0.6] \times 10^{-3}$) substitutions per nucleotide, with no significant differences between G sites located at constant regions of the 5' UTR, or 3D-, 3C-, or 2B-coding regions, and G sites located at variable sites of the capsid-coding region.

Error rates determined either with purified enzymes or by biochemical methods tend to be larger than error rates based on genetic analyses such as the reversion of viable mutants. Reversion of a temperature-sensitive mutant of poliovirus type 1 depended on a nonsynonymous transition U $\rightarrow$ C within the 3AB-coding region; the frequency of this specific mutation averaged 2×10^{-5} substitutions per nucleotide (37). In this study, 7 out of 10 revertants analyzed exhibited complete reversion of four additional silent mutations that had been introduced into the temperature-sensitive clone. This result emphasizes the potential for variation of poliovirus even within a stable cell culture environment (37).

Several estimates of error frequencies for poliovirus have been strikingly low (146, 168) not only in comparison with most other estimates for poliovirus but also in comparison with determinations for other RNA viruses. Based on the absence of mutations during repetitive sequencing of 105 VP1 genes from biological clones derived from a single poliovirus plaque, a mutation frequency of less than 2×10^{-6} mutations per nucleotide per infectious cycle was calculated (146). It is obvious that this must be a measure, not of all mutants that arose, but of advantageous or neutral mutants arising early during plaque development. Even slightly deleterious mutations would not have been scored. It would be interesting to repeat this experiment in HeLa cells using a wild-type poliovirus newly isolated from an infected person rather than the type 1 Mahoney strain employed (which was well adapted to cell culture). In another such set of measurements, Sedivy et al. (168) studied the reversion of an *amber* mutation in the poliovirus polymerase (3D) gene. A specific transversion (A → C) was required to revert the *amber* codon to a serine codon present in the functional 3D, and this occurred at a frequency of 2.5×10^{-6} revertants per *amber* plaque-forming unit. In addition to the probability of losing late-arising revertants in this multiday screen, the specific transversion required would not reflect the true, overall mutation rate at this site. This possibility is reinforced by the observations of Kuge et al. (105) that the transition-to-transversion ratio in a highly mutation-tolerant region of the poliovirus genome approached 50. If this bias applied to the triplet analyzed by Sedivy et al. (168), and the specific transversion A → C was needed for functional reversion of the polymerase, then the true mutation rate at this site would be about 1×10^{-4} substitutions per nucleotide, even if we ignore the likely failure to detect late-arising revertants.

Results of drug- or antibody-escape mutants, as well as estimates of error rates and mutation frequencies derived from biochemical and genetic studies, suggest that picornaviral populations will hide a rich repertoire of variants. As emphasized by Holland et al. (94), low mutation frequencies in even half of the genome sites of a virus should still generate quasispecies populations, and extremely low frequencies (10^{-7} to 10^{-8} substitutions per nucleotide) should provoke the search for a proofreading function. The heterogeneity of quasispecies populations, combined with the potential for rapid variation in the consensus (and dominant) genomic sequences, has a number of biological implications regarding phenotypic alterations (notably in host tropism and virulence), emergence of new picornaviral pathogens, and complications for control and eradication of picornaviruses.

Biological Implications of High Mutation Rates and Frequencies for Picornaviruses: Coevolution of Antigenic Sites and Receptor-Recognition Sites

Different extents of overlap between residues and structures involved in receptor recognition and interaction with antibodies exist in picornaviruses (85, 89, 175, 190–192). A manifest example is the direct participation of the integrin receptor-recognition triplet RGD (Arg-Gly-Asp in the G-H loop of capsid protein VP1 of FMDV) in the interaction with neutralizing antibodies (89, 190–192). Such an overlap predicts a possible coevolution of antigenicity and receptor specificity, given the extensive sequence explorations during the natural evolution of picornaviruses, with rates of evolution that can approach 10^{-2} substitutions per nucleotide and year either within individual infected hosts or in the course of disease episodes (24, 75, 100, 101, 117).

Model cell culture experiments carried out with FMDV suggest one of the possible mechanisms by which a mutual influence of alterations in cell receptor recognition and antigenic variation could come about. Using a monoclonal antibody that defines an epitope at the major antigenic site of FMDV, the basal MAR mutant frequency in the standard FMDV clone C-S8c1 was $(8.5 \pm 1.0) \times 10^{-4}$, while in populations and clones derived after 100 passages of C-S8c1 in BHK-21 cells the frequencies increased to $(4.1 \pm 0.5) \times 10^{-3}$ to $(8.7 \pm 0.3) \times 10^{-3}$ (119). The relevant epitope involved the RGD integrin-recognition triplet. The reason for the increase in MAR mutant frequency was the use of alternative receptors by the multiply passaged virus that rendered dispensable the RGD triplet (10, 119). Thus, the MAR phenotype could be attained not only with amino acid replacements around the RGD but also within the RGD (119). By using infectious transcripts, it was shown that at least some replacements at the RGD triplet are lethal in the sequence context of the C-S8c1 capsid, but not in the context of the capsid of C-S8c1 passaged 100 times in BHK-21 cells (10). The capsid of this passaged virus differed from that of the parental C-S8c1 in six amino acid replacements (three in VP1 and three in VP3). Dispensability of the RGD has allowed the isolation of interesting variants such as those with RED, RGG, or even GGG instead of RGD (161). Several cell culture-adapted FMDVs enter cells via heparan sulfate (HS), a molecule regarded as a second, alternative receptor for the virus (72, 98, 162). In contrast, the C-S8c1 mutants lacking RGD may use a third mechanism for entry into the cell, and, interestingly, they could shift receptor choice depending on environmental pressures, providing evidence that a virus may harbor the potential to use alternative receptors for entry even into the same cell type (10). This putative receptor for FMDV has not yet been identified. Not unexpectedly from what we know of the interaction of the RGD with neutralizing antibodies, mutants lacking RGD show profound alterations with regard to antigenicity (161; unpublished results).

Cytolytic FMDV can persist in cell culture (36), and during persistence the virus acquires a number of genetic and phenotypic modifications (38, 40). When persistent virus was subjected to serial cytolytic passages, some of these phenotypic traits reverted despite continued genetic diversification (169). In these cytolytic passages the repertoire of antigenic variants that became dominant in the populations was greatly influenced by the population size of the virus (169, 171). Probably, very subtle modifications in the FMDV-receptor interactions, brought about by amino acid substitutions at the major antigenic site of the virus, were responsible for the striking observation that FMDV can adapt to the multiplicity of infection in cell culture: indeed, an FMDV population grown at low multiplicity of infection for several generations acquired a selective advantage over another population, provided the competition passages were carried out at low multiplicity of infection (170).

Theiler's virus adapted to penetrate efficiently into L929 cells exhibited replacements at VP1 and VP2 sites, which are part of neutralization epitopes. The adaptation to L929 resulted in attenuation for mice, providing an example of a close relationship between antigenic changes, receptor binding, and an important in vivo phenotypic alteration of the virus (99). Structural, biochemical, and genetic investigations increasingly indicate that possible links between antigenic variation and changes in cell tropism and virulence must be very complex. Antigenic variation may be modulated by different degrees of surface exposure of amino acid residues involved in receptor recognition (203). Also, even under carefully controlled laboratory conditions, the repertoire of amino acid substitutions (and their effects on fitness) selected in FMDV propagated in the presence of polyclonal antibodies (raised against a chemically defined peptide) varied depending on the individual guinea pig employed in antibody production (22). Obviously, the concentration of neutralizing antibodies and their affinities for different antigenic variants arising during viral replication must have an influence in the selection of antigenic variants of viruses within infected hosts. The partial protection of cattle afforded by peptide vaccines led to selection of FMDV escape mutants harboring amino acid replacements at the antigenic site represented in the synthetic peptide (184). Conversely, there was a delay in the rise to dominance of antigenic variants of poliovirus in a hypogammaglobulinemic patient, as compared with poliovirus replicating in immunocompetent individuals (117). Thus, the extent of overlap between antigenic sites and receptor recognition sites, their tolerance to accept amino acid replacements while remaining functional (with regard to viral stability, uncoating, assembly), and the quality of the immune response all must have some contribution to maintaining antigenic stability versus favoring diversification of picornaviruses (46, 82, 124).

Picornaviruses use a remarkable variety of molecules as cellular receptors, and most of them play a role in the host immune response; some are members of the same superfamily of macromolecules (9a, 65). Yet the key residues that provide receptor specificity for different viruses are not the same for members of the same receptor superfamily and, conversely, related viruses (such as rhinovirus serotypes or cluster B enteroviruses) may recognize receptors belonging to different superfamilies (9a, 18, 65, 86, 104). Since the capsid sites involved in receptor recognition (or neighboring sites) are likely to be involved also in other key processes such as viral uncoating and capsid stability, it is not surprising that different picornavirus genera may attain different degrees of antigenic diversification in spite of being subjected to similar mutational pressure during RNA genome replication (discussions in references 82, 85, 124, 174, and 200). Taken together, these results suggest that receptor specificity of picornaviruses may be influenced by variations in a limited number of capsid residues. Poliovirus variants capable of recognizing the wild-type and mutated forms of the poliovirus receptor were readily selected, and one or few amino acid replacements were sufficient for adaptation to utilize an expanded receptor repertoire (111).

There is no reason to suspect that during the natural evolution of some picornaviruses, amino acid replacements that favor changes in host cell tropism should be forbidden. During acute and persistent picornaviral infections, multiple evolutionary sublines develop as an outcome of diversification of quasispecies swarms (9). A recent model proposed for the evolutionary forces acting on poliovirus points, as a key feature, to selection and random sampling events acting on basically heterogeneous viral populations (74), a model that is in agreement with current views on RNA virus evolution in general. These models emphasize the viral capacity to explore large portions of sequence space (59), which in concrete virological terms means production of many variants to increase the chances of adaptation.

In spite of the above considerations, there is also evidence that viruses may reach a strong degree of specialization to use one type of cellular receptor, and may be constrained to a defined cellular tropism. This may be the case for hepatitis A virus and other hepatotropic viruses that grow poorly or not at all in cell culture; it has been suggested that evolutionary constraints controlling viral transmission and propagation could restrict replication of the hepatitis viruses (109).

The tissue distribution of picornavirus receptors is often broader than the infectable tissues (9a), suggesting that additional determinants of host range and virulence may be involved. Indeed, studies with several picornaviruses, summarized in the next section, indicate that this is the case.

Replacements in Viral Regulatory Regions and in Nonstructural and Structural Proteins Can Affect Picornavirus Host Cell Tropism and Virulence

Viral attenuation for live vaccines is a process of genetic change followed by selection of subpopulations that maintain infectivity for the target host but do not cause disease. This process led soon to preparation of attenuated poliovirus strains that were the basis of an extremely successful live vaccine for the control of poliomyelitis (reviews in references 109, 129, and 200). Once genomic nucleotide sequences for virulent and attenuated strains of the three poliovirus serotypes became known, a search for genes and mutations associated with attenuation began, taking advantage of the rescue of infectious poliovirus from cDNA copies cloned into plasmids (155). Not unexpectedly (see fragment of a letter by A. Sabin transcribed in reference 200), it turned out that different degrees of virulence are found among natural poliovirus isolates and that mutations in both noncoding regulatory regions and in structural and nonstructural proteins may affect poliovirus virulence phenotypes. In poliovirus types 1 and 3, 11 to 55 nucleotide differences distinguish the vaccine strains from the corresponding parental strains, and the mutations are fairly widely distributed along the genome (129, 140, 178, 200). Of course, many rounds of genome replication distance vaccine from parental strains, and several of the mutations recorded may be irrelevant to attenuation or have a very marginal contribution to this phenotype. Site-directed mutagenesis and the construction of recombinant, chimeric viruses have highlighted the contribution of certain mutations to poliovirus attenuation. For example, three mutations have been associated with attenuation of poliovirus type 1 (amino acid replacements in VP1 and VP3 [185, 200]). However, poliovirus is in continuous evolution (74), and combinations of different mutations may arise unpredictably to cause alterations in virulence. Unfortunately, this can happen not only with poliovirus but also with less closely related enteroviruses that may acquire neurovirulent tendencies, since limited numbers of mutations, not reflected in the grand picornavirus phylogenetic classifications (97, 158), may influence pathogenesis in a decisive manner (82).

The quasispecies nature of RNA viruses is directly relevant to vaccine preparation and usage since many viral vaccines have been found to consist of mixtures of mutant viruses. Chumakov and his colleagues documented that failure in the monkey safety test of live attenuated poliovirus vaccines related to the proportion of mutant sequences that decrease attenuation (30).

Viral virulence may be modulated by partial resistance of a cell to infection. A population replacement experiment was used to document that a virulent viral phenotype was a trait needed for an FMDV population to replace the FMDV that persisted in modified (partially virus-resistant) BHK-21 cells (163). Thus, paradoxically, virulence can be a positive factor in viral persistence. Moreover, the partially resistant BHK-21 cells can rapidly (in a single infection!) select for FMDV variants of higher virulence for standard BHK-21 cells, and the variants are able to overcome the resistance of modified BHK-21 cells (62). This selection of virulent FMDV occurred in a highly reproducible manner, and it was associated with two amino acid replacements in the capsid, with no other mutations in the consensus sequence of the viral genome (62).

An often disconcerting observation made with many virus groups, including the picornaviruses, is that taxonomical classifications based on genomic nucleotide sequences do not necessarily parallel biological features. Dramatic examples are the comparisons between virulent and avirulent coxsackieviruses and the aphthovirus-like genome of some respiratory rhinoviruses. In coxsackievirus B3 a single nucleotide replacement at the 5' nontranslated region had an important participation in the cardiovirulent phenotype of the virus in mice (29, 186). This was also influenced by immune mechanisms and the genetic background of the host (73, 167). This same extracistronic mutation, together with five additional mutations elsewhere in the genome, was regularly found to result from the evolution of avirulent to cardiovirulent virus that occurs in selenium-deficient mice (15, 16).

The equine rhinovirus 1 is a respiratory pathogen of horses, and its genome is more closely related to the aphthoviruses than to other picornaviruses (110, 201). Avian encephalomyelitis virus is a picornavirus whose polyprotein displays 39% amino acid sequence identity with hepatitis A virus and only 19 to 21% with representatives of the other five picornavirus genera (122). Host barriers among picornaviruses seem rather volatile. Molecular recombination may have contributed to create a variant of human coxsackievirus B5, the agent of hand-foot-and-mouth disease, capable of infecting swine. Indeed, the structural and nonstructural proteins of coxsackievirus B5 and those of swine vesicular disease virus show amino acid sequence identities ranging from 86.7 to 100% while noncoding regions are more divergent (207).

Minimal genetic change can effect changes in virulence and host range. The acquisition of the virulent phenotype for mice, reflected in pancreatitis associated with coxsackievirus B4 infection, is determined by a single amino acid replacement in VP1 (25), and to a lesser extent also by a substitution in VP4 (156). Disease severity was modulated by T-cell-mediated immunity (157). The EMC-D variant of encephalomyocarditis virus can induce diabetes in mice, and the diabetogenic character was dependent on a single amino acid replacement (8, 204). In this case, the host contribution to disease appears to involve virus-induced macrophage activation and macrophage-mediated destruction of beta cells in the pancreas (90).

Amino acid deletions and point mutations in nonstructural protein 3A were associated with attenuation for cattle of several FMDV isolates (12, 78). A single amino acid replacement in 3A could mediate adaptation of FMDV to guinea pig (145a).

The inescapable conclusion of the unavoidably incomplete account of observations summarized in previous paragraphs is that picornavirus quasispecies evolution in its many facets (population heterogeneity, adaptability, potential for rapid genetic change, etc.) is an important element of picornaviral pathogenesis and probably also a factor contributing to picornaviral disease emergence.

Additional Implications of High Mutation Rates and Frequencies in Picornavirus Populations: Complexity, Memory, and New Antiviral Strategies

The quasispecies structure of RNA viruses and very especially of picornaviruses—given their extensive diversity in genomic sequences and disease associations—has gradually introduced a change in emphasis on how we understand individual viruses and their behavior. One of the key words in this new accent is complexity, a concept originated in physics but with important ramifications in a variety of disciplines including biology (for reviews on several facets of complexity see reference 32, and as an introduction to its application to viral evolution, see references 44 and 45). Perhaps the most descriptive definition of a complex system is that in which changes in behavior are not linearly related to changes occurring in the surroundings (116). Complex processes affect systems with many components subjected to multiple influences. For example, the emergence of a new viral pathogen is the result of many ill-defined influences (probably genetic modifications of the virus; chance encounter of a modified virus with a potentially susceptible new host species, whose presence is in turn affected by environmental and ecological factors, in turn affected by human activity, and so on). This chain of interconnected chance events renders viral emergences highly unpredictable occurrences (94, 137).

How can concepts related to complexity be useful to virologists? We suspect that, although this field of research is truly in its early infancy, complexity will be of practical use to virology. First, several workers have calculated Shannon entropies (194) to describe the number of different genomic sequences that compose the mutant spectrum of a viral quasispecies. Shannon entropy complements, and does not duplicate, the information derived from the calculation of mutation frequencies. Shannon entropy and mutation frequency provide a parallel concept to that of effective algorithmic complexity described by Gell-Mann (76) (see also discussion in reference 44). It is clear that levels of algorithmic complexity, by reflecting the abundance of variants in a viral population, may be indicative of adaptive potential. There is now good evidence that the complexity of hepatitis C genome populations can be a predictor of response to treatment with a combination of interferon and ribavirin (149a, 150), and of probability of development of chronic infection (66). We see no reason why some related predictions eventually could not be established with picornaviruses, given the rapid progress in nucleotide sequencing techniques and other genome sampling procedures required to assess viral genome complexity.

Viral quasispecies show features of complex adaptive systems such as mobilization of minority components (individual genomes from the mutant spectrum) in response to external stimuli. Recently the presence of memory in FMDV quasispecies has been documented (160, 160a) by using two genetic markers: a MAR mutation and an internal polyadenylate present in FMDV clones subjected to Muller's ratchet (plaque-to-plaque transfers). An FMDV MAR mutant containing an RED triplet (instead of the RGD in VP1), subjected to serial passages in BHK-21 cells, was outcompeted by RGD-containing revertants. Even though the consensus sequence of this multiply passaged population did not reveal the presence of RED, mutant frequencies reached values up to 100 times larger than those observed with clones containing RGD (passaged in parallel), and mutants with RED were systematically selected by the relevant monoclonal antibody (160, 160a). Therefore, past evolutionary history influenced both the nature and the intensity of the response of FMDV to the selective pressure of a neutralizing antibody. The second marker used was an internal polyadenylate preceding the second functional AUG of FMDV that forms upon serial plaque-to-plaque transfers of FMDV clones (63). While the poly(A) is already absent following 20 large population passages, the mutant spectrum of the evolving FMDV population maintains it at least up to passage 150 (3a, 160)! As expected, with both markers, the introduction of a genetic bottleneck erased quasispecies memory, demonstrating that this memory was a property of the quasispecies as a whole and not merely a tendency of individual genomes to produce variants with the memory markers (160; review in reference 45). Therefore, quasispecies dynamics dictates that frequencies of specific mutant types may vary, in a rather unpredictable manner, depending on past and present physical and biological environments in which virus replication takes place, nucleotide sequence context in myriad genomes that compose the mutant spectra, and quasispecies memory, among many other influences; this undoubtedly provides a good case for complexity.

The quasispecies nature of RNA viruses has opened the possibility for an entirely new antiviral strategy based on loss of infectivity brought about by enhanced mutagenesis. The theoretical developments of Eigen, Schuster, and their colleagues led to the conclusion that the maximum length of a genome that can be maintained during extensive replication is inversely proportional to the average error rate per nucleotide and replication round (review and mathematical formulation in reference 59). Several studies have demonstrated decreases in viral infectivity associated with slightly increased levels of mutagenesis during RNA genome replication (96, 112, 113, 147, 173). A recent study with many FMDV clones and populations has documented that low viral loads and low viral fitness favor loss of infectivity by enhanced mutagenesis (145b, 173). Thus, attempts to identify effective, virus-specific mutagenic agents may become an important approach for development of new antiviral agents. This approach is based on the concept of error catastrophe, which is inherent to quasispecies dynamics (45, 59).

In a promising new development using purified poliovirus polymerase, the antiviral agent ribavirin has been shown to cause increased mutation frequencies during poliovirus replication (33). Both cytidine and uridine in template RNA directed low-level ribavirin incorporation and, conversely, template ribavirin monophosphate directed the incorporation of CMP and UMP into the RNA product with similar efficiency. If ribavirin is proven mutagenic for other viruses, it may well be that its broader antiviral activity (against hepatitis C virus, some arenaviruses, and respiratory syncytial virus infections) is due largely to its mutagenic activity. This must await confirmation in the near future (see also chapter 21, this volume).

Clearly, we live in exciting times for picornavirology. New developments in biochemistry and structural biology, and a deeper understanding of the principles governing viral evolution can now be combined to produce practical developments following an extensive (and necessary) accumulation of results from basic research. Purified picornaviral polymerase preparations can now help in the development and testing of new inhibitors and mutagenic agents. We are beginning to understand how viruses evolve high-fitness populations and how we might impede this. Error catastrophe of quasispecies, which was an exquisitely theoretical concept just a decade ago, can now be put into practice. A number of opportunities for practical application of the emerging principles of quasispecies evolution can now be envisioned. Picornaviruses will undoubtedly play a key role in such research efforts. Never again will it be appropriate to approach the prevention, therapy, and control of RNA virus diseases in a manner that assumes that the causative agents are stable genetic elements of defined genome sequence.

We are indebted to C. M. Ruiz-Jarabo, A. Arias, S. Sierra, N. Pariente, E. Yuste, A. Mas, P. Lowenstein, and L. Menéndez-Arias for interesting contributions to research related to the present review. Work in Madrid was supported by grants PM97-0060-C02-01, FIS 98/0054-01, EU FAIR5 PL97-3665, and Fundación Ramón Areces.

REFERENCES

1. **Ahmad, A. L., A. B. Dowsett, and D. A. Tyrrell.** 1987. Studies of rhinovirus resistant to an antiviral chalcone. *Antiviral Res.* **8:**27–39.
2. **Albiach-Marti, M. R., M. Mawassi, S. Gowda, T. Satyanarayana, M. E. Hilf, S. Shanker, E. C. Almira, M. C. Vives, C. Lopez, J. Guerri, R. Flores, P. Moreno, S. M. Garnsey, and W. O. Dawson.** 2000. Sequences of Citrus Tristeza Virus separated in time and space are essentially identical. *J. Virol.* **74:**6856–6865.
3. **Anderson-Sillman, K., S. Bartal, and D. R. Tershak.** 1984. Guanidine-resistant poliovirus mutants produce modified 37-kilodalton proteins. *J. Virol.* **50:**922–928.
3a. **Arias, A. E. Lázaro, C. Escarmís, and E. Domingo.** 2001. Molecular intermediates of fitness gain of an RNA virus: characterization of a mutant spectrum by biological and molecular cloning. *J. Gen. Virol.* **82:**1049–1060.
4. **Arion, D., N. Kaushik, S. McCormick, G. Borkow, and M. A. Parniak.** 1998. Phenotypic mechanism of HIV-1 resistance to 3'-azido-3'-deoxythymidine (AZT): increased polymerization processivity and enhanced sensitivity to pyrophosphate of the mutant viral reverse transcriptase. *Biochemistry* **37:**15908–15917.
5. **Arnold, J. J., and C. E. Cameron.** 2000. Poliovirus RNA-dependent RNA polymerase (3D^{pol}). Assembly of stable, elongation-competent complexes by using a symmetrical primer-template substrate (sym/sub). *J. Biol. Chem.* **275:**5329–5336.
6. **Arnold, J. J., S. K. Ghosh, and C. E. Cameron.** 1999. Poliovirus RNA-dependent RNA polymerase (3D^{pol}). Divalent cation modulation of primer, template, and nucleotide selection. *J. Biol. Chem.* **274:**37060–37069.
7. **Arts, E. J., and S. F. Le Grice.** 1998. Interaction of retroviral reverse transcriptase with template-primer duplexes during replication. *Prog. Nucleic Acid Res. Mol. Biol.* **58:**339–393.
8. **Bae, Y. S., and J. W. Yoon.** 1993. Determination of diabetogenicity attributable to a single amino acid, Ala776, on the polyprotein of encephalomyocarditis virus. *Diabetes* **42:**435–443.
9. **Bailly, J. L., M. Chambon, C. Henquell, J. Icart, and H. Peigue-Lafeuille.** 2000. Genomic variations in echovirus 30 persistent isolates recovered from a chronically infected immunodeficient child and comparison with the reference strain. *J. Clin. Microbiol.* **38:**552–557.
9a. **Baranowski, E., C. M. Ruíz-Jarabo, and E. Domingo.** 2001. Evolution of cell recognition by viruses. *Science* **292:**1102–1105.
10. **Baranowski, E., C. M. Ruíz-Jarabo, N. Sevilla, D. Andreu, E. Beck, and E. Domingo.** 2000. Cell recognition by foot-and-mouth disease virus that lacks the RGD integrin-binding motif: flexibility in aphthovirus receptor usage. *J. Virol.* **74:**1641–1647.
11. **Batschelet, E., E. Domingo, and C. Weissmann.** 1976. The proportion of revertant and mutant phage in a growing population, as a function of mutation and growth rate. *Gene* **1:**27–32.

12. Beard, C. W., and P. W. Mason. 2000. Genetic determinants of altered virulence of Taiwanese foot-and-mouth disease virus. *J. Virol.* **74:**987–991.
13. Bebenek, K., and T. A. Kunkel. 1993. The fidelity of retroviral reverse transcriptases, p. 85–102. *In* A. M. Skalka and S. P. Goff (ed.), *Reverse Transcriptase*. Cold Spring Harbor Laboratory Press, Cold Spring Harbor, N.Y.
14. Beck, E., and K. Strohmaier. 1987. Subtyping of European foot-and-mouth disease virus strains by nucleotide sequence determination. *J. Virol.* **61:**1621–1629.
15. Beck, M. A., and O. A. Levander. 1997. Effects of nutritional antioxidants and other dietary constituents on coxsackievirus-induced myocarditis. *Curr. Top. Microbiol. Immunol.* **223:**81–96.
16. Beck, M. A., Q. Shi, V. C. Morris, and O. A. Levander. 1995. Rapid genomic evolution of a non-virulent coxsackievirus B3 in selenium-deficient mice results in selection of identical virulent isolates. *Nat. Med.* **1:**433–436.
17. Bellmunt, A., G. May, R. Zell, P. Pring-Akerblom, W. Verhagen, and A. Heim. 1999. Evolution of poliovirus type I during 5.5 years of prolonged enteral replication in an immunodeficient patient. *Virology* **265:**178–184.
18. Belnap, D. M., B. M. McDermott, Jr., D. J. Filman, N. Cheng, B. L. Trus, H. J. Zuccola, V. R. Racaniello, J. M. Hogle, and A. C. Steven. 2000. Three-dimensional structure of poliovirus receptor bound to poliovirus. *Proc. Natl. Acad. Sci. USA* **97:**73–78.
19. Bernad, A., L. Blanco, J. M. Lazaro, G. Martin, and M. Salas. 1989. A conserved 3′ → 5′ exonuclease active site in prokaryotic and eukaryotic DNA polymerases. *Cell* **59:**219–228.
20. Biebricher, C. K. 1999. Mutation, competition and selection as measured with small RNA molecules, p. 65–85. *In* E. Domingo, R. G. Webster, and J. J. Holland (ed.), *Origin and Evolution of Viruses*. Academic Press, San Diego, Calif.
21. Boege, U., D. Kobasa, S. Onodera, G. D. Parks, A. C. Palmenberg, and D. G. Scraba. 1991. Characterization of mengo virus neutralization epitopes. *Virology* **181:**1–13.
22. Borrego, B., I. S. Novella, E. Giralt, D. Andreu, and E. Domingo. 1993. Distinct repertoire of antigenic variants of foot-and-mouth disease virus in the presence or absence of immune selection. *J. Virol.* **67:**6071–6079.
23. Boyer, J. C., K. Bebenek, and T. A. Kunkel. 1996. Analyzing the fidelity of reverse transcription and transcription. *Methods Enzymol.* **275:**523–537.
24. Brown, B. A., M. S. Oberste, J. P. Alexander, Jr., M. L. Kennett, and M. A. Pallansch. 1999. Molecular epidemiology and evolution of enterovirus 71 strains isolated from 1970 to 1998. *J. Virol.* **73:**9969–9975.
25. Caggana, M., P. Chan, and A. Ramsingh. 1993. Identification of a single amino acid residue in the capsid protein VP1 of coxsackievirus B4 that determines the virulent phenotype. *J. Virol.* **67:**4797–4803.
26. Carrillo, C., M. Borca, D. M. Moore, D. O. Morgan, and F. Sobrino. 1998. In vivo analysis of the stability and fitness of variants recovered from foot-and-mouth disease virus quasispecies. *J. Gen. Virol.* **79:**1699–1706.
27. Carrillo, C., J. Plana, R. Mascarella, J. Bergada, and F. Sobrino. 1990. Genetic and phenotypic variability during replication of foot-and-mouth disease virus in swine. *Virology* **179:**890–892.
28. Chao, L. 1990. Fitness of RNA virus decreased by Muller's ratchet. *Nature* **348:**454–455.
29. Chapman, N. M., A. I. Ramsingh, and S. Tracy. 1997. Genetics of coxsackievirus virulence. *Curr. Top. Microbiol. Immunol.* **223:**227–258.
30. Chumakov, K. M., L. B. Powers, K. E. Noonan, I. B. Roninson, and I. S. Levenbook. 1991. Correlation between amount of virus with altered nucleotide sequence and the monkey test for acceptability of oral poliovirus vaccine. *Proc. Natl. Acad. Sci. USA* **88:**199–203.
31. Clarke, D. K., E. A. Duarte, A. Moya, S. F. Elena, E. Domingo, and J. Holland. 1993. Genetic bottlenecks and population passages cause profound fitness differences in RNA viruses. *J. Virol.* **67:**222–228.
32. Cowan, G. A., D. Pines, and D. Meltzer (ed.). 1994. *Complexity. Metaphors, Models and Reality*. Addison-Wesley Publishing Company, Reading, Mass.
32a.Crotty, S., C. E. Cameron, and R. Andino. 2001. RNA virus error catastrophe: direct molecular test by using ribavirin. *Proc. Natl. Acad. Sci. USA* **98:**6895–6900.
33. Crotty, S., D. Maag, J. J. Arnold, W. Zhong, J. Y. N. Lau, Z. Hong, R. Andino, and C. E. Cameron. The broad-spectrum antiviral ribonucleotide, ribavirin, is an RNA virus mutagen. *Nat. Med.*, in press.
34. Dasgupta, A., M. H. Baron, and D. Baltimore. 1979. Poliovirus replicase: a soluble enzyme able to initiate copying of poliovirus RNA. *Proc. Natl. Acad. Sci. USA* **76:**2679–2683.
35. Dearden, C., W. al-Nakib, K. Andries, R. Woestenborghs, and D. A. Tyrrell. 1989. Drug resistant rhinoviruses from the nose of experimentally treated volunteers. *Arch. Virol.* **109:**71–81.
36. de la Torre, J. C., M. Dávila, F. Sobrino, J. Ortín, and E. Domingo. 1985. Establishment of cell lines persistently infected with foot-and-mouth disease virus. *Virology* **145:**24–35.
37. de la Torre, J. C., C. Giachetti, B. L. Semler, and J. J. Holland. 1992. High frequency of single-base transitions and extreme frequency of precise multiple-base reversion mutations in poliovirus. *Proc. Natl. Acad. Sci. USA* **89:**2531–2535.
38. de la Torre, J. C., E. Martínez-Salas, J. Diez, A. Villaverde, F. Gebauer, E. Rocha, M. Dávila, and E. Domingo. 1988. Coevolution of cells and viruses in a persistent infection of foot-and-mouth disease virus in cell culture. *J. Virol.* **62:**2050–2058.
39. de la Torre, J. C., E. Wimmer, and J. J. Holland. 1990. Very high frequency of reversion to guanidine resistance in clonal pools of guanidine-dependent type 1 poliovirus. *J. Virol.* **64:**664–671.
40. Díez, J., M. Dávila, C. Escarmís, M. G. Mateu, J. Dominguez, J. J. Pérez, E. Giralt, J. A. Melero, and E. Domingo. 1990. Unique amino acid substitutions in the capsid proteins of foot-and-mouth disease virus from a persistent infection in cell culture. *J. Virol.* **64:**5519–5528.
41. Díez, J., M. G. Mateu, and E. Domingo. 1989. Selection of antigenic variants of foot-and-mouth disease virus in the absence of antibodies, as revealed by an in situ assay. *J. Gen. Virol.* **70:**3281–3289.
42. Domingo, E. 1999. Quasispecies, p. 1431–1436. *In* A. Granoff and R. G. Webster (ed.), *Encyclopedia of Virology*. Academic Press, London, United Kingdom.
43. Domingo, E. 1989. RNA virus evolution and the control of viral disease. *Prog. Drug Res.* **33:**93–133.
44. Domingo, E. 1999. RNA virus quasispecies as models of biological complexity, p. 79–90. *In* R. A. Dixon, M. J. Harrison, and M. J. Roossinck (ed.), *Proceedings 10th Anniversary Symposium. The Samuel Roberts Noble Foundation, Plant Biology Division*. The Samuel Roberts Foundation, Ardmore, Okla.
45. Domingo, E., C. Biebricher, M. Eigen, and J. J. Holland. 2001. *Quasispecies and RNA Virus Evolution: Principles and Consequences*. Landes Bioscience, Austin, Tex.
46. Domingo, E., J. Díez, M. A. Martínez, J. Hernández, A. Holguín, B. Borrego, and M. G. Mateu. 1993. New ob-

servations on antigenic diversification of RNA viruses. Antigenic variation is not dependent on immune selection. *J. Gen. Virol.* **74:**2039–2045.
47. **Domingo, E., C. Escarmís, L. Menéndez-Arias, and J. J. Holland.** 1999. Viral quasispecies and fitness variations, p. 141–161. *In* E. Domingo, R. G. Webster, and J. J. Holland (ed.), *Origin and Evolution of Viruses*. Academic Press, San Diego, Calif.
48. **Domingo, E., and J. J. Holland.** 1994. Mutation rates and rapid evolution of RNA viruses, p. 161–184. *In* S. S. Morse (ed.), *Evolutionary Biology of Viruses*. Raven Press, New York, N.Y.
49. **Domingo, E., D. Sabo, T. Taniguchi, and C. Weissmann.** 1978. Nucleotide sequence heterogeneity of an RNA phage population. *Cell* **13:**735–744.
50. **Domingo, E., R. G. Webster, and J. J. Holland (ed.).** 1999. *Origin and Evolution of Viruses*. Academic Press, San Diego, Calif.
51. **Drake, J. W.** 1969. Comparative rates of spontaneous mutation. *Nature* **221:**1132.
52. **Drake, J. W.** 1991. A constant rate of spontaneous mutation in DNA-based microbes. *Proc. Natl. Acad. Sci. USA* **88:**7160–7164.
53. **Drake, J. W., and J. J. Holland.** 1999. Mutation rates among RNA viruses. *Proc. Natl. Acad. Sci. USA* **96:**13910–13913.
54. **Duarte, E., D. Clarke, A. Moya, E. Domingo, and J. Holland.** 1992. Rapid fitness losses in mammalian RNA virus clones due to Muller's ratchet. *Proc. Natl. Acad. Sci. USA* **89:**6015–6019.
55. **Duarte, E. A., D. K. Clarke, A. Moya, S. F. Elena, E. Domingo, and J. Holland.** 1993. Many-trillionfold amplification of single RNA virus particles fails to overcome the Muller's ratchet effect. *J. Virol.* **67:**3620–3623.
56. **Eggers, H. J., and I. Tamm.** 1965. Coxsackie A9 virus: mutation from drug dependence to drug independence. *Science* **148:**97–98.
57. **Eigen, M.** 1996. On the nature of virus quasispecies. *Trends Microbiol.* **4:**216–218.
58. **Eigen, M.** 1971. Self-organization of matter and the evolution of biological macromolecules. *Naturwissenschaften* **58:**465–523.
59. **Eigen, M., and C. K. Biebricher.** 1988. Sequence space and quasispecies distribution, p. 211–245. *In* E. Domingo, P. Ahlquist, and J. J. Holland (ed.), *RNA Genetics*, vol. 3. CRC Press, Boca Raton, Fla.
60. **Elena, S. F., F. González-Candelas, I. S. Novella, E. A. Duarte, D. K. Clarke, E. Domingo, J. J. Holland, and A. Moya.** 1996. Evolution of fitness in experimental populations of vesicular stomatitis virus. *Genetics* **142:**673–679.
61. **Emini, E. A., B. A. Jameson, A. J. Lewis, G. R. Larsen, and E. Wimmer.** 1982. Poliovirus neutralization epitopes: analysis and localization with neutralizing monoclonal antibodies. *J. Virol.* **43:**997–1005.
62. **Escarmís, C., E. C. Carrillo, M. Ferrer, J. F. Arriaza, N. Lopez, C. Tami, N. Verdaguer, E. Domingo, and M. T. Franze-Fernández.** 1998. Rapid selection in modified BHK-21 cells of a foot-and-mouth disease virus variant showing alterations in cell tropism. *J. Virol.* **72:**10171–10179.
63. **Escarmís, C., M. Dávila, N. Charpentier, A. Bracho, A. Moya, and E. Domingo.** 1996. Genetic lesions associated with Muller's ratchet in an RNA virus. *J. Mol. Biol.* **264:**255–267.
64. **Escarmís, C., M. Dávila, and E. Domingo.** 1999. Multiple molecular pathways for fitness recovery of an RNA virus debilitated by operation of Muller's ratchet. *J. Mol. Biol.* **285:**495–505.

65. **Evans, D. J., and J. W. Almond.** 1998. Cell receptors for picornaviruses as determinants of cell tropism and pathogenesis. *Trends Microbiol.* **6:**198–202.
66. **Farci, P., A. Shimoda, A. Coiana, G. Diaz, G. Peddis, J. C. Melpolder, A. Strazzera, D. Y. Chien, S. J. Munoz, A. Balestrieri, R. H. Purcell, and H. J. Alter.** 2000. The outcome of acute hepatitis C predicted by the evolution of the viral quasispecies. *Science* **288:**339–344.
67. **Flanegan, J. B., and D. Baltimore.** 1977. Poliovirus-specific primer-dependent RNA polymerase able to copy poly(A). *Proc. Natl. Acad. Sci. USA* **74:**3677–3680.
68. **Flanegan, J. B., and T. A. Van Dyke.** 1979. Isolation of a soluble and template-dependent poliovirus RNA polymerase that copies virion RNA in vitro. *J. Virol.* **32:**155–161.
69. **Flint, S. J., L. W. Enquist, R. M. Krug, V. R. Racaniello, and A. M. Skalka.** 2000. *Virology. Molecular Biology, Pathogenesis and Control*. ASM Press, Washington, D.C.
70. **Forns, X., R. H. Purcell, and J. Bukh.** 1999. Quasispecies in viral persistence and pathogenesis of hepatitis C virus. *Trends Microbiol.* **7:**402–410.
71. **Fox, M. P., M. J. Otto, and M. A. McKinlay.** 1986. The prevention of rhinovirus and poliovirus uncoating by WIN 51711: a new antiviral drug. *Antimicrob. Agents Chemother.* **30:**110–116.
72. **Fry, E. E., S. M. Lea, T. Jackson, J. W. Newman, F. M. Ellard, W. E. Blakemore, R. Abu-Ghazaleh, A. Samuel, A. M. King, and D. I. Stuart.** 1999. The structure and function of a foot-and-mouth disease virus-oligosaccharide receptor complex. *EMBO J.* **18:**543–554.
73. **Gauntt, C. J.** 1997. Roles of the humoral response in coxsackievirus B-induced disease. *Curr. Top. Microbiol. Immunol.* **223:**259–282.
74. **Gavrilin, G. V., E. A. Cherkasova, G. Y. Lipskaya, O. M. Kew, and V. I. Agol.** 2000. Evolution of circulating wild poliovirus and of vaccine-derived poliovirus in an immunodeficient patient: a unifying model. *J. Virol.* **74:**7381–7390.
75. **Gebauer, F., J. C. de la Torre, I. Gomes, M. G. Mateu, H. Barahona, B. Tiraboschi, I. Bergmann, P. A. de Mello, and E. Domingo.** 1988. Rapid selection of genetic and antigenic variants of foot-and-mouth disease virus during persistence in cattle. *J. Virol.* **62:**2041–2049.
76. **Gell-Mann, M.** 1994. *The Quark and the Jaguar*. Freeman, New York, N.Y.
77. **Gibbs, A., C. Calisher, and F. García-Arenal (ed.).** 1995. *Molecular Basis of Virus Evolution*. Cambridge University Press, Cambridge, United Kingdom.
78. **Giraudo, A. T., E. Beck, K. Strebel, P. A. de Mello, J. L. La Torre, E. A. Scodeller, and I. E. Bergmann.** 1990. Identification of a nucleotide deletion in parts of polypeptide 3A in two independent attenuated aphthovirus strains. *Virology* **177:**780–783.
79. **Gohara, D. W., S. Crotty, J. J. Arnold, J. D. Yoder, R. Andino, and C. E. Cameron.** 2000. Poliovirus RNA-dependent RNA polymerase (3D^{pol}). Structural, biochemical, and biological analysis of conserved structural motifs A and B. *J. Biol. Chem.* **275:**25523–25532.
80. **González, M. J., J. C. Sáiz, O. Laor, and D. M. Moore.** 1981. Antigenic stability of foot-and-mouth disease virus variants on serial passage in cell culture. *J. Virol.* **65:**3949–3953.
81. **Goodman, M. F., and K. D. Fygenson.** 1998. DNA polymerase fidelity: from genetics toward a biochemical understanding. *Genetics* **148:**1475–1482.
82. **Gromeier, M., E. Wimmer, and A. E. Gorbalenya.** 1999. Genetics, pathogenesis and evolution of picornaviruses, p. 287–343. *In* E. Domingo, R. G. Webster, and J. J. Holland (ed.), *Origin and Evolution of Viruses*. Academic Press, San Diego, Calif.

83. Hadfield, A. T., M. A. Oliveira, K. H. Kim, P. Minor, M. Kremer, B. A. Heinz, D. Shepard, D. C. Pevear, R. R. Rueckert, and M. G. Rossmann. 1995. Structural studies on human rhinovirus 14 drug-resistant compensation mutants. *J. Mol. Biol.* **253**:61–73.
84. Hansen, J., A. M. Long, and S. Schultz. 1997. Structure of the RNA-dependent RNA polymerase of poliovirus. *Structure* **15**:1109–1122.
85. Harber, J., G. Bernhardt, H. H. Lu, J. Y. Sgro, and E. Wimmer. 1995. Canyon rim residues, including antigenic determinants, modulate serotype-specific binding of polioviruses to mutants of the poliovirus receptor. *Virology* **214**:559–570.
86. He, Y., V. D. Bowman, S. Mueller, C. M. Bator, J. Bella, X. Peng, T. S. Baker, E. Wimmer, R. J. Kuhn, and M. G. Rossmann. 2000. Interaction of the poliovirus receptor with poliovirus. *Proc. Natl. Acad. Sci. USA* **97**:79–84.
87. Heinz, B. A., R. R. Rueckert, D. A. Shepard, F. J. Dutko, M. A. McKinlay, M. Fancher, M. G. Rossmann, J. Badger, and T. J. Smith. 1989. Genetic and molecular analyses of spontaneous mutants of human rhinovirus 14 that are resistant to an antiviral compound. *J. Virol.* **63**:2476–2485.
88. Hernández, J., M. A. Martínez, E. Rocha, E. Domingo, and M. G. Mateu. 1992. Generation of a subtype-specific neutralization epitope in foot-and-mouth disease virus of a different subtype. *J. Gen. Virol.* **73**:213–216.
89. Hewat, E. A., N. Verdaguer, I. Fita, W. Blakemore, S. Brookes, A. King, J. Newman, E. Domingo, M. G. Mateu, and D. I. Stuart. 1997. Structure of the complex of an Fab fragment of a neutralizing antibody with foot-and-mouth disease virus: positioning of a highly mobile antigenic loop. *EMBO J.* **16**:1492–1500.
90. Hirasawa, K., H. S. Jun, H. S. Han, M. L. Zhang, M. D. Hollenberg, and J. W. Yoon. 1999. Prevention of encephalomyocarditis virus-induced diabetes in mice by inhibition of the tyrosine kinase signalling pathway and subsequent suppression of nitric oxide production in macrophages. *J. Virol.* **73**:8541–8548.
91. Holland, J., K. Spindler, F. Horodyski, E. Grabau, S. Nichol, and S. VandePol. 1982. Rapid evolution of RNA genomes. *Science* **215**:1577–1585.
92. Holland, J. J. (ed.). 1992. Genetic diversity of RNA viruses. *Curr. Top. Microbiol. Immunol.*, vol. 176.
93. Holland, J. J., J. C. de la Torre, D. K. Clarke, and E. Duarte. 1991. Quantitation of relative fitness and great adaptability of clonal populations of RNA viruses. *J. Virol.* **65**:2960–2967.
94. Holland, J. J., J. C. de La Torre, and D. A. Steinhauer. 1992. RNA virus populations as quasispecies. *Curr. Top. Microbiol. Immunol.* **176**:1–20.
95. Holland, J. J., J. C. de la Torre, D. A. Steinhauer, D. Clarke, E. Duarte, and E. Domingo. 1989. Virus mutation frequencies can be greatly underestimated by monoclonal antibody neutralization of virions. *J. Virol.* **63**:5030–5036.
96. Holland, J. J., E. Domingo, J. C. de la Torre, and D. A. Steinhauer. 1990. Mutation frequencies at defined single codon sites in vesicular stomatitis virus and poliovirus can be increased only slightly by chemical mutagenesis. *J. Virol.* **64**:3960–3962.
97. Hyypiä, T., T. Hovi, N. J. Knowles, and G. Stanway. 1997. Classification of enteroviruses based on molecular and biological properties. *J. Gen. Virol.* **78**:1–11.
98. Jackson, T., F. M. Ellard, R. A. Ghazaleh, S. M. Brookes, W. E. Blakemore, A. H. Corteyn, D. I. Stuart, J. W. Newman, and A. M. King. 1996. Efficient infection of cells in culture by type O foot-and-mouth disease virus requires binding to cell surface heparan sulfate. *J. Virol.* **70**:5282–5287.
99. Jnaoui, K., and T. Michiels. 1998. Adaptation of Theiler's virus to L929 cells: mutations in the putative receptor binding site on the capsid map to neutralization sites and modulate viral persistence. *Virology* **244**:397–404.
100. Kew, O. M., R. W. Sutter, B. K. Nottay, M. J. McDenough, R. Prevots, L. Quick, and M. A. Pallansch. 1995. Molecular epidemiology of poliovirus. *Semin. Virol.* **6**:401–414.
100a. Kew, O., V. Morris-Glasgow, M. Landaverde, C. Burns, J. Shaw, Z. Garib, J. Andre, E. Blackman, C. J. Freeman, J. Jorba, R. Sutter, G. Tambini, L. Venczel, C. Perdreira, F. Laender, H. Shimizu, T. Yoneyama, T. Miyamura, H. van der Avoort, M. S. Oberste, D. Kilpatrick, S. Cochi, M. Pallansch, and C. de Quadros. 2002. Outbreak of poliomyelitis in Hispaniola associated with circulating type 1 vaccine-derived poliovirus. *Science* **296**:356–359.
101. Kew, O. M., R. W. Sutter, B. K. Nottay, M. J. McDonough, D. R. Prevots, L. Quick, and M. A. Pallansch. 1998. Prolonged replication of a type 1 vaccine-derived poliovirus in an immunodeficient patient. *J. Clin. Microbiol.* **36**:2893–2899.
102. Kilbourne, E. D. 1994. Host determination of viral evolution: a variable tautology, p. 253–271. *In* S. S. Morse (ed.), *The Evolutionary Biology of Viruses*. Raven Press, New York, N.Y.
103. King, A. M., D. McCahon, W. R. Slade, and J. W. Newman. 1982. Recombination in RNA. *Cell* **29**:921–928.
104. Kolatkar, P. R., J. Bella, N. H. Olson, C. M. Bator, T. S. Baker, and M. G. Rossmann. 1999. Structural studies of two rhinovirus serotypes complexed with fragments of their cellular receptor. *EMBO J.* **18**:6249–6259.
105. Kuge, S., N. Kawamura, and A. Nomoto. 1989. Strong inclination toward transition mutation in nucleotide substitutions by poliovirus replicase. *J. Mol. Biol.* **207**:175–182.
106. Lai, M. M. C. 1995. Recombination and its evolutionary effects on viruses with RNA genomes, p. 119–132. *In* A. Gibbs (ed.), *Molecular Basis of Virus Evolution*. Cambridge University Press, Cambridge, United Kingdom.
107. Lea, S., J. Hernández, W. Blakemore, E. Brocchi, S. Curry, E. Domingo, E. Fry, R. Abu-Ghazaleh, A. King, J. Newman, D. Stuart, and M. G. Mateu. 1994. The structure and antigenicity of a type C foot-and-mouth disease virus. *Structure* **2**:123–139.
108. Ledinko, N. 1963. Genetic recombination with poliovirus type 1. Studies of crosses between a normal horse serum-resistant mutant and several guanidine-resistant mutants of the same strain. *Virology* **20**:107–119.
109. Lemon, S. M., L. Whetter, K. H. Chang, and E. A. Brown. 1992. Why do human hepatitis viruses replicate so poorly in cell cultures? *FEMS Microbiol. Lett.* **79**:455–459.
110. Li, F., G. F. Browning, M. J. Studdert, and B. S. Crabb. 1996. Equine rhinovirus 1 is more closely related to foot-and-mouth disease virus than to other picornaviruses. *Proc. Natl. Acad. Sci. USA* **93**:990–995.
111. Liao, S., and V. Racaniello. 1997. Allele-specific adaptation of poliovirus VP1 B-C loop variants to mutant cell receptors. *J. Virol.* **71**:9770–9777.
112. Loeb, L. A., J. M. Essigmann, F. Kazazi, J. Zhang, K. D. Rose, and J. I. Mullins. 1999. Lethal mutagenesis of HIV with mutagenic nucleoside analogs. *Proc. Natl. Acad. Sci. USA* **96**:1492–1497.
113. Loeb, L. A., and J. I. Mullins. 2000. Lethal mutagenesis of HIV by mutagenic ribonucleoside analogs. *AIDS Res. Hum. Retrovir.* **13**:1–3.

114. **Mansky, L. M.** 1996. The mutation rate of human immunodeficiency virus type 1 is influenced by the *vpr* gene. *Virology* **222:**391–400.
115. **Mansky, L. M., S. Preveral, L. Selig, R. Benarous, and S. Benichou.** 2000. The interaction of Vpr with uracil DNA glycosylase modulates the human immunodeficiency virus type 1 in vivo mutation rate. *J. Virol.* **74:**7039–7047.
116. **Martin, B.** 1994. The schema, p. 263–285. *In* G. A. Cowan, D. Pines, and D. Meltzer (ed.), *Complexity. Metaphors, Models and Reality.* Addison Wesley Publishing Co., Reading, Mass.
117. **Martin, J., G. Dunn, R. Hull, V. Patel, and P. D. Minor.** 2000. Evolution of the Sabin strain of type 3 poliovirus in an immunodeficient patient during the entire 637-day period of virus excretion. *J. Virol.* **74:**3001–3010.
118. **Martínez, M. A., C. Carrillo, F. González-Candelas, A. Moya, E. Domingo, and F. Sobrino.** 1991. Fitness alteration of foot-and-mouth disease virus mutants: measurement of adaptability of viral quasispecies. *J. Virol.* **65:**3954–3957.
119. **Martínez, M. A., N. Verdaguer, M. G. Mateu, and E. Domingo.** 1997. Evolution subverting essentiality: dispensability of the cell attachment Arg-Gly-Asp motif in multiply passaged foot-and-mouth disease virus. *Proc. Natl. Acad. Sci. USA* **94:**6798–6802.
120. **Martínez-Salas, E., J. Ortín, and E. Domingo.** 1985. Sequence of the viral replicase gene from foot-and-mouth disease virus C1-Santa Pau (C-S8). *Gene* **35:**55–61.
121. **Martín-Hernández, A. M., E. Domingo, and L. Menéndez-Arias.** 1996. Human immunodeficiency virus type 1 reverse transcriptase: role of Tyr115 in deoxynucleotide binding and misinsertion fidelity of DNA synthesis. *EMBO J.* **15:**4434–4442.
122. **Marvil, P., N. J. Knowles, A. P. Mockett, P. Britton, T. D. Brown, and D. Cavanagh.** 1999. Avian encephalomyelitis virus is a picornavirus and is most closely related to hepatitis A virus. *J. Gen. Virol.* **80:**653–662.
123. **Mas, A., M. Parera, C. Briones, V. Soriano, M. A. Martínez, E. Domingo, and L. Menéndez-Arias.** 2000. Role of a dipeptide insertion between codons 69–70 of HIV-1 reverse transcriptase in the mechanism of AZT resistance. *EMBO J.* **19:**5752–5761.
124. **Mateu, M. G.** 1995. Antibody recognition of picornaviruses and escape from neutralization: a structural view. *Virus Res.* **38:**1–24.
125. **Mateu, M. G., C. Escarmís, and E. Domingo.** 1998. Mutational analysis of discontinuous epitopes of foot-and-mouth disease virus using an unprocessed capsid protomer precursor. *Virus Res.* **53:**27–37.
126. **Melnick, J. L., D. Crowther, and J. Barrera-Oro.** 1961. Rapid development of drug-resistant mutants of poliovirus. *Science* **134:**557.
127. **Meyer, P. R., S. E. Matsuura, A. M. Mian, A. G. So, and W. A. Scott.** 1999. A mechanism of AZT resistance: an increase in nucleotide-dependent primer unblocking by mutant HIV-1 reverse transcriptase. *Mol. Cell* **4:**35–43.
128. **Meyerhans, A., and J.-P. Vartanian.** 1999. The fidelity of cellular and viral polymerases and its manipulation for hypermutagenesis, p. 87–114. *In* E. Domingo, R. G. Webster, and J. J. Holland (ed.), *Origin and Evolution of Viruses.* Academic Press, San Diego, Calif.
129. **Minor, P. D.** 1992. The molecular biology of poliovaccines. *J. Gen. Virol.* **73:**3065–3077.
130. **Minor, P. D., M. Ferguson, D. M. Evans, J. W. Almond, and J. P. Icenogle.** 1986. Antigenic structure of polioviruses of serotypes 1, 2 and 3. *J. Gen. Virol.* **67:**1283–1291.
131. **Minor, P. D., G. C. Schild, J. Bootman, D. M. Evans, M. Ferguson, P. Reeve, M. Spitz, G. Stanway, A. J. Cann, R. Hauptmann, L. D. Clarke, R. C. Mountford, and J. W. Almond.** 1983. Location and primary structure of a major antigenic site for poliovirus neutralization. *Nature* **301:**674–679.
132. **Misbah, S. A., G. P. Spickett, P. C. Ryba, J. M. Hockaday, J. S. Kroll, C. Sherwood, J. B. Kurtz, E. R. Moxon, and H. M. Chapel.** 1992. Chronic enteroviral meningoencephalitis in agammaglobulinemia: case report and literature review. *J. Clin. Immunol.* **12:**266–270.
133. **Morse, S. S. (ed.).** 1993. *Emerging Viruses.* Oxford University Press, Oxford, United Kingdom.
134. **Morse, S. S. (ed.).** 1994. *The Evolutionary Biology of Viruses.* Raven Press, New York, N.Y.
135. **Mosser, A. G., and R. R. Rueckert.** 1996. Capsid-binding agents, p. 13–40. *In* D. D. Richman (ed.), *Antiviral Drug Resistance.* John Wiley and Sons Ltd., Chichester, United Kingdom.
136. **Mosser, A. G., J. Y. Sgro, and R. R. Rueckert.** 1994. Distribution of drug resistance mutations in type 3 poliovirus identifies three regions involved in uncoating functions. *J. Virol.* **68:**8193–8201.
137. **Murphy, F. A., and N. Nathanson.** 1994. The emergence of new virus diseases: an overview. *Semin. Virol.* **5:**87–102.
138. **Nagy, P. D., and A. E. Simon.** 1997. New insights into the mechanisms of RNA recombination. *Virology* **235:**1–9.
139. **Nájera, I., A. Holguín, M. E. Quiñones-Mateu, M. A. Muñoz-Fernández, R. Nájera, C. López-Galíndez, and E. Domingo.** 1995. Pol gene quasispecies of human immunodeficiency virus: mutations associated with drug resistance in virus from patients undergoing no drug therapy. *J. Virol.* **69:**23–31.
140. **Nomoto, A., T. Omata, H. Toyoda, S. Kuge, H. Horie, Y. Kataoka, Y. Genba, Y. Nakano, and N. Imura.** 1982. Complete nucleotide sequence of the attenuated poliovirus Sabin 1 strain genome. *Proc. Natl. Acad. Sci. USA* **79:**5793–5797.
141. **Novella, I. S., E. A. Duarte, S. F. Elena, A. Moya, E. Domingo, and J. J. Holland.** 1995. Exponential increases of RNA virus fitness during large population transmissions. *Proc. Natl. Acad. Sci. USA* **92:**5841–5844.
142. **Novella, I. S., S. F. Elena, A. Moya, E. Domingo, and J. J. Holland.** 1995. Size of genetic bottlenecks leading to virus fitness loss is determined by mean initial population fitness. *J. Virol.* **69:**2869–2872.
143. **Novella, I. S., C. L. Hershey, C. Escarmis, E. Domingo, and J. J. Holland.** 1999. Lack of evolutionary stasis during alternating replication of an arbovirus in insect and mammalian cells. *J. Mol. Biol.* **287:**459–465.
144. **Novella, I. S., J. Quer, E. Domingo, and J. J. Holland.** 1999. Exponential fitness gains of RNA virus populations are limited by bottleneck effects. *J. Virol.* **73:**1668–1671.
145. **Nowak, M. A.** 1992. What is a quasispecies? *Trends Ecol. Evol.* **4:**118–121.
145a.**Núñez, J. I., E. Baranowski, N. Molina, C. M. Ruíz-Jarabo, C. Sanchez, E. Domingo, and F. Sobrino.** 2001. A single amino acid substitution in nonstructural protein 3A can mediate adaptation of foot-and-mouth disease virus to the guinea pig. *J. Virol.* **75:**3977–3983.
145b.**Pariente, N., S. Sierra, P. R. Lowenstein, and E. Domingo.** 2001. Efficient virus extinction by combinations of a mutagen and antiviral inhibitors. *J. Virol.* **75:**9723–9730.
146. **Parvin, J. D., A. Moscona, W. T. Pan, J. M. Leider, and P. Palese.** 1986. Measurement of the mutation rates

of animal viruses: influenza A virus and poliovirus type 1. *J. Virol.* **59:**377–383.
147. **Pathak, V. K., and H. M. Temin.** 1992. 5-Azacytidine and RNA secondary structure increase the retrovirus mutation rate. *J. Virol.* **66:**3093–3100.
148. **Patterson, L. J., and V. V. Hamparian.** 1997. Hyperantigenic variation occurs with human rhinovirus type 17. *J. Virol.* **71:**1370–1374.
149. **Paul, A. V., J. H. van Boom, D. Filippov, and E. Wimmer.** 1998. Protein-primed RNA synthesis by purified poliovirus RNA polymerase. *Nature* **393:**280–284.
149a.**Pawlotsky, J. M.** 2000. Hepatitis C. virus resistance to antiviral therapy. *Hepatology* **32:**889–896.
150. **Pawlotsky, J. M., G. Germanidis, A. U. Neumann, M. Pellerin, P. O. Frainais, and D. Dhumeaux.** 1998. Interferon resistance of hepatitis C virus genotype 1b: relationship to nonstructural 5A gene quasispecies mutations. *J. Virol.* **72:**2795–2805.
151. **Pfister, T., and E. Wimmer.** 1999. Characterization of the nucleoside triphosphatase activity of poliovirus protein 2C reveals a mechanism by which guanidine inhibits poliovirus replication. *J. Biol. Chem.* **274:**6992–7001.
152. **Pincus, S. E., and E. Wimmer.** 1986. Production of guanidine-resistant and -dependent poliovirus mutants from cloned cDNA: mutations in polypeptide 2C are directly responsible for altered guanidine sensitivity. *J. Virol.* **60:**793–796.
153. **Prabhakar, B. S., V. M. Haspel, P. R. McClintock, and A. L. Notkins.** 1982. High frequency of antigenic variants among naturally occurring human coxsackie B4 virus isolates identified by monoclonal antibodies. *Nature* **300:**374–376.
154. **Prabhakar, B. S., M. A. Menegus, and A. L. Notkins.** 1985. Detection of conserved and nonconserved epitopes on coxsackievirus B4: frequency of antigenic change. *Virology* **146:**302–306.
155. **Racaniello, V. R., and D. Baltimore.** 1981. Cloned poliovirus complementary DNA is infectious in mammalian cells. *Science* **214:**916–919.
156. **Ramsingh, A. I., and D. N. Collins.** 1995. A point mutation in the VP4 coding sequence of coxsackievirus B4 influences virulence. *J. Virol.* **69:**7278–7281.
157. **Ramsingh, A. I., W. T. Lee, D. N. Collins, and L. E. Armstrong.** 1999. T cells contribute to disease severity during coxsackievirus B4 infection. *J. Virol.* **73:**3080–3086.
158. **Rodrigo, M. J., and J. Dopazo.** 1995. Evolutionary analysis of the picornavirus family. *J. Mol. Evol.* **40:**362–371.
159. **Rossmann, M. G., J. Bella, P. R. Kolatkar, Y. He, E. Wimmer, R. Kuhn, and T. S. Baker.** 2000. Cell recognition and entry by rhino- and enteroviruses. *Virology* **269:**239–247.
160. **Ruiz-Jarabo, C. M., A. Arias, E. Baranowski, C. Escarmís, and E. Domingo.** 2000. Memory in viral quasispecies. *J. Virol.* **74:**3543–3547.
160a.**Ruiz-Jarabo, C. M., A. Arias, C. Molina-Paris, C. Briones, E. Baranowski, C. Escarmís, and E. Domingo.** 2002. Duration and fitness dependence of quasispecies memory. *J. Mol. Biol.* **315:**285–296.
161. **Ruiz-Jarabo, C. M., N. Sevilla, M. Davila, G. Gomez-Mariano, E. Baranowski, and E. Domingo.** 1999. Antigenic properties and population stability of a foot-and-mouth disease virus with an altered Arg-Gly-Asp receptor-recognition motif. *J. Gen. Virol.* **80:**1899–1909.
162. **Sa-Carvalho, D., E. Rieder, B. Baxt, R. Rodarte, A. Tanuri, and P. W. Mason.** 1997. Tissue culture adaptation of foot-and-mouth disease virus selects viruses that bind to heparin and are attenuated in cattle. *J. Virol.* **71:**5115–5123.
163. **Sáiz, J. C., and E. Domingo.** 1996. Virulence as a positive trait in viral persistence. *J. Virol.* **70:**6410–6413.
164. **Sankar, S., and A. G. Porter.** 1992. Point mutations which drastically affect the polymerization activity of encephalomyocarditis virus RNA-dependent RNA polymerase correspond to the active site of *Escherichia coli* DNA polymerase I. *J. Biol. Chem.* **267:**10168–10176.
165. **Saunders, K., and A. M. King.** 1982. Guanidine-resistant mutants of aphthovirus induce the synthesis of an altered nonstructural polypeptide, P34. *J. Virol.* **42:**389–394.
166. **Schrag, S. J., P. A. Rota, and W. J. Bellini.** 1999. Spontaneous mutation rate of measles virus: direct estimation based on mutations conferring monoclonal antibody resistance. *J. Virol.* **73:**51–54.
167. **Schwimmbeck, P. L., S. A. Huber, and H. P. Schultheiss.** 1997. Roles of T cells in coxsackievirus B-induced disease. *Curr. Top. Microbiol. Immunol.* **223:**283–303.
168. **Sedivy, J. M., J. P. Capone, U. L. RajBhandary, and P. A. Sharp.** 1987. An inducible mammalian amber suppressor: propagation of a poliovirus mutant. *Cell* **50:**379–389.
169. **Sevilla, N., and E. Domingo.** 1996. Evolution of a persistent aphthovirus in cytolytic infections: partial reversion of phenotypic traits accompanied by genetic diversification. *J. Virol.* **70:**6617–6624.
170. **Sevilla, N., C. M. Ruiz-Jarabo, G. Gómez-Mariano, E. Baranowski, and E. Domingo.** 1998. An RNA virus can adapt to the multiplicity of infection. *J. Gen. Virol.* **79:**2971–2980.
171. **Sevilla, N., N. Verdaguer, and E. Domingo.** 1996. Antigenically profound amino acid substitutions occur during large population passages of foot-and-mouth disease virus. *Virology* **225:**400–405.
172. **Sherry, B., A. G. Mosser, R. J. Colonno, and R. R. Rueckert.** 1986. Use of monoclonal antibodies to identify four neutralization immunogens on a common cold picornavirus, human rhinovirus 14. *J. Virol.* **57:**246–257.
173. **Sierra, S., M. Dávila, P. R. Lowenstein, and E. Domingo.** 2000. Response of foot-and-mouth disease virus to increased mutagenesis. Influence of viral load and fitness in loss of infectivity. *J. Virol.* **74:**8316–8323.
174. **Smith, T. J., and T. Baker.** 1999. Picornaviruses: epitopes, canyons, and pockets. *Adv. Virus Res.* **52:**1–23.
175. **Smith, T. J., E. S. Chase, T. J. Schmidt, N. H. Olson, and T. S. Baker.** 1996. Neutralizing antibody to human rhinovirus 14 penetrates the receptor-binding canyon. *Nature* **383:**350–354.
176. **Smith, T. J., M. J. Kremer, M. Luo, G. Vriend, E. Arnold, G. Kamer, M. G. Rossmann, M. A. McKinlay, G. D. Diana, and M. J. Otto.** 1986. The site of attachment in human rhinovirus 14 for antiviral agents that inhibit uncoating. *Science* **233:**1286–1293.
177. **Sousa, R.** 1996. Structural and mechanistic relationships between nucleic acid polymerases. *Trends Biochem. Sci.* **21:**186–190.
178. **Stanway, G., P. J. Hughes, R. C. Mountford, P. Reeve, P. D. Minor, G. C. Schild, and J. W. Almond.** 1984. Comparison of the complete nucleotide sequences of the genomes of the neurovirulent poliovirus P3/Leon/37 and its attenuated Sabin vaccine derivative P3/Leon 12a1b. *Proc. Natl. Acad. Sci. USA* **81:**1539–1543.
179. **Stapleton, J. T., and S. M. Lemon.** 1987. Neutralization escape mutants define a dominant immunogenic neutralization site on hepatitis A virus. *J. Virol.* **61:**491–498.
180. **Steinhauer, D. A., J. C. de la Torre, and J. J. Holland.** 1989. High nucleotide substitution error frequencies in clonal pools of vesicular stomatitis virus. *J. Virol.* **63:**2063–2071.

181. Steinhauer, D. A., E. Domingo, and J. J. Holland. 1992. Lack of evidence for proofreading mechanisms associated with an RNA virus polymerase. *Gene* **122:**281–288.
182. Steinhauer, D. A., and J. J. Holland. 1986. Direct method for quantitation of extreme polymerase error frequencies at selected single base sites in viral RNA. *J. Virol.* **57:**219–228.
183. Steitz, T. A. 1999. DNA polymerases: structural diversity and common mechanisms. *J. Biol. Chem.* **274:**17395–17398.
184. Taboga, O., C. Tami, E. Carrillo, J. I. Núñez, A. Rodríguez, J. C. Saíz, E. Blanco, M. L. Valero, X. Roig, J. A. Camarero, D. Andreu, M. G. Mateu, E. Giralt, E. Domingo, F. Sobrino, and E. L. Palma. 1997. A large-scale evaluation of peptide vaccines against foot-and-mouth disease: lack of solid protection in cattle and isolation of escape mutants. *J. Virol.* **71:**2606–2614.
185. Tatem, J. M., C. Weeks-Levy, A. Georgiu, S. J. DiMichele, E. J. Gorgacz, V. R. Racaniello, F. R. Cano, and S. J. Mento. 1992. A mutation present in the amino terminus of Sabin 3 poliovirus VP1 protein is attenuating. *J. Virol.* **66:**3194–3197.
186. Tu, Z., N. M. Chapman, G. Hufnagel, S. Tracy, J. R. Romero, W. H. Barry, L. Zhao, K. Currey, and B. Shapiro. 1995. The cardiovirulent phenotype of coxsackievirus B3 is determined at a single site in the genomic 5′ nontranslated region. *J. Virol.* **69:**4607–4618.
187. Tyrrell, D. A. 1988. Hot news on the common cold. *Annu. Rev. Microbiol.* **42:**35–47.
188. Usherwood, E. J., and A. A. Nash. 1995. Lymphocyte recognition of picornaviruses. *J. Gen. Virol.* **76:**499–508.
189. Valcarcel, J., and J. Ortin. 1989. Phenotypic hiding: the carryover of mutations in RNA viruses as shown by detection of *mar* mutants in influenza virus. *J. Virol.* **63:**4107–4109.
190. Verdaguer, N., M. G. Mateu, D. Andreu, E. Giralt, E. Domingo, and I. Fita. 1995. Structure of the major antigenic loop of foot-and-mouth disease virus complexed with a neutralizing antibody: direct involvement of the Arg-Gly-Asp motif in the interaction. *EMBO J.* **14:**1690–1696.
191. Verdaguer, N., M. G. Mateu, J. Bravo, E. Domingo, and I. Fita. 1996. Induced pocket to accommodate the cell attachment Arg-Gly-Asp motif in a neutralizing antibody against foot-and-mouth-disease virus. *J. Mol. Biol.* **256:**364–376.
192. Verdaguer, N., N. Sevilla, M. L. Valero, D. Stuart, E. Brocchi, D. Andreu, E. Giralt, E. Domingo, M. G. Mateu, and I. Fita. 1998. A similar pattern of interaction for different antibodies with a major antigenic site of foot-and-mouth disease virus: implications for intratypic antigenic variation. *J. Virol.* **72:**739–748.
193. Villaverde, A., E. Martínez-Salas, and E. Domingo. 1988. 3D gene of foot-and-mouth disease virus. Conservation by convergence of average sequences. *J. Mol. Biol.* **204:**771–776.
194. Volkenstein, M. V. 1994. *Physical Approaches to Biological Evolution.* Springer-Verlag, Berlin, Germany.
195. Wainberg, M. A., W. C. Drosopoulos, H. Salomon, M. Hsu, G. Borkow, M. Parniak, Z. Gu, Q. Song, J. Manne, S. Islam, G. Castriota, and V. R. Prasad. 1996. Enhanced fidelity of 3TC-selected mutant HIV-1 reverse transcriptase. *Science* **271:**1282–1285.
196. Ward, C. D., and J. B. Flanegan. 1992. Determination of the poliovirus RNA polymerase error frequency at eight sites in the viral genome. *J. Virol.* **66:**3784–3793.
197. Ward, C. D., M. A. Stokes, and J. B. Flanegan. 1988. Direct measurement of the poliovirus RNA polymerase error frequency in vitro. *J. Virol.* **62:**558–562.
198. Weaver, S. C., A. C. Brault, W. Kang, and J. J. Holland. 1999. Genetic and fitness changes accompanying adaptation of an arbovirus to vertebrate and invertebrate cells. *J. Virol.* **73:**4316–4326.
199. Webster, R. G. 1999. Antigenic variation in influenza viruses, p. 377–390. *In* E. Domingo, R. G. Webster, and J. J. Holland (ed.), *Origin and Evolution of Viruses*. Academic Press, San Diego, Calif.
199a. Wells, V. R., S. J. Plotch, and J. J. DeStefano. 2001. Determination of the mutation rate of poliovirus RNA-dependent RNA polymerase. *Virus Res.* **74:**119–132.
200. Wimmer, E., C. U. Hellen, and X. Cao. 1993. Genetics of poliovirus. *Annu. Rev. Genet.* **27:**353–436.
201. Wutz, G., H. Auer, N. Nowotny, B. Grosse, T. Skern, and E. Kuechler. 1996. Equine rhinovirus serotypes 1 and 2: relationship to each other and to aphthoviruses and cardioviruses. *J. Gen. Virol.* **77:**1719–1730.
202. Xie, Q.-C., D. McCahon, J. R. Crowther, G. J. Belsham, and K. C. McCullough. 1987. Neutralization of foot-and-mouth disease virus can be mediated through any of at least three separate antigenic sites. *J. Gen. Virol.* **68:**1637–1647.
203. Xing, L., K. Tjarnlund, B. Lindqvist, G. G. Kaplan, D. Feigelstock, R. H. Cheng, and J. M. Casasnovas. 2000. Distinct cellular receptor interactions in poliovirus and rhinoviruses. *EMBO J.* **19:**1207–1216.
204. Yoon, J. W., and H. S. Jun. 1998. Insulin-dependent diabetes mellitus, p. 1390–1398. *In* I. M. Roitt and P. J. Delves (ed.), *Encyclopedia of Immunology*, 2nd ed. Academic Press, London, United Kingdom.
205. Yuste, E., C. López-Galíndez, and E. Domingo. 2000. Unusual distribution of mutations associated with serial bottleneck passages of human immunodeficiency virus type 1. *J. Virol.* **74:**9546–9552.
206. Yuste, E., S. Sánchez-Palomino, C. Casado, E. Domingo, and C. López-Galíndez. 1999. Drastic fitness loss in human immunodeficiency virus type 1 upon serial bottleneck events. *J. Virol.* **73:**2745–2751.
207. Zhang, G., G. Wilsden, N. J. Knowles, and J. W. McCauley. 1993. Complete nucleotide sequence of a coxsackie B5 virus and its relationship to swine vesicular disease virus. *J. Gen. Virol.* **74:**845–853.
208. Zimmern, D. 1988. Evolution of RNA viruses, p. 211–240. *In* E. Domingo, J. J. Holland, and P. Ahlquist (ed.), *RNA Genetics*, vol. 2. CRC Press Inc., Boca Raton, Fla.

SHUTOFF OF HOST CELL TRANSLATION AND TRANSCRIPTION

Molecular Biology of Picornaviruses
Editors, B. L. Semler and E. Wimmer
©2002 ASM Press, Washington, DC 20036-2904

Picornavirus Proteinase-Mediated Shutoff of Host Cell Translation: Direct Cleavage of a Cellular Initiation Factor

ERNST KUECHLER, JOACHIM SEIPELT, HANS-DIETER LIEBIG, AND WOLFGANG SOMMERGRUBER

24

In the course of evolution picornaviruses, like other viruses, have developed subtle strategies to interfere with host cell metabolism and to promote simultaneously the expression of their own genome. Picornaviruses are a family of small RNA viruses that includes various pathogens such as poliovirus, coxsackievirus, human rhinovirus (HRV), foot-and-mouth disease virus (FMDV), encephalomyocarditis virus, and hepatitis A virus. For poliovirus, the best studied picornavirus, it has long been known that infected cells lose the capability of synthesizing cellular proteins within 2 to 3 h after infection (designated as "host cell shutoff") while translation of viral proteins increases progressively. Nevertheless, infected cells maintain their complement of cellular mRNAs during the host cell shutoff (for reviews, see references 28, 107, and 108). When isolated from infected cells, these mRNAs can be translated in vitro in extracts from uninfected cells indicating that they are functionally preserved. Thus, despite their small size, polioviruses, like most other picornaviruses, must have a means to divert the cellular translational machinery to effectively block host cell protein synthesis while viral protein synthesis remains unabated and/or is even stimulated.

Picornaviruses contain a single-stranded genomic RNA of positive polarity from about 7,000 to more than 8,000 nucleotides in length. The RNA is polyadenylated at its 3' end and has at its 5' terminus a small, virally encoded, genome-linked protein (VPg) attached by a tyrosine-O^4-phosphodiester bond to the 5'-nucleotide of the RNA (3, 66, 80, 92). Following infection and uncoating of the virus, VPg is removed by a cellular enzyme that cleaves the phosphodiester bond (4, 5, 119). As a result, the picornaviral RNA is left with a free phosphate residue at its 5' terminus. This is in contrast to cellular mRNAs and mRNAs of other viruses that carry a 7-methyl-guanosine (m^7G) cap at their 5' end. The m^7G cap is considered the canonical signal for ribosomal binding to the 5' terminus of cellular mRNA followed by scanning of the 5' untranslated region (109). However, picornaviral RNAs not only lack this m^7G cap but, in addition, have an extensive 5' untranslated region of about 600 to more than 1,200 nucleotides in length that contains regions of high secondary structure and multiple AUGs before the authentic polyprotein AUG initiation codon (22, 54, 88, 101). Secondary structure elements are known to constitute a severe obstacle to ribosomal scanning. It was thus proposed that initiation of protein synthesis of picornaviruses does not occur by recognition of the 5' terminus as in most other mRNAs (56) but occurs by a different mechanism.

In this chapter, we discuss the strategy used by picornaviruses belonging to the genera of enteroviruses, rhinoviruses, and aphthoviruses to interfere with host cell protein synthesis. For this purpose, we will at first describe the mechanism of initiation of capped mRNA and compare it with that of uncapped mRNA. We will then discuss the role of the viral proteinases and their cellular targets. Finally, we will focus on the effect of specific proteolytic cleavage and its function in the initiation of protein synthesis. For clarity, only those steps of initiation will be addressed that are relevant for the shutoff of host cell translation.

MECHANISM OF INITIATION OF PROTEIN SYNTHESIS ON CAPPED mRNA

According to the model of Kozak (57), initiation of translation starts by recognition of the 5'-terminal m^7G cap structure followed by recruitment of the 43S preinitiation complex. The 43S preinitiation complex consists of the 40S ribosomal subunit, Met-tRNA$_f$, GTP, and several associated initiation factors. The ribosomal subunit then scans the mRNA in the 3' direction until it reaches the first initiation codon. An AUG codon alone is, however, usually not sufficient to act as a site for initiation. The efficiency of initiation is greatly influenced by the codon context. Protein synthesis commences preferentially at an A/GNNAUGG sequence (N can be any nucleotide [56–58]). For this reason, the ribosomal subunit may skip the first AUG during the scanning process and start at a subsequent initiation codon. After the 60S subunit has joined

---

Ernst Kuechler, Joachim Seipelt, and Hans-Dieter Liebig ■ Institute of Medical Biochemistry, University of Vienna, Vienna A-1030, Austria.
Wolfgang Sommergruber ■ Boehringer Ingelheim Austria, Vienna A-1121, Austria.

the initiation complex, the 80S ribosome assumes translation of the mRNA.

The whole process is guided by initiation factors that mediate ribosomal binding to the mRNA by protein-RNA and/or protein-protein interactions. The mechanism of initiation of eukaryotic translation and the role of the various factors involved have been intensively investigated (for reviews, see references 43, 48, 76, and 95). Recognition of the m^{7}G cap is brought about by the initiation factor eIF4E, also known as cap-binding protein (109). Its affinity for capped mRNA is significantly increased by addition of another initiation factor, eIF4G (37). These factors can be isolated in complexed form from cellular extracts together with eIF4A, an RNA-dependent ATPase, which, in combination with eIF4B, exhibits RNA helicase activity (90, 93). eIF4G is a large polypeptide that migrates on sodium dodecyl sulfate-polyacrylamide gel electrophoresis (SDS-PAGE) with an apparent molecular weight of 220 kDa. Given its unknown function at the time of its discovery, it was simply designated as p220 (29). Later its name was changed to eIF4γ and more recently to eIF4G. The initiation factor complex consisting of eIF4A, eIF4E, and eIF4G is termed eIF4F. As shown schematically in Fig. 1, eIF4G acts as an alignment factor connecting eIF4E bound to the N-terminal domain and eIF4A bound to the C-terminal domain of eIF4G (61, 73). eIF4G also has affinity for RNA and is believed to mediate nonspecific RNA binding of the eIF4F complex (49). Following cap recognition, eIF4F in conjunction with eIF4B is believed to promote unwinding of the secondary structure of the mRNA to facilitate recruitment of the 43S preinitiation complex (43, 48, 77, 95). In addition, eIF4G was found to harbor a binding site for eIF3 that can attach to the 40S ribosomal subunit (61). eIF4G also has an additional binding site for the poly(A)-binding protein, which is attached to the 3'-terminal poly(A) of mRNA (45, 113). This interaction results in the circularization of the functional mRNA in the state of translation and reinitiation (Fig. 1). eIF4G thus acts as a central scaffold in the assembly of the various components participating in complex formation between the capped mRNA and the ribosome during initiation of protein synthesis (75).

PICORNAVIRAL TRANSLATION AND POLYPROTEIN PROCESSING

In contrast to most cellular and viral mRNAs, picornaviral translation is initiated from an internal ribosome entry site (IRES) located in the 5' untranslated region. The IRES is a well-defined, highly structured element of about 450 nucleotides upstream of the start AUG (for reviews, see references 12, 28, 48, and 79; chapter 14, this volume). There are three types of IRES elements in picornaviruses that can be discriminated by their secondary structure. Enteroviruses (such as polio- and coxsackieviruses) and rhinoviruses share one type of IRES (type I), whereas cardioviruses and aphthoviruses (such as FMDV) have a different type of IRES (type II). Hepatitis A virus contains a type III IRES. There is little similarity among the different types of IRES elements.

Following IRES-dependent binding, the 40S ribosomal subunit moves to the AUG start codon and the 60S subunit joins the initiation complex. As eukaryotic mRNAs are functionally monocistronic, the start AUG is followed by a single open reading frame; in the case of picornaviruses, the monocistronic RNA is translated into a large precursor polyprotein of about 2,100 amino acids. The primary translation product is subsequently processed by a series of proteolytic cleavages into the different viral proteins (59). The enzymes responsible for the various processing steps are encoded by the virus itself. In enteroviruses and rhinoviruses, the first scission of the polyprotein is performed by the 2A proteinase (2A^{pro}), which is located downstream of the polypeptide precursor comprising the viral capsid proteins VP4, VP2, VP3, and VP1. 2A^{pro} cleaves between the C terminus of VP1 and its own N terminus, thereby separating the capsid protein precursor from that of the nonstructural proteins (106, 114; chapter 16). In contrast, in cardio- and aphthoviruses the cleavage occurs between 2A and 2B by a novel self-cleavage mechanism (27, 94; chapter 18). In addition, aphthoviruses also encode two forms of a leader proteinase (Lab^{pro} and Lb^{pro}) that are generated by initiation of the polyprotein synthesis at one of two in-frame AUG codons located 84 nucleotides apart. Both L^{pro} forms possess the same enzymatic properties and are released from the polyprotein precursor by autoprocessing at their own C terminus (11, 20, 74).

The complete primary translation product of the picornaviral RNA is never found in infected cells unless proteinase action is inhibited. It is therefore assumed that cleavage takes place already in the nascent state of the viral polyprotein precursor. The mechanism has been studied most extensively for 2A^{pro} of poliovirus (78, 114). It is generally assumed that 2A^{pro} acts intramolecularly (in *cis*), which requires the 2A^{pro} to fold into the active conformation while still being part of the growing polypeptide chain. 2A^{pro} also mediates *trans*-cleavage in entero- and rhinoviruses. The viral substrate for *trans*-cleavage is the 3CD precursor, which is split into the 3C' and 3D' poly-

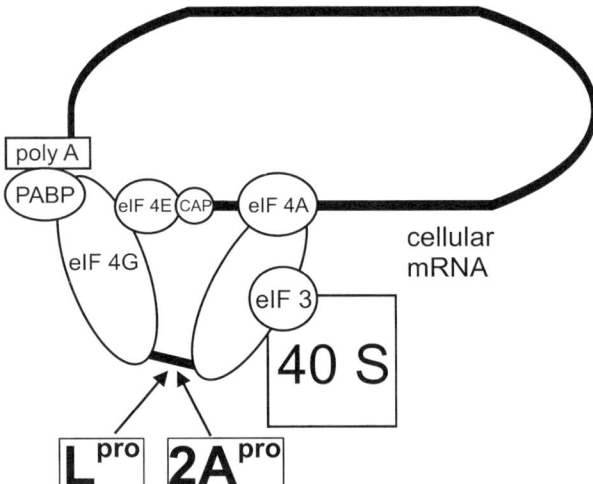

FIGURE 1 Effect of proteolytic cleavage of eIF4G by 2A^{pro} and Lb^{pro}: sequestration of the cap-binding domain of eIF4F from the ribosomal initiation complex. The two domains of the eIF4G structure are connected by the hinge region, which is the target of 2A^{pro} and L^{pro}. Cleavage by both enzymes sequesters the N-terminal domain comprising the binding sites for eIF4E (attached to the 5'-terminal m^{7}G cap structure) and for PABP ([poly(A) binding protein]. The C-terminal domain of eIF4G harboring the eIF4A- and eIF3-binding sites remains attached to the 40S ribosomal complex. Reprinted from reference 97 with permission from Elsevier Science.

peptides. The functional significance of this reaction is, however, not clear since mutations leading to a loss of the cleavage site in poliovirus do not affect virus viability (63). Most of the other processing steps are carried out by the 3C proteinase or its precursor 3CD (40; chapter 16). A further cleavage reaction occurs late in the infection cycle during assembly of the virus when VP0 is cleaved into the mature coat proteins VP4 and VP2, but the enzymatic activity responsible has not yet been defined (39).

eIF4G Cleavage in Picornavirus-Infected Cells

To promote the expression of their genomes, entero-, rhino-, and aphthoviruses have developed strategies to shut off cellular protein synthesis by inhibiting cap-dependent translation. As initiation of picornaviral protein synthesis occurs by a cap-independent mechanism via the IRES region in the 5' noncoding tract of the RNA, translation of viral proteins is not impaired. In rhino- and enteroviruses it has been demonstrated that viral protein synthesis is in fact increased (16, 67, 83, 86, 124, 125). This effect is only partly due to the increase of free ribosomes and translation initiation factors. There is evidence that additional factors are responsible for the specific rise in viral protein synthesis (chapter 15).

An early event preceding the shutoff of host cell protein synthesis is the cleavage of eIF4G. In poliovirus-infected cells eIF4G was shown to be cleaved into an N-terminal fragment, which migrates on SDS-PAGE as a set of two to three polypeptides of 110 to 130 kDa, and a C-terminal fragment of about 100 kDa (29, 65, 69). Furthermore, a modified cap-binding complex containing the proteolytic cleavage products of eIF4G was purified from poliovirus-infected cells (19, 64). Cleavage of eIF4G results in the sequestration of the N-terminal domain, which binds eIF4E (Fig. 1). This leads to the loss of the cap-binding function of eIF4F and prevents the recruitment of cellular mRNA to the ribosomal initiation complex. The remaining C-terminal fragment of eIF4G has been shown to be more effective in promoting IRES-dependent translation than intact eIF4G (16, 67, 83, 86, 124, 125). This stimulatory effect is additive to that of specific factors required for IRES-mediated initiation (44, 91).

A wealth of evidence supports the notion that the enzymes responsible for eIF4G cleavage are 2A^{pro} of entero- and rhinoviruses and L^{pro} of aphthoviruses. Early experiments have indicated that mutations in the 2A^{pro} gene of poliovirus lead to the production of a virus unable to inhibit host cell protein synthesis and to cleave eIF4G (13, 84). In addition, expression of portions of the poliovirus genome comprising the intact coding region of 2A^{pro} was shown to induce cleavage of eIF4G (60, 68). Similar results were obtained with the region encoding L^{pro} of FMDV (26). Transfection of cells with expression vectors containing the poliovirus 2A^{pro} gene inhibited cap-dependent translation and also induced cleavage of eIF4G (1, 25, 111). Similarly, expression of 2A^{pro} of poliovirus using a vaccinia virus vector caused cleavage of eIF4G and shutoff of host cell protein synthesis, whereas expression of a truncated inactive 2A^{pro} had no effect (28, 50). Further evidence for the role of 2A^{pro} came from in vitro experiments. Incubation of extracts of *Escherichia coli* expressing recombinant 2A^{pro} with an extract from uninfected HeLa cells caused cleavage of eIF4G (2), whereas expression of 2A^{pro} bearing inactivating single amino acid substitutions did not result in cleavage of the VP1-2A precursor nor did it induce cleavage of eIF4G in HeLa cell extracts (41). Interestingly, hybrid proteins between *Pseudomonas aeruginosa* exotoxin A and poliovirus 2A^{pro} still retain the proteolytic activity and were capable of cleaving eIF4G when expressed in COS cells and in HeLa cells (81, 82). Thus, there is ample evidence that 2A^{pro} is the viral proteinase responsible for eIF4G cleavage, which results in the inactivation of cap-dependent translation leading to the shutoff of cellular protein synthesis.

Early Studies on the Mechanism of 2A^{pro} Cleavage of eIF4G

Although there is general agreement on the role of 2A^{pro} of entero- and rhinoviruses in eIF4G cleavage, the actual molecular mechanism of this cleavage has been a matter of much debate. Original findings on poliovirus seemed to favor an indirect mode of action rather than a direct cleavage of eIF4G by 2A^{pro}: Antibodies directed against 2A^{pro} failed to inhibit in vitro cleavage of eIF4G when incubated with extracts from poliovirus-infected cells. On size exclusion column chromatography, the eIF4G cleavage activity did not copurify with the bulk of poliovirus 2A^{pro} (70). Furthermore, translation of 2A^{pro} mRNA in HeLa cell extract resulted in cleavage of eIF4G, which could be inhibited by an antibody against 2A^{pro}, but only when the antiserum was present before or during translation. However, when the anti-2A^{pro} antiserum was added after translation of the 2A^{pro} mRNA, no inhibition of eIF4G cleavage was observed (60, 68). Other studies indicated that poliovirus 2A^{pro} requires eIF3 for cleavage of purified eIF4G (120). Nevertheless, no modification of any of the polypeptide components of eIF3 was detected upon incubation with poliovirus 2A^{pro}. The putative eIF4G cleavage activity had an apparent molecular mass of 50 to 60 kDa and was thus separable from the 17-kDa 2A^{pro} and from eIF3 (18, 121). To explain these data it was proposed that 2A^{pro} might modify the specificity of a host proteinase or might activate a latent cellular proteinase, resulting in the generation of a novel proteolytic activity that would subsequently cleave eIF4G (60, 120, 121). However, as most of these studies were carried out with crude cell extracts or partially purified proteins, no definite conclusion could be drawn about the molecular mechanism of eIF4G cleavage. It is also important to emphasize that despite many attempts, no cellular eIF4G-specific proteinase activated by 2A^{pro} has been isolated. As will be described below, elucidation of the cleavage mechanism of eIF4G by 2A^{pro} required the availability of purified viral proteinases.

Evidence for a Direct Cleavage of eIF4G

Both 2A^{pro} of HRV serotype 2 (HRV2 2A^{pro}) and 2A^{pro} of coxsackievirus B4 have been expressed in *E. coli* and purified to homogeneity (67). Upon incubation of highly purified eIF4F with either of the two recombinant 2A^{pro} proteins, complete cleavage of eIF4G was obtained without addition of any other cellular protein. Sequencing of the cleavage product revealed that the cleavage had occurred at an amino acid sequence of eIF4G that resembles the cleavage site in the HRV2 polyprotein (Fig. 2). These results were clearly at variance with the previous hypothesis that the eIF4G cleavage is mediated by a cellular enzyme. There was also no eIF3 requirement for eIF4G cleavage by recombinant 2A^{pro} (62). It was therefore postulated that 2A^{pro} proteins of rhino- and coxsackieviruses cleave eIF4G directly without activation of a latent host cell enzyme or modification of the specificity of a preexisting cellular proteinase (Fig. 1). In addition, based on the known cleavage

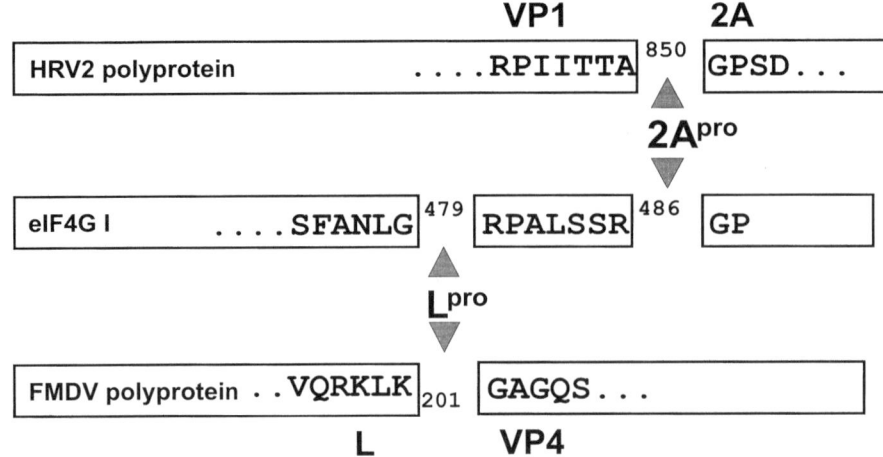

FIGURE 2 Comparison of 2A^{pro} and of Lb^{pro} cleavage sites in rabbit eIF4G with that of the respective viral polyproteins. Amino acid sequences at the eIF4GI cleavage sites of 2A^{pro} and of Lb^{pro} are indicated. 2A^{pro} cleavage in the HRV2 polyprotein occurs between the C terminus of the capsid protein VP1 and the N terminus of 2A^{pro}. L^{pro} cleaves the FMDV polyprotein between the C terminus of L^{pro} and the N terminus of the capsid protein VP4.

sites of 2A^{pro} of HRV2 and 2A^{pro} of coxsackievirus B4 in the viral polyprotein, sequence comparisons allowed the prediction of three potential cleavage sites in eIF4G (100, 102, 103). The corresponding peptides containing the common motif P4(Ile/Leu)–P3(X)–P2(Thr/Ser)–P1(X)*P1'(Gly)–P2'(Pro) were synthesized (X indicates amino acids that do not contribute significantly to cleavage specificity [100, 102, 103, 106]). The nomenclature Pn-P1* P1'-Pn' is that of Schechter and Berger (96), with the scissile peptide bond occurring between P1 and P1'. Indeed two peptide substrates derived from these sequences were cleaved by both proteinases (102). One of these corresponded to the cleavage site for 2A^{pro} mapped on eIF4G (62), which provides further support for a direct cleavage mechanism.

A similar result was obtained when recombinant Lb^{pro} of FMDV was incubated with highly purified eIF4F (53). Sequence analysis of the cleavage products of eIF4G generated by 2A^{pro} and Lb^{pro} revealed that the cleavage sites are close to each other but they are not identical (Fig. 2). This is not surprising since Lb^{pro} exhibits a different cleavage specificity (36, 97). For comparison, the L^{pro} cleavage site on the FMDV polyprotein is also shown. As indicated in Fig. 2, Lb^{pro} cleaves 7 amino acids upstream of the bond hydrolyzed by 2A^{pro} in eIF4G (53, 62). Nevertheless, the effect of both proteolytic events is the same (Fig. 1), as the N-terminal part of eIF4G harboring the eIF4E-binding site is separated from the C-terminal part responsible for binding of eIF3 and eIF4A (61, 73). Apparently the region of eIF4G connecting the N-terminal eIF4E cap-binding domain and the C-terminal ribosome attachment domain is particularly sensitive to proteolytic attack (Fig. 1). The fact that both 2A^{pro} and Lb^{pro} cleave at distinct sites provides an additional argument for a direct cleavage mechanism. If cleavage were indirect, one would have to postulate that there are two different latent host cell proteinases potentially capable of cleaving eIF4G at two different sites. One of these would have to be activated by 2A^{pro} of entero- and rhinoviruses, the other one by Lab^{pro} and/or Lb^{pro} of FMDV. Alternatively, one would have to assume that a single cellular proteinase is modified to induce two different cleavage specificities for eIF4G.

The eIF4G-eIF4E Complex is the Target for Direct Cleavage by 2A^{pro}

There are several possible explanations to account for the discrepancies between the results obtained by the different authors (17, 18, 21, 41, 53, 60, 61, 65, 67, 70, 102, 121, 122). Most of the early studies on eIF4G cleavage favoring an indirect mode of action were carried out with poliovirus 2A^{pro}. In contrast, experiments supporting a direct mode of eIF4G cleavage were performed with recombinant 2A^{pro} of HRV2 and/or 2A^{pro} of coxsackievirus B4. Nevertheless, considering the high degree of conservation of the amino acid sequence of 2A^{pro} of entero- and rhinoviruses (68), it is unlikely that these viruses actually use completely different modes of eIF4G cleavage to achieve host cell shutoff of protein synthesis. An alternative explanation for the apparent contradiction of the results is that the experimental conditions employed by the various authors for in vitro cleavage of eIF4G by 2A^{pro} were substantially different. Indeed, comparison of the purification schemes showed that Wyckoff et al. (120, 121) utilized a partially purified eIF4G preparation essentially lacking the other polypeptides of the eIF4F complex for incubation with poliovirus 2A^{pro}. In contrast, digestions with recombinant 2A^{pro} of HRV2 and/or 2A^{pro} of coxsackievirus B4 and with Lb^{pro} were performed with eIF4G in the form of the purified eIF4F complex (53, 62). To test whether the other components of eIF4F, i.e., eIF4A and eIF4E, were required for efficient cleavage, the digestion experiments with 2A^{pro} of HRV2 were repeated with eIF4G, eIF4A, and eIF4E in recombinant form. Indeed, it was demonstrated that pure eIF4G is a poor substrate for 2A^{pro}. However, addition of eIF4E but not of eIF4A increased the susceptibility by about 100-fold (38). As eIF3 preparations frequently contain eIF4E as a contaminant (109), this would explain why there was stimulation by eIF3 in the experiments with purified eIF4G (120, 121) but not in those employing eIF4G as part of the eIF4F complex (62). Apparently, isolated eIF4G is either misfolded and requires the presence of eIF4E to fold into the proper conformation or 2A^{pro} may simply require the eIF4G-eIF4E complex as a minimal structure for binding. Although eIF4A does not stimulate cleavage, it is nevertheless conceivable that in the infected cell the complete eIF4F complex may constitute the substrate for 2A^{pro} (28, 38). Recently, Ventoso et al. (116) reported that a recombinant form of poliovirus 2A^{pro} fused to the maltose-binding protein cleaves human eIF4G directly when supplied as a highly purified eIF4F complex. Similarly, an eIF4G cleavage site-derived synthetic peptide was cleaved by the poliovirus 2A^{pro} fusion protein. It can, therefore, be concluded that complex formation of eIF4G with eIF4E (as contained in eIF4F) is required for direct cleavage of eIF4G by 2A^{pro} of rhino- and enteroviruses.

Comparison of in vitro eIF4G cleavage (employed as eIF4F complex) by 2A^{pro} of poliovirus with that in the infected cell has demonstrated that in vivo cleavage is by far more efficient (17, 18). Quantitation of the ratios necessary for complete in vitro cleavage of eIF4G yielded similar results both for 2A^{pro} of poliovirus and for 2A^{pro} of coxsackievirus B4. The data are also comparable to those obtained previously with 2A^{pro} of HRV2 (38). Furthermore, the addition to poliovirus-infected cells of guanidine-HCl, which inhibits viral RNA replication and thus reduces the cellular concentration of 2A^{pro} by at least 20-fold, caused only a slight delay in eIF4G cleavage (17). Thus, the stimulation of eIF4G cleavage by complex formation with eIF4E alone cannot account for the discrepancy between in vitro and in vivo data. There must be additional factors required for rapid and efficient eIF4G cleavage in the infected cell.

eIF4G Cleavage Occurs during Translation of the Picornaviral Proteinases

During synthesis of the viral polyprotein, 2A^{pro} is active in its nascent state, indicating that the self-cleavage reaction separating the viral capsid protein precursor from the nonstructural proteins occurs on ribosomal complexes. As most of the eIF4G in the cell is complexed with eIF4E and is bound to ribosomes (89), it was of interest to determine whether eIF4G cleavage also takes place on ribosomal complexes. It has recently been demonstrated using an in vitro translation system that newly synthesized 2A^{pro} of HRV2 is highly efficient in eIF4G cleavage (31). Similar results have also been obtained upon in vitro translation of Lb^{pro} of FMDV. Estimation of the relative ratios indicated that the amounts of 2A^{pro} and/or Lb^{pro} required for rapid eIF4G cleavage are comparable to those found in vivo in the infected cell (17). Several factors may be responsible for creating a more favorable microenvironment for cleavage: (i) rapid cleavage of eIF4G may simply be a consequence of the close proximity between the initiation factors and the viral proteinases on the ribosomal complex, (ii) eIF4F bound to ribosomes may assume a conformation allowing a better presentation of eIF4G as a proteinase substrate, or (iii) newly synthesized viral proteinases may be more active than the recombinant proteinases used in the in vitro cleavage studies. Whatever the reason is, eIF4G cleavage apparently starts at an early stage of viral infection even before mature viral proteins are detectable. It thus appears that both the cis-cleavage of the viral polyprotein and the trans-cleavage of eIF4G occur on ribosomal complexes. The fact that the switch from cap-dependent to cap-independent initiation takes place early in the infection is of particular interest in the light of recent findings that several cellular mRNAs implicated in stress responses, inflammation, angiogenesis, and serum response are translated under conditions of reduced eIF4F concentrations (51).

Differential Cleavage of the Two Homologues eIF4GI and eIF4GII by 2A^{pro}

Although conceptually the connection between cleavage of eIF4G and the inhibition of cap-dependent protein synthesis appears evident, a considerable difference was observed experimentally when the kinetics of eIF4G cleavage were determined and compared with the rate of shutoff of host cell protein synthesis. The discrepancy was particularly dramatic when viral replication was partially inhibited by guanidine-HCl, 3-methyl quercetin, monensin, or nigericin (15, 21, 47, 85). In the presence of these inhibitors, eIF4G cleavage was found to be essentially complete, whereas cellular protein synthesis was only partially inhibited. This apparent contradiction was resolved when it was discovered that there is a homologue of eIF4G that shares 46% amino acid identity (34). This homologue has been termed eIF4GII, with eIF4G therefore being renamed eIF4GI. eIF4GII shares all the factor-binding properties with eIF4GI. The N-terminal part contains an eIF4E-binding site; the C-terminal fragment is capable of binding eIF3 and eIF4A. It can thus be assumed that eIF4GII is equally capable of forming an eIF4F complex and can participate in cap-dependent translation just like eIF4GI. However, eIF4GI and eIF4GII may have different specificities for translation of certain groups of mRNA. Interestingly, eIF4GII is much more refractory to poliovirus 2A^{pro} cleavage than eIF4GI is. Comparison of the kinetics of eIF4GII cleavage indicated a close correlation between the disappearance of intact eIF4GII and the inhibition of cap-dependent translation (35). Both eIF4G homologues have to be cleaved to achieve the shutoff of host cell protein synthesis. Similar results have also been obtained with HRV14 (112). In contrast, infection of HeLa cells with HRV2 or HRV16 indicated that cleavage of eIF4GI and of eIF4GII occurs at the same rate (98; A. Gradi and Y. V. Svitkin, personal communication). Thus, there are differences in the susceptibilities of the two eIF4G homologues for the various 2A^{pro} proteins.

The ultimate proof for direct cleavage of eIF4GI and eIF4GII comes from recent studies employing a temperature-sensitive variant of HRV2 2A^{pro} (ts 2A^{pro}). In ts 2A^{pro} the Phe residue 130 was replaced by Tyr, resulting in an enzyme that is active at 20°C but is rapidly inactivated at 42°C (72). In vitro incubation of HeLa cell extract with ts 2A^{pro} at 20°C resulted in complete cleavage of both eIF4GI and eIF4GII. However, following heat inactivation of ts 2A^{pro} at 42°C and addition of fresh HeLa cell extract, no further cleavage of eIF4GI and eIF4GII was obtained upon incubation at 20°C. In contrast, complete cleavage was observed in a parallel experiment with wild-type 2A^{pro}. The loss of cleavage activity for both eIF4GI and eIF4GII was thus shown to correlate with the inactivation profile of ts 2A^{pro} (H.-D. Liebig et al., submitted). It was concluded that no activation of a latent cellular proteinase occurred during the initial incubation with ts 2A^{pro} at 20°C. Taken together, these data demonstrate that 2A^{pro} cleaves both eIF4GI and eIF4GII by a direct cleavage mechanism.

Structure and Cleavage Specificity of 2A^{pro}

Understanding of the mechanism of eIF4G cleavage requires the knowledge of the three-dimensional structure of 2A^{pro}. Indeed, entero- and rhinoviral 2A^{pro} enzymes are of interest not only as important players in viral gene expression and in virus-host cell interactions, but also as enzymes that are members of an unusual class of proteinases. Like the 3C^{pro} of picornaviruses, they have a cysteine residue as the active site nucleophile, but at the amino acid sequence level they show no significant homology to the other known cysteine proteinases (23, 32, 33). Instead, the active site cysteine is flanked by sequences similar to those of serine proteinases (6, 33, 106). On the basis of these sequence similarities, 2A^{pro} was proposed to have a three-dimensional structure similar to those of the small bacterial serine proteinases, e.g., α-lytic proteinase from *Lysobacter enzymogenes* (10, 32, 105). Site-directed mutagenesis studies of polio- and rhinovirus 2A^{pro} were used to identify the putative catalytic triad as well as amino acids essential for *cis*- and/or *trans*-cleavage activity (41, 71, 99, 100, 105, 106, 115, 122, 123). Detailed studies of the substrate requirement of 2A^{pro} of HRV2 for *cis*- and for *trans*-cleavage activities have shown that the occupancy of P4 (Ile/Leu), P2 (Thr/Ser), P1' (Gly), and P2' (Pro) is critical for efficient cleavage (99, 102, 103, 106). A similar cleavage specificity was shown for poliovirus 2A^{pro} (42). A further unusual aspect of HRV2 2A^{pro} (and presumably of 2A^{pro} enzymes of other rhino- and enteroviruses as well) is that it contains Zn bound in an equimolar ratio, even though the enzyme is not inhibited by chelating agents (104, 106, 118). A similar but not identical Zn-binding motif was also detected in proteinase NS3 of hepatitis C virus, a member of the *Flaviviridae* (52). Spectroscopic characterization and three-dimensional modeling suggested that the Zn ion is part of a structural motif found in all 2A^{pro} enzymes of entero- and rhinoviruses examined so far (104, 105, 117). The importance of the C terminus for the overall stability and integrity of HRV2 2A^{pro} has also been demonstrated (72). Recently, the crystal structure of HRV2 2A^{pro} has been solved at 1.95 Å resolution (87). As proposed in the three-dimensional model (105), the active site consists of the catalytic triad formed by His-18, Asp-35, and Cys-106. It also shows that the Zn-binding motif is indeed a structural element required for stabilization. The Zn-binding site is located in a position comparable to that of an S-S bridge in chymotrypsin. Modeling studies reveal a substrate-induced fit in the 2A^{pro} substrate-binding site that explains the cleavage specificity and illustrates the potential of 2A^{pro} for both *cis*- and *trans*-cleavage activity (chapter 17).

As expected, 2A^{pro} enzymes of rhino- and enteroviruses exhibit a unique inhibitor profile that reflects the unusual structure of the active site of these enzymes (42, 55, 76, 103, 106, 123). As cysteine is the active site nucleophile, the enzyme is inhibited by nonspecific SH reagents such as iodoacetamide and N-ethylmaleimide. It is, however, not inhibited by specific inhibitors for papain-like cysteine proteinases such as E-64 or by inhibitors of metalloproteinases, indicating that the Zn ion is not directly involved in the enzymatic activity. In contrast, classical serine-proteinase inhibitors such as elastatinal and chymostatin and cysteine/serine-proteinase inhibitors such as antipain and tosyl-lysyl-chloromethyl ketone are very effective on 2A^{pro}. The inhibitor profile was the same independent of whether synthetic peptides corresponding to the 2A^{pro} cleavage site or eIF4G were used as substrates (67, 103). Interestingly, the 50- to 60-kDa eIF4G cleavage activity isolated from poliovirus-infected HeLa cells by Wyckoff et al. (120, 121) also exhibited an inhibition profile similar to that of purified 2A^{pro} of poliovirus, coxsackievirus, and/or HRV (42, 55, 76, 103, 106, 123). These data are consistent with the assumption that the 50- to 60-kDa eIF4G cleavage activity isolated from poliovirus-infected cells might represent a multimeric form of 2A^{pro} or an aggregate of 2A^{pro} with some other polypeptide, rather than an activated form of a latent cellular proteinase.

Direct Cleavage of Cytoskeletal Proteins by 2A^{pro}

There is recent evidence that 2A^{pro} is not only involved in the shutoff of host cell protein synthesis, but it is also responsible for cytoskeletal alterations in the infected cell. Badorff et al. (8, 9) have reported that purified recombinant coxsackievirus 2A^{pro} cleaves dystrophin in cell lysates of myocytes. Dystrophin is also cleaved in coxsackievirus B3-infected cultured myocytes and in the hearts of coxsackievirus B3-infected mice. The proteolytic processing takes place at a sequence motif predicted earlier as a potential recognition site for 2A^{pro} of entero- and rhinoviruses (14, 102). As dystrophin connects the actin filaments with the β-dystroglycan on the sarcolemma, cleavage of dystrophin disrupts the interaction of actin with the membrane, leading to myocyte dysfunction characteristic of cardiomyopathy.

A more general effect of picornavirus infection on cytoskeletal proteins was discovered when HeLa cells were infected with HRV2 (98). Late in infection 2A^{pro} was found to cleave cytokeratin 8, a member of the intermediate filament proteins. The same proteolytic cleavage occurred in vitro with purified recombinant 2A^{pro} from HRV2 and/or 2A^{pro} from coxsackievirus B4. Cleavage resulted in the removal of 14 amino acids from the N-terminal head domain of cytokeratin 8. The site matches the consensus cleavage site sequence of HRV2 2A^{pro}, implying that it is also caused by a direct cleavage event. Other intermediate filament proteins such as cytokeratins 7 and 18 and vimentin were not affected by 2A^{pro} in the course of HRV2 infection. Cleavage of cytokeratin 8 occurs much later during infection than that of eIF4GI and of eIF4GII, at the time of the onset of the cytopathic effect when cells round up and begin to detach from the surface. At this point major morphological changes take place in the infected cell, leading to a collapse of the cytoskeletal network. Interestingly, a similar cleavage occurs late in adenovirus infection when the L3 23-kDa proteinase removes 73 amino acids from the N terminus of cytokeratin 18 (24). Cytokeratins 8 and 18 are heterodimeric binding partners in HeLa cells that form the basic unit of the cytokeratin network. N-terminal deletion of 83 amino acids of cytokeratin 18 has been shown to prevent filament elongation (7). It is tempting to assume that a similar effect may be caused by the cleavage in the head domain of cytokeratin 8. Alternatively, N-terminal truncation of cytokeratin 8 may affect cytoskeletal scaffolding by disrupting the interaction with cytolinker proteins that cross-link cytokeratin filaments with other cytoskeletal components (30, 110). This may either be a direct effect or it may be the consequence of a change in the phosphorylation pattern of cytokeratin 8, as there are several potential phosphorylation sites in the cytokeratin 8 head domain located close to the 2A^{pro} cleavage site (46).

CONCLUDING REMARKS

As might be expected, many of the steps of protein synthesis are similar or identical between capped and uncapped mRNAs. Furthermore, generally the same initiation factors are involved in the translation of both types of mRNAs. However, there are some critical differences that provide a plausible explanation for the dramatic changes in protein synthesis occurring after picornavirus infection. These new discoveries have given us important insights into the tricks picornaviruses play to interfere with protein synthesis of the host cell. Not surprisingly, the primary target of the viral attack is a cellular initiation factor, i.e., eIF4G, which is intimately associated with the process of ribosomal binding to the m⁷G cap of the mRNA.

The mode of cleavage of eIF4G has been the subject of considerable controversy. Several authors originally favored the concept of the activation of a latent cellular proteinase by 2A^{pro}. However, such a cellular proteinase has never been isolated. As several picornaviral proteinases and initiation factors of protein synthesis have now been obtained as recombinant proteins, a detailed study of the molecular mechanism of cleavage of eIF4G has been possible using all components in highly purified form. Indeed, these data prove that 2A^{pro} of rhino- and enteroviruses and L^{pro} of FMDV are able to cleave eIF4G directly. Most of the apparent discrepancies between the different results obtained in the past can now be explained by the fact that eIF4G itself is a poor substrate for 2A^{pro}. To be cleaved efficiently, eIF4G has to be complexed with the cap-binding protein eIF4E. Furthermore, cleavage of eIF4G on ribosomal complexes occurs very rapidly at 2A^{pro} and Lb^{pro} concentrations comparable to those found in vivo. Both homologues eIF4GI and eIF4GII have to be cleaved to achieve the shutoff of cap-dependent host cell protein synthesis.

eIF4G constitutes an ideal target as it is a central player in the initiation mechanism of translation. It serves as the basic scaffold for mRNA-ribosome complex formation since it has binding sites for the cap-binding protein eIF4E, for the helicase eIF4A, for eIF3 (which binds to the ribosome), and for the poly(A)-binding protein (which binds the 3' terminus of mRNAs). As a consequence of the direct proteolytic cleavage, the eIF4E-binding domain is sequestered from the ribosome-binding domain and the recruitment of m⁷G-capped mRNAs to the initiation complexes is prevented. At the same time the capacity to support cap-independent translation by IRES-mediated initiation is increased. The details of this enhancement of initiation activity are still not fully understood. The mechanism of IRES-dependent initiation of picornaviral translation thus remains a fascinating subject for future research.

This work was supported by grants from the Austrian Science Foundation (P12193-MOB and SFB 005/8 to E. Kuechler). We thank T. Skern for critical reading of the manuscript. The technical help of M. Langer and F. Fessl is gratefully acknowledged.

REFERENCES

1. **Aldabe, R., E. Feduchi, I. Novoa, and L. Carrasco.** 1995. Expression of 2A^{pro} in mammalian cells: effects on translation. *FEBS Lett.* **377:**1–5.
2. **Alvey, I. C., E. E. Wyckoff, S. F. Yu, R. Lloyd, and E. Ehrenfeld.** 1991. cis and trans activities of poliovirus 2A protease expressed in *Escherichia coli. J. Virol.* **65:**6077–6083.
3. **Ambros, V., and D. Baltimore.** 1978. Protein is linked to the 5' end of poliovirus RNA by phosphodiester linkage to tyrosine. *J. Biol. Chem.* **253:**5263–5266.
4. **Ambros, V., and D. Baltimore.** 1980. Purification and properties of a HeLa cell enzyme able to remove the 5'-terminal protein from poliovirus RNA. *J. Biol. Chem.* **255:**6739–6744.
5. **Ambros, V., R. F. Petterson, and D. Baltimore.** 1978. An enzymatic activity in uninfected cells that cleaves the linkage between poliovirion RNA and the 5' terminal protein. *Cell* **15:**1439–1446.
6. **Argos, P., G. Kamer, M. J. H. Nicklin, and E. Wimmer.** 1984. Similarity in gene organization and homology between proteins of animal picornaviruses and a plant comovirus suggest common ancestry of these virus families. *Nucleic Acids Res.* **12:**7251–7267.
7. **Bader, B., T. Magin, S. Freudenmann, and W. Franke.** 1991. Intermediate filaments formed de novo from tailless cytokeratins in the cytoplasm and in the nucleus. *J. Cell Biol.* **115:**1293–1307.
8. **Badorff, C., N. Berkely, S. Mehrotra, J. W. Talhouk, R. E. Rhoads, and K. U. Knowlton.** 2000. Enteroviral protease 2A directly cleaves dystrophin and is inhibited by a dystrophin-based substrate analogue. *J. Biol. Chem.* **275:**11191–11197.
9. **Badorff, C., G. H. Lee, B. J. Lamphear, M. E. Martone, K. P. Campbell, R. E. Rhoads, and K. U. Knowlton.** 1999. Enteroviral protease 2A cleaves dystrophin: evidence of cytoskeletal disruption in an acquired cardiomyopathy. *Nat. Med.* **5:**320–326.
10. **Bazan, J. F., and R. J. Fletterick.** 1988. Viral cysteine proteases are homologous to the trypsin-like family of serine proteases: structural and functional implications. *Proc. Natl. Acad. Sci. USA* **85:**7872–7876.
11. **Belsham, G. J., J. K. Brangwyn, M. D. Ryan, C. C. Abrams, and A. M. King.** 1990. Intracellular expression and processing of foot-and-mouth disease virus capsid precursors using vaccinia virus vectors: influence of the L protease. *Virology* **176:**524–530.
12. **Belsham, G. J., and N. Sonenberg.** 1996. RNA-protein interactions in regulation of picornavirus RNA translation. *Microbiol. Rev.* **60:**499–511.
13. **Bernstein, H. D., N. Sonenberg, and D. Baltimore.** 1985. Poliovirus mutant that does not selectively inhibit host cell protein synthesis. *Mol. Cell. Biol.* **5:**2913–2923.
14. **Blom, N., J. Hansen, D. Blaas, and S. Brunak.** 1996. Cleavage site analysis in picornaviral polyproteins: discovering cellular targets by neural networks. *Protein Sci.* **5:**2203–2216.
15. **Bonneau, A. M., and N. Sonenberg.** 1987. Proteolysis of the p220 component of the cap-binding protein complex is not sufficient for complete inhibition of host cell protein synthesis after poliovirus infection. *J. Virol.* **61:**986–991.
16. **Borman, A. M., R. Kirchweger, E. Ziegler, R. E. Rhoads, T. Skern, and K. M. Kean.** 1997. eIF4G and its proteolytic cleavage products: effect on initiation of protein synthesis from capped, uncapped, and IRES-containing mRNAs. *RNA* **3:**186–196.
17. **Bovee, M. L., B. J. Lamphear, R. E. Rhoads, and R. E. Lloyd.** 1998. Direct cleavage of eIF4G by poliovirus 2A protease is inefficient in vitro. *Virology* **245:**241–249.
18. **Bovee, M. L., W. E. Marissen, M. Zamora, and R. E. Lloyd.** 1998. The predominant eIF-4G-specific activity in poliovirus-infected HeLa cells is distinct from 2A protease. *Virology* **245:**229–240.
19. **Buckley, B., and E. Ehrenfeld.** 1987. The cap-binding protein complex in uninfected and poliovirus-infected HeLa cells. *J. Biol. Chem.* **262:**13599–13606.
20. **Burroughs, J. N., D. V. Sangar, B. E. Clarke, D. J. Rowlands, A. Billiau, and D. Collen.** 1984. Multiple proteases in foot-and-mouth disease virus replication. *J. Virol.* **50:**878–883.
21. **Carrasco, L., and J. L. Castrillo.** 1987. The regulation of translation in picornavirus-infected cells, p. 115–146. *In* L. Carrasco (ed.), *Mechanisms of Viral Toxicity in Animal Cells.* CRC Press, Boca Raton, Fla.
22. **Carroll, A. R., D. J. Rowlands, and B. E. Clarke.** 1984. The complete nucleotide sequence of the RNA coding for

the primary translation product of foot and mouth disease virus. *Nucleic Acids Res.* **12**:2461–2472.
23. **Cheah, K.-C., L. E.-C. Leong, and A. G. Porter.** 1990. Site-directed mutagenesis suggests close functional relationship between a human rhinovirus 3C cysteine protease and cellular trypsin-like serine proteases. *J. Biol. Chem.* **265**:7180–7187.
24. **Chen, P. H., D. A. Ornelles, and T. Shenk.** 1993. The adenovirus L3 23-kilodalton proteinase cleaves the amino-terminal head domain from cytokeratin 18 and disrupts the cytokeratin network of HeLa cells. *J. Virol.* **67**:3507–3514.
25. **Davies, M., J. Pelletier, L. Meerovitch, N. Sonenberg, and R. J. Kaufman.** 1991. The effect of poliovirus protease 2A^{pro} expression on cellular metabolism. *J. Biol. Chem.* **266**:14714–14720.
26. **Devaney, M. A., V. N. Vakharia, R. E. Lloyd, E. Ehrenfeld, and M. J. Grubman.** 1988. Leader protein of foot-and-mouth disease virus is required for cleavage of the p220 component of the cap-binding protein complex. *J. Virol.* **62**:4407–4409.
27. **Donnelly, M. L. L., D. Gani, S. Monaghan, and M. D. Ryan.** 1997. The cleavage activities of aphthovirus and cardiovirus 2A proteins. *J. Gen. Virol.* **78**:13–21.
28. **Ehrenfeld, E.** 1996. Initiation of translation by picornavirus RNAs, p. 549–573. *In* J. W. B. Hershey, M. B. Mathews, and N. Sonenberg (ed.), *Translational Control*. Cold Spring Harbor Laboratory Press, Plainview, N.Y.
29. **Etchison, D., S. C. Milburn, I. Edery, N. Sonenberg, and J. W. Hershey.** 1982. Inhibition of HeLa cell protein synthesis following poliovirus infection correlates with proteolysis of a 220,000 dalton polypeptide associated with eucaryotic initiation factor 3 and a cap binding protein complex. *J. Biol. Chem.* **257**:14806–14810.
30. **Fuchs, E., and D. W. Cleveland.** 1998. A structural scaffolding of intermediate filaments in health and disease. *Science* **279**:514–519.
31. **Glaser, W., and T. Skern.** 2000. Extremely efficient cleavage of eIF4G by picornaviral proteinases L and 2A in vitro. *FEBS Lett.* **480**:151–155.
32. **Gorbalenya, A. E., V. M. Blinov, and A. M. Donchenko.** 1986. Poliovirus-encoded proteinase 3C: a possible evolutionary link between cellular serine and cysteine proteinase families. *FEBS Lett.* **194**:253–257.
33. **Gorbalenya, A. E., A. P. Donchenko, V. M. Blinov, and E. V. Koonin.** 1989. Cysteine proteases of positive strand RNA viruses and chymotrypsin-like serine proteases: a distinct protein superfamily with a common structural fold. *FEBS Lett.* **243**:103–114.
34. **Gradi, A., H. Imataka, Y. V. Svitkin, E. Rom, B. Raught, S. Morino, and N. Sonenberg.** 1998. A novel functional human eukaryotic translation initiation factor 4G. *Mol. Cell. Biol.* **18**:334–342.
35. **Gradi, A., Y. V. Svitkin, H. Imataka, and N. Sonenberg.** 1998. Proteolysis of human eukaryotic translation initiation factor eIF4GII, but not eIF4GI, coincides with the shut off of host protein synthesis after poliovirus infection. *Proc. Natl. Acad. Sci. USA* **95**:11089–11094.
36. **Guarné, A., J. Tormo, R. Kirchweger, D. Pfistermüller, I. Fita, and T. Skern.** 1998. Structure of the foot-and-mouth disease virus leader protease: a papain-like fold adapted for self-processing and eIF4G recognition. *EMBO J.* **17**:7469–7479.
37. **Haghigat, A., and N. Sonenberg.** 1997. eIF4G dramatically enhances the binding of eIF4E to the mRNA 5'-cap structure. *J. Biol. Chem.* **272**:21677–21680.
38. **Haghigat, A., Y. Svitkin, I. Novoa, E. Kuechler, T. Skern, and N. Sonenberg.** 1996. The eIF4G-eIF4E complex is the target for direct cleavage by the rhinovirus 2A proteinase. *J. Virol.* **70**:8444–8450.

39. **Harber, J. J., J. Bradley, C. W. Anderson, and E. Wimmer.** 1991. Catalysis of poliovirus VP0 maturation cleavage is not mediated by serine 10 of VP2. *J. Virol.* **65**:326–334.
40. **Harris, K. S., C. U. T. Hellen, and E. Wimmer.** 1990. Proteolytic processing in the replication of picornaviruses. *Semin. Virol.* **1**:323–333.
41. **Hellen, C. U. T., M. Fäcke, H.-G. Kräusslich, C.-K. Lee, and E. Wimmer.** 1991. Characterization of poliovirus 2A proteinase by mutational analysis: residues required for autocatalytic activity are essential for induction of cleavage of eukaryotic initiation factor 4F polypeptide p220. *J. Virol.* **65**:4226–4231.
42. **Hellen, C. U. T., C. K. Lee, and E. Wimmer.** 1992. Determinants of substrate recognition by poliovirus 2A proteinase. *J. Virol.* **66**:3330–3336.
43. **Hentze, M. W.** 1997. eIF4G: a multipurpose ribosome adapter? *Science* **275**:500–501.
44. **Hunt, S. L., T. Skern, H.-D. Liebig, E. Kuechler, and R. J. Jackson.** 1999. Rhinovirus 2A proteinase mediated stimulation of rhinovirus RNA translation is additive to the stimulation effected by cellular RNA binding proteins. *Virus Res.* **62**:119–128.
45. **Imataka, H., A. Gradi, and N. Sonenberg.** 1998. A newly identified N-terminal amino acid sequence of human eIF4G binds poly(A)-binding protein and functions in poly(A)-dependent translation. *EMBO J.* **17**:7480–7489.
46. **Inagaki, M., Y. Matsuoka, K. Tsujimura, S. Ando, T. Tokui, T. Takahashi, and N. Inagaki.** 1996. Dynamic property of intermediate filaments: regulation by phosphorylation. *Bioessays* **18**:481–487.
47. **Irurzun, A., S. Sanchez-Palomino, I. Novoa, and L. Carrasco.** 1995. Monensin and nigericin prevent the inhibition of host translation by poliovirus, without affecting p220 cleavage. *J. Virol.* **69**:7453–7460.
48. **Jackson, R. J., and M. Wickens.** 1997. Translational controls impinging on the 5'-untranslated region and initiation factor proteins. *Curr. Opin. Genet. Dev.* **7**:233–241.
49. **Jaramillo, M., T. E. Dever, W. C. Merrick, and N. Sonenberg.** 1991. RNA unwinding in translation: assembly of helicase complex intermediates comprising eukaryotic initiation factors eIF-4F and eIF-4B. *Mol. Cell. Biol.* **11**:5992–5997.
50. **Jewell, J. E., L. A. Ball, and R. Rueckert.** 1990. Limited expression of poliovirus by vaccinia virus recombinants due to inhibition of the vector by proteinase 2A. *J. Virol.* **64**:1388–1393.
51. **Johannes, G., M. S. Carter, M. B. Eisen, P. O. Brown, and P. Sarnow.** 1999. Identification of eukaryotic mRNAs that are translated at reduced cap binding complex eIF4F concentrations using a cDNA microarray. *Proc. Natl. Acad. Sci. USA* **96**:13118–13123.
52. **Kim, J. L., K. A. Morgenstern, C. Lin, T. Fox, M. D. Dwyer, J. A. Landro, S. P. Chambers, W. Markland, C. A. Lepre, E. T. O'Malley, S. L. Harberson, C. M. Rice, M. A. Murcko, P. R. Caron, and J. A. Thomson.** 1996. Crystal structure of the hepatitis C virus NS3 protease domain complexed with a synthetic NS4A cofactor peptide. *Cell* **87**:343–355.
53. **Kirchweger, R., E. Ziegler, B. J. Lamphear, D. Waters, H.-D. Liebig, W. Sommergruber, F. Sobrino, C. Hohenadl, D. Blaas, R. E. Rhoads, and T. Skern.** 1994. Foot-and-mouth disease virus leader proteinase: purification of the Lb form and determination of its cleavage site on eIF-4γ. *J. Virol.* **68**:5677–5684.
54. **Kitamura, N., B. L. Semler, P. G. Rothberg, G. R. Larsen, C. J. Adler, A. J. Dorner, E. A. Emini, R. Hanecak, J. J. Lee, S. Van Der Werf, C. W. Anderson, and E.**

Wimmer. 1981. Primary structure, gene organization, polypeptide expression of poliovirus RNA. *Nature* **291:** 547–553.
55. **Koenig, H., and B. Rosenwirth.** 1988. Purification and partial characterization of poliovirus protease 2A by means of a functional assay. *J. Virol.* **62:**1243–1250.
56. **Kozak, M.** 1978. How do eukaryotic ribosomes select initiation regions in messenger RNA? *Cell* **15:**1109–1123.
57. **Kozak, M.** 1989. The scanning model for translation: an update. *J. Cell Biol.* **108:**229–241.
58. **Kozak, M.** 1997. Recognition of AUG and alternative initiator codons is augmented by G in position +4 but is not generally affected by the nucleotides in positions +5 and +6. *EMBO J.* **16:**2482–2492.
59. **Kräusslich, H. G., and E. Wimmer.** 1988. Viral proteinases. *Ann. Rev. Biochem.* **57:**701–754.
60. **Kräusslich, H.-G., M. J. H. Nicklin, H. Toyoda, D. Etchison, and E. Wimmer.** 1987. Poliovirus proteinase 2A induces cleavage of eukaryotic initiation factor 4F polypeptide p220. *J. Virol.* **61:**2711–2718.
61. **Lamphear, B. J., R. Kirchweger, T. Skern, and R. E. Rhoads.** 1995. Mapping of functional domains in eukaryotic protein synthesis initiation factor 4G (eIF4G) with picornaviral proteases. Implications for cap-dependent and cap-independent translational initiation. *J. Biol. Chem.* **270:**21975–21983.
62. **Lamphear, B. J., R. Yan, F. Yang, D. Waters, H.-D. Liebig, H. Klump, H. Kuechler, T. Skern, and R. E. Rhoads.** 1993. Mapping the cleavage site in protein synthesis initiation factor eIF-4γ of the 2A proteases from human coxsackievirus and rhinovirus. *J. Biol. Chem.* **268:**19200–19203.
63. **Lee, C. K., and E. Wimmer.** 1988. Proteolytic processing of poliovirus polyprotein: elimination of 2A^{pro}-mediated, alternative cleavage of polypeptide 3CD by in vitro mutagenesis. *Virology* **166:**405–414.
64. **Lee, K. A. W., I. Edery, and N. Sonenberg.** 1985. Isolation and structural characterization of cap-binding proteins from poliovirus-infected HeLa cells. *J. Virol.* **54:** 515–524.
65. **Lee, K. A. W., I. Edery, R. Hanecak, E. Wimmer, and N. Sonenberg.** 1985. Poliovirus protease 3C (P3-7c) does not cleave p220 of eukaryotic mRNA cap-binding protein complex. *J. Virol.* **55:**489–493.
66. **Lee, Y. F., A. Nomoto, B. M. Detjen, and E. Wimmer.** 1977. A protein covalently linked to poliovirus genome RNA. *Proc. Natl. Acad. Sci. USA* **74:**59–63.
67. **Liebig, H.-D., E. Ziegler, R. Yan, K. Hartmuth, H. Klump, H. Kowalski, D. Blaas, W. Sommergruber, L. Frasel, B. J. Lamphear, R. E. Rhoads, E. Kuechler, and T. Skern.** 1993. Purification of two picornaviral 2A proteinases: interaction with eIF-4γ and influence on in vitro translation. *Biochemistry* **32:**7581–7588.
68. **Lloyd, R. E., M. J. Grubman, and E. Ehrenfeld.** 1988. Relationship of p220 cleavage during picornavirus infection to 2A proteinase sequencing. *J. Virol.* **62:**4216–4223.
69. **Lloyd, R. E., H. G. Jense, and E. Ehrenfeld.** 1987. Restriction of translation of capped mRNA in vitro as a model for poliovirus-induced inhibition of host cell protein synthesis: relationship to p220 cleavage. *J. Virol.* **61:** 2480–2488.
70. **Lloyd, R. E., H. Toyoda, D. Etchison, E. Wimmer, and E. Ehrenfeld.** 1986. Cleavage of the cap binding protein complex polypeptide p220 is not effected by the second poliovirus protease 2A. *Virology* **150:**299–303.
71. **Lu, H. H., X. Li, A. Cuconati, and E. Wimmer.** 1995. Analysis of picornavirus 2A(pro) proteins: separation of proteinase from translation and replication functions. *J. Virol.* **69:**7445–7452.
72. **Luderer-Gmach, M., H.-D. Liebig, W. Sommergruber, T. Voss, F. Fessl, T. Skern, and E. Kuechler.** 1996. A human rhinovirus 2A proteinase mutant and its second site revertants. *Biochem. J.* **318:**213–218.
73. **Mader, S., H. Lee, A. Pause, and N. Sonenberg.** 1995. The translation initiation factor eIF4E binds to a common motif shared by the translation factor eIF-4γ and the translational repressors 4E-binding proteins. *Mol. Cell. Biol.* **15:**4990–4997.
74. **Medina, M., E. Domingo, J. K. Brangwyn, and G. J. Belsham.** 1993. The two species of the foot-and-mouth disease virus leader protein, expressed individually, exhibit the same activities. *Virology* **194:**355–359.
75. **Michel, Y. M., D. Poncet, M. Piron, K. M. Kean, and A. M. Borman.** 2000. Cap-poly(A) synergy in mammalian cell-free extracts: investigation of the requirements for poly(A)-mediated stimulation of translation initiation. *J. Biol. Chem.* **275:**32268–32276.
76. **Molla, A., C. U. T. Hellen, and E. Wimmer.** 1993. Inhibition of proteolytic activity of poliovirus and rhinovirus 2A proteinases by elastase-specific inhibitors. *J. Virol.* **76:**4688–4695.
77. **Morley, S. J., P. S. Curtis, and V. M. Pain.** 1997. eIF4G: translation's mystery factor begins to yield its secrets. *RNA* **3:**1085–1104.
78. **Nicklin, M. J., H.-G. Kräusslich, H. Toyoda, J. J. Dunn, and E. Wimmer.** 1987. Poliovirus polypeptide precursors: expression in vitro and processing by exogenous 3C and 2A proteinases. *Proc. Natl. Acad. Sci. USA* **84:**4002–4006.
79. **Niepmann, M.** 1999. Internal initiation of translation of picornaviruses, hepatitis C virus and pestiviruses. *Recent Res. Devel. Virol.* **1:**229–250.
80. **Nomoto, A., Y. F. Lee, and E. Wimmer.** 1976. The 5'-end of poliovirus mRNA is not capped with m^{7}G(5')ppp(5')Np. *Proc. Natl. Acad. Sci. USA* **73:**375–380.
81. **Novoa, I., M. Cotton, and L. Carrasco.** 1996. Hybrid proteins between *Pseudomonas aeruginosa* exotoxin A and poliovirus 2A^{pro} cleave p220 in HeLa cells. *J. Virol.* **70:** 3319–3324.
82. **Novoa, I., E. Feduchi, and L. Carrasco.** 1994. Hybrid proteins between *Pseudomonas* exotoxin A and poliovirus protease 2A^{pro}. *FEBS Lett.* **355:**45–48.
83. **Ohlmann, T., M. Rau, V. M. Pain, and S. J. Morley.** 1996. The C-terminal domain of eukaryotic protein synthesis initiation factor (eIF) 4G is sufficient to support cap-independent translation in the absence of eIF4E. *EMBO J.* **15:**1371–1382.
84. **O'Neil, R. E., and V. R. Racaniello.** 1989. Inhibition of translation in cells infected with a poliovirus 2A^{pro} mutant correlates with phosphorylation of the alpha subunit of eukaryotic initiation factor 2. *J. Virol.* **63:**5069–5075.
85. **Perez, L., and L. Carrasco.** 1992. Lack of correlation between p220 cleavage and the shutoff of host translation after poliovirus infection. *Virology* **189:**178–186.
86. **Pestova, T. V., I. N. Shatsky, and C. U. T. Hellen.** 1996. Functional dissection of eukaryotic initiation factor 4F: the 4A subunit and the central domain of the 4G subunit are sufficient to mediate internal entry of 43S preinitiation complexes. *Mol. Cell. Biol.* **16:**6870–6878.
87. **Petersen, J. F. W., M. M. Cherney, H.-D. Liebig, T. Skern, E. Kuechler, and M. N. G. James.** 1999. The structure of the 2A proteinase from a common cold virus: a proteinase responsible for the shut-off of host-cell protein synthesis. *EMBO J.* **18:**5463–5475.
88. **Racaniello, V. R., and D. Baltimore.** 1981. Molecular cloning of poliovirus cDNA and determination of the complete nucleotide sequence of the viral genome. *Proc. Natl. Acad. Sci. USA* **78:**4887–4891.

89. **Rau, M., T. Ohlmann, S. J. Morley, and V. M. Pain.** 1996. A reevaluation of the cap-binding protein, eIF4E, as a rate-limiting factor for initiation of translation in reticulocyte lysate. *J. Biol. Chem.* **271:**8983–8990.
90. **Ray, B. K., T. G. Lawson, J. C. Kramer, M. H. Cladaras, J. A. Grifo, R. D. Abramson, W. C. Merrick, and R. E. Thach.** 1985. ATP-dependent unwinding of messenger RNA structure by eukaryotic initiation factors. *J. Biol. Chem.* **260:**7651–7658.
91. **Roberts, L. O., R. A. Seamons, and G. J. Belsham.** 1998. Recognition of picornavirus internal ribosome entry sites within cells; influence of cellular and viral proteins. *RNA* **4:**520–529.
92. **Rothberg, P. G., T. J. R. Harris, A. Nomoto, and E. Wimmer.** 1978. The genome-linked protein of picornaviruses. V. O^4-(5'-uridinyl)-tyrosine is the bond between the genome-linked protein and the RNA of poliovirus. *Proc. Natl. Acad. Sci. USA* **75:**4868–4872.
93. **Rozen, F., I. Edery, K. Meerovitch, T. E. Dever, W. C. Merrick, and N. Sonenberg.** 1990. Bidirectional RNA helicase activity of eukaryotic translation factors 4A and 4F. *Mol. Cell. Biol.* **10:**1134–1144.
94. **Ryan, M. D., A. M. Q. King, and G. P. Thomas.** 1991. Cleavage of foot-and-mouth disease virus polyprotein is mediated by residues located within a 19 amino acid sequence. *J. Gen. Virol.* **72:**2727–2732.
95. **Sachs, A. B., P. Sarnow, and M. W. Hentze.** 1997. Starting at the beginning, middle, and end: translation initiation in eukaryotes. *Cell* **89:**831–838.
96. **Schechter, I., and A. Berger.** 1967. On the size of the active site in proteases. I. Papain. *Biochem. Biophys. Res. Commun.* **27:**157–162.
97. **Seipelt, J., A. Guarné, E. Bergmann, M. James, W. Sommergruber, I. Fita, and T. Skern.** 1999. The structures of picornaviral proteinases. *Virus Res.* **62:**159–168.
98. **Seipelt, J., H.-D. Liebig, W. Sommergruber, C. Gerner, and E. Kuechler.** 2000. 2A proteinase of human rhinovirus cleaves cytokeratin 8 in infected HeLa cells. *J. Biol. Chem.* **275:**20084–20089.
99. **Skern, T.** 1998. Picornain 2A, p. 713–715. *In* A. J. Barrett, N. D. Rawlings, and J. F. Woessner (ed.), *Handbook of Proteolytic Enzymes.* Academic Press, London, United Kingdom.
100. **Skern, T., W. Sommergruber, H. Auer, P. Volkmann, M. Zorn, H.-D. Liebig, F. Fessl, D. Blaas, and E. Kuechler.** 1991. Substrate requirements of a human rhinoviral 2A proteinase. *Virology* **181:**46–54.
101. **Skern, T., W. Sommergruber, D. Blaas, P. Gruendler, F. Fraundorfer, C. Pieler, I. Fogy, and E. Kuechler.** 1985. Human rhinovirus 2: complete nucleotide sequence and proteolytic processing signals in the capsid protein region. *Nucleic Acids Res.* **13:**2111–2126.
102. **Sommergruber, W., H. Ahorn, H. Klump, A. Zoephel, F. Fessl, D. Blaas, E. Kuechler, H.-D. Liebig, and T. Skern.** 1994. 2A proteinases of coxsackie- and rhinovirus cleave peptides derived from eIF-4γ via a common recognition motif. *Virology* **198:**741–745.
103. **Sommergruber, W., H. Ahorn, A. Zoephel, I. Maurer-Fogy, F. Fessl, G. Schnorrenberg, H.-D. Liebig, D. Blaas, E. Kuechler, and T. Skern.** 1992. Cleavage specificity on synthetic peptide substrates of human rhinovirus 2 proteinase 2A. *J. Biol. Chem.* **267:**22639–22644.
104. **Sommergruber, W., G. Casari, F. Fessl, J. Seipelt, and T. Skern.** 1994. The 2A proteinase of human rhinovirus is a zinc containing enzyme. *Virology* **204:**815–818.
105. **Sommergruber, W., J. Seipelt, F. Fessl, T. Skern, H.-D. Liebig, and G. Casari.** 1997. Mutational analyses support a model for the HRV2 2A proteinase. *Virology* **234:**203–214.
106. **Sommergruber, W., M. Zorn, D. Blaas, F. Fessl, P. Volkmann, I. Maurer-Fogy, P. Pallai, V. Merluzzi, M. Matteo, T. Skern, and E. Kuechler.** 1989. Polypeptide 2A of human rhinovirus type 2: identification as a protease and characterisation by mutational analysis. *Virology* **169:**68–77.
107. **Sonenberg, N.** 1990. Poliovirus translation. *Curr. Top. Microbiol. Immunol.* **161:**23–47.
108. **Sonenberg, N.** 1996. mRNA 5'cap-binding protein eIF4E and control of cell growth, p. 245–269. *In* J. W. B. Hershey, M. B. Mathews, and N. Sonenberg (ed.), *Translational Control.* Cold Spring Harbor Laboratory Press, Plainview, N.Y.
109. **Sonenberg, N., M. A. Morgan, W. C. Merrick, and A. J. Shatkin.** 1978. A polypeptide in eukaryotic initiation factors that crosslinks specifically to the 5'-terminal cap in mRNA. *Proc. Natl. Acad. Sci. USA* **75:**4843–4847.
110. **Steinböck, F. A., B. Nikolic, P. A. Coulombe, E. Fuchs, P. Traub, and G. Wiche.** 2000. Dose-dependent linkage, assembly inhibition and disassembly of vimentin and cytokeratin 5/14 filaments through plectin's intermediate filament-binding domain. *J. Cell Sci.* **113:**483–491.
111. **Sun, X.-H., and D. Baltimore.** 1989. Human immunodeficiency virus tat-regulated expression of poliovirus protein 2A inhibits mRNA translation. *Proc. Natl. Acad. Sci. USA* **86:**2143–2146.
112. **Svitkin, Y. V., A. Gradi, H. Imataka, S. Morino, and N. Sonenberg.** 1999. eIF4GII, but not eIF4GI, cleavage correlates with the inhibition of host cell protein synthesis after human rhinovirus infection. *J. Virol.* **73:**3467–3472.
113. **Tarun, S. Z., and A. B. Sachs.** 1996. Association of the yeast poly(A) tail binding protein with translation initiation factor eIF-4G. *EMBO J.* **15:**7168–7177.
114. **Toyoda, H., M. J. H. Nicklin, M. G. Murray, C. W. Anderson, J. J. Dunn, F. W. Studier, and E. Wimmer.** 1986. A second virus-encoded proteinase involved in proteolytic processing of poliovirus polyprotein. *Cell* **45:**761–770.
115. **Ventoso, I., A. Barco, and L. Carrasco.** 1998. Mutational analysis of poliovirus 2A[pro]. Distinct inhibitory functions of 2A[pro] on translation and transcription. *J. Biol. Chem.* **273:**27960–27970.
116. **Ventoso, I., S. E. MacMillan, J. W. Hershey, and L. Carrasco.** 1998. Poliovirus 2A proteinase cleaves directly the eIF-4G subunit of eIF-4F complex. *FEBS Lett.* **435:**79–83.
117. **Voss, T., R. Meyer, and W. Sommergruber.** 1995. Spectroscopic characterization of rhinoviral protease 2A: Zn is essential for the structural integrity. *Protein Sci.* **4:**2526–2531.
118. **Wang, Q. M., R. B. Johnson, W. Sommergruber, and T. A. Shepherd.** 1998. Development of in vitro peptide substrates for human rhinovirus-14 2A protease. *Arch. Biochem. Biophys.* **356:**12–18.
119. **Wimmer, E.** 1982. Genome-linked proteins of viruses. *Cell* **28:**199–201.
120. **Wyckoff, E. E., J. W. B. Hershey, and E. Ehrenfeld.** 1990. Eukaryotic initiation factor 3 is required for poliovirus 2A protease-induced cleavage of the p220 component of eucaryotic initiation factor 4F. *Proc. Natl. Acad. Sci. USA* **87:**9529–9533.
121. **Wyckoff, E. E., R. E. Lloyd, and E. Ehrenfeld.** 1992. Relationship of eukaryotic initiation factor 3 to poliovirus-induced p220 cleavage activity. *J. Virol.* **66:**2943–2951.
122. **Yu, S. F., and R. E. Lloyd.** 1991. Identification of es-

sential amino acid residues in the functional activity of poliovirus 2A protease. *Virology* **182:**615–625.
123. **Yu, S. F., and R. E. Lloyd.** 1992. Characterization of the roles of conserved cysteine and histidine residues in poliovirus 2A protease. *Virology* **186:**725–735.
124. **Ziegler, E., A. M. Borman, F. G. Deliat, H.-D. Liebig, D. Jugovic, K. M. Kean, T. Skern, and E. Kuechler.** 1995. Picornavirus 2A proteinase-mediated stimulation of internal initiation of translation is dependent on enzymatic activity and the cleavage products of cellular proteins. *Virology* **213:**549–557.
125. **Ziegler, E., A. M. Borman, R. Kirchweger, T. Skern, and K. M. Kean.** 1995. Foot-and mouth disease virus Lb proteinase can stimulate rhinovirus and enterovirus IRES-driven translation and cleaves several proteins of cellular and viral origin. *J. Virol.* **69:**3465–3474.

Poliovirus-Mediated Shutoff of Host Translation: an Indirect Effect

MIGUEL ZAMORA, WILFRED E. MARISSEN, AND RICHARD E. LLOYD

25

The inhibition of host cell translation by poliovirus, also called host cell shutoff, occurs early in the infectious cycle, typically only 1.5 to 2.5 h postinfection in HeLa cells. However, only cap-dependent host translation, comprising over 95% of total translation activity in the cell (19), is blocked by poliovirus. The virus itself utilizes a cap-independent translation initiation mechanism to bind ribosomes directly to its large internal ribosome entry site (IRES) (reviewed in this volume). The defect in cap-dependent translation imposed by the virus occurs at the initiation step of translation, since polysomes have been shown to dissaggregate from cellular mRNA, then reform on viral mRNA (21, 35, 40). A landmark discovery was made by Etchison et al. in 1982 when cleavage of eukaryotic translation initiation factor 4GI (eIF4GI; formerly known as p220) was shown to occur nearly coincident with translation shutoff (shutoff lagged behind slightly). Although it was initially not known how eIF4GI cleavage could affect translation, we have since learned that eIF4GI is the large subunit of the eIF4F complex that is required for 40S ribosomal subunits to bind to the 5' end of mRNA. eIF4GI is a large scaffolding protein that furnishes binding sites for several proteins that function in translation (eIF4E, eIF4A, eIF3, mnk-1 kinase, eIF4B, and poly(A)-binding protein [PABP]) (16, 25, 33, 36). By its ability to simultaneously bind to both the cap-binding protein eIF4E and eIF3 (situated on 40S ribosomal subunits), eIF4G provides the molecular link between the 5' end of mRNA and the ribosome. This interaction is disrupted by 2A proteases of poliovirus (PV), coxsackievirus B (CVB), human rhinovirus (HRV), and the L protease of foot-and-mouth disease virus (FMDV). Each of these proteases cleaves eIF4GI at sites located between the eIF4E binding domain and the eIF3 binding domain, thus separating them (4, 23, 25, 26). Therefore, mRNA is no longer capable of efficiently binding to 40S ribosomes at this early step in initiation. Even though this seminal discovery of eIF4GI cleavage by virus infection has dominated all hypotheses of enterovirus-translation control for years, and is a major part of the translation shutoff mechanism, it alone does not account for the nearly complete block in cap-dependent translation that is observed in infected HeLa cells.

Investigation of the molecular basis of specific inhibition of cap-dependent translation in poliovirus-infected cells has been ongoing for many years, generating many breakthroughs in the understanding of translation initiation and its regulation. Despite these advances, a thoroughly satisfactory biochemical explanation for the mechanism of host shutoff that fits all experimental data is still lacking. Part of the explanation undoubtedly stems from the fact that new fundamental features of the translation process are still being uncovered and that enteroviruses have recently been shown to target new translation factors that were not previously known or thought to function in translation initiation. For instance, it has only recently been recognized that crucial cross-talk between 5' and 3' ends of mRNA mediated by proteins bound to each end of the RNA arranges mRNA into quasicircular structures. These 5'-3' interactions may mediate ribosome reinitiation at the start codon of the same mRNA after encountering a stop codon (11, 43, 44, 46). Further, there is evidence that ribosome reinitiation may occur via a fundamentally different process than de novo initiation at the cap structure (2). Most hypotheses of translation shutoff mechanisms in PV-infected cells only apply to de novo ribosome initiation, but new processes must be invoked to explain interruption of all cap-dependent translation that occurs in cells. Further, the use of different experimental approaches has led to confusion concerning whether virus-induced cleavage of translation factors is mediated by viral proteases or cellular proteases that become activated upon virus infection. In this chapter, we will first explore information regarding cleavage of new initiation factors and then discuss information relevant to whether these factors, particularly eIF4GI, are cleaved in vivo by viral or cellular proteases or both.

OTHER TRANSLATION FACTORS INVOLVED IN TRANSLATION SHUTOFF

Several groups have shown that when HeLa cells are infected in the presence of 1 to 2 mM of guanidine-HCl or other agents that selectively block viral RNA replica-

---

Miguel Zamora, Wilfred E. Marissen, and Richard E. Lloyd ■ Department of Molecular Virology and Microbiology, Baylor College of Medicine, One Baylor Plaza, Houston, TX 77030.

tion, complete cleavage of eIF4GI is observed, yet cap-dependent translation is blocked only 40 to 50%. Thus, cap-dependent translation can somehow proceed for hours in the absence of intact eIF4GI. Continued translation for such lengths of time may be due largely to repeated ribosome reinitiation mediated by 5'-3' interactions rather than ribosome runoff since transit times for ribosomes through typical open reading frames are in the order of a few minutes and virus infection does not slow ribosome elongation rates (27, 34).

Recently, the virus-induced cleavage of two translation factors has been shown to be blocked by addition of guanidine, thus implicating the cleavage of both factors as requirements in the mechanism of translation shutoff. First, the new functional homologue of eIF4GI, termed eIF4GII, was shown to be cleaved in normal infections, albeit more slowly than eIF4GI. Importantly, cleavage of eIF4GII was blocked in PV or HRV infections in the presence of guanidine (13, 42). Cleavage of eIF4GII, which could be induced by HRV 2A^{pro}, was found to correlate very well with translation shutoff during virus infection, and addition of purified eIF4GII partly restored translation in extracts in vitro (12). eIF4GII is found in a small subset of eIF4F complexes, by our estimates comprising approximately 10 to 15% of the total eIF4G in HeLa cells, which explains how eIF4GII and its cleavage products (which are distinct from eIF4GI cleavage products) had previously eluded discovery in silver stains of eIF4F preparations (4). Thus, eIF4GII would be expected to catalyze approximately 10 to 15% of total de novo initiation reactions in the cell, which does not easily account for the 50% translation still ongoing in infected cells in the presence of guanidine.

Second, two groups independently showed that PABP, which binds to eIF4GI and eIF4GII and facilitates 5'-3' interactions of mRNA, was cleaved by PV and CVB3 and CVB4 2A^{pro} (18, 22). In addition, our laboratory showed that PABP was also cleaved by PV 3C^{pro}. Recent evidence from our laboratory indicates that 3C^{pro}-mediated cleavage of PABP occurs at three cleavage sites, each distinct from the 2A^{pro} cleavage site, and 3C^{pro} preferentially cleaves ribosome-associated PABP (24a). The impact of PABP cleavage on translation in vivo is unclear since the bulk of PABP cleavage occurs relatively late in the infectious cycle and only a portion of total cellular PABP is cleaved during infection (approximately 70%). However, the importance of PABP cleavage, though currently unknown, is tantalizing since it invokes disruption of 5'-3' interactions and enteroviruses have evolved to a state where both viral proteases cleave this host target protein.

Cleavage of Most Cellular Target Proteins Requires High-Level Virus Expression; eIF4GI Cleavage Does Not

Many host proteins have been determined to be substrates of poliovirus proteases. 3C^{pro} has been shown to cleave TATA-binding protein (8), transcription factors Creb and Oct-1 (50, 51), PABP (18, 24a), and microtubule-associated protein 4 (MAP-4) (17). 2A^{pro} has been shown to cleave TATA-binding protein (49) in addition to PABP and both forms of eIF4G. When one compares these cleavage events in vivo, it can be seen that cleavage of these proteins occurs significantly later in the viral infection cycle than eIF4GI cleavage, at times when cytoplasmic concentrations of 3C^{pro} and 2A^{pro} reach high levels. We have shown that inclusion of guanidine in PV-infected HeLa cells results in at least a 20-fold decrease, more likely a 100-fold decrease, in intracellular concentrations of 2A^{pro} in infected cells at 4 h postinfection (h pi) (5) compared to normal infections. This reduction in intracellular viral protease concentration by guanidine has been shown to block cleavage of MAP-4, eIF4GII, and PABP but not eIF4GI in vivo (13, 17, 18). Since the degree of cleavage of most of these factors is dependent on the concentration of viral protease in the cell, it is generally agreed that eIF4GII, PABP, and MAP-4 cleavage is directly catalyzed by 2A^{pro} or 3C^{pro} in vivo. However, it also suggests that the mechanism of cleavage of eIF4GI in vivo, which is uniquely insensitive to guanidine addition, is somehow different from cleavage of eIF4GII and PABP. Two mechanisms that have been proposed are that 2A^{pro} directly cleaves eIF4GI in cotranslational reactions that are extremely efficient or that eIF4GI cleavage by 2A^{pro} is supplemented by activation of latent cellular proteases.

EXPERIMENTAL APPROACHES TO ELUCIDATE eIF4GI CLEAVAGE MECHANISM

Although there is general agreement that cleavage of eIF4GII and PABP is likely mediated directly by 2A^{pro} (and 3C^{pro} in the case of the latter), confusion has resulted from studies of eIF4GI cleavage as to whether direct cleavage by 2A^{pro} occurs or whether 2A^{pro} indirectly cleaves eIF4GI via activation of a cellular protease. Two approaches have been taken to understand the mechanism of eIF4GI cleavage in enterovirus-infected cells. The first was to purify the protease or protease-substrate complex from infected cells to identify the protease responsible and its substrate determinants. The rationale for this approach is that all the species found in infected cells will be present in their native configurations, allowing for any cofactors and/or conformational restrictions to be retained. As soon as cleavage of eIF4GI was discovered, it was assumed that this reaction was likely catalyzed directly by one of the viral proteases. An in vitro assay was developed to measure eIF4GI cleavage activity present in PV-infected cell extracts, which could catalyze cleavage of eIF4GI present in whole S10 lysates or ribosomal salt washes (crude initiation factor preparations). This assay was used to partially purify eIF4GI cleavage activity (which will be called eIF4Gase here), and it was shown that 3C^{pro} did not copurify with eIF4Gase and antisera against 3C^{pro} that inhibited its trans-cleavage activity did not inhibit eIF4Gase activity (28). Similarly, 2A^{pro} was found to not copurify in crude fractionation steps with cleavage activity and again, an antibody that inhibited 2A^{pro}-mediated cleavage did not inhibit eIF4Gase activity in vitro (24, 30). However, expression of 2A^{pro} in vitro or in cells was found to result in cleavage of eIF4GI (24, 29, 41); thus, 2A^{pro} was shown to be responsible for eIF4GI cleavage. Further purification of the eIF4G cleavage activity to high levels produced fractions with no detectable viral protease; however, insufficient protein was available to identify the putative cellular protease in fractions (5, 48). The prevailing conclusion from these studies was that 2A^{pro} may activate a cellular activity that cleaves eIF4GI and may cleave some eIF4GI itself, yet 2A^{pro} does not comprise the major eIF4GI-specific cleavage activity in PV-infected HeLa cells.

The second approach to attempt to understand the mechanism of eIF4G cleavage has been to purify separately the viral 2A^{pro} and eIF4G substrates, which were then incubated together in vitro. This rationale allows identification of the minimal viral and/or cellular proteins required to reconstitute cleavage reactions. This approach, which is examined in detail in chapter 24, has conclusively demonstrated that first rhinovirus and CVB4 2A^{pro} (26, 38), then PV 2A^{pro} (4), can utilize highly purified eIF4GI or peptides derived from eIF4GI as substrates in direct cleavage reactions. Related studies have also shown that eIF4G is a poor substrate of 2A^{pro} unless it is bound to eIF4E (14). Thus eIF4E can be viewed as a cofactor that likely holds eIF4G in a conformation more suitable for cleavage by 2A^{pro}. However, careful analysis of these reactions also revealed that CVB4 and PV 2A^{pro} were very inefficient at cleaving eIF4G in vitro, usually requiring near-molar equivalency of substrate and enzyme, whereas the same 2A^{pro} cleaved substrate derived from viral polyprotein at 1,000-fold higher efficiency. The poor cleavage of purified eIF4F preparations by PV 2A^{pro} and CVB4 2A^{pro} in these studies cannot be explained by lack of eIF4E cofactor since eIF4E was bound to eIF4G in all eIF4F preparations used in those studies (4). One conclusion from these studies is that 2A^{pro} itself cleaves eIF4GI; therefore, there was no requirement for virus induction of cellular activities to perform the same cleavage. Further, it has been argued that inefficient cleavage by 2A^{pro} measured in in vitro assays may not accurately reflect conditions within the cell where microenvironments may highly concentrate 2A^{pro} together with eIF4G or special conditions such as cotranslational cleavage may activate eIF4GI cleavage potential by 2A^{pro} (11a).

Thus, confusion continues to exist concerning whether cellular protease(s) or viral 2A^{pro} cleave eIF4GI in vivo and about the identity of any cellular eIF4GI-specific protease(s). So what is eIF4Gase? Work has continued in this laboratory to characterize and identify eIF4Gase activities present in both PV-infected and uninfected cells. We have discovered evidence for several eIF4Gase activities that cleave eIF4GI at different sites to produce distinct types of eIF4G cleavage products. Throughout the discussion below, we define eIF4Gase activities based on the size of cleavage products generated (which results from use of alternate cleavage sites) and the mode of induction of the activity. While it is likely that cleavage at different sites is mediated by different enzymes, it is also possible that conditions can be altered to allow one enzyme to cleave different sites under different conditions. These possibilities cannot be distinguished at this time.

eIF4Gase Activities in Uninfected Cells

One approach to identify cellular eIF4Gase is to activate this activity in uninfected cells or extracts, followed by biochemical purification of the cleavage activity. There is no doubt that several cellular proteases exist that process eIF4GI, and many laboratories have discovered that failure to include several protease inhibitors in cell extracts will result in substantial eIF4Gase degradation. In fact, the habitual inclusion of PMSF, TPCK, and other inhibitors in eIF4G substrate preparations to prevent degradation has likely inhibited progress in identification of these enzymes. Interestingly, "degradation" of eIF4GI in uninfected cell extracts often results in cleavage products that comigrate exactly with 2A^{pro}-generated cleavage products. We have identified three types of eIF4Gase activities (termed eIF4Gase-α, eIF4Gase-β, eIF4Gase-γ) that can be generated without PV infection; two of these appear similar to activities also present in infected cells. Figure 1 shows a schematic diagram of the relevant cleavage sites mapped on eIF4G. In related work, we have recently obtained the complete sequence of eIF4G, revealing yet another 40-amino-acid N-terminal extension (past the previous N-terminal methionine [20]) that was not previously reported (6a). By expressing multiple constructs containing these new upstream eIF4GI sequences, we now have evidence that the characteristic multiple banding pattern of eIF4GI results from translation initiation at multiple AUG codons, not posttranslational modifications such as phosphorylation that have been shown to occur in the C-terminal domain of the protein (6a, 37). Thus, cleavage of eIF4GI produces a set of N-terminal cleavage products that differ in defined lengths that are now known, making it easier to map protease cleavage sites.

We previously have shown that generation of apoptosis by several means of induction results in cleavage of eIF4GI (32). In these studies, two types of N-terminal eIF4GI cleavage products were detected. A transient, relatively weak cleavage activity generates cleavage products similar to 2A^{pro} cleavage products and is overtaken by a dominant activity, which generates faster-migrating N-terminal cleavage products. The latter, more vigorous activity was subsequently identified as caspase 3 (32). In collaboration with the Morley lab, we have used microsequencing to identify the two caspase cleavage sites on eIF4GI. The sites, which generate the three major N-terminal cleavage products seen on our immunoblots, are 149 amino acids (aa) upstream of the 2A^{pro} cleavage site and 106 aa upstream of the putative eIF4Gase-β cleavage site described below (6). Figure 2 shows an experiment in which cell extracts taken at time points from cisplatin-treated HeLa cells contain a cleavage activity (termed eIF4Gase-α) whose products comigrate with cleavage products from PV-infected cells. As seen previously, by later time points, caspase 3 cleavage activity becomes dominant over eIF4Gase-α, and only

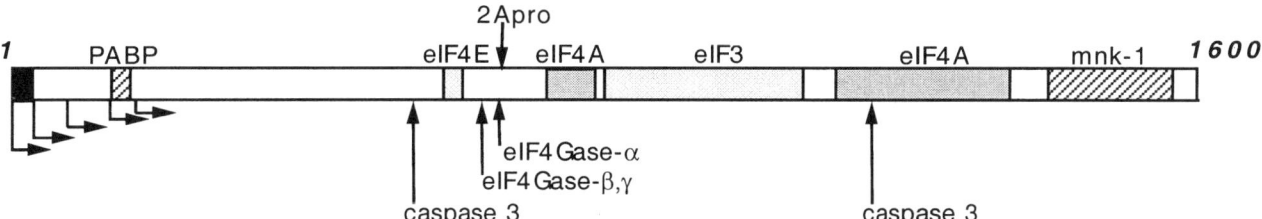

FIGURE 1 Schematic diagram of eIF4GI. Locations of known binding sites for other polypeptides are indicated by shaded or hatched areas and identified above the region. The new N-terminal extension is indicated in black. Locations of methionine residues that serve as N termini of eIF4GI isoforms are indicated by bent arrows. Arrows denote mapping of protease cleavage sites.

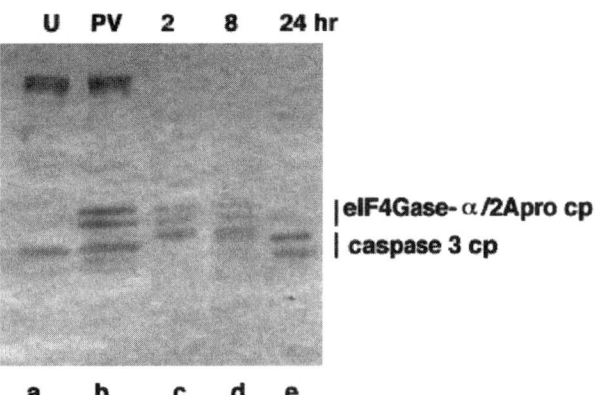

FIGURE 2 In vitro assay for eIF4Gase-α. Uninfected ribosomal salt wash preparations (RSW) containing eIF4GI were incubated alone (lane a) or with S10 extracts from HeLa cells treated with 25 cisplatin for the indicated number of hours before sample preparation (lanes c to e). Lane b contains S10 extract from PV-infected cells to show migration of 2A^{pro}/eIF4Gase-α cleavage products. Intact and cleaved eIF4G was detected by immunoblot analysis using polyclonal antiserum specific for epitopes located in the N-terminal domain of eIF4GI.

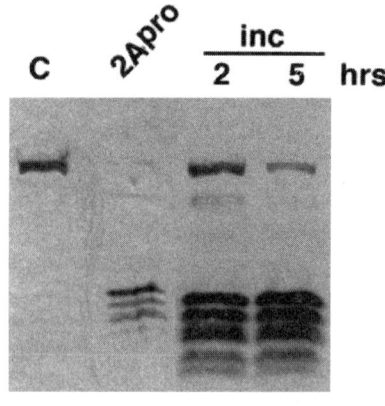

FIGURE 3 Generation of eIF4Gase-γ cleavage products. An uninfected HeLa S10 extract was incubated for 2 or 5 h at 34°C or unincubated (C). A separate S10 extract was incubated with CVB3 2A^{pro} and included in the gel as a marker. Intact and carved eIF4G was detected by immunoblot analysis.

faster-migrating caspase 3 N-terminal cleavage products are generated. This provides evidence that a PV infection is not required to generate characteristic PV-type cleavage products. It should also be mentioned that in many experiments using high levels of cisplatin or other apoptosis inducers, caspase 3 is induced so rapidly that it obscures any eIF4Gase-α activity that may be present. We have also discovered from protease inhibitor studies that eIF4Gase-α activity generated this way often also contains a calpain-like protease activity that is uniquely sensitive to calpain inhibitors. This extra cleavage activity does not generate discrete high-molecular-weight cleavage products, similar to calpain itself (47), but rather results in complete degradation of eIF4G to smaller peptides that do not contain antibody epitopes (data not shown). The lysate shown in Fig. 2 contained both protease activities, which accounted for the overall loss of eIF4G antigen.

In another experiment, we followed a lead from Hsiao Kakegawa of the Wimmer lab and were able to generate a new spontaneous eIF4GI cleavage activity in HeLa cell S10 extracts (called eIF4Gase-γ) by incubating 3 to 5 h at 34°C. We have screened many S10 extracts with this procedure and found that this specific cleavage activity, which is often weak, appeared in approximately 40% of the extracts tested. Apparently, undetermined conditions of cell growth or the cell cycle allow activation of this protease in certain cells only. When the cleavage products generated by this activity are compared with those induced by PV infection, they are found to migrate slightly faster, so that the largest cleavage fragment overlaps with the second-largest cleavage fragment produced by 2A^{pro} (see Fig. 3). Since we now know the separation in sodium dodecyl sulfate-polyacrylamide gel electrophoresis gels between the largest two eIF4GI isoforms is due to the presence of an additional 40 aa on the slower migrating isoform, this suggests that eIF4Gase-γ likely cleaves eIF4G approximately 40 to 45 aa upstream of cleavage sites used by 2A^{pro} and eIF4Gase-α. In our experiments, cleavage products of eIF4Gase-γ are indistinguishable from products generated by another activity (eIF4Gase-β, discussed below), raising the possibility that both activities may be due to the same cellular protease.

eIF4Gase Activities in Infected Cells and Cell Extracts

We have previously shown that eIF4Gase can be highly purified from infected cell extracts, and this activity contains no detectable 2A^{pro}. In data that will be reported elsewhere in detail, we have found that the C-terminal cleavage product of eIF4GI appears in gels as a closely migrating doublet, particularly early in infection. We have purified and microsequenced both of the C-terminal eIF4GI cleavage products and determined that late in infection (e.g., 4 h pi) most of the eIF4GI cleavage product has the previously published 2A^{pro} cleavage site as its N terminus. Interestingly, however, at 2 h pi, the larger band of the doublet was more prevalent, and microsequencing suggested a new N terminus 43 aa upstream beginning at the sequence VVLDKA (52). This putative new cleavage site bears no resemblance to substrate recognition sites of 2A^{pro}, but since truncation apparently occurs at the C-terminal peptide bond of an aspartic acid, this site potentially could be used by a caspase. This suggested that multiple eIF4Gase activities may be present in PV-infected cells.

The evidence for multiple cleavage activities has been further supported by chromatographic purification of eIF4Gase activity itself. Figure 4 shows that when eIF4Gase material from infected cells is applied to m^{7}GTP cap columns, an eIF4Gase activity (termed eIF4Gase-α) is eluted with low EDTA, which generates cleavage products (detected with antibody reactive with an epitope in the N-terminal third of eIF4G) indistinguishable from cleavage products generated by 2A^{pro}. At higher EDTA concentrations, a new activity elutes from the column that produces eIF4G cleavage products that migrate faster in gels (called eIF4Gase-β). Thus, generation of a set of faster-migrating bands most likely results from cleavage at a site upstream of the 2A^{pro} cleavage site. The distance of the putative new eIF4Gase-β cleavage site 43 aa upstream from the 2A^{pro} cleavage site (mentioned above) is consistent with the shift in band migration in gels observed here, which is estimated

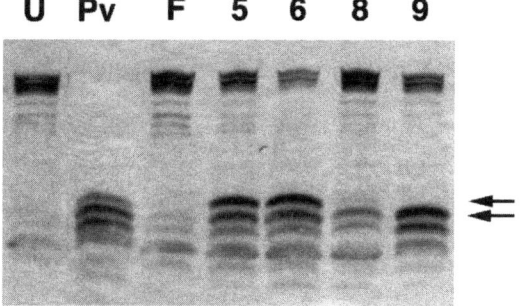

FIGURE 4 Separation of eIF4Gase-α and eIF4Gase-β activities present in infected cell extracts. RSW material from PV-infected cells was highly purified by sequential chromatography on Sephacryl S300, Fast Q Sepharose, and then applied to an m⁷GTP agarose column. Material eluting in the flow (F) or fractions containing low EDTA (5 mM) or high EDTA (25 mM) was dialyzed and incubated with RSW from uninfected cells. Fractions 5 and 6 contain eIF4Gase-α activity, which generates slow-migrating cleavage products. Fractions 8 and 9 contain eIF4Gase-β activity, which generates faster-migrating cleavage products (arrows). Lanes U and Pv contain RSW incubated alone or PV-RSW, respectively.

to be from loss of about 40 aa (the number of amino acids between the first and second methionine [start codon] in the eIF4G sequence). We have also discovered that although they comigrate on many chromatography steps, several other types of chromatographic media can separate these two activities (data not shown). Further, when radiolabeled eIF4G derived from in vitro translation of a truncated eIF4GI mRNA is used as substrate, clearly different N- and C-terminal fragments are generated by recombinant 2A^{pro} and eIF4Gase-β (data not shown), providing strong evidence for cleavage at alternate sites on eIF4G. To date, we have not been able to identify eIF4Gase-α or eIF4Gase-β, as both activities can be highly purified but result in material that contains insufficient protein for microsequencing.

Evidence is accumulating that PV infection rapidly begins induction of apoptosis, which is quickly arrested from further development by unknown viral processes (1, 45). We have shown that caspase 3 is distinct from eIF4Gase-α and eIF4Gase-β, and we have tested caspases 6, 8, 9, and 10 for the ability to cleave eIF4GI and found little to no cleavage (31). However, many proteases, including noncaspases, are activated during apoptosis signaling cascades (7, 9, 39). Further, we have also uncovered evidence for an eIF4Gase-like activity in apoptotic cell lysates (see above) (Fig. 2). We reasoned that even if several known caspases clearly do not contain eIF4Gase-α- or eIF4Gase-β-like cleavage activity, a caspase or caspase-dependent activity may still activate the enzymes that do. We also reasoned that a portion of the eIF4GI-specific cleavage activity in PV-infected HeLa cells is directly due to 2A^{pro}. However, the cleavage activity in PV infections carried out in the presence of guanidine would be skewed to contain much less 2A^{pro} and contain a higher proportion of cellular eIF4Gase. Thus, we tested whether eIF4G-specific cleavage activity produced in the presence of guanidine during PV infection could be inhibited by a broad-specificity, cell-permeable caspase inhibitor such as zVAD-fmk. In this set of experiments cells were simultaneously infected and treated with 2 mM of guanidine-HCl and/or 75 μM zVAD-fmk. At different times after infection/treatment, cells were lysed and assayed for eIF4GI cleavage by immunoblot. The data show (Fig. 5) that addition of guanidine did not block eIF4GI cleavage, as has been reported many times previously. Similarly, zVAD alone did not inhibit eIF4GI cleavage in most experiments but did delay cleavage in some (data not shown). In these cells, PV polyprotein processing was normal, suggesting that zVAD did not inhibit 2A^{pro} or 3C^{pro} activity (data not shown). In addition, direct in vitro cleavage reactions containing 75 or 150 μM of zVAD did not block 2A^{pro} cleavage of partly purified eIF4GI but did block caspase 3 cleavage of the same substrate (51). Since zVAD has no detectable effect on 2A^{pro} at these concentrations, this suggests that the majority of the cleavage activity in guanidine/PV-infected cells must be from a distinct cellular activity (eIF4Gase-α) that is sensitive to zVAD. This experiment does not demonstrate that eIF4Gase-α is a caspase, however, since the activity could be induced by a zVAD-sensitive caspase. Experiments are under way to further characterize this activity. It is important to recognize that this zVAD-sensitive eIF4Gase activity may be induced by processes or products of virus infection other than 2A^{pro}. Interestingly, it was recently reported that zVAD has no effect on eIF4G cleavage during PV infection (similar to Fig. 5, lanes 6 and 7); however, those authors did not use guanidine in their experiments, which would generate higher levels of 2A^{pro} in vivo than the experiments described here (38).

Can a Unified Mechanism of eIF4GI Cleavage Be Described?

The data presented above provide evidence for multiple cellular protease activities that process eIF4GI into high-molecular-weight products that are similar to those produced by 2A^{pro} itself. But what happens in infected cells? Actions by 2A^{pro} and cellular eIF4Gases are not mutually exclusive, and we assume that both direct and indirect cleavage reactions are involved in processing eIF4GI during virus infection. What now becomes the difficult question to determine is the relative physiological role played by these competing proteases in eIF4GI processing in vivo. Further, the relative importance of each protease may differ significantly depending on cell type infected and multiplicity of infection.

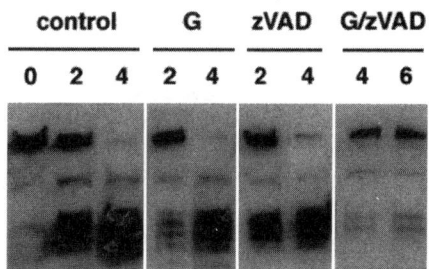

FIGURE 5 eIF4G-specific protease activity sensitive to zVAD is present in PV-infected cells. Shown is an immunoblot using eIF4GI-specific antisera of S10 extracts from four parallel PV infections initiated at a multiplicity of infection of 25 PFU/cell. Cells were collected for processing at indicated time points (h pi) from a control PV infection or PV infections supplemented with 2 mM of guanidine-HCl (G), 75 mM of zVAD-fmk, or both reagents.

It is likely that $2A^{pro}$ is more efficient at cleaving eIF4GI in vivo than in the in vitro assays described by many investigators. Since $2A^{pro}$ is first introduced to the cell via translation on a polyribosome in the immediate proximity of eIF4G, it is likely that the ongoing translation process greatly facilitates $2A^{pro}$ cleavage of eIF4GI. This could occur both by concentrating $2A^{pro}$ in the microenvironment of the ribosome and providing novel transient eIF4GI conformations that are highly susceptible to $2A^{pro}$ during the translation process. Such supersusceptible eIF4G conformations may not be present in purified eIF4F preparations. Indeed, our own experiments have often suggested that $2A^{pro}$ produced de novo by translation in vitro results in disproportionately efficient eIF4GI cleavage compared to the actual amount of $2A^{pro}$ synthesized. However, it was not possible to determine whether $2A^{pro}$ also activated cellular eIF4Gase in these types of experiments. On the other hand, a cotranslational enhancement of $2A^{pro}$ activity does not explain why cleavage of ribosome-associated PABP and eIF4GII, which should also be cotranslationally enhanced, occurs so much more slowly and is so easily blocked by guanidine. The ability of guanidine (which reduces viral protease concentrations drastically) to block cleavage of a cellular target demonstrates dependence on intracellular concentrations of $2A^{pro}$ or $3C^{pro}$ and provides some evidence for direct cleavage of those substrates by viral proteases.

Part of the quest for a unified mechanism of eIF4GI cleavage will be achieved by determining why cells contain eIF4Gase activities and to what extent these proteases regulate translation. We have observed partial regulated cleavage of eIF4GI during apoptosis (52) and also during mitosis in synchronized cells (data not shown). This illustrates at least two physiological situations in which translation rates are slowed and eIF4GI cleavage occurs.

So if eIF4G can be cleaved by cellular proteases, why did enteroviruses evolve to encode $2A^{pro}$ that could also cleave eIF4GI? Why do enteroviruses encode what is essentially a duplicate cleavage function? The answer to this question, though unknown, may lie in differential tissue-specific expression of the key cellular proteases that process eIF4GI. It is possible that enteroviruses may have adapted to grow in cell types in which these enzymes are not expressed or have low activities; thus, the ability to directly cleave eIF4GI may aid viral pathogenesis or virus spread. Some support for this notion arises from comparison of PV infections in HeLa and K562-Mu erythroblastoid cells, in which comparable $2A^{pro}$ was produced in both cell types, yet levels of eIF4GI cleavage were significantly reduced in the K562 cells and never reached completion (3). Such a result could be explained by lower expression of eIF4Gase in K562 cells. Alternatively, apparent functional duplication of $2A^{pro}$ and eIF4Gase may be illusory. It is possible that $2A^{pro}$ and eIF4Gase cleave different subcellular pools of eIF4GI in vivo. eIF4GI exists in multiple subcellular fractions and functions as a scaffolding protein that binds a growing assortment of proteins; thus, eIF4GI likely exists in distinct types of multiprotein complexes that could easily influence protease cleavages. It has already been demonstrated that $2A^{pro}$ can only cleave eIF4GI found in eIF4F complexes where it is tightly complexed with eIF4E (14). This naturally targets an eIF4GI pool intimately associated with polyribosomes. However, it has been suggested that as much as half of eIF4GI in the cell is not complexed with eIF4E, which exists in lower stoichiometric amounts (10, 15). Such pools of eIF4GI would be resistant to $2A^{pro}$ cleavage. Conversely, it is possible that individual eIF4Gases also display restricted cleavage of certain subcellular pools of eIF4GI and that a combination of activated eIF4Gase and $2A^{pro}$ is the most efficient at cleaving all eIF4GI in the cell.

It is interesting to note that poliovirus has evolved such that both $2A^{pro}$ and $3C^{pro}$ cleave the same cellular target, PABP (18, 24a). This is another, even more striking, example of apparent duplication of function. However, a clue to explain this duplication may lie in new experimental data that show that $2A^{pro}$ and $3C^{pro}$ preferentially cleave different cellular pools of PABP (24a). A similar relationship may exist between $2A^{pro}$ and any cellular eIF4Gase enzymes activated by virus infection. Thus, the curious appearance of duplication illustrates our poor understanding of the complex functions of these translation proteins and the complicated relationship of the virus with the host cell. Clearly much more research will be required before the answers to these important questions are completely elucidated.

This work was supported by NIH grants AI 27914 and GM 59803.

REFERENCES

1. **Agol, V. I., G. A. Belov, K. Bienz, D. Egger, M. S. Kolesnikova, L. I. Romanova, L. V. Sladkova, and E. A. Tolskaya.** 2000. Competing death programs in poliovirus-infected cells: commitment switch in the middle of the infectious cycle. *J. Virol.* **74:**5534–5541.
2. **Asselbergs, F., W. Peters, W. van Venrooij, and H. Bloemendal.** 1978. Diminished sensitivity of re-initiation of translation to inhibition by cap analogues in reticulocyte lysates. *Eur. J. Biochem.* **88:**483–488.
3. **Benton, P. A., J. W. Murphy, and R. E. Lloyd.** 1995. K562 cell strains differ in their response to poliovirus infection. *Virology* **213:**7–18.
4. **Bovee, M. L., B. Lamphear, R. E. Rhoads, and R. E. Lloyd.** 1998. Direct cleavage of eIF4G by poliovirus 2A protease is inefficient in vitro. *Virology* **245:**241–249.
5. **Bovee, M. L., W. E. Marissen, M. Zamora, and R. E. Lloyd.** 1998. The predominant eIF4G-specific cleavage activity in poliovirus-infected HeLa cells is distinct from 2A protease. *Virology* **245:**229–240.
6. **Bushell, M., D. Poncet, W. W. Marissen, H. Flotow, R. E. Lloyd, M. J. Clemens, and S. J. Morley.** 2000. Cleavage of polypeptide chain initiation factor eIF4GI during apoptosis in lymphoma cells: characterisation of an internal fragment generated by caspase-3-mediated cleavage. *Cell Death Different.* **7:**628–636.
6a. **Byrd, M. P., M. Zamora, and R. E. Lloyd.** 2002. Generation of multiple isoforms of eukaryotic translation initiation factor 4GI by use of alternate translation initiation codons. *Mol. Cell. Biol.* **22:**4499–4511.
7. **Chow, S. C., M. Weis, G. Kass, T. H. Holmstrom, J. E. Eriksson, and S. Orrenius.** 1995. Involvement of multiple proteases during fas-mediated apoptosis in T-lymphocytes. *FEBS Lett.* **364:**134–138.
8. **Das, S., and A. Dasgupta.** 1993. Identification of the cleavage site and determinants required for poliovirus 3CPro-catalyzed cleavage of human TATA-binding transcription factor TBP. *J. Virol.* **67:**3326–3331.
9. **Deiss, L. P., H. Galinka, H. Berissi, O. Cohen, and A. Kimchi.** 1996. Cathepsin d protease mediates programmed cell death induced by interferon-gamma, Fas/Apo1 and TNF-alpha. *EMBO J.* **15:**3861–3870.
10. **Duncan, R., S. C. Milburn, and J. W. B. Hershey.** 1987. Regulated phosphorylation and low abundance of HeLa

cell initiation factor eIF-4F suggest a role in translational control. Heat shock effects on eIF-4F. *J. Biol. Chem.* **262:** 380–388.
11. Gallie, D. R. 1998. A tale of two termini—a functional interaction between the termini of an mRNA is a prerequisite for efficient translation initiation. *Gene* **216:**1–11.
11a. Glaser, W., and T. Skern. 2000. Extremely efficient cleavage of eIF4G by picornaviral proteinases L and 2A in vitro. *FEBS Lett.* **480:**151–155.
12. Gradi, A., H. Imataka, Y. V. Svitkin, E. Rom, B. Raught, S. Morino, and N. Sonenberg. 1998. A novel functional human eukaryotic translation initiation factor 4G. *Mol. Cell. Biol.* **18:**334–342.
13. Gradi, A., Y. V. Svitkin, H. Imataka, and N. Sonenberg. 1998. Proteolysis of human eukaryotic translation initiation factor eIF4GII, but not eIF4GI, coincides with the shutoff of host protein synthesis after poliovirus infection. *Proc. Natl. Acad. Sci. USA* **95:**11089–11094.
14. Haghighat, A., Y. Svitkin, I. Novoa, E. Kuechler, T. Skern, and N. Sonenberg. 1996. The eIF4G-eIF4E complex is the target for direct cleavage by the rhinovirus 2A proteinase. *J. Virol.* **70:**8444–8450.
15. Hiremath, L. S., N. R. Webb, and R. E. Rhoads. 1985. Immunological detection of the messenger RNA cap-binding protein. *J. Biol. Chem.* **260:**7843–7849.
16. Imataka, H., A. Gradi, and N. Sonenberg. 1998. A newly identified N-terminal amino acid sequence of human eIF4G binds poly(A)-binding protein and functions in poly(A)-dependent translation. *EMBO J.* **17:**7480–7489.
17. Joachims, M., K. S. Harris, and D. Etchison. 1995. Poliovirus protease 3C mediates cleavage of microtubule-associated protein 4. *Virology* **211:**451–461.
18. Joachims, M., P. C. van Breugel, and R. E. Lloyd. 1999. Cleavage of poly(A)-binding protein by enterovirus proteases concurrent with inhibition of translation in vitro. *J. Virol.* **73:**718–727.
19. Johannes, G., M. Carter, M. Eisen, P. Brown, and P. Sarnow. 1999. Identification of eukaryotic mRNA that are translated at reduced cap binding complex eIF4F concentrations using a cDNA microarray. *Proc. Natl. Acad. Sci. USA* **96:**13118–13123.
20. Johannes, G., and P. Sarnow. 1998. Cap-independent polysomal association of natural mRNAs encoding c-myc, BiP and eIF4G conferred by internal ribosome entry sites. *RNA* **4:**1500–1513.
21. Kaufman, Y., E. Goldstein, and S. Penman. 1976. Poliovirus induced inhibition of polypeptide initiation in vitro on native polysomes. *Proc. Natl. Acad. Sci. USA* **73:** 1834–1838.
22. Kerekatte, V., B. D. Keiper, C. Bradorff, A. Cai, K. U. Knowlton, and R. E. Rhoads. 1999. Cleavage of poly(A)-binding protein by coxsackievirus 2A protease in vitro and in vivo: another mechanism for host protein synthesis shutoff? *J. Virol.* **73:**709–717.
23. Kirchweger, R., E. Ziegler, B. J. Lamphear, D. Waters, H. D. Liebig, W. Sommergruber, F. Sobrino, C. Hohenadl, D. Blaas, R. E. Rhoads, and T. Skern. 1994. Foot-and-mouth disease virus leader proteinase: purification of the Ib form and determination of its cleavage site on eIF-4 gamma. *J. Virol.* **68:**5677–5684.
24. Kräusslich, H. G., M. J. H. Nicklin, H. Toyoda, D. Etchison, and E. Wimmer. 1987. Poliovirus proteinase 2A induces cleavage of eukaryotic initiation factor 4F polypeptide p220. *J. Virol.* **61:**2711–2718.
24a. Kuyumcu-Martinez, N. M., M. Joachims, and R. E. Lloyd. 2002. Efficient cleavage of ribosome-associated poly(A)-binding protein by enterovirus 3C protease. *J. Virol.* **76:**2062–2074.
25. Lamphear, B. J., R. Kirchweger, T. Skern, and R. E. Rhoads. 1995. Mapping of functional domains in eukaryotic protein synthesis initiation factor 4G (eIF4G) with picornaviral proteases—implications for cap-dependent and cap-independent translational initiation. *J. Biol. Chem.* **270:**21975–21983.
26. Lamphear, B. J., R. Q. Yan, F. Yang, D. Waters, H. D. Liebig, H. Klump, E. Kuechler, T. Skern, and R. E. Rhoads. 1993. Mapping the cleavage site in protein synthesis initiation factor-eIF-4γ of the 2A proteases from human coxsackievirus and rhinovirus. *J. Biol. Chem.* **268:** 19200–19203.
27. Leibowitz, R., and S. Penman. 1971. Regulation of protein synthesis in HeLa cells. III. Inhibition during poliovirus infection. *J. Virol.* **8:**661–668.
28. Lloyd, R. E., D. Etchison, and E. Ehrenfeld. 1985. Poliovirus protease does not mediate cleavage of the 220,000-Da component of the cap binding protein complex. *Proc. Natl. Acad. Sci. USA* **82:**2723–2727.
29. Lloyd, R. E., M. J. Grubman, and E. Ehrenfeld. 1988. Relationship of p220 cleavage during picornavirus infection to 2A proteinase sequences. *J. Virol.* **62:**4216–4223.
30. Lloyd, R. E., H. Toyoda, D. Etchison, E. Wimmer, and E. Ehrenfeld. 1986. Cleavage of the cap binding protein complex polypeptide p220 is not effected by the second poliovirus protease 2A. *Virology* **150:**229–303.
31. Marissen, W. E., A. Gradi, N. Sonenberg, and R. E. Lloyd. 2000. Cleavage of eukaryotic translation initiation factor 4GII correlates with translation inhibition during apoptosis. *Cell Death Different.* **7:**1234–1243.
32. Marissen, W. E., and R. E. Lloyd. 1998. Eukaryotic translation initiation factor 4G is targeted for proteolytic cleavage by caspase 3 during inhibition of translation in apoptotic cells. *Mol. Cell. Biol.* **18:**7565–7574.
33. Morley, S. J., P. S. Curtis, and V. M. Pain. 1997. eIF4G —translation's mystery factor begins to yield its secrets [review]. *RNA* **3:**1085–1104.
34. Nielson, P. J., and E. H. McConkey. 1980. Evidence for the control of protein synthesis in HeLa cells via elongation rate. *J. Cell. Physiol.* **104:**269–277.
35. Penman, S., K. Scherrer, Y. Becker, and J. E. Darnell. 1963. Polyribosomes in normal and poliovirus-infected HeLa cells and their relationship to messenger RNA. *Proc. Natl. Acad. Sci. USA* **49:**654–662.
36. Pyronnet, S., H. Imataka, A. C. Gingras, R. Fukunaga, T. Hunter, and N. Sonenberg. 1999. Human eukaryotic translation initiation factor 4G (eIF4G) recruits mnk1 to phosphorylate eIF4E. *EMBO J.* **18:**270–279.
37. Raught, B., A.-C. Gingras, S. P. Gygi, H. Imataka, S. Morino, A. Gradi, R. Aebersold, and N. Sonenberg. 2000. Serum-stimulated, rapamycin-sensitive phosphorylation sites in the eukaryotic translation initiation factor 4GI. *EMBO J.* **19:**434–444.
37a. Roberts, L. O., A. J. Boxall, L. J. Lewis, G. J. Belsham, and G. E. Koss. 2000. Caspases are not involved in the cleavage of translation initiation factor eIF4GI during picornavirus infection. *J. Gen. Virol.* **81:**1703–1707.
38. Sommergruber, W., H. Ahron, H. Klump, J. Seipelt, A. Zoephel, F. Fessl, E. Krystek, D. Blaas, E. Kuechler, H. D. Liebig, and T. Skern. 1994. 2A proteinases of coxsackie- and rhinovirus cleave peptides derived from eIF-4 γ via a common recognition motif. *Virology* **198:** 741–745.
39. Squier, M. K. T., and J. J. Cohen. 1997. Calpain, an upstream regulator of thymocyte apoptosis. *J. Immunol.* **158:**3690–3697.

40. **Summers, D., J. V. Maizel, and J. E. Darnell.** 1965. Evidence for virus-specific noncapsid proteins in poliovirus-infected cells. *Proc. Natl. Acad. Sci. USA* **54:** 505–509.
41. **Sun, X.-H., and D. Baltimore.** 1989. Human immunodeficiency virus tat-activated expression of poliovirus protein 2A inhibits mRNA translation. *Proc. Natl. Acad. Sci. USA* **86:**2143–2146.
42. **Svitkin, Y. V., A. Gradi, H. Imataka, S. Morino, and N. Sonenberg.** 1999. Eukaryotic initiation factor 4GII (eIF4GII), but not eIF4GI, cleavage correlates with inhibition of host cell protein synthesis after human rhinovirus infection. *J. Virol.* **73:**3467–3472.
43. **Tarun, S. Z., and A. B. Sachs.** 1996. Association of the yeast poly(A) tail binding protein with translation initiation factor eIF-4G. *EMBO J.* **15:**7168–7177.
44. **Tarun, S. Z., Jr., S. E. Wells, J. A. Deardorff, and A. B. Sachs.** 1997. Translation initiation factor eIF4G mediates in vitro poly(A) tail-dependent translation. *Proc. Natl. Acad. Sci. USA* **94:**9046–9051.
45. **Tolskaya, E. A., L. I. Romanova, M. S. Kolesnikova, T. A. Ivannikova, E. A. Smirnova, N. T. Raikhlin, and V. I. Agol.** 1995. Apoptosis-inducing and apoptosis-preventing functions of poliovirus. *J. Virol.* **69:**1181–1189.
46. **Wells, S. E., P. E. Hillner, R. D. Vale, and A. B. Sachs.** 1998. Circularization of mRNA by eukaryotic translation initiation factors. *Mol. Cell* **2:**135–140.
47. **Wyckoff, E. E., D. E. Croall, and E. Ehrenfeld.** 1990. The p220 component of eukaryotic initiation factor-4F is a substrate for multiple calcium-dependent enzymes. *Biochemistry* **29:**10055–10061.
48. **Wyckoff, E. E., R. E. Lloyd, and E. Ehrenfeld.** 1992. Relationship of eukaryotic initiation factor 3 to poliovirus-induced p220 cleavage activity. *J. Virol.* **66:** 2943–2951.
49. **Yalamanchili, P., R. Banerjee, and A. Dasgupta.** 1997. Poliovirus-encoded protease 2Apro cleaves the TATA-binding protein but does not inhibit host cell RNA polymerase II transcription in vitro. *J. Virol.* **71:**6881–6886.
50. **Yalamanchili, P., U. Datta, and A. Dasgupta.** 1997. Inhibition of host cell transcription by poliovirus: cleavage of transcription factor CREB by poliovirus-encoded protease 3C(Pro). *J. Virol.* **71:**1220–1226.
51. **Yalamanchili, P., K. Weidman, and A. Dasgupta.** 1997. Cleavage of transcriptional activator oct-1 by poliovirus encoded protease 3c(pro). *Virology* **239:**176–185.
52. **Zamora, M., W. E. Morrisen, and R. E. Lloyd.** 2002. Multiple eIF4GI-specific protease activities present in uninfected and poliovirus-infected cells. *J. Virol.* **76:**165–177.

Effects of Picornavirus Proteinases on Host Cell Transcription

ASIM DASGUPTA, PADMAJA YALAMANCHILI, MELODY CLARK,
STEVEN KLIEWER, LEE FRADKIN, SHERYL RUBINSTEIN, SAUMITRA DAS,
YUHONG SHEN, MARY K. WEIDMAN, RAJEEV BANERJEE, UTPAL DATTA,
MEGAN IGO, PALLOB KUNDU, BHASWATI BARAT, AND ARNOLD J. BERK

26

Viruses are obligate intracellular parasites and thus they are dependent on the host cell machinery for replication, transcription, and translation of viral genes. Many viruses are known to shut off transcription or translation or both of host cell genes to increase expression of their own genes (27). The shutoff of host cell functions also leads to some of the pathogenesis of viral infections. Poliovirus (PV) is known to shut off both host cell transcription and translation. It is believed that the shutoff of host cell transcription in PV-infected cells increases the pool of free ribonucleotides that the PV-encoded RNA-dependent RNA polymerase (Pol) uses to transcribe and replicate the viral genomic RNA. In support of this theory, PV first shuts off Pol I-mediated transcription in the cell that accounts for greater than 50% of all host cell transcription. Pol II transcription is inhibited next, followed by inhibition of Pol III transcription. We have used in vitro transcription systems for understanding the mechanism by which PV shuts off host cell transcription catalyzed by RNA Pol I, II, and III.

PV

PV is the prototype agent of a large group of medically important viruses (picornaviruses) that include those inducing infectious hepatitis (hepatitis A), common cold (rhinoviruses), encephalitis, and mycocarditis (coxsackieviruses). The single-stranded, plus-polarity RNA genome (~7,500 nucleotides) of PV is translated into one large polyprotein, which is cotranslationally processed by virus-encoded proteases $2A^{pro}$, $3C^{pro}$, and $3CD^{pro}$ to release the mature viral structural and nonstructural proteins (53). The nonstructural proteins include viral proteases, the viral RNA-dependent RNA polymerase ($3D^{pol}$), the genome-linked protein (VPg or 3B), an RNA-binding protein containing NTPase activity (2C), and protein 2B. Both biochemical and genetic evidence suggests that most of the nonstructural proteins (and some of their precursors) of PV are involved in viral RNA replication (35, 53). The viral proteases have been extensively studied and found to be very specific in polyprotein cleavage; $3C^{pro}$ and $3CD^{pro}$ cleave the polyprotein at glutamine-glycine (QG) bonds while the $2A^{pro}$ cleaves only at tyrosine-glycine (YG) bonds (35). The proteases do not cleave every potential cleavage site within the polyprotein; other determinants such as accessibility and context of the cleavage site are also important. Soon after infection, PV shuts off host cell RNA and protein synthesis. The two processes are unrelated, i.e., inhibition of host cell translation is not the cause of host cell transcription shutoff (27). Although host cell transcription is shut off in infected cells, the viral RNA needed both for encapsidation and use as a messenger RNA is synthesized by $3D^{pol}$ (3). Unlike 5'-capped host cell mRNAs, the uncapped PV RNA is translated by a mechanism known as internal ribosome entry site-mediated translation, which involves ribosome binding within the 5' untranslated region of viral RNA, upstream of the initiator AUG codon (62). This provides the virus with the opportunity of shutting off cellular mRNA translation by proteolytic cleavage of a component (eIF4G) of the cap-binding protein (CBP) complex required for capped mRNA translation, without compromising its own protein synthesis (6, 19, 34, 38, 69).

HOST CELL TRANSCRIPTION SHUTOFF BY PV

Infection of susceptible cells with PV results in rapid and dramatic changes in macromolecular metabolism, including the shutoff of host cell transcription. Infection of HeLa cells with PV, for example, causes a severe decrease in transcription catalyzed by RNA Pol I, II, and III. Transcription mediated by Pol I is inhibited first, at 1 to 2 h postinfection, followed by the inhibition of Pol II- and Pol III-mediated transcription at approximately 3 and 4 h postinfection, respectively. Two observations suggest that the synthesis of viral proteins is required for transcriptional in-

---

Asim Dasgupta, Padmaja Yalamanchili, Melody Clark, Steven Kliewer, Lee Fradkin, Sheryl Rubinstein, Saumitra Das, Yuhong Shen, Mary K. Weidman, Rajeev Banerjee, Utpal Datta, Megan Igo, Pallob Kundu, Bhaswati Barat, and Arnold J. Berk ■ Department of Microbiology, Immunology and Molecular Genetics, UCLA School of Medicine, and The Molecular Biology Institute, UCLA, Los Angeles, CA 90095-1747.

hibition: first, an intact viral genome is required for the inhibition of transcription; ultraviolet-irradiated PV is unable to inhibit transcription; second, drugs that block translation prevent the inhibition of transcription (27).

Early attempts to identify the cellular components of the transcriptional machinery inactivated by picornavirus infection focused on the polymerases. However, RNA Pol I, II, and III solubilized from infected cell extracts were shown to be fully active when assayed under conditions requiring only nonspecific initiation. Furthermore, no differences were seen in the chromatographic properties of the polymerases partially purified from mock-infected or virus-infected cells. These data suggested that transcriptional components other than the elongation-competent polymerases were inactivated by viral infection (2, 56). More recent studies, however, have shown that the IIO subspecies of RNA Pol II is modified after infection of cells with PV and that this modification is prevented by cycloheximide and zinc (48). Although these results suggest that one or more viral proteins are responsible for the modification of the IIO polypeptide, the functional relevance of this modification is not known.

Crawford et al. first showed that the PV-induced inhibition of transcription observed in vivo could be recapitulated in vitro (12). Unlike whole-cell extracts prepared from mock-infected cells, extracts prepared from PV-infected HeLa cells at 3 h postinfection were unable to catalyze specific transcription from the adenovirus major late promoter. Addition of partially purified Pol II failed to restore transcription in infected cell extracts. However, addition of a chromatographic fraction containing a subset of the Pol II transcription factors (TFs) efficiently restored transcription from the major late promoter in vitro. These data suggested that one or more transcription factors required for Pol II transcription in vitro were inactivated by PV infection. In addition to the Pol II data, Crawford et al. also showed that inhibition from the Pol III-transcribed adenovirus VA promoter was inhibited in extracts prepared from PV-infected cells at 5 h postinfection.

The ability to reproduce PV-mediated inhibition of transcription in vitro provided a powerful tool with which to study the mechanism of transcriptional inhibition. Our laboratory has focused its efforts during the last several years on determining which TFs required for specific transcription in vitro by Pol I, II, and III are inactivated by PV infection and the mechanism(s) of this inactivation. Fradkin et al. first showed that the inhibition of Pol III-mediated transcription by PV infection was the result of inactivation of specific transcription factors (22). The activities of Pol III and TFIIIA were unaffected by PV infection. However, the transcriptional activity of TFIIIC was severely reduced in infected cell extracts; the activity of TFIIIB was also reduced, though to a lesser degree. Interestingly, the reduction in TFIIIC transcriptional activity was not reflected by a concomitant reduction in the DNA-binding activity of TFIIIC, indicating that domains other than those involved in DNA binding were affected by viral infection. The inhibition of Pol I- and Pol II-mediated transcription has also been shown to be the result of the inactivation of specific transcription factors. We will briefly describe the cellular RNA Pol I, II, and III transcription machineries and discuss shutoff of transcription by PV in those contexts.

RNA Pol II Machinery and Shutoff by PV

Eukaryotic DNA-dependent RNA polymerases cannot locate promoters on their own. Promoter recognition is imparted by basal (general) transcription factors that can be separated easily from the RNA polymerase during purification (5, 55). For Pol II, a crucial basal factor is the TATA-binding protein (TBP), which interacts with the TATA box located approximately 25 bp upstream of the transcription start site (Fig. 1). Once bound to the DNA, TBP recruits transcription factor B (TFIIB), which, in turn, recruits Pol II and other basal factors such as TFIIA, TFIIE, TFIIF, TFIIG, and TFIIH (77). This leads to basal transcription from simple Pol II promoters (core promoters). Activator-dependent transcription from more complex promoters (those containing cis-acting, upstream binding sites such as AP-1, SP-1, CREB, Oct-1, etc.), however, requires additional proteins, called TBP-associated factors (TAFs) (47). In such transcription, TBP is tightly associated with TAFs to form a multiprotein complex called TFIID (Fig. 1). In activated Pol II transcription, transcriptional activators bound to cis-acting sequences stimulate the activity of the basal transcription complex by mediating interactions with basal transcription factors and TAFs (Fig. 1) (18–46).

Proteolytic Cleavage and Inactivation of Basal Transcription Factor TBP by 3C^{pro}

It is now clear that the TBP, first identified as a component of the Pol II factor, TFIID, is not only required for transcription by RNA Pol II, but also is required for RNA Pol I and III (11, 41, 50, 58). TBP associates with different sets of TAFs of 250, 125, 95, 78, and 50 kDa in HeLa cells (78). A TBP-TAF complex (SL1) is a Pol I factor, and these TAFs are different from those in TFIID, having polypeptides of 110, 63, and 43 kDa (11). Pol III transcription factor TFIIIB consists of three subunits in yeast: the TBP and two TAFs having molecular masses of 70 and 90 kDa (64) (Fig. 1).

Two lines of evidence from our laboratory suggested that TFIID was inactivated in PV-infected HeLa cells. The specific activity of TFIID was fivefold less when isolated from PV-infected cells compared with that from uninfected (or mock-infected) cells (31). Also, only TFIID, but no other TF, could specifically restore Pol II transcription in virus-infected cell extracts. Both TATA- and initiator-mediated basal transcription is inhibited in HeLa cell extracts prepared at approximately 4 h postinfection (72). As a consequence of inhibition of basal transcription, SP1-mediated activated transcription from both the TATA and initiator was inhibited at the same time postinfection (72). Inhibition of basal transcription could be reproduced by incubation of uninfected HeLa cell extracts with purified recombinant 3C^{pro} but not with an enzymatically inactive point mutant of 3C^{pro} (Fig. 2). We also demonstrated that TBP was proteolytically cleaved in PV-infected cells, generating two cleaved products (10). The two cleaved forms of TBP in PV-infected cell extract can be reproduced in vitro by incubating TBP with 3C^{pro} and 2A^{pro} (Fig. 3B) (70). Site-directed mutagenesis showed that while 3C^{pro} cleaves at the N-terminal 18th QG site, 2A^{pro} cleaves TBP at the 34th YG bond (14) (Fig. 3A). However, only 3C^{pro} but not 2A^{pro} was able to inhibit TATA-mediated Pol II transcription in vitro (70). A mutant PV (Sel 3C-02), which has a valine-to-alanine substitution at amino acid 54 of 3C^{pro}, was used to determine whether it was defective in inhibiting basal transcription. This mutant virus produces a small plaque phenotype; however, it grows to nearly wild-type titers because PV overproduces 3C^{pro} and other viral proteins. The mutant protease is not totally defective

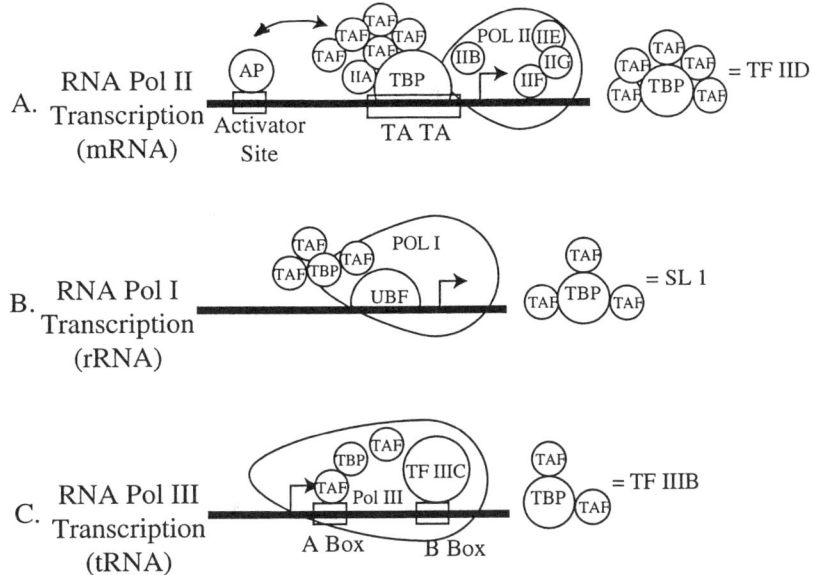

FIGURE 1 Schematic diagram of preinitiation complex assembly for RNA Pol II, Pol I, and Pol III transcription. (A) Basal and activated transcription complex formation at the TATA box is shown. TBP plus five TAFs constitute TFIID. TFIIA through TFIIF are general transcription factors. Pol II is RNA polymerase II. Activator proteins (AP) bind to upstream activator sites and interact with the basal complex (indicated by two-headed arrow) to promote activated transcription. Single-headed arrow shows transcription start site. (B) RNA Pol I transcription requires cooperative binding of UBF and SL1 (TBP plus three TAFs) to rRNA promoter. (C) RNA Pol III transcription requires binding of TFIIIC to B-box internal promoter and recruitment of TFIIIB (TBP plus TAFs) and Pol III.

but is much less active than the wild-type protease. The mutant virus was found to be much less effective in inhibiting basal transcription from both TATA and initiator promoters (72) (Fig. 4).

To examine whether $3C^{pro}$ is sufficient to cause inhibition of host cell transcription seen in virus-infected cells, $3C^{pro}$ was cloned into the eukaryotic expression vector pCDNA. Two reporter plasmids that support SP1-activated TATA and initiator-mediated RNA Pol II transcription in vivo were used in transient transfection assays. Transcription from both TATA and initiator promoters was drastically inhibited by $3C^{pro}$ in cotransfected cells (72). Thus, $3C^{pro}$ alone in the absence of other viral proteins was able to shut off Pol II transcription in vivo. A number of observations strongly suggested that inactivation of TBP (by $3C^{pro}$) was the major cause of transcription shutoff by PV.

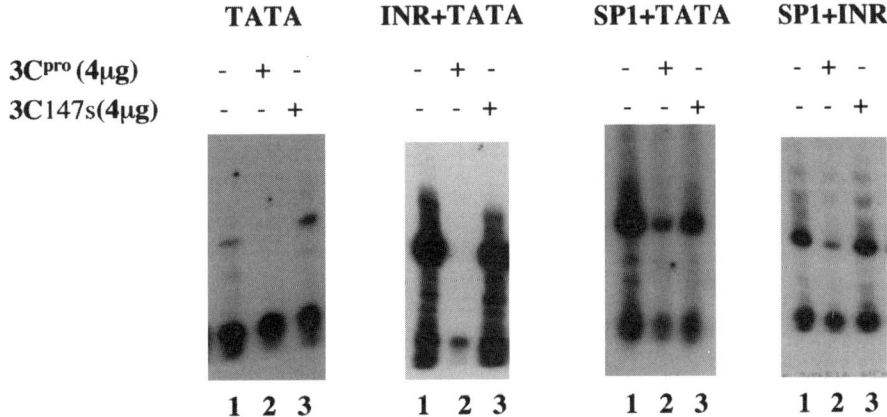

FIGURE 2 Effect of purified $3C^{pro}$ on basal and activated transcription. Nuclear extracts prepared from uninfected HeLa cells were treated with *Escherichia coli*-expressed and purified $3C^{pro}$ before being used in an in vitro transcription reaction. (A) TATA-, (B) TATA-plus-INR-, (C) SP1-plus-TATA-, and (D) SP1-plus-INR-mediated transcription was determined in the absence (lanes 1) or presence of bacterially expressed purified wild-type $3C^{pro}$ (lanes 2) or an inactive protease mutant, 3C-147S (lanes 3).

A MDDQNNSLPPYA<u>QG</u>LASP<u>QG</u>AMTPGIPIGSPMMR(YG)TGLTPQPIQNTNSLSILEEQQR
QQQQQQQQQQQQQQQQQQQQQQQQQQQQQQQQQQQQQQQAVAAAAVQQSTSQQ
A<u>QG</u>GTSGQAPQLFHSQTLTTAPLPGTTPLYPSPMTPMTPITPATPASESSGIVPQLQNI
VSTVNLGCKLDLKTIIALRRRRNAEYNPPKRRFFAAVIIMRIREPRTTALIIFFSSGKMVCTG
AKSEEQSRRLAARKYARVVQKLGFPAKFLDFKIQNMVGSSCDVKFPIRLEGLVLTHQQ
FSSYEPELFFPGLIYYRMIRRRIVLLIIFVSGKVVLTGAKVRAEIYEAFENIYPILKGFRKTTZ

Potential Cleavage at:	Protease	Expected Apparent MW
amino acid 12	3C	39 kD
amino acid 18	3C	38
amino acid 34	2A	36
amino acid 115	3C	28
full length TBP	(37.4)	41

B

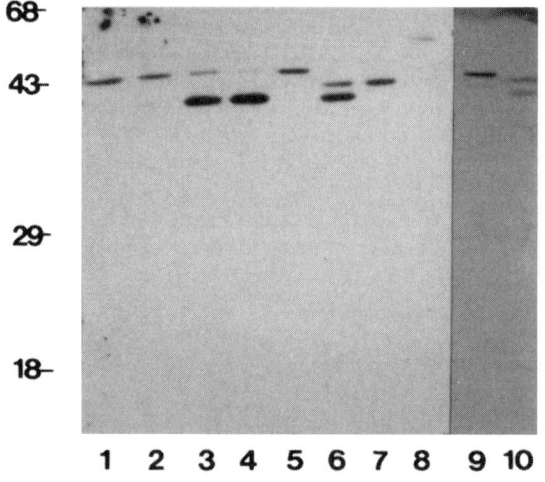

FIGURE 3 Sequence and potential poliovirus protease cleavage sites in TBP. (A) Predicted amino acid sequence of human TBP is shown. Three glutamine-glycine (QG) sites are boxed, and a tyrosine-glycine (YG) site is circled. The lower panel shows predicted size of TBP if it is cleaved by $3C^{pro}$ at the QG sites and by $2A^{pro}$ at the YG site. The predicted molecular mass of TBP is 37.4 kDa, but the apparent molecular mass in our sodium dodecyl sulfate gels is 41 kDa. (B) Western blot analysis of recombinant purified TBP treated with recombinant purified $2A^{pro}$ and $3C^{pro}$. Bacterially expressed and purified TBP (lane 1) was incubated with increasing amounts of $2A^{pro}$ (lanes 2 to 4) or $\Delta 2A^{pro}$ (lane 5), $3C^{pro}$ (lane 7), or both $2A^{pro}$ and $3C^{pro}$ (lane 6). $2A^{pro}$ alone was also run alongside as a control (lane 8). Mock- and PV-infected HeLa cell extracts (lanes 9 and 10, respectively) were also analyzed. The position of full-length TBP is indicated by an arrow. The positions of $3C^{pro}$- and $2A^{pro}$-cleaved TBP are indicated by a square and an asterisk, respectively.

First, both basal and SP1-activated RNA Pol II transcription in PV-infected cell extract was fully restored by exogenously added bacterially expressed TBP (Fig. 5) (72). Second, infection of cells with a mutant PV defective in $3C^{pro}$ function did not result in shutoff of Pol II transcription (72). Third, addition of purified TBP restored transcription in heat-treated nuclear extracts from mock- and virus-infected cells to identical levels (Fig. 6). As TBP is the only component that is preferentially inactivated by heating transcription extracts at 47° for 10 min (31, 68), the ability of recombinant TBP to restore transcription in both mock- and virus-infected extracts to identical levels suggests that the only basal component inactivated in PV-infected cells is TBP. Finally, incubation of TBP with $3C^{pro}$ inhibited its ability to form a complex with the TATA box (Fig. 7) (72). Thus, $3C^{pro}$-modified TBP was unable to bind the TATA box. The conundrum was why removal of 18 N-terminal amino acids of TBP by $3C^{pro}$ led to inhibition of transcription, yet removal of 34 N-terminal amino acids by $2A^{pro}$ did not result in transcription inhibition (70).

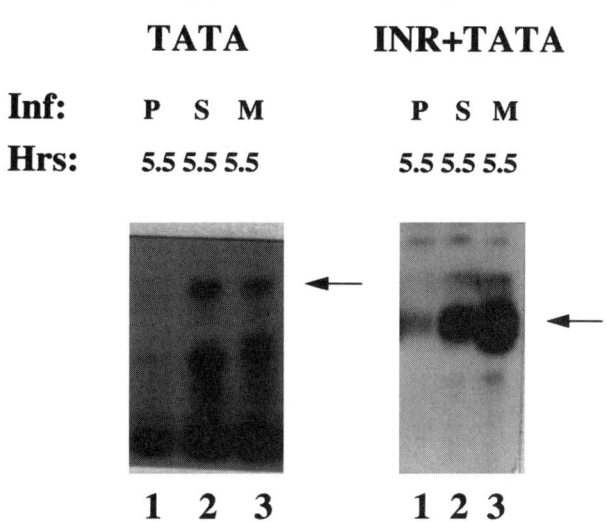

FIGURE 4 Inhibition of basal transcription by PV. Transcription from the (A) TATA and (B) TATA plus INR in cell extracts prepared from mock-infected (M), wild-type PV-infected (P), and PV Sel 3C-02 mutant-infected (S) cells is shown.

Later studies with NΔ18 TBP (truncated TBP in which the N-terminal 18 amino acids were deleted) showed that NΔ18 TBP was fully transcriptionally active (data not shown). Thus, the cleavage of TBP at the 18th QG site by 3C^{pro} was probably not the cause for transcription inhibition. We recently found that 3C^{pro} can cleave TBP at a site that lies between amino acids 105 and 115, and this cleavage appears to be responsible for TATA-mediated Pol II transcription shutoff (to be published elsewhere).

The role of N-terminal amino acids to TBP is poorly understood. The C-terminal half of TBP appears to be important for TATA-mediated transcription from Pol II promoters. Recently it has been reported that the N-terminal amino acids of TBP are essential for RNA Pol III transcription from the small nuclear RNA (SnRNA) promoters (42). An interesting question is whether removal of N-terminal 18 and 34 amino acids of TBP by 3C^{pro} and 2A^{pro}, respectively, would lead to inhibition of SnRNA transcription. Thus, both 3C^{pro} and 2A^{pro} could potentially inhibit SnRNA transcription.

Cleavage and Inactivation of Activated Transcription Factors by 3C^{pro}

In addition to basal factor TBP, three activator proteins, CREB (cyclic AMP-responsive element-binding protein required for activation of cAMP-regulated genes), Oct-1 (octamer-binding protein that activates SnRNA transcription), and tumor suppressor p53, are also cleaved by 3C^{pro} in vitro and in PV-infected cells. Both CREB and Oct-1 cleavage by 3C^{pro} results in altered binding of these factors to the target sequence (71, 73). While both CREB and Oct-1 are directly cleaved by 3C^{pro}, degradation of p53 appears to require both 3C^{pro} and a cellular activity (P. Yalamanchili, M. K. Weidman, and A. Dasgupta, unpublished data). Recent results from our laboratory suggest that 3C^{pro} activates a latent cellular protease, which in turn cleaves (or degrades) p53 in virus-infected cells. The nature of the cellular component(s) required along with 3C^{pro} for cleavage of p53 remains to be determined.

Previous results from our laboratory demonstrated dephosphorylation and transcription inactivation of CREB in PV-infected cells (32). Because basal transcription is inhibited by infection of cells with PV, it was necessary to dissociate CREB-mediated activated transcription from basal transcription to examine the role of 3C^{pro} in CREB-activated transcription. This was achieved by purifying CREB away from other transcription factors that are af-

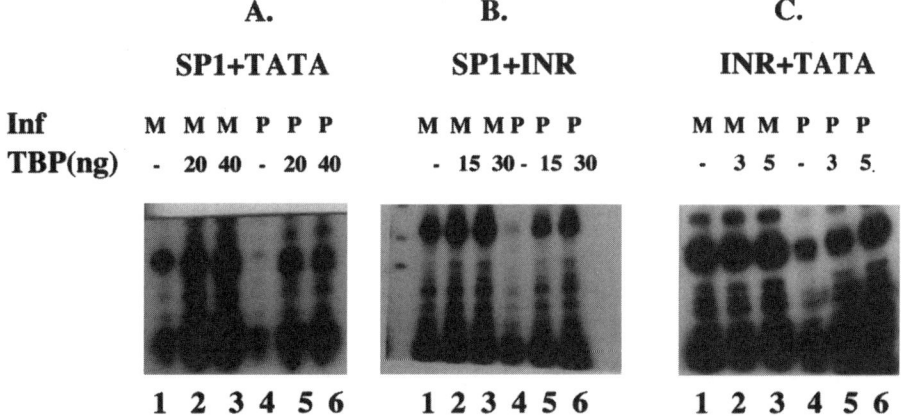

FIGURE 5 Restoration of transcription by TBP. Recombinant TBP was added to mock-infected and PV-infected cell extracts. These TBP-supplemented extracts were then used for in vitro transcriptional analysis. The DNA templates used for transcription contained (A) SP1 plus TATA, (B) SP1 plus INR, and (C) INR plus TATA sequence elements. Transcription reactions were performed with mock-infected nuclear extract (lanes 1) and mock-infected nuclear extracts supplemented with increasing amounts of TBP (lanes 2 and 3). Transcription reactions were also performed with PV-infected extracts prepared 4 h postinfection (lanes 4) and PV-infected extracts supplemented with increasing amounts of TBP (lanes 5 and 6). The amount of TBP added is indicated at the top. Panel B has the pBR/HpaII marker in the far-left lane.

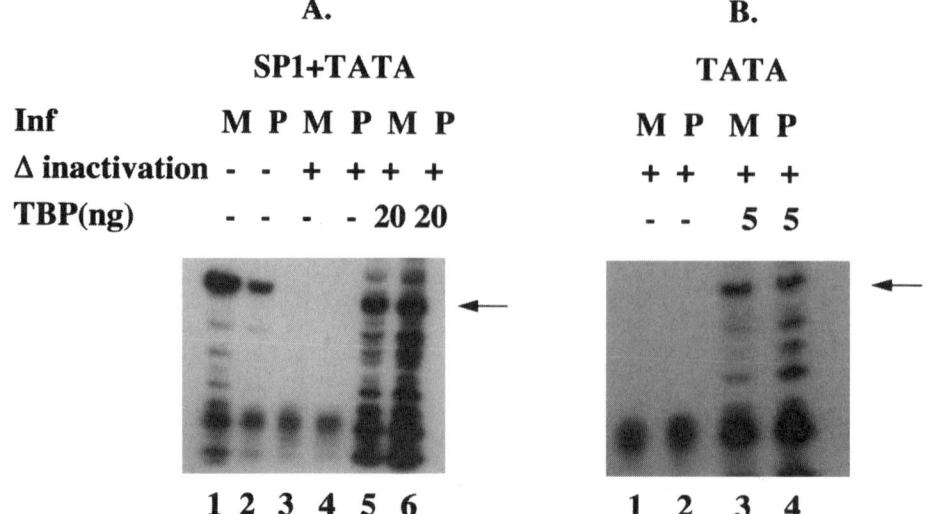

FIGURE 6 Restoration of transcription by TBP in heat-inactivated PV-infected extracts. Transcription from (A) TATA + SP1 and (B) TATA promoter was carried out in either unheated or heated (47°C for 15 min) mock-infected (M) or PV-infected (PV) cell extract in the presence or absence of purified TBP as indicated.

fected by virus infection (e.g., TBP). The activities of purified CREB isolated from mock- and virus-infected cells were studied in CREB-depleted transcription extracts derived from mock-infected cells (71). This system allowed us to directly study the effects of PV infection (and 3C^{pro}) on CREB. We demonstrated that CREB was specifically cleaved by the viral protease 3C^{pro} both in vivo and in vitro (Fig. 8). The QG bond at position 172 was cleaved by 3C^{pro}. The 3C^{pro}-mediated cleavage of CREB led to a significant loss of its DNA binding as well as transcriptional activity (71). The phosphorylated, transcriptionally active form of CREB was cleaved by the viral protease 3C^{pro}. These results suggested that a direct cleavage of CREB by 3C^{pro} leads to inhibition of CREB-activated transcription in PV-infected HeLa cells.

The octamer-binding transcription factor, Oct-1, was also found to be specifically cleaved by 3C^{pro} in vitro and in virus-infected cells (73). PV infection led to the formation of altered Oct-1-DNA complexes that could also be generated by incubation of Oct-1 with purified 3C^{pro}. We demonstrated that the 3C^{pro}-cleaved Oct-1 lost its ability to inhibit transcriptional activation by the simian virus 40 B enhancer. The Oct-1 protein is modular and contains three distinct domains (Fig. 9). The N-terminal domain is essential for activation of transcription. It extends from amino acids 1 to 280. The homeodomain from amino acids 280 to 440 is essential for DNA binding. The C-terminal domain extends from amino acids 440 to 766. The Oct-1 protein contains four QG sites at positions 236, 239, 330, and 602. The molecular weight of the 3C^{pro}-catalyzed cleaved product (55 kDa) (compared to the full-length 94-kDa Oct-1) is consistent with the cleavage at position 330. The 55-kDa cleaved product seen in PV-infected cells must have an N-terminal deletion, since the N terminus is essential for activated transcription and the cleaved Oct-1 would no longer support activated transcription.

We have shown recently that the transcriptional activator (tumor suppressor) p53 is degraded in HeLa cells when infected with the wild-type PV but not with a mutant PV (Sel 3C-02) defective in 3C^{pro} function (Yalamanchili et al., unpublished). Degradation of p53 can be achieved in vitro by incubating mock-infected HeLa extracts with recombinant 3C^{pro}. The recombinant, purified p53, however, is not cleaved by 3C^{pro} in vitro unless the reactions are supplied with an uninfected HeLa cell extract. It, therefore, appears that 3C^{pro}-catalyzed degradation of p53 requires one or more cellular activities. HeLa cells and rabbit reticulocyte lysates contain this activity; however, wheat germ extracts lack this activity. The activity from HeLa cells is heat labile and is also inactivated by infection

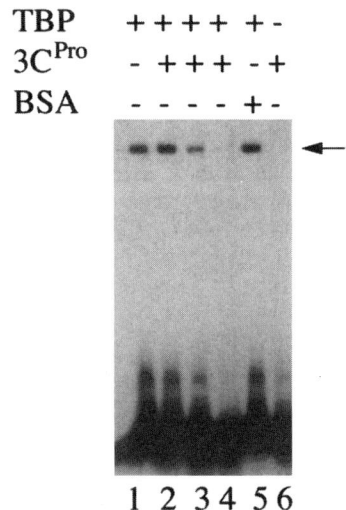

FIGURE 7 Gel retardation analysis of TBP binding to the TATA box following 3C^{pro} treatment. Gel retardation assays were performed with purified TBP without 3C^{pro} (lane 1) or treated with 1, 4, or 8 µg of 3C^{pro} (lanes 2 through 4) or 8 µg of bovine serum albumin (BSA) (lane 5). Lane 6 contained 8 µg of 3C^{pro} but not TBP.

A.

MTMESGAENQQSGDAAVTEAENQQMTVQAPQIATLAQVS
MPAAHATSSAPTVTLVRCPMGNSQVHGVIQAAQPSVIQSP
QVQTVQISTIAESEDSQESVDSVTDSQKRREILSRRPSYR
KILNDLSSDAPGVPRIEEEKSEEETSAPAITTVTVPTPIY
QTSSGQYIAIT**QG**GAIQLANNGTDGV**QG**LQTLTMTNAAAT
QPGTTILQYAQTTDGQQILVPSNQVVVQAASGDVQTYQIR
TAPTSTIAPGVVMASSPALPTQPAEEAARKREVRLMKNRE
AARECRRKKKEYVKCLENRVAVLENQNKTLIEELKALKDLY
CHKSD

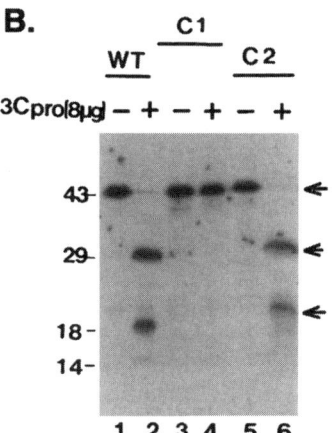

FIGURE 8 (A) Predicted amino acid sequence and potential 3C^{pro} cleavage sites in CREB. Two glutamine-glycine (QG) sites are boxed. (B) Identification of the 3C^{pro} cleavage site in CREB. Site-directed mutagenesis was used to replace the QG pairs at positions 172 and 187 with valine-aspartate pairs. The wild type (WT; lanes 1 and 2) and mutants C1 (position 172; lanes 3 and 4) and C2 (position 187; lanes 5 and 6) were translated in the presence of [^{35}S]methionine. The in vitro translated proteins were incubated with buffer (−; lanes 1, 3, and 5) or purified 3C^{pro} (+; lanes 2, 4, and 6). Labeled products were analyzed by sodium dodecyl sulfate-polyacrylamide gel electrophoresis. The positions of molecular mass (in kilodaltons) markers are indicated on the left, and the positions of full-length CREB and cleaved products are indicated by arrows on the right.

of HeLa cells with vaccinia virus. These results suggest that PV-encoded protease 3C^{pro} does not directly cleave p53 and possibly activates a cellular enzyme that in turn degrades p53.

The homologous 3C^{pro} from another picornavirus, foot-and-mouth disease virus, also inhibits gene expression when transiently transfected into HeLa cells (66). This inhibition is believed to be caused by cleavage of histone H3, a phenomenon not detected in PV-infected cells (20). Another animal RNA virus, vesicular stomatitis virus (VSV), also shuts off host cell RNA transcription (1). The matrix protein M appears to be responsible for RNA Pol II shutoff by VSV. The same transcription factor (TBP) targeted by PV is also targeted by VSV (76). However, unlike proteolytic cleavage of TBP by PV, VSV-induced inhibition of Pol II transcription does not involve reduction of intact TBP. The mechanism of TBP inactivation in VSV-infected cells remains to be determined. The delta antigen of the hepatitis delta virus (HDV), a replication-defective RNA-containing virus, also inhibits cellular RNA Pol II-mediated transcription (39). Evidence suggests that HDV RNA is replicated by the cellular DNA-dependent RNA polymerase, which is programmed by the delta antigen to copy HDV RNA specifically. Thus, it is believed that the delta antigen participates in a complex with host cell Pol II transcription factors to mediate Pol III-dependent HDV RNA replication, concomitantly inhibiting cellular Pol II transcription.

PV inhibits basal transcription by inactivating TBP. Since basal transcription is up-regulated by activators such as CREB, Oct-1, and p53, why does the virus also target activated transcription? The inhibition of basal transcription is never complete in infected cells, and the residual level of basal transcription can be stimulated by the activators. Inactivating both basal and activated transcription ensures that there is maximal level of inhibition of transcription in PV-infected cells.

RNA Pol III Transcription and Shutoff by PV

RNA Pol III transcribes a set of genes giving rise to small RNAs. This family includes the 5S RNA, tRNAs, the VA genes of adenovirus, and the EBER genes of Epstein-Barr virus. Two transcription factors, TFIIIB and TFIIIC, are required in addition to RNA Pol III for transcription of tRNA and adenovirus VA genes in vitro (57). Another transcription factor, TFIIIA, is required solely for transcription of 5S rRNA genes. The first step in formation of a stable transcription complex on a tRNA or VA RNA gene is the sequence-specific binding of TFIIIC to B-box internal Pol III promoter element. This binding is necessary to position TFIIIB at the start site of the gene. Subsequently, RNA Pol III is assembled on the promoter by recognition of TFIIIB (23). Once assembled on the promoter by TFIIIC, TFIIIB will remain associated with the DNA template and promote initiation of Pol III transcription after dissociation of the TFIIIC factor (29, 30) (Fig. 1). TFIIIB is best characterized from the yeast *Saccharomyces cerevisiae* (29). It contains TBP and two TAFs (called BRF and B″) having apparent molecular masses of 70 and 90 kDa. Human TBP interacts with yeast BRF and B″ to form functional TFIIIB (64). The DNA binding component of TFIIIC contains five polypeptides of 240, 110, 100, 80, and 60 kDa, referred to as α, β, γ, δ, and ε subunits, respectively (33, 75). The α subunit of both yeast and human TFIIIC can be specifically cross-linked to B-box DNA (75).

Earlier studies showed that transcriptional activity of TFIIIA and RNA Pol III was not affected by infection of HeLa cells with PV (22). Transcriptional activity of TFIIIC was drastically reduced (six- to eightfold) by PV infection compared to TFIIIC isolated from mock-infected cells (22). When TFIIIC DNA-binding activity was assayed in extracts of infected cells by gel retardation assay, transcriptionally inactive forms of B-box binding activity that had mobilities much greater than that of (mock-infected cell-derived) TFIIIC-DNA complex were detected (Fig. 10B).

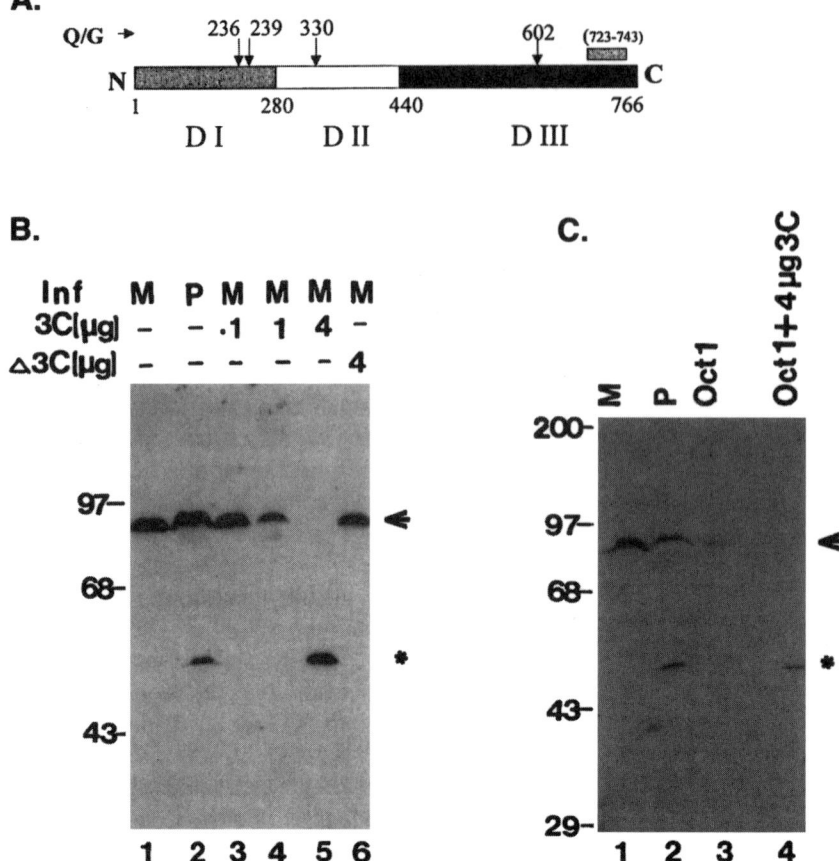

FIGURE 9 (A) Modular structure of the transcriptional activator, Oct-1. Three domains, the N-terminal transcription-activation domain (DI), the DNA-binding domain (homeodomain) (DII), and the C-terminal domain (DIII), are shown. The numbers at the bottom indicate positions of amino acids constituting each domain. Numbers at the top indicate potential QG cleavage sites. The position of Oct-1 (amino acids 723 to 743) shown near the C terminus was used for the preparation of antibodies to Oct-1. (B) Western blot analysis of Oct-1 treated with $3C^{pro}$. Mock-infected nuclear extracts (M) were incubated with 0.1, 1, and 4 μg of $3C^{pro}$ (lanes 3, 4, and 5, respectively) or 4 μg of heat-treated $3C^{pro}$ (lane 6) at 30°C for 4 h. Mock-infected and PV-infected extracts prepared 3 h postinfection were also run on the same gel (lanes 1 and 2, respectively). Position of the full-length Oct-1 is indicated by an arrow and that of cleaved Oct-1 is indicated by an asterisk. The sizes of the molecular weight markers are on the left in kilodaltons. (C) Western blot analysis of purified Oct-1 treated with recombinant, purified $3C^{pro}$. Purified Oct-1 was treated with buffer (lane 3) or 4 μg of $3C^{pro}$ (lane 4). Lanes 1 and 2 show Western blot analysis of mock-infected or PV-infected extracts prepared 3 h postinfection.

A poliovirus with a point mutation in the 3C gene failed to produce the faster-migrating complex and was unable to inhibit Pol III transcription (8, 9) (Fig. 10A and B). B-box DNA-protein complexes with similar faster mobilities could be generated in vitro by treating partially purified TFIIIC with recombinant 3C protease, indicating that the more rapidly migrating TFIIIC-DNA complexes are generated by the cleavage of TFIIIC by the 3C protease. Addition of wild-type $3C^{pro}$ but not an enzymatically inactive point mutant to the in vitro transcription reaction inhibited Pol III transcription (Fig. 10C). Introduction of the $3C^{pro}$ gene alone into HeLa cells inhibited Pol III transcription from the VA gene (Fig. 10D).

Recently we have shown that the α-subunit of TFIIIC (the DNA-binding subunit) is cleaved by $3C^{pro}$ (59). To assess whether the Q732-G733 or Q740-G741 site was cleaved by $3C^{pro}$, PCR was used to introduce stop codons into cDNA clones of the α-subunit after Q732 or Q740. These mutant cDNAs were transcribed and translated in vitro. Then translation products were analyzed by immunoblotting with a TFIIICα antibody and TFIIIC cleavage products generated by $3C^{pro}$ digestion as markers. Fragment Q732 of TFIIIC comigrated with the $3C^{pro}$ cleavage product, strongly suggesting that $3C^{pro}$ cleaves TFIIIC between Q732 and G733 to generate the N-terminal fragment (Fig. 11) (59).

No obvious known DNA-binding motif can be identified in the α-subunit of TFIIIC. To determine which portion of TFIIICα forms the B-box DNA-binding domain, we analyzed the specific DNA-binding subcomplexes generated from TFIIIC by $3C^{pro}$ digestion. The different TFIIIC complexes generated during PV infection were sep-

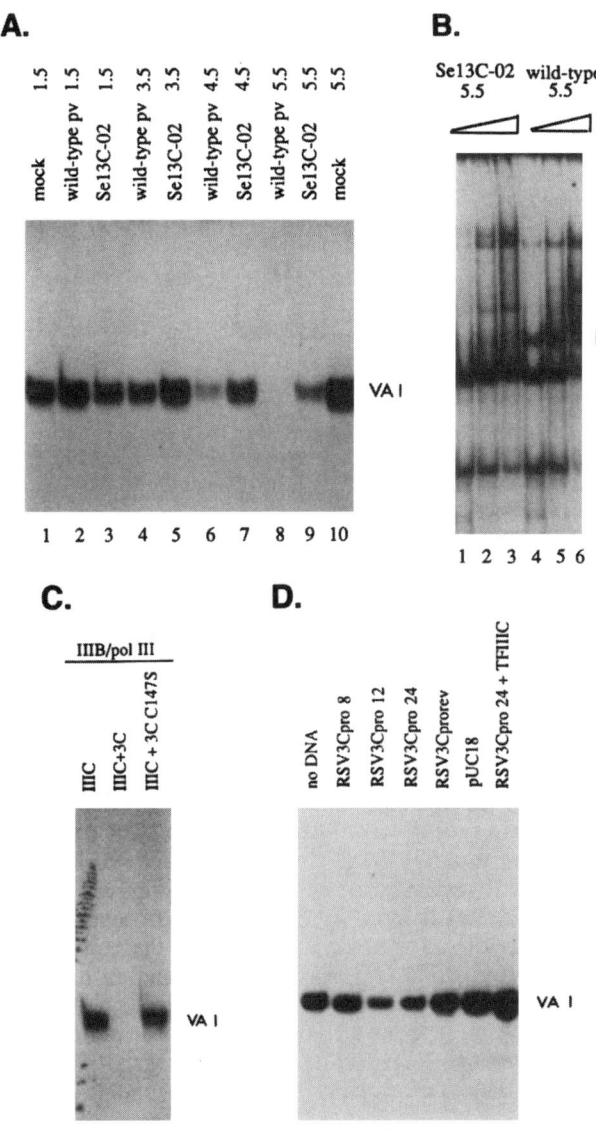

FIGURE 10 Poliovirus 3C protease mediates shutoff of RNA Pol III transcription. (A) In vitro transcription analysis of cell extracts prepared at different times after infection of cells with wild-type or Sel 3C-02 mutant PV. The numbers at the top indicate time of infection or mock infection. The correctly initiated VA I transcript position is indicated. (B) Gel retardation analysis of B-box binding activity of extracts (4, 8, and 12 μg) from HeLa cells infected for 5.5 h with wild-type or the $3C^{pro}$ mutant virus Sel 3C-02. (C) In vitro transcriptional analysis of TFIIIC treated directly with $3C^{pro}$. Untreated, $3C^{pro}$-treated, or mutant (C147S) $3C^{pro}$-treated TFIIIC was added to reactions containing TFIIIB and Pol III. The VA I transcript is shown. (D) Transcription analysis of TFIIIC recovered from nuclear extracts of cells transfected with no DNA (lane 1), $3C^{pro}$ DNA (lanes 2, 3, and 4), $3C^{pro}$ DNA in reverse orientation (lane 5), and pUC18 vector (lane 6). Lane 7 is the same as lane 4 except purified TFIIIC was added to the reaction before the start of transcription.

arated by salt gradient elution of nuclear extracts bound to a phosphocellulose column. As assayed by B-box DNA-binding activity in a gel retardation assay, the two proteolyzed fragments (called $TFIIIC_{polio}$ and $TFIIIC_{polio*}$) were purified, and their ability to form DNA-protein complexes following incubation with preimmune and anti-TFIIIα serum was examined. While one antibody (against amino acids 302-585 of TFIIICα) specifically inhibited complex formation by uncleaved TFIIIC as well as $TFIIIC_{polio}$ and $TFIIIC_{polio*}$, the two other antibodies (against peptides corresponding to amino acids 753-1082 and 1745-2110 of the α-subunit) inhibited complex formation by uncleaved TFIIIC but not by $TFIIIC_{polio}$ and $TFIIIC_{polio*}$. These results indicate that $TFIIIC_{polio}$ and $TFIIIC_{polio*}$ contain the N-terminal 90-kDa fragment of the α-subunit generated by $3C^{pro}$ cleavage but not the large fragment of the α-subunit (125 kDa) that would interact with antibodies against 753-1082 and 1745-2110 TFIIICα peptides. Direct analysis of the polypeptide composition of $TFIIIC_{polio}$ and $TFIIIC_{polio*}$ showed that while $TFIIIC_{polio}$ was composed of only the 90-kDa N-terminal fragment of TFIIICα, the $TFIIIC_{polio*}$ contained the 90-kDa fragment in association with the 110-kDa β-subunit of TFIIIC (59). Thus, $3C^{pro}$ cleavage identified a TFIIIC DNA-binding domain with portions of α- and β-subunits.

RNA Pol I Machinery and Shutoff by PV

RNA Pol I directs RNA synthesis from a single class of genes, the rRNA genes, which are found in multiple, tandemly arrayed copies in the nucleoli of eukaryotic cells (26, 43, 49). rRNA transcription plays a critical role in ribosome biogenesis, and changes in Pol I transcription rate are associated with profound alterations in the growth rate of the cell (60, 61). rRNA transcription is the first to be shut off by PV infection (90 to 120 min of infection). In humans, transcription initiation by Pol I requires at least two TFs in addition to Pol I: the upstream binding factor (UBF) and the species-specific factor, SL1 (see Fig. 1) (36, 37). Human UBF consists of two distinct polypeptides of 97 and 94 kDa. The 94-kDa form results from a 37-amino-acid deletion due to differential splicing (7, 45). UBF, a sequence-specific DNA-binding protein, interacts with two regions of the template: the upstream control element (UCE) located between nucleotides −200 and −170 on the human rRNA gene and the core promoter element located between nucleotides +20 and −45 relative to the site of transcription initiation. The human SL1 is a species-specific factor that, when added to a mouse cell-free transcription extract, has the ability to reprogram that extract to recognize a human rRNA promoter. Human SL1 is composed of TBP and three distinct TAFs of 110, 63, and 48 kDa (11). The SL1 complex cooperatively binds with UBF to the promoter of rRNA genes; however, SL1 does not bind to rRNA genes by itself (4).

Initial studies performed with partially purified fractions of Pol I factors showed that a UBF-containing fraction specifically restored Pol I transcription in PV-infected HeLa cell extract (51). We also showed that addition of purified $3C^{pro}$ to the in vitro transcription reaction resulted in almost total inhibition of Pol I transcription (52). Using a gel retardation assay with an oligonucleotide containing the Pol I promoter sequence, we showed that a transcriptionally active DNA-protein complex can be formed using mock-infected cell extract (52) (Fig. 12). However, a faster-migrating complex was detected with extracts prepared from virus-infected cells (Fig. 12). When an unin-

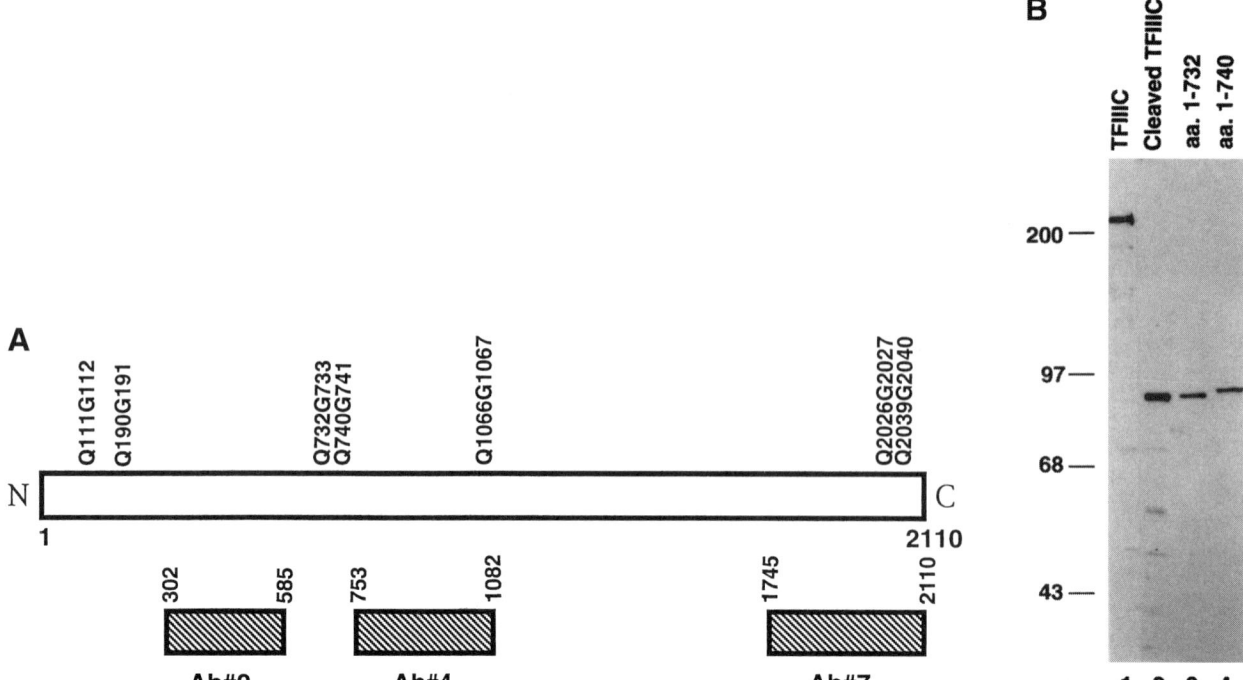

FIGURE 11 (A) Fragments of TFIIIC used to generate antisera. The TFIIICα amino acid sequence is diagrammed; the fragments shown below were expressed as His-tagged polypeptides in E. coli and used to generate antisera. The positions of QG bonds, preferred cleavage sites for PV 3C^{pro}, are indicated above the diagram. (B) Mapping of the N-terminal 3C^{pro} cleavage site in TFIIICα. Immunoblots were performed with Ab2 on uncleaved PC-C (lane 1), 3C^{pro}-cleaved PC-C (lane 2), and in vitro transcribed and translated pTMIIICα1-732 (lane 3) and pTMIIICα1-740 (lane 4).

fected extract was treated with purified 3C^{pro}, the same rapidly migrating complex seen with virus-infected cell extracts was formed (52). Although these extracts contained UBF, in vitro translated or bacterially expressed UBF could not be cleaved by very high concentrations of 3C^{pro} (52). These results suggested that a polypeptide other than UBF was being cleaved by 3C^{pro}. Recently we have shown that the 110-kDa TAF (TAF$_{110}$) of the SL1 complex is efficiently cleaved by 3C^{pro} in vitro. It remains to be seen, however, whether the cleavage of TAF$_{110}$ by 3C^{pro} is responsible for inhibition of Pol I transcription in PV-infected cells.

SnRNA Transcription Machinery

The promoters of human SnRNA genes are similar in structure even though some of them are recognized by RNA Pol II, whereas others are recognized by RNA Pol III. The human U1 and U2 SnRNA (involved in pre-mRNA splicing) promoters are recognized by RNA Pol II and consist essentially of two elements: a proximal sequence element (PSE) located upstream of position −40 that is essential and sufficient to direct basal levels of transcription, and a distal sequence element (DSE) located upstream of position −200 that serves as a transcriptional enhancer and is characterized by the presence of an octamer motif (13, 25) (Fig. 13). The human U6 SnRNA promoter, which is recognized by RNA Pol III, differs from most other Pol III promoters in that it does not contain any essential promoter elements that are internal (like B box) to the gene. Instead, it contains, like U1 and U2 promoters, PSE and DSE, and in addition, a TATA box located between positions −24 and −31 (Fig. 13). The TATA box is a dominant element that defines the U6 promoter as an RNA Pol III promoter. If this TATA box is inactivated by mutation, it predominantly directs Pol II transcription. Conversely, if the U6 TATA box is introduced into the U2 promoter, the U2 promoter directs RNA Pol III transcription (40).

The PSE elements of both U2 and U6 promoters bind a multisubunit protein complex called SnRNA-activating protein complex (SNAPc) containing polypeptides of molecular masses of 43, 45, 50, and 190 kDa (54). In addition, SNAPc contains variable amounts of TBP. Binding of Pol II general factors and RNA Pol II to this complex directs basal transcription from the U2 promoter. Activated transcription from the U2 promoter is carried out by interaction of the basal complex with Oct-1 bound at the DSE element (Fig. 13) (65). We have recently shown cleavage of Oct-1 by 3C^{pro} in PV-infected cells. However, it remains to be seen whether 3C^{pro} would abrogate Oct-1-mediated transcriptional activation from the U2 promoter.

On the TATA-containing RNA Pol III U6 promoter, SNAPc and TBP can both bind directly to the DNA. The combination of the two factors then recruits RNA Pol III and possibly TFIIIB to start Pol III transcription (54). It has recently been shown that the N-terminal (1–55) amino acids of TBP play an important role in U6 RNA transcription (42). Because both the 18th QC and the 34th YG bonds in TBP are cleaved by the PV proteases 3C^{pro} and 2A^{pro}, respectively, it is likely that both proteases

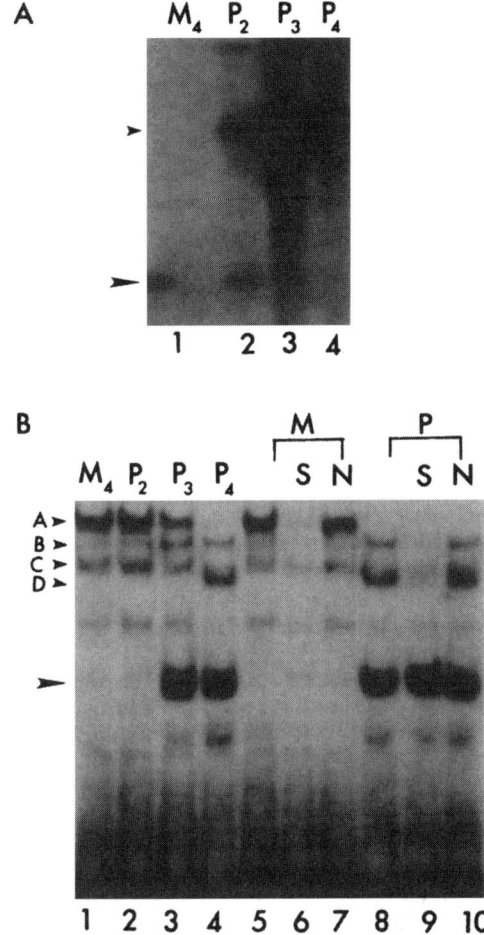

FIGURE 12 Kinetics of inhibition of rRNA transcription correlates with alteration in UCE complex mobility. (A) Pol I transcription (indicated by large arrowhead) was examined in extracts prepared from mock-infected (4 h, M_4) and PV-infected HeLa cells at 2, 3, and 4 h postinfection (P_2, P_3, P_4). (B) Gel retardation analysis was performed using cell-free extracts and [^{32}P]UMP-labeled promoter sequence (lanes 1 to 4). Specificity of protein binding to the promoter was examined by competition gel retardation analysis with mock (lanes 5 to 7) and PV-infected extract (lanes 8 to 10) and addition of no RNA (lanes 5 and 8), unlabeled UCE RNA (lanes 6 and 9), and nonspecific RNA (lanes 7 and 10).

would inhibit SnRNA transcription. The experiments are in progress to determine whether both $3C^{pro}$ and $2A^{pro}$ are able to block SnRNA transcription.

SUMMARY

In the Pol II system, we have shown that both basal and activated transcription were affected by PV infection and demonstrated that transcription inhibition was due to the inability of $3C^{pro}$-modified TBP to form the TBP-TATA box complex (72). In addition, three other TFs required for activated transcription, CREB, Oct-1, and p53, were cleaved and inactivated by $3C^{pro}$ (71, 73). We have shown that the other viral protease, $2A^{pro}$, also cleaves TBP at the 34th YG residue; however, this cleavage does not inhibit TATA-mediated Pol II transcription in vitro (70). In the Pol III system, we demonstrated that the 243-kDa, DNA-binding α-subunit of Pol III factor TFIIIC was cleaved by $3C^{pro}$ and was transcriptionally inactivated (59). Furthermore, characterization of subcomplexes generated by $3C^{pro}$ cleavage of the TFIIIC complex containing five subunits identified the DNA-binding domain and subunit interactions of TFIIIC. This is a very good example of how a viral protease could be utilized to dissect the structure of a multisubunit transcription factor. In the Pol I system, we have shown that one of the Pol I factors (SL1) is the target of the viral protease. SL1 consists of TBP and three TAFs (110, 63, and 48 kDa). The TAF_{110} is cleaved by $3C^{pro}$, and this appears to be the cause for inactivation of Pol I transcription.

UNANSWERED QUESTIONS AND FUTURE RESEARCH

Although many basic questions such as the nature of transcription factors inactivated and the viral components necessary for transcription factor inactivation have been successfully addressed (Table 1), a number of questions regarding the details of transcription shutoff by PV remain unanswered. The precise location of TBP cleavage by $3C^{pro}$ (between amino acid residues 105 and 116) needs to be determined. The amino acid sequence of this region of TBP is ^{105}VQQSTSQQATQG^{116}. Because the primary specificity of the 3C protease is the bond between Q and G, it is probable that the Q115-G116 bond is being cleaved by $3C^{pro}$. Alternatively, the Q107-S108 or the Q112-A113 bond may also be cleaved by $3C^{pro}$. Once the precise cleavage site of TBP that is responsible for Pol II transcriptional inactivation is determined, an interesting experiment would be to determine whether Pol II transcription shutoff in a cell line expressing a mutant TBP that is not cleaved by $3C^{pro}$ would be as complete as that seen in the HeLa cells containing the wild-type TBP. If the sole reason for inactivation of TBP basal transcriptional activity is the cleavage of a particular QG (or other) bond by $3C^{pro}$, it is expected that a TBP with an altered cleavage site would not lead to inhibition of basal transcription.

We have shown that the tumor suppressor, p53, is degraded in PV-infected cells and that this degradation requires both $3C^{pro}$ and a cellular activity. Preliminary experiments have shown that the cellular activity can be partially purified from HeLa cells. It would be interesting to determine the mechanism by which both $3C^{pro}$ and the cellular activity participate in p53 degradation. One possibility is that the interaction of p53 with the cellular protein(s) exposes one or more cleavage sites (possibly QG) in p53 that are then cleaved by $3C^{pro}$. Alternatively, $3C^{pro}$ may activate a cellular protease, which in turn cleaves (or degrades) p53.

One of the questions that remains to be answered is the mechanism by which PV infection shuts off RNA Pol I transcription. Available results suggest that SL1 (TBP plus Pol I TAFs) is cleaved by $3C^{pro}$ in virus-infected cells. What remains to be seen is whether this cleavage is responsible for Pol I transcription shutoff. This question can be best approached by determining whether the transcriptional activity of SL1 that has been treated with $3C^{pro}$ is significantly reduced in a reconstituted transcription assay consisting of UBF, SL1, and Pol I. In addition, an interesting experiment would be to examine whether addition of purified SL1 to PV-infected cell extract would restore polymerase transcription in vivo.

332 ■ SHUTOFF OF HOST CELL TRANSLATION AND TRANSCRIPTION

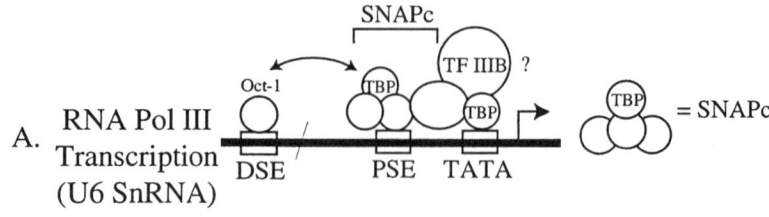

A. RNA Pol III Transcription (U6 SnRNA)

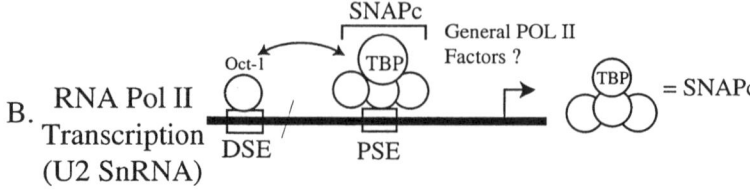

B. RNA Pol II Transcription (U2 SnRNA)

FIGURE 13 Schematic diagram of preinitiation complex assembly for RNA Pol III- and Pol II-catalyzed SnRNA transcription. (A) Basal transcription from Pol III-catalyzed U6 SnRNA transcription requires cooperative binding of TBP to TATA box and SNAPc to the PSE. Activated transcription requires interaction (shown by double-headed arrow) of the basal complex formed at the PSE with the activator Oct-1 bound at the DSE. Single-headed arrow shows transcription start site. (B) RNA Pol II-catalyzed basal transcription from the U2 SnRNA promoter requires binding of SNAPc to PSE and possibly binding of other general Pol II factors. Activated transcription requires interaction (double-headed arrow) between Oct-1 bound to DSE with the basal complex at PSE.

The role of the 3C protease in host cell transcription shutoff is clear from both genetic and biochemical analyses (8–10, 52, 71–74; Yalamanchili et al., unpublished). In contrast, there is no direct evidence that 2A^{pro} can inhibit cellular transcription. Results from a number of laboratories have shown that RNA Pol II transcription is significantly reduced in cells transfected with 2A^{pro} (15, 44). This is in contrast to the result that showed that 2A^{pro}, even at very high concentrations, was unable to inhibit RNA Pol II transcription in vitro (70). Thus, it is highly unlikely that 2A^{pro} directly inhibits Pol II transcription. One likely possibility is that 2A^{pro} may be blocking the synthesis of SnRNA by cleavage of the 34th YG in TBP. In view of the recent result that the N-terminal amino acids to TBP play a crucial role in SnRNA synthesis, 2A^{pro} would be expected to inhibit SnRNA synthesis. Inhibition of Pol II transcription observed in 2A^{pro} transfected cells could be a secondary effect caused by translation shutoff, SnRNA transcription shutoff, or both.

PV is an RNA virus, which replicates in the cytoplasm of infected cells. To shut off host cell transcription, one or more viral gene products must enter the nucleus of the infected host cell. A previous study reported detection of PV precursor protein 3CD (protease 3C and polymerase 3D precursor) in the nuclei of infected cells prior to onset of inhibition of cellular transcription (21). The viral precursor 3CD has protease activity and is able to autocatalyze the formation of 3C and 3D polypeptides (67). These results suggested that 3C^{pro} (and/or 3CD) could interact with transcription factors in the nucleus of infected cells. A computer search of the amino acid sequence of 3C^{pro} did not reveal a nuclear localization signal. Amino acid sequence examination of 3D^{pol}, however, identified a potential "single basic type nuclear localization signal (NLS)" within this polypeptide (KKKRD at positions 125 to 129) (17, 74). This sequence is well conserved among enteroviruses and is present within the finger subdomain of poliovirus 3D^{pol}, whose crystal structure has been resolved recently (24). Triple alanine substitution of the 3D^{pol} residues $K_{125}K_{126}K_{127}$ or $K_{127}R_{128}D_{129}$ produced no viable virus (16). It is possible to envision a scenario in which 3C^{pro} enters the nucleus in the form of its precursor 3CD, which is then

TABLE 1 Summary of transcription factors cleaved by poliovirus proteases 3C^{pro} and 2A^{pro} [a]

Factor	Protease	Cleavage site	Transcription affected	References
TBP	3C^{pro}	18 QG	SnRNA (?), Pol II (?)	10, 42
TBP	3C^{pro}	115 QG (?)	Pol II	Unpublished (Dasgupta lab)
CREB	3C^{pro}	172 QG	Pol II	71
Oct-1	3C^{pro}	330 QG	Pol II, SnRNA (?)	73
p53	3C^{pro}/cellular protease	ND	Pol II	Unpublished (Dasgupta lab)
TFIIICα	3C^{pro}	732 QG	Pol III	8, 9, 59
		1067 QG (?)		
SL1 (TAF$_{100}$)	3C^{pro}	265 QG	Pol I	51, 52
		805 QG		Unpublished (Dasgupta lab)

[a] ND, not determined.

autocatalyzed to generate 3C^{pro} inside the nucleus. Future studies should determine (i) whether 3D^{pol} or 3CD enters the nucleus, and (ii) whether mutagenesis of the putative NLS in 3D^{pol} would interfere with nuclear localization of 3D^{pol} and 3CD. Would 3D^{pol} sequences containing the putative NLS target a soluble protein to the nucleus? Would transfection of HeLa cells with 3CD bearing the NLS mutation that interferes with its nuclear localization lead to shutoff of host cell transcription? Would full-length viral RNA bearing this mutation be infectious, and if so, would it efficiently shut off host cell transcription? It is also possible that 3C^{pro} itself could diffuse into the nucleus due to its small size.

This work was supported by NIH grants AI-18272 and AI-27451 to A. Dasgupta and CA 25235 to A. J. Berk. We are grateful to E. Wimmer and B. Semler for reagents.

REFERENCES

1. **Ahmed, M., and D. S. Lyles.** 1988. Effect of vesicular stomatitis virus matrix protein on transcription directed by host RNA polymerase I, II and III. *J. Virol.* **72:**8413–8419.
2. **Apriletti, J. W., and E.-E. Penhoet.** 1978. Cellular RNA synthesis in normal and mengovirus infected L-929 cells. *J. Biol. Chem.* **253:**603–611.
3. **Baltimore, D., H. J. Egger, R. M. Franklin, and I. Tamm.** 1963. Poliovirus-induced RNA polymerase and the effects of virus-specific inhibitors on its production. *Proc. Natl. Acad. Sci. USA* **49:**834–849.
4. **Bell, S. P., R. M. Lerned, H.-M. Jantzen, and R. Tjian.** 1988. Functional cooperativity between transcription factors UBFI and SL1 mediates human ribosomal RNA synthesis. *Science* **241:**1102–1197.
5. **Berk, A. J.** 1989. Regulation of eukaryotic transcription factors by post-translation modification. *Biochim. Biophys. Acta* **1009:**103–109.
6. **Bernstein, H. D., N. Sonenberg, and D. Baltimore.** 1985. Poliovirus mutant that does not selectively inhibit host cell protein synthesis. *Mol. Cell. Biol.* **5:**2913–2923.
7. **Chan, E. K. L., H. Imai, J. C. Hamel, and E. M. Tan.** 1991. Human autoantibody to RNA pol I transcription factor hUBF: molecular identity of nucleolus organizer region autoantigen NOR-90 and ribosomal RNA transcription upstream binding factor. *J. Exp. Med.* **174:**1239–1244.
8. **Clark, M. E., and A. Dasgupta.** 1990. A transcriptionally active form of TFIIIC is modified in poliovirus-infected cells. *Mol. Cell. Biol.* **10:**5106–5113.
9. **Clark, M. E., T. Hammerle, E. Wimmer, and A. Dasgupta.** 1991. Poliovirus proteinase 3C converts an active form of transcription factor IIIC to an inactive form: a mechanism for inhibition of host cell pol III transcription by poliovirus. *EMBO J.* **10:**2941–2947.
10. **Clark, M. E., P. M. Lieberman, A. J. Berk, and A. Dasgupta.** 1993. Direct cleavage of human TATA-binding protein by poliovirus protease 3C in vivo and in vitro. *Mol. Cell. Biol.* **13:**1232–1237.
11. **Comai, L., N. Tenese, and R. Tjian.** 1992. The TATA-binding protein and associated factors are integral components of the RNA polymerase I transcription factor, SL1. *Cell* **68:**965–976.
12. **Crawford, N., A. Fires, M. Samuels, P. A. Sharp, and D. Baltimore.** 1981. Inhibition of transcription factor activity by poliovirus. *Cell* **27:**555–561.
13. **Dahlberg, J. E., and E. Lund.** 1988. The genes and transcription of the major small nuclear RNAs, p. 38–70. *In* M. L. Birnstiel (ed.), *Structure and Function of Major and Minor Small Nuclear Ribonucleoprotein Particles*. Springer-Verlag, Berlin, Germany.
14. **Das, S., and A. Dasgupta.** 1993. Identification of the cleavage site and determinants required for poliovirus 3C^{pro}-catalyzed cleavage of human TBP. *J. Virol.* **67:**3326–3331.
15. **Davies, M. V., J. Pelletier, K. Meerovitich, N. Sonenberg, and R. J. Kaufman.** 1991. The effect of poliovirus proteinase 2A^{pro} expression on cellular metabolism. *J. Biol. Chem.* **266:**14714–14721.
16. **Diamond, S., and K. Kirkegaard.** 1994. Clustured charged-to-alanine mutagenesis of poliovirus RNA-dependent RNA polymerase yields multiple ts mutants defective in RNA synthesis. *J. Virol.* **68:**863–876.
17. **Dingwall, C., and R. A. Laskey.** 1991. Nuclear targeting sequences a consensus? *Trends Biochem. Sci.* **16:**478–491.
18. **Dynalact, B. D., T. Hoey, and R. Tjian.** 1991. Isolation of coactivators associated with the TATA-binding protein that mediate transcriptional activation. *Cell* **66:**563–576.
19. **Etchison, D., S. C. Mulburn, I. Edery, N. Sonenberg, and J. W. B. Hershey.** 1988. Inhibition of HeLa cell protein synthesis following poliovirus infection correlates with the proteolysis of a 220,000-dalton polypeptide associated with eukaryotic initiation factor 3 and a cap binding protein complex. *J. Biol. Chem.* **257:**14806–14810.
20. **Falk, M. M., P. R. Grigera, I. E. Bergman, A. Zibert, G. Multhaup, and E. Beck.** 1990. Foot-and-mouth disease virus protease 3C induces specific proteolytic cleavage of host cell histone H3. *J. Virol.* **64:**748–756.
21. **Fernandez-Tomas, C.** 1982. The presence of viral induced proteins in nuclei from poliovirus-infected HeLa cells. *Virology* **116:**629–634.
22. **Fradkin, L. G., S. K. Yoshinaga, A. J. Berk, and A. Dasgupta.** 1987. Inhibition of host cell RNA polymerase III-mediated transcription by poliovirus: inactivation of specific transcription factor. *Mol. Cell. Biol.* **7:**3880–3887.
23. **Geiduschek, E. P., and G. P. Tocchini-Valentini.** 1988. Transcription by RNA pol III. *Annu. Rev. Biochem.* **57:**873–914.
24. **Hansen, J., A. Long, and S. Schultz.** 1997. Structure of the RNA-dependent RNA polymerase of poliovirus. *Structure* **5:**1109–1122.
25. **Hernandez, N.** 1992. Transcription of vertebrate snRNA genes and related genes, p. 281–313. *In* S. L. McKnight and K. R. Yamamoto (ed.), *Transcriptional Regulation*. Cold Spring Harbor Laboratory Press, Cold Spring Harbor, N.Y.
26. **Jacob, S. T.** 1995. Regulation of ribosomal gene transcription. *Biochem. J.* **306:**617–626.
27. **Kaariainen, L., and M. Ranki.** 1984. Inhibition of cell functions by RNA virus infections. *Annu. Rev. Microbiol.* **38:**91–109.
28. **Kao, C. C., P. M. Lieberman, M. C. Schmidt, Q. Zhou, R. Pei, and A. J. Berk.** 1990. Cloning of a transcriptionally active human TATA-binding factor. *Science* **248:**1646–1650.
29. **Kassavetis, G. A., B. R. Braun, L. H. Nguyen, and E. P. Geiduschek.** 1990. *Saccharomyces cerevisiae* TFIIIB is the transcription initiation factor proper of RNA polymerase III while TFIIIA and TFIIIC are assembly factors. *Cell* **60:**235–245.
30. **Kassavetis, G. A., D. L. Riggs, R. Negri, L. H. Nguyen, and E. P. Geiduschek.** 1989. Transcription factor TFIIIB generates extended DNA interactions in RNA pol III transcription complexes on tRNA genes. *Mol. Cell. Biol.* **9:**2551–2566.
31. **Kliewer, S., and A. Dasgupta.** 1988. An RNA polymerase II transcription factor inactivated in poliovirus-infected

cells copurifies with transcription factor TFIID. *Mol. Cell. Biol.* **8:**3175–3182.
32. Kliewer, S., C. Muchardt, R. B. Gaynor, and A. Dasgupta. 1990. Loss of a phosphorylated form of transcription factor CREB/ATF in poliovirus-infected cells. *J. Virol.* **64:**4507–4515.
33. Kovelman, R., and R. G. Roeder. 1992. Purification and characterization of two forms of human transcription factor IIIC. *J. Biol. Chem.* **267:**24446–24456.
34. Krausslich, H.-G., M. J. Nicklin, H. Toyoda, D. Etchison, and E. Wimmer. 1987. Poliovirus proteinase 2A induces cleavage of eukaryotic initiation factor 4F polypeptide p 220. *J. Virol.* **61:**2711–2718.
35. Krausslich, H.-G., and E. Wimmer. 1988. Viral proteinases. *Annu. Rev. Biochem.* **57:**701–754.
36. Learned, R. M., S. Cordes, and R. Tjian. 1985. Purification and characterization of a transcription factor that confers promoter specificity to human RNA polymerase I. *Mol. Cell. Biol.* **5:**1358–1369.
37. Learned, R. M., T. K. Learned, M. M. Haltiner, and R. Tjian. 1986. Human rRNA transcription is modulated by the coordinate binding of two factors to an upstream control element. *Cell* **45:**847–857.
38. Lloyd, R. E., M. J. Grubman, and E. Ehrenfeld. 1988. Relationship of p220 cleavage during picornavirus infection to 2A protease sequences. *J. Virol.* **62:**4216–4223.
39. Lo, K., G. T. Sheu, and M. M. Lai. 1998. Inhibition of cellular RNA polymerase II transcription by delta antigen of hepatitis delta virus. *Virology* **247:**178–188.
40. Lobo, S. M., and N. Hernandez. 1989. A 7 bp mutation converts a human Rna polymerase II snRNA promoter into an RNA polymerase III promoter. *Cell* **58:**55–67.
41. Margottin, F., G. Dujardin, M. Gerard, J.-M. Egly, J. Huet, and A. Sentenac. 1991. Participation of the TATA factor in transcription of the yeast U6 gene by RNA polymerase C. *Science* **252:**424–426.
42. Mittal, V., and N. Hernandez. 1997. Role of the amino terminal region of human TBP in U6 SnRNA transcription. *Science* **275:**1136–1139.
43. Moss, T., and V. Y. Stetanovaky. 1995. Promotion and regulation of ribosomal transcription in eukaryotes by RNA polymerase I. *Prog. Nucleic Acids Res. Mol. Biol.* **50:**25–66.
44. Novoa, I., and L. Carrasco. 1999. Cleavage of eukaryotic translation factor 46 by exogenously added hybrid proteins containing poliovirus 2^{pro} in HeLa cells: effects on gene expression. *Mol. Cell. Biol.* **19:**2445–2454.
45. O'Mahoney, D. J., and L. I. Rothblum. 1991. Identification of two forms of the RNA pol I transcription factor, UBF. *Proc. Natl. Acad. Sci. USA* **88:**3180–3184.
46. Pugh, B. F., and R. Tjian. 1991. Transcription from a TATA-less promoter requires a multisubunit TFIID complex. *Genes Dev.* **5:**1935–1945.
47. Pugh, B. F., and R. Tjian. 1992. Diverse transcriptional functions of the multisubunit eukaryotic TFIID complex. Minireview. *J. Biol. Chem.* **267:**679–682.
48. Rangel, L. M., C. Fernandez-Thomas, M. E. Dahmas, and P. Gariglio. 1988. Poliovirus-induced modification of host cell RNA polymerase IIO is prevented by cycloheximide and zinc. *J. Biol. Chem.* **23:**19267–19269.
49. Reeder, R. H. 1994. *Regulation of Transcription by RNA Polymerase I.* Cold Spring Harbor Laboratory Press, Cold Spring Harbor, N.Y.
50. Rigby, P. W. 1993. Three on one and one in three: it all depends on TBP. *Cell* **72:**7–10.
51. Rubinstein, S. J., and A. Dasgupta. 1989. Inhibition of rRNA synthesis by poliovirus: specific inactivation of transcription factors. *J. Virol.* **63:**4689–4696.
52. Rubinstein, S. J., T. Hammerle, E. Wimmer, and A. Dasgupta. 1992. Infection of HeLa cells with poliovirus results in modification of a complex that binds to the rRNA promoter. *J. Virol.* **66:**3062–3068.
53. Rueckert, R. R. 1990. Picornaviridae and their replication, p. 507–547. *In* B. N. Fields, D. Knipe, et al. (ed.), *Virology.* Raven, New York, N.Y.
54. Sadowski, C., R. Henry, S. Lobo, and N. Hernandez. 1993. Targeting TBP to a non TATA-box cis-regulatory element: a TBP containing complex activates transcription from SnRNA promoters through the PSE. *Genes Dev.* **7:**1535–1548.
55. Sawadogo, M., and A. Senenac. 1990. RNA polymerase B (II) and general transcriptional factors. *Annu. Rev. Biochem.* **759:**711–754.
56. Schwartz, L. B., C. Lawrence, R. E. Thach, and R. G. Roeder. 1974. Encephalomyocarditis virus infection of mouse plasmacytoma cells. II. Effect on host RNA synthesis and RNA polymerases. *J. Virol.* **14:**611–619.
57. Segall, J., T. Matsu, and R. G. Roeder. 1980. Multiple factors are required for accurate transcription of purified genes by RNA pol III. *J. Biol. Chem.* **255:**11986–11991.
58. Sharp, P. A. 1992. TATA-binding protein is a classless factor. *Cell* **68:**819–821.
59. Shen, Y., M. Igo, P. Yalamanchili, A. Berk, and A. Dasgupta. 1996. DNA-binding domain and subunit interaction of transcription factor TFIIIC revealed by dissection with poliovirus 3C protease. *Mol. Cell. Biol.* **16:**4163–4171.
60. Sollner-Webb, B., and J. Tower. 1986. Transcription of cloned eukaryotic ribosomal RNA genes. *Annu. Rev. Biochem.* **55:**801–830.
61. Sommerville, J. 1986. Nucleolar structure and ribosome biogenesis. *Trends Biochem. Sci.* **11:**438–442.
62. Sonenberg, N. 1990. Poliovirus translation. *Curr. Top. Microbiol. Immunol.* **161:**23–47.
63. Sorger, P., and H. R. B. Pelham. 1988. Yeast heat shock factor is an essential DNA-binding protein that exhibits temperature-dependent phosphorylation. *Cell* **54:**855–864.
64. Taggart, A. K. P., T. S. Fisher, and B. F. Pugh. 1992. The TATA-binding protein and associated factors are components of pol III transcription factor TAFIIIB. *Cell* **71:**1015–1028.
65. Tanaka, M., J. S. Lai, and W. Herr. 1992. Promoter-selective activation domains in Oct-1 and Oct-2 direct differential activation of an SnRNA and mRNA promoter. *Cell* **68:**755–767.
66. Tesar, M., and O. Marquardt. 1990. Foot-and-mouth disease virus protease 3C inhibits cellular transcription and mediates cleavage of histone H3. *Virology* **174:**364–374.
67. Wimmer, E., C. U. T. Hellen, and X. Cao. 1993. Genetics of poliovirus. *Annu. Rev. Genet.* **27:**353–436.
68. Workman, J. L., and R. G. Roeder. 1987. Binding of transcription factor TFIID to the major late promoter during in vitro nucleosome assembly protentiates subsequent initiation by RNA polymerase II. *Cell* **51:**613–622.
69. Wyckoff, E. E., J. W. B. Hershey, and E. Ehrenfeld. 1990. Eukaryotic initiation factor 3 is required for poliovirus 2A protease-induced cleavage of the p220 component of eukaryotic initiation factor 4F. *Proc. Natl. Acad. Sci. USA* **87:**9529–9533.
70. Yalamanchili, P., R. Banerjee, and A. Dasgupta. 1997. Poliovirus-encoded protease $2A^{pro}$ cleaves the TATA-binding protein but does not inhibit host cell RNA polymerase II transcription in vitro. *J. Virol.* **71:**6881–6886.
71. Yalamanchili, P., U. Datta, and A. Dasgupta. 1997. Inhibition of host cell transcription by poliovirus: cleavage of transcription factor CREB by poliovirus-encoded protease $3C^{pro}$. *J. Virol.* **71:**1220–1226.
72. Yalamanchili, P., K. Harris, E. Wimmer, and A. Dasgupta. 1996. Inhibition of basal transcription by poliovi-

rus: a virus-encoded protease (3C^{pro}) inhibits formation of TBP-TATA box complex in vitro. *J. Virol.* **70:**2922–2929.
73. **Yalamanchili, P., K. Weidman, and A. Dasgupta.** 1997. Cleavage of transcriptional activator Oct-1 by poliovirus-encoded protease 3C^{pro}. *Virology* **239:**176–185.
74. **Yoneda, Y.** 1996. Nuclear export and its significance in retroviral infection. *Trends Microbiol.* **4:**1–2.
75. **Yoshinaga, S. K., N. D. L'Etoile, and A. J. Berk.** 1989. Purification and characterization of transcription factor IIIC2. *J. Biol. Chem.* **264:**10726–10731.
76. **Yuan, H., B. K. Yoza, and D. S. Lyles.** 1998. Inhibition of host RNA polymerase II-dependent transcription by VSV results from inactivation of TFIIID. *Virology* **251:**383–392.
77. **Zawel, L., and D. Rienberg.** 1992. Advances in RNA polymerase II transcription. *Curr. Opin. Cell Biol.* **4:**488–495.
78. **Zhou, Q., P. M. Lieberman, T. J. Boyer, and A. J. Berk.** 1992. Holo TFIID supports transcriptional stimulation by diverse activators and from a TATA-less promoter. *Genes Dev.* **6:**1964–1974.

Effects of Viral Replication on Cellular Membrane Metabolism and Function

LUIS CARRASCO, ROSARIO GUINEA, ALICIA IRURZUN, AND ÁNGEL BARCO

27

As with the majority of cytolytic animal viruses, picornavirus infection leads to profound alterations in cellular membranes. Both the morphology and the functioning of cell membranes are modified upon infection (44, 46). These alterations occur at two well-defined moments during the picornavirus cycle: at early times, when virus particles penetrate into cells, and late during infection, when the majority of viral products are being synthesized (Fig. 1) (44, 46).

The initial attachment of the virus particle to the receptor located at the cell surface soon leads to the interaction of structural proteins with the lipid bilayer (21), followed by membrane permeabilization. In fact, the interaction of poliovirus (PV) particles with artificial membranes induces the formation of ion channels (206). This early membrane permeabilization precedes the delivery of the virus genome to the cytoplasm and does not require virus gene expression (42, 80). Low-molecular-weight compounds and macromolecules enter cells together with virus particles (63, 80).

Three types of changes are observed at late times of infection in cellular membranes: enhanced membrane permeability, proliferation of intracellular membranous vesicles, and inhibition of vesicular trafficking with the consequent blockage of protein glycosylation. Late membrane leakiness requires viral gene expression and involves the diffusion of ions and small molecules, but not macromolecules, through the plasma membrane (41, 48, 137, 155). In addition, at late times of infection, cell morphology is profoundly altered (84). Proliferation of cytoplasmic membrane vesicles is a common phenomenon observed during the replication of picornaviruses (44, 84). Some of the newly made vesicles interact tightly with viral replication complexes, in such a way that viral genome replication depends on the synthesis of membranous vesicles (44, 84). Thus, inhibition of membrane proliferation blocks the synthesis of viral genomes (43, 97, 166, 167). Viral macromolecular synthesis, such as translation and particularly the replication of viral genomes, and the morphogenesis of new virions occur in tight association with membranes. The appearance of the picornavirus replication complexes involves not only the synthesis of several viral nonstructural proteins, but also de novo formation of specialized cytoplasmic membranes. The generation of these membranous structures where viral replication takes place involves drastic alterations in vesicular traffic. As a result, protein glycosylation is blocked in picornavirus-infected cells.

This review focuses on both the structural and functional modifications that membranes of picornavirus-infected cells undergo during virus replication.

MODIFICATION OF MEMBRANE FUNCTION AT LATE TIMES OF INFECTION

Enhancement of Plasma Membrane Permeability during Picornavirus Replication

At the beginning of the late phase of picornavirus infection, when viral RNA replication occurs, drastic changes in membrane permeability start to be apparent. Virus gene expression is required for these phenomena to take place, suggesting that one or several virus gene products are responsible for these changes.

The progressive membrane damage induced by picornaviruses is reflected in the following parameters.

(i) Monovalent cations (6, 155). There is a marked change in the intracellular content of both sodium and potassium ions at about 4 h postinfection (hpi) with encephalomyocarditis virus (EMCV) (48, 79), mengovirus (75), human rhinovirus (155), coxsackievirus (146), and PV (127, 137, 154). The increased entry of sodium and the leakage of potassium ions from cells seem to be the consequence of an increased passive permeability of the cell membrane, since movement of these ions is not affected by ouabain, quinidine, or furosemide (137, 154). However, inhibition of Na^+/K^+ ATPase was reported in PV-infected cells 3 hpi (189, 190). As a result, transport of amino acids

---

Luis Carrasco, Rosario Guinea, and Alicia Irurzun ■ Centro de Biología Molecular "Severo Ochoa," Universidad Autónoma de Madrid, Campus de Cantoblanco, 28049 Madrid, Spain. *Ángel Barco* ■ Center for Neurobiology and Behavior, Columbia University, 722 West 168th Street, 6th floor, New York, NY 10032.

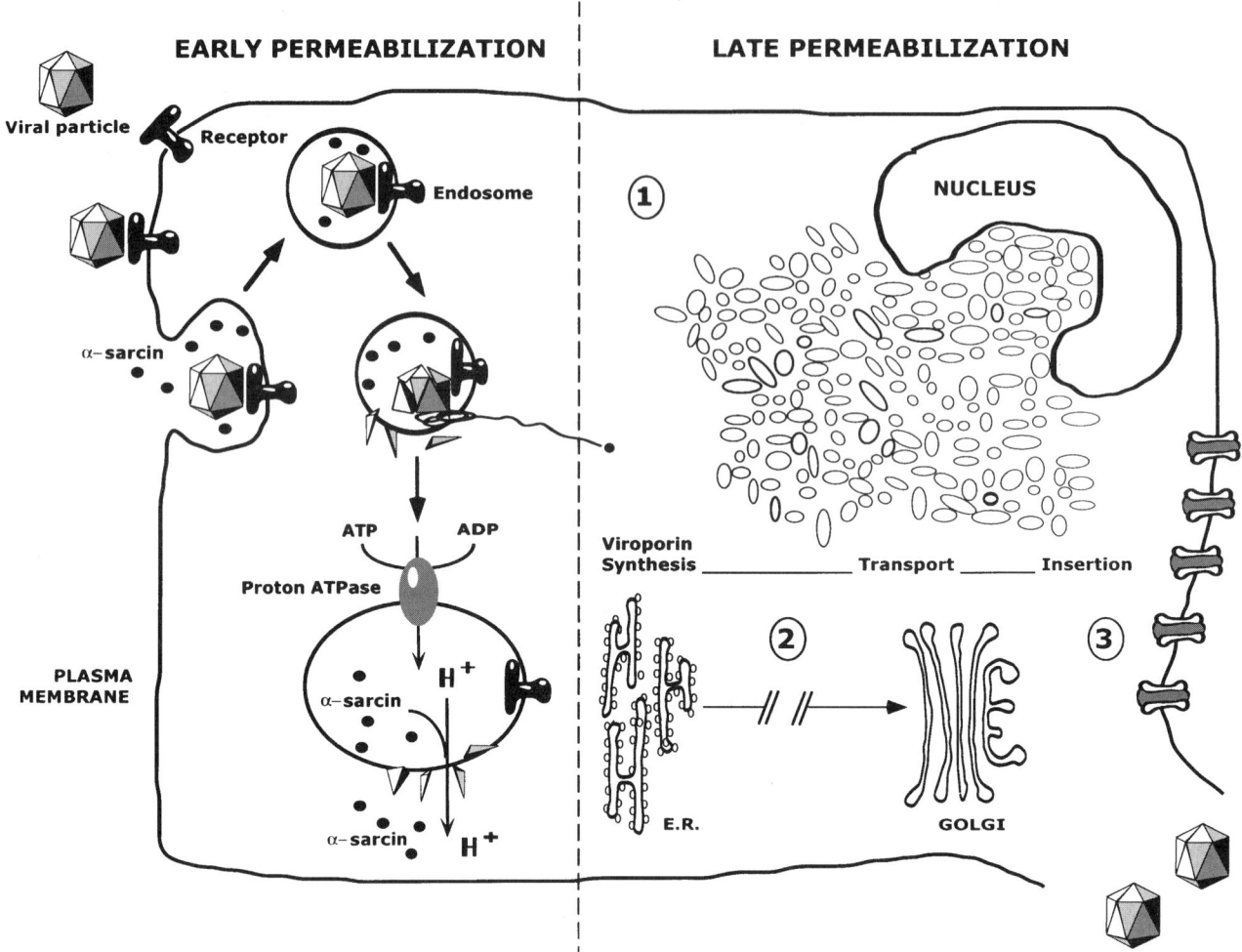

FIGURE 1 Schematic depiction of membrane modifications induced by picornavirus at early and late stages of infection. During viral entry, early membrane permeabilization is directed to locate the virus genome in the cytoplasm. Low-molecular-weight compounds, as well as macromolecules such as α-sarcin, enter cells together with virus particles. At late times of infection three types of changes are observed in cellular membranes: (1) proliferation of intracellular membranous vesicles, (2) inhibition of vesicular trafficking with the consequent blockage of protein glycosylation, and (3) enhanced membrane permeability.

that require a sodium gradient (alanine and methionine) is impaired (127).

(ii) Membrane potential. Depolarization of the membrane occurs 4 hpi (40, 46, 51, 86, 127, 146, 189, 190), probably due to the leakage of monovalent cations.

(iii) pH. An intracellular alkalinization has been reported in PV-infected cells. This change might promote viral replication (105, 106, 221); however, little is known about the origin of this change in cytoplasmic proton concentration.

(iv) Divalent cations. Cytoplasmic free calcium increases from 2 to 3 hpi, and by 5 hpi there is a 5- to 10-fold increase of $[Ca^{2+}]$ in PV-infected and coxsackievirus B3 (CVB3)-infected cells (110, 214). Modification of divalent cations, as measured by depletion of magnesium from the cells and decrease in polyamine content, was also apparent in mengovirus-infected Ehrlich ascites tumor cells (75).

(v) Other metabolites. A decrease of ATP content in several picornavirus-infected cells has been described from 3 hpi (75, 127, 146). This might reflect an interference of picornaviruses with mitochondrial function. Nucleotides, sugars, and amino acids such as methionine (127), as well as other small molecules, e.g., choline, betaine, and phosphorylcholine, are released from intracellular pools to the medium during infections with PV and mengovirus (49, 112, 175).

(vi) Several enzymes are detected in the culture medium at late times of infection as a consequence of cell lysis. This leakage depends on the picornavirus analyzed (88). Thus, echovirus 12 releases lactic dehydrogenase 4 hpi of monkey cells. In addition, the permeability of the lysosomal membrane also becomes altered in PV infection (7, 8), allowing the enzymes to leak out (31, 33, 82, 204).

(vii) Low-molecular-weight inhibitors. Hydrophilic compounds of less than about 1,500 Da, such as hygromycin B, GTP analogue GppCH$_2$p, gougerotin, blasticidin S, edeine, and anthelmycin, pass through the plasma membrane and exert their inhibitory effect upon infection with EMCV and PV (41, 46, 47, 61). The transcription inhibitor α-amanitin also diffuses into infected cells (50). This entry of compounds is the result of an increased membrane permeability at 3 hpi. The use of nonpermeant inhibitors provides a sensitive assay to estimate changes in membrane permeability induced by virus infection or by membrane-disrupting compounds. They give an accurate indication of the moment when changes in permeability start (4, 5, 128).

These phenomena, together with other morphological alterations induced by the virus, such as nuclear modifications, disruption of the cytoskeletal network (50, 70, 165), and the appearance of membrane vesicles (53, 163), have been collectively referred to as the cytopathic effect (CPE). Under the phase contrast microscope, cells are rounded, shrunk, and refringent. Appearance of CPE includes a number of morphological and physiological alterations that culminate in cell lysis and the release of the new progeny (45, 122). At the same time, late membrane leakiness alters the internal milieu and has important consequences for both cellular and viral macromolecular synthesis.

The phenomenology of the increase in membrane permeability during PV infection is fairly well known (47); more recently, the viral proteins involved in this phenomenon have been identified. Several picornaviral proteins have been proposed as "viroporins" or proteins with membrane-damaging properties (44, 54, 207, 214). Three PV proteins, 2B, 3A, and 3AB, expressed in *Escherichia coli* cells induced changes in membrane permeability to low-molecular-weight compounds (128). The most permeabilizing protein in this system was 2B. Later, two picornaviral proteins have been identified as major factors responsible for the plasma membrane permeability changes observed at late time of infection of mammalian cells: proteins 2BC and 2B (1, 72, 115, 207).

Rearrangement and Proliferation of Intracellular Membranes

The pioneering work of Dales et al. in 1965 revealed the existence of a large number of membrane vesicles in the perinuclear region of PV-infected cells (67). These structures are apparent 3 hpi and proliferate extensively, occupying almost all of the cytoplasm by 7 hpi (Fig. 2A). Accumulation of dense aggregates designated as "viroplasm," consisting of aggregated membranous structures, is observed in the cytoplasmic matrix (141). The proliferation of these membranous structures is a common morphological change induced by picornaviruses, including echovirus 9 (91, 92, 196), enterovirus 71 (178), coxsackievirus (116), mengovirus (7, 8, 175, 210), EMCV (68, 104), Theiler virus (85), and foot-and-mouth disease virus (FMDV) (224).

The virus-induced vesicles are very heterogeneous in size; their diameters range from 50 to 400 nm. Many of them contain material of a texture similar to that of the cytoplasmic matrix (122). Distinct portions of the vesicle membranes are very densely stained and thicker than typical intracellular membranes. Some vesicles appear to adhere but retain their integrity, although the region between two vesicles may appear as a single membrane (28, 29). Single vesicles usually present rounded or rather smooth elongated contours, whereas the "sticky vesicles" within clusters often have awkward irregular contours. At the beginning of poliovirus infection small vesicles accumulate in the central region of the cytoplasm, while at the end of the replication cycle the vesicles are bigger, resembling autolytic vacuoles. The use of cryofixation and electron microscopy has shown recently that the vesicles have a double lipid bilayer, suggesting a double-budding mechanism or a wrapping of the cytosol by membranous compartments (192). For some time it was considered that these cytoplasmic structures originated by budding from the endoplasmic reticulum (ER) (25), but some studies suggest that the ER constitutes a significant but not exclusive source of the intracellular membranes induced by PV infection. Markers from the Golgi apparatus and lysosomes are also found in these membranes (192). The generation of these vesicles requires at least in part de novo synthesis of phospholipids (97).

The microscopic observations were confirmed by biochemical studies. After infection with PV, cells incorporate increasing amounts of ^{32}P-phosphate and ^{3}H-choline into cellular phospholipids (62, 144, 163). The stimulation of phospholipid synthesis leads to the proliferation of membrane structures (56, 219). Incorporation of radioactive phospholipid precursors followed by fractionation of the cytoplasmic extracts in sucrose gradients revealed that the distribution of the cytoplasmic membranes changes during PV infection (37, 38, 152, 153). There is a preferential synthesis of smooth membranes of low density in PV-infected cells that are absent in uninfected cells. This membrane fraction obtained by centrifugation of cell extracts corresponds to the vesicles observed by electron microscopy (29, 30). Kinetic studies of ^{3}H-uridine incorporation indicate that PV RNA replication is associated with these smooth membranes (36–38) and the viral RNA replicase activity is found in this fraction (34, 89). Viral RNA synthesis also occurs in close association with membranous vesicles in cells infected with FMDV (177) and mengovirus (210). High-resolution autoradiography confirms that viral RNA synthesis takes place on virus-induced membranes (25, 26, 28, 29, 32, 76).

The mechanism used by PV to generate these intracellular vesicles remains unclear although protein 2BC seems to play an important part in this process. The requirement of these membranes for viral RNA replication will be discussed below.

Changes in Lipid Composition and Phospholipase Activity

During the picornavirus replication cycle cellular lipid molecules are involved in at least two stages: proliferation of cytoplasmic membranous vesicles and changes in membrane permeability. Both phenomena are the result of a very profound alteration in the metabolism, structure, and trafficking of cellular lipids induced by the virus.

Lipid Metabolism

The presence of the novel vesicles involved in picornavirus RNA replication (20, 37, 38, 164) requires an increased rate of incorporation of lipid precursors (such as phosphate, choline, or glycerol) into phospholipids of picornavirus-infected cells including PV, mengovirus, EMCV, and FMDV (7, 8, 36, 60, 144, 146, 152, 153, 210). Virus-induced enhancement in radioactive choline incorporation reflects an increase in de novo synthesis of phosphatidylcholine (175). Thus, this augmentation in choline uptake is an indirect measure of virus-induced membrane proliferation (60). Notably, these are the only cellular processes that are stimulated during PV infection, because metabolite transport as well as the synthesis of proteins, ATP, DNA, and RNA polymerase I-, II-, and III-mediated transcription are impaired in PV-infected cells (52, 58, 59, 83, 120, 121, 183, 184).

In general, the phospholipid composition of membranes from picornavirus-infected and uninfected cells is similar (152). In PV replication vesicles, the ratio of phospholipid:protein is doubled, whereas sphingomyelin content decreases (146, 152). In addition, Cornatzer et al. suggested that phosphatidylserine synthesis was not stimulated by PV (62). Mengovirus infection, however, produces a decrease in the rate of phosphatidylethanolamine synthesis and an increase of phosphatidylinositol synthesis (210). The bulk of phospholipids increases throughout infection in PV-infected HeLa cells, as measured by phosphorus content, lipid:phosphorus protein ratio, and incorporation of radioactive precursors (62, 112, 144). CTP:phosphorylcholine cytidylyl transferase (CCT) is the regulatory enzyme involved in the limiting step of de novo synthesis of the major phospholipid, phosphatidylcholine, in HeLa cells (114, 223). The reaction is regulated by the concentration of CTP, the amount of calcium, and the translocation of the soluble form of the enzyme CCT to the ER membranes (114, 186, 218, 222, 225, 228). Recently, a second and distinct human CCT has been described (138, 139). During PV infection, there is a rise in the amount of free CTP and calcium (56, 110, 219). However, incomplete turnover of neutral lipids is also favored in PV-infected cells and the analysis of lipid turnover suggests that all lipid metabolism in mengovirus- or PV-infected cells is directed to the synthesis of phospholipids (112, 175, 210).

There are very few data available about the metabolism of neutral lipids during a picornaviral infectious cycle. Cholesterol esters are decreased during mengovirus infection while the formation of triacylglycerols is significantly enhanced (210). PV infection induces an increased generation of diacylglycerols. At the same time, a higher uptake of this metabolite into new phospholipids takes place (112). In addition, production of arachidonic acid might be inhibited (100). Although PV VP4 capsid protein is covalently modified with a C14 saturated acid (myristic acid) (161), no increase in this fatty acid has been described. Myristoylation of VP4 is an important process at

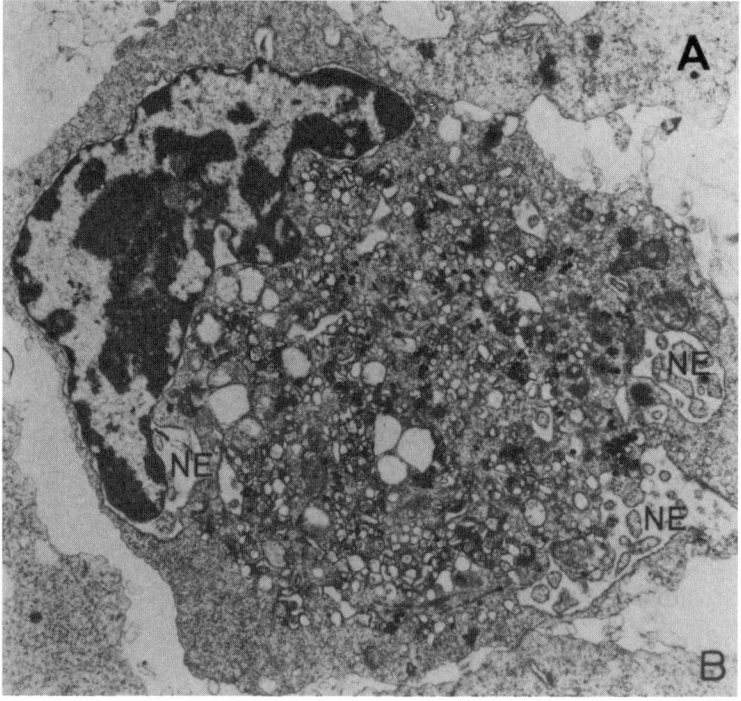

FIGURE 2 (A) Membranes generated in PV-infected cells. Electron microscopic autoradiograph of a PV-infected, actinomycin D-treated and ^{3}H-uridine-labeled HEp-2 cell at 4 hpi. Note the different types of vesicles filling the cytoplasm. Silver grains show different centers of viral RNA synthesis fused into a large area of vacuoles. The cell shows a typical PV CPE. The nucleus assumes the typical crescent shape and is pushed aside by the mass of vacuolated membranes. The outer part of the cytoplasm is devoid of ER and contains single ribosomes; it shows no silver grain indicative of viral RNA synthesis. Also free of silver grains are the "nuclear extrusions" that appear and tend to surround the central vacuolated region (×11,000). Reprinted from Virology (28), with permission. (B) Structure of the PV replication complex. Electron micrograph of a PV replication complex surrounded by and attached to a rosette of virus-induced membrane vesicles (V) and containing a second, compact membrane system (arrowheads). Immunocytochemical labeling with 2C-Mab and 5-nm colloidal gold. Bar: 100 nm. Reprinted from Journal of Virology (27), with permission.

multiple stages of the PV cycle (123, 151); recently, the capacity of the NH_2-terminal 9-amino-acid sequence of VP4 to confer both myristoylation and targeting to specialized membranes to different chimeras has been reported (140). During coxsackievirus B6 infection of Vero cells, a drastic increase in saturated C18 (stearic acid) but not in C16 fatty acids has been reported preceding the enhancement in membrane leakiness. However, stearic acid is under a strong cellular control because it returns to normal values later in infection. This increase could be sufficient to induce a physical change in the lipid bilayer of membranes (157).

Effects on Lipase Activities

Picornavirus infection gives rise to alteration of several phospholipase activities. Phosphatidylinositol-phospholipase C is enhanced during PV infection as measured by the increase of inositol trisphosphate (IP_3) formation (100). Both IP_3 and the other metabolite generated, diacylglycerol, might act as second messengers (24). Phosphatidylcholine-phospholipase C is also activated (112), while phospholipase A_2 becomes inhibited in PV-infected cells (100) (Fig. 3). Unlike PV, mengovirus infection provokes an activation of phospholipase D (210) and CVB3 induces phosphorylation and activation of phospholipase A_2 (109). Release of phospholipase A, as well as other enzymes, from lysosomes to the membranous cisternae has been reported for HEp-2 cells infected with PV (179).

The exact contribution of lipase activation to membrane leakiness remains to be established, but it seems that a general disorganization of the plasma membrane takes place at late times of infection (44, 46). The activation of phospholipases could be involved in several phenomena taking place during PV infection, e.g., increased phospholipid synthesis, CPE, and the increase of cytosolic calcium (3, 110, 112). The stimulation of CCT activity by degraded phospholipids was suggested to represent a positive feedback mechanism for the control of the synthesis of phospholipids (81). Thus, activation of phosphatidylcholine-phospholipase C activity in PV-infected cells could contribute to the stimulation of phospholipid synthesis. In this regard, an increased incorporation of diacylglycerol into phosphatidylcholine has been reported in PV-infected cells (112). During mengovirus infection, lipase activation has been implicated in virus release (108) and in lipid turnover (210), whereas lysophospholipids have been identified as natural detergents during infection (15, 210). CVB3 replication in Vero cells increases stearic acid levels, suggesting an involvement of this fatty acid in the CPE (157).

Inhibition of Vesicular Trafficking and Glycoprotein Processing

Concomitant with the formation of novel vesicles there is an important rearrangement of the intracellular membranous organelles of the secretory system, the disappearance of the Golgi complex, and a swelling of the ER together with a reorganization of the cytoskeletal framework (117,

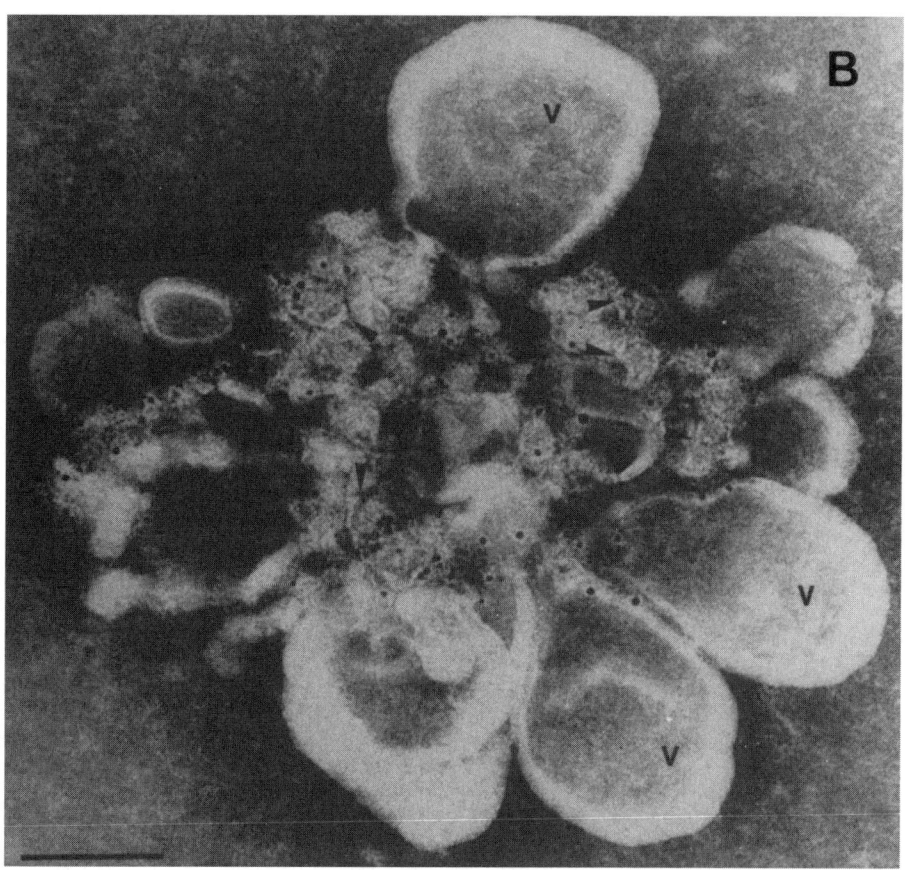

FIGURE 2 *Continued*

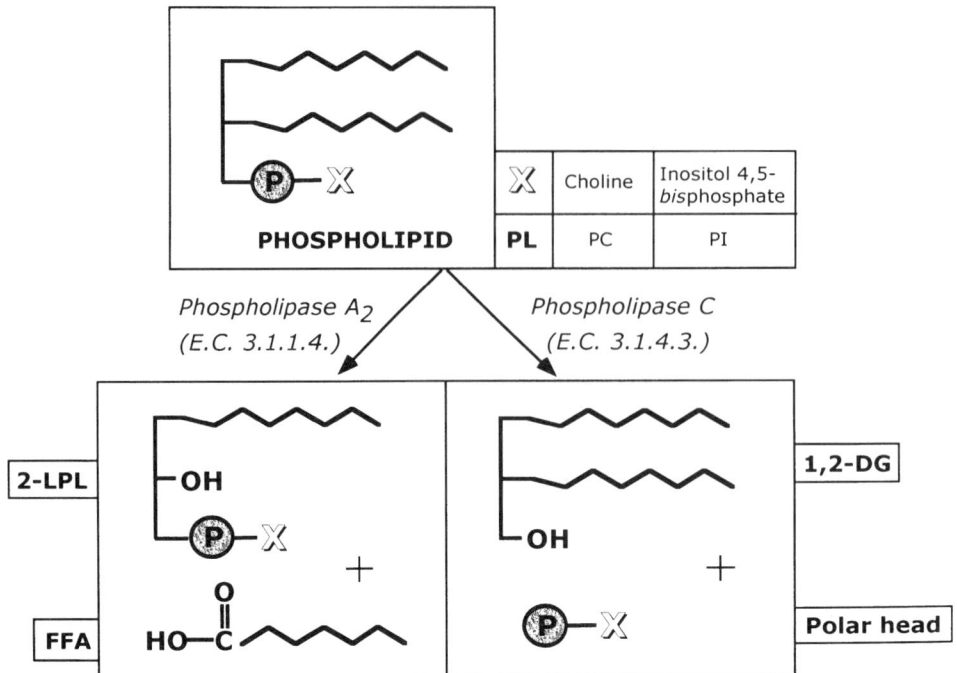

FIGURE 3 Modifications of lipase activity by picornavirus. Schematic representation of the action of phospholipases A₂ and C on a phospholipid. All phospholipids have a common backbone of sn-glycerol. The wavy lines denote fatty acyl esters or fatty acids; phosphate oxygens have been omitted for simplicity. "X" represents a polar head. The structures shown do not reflect the actual stereoconfiguration of a phospholipid. PL, phospholipid; PC, phosphatidylcholine; PI, phosphatidylinositol; 2-LPL, 2-lysophospholipid; FFA, free fatty acid; 1,2-DG, 1,2-diacylglycerol.

134). PV infection provokes the disassembly of the Golgi complex, an effect attributed to the expression of 2B protein (185). However, the recruitment of new vesicles by PV depends on a functional vesicular system because brefeldin A (BFA), an inhibitor of membrane traffic, blocks viral RNA replication (65, 111, 142). Certain selective inhibitors of PV replication such as Ro-090179 or ionophores (95, 113) exert their action by interfering with the proper functioning of the cellular vesicular system (185).

In addition, PV infection causes a powerful block in the secretion and transport of glycoproteins (70–72, 214). PV 2B, 2BC, and 3A proteins are able to block glycoprotein transport when they are expressed individually in mammalian cells (71, 72, 185), although the sites of action of these proteins may differ (71, 72, 185, 215). Thus, 3A seems to block transport from the ER to the Golgi apparatus, while 2B and 2BC appear to act on a later step in the exocytic pathway (72). Notably, PV 2BC exhibits the same blocking activity of the exocytic pathway in both yeast and mammalian cells (16, 18). A detailed analysis of this process in yeast cells using different protein markers revealed that 2BC interferes with vesicular system trafficking at the level of the vesicles that arise from the ER and fuse with the cis-Golgi or at the cis-Golgi itself (Fig. 4) (16). The individual expression of 3AB in mammalian cells also inhibits the transport of proteins out of the ER and induces an accumulation and swelling of ER membranes (71).

The inhibition of protein secretion observed during PV infection might help the virus evade the host immune response by interfering with secretion of interferon and other cytokines and by blocking antigen presentation in the context of major histocompatibility complex class I molecules (72).

PROLIFERATION OF INTRACELLULAR MEMBRANES IS NECESSARY FOR REPLICATION OF VIRAL GENOMES

Proliferation of cytoplasmic membranous vesicles is observed in cells infected by viruses that replicate their genomes in the cytoplasm (44, 84). Regarding picornaviruses, these vesicles have not only been associated with RNA replication, but also with virus morphogenesis and with development of the CPE, e.g., coxsackievirus, echovirus, EMCV, FMDV, and mengovirus (7, 8, 11, 68, 85, 116, 159, 210). In PV-, mengovirus-, and mouse Elberfeld virus-infected cells both phenomena (cytoplasmic membrane proliferation and viral replication) are coupled (146, 153, 175, 210, 230, 231).

Picornaviruses synthesize their genomes in association with newly generated membranous vesicles that proliferate from the mid-phase of infection (36–38). Sedimentation of cytoplasmic extracts in sucrose gradients yielded viral RNA polymerase activity associated with the smooth membranes (89). Viral replication complexes from this fraction contain all types of PV RNA and several viral proteins involved in RNA replication (77, 78, 201). High-resolution autoradiography also indicated that viral RNA synthesis is associated with these vesicles (27, 29, 32, 76, 211). Indeed, encapsidation of PV RNA starts in these complexes (168) in such a way that only newly synthesized PV RNA molecules are packaged (158). The replication

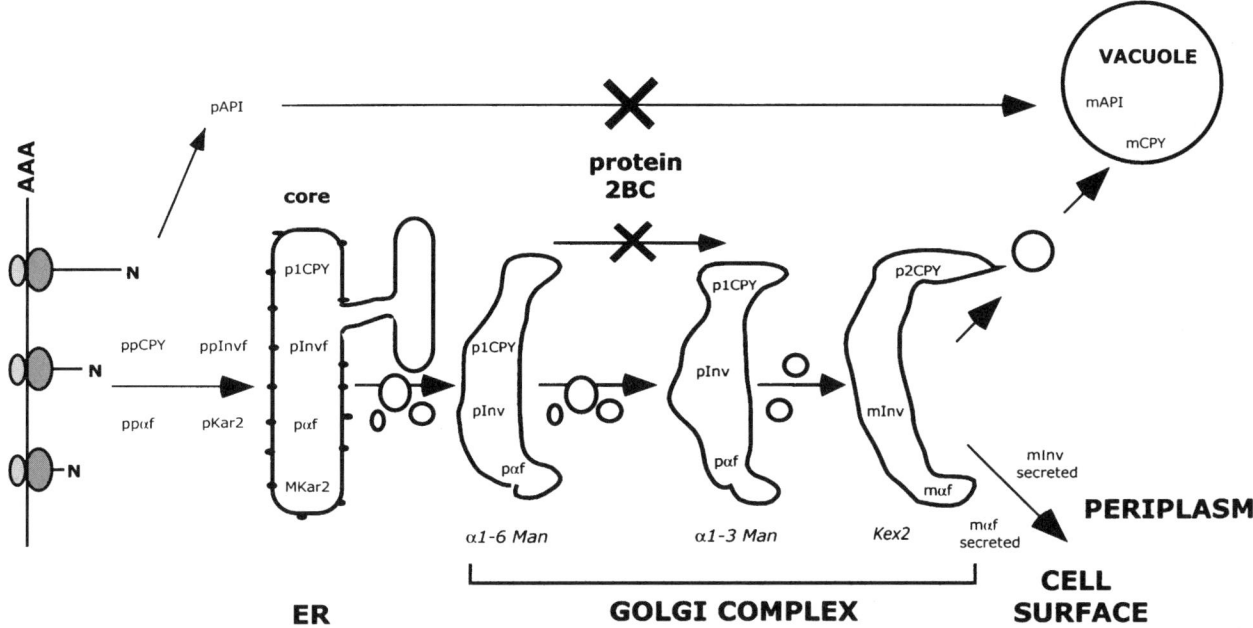

FIGURE 4 Schematic representation of protein transport in *Saccharomyces cerevisiae* and the sites of action of PV 2BC. Synthesis and maturation of four yeast proteins, vacuolar carboxypeptidase Y (CPY), aminopeptidase I (API), KAR2, and α-mating factor in the presence of PV protein 2BC. Reprinted from *The EMBO Journal* (16), with permission.

complex was identified on the surface of the membrane structures, which are arranged in a rosette-like fashion (Fig. 2B) (26, 28). Recently, structures similar to these rosette-like vesicles have been described in poliovirus-infected cells, the so-called detergent-insoluble membranes (DIM) to which some specific viral proteins are attached (140).

Several observations indicate that the membranous environment is necessary for viral RNA synthesis: (i) Initiation of RNA synthesis in vitro is abolished after treatment of crude replication complexes with detergents (199). (ii) Several viral proteins essential for RNA replication are physically associated with these membranes (193, 200). (iii) Inhibitors of the synthesis of the membranes or their rearrangements such as cerulenin or BFA block viral RNA synthesis (97, 111, 142).

For many years attempts to reconstitute membrane-free replication complexes that would synthesize single-stranded RNA with purified proteins and viral RNA were unsuccessful. Only the endogenous membrane-bound RNA replication complex, known as crude replication complex, present in cytoplasmic extracts from PV-infected cells was able to synthesize single-stranded RNA (197, 198, 209). The in vitro synthesis of VPg-pUpU, which is the primer for both positive- and negative-strand RNA initiation (119), is strictly dependent on the presence of membranes. Formation of VPg-pUpU is totally abolished by addition of detergent (199, 200), while minus-strand RNA generation could take place (229), indicating two different types of initiation of RNA synthesis. In good agreement with these findings, colocalization experiments show minus- and plus-strand viral RNA in different compartments (32). It has been shown that VPg can be uridylylated by the PV polymerase 3D in vitro to prime transcription by 3D polymerase (162). In this case, the addition of detergent does not affect the uridylylation of VPg or the elongation of RNA synthesis. However, the yield of products was low, indicating that efficient uridylylation may require additional factors, such as a hydrophobic membranous environment to stabilize protein-RNA complexes (162).

Additional evidence for the involvement of membranes in viral RNA replication comes from the fact that the replication complexes are physically associated with vesicles. The vesicles play a structural role in maintaining the complexes in the correct configuration for RNA synthesis and to provide the necessary viral proteins. PV 2B, 2C, and 3AB proteins could mediate the association between the replication complexes and membranes, all being essential for RNA replication (19, 25, 102, 103, 118, 124, 188). Astonishingly, a cell-free extract from uninfected cells is able to replicate, translate, and package RNA of PV (19, 148). However, the cell extract employed probably contains sufficient amounts of membrane material to allow viral RNA synthesis and assembly.

There is not only a physical connection between membranes and viral replication. Cerulenin, an inhibitor of phospholipid metabolism, blocks viral RNA synthesis soon after its addition, indicating that continuous phospholipid formation is needed for viral replication to occur and that preexisting membranes do not fulfill this requirement (97). Two mechanisms can be put forward to explain these results: (i) continuous synthesis of phospholipid molecules directly regulates the activity of a viral protein involved in PV genome replication without the need for newly made membranes; and (ii) maturation and organization of new membranes containing PV proteins are necessary to replicate viral genomes. Cerulenin inhibits viral production in vitro but does not affect virus-specific translation or protein processing (149). Moreover, modification of the physical characteristics of membranes by oleic acid selectively blocks PV RNA synthesis, suggesting that not only membrane formation but also the integrity of the mature membrane is required for replication of the PV genome (98).

Finally, evidence for the requirement of a membranous environment for viral RNA synthesis comes from the ability of BFA, an inhibitor of vesicular trafficking, to potently block PV RNA replication in infected cells (111, 142). Not all picornaviruses are equally susceptible to BFA; replication of enteroviruses and rhinoviruses is strongly blocked by the antibiotic whereas a cardiovirus (EMCV) is insensitive to its action (111). Therefore, PV-induced membranous vesicles are a process inhibited by BFA. Notably, the inhibition of PV replication by BFA can be reproduced in a cell-free replication system (65). N-terminal peptides corresponding to sequences of ADP-ribosylation factors (ARFs) that compete with ARF interaction during coated vesicle formation are inhibitors of cell-free RNA replication. These findings suggest that the activity of ARF proteins is somehow required for viral RNA replication (65).

PROTEINS INVOLVED IN MEMBRANE EFFECTS AND THEIR MECHANISMS OF ACTION

2B Is a Potential Viroporin

The sequence of protein 2B is one of the least conserved among picornaviruses. Picornavirus 2B is a rather small protein of about 100 amino acids (Fig. 5A) that contains two hydrophobic regions (Fig. 5B), one amphipathic α-helix (amino acids 34 to 53 in PV) (Fig. 5C) and a potential transmembrane domain with a β-sheet configuration (amino acids 61 to 78 in PV); closely following this domain are several positively charged amino acids. This general structure is true for the 2B molecule of most picornaviruses (213), although in members more distant from enteroviruses, such as FMDV, 2B contains 170 amino acids and a second transmembrane domain at the C terminus.

The precise function of 2B in the picornavirus replication cycle remains to be defined. It was shown that PV with mutations in the 2B gene is defective in genome replication (118, 188). Moreover, some 2B mutants cannot be complemented in trans and even interfere with wild-type PV (118). Recently, some biochemical activities have been reported. Different data indicate that the 2B proteins of CVB3 and PV may represent the first examples of viroporin from naked viruses (1, 18, 213–215). Viroporins are hydrophobic proteins encoded by animal viruses that are able to disturb membrane integrity, favoring the release of viral progeny (12, 54, 94, 99, 187, 214). Other protein families (holins, hemolysins, defensins) or peptides (cecropines, magainins) also destabilize the lipid bilayer (64).

The presence of amphipathic α-helices is a general feature of these membrane-disrupting proteins. Two models of action have emerged from structural and functional studies of these proteins: (i) the helices form oligomers and constitute an aqueous pore by spanning the membrane, exposing their hydrophobic sides to the lipid bilayer and their hydrophilic faces to the inner aqueous pore (Fig. 5D); (ii) the amphipathic helices lie parallel to the membrane plane and partially penetrate it. This interaction disturbs the structure of the lipid bilayer, making the phospholipids more susceptible to degradation by phospholipases. These two models are not mutually exclusive (213, 215).

In the case of enterovirus 2B, different lines of evidence support the first model, as follows. (i) Studies using the two-hybrid system and in vitro assays have shown that 2BC and its cleavage products, 2B and 2C, interact in all possible combinations, and at least the 2B-2B interaction is required for PV replication (66). It should, therefore, be considered that multimers of 2B form membrane-embedded pores. (ii) Analysis of mutations in CVB3 2B and PV 2B and 2BC confirmed that the predicted cationic amphipathic α-helix in 2B is a major determinant for its ability to increase permeability (18, 213, 215) and, in turn, to allow RNA replication (212, 216).

Studies examining the localization of CVB3 2B showed that this protein associates directly with the plasma membrane, suggesting that its disrupting action might be direct. A mutant containing poorly processed 2B-2C cleavage sites exhibited a reduced ability to modify plasma membrane permeabilization (217). The permeabilizing activity of CVB3 2B has been implicated in virus release, since viruses carrying a mutant 2B protein exhibited a defect in virus yield (214). However, in the case of PV 2B, it has been reported that this protein is located mainly in the central portion of the cytoplasm, associated with the membranous vesicles that surround the viral replication complexes. Therefore, the changes in plasma membrane permeability induced by PV 2B could be an indirect effect of internal membrane alterations (185). The 2BC proteins of PV and hepatitis A virus (HAV) also exhibit a permeabilizing activity that is even stronger than that of the 2B protein (see below).

The expression of 2B from CVB3 produces an increase of cytoplasmic calcium ions (214), whereas PV 2B is devoid of this activity (3). This increase in intracellular calcium might be a consequence of calcium influx from the exterior and/or from intracellular pools (214). The enhanced calcium concentration could activate phospholipases, giving rise to diacylglycerol that, in turn, activates protein kinase C. Modification of the lipid bilayer might stimulate capacitative calcium entry across the plasma membrane. Moreover, lowering the calcium level in the lumen causes vesiculation of the ER (143); this budding from the ER could in part explain the origin of new membranous structures induced by picornaviruses (25).

An initial consequence of membrane modifications seems to be a prerequisite for viral RNA replication since mutations that disrupt the cationic amphipathic α-helix in protein 2B cause defects in viral replication (213). Other activities for protein 2B have been described. The expression of PV protein 2B showed a disassembly of the Golgi complex and a block in protein secretion (72, 185). In addition, protein 2B from HAV has been implicated in the rearrangement of cellular membranes, since it is closely associated with the altered membranes (96).

2C, a Link between Cellular Membranes and Viral Nucleic Acids

PV protein 2C is a 329-amino-acid polypeptide that contains a typical nucleoside triphosphate (NTP)-binding domain (Fig. 6) (69). Its sequence is one of the most highly conserved among all picornaviruses. A tentative model of domain organization has recently been proposed for this protein. According to this model, 2C would have three differentiated regions: the central portion includes the NTP-binding domain, while the N- and C-terminal ends show an α-helix configuration and might contain amphipathic helices (203). A cysteine-rich region near the carboxy terminus displays a zinc finger motif that is conserved

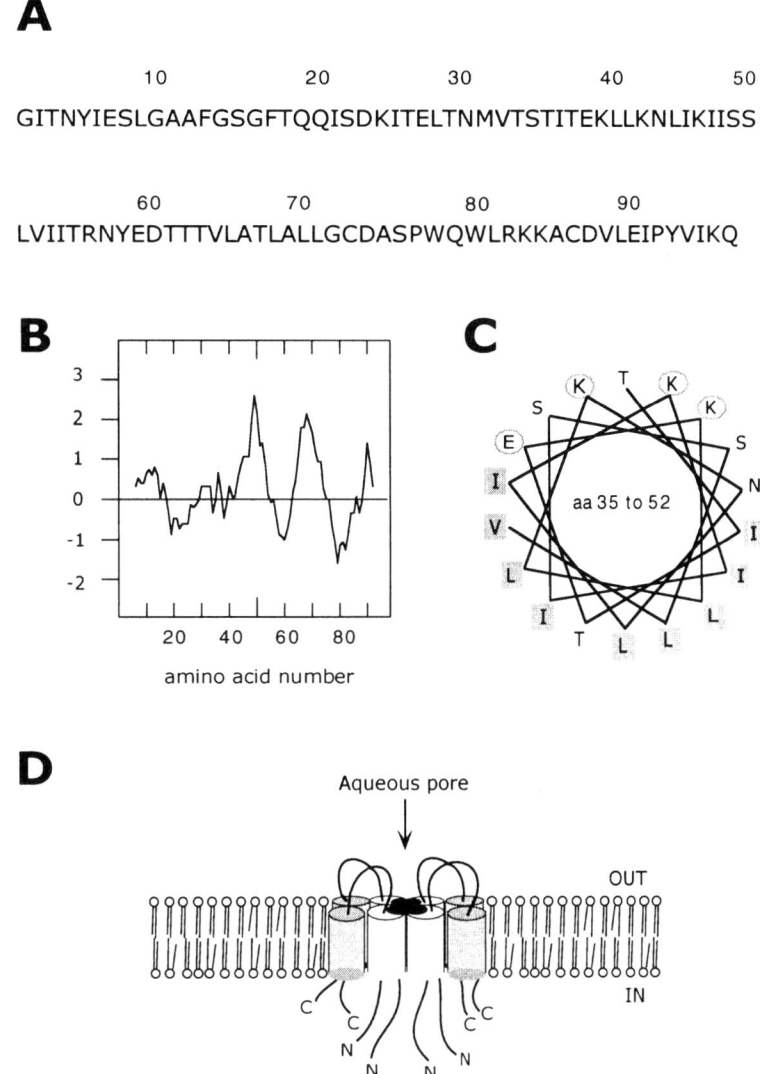

FIGURE 5 Structure of PV 2B. (A) Amino acid sequence of PV 2B protein. (B) Hydropathy plot according to Kyte and Doolittle (126). (C) Helical wheel diagram of a putative amphipathic helix found according to the method of Schiffer and Edmundson (191). The distribution of charged residues on the hydrophilic face is well conserved among all enteroviruses. Hydrophobic residues are boxed; charged amino acids are circled. (D) Model of 2B insertion into membranes. Cylinders represent helices, the amphipathic one (nearer the N terminus) and the hydrophobic one (nearer the C terminus). Hydrophilic α-helix face is darkly shaded. Reprinted from *Virology* (215), with permission.

in enteroviruses and rhinoviruses and is essential for viral replication (169).

Protein 2C is needed for viral RNA synthesis since viruses with linker insertion mutations in the 2C-coding genomic region were found to be defective in viral RNA synthesis (135). Moreover, picornavirus mutants dependent on or resistant to RNA synthesis inhibitors such as guanidine, hydroxybenzyl-benzimidazole, or benzimidazole derivatives have lesions that map to the 2C gene (13, 101, 170–173, 188, 195, 205). On the other hand, mutations in the PV genome that confer resistance to hydantoin, a compound that inhibits morphogenesis but not replication, also map at the 2C region (220). Other functions such as ATPase and GTPase activities (145, 170, 180) and interaction with RNA (14, 181) have also been assigned to 2C protein. Oligomerization of 2C seems to be an essential step in the replication of the viral genome (205).

The 2C protein has been localized to the surface of the vesicles and in association with viral RNA (25). When this protein is expressed in a baculovirus system, it appears with a fraction enriched in plasma membrane and smooth ER (145). 2C might interact with membranes through its N-terminal region, which contains a putative amphipathic helix sufficient for membrane association (73, 74, 160, 203). More recently, a second amphipathic α-helix located at the C terminus has also been implicated in membrane interaction (203). Regarding the role of 2C, it has been shown that addition of guanidine causes the replication complex to detach from the membranes, probably due to its inhibitory effect on the ATPase activity of 2C (170), suggesting that 2C is responsible for maintaining a correct spatial organization of the replication machinery (30). This dissociation of the replication complex would inhibit the initiation of the viral RNA synthesis (35, 39). Finally, the individual expression of PV 2C induces the formation of tubular swirls of ER membranes and some vesicles with a myelin-like arrangement (2, 55). A detailed analysis of 2C regions involved in membrane rearrangement has been carried out in human and yeast cells. In both systems, progressive deletions at the N or C terminus of 2C dictate the type of membrane generated (18, 203). Some of these activities, e.g., RNA binding, membrane association, or membrane rearrangement, have been also reported for HAV 2C (125, 202).

Therefore, genetic evidence and biochemical data indicate that 2C is a multifunctional protein involved in several processes during virus replication (136, 220, 226). It can be hypothesized that 2C is responsible for binding of poliovirus RNA to the induced cytoplasmic vesicles and participates in the spatial organization of the replicative complexes (14, 181, 203). In addition, 2C may participate in other processes, such as RNA packaging (135, 145, 180, 220).

2BC, the Most Potent Membrane-Active Protein of Picornaviruses

The precursor 2BC remains largely uncleaved in picornavirus-infected cells (Fig. 6) and exerts some of the activities described for the mature products 2B and 2C (226). 2BC participates by itself in certain processes of the replication cycle; thus, the insertion of the EMCV 5′ untranslated region between the 2B and 2C genes is lethal for PV. In contrast, if the same region is inserted between 2A^{pro} and 2B, a viable PV-EMCV hybrid is formed (147, 226). This suggests that 2BC should be present as such, and the synthesis of 2B and 2C separately is not sufficient to support the PV replication cycle.

PV 2BC has been implicated in the induction of membrane proliferation (188). The vesicle proliferation induced by 2BC in mammalian cells is similar to that observed in PV-infected cells (2, 55). Notably, the inducible expression of protein 2BC in yeast cells also provokes membrane proliferation (Fig. 7) in a manner similar to that seen in PV-infected human cells, despite the evolutionary distance between the vesicular systems of these cell types (16). In the case of HAV, 2BC can also induce rearrangement of intracellular membranes although this virus shows no CPE in cultures of mammalian cells (96, 202). The structures generated by HAV 2C and 2BC proteins from a cytopathic HAV strain seem to be more similar to those generated by PV 2C and 2BC (202). Therefore, there is a correlation between the ability of these proteins to induce proliferation of membranes and the ability of HAV to induce the CPE.

The permeabilizing activity of poliovirus 2BC protein is much greater than 2B alone (1, 18, 72). In addition, PV 2BC, but not 2B, increases cytosolic free calcium levels (3) and releases intracellular nucleotides to the medium (1) in mammalian cells. The HAV 2BC protein also exhibits this permeabilization activity (115). The inhibition of the exocytic pathway between ER and Golgi described for 2B is also seen with 2BC (see Fig. 4) (16, 72).

It is possible that the activity of 2BC itself could account for part of the cytopathic phenotype observed in PV-infected cells, such as membrane permeabilization and intracellular vesicle proliferation. In this regard, it is interesting to keep in mind the results obtained in yeast. Characterization of a number of site-directed and random mutants identified the initial N-terminal amino acids of 2C as a major determinant of the 2BC cytotoxic activity. Moreover, deletion of the C terminus of 2B generated a more cytotoxic 2B protein. Therefore, the intramolecular interaction of the C-terminal region of 2B with the N-terminal region of 2C in 2BC might make this protein more active than its processing products, 2B and 2C (18). The processing of 2BC by 3C^{pro} could then induce a conformational change both in the C terminus of 2B and in the N terminus of 2C that generates two new proteins, 2B and 2C, with different locations and different roles compared with those of 2BC (Fig. 6) (217). This putative intramolecular interaction between 2B and 2C regions in the 2BC protein has also been inferred from an extensive analysis of PV protein interactions using the two-hybrid system (66).

3A Anchors 3B to Membranes To Allow Priming of Viral RNA Synthesis

A number of genetic and biochemical studies on 3A, VPg, and 3AB implicate these proteins in RNA replication (9, 10, 22, 107, 162, 176, 193, 200, 227). The main role for 3AB is as the donor of VPg (3B) to RNA chains, thereby participating in viral genome replication. Since these studies have been reviewed in chapter 19 of this volume, we will discuss here only the effects of these proteins in membrane function.

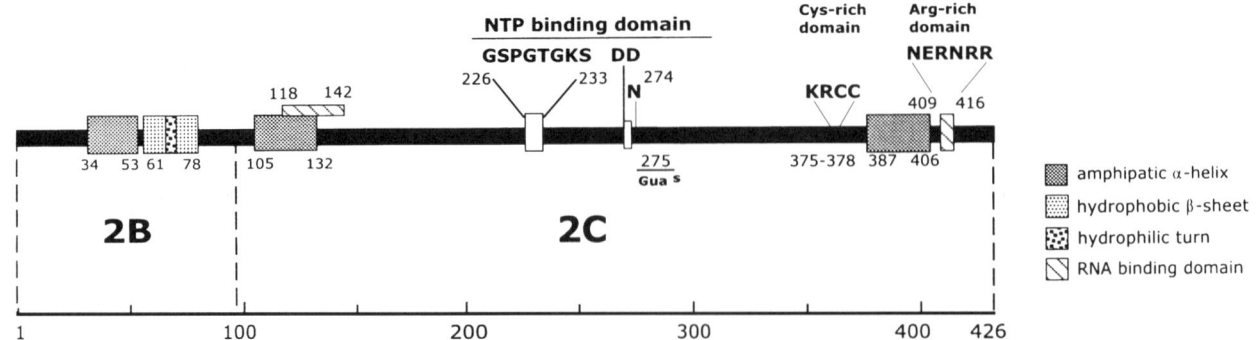

FIGURE 6 PV 2BC motifs. Linear map of PV protein 2BC. Functional domains for RNA and NTP binding are depicted for 2C. Reprinted from *The EMBO Journal* (16), with permission.

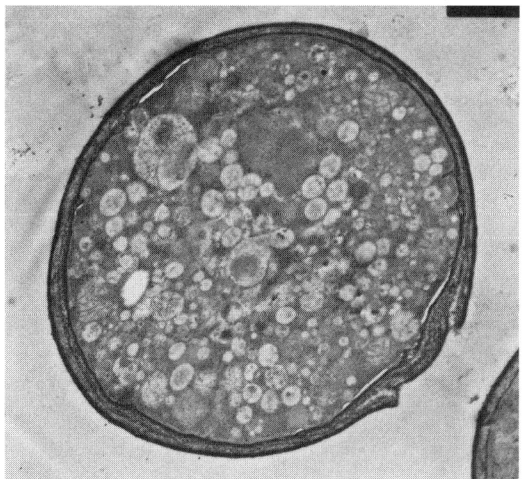

FIGURE 7 Intracellular vesicle proliferation induced by PV 2BC in yeast. Thin-section electron microscopy of yeast cells expressing 2BC. Cells were fixed at 20 hpi and were processed for electron microscopy. Bar = 1 μM. Reprinted from *EMBO Journal* (16), with permission.

Protein 3AB interacts with membranes both in vivo and in vitro (174, 193, 208) and behaves as an integral membrane protein (57). 3A protein contains a conserved hydrophobic region of 22 amino acids (residues 60 to 80) near its C terminus (130, 194), which is responsible for association with membranes (Fig. 8A) (124, 208). The introduction of charged residues into this hydrophobic sequence disrupts the 3AB membrane interaction (57). Separated by only 7 amino acids from that region, the 22-amino-acid sequence of PV protein VPg (3B) acts as a primer in PV RNA replication and is covalently linked to genomic RNA in virus particles (93, 182, 193). Thus, the hydrophobic region might serve to anchor 3AB to the membranous replication complex, at the same time providing the VPg needed to initiate viral replication. In addition, amino acid substitution in the 3AB hydrophobic region drastically altered the pattern of proteolytic processing of the viral polyprotein (87). Membrane insertion of PV precursor polypeptides, probably through the 3AB domain, might be required for correct polyprotein processing (132, 156, 227).

The cloning and inducible expression of PV nonstructural proteins in *E. coli* led to the identification of two polypeptides, namely, 2B and 3A/3AB, that are toxic for bacterial cells (128, 131). A genetic screening led to the identification of amino acid substitutions in the membrane-spanning region of 3A protein that blocked membrane permeabilization in *E. coli* (Fig. 8A) (129, 130). Full-length PV cDNA carrying these mutations has been obtained (133). Most of the changes produced nonviable viruses, probably due to the multifunctional character of the protein. However, a single amino acid substitution (I46T) leads to a mutant virus with a dramatic reduction in cytotoxic activity in Vero cells, but not in HeLa cells. This result indicates a role for 3A/3AB in virus-induced CPE.

A relationship between protein 3A and the cytopathic phenotype is also suggested in HAV and FMDV. In the case of HAV, most wild-type isolates replicate without inducing visible CPE; however, some HAV variants induce

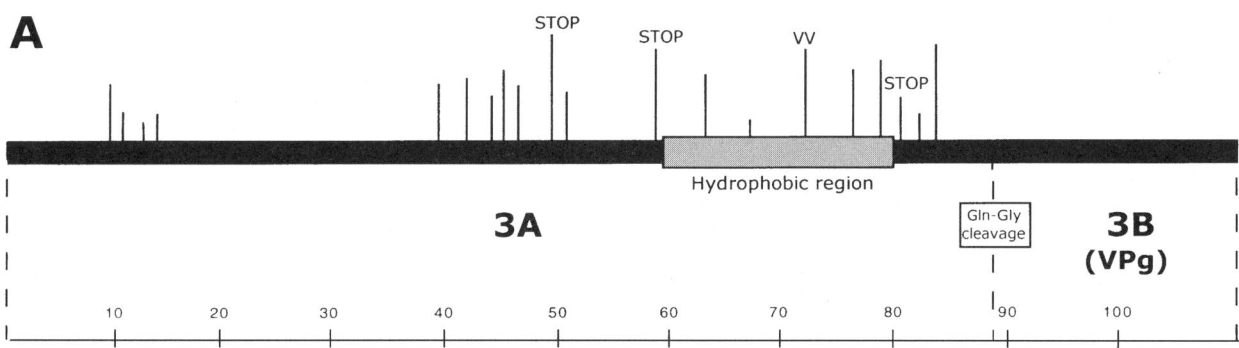

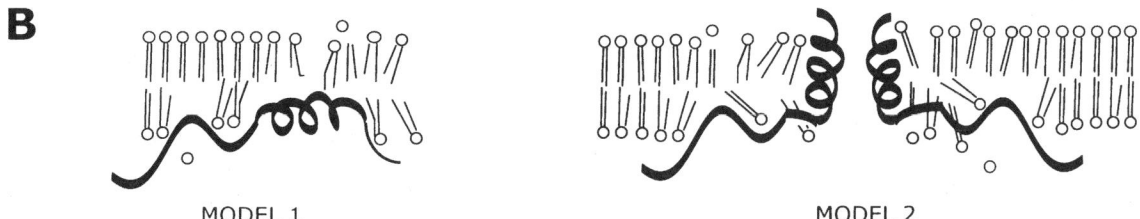

FIGURE 8 Structure of PV 3AB. (A) Schematic representation of the 3AB protein showing the conserved hydrophobic region (amino acids 60 to 80) and the positions of the different amino acid changes. The length of the line showing each variant represents the degree of change as measured by the lack of permeabilization to hygromycin B in *E. coli*. The largest line corresponds to the lowest permeabilizing capacity. (B) Two alternative models are represented to explain the mode of action of 3AB as a membrane permeabilizer in *E. coli* cells. Reprinted from *Journal of General Virology* (130), with permission.

CPE. The genome sequence of these variants indicates a deletion in the 3A gene near the N terminus that might be responsible for the CPE phenotype (150). The 3AB proteins of two HAV strains (FG and HM175), which, respectively, cause CPE or persistent replication in cell culture, were expressed in *E. coli*. The protein 3AB of the cytopathogenic HAV strain induced a pronounced increase in membrane permeability leading to cytolysis, whereas 3AB of the attenuated HAV strain HM175 did not affect bacterial membrane integrity. A putative amphipathic helix is present in the N-terminal tract of HAV 3A FG, which could be responsible for the pore-forming ability, inducing the membrane leakiness observed in bacteria (174). To assess the structure-function relationship of HAV protein 3A, site-specific mutations were introduced. The changes did not affect membrane binding but altered or blocked the ability to permeabilize bacterial membranes. This result suggests that the formation of a putative amphipathic helix and the presence of negative charges at the N terminus are crucial for the cytotoxic feature of 3A FG (23). Studies in mammalian cells should be made to test the role of the protein during virus infection.

Sequence analysis of wild-type and attenuated strains of FMDV revealed nucleotide deletions in the 3A coding regions of the attenuated strains, suggesting that this polypeptide may contribute to virulence in cattle (90). The membrane-modifying capacity of FMDV 3A has been revealed by its ability to promote a dramatic intracellular membrane proliferation in *E. coli* (224).

Finally, the synthesis of PV 3A in mammalian cells alters the location of intracellular membrane markers and blocks the exocytic pathway in tissue culture cells (72). The electron microscopic analysis of cells expressing 3A showed a distinct accumulation of dilated tubular and whirled membranes derived from the ER (71).

Structural characteristics of 3A/3AB might implicate a pore-forming capacity for these proteins. However, attempts to localize 3A/3AB at the plasma membrane have been unsuccessful, and the individual expression of 3A/3AB proteins in mammalian or yeast cells did not increase plasma membrane permeability (1, 17). The inability of 3A to permeabilize mammalian cells may be due to its remaining in internal membranes when it is expressed individually. Additional experiments should be aimed at testing directly the potential pore-forming capacity of 3A in model membranes.

The financial support of DGICYT project no. PM99-0002 and CAM project no. 08.2/0024.2/2000 is acknowledged. Further support to Centro de Biología Molecular was provided by an institutional grant from the Fundación Ramón Areces.

REFERENCES

1. **Aldabe, R., A. Barco, and L. Carrasco.** 1996. Membrane permeabilization by poliovirus proteins 2B and 2BC. *J. Biol. Chem.* **271:**23134–23137.
2. **Aldabe, R., and L. Carrasco.** 1995. Induction of membrane proliferation by poliovirus proteins 2C and 2BC. *Biochem. Biophys. Res. Commun.* **206:**64–76.
3. **Aldabe, R., A. Irurzun, and L. Carrasco.** 1997. Poliovirus protein 2BC increases cytosolic free calcium concentrations. *J. Virol.* **71:**6214–6217.
4. **Alonso, M. A., and L. Carrasco.** 1981. Selective inhibition of cellular protein synthesis by amphotericin B in EMC virus-infected cells. *Virology* **114:**247–251.
5. **Alonso, M. A., and L. Carrasco.** 1981. Relationship between membrane permeability and the translation capacity of human HeLa cells studied by means of the ionophore nigericin. *Eur. J. Biochem.* **118:**289–294.
6. **Alonso, R., J. I. Andres, M. T. García-Lopez, F. G. de las Heras, R. Herranz, B. Alarcón, and L. Carrasco.** 1985. Synthesis and antiviral evaluation of nucleosides of 5-methylimidazole-4-carboxamide. *J. Med. Chem.* **28:**834–838.
7. **Amako, K., and S. Dales.** 1962. Cytopathology of mengovirus infection. I. Relationship between cellular disintegration and virulence. *Virology* **32:**184–200.
8. **Amako, J., and S. Dales.** 1962. Cytopathology of mengovirus infection. II. Proliferation of membranous cisternae. *Virology* **32:**201–205.
9. **Andino, R., G. E. Rieckhof, P. L. Achacoso, and D. Baltimore.** 1993. Poliovirus RNA synthesis utilizes an RNP complex formed around the 5′-end of viral RNA. *EMBO J.* **12:**3587–3598.
10. **Andino, R., G. E. Rieckhof, and D. Baltimore.** 1990. A functional ribonucleoprotein complex forms around the 5′ end of poliovirus RNA. *Cell* **63:**369–380.
11. **Arlinghaus, R. B., and J. Polatnick.** 1967. Detergent-solubilized RNA polymerase from cells infected with foot-and-mouth disease virus. *Science* **158:**1320–1322.
12. **Arroyo, J., M. Boceta, M. E. González, M. Michel, and L. Carrasco.** 1995. Membrane permeabilization by different regions of the human immunodeficiency virus type 1 transmembrane glycoprotein gp41. *J. Virol.* **69:**4095–4102.
13. **Baltera, R. F. J., and D. R. Tershak.** 1989. Guanidine-resistant mutants of poliovirus have distinct mutations in peptide 2C. *J. Virol* **63:**4441–4444.
14. **Banerjee, R., A. Echeverri, and A. Dasgupta.** 1997. Poliovirus-encoded 2C polypeptide specifically binds to the 3′-terminal sequences of viral negative-strand RNA. *J. Virol.* **71:**9570–9578.
15. **Barbanti-Brodano, G., L. Possati, and M. La Placa.** 1971. Inactivation of polykaryocytogenic and hemolytic activities of Sendai virus by phospholipase B (lysolecithinase). *J. Virol.* **8:**796–800.
16. **Barco, A., and L. Carrasco.** 1995. A human virus protein, poliovirus protein 2BC, induces membrane proliferation and blocks the exocytic pathway in the yeast *Saccharomyces cerevisiae*. *EMBO J.* **14:**3349–3364.
17. **Barco, A., and L. Carrasco.** 1995. Cloning and inducible synthesis of poliovirus non-structural proteins in *Saccharomyces cerevisiae*. *Gene* **156:**19–25.
18. **Barco, A., and L. Carrasco.** 1998. Identification of regions of poliovirus 2BC protein that are involved in cytotoxicity. *J. Virol.* **72:**3560–3570.
19. **Barton, D. J., E. P. Black, and J. B. Flanegan.** 1995. Complete replication of poliovirus in vitro: preinitiation RNA replication complexes require soluble cellular factors for the synthesis of VPg-linked RNA. *J. Virol.* **69:**5516–5527.
20. **Becker, Y., S. Penman, and J. E. Darnell.** 1963. A cytoplasmic particulate involved in poliovirus synthesis. *Virology* **21:**274–276.
21. **Belnap, D. M., D. J. Filman, B. L. Trus, N. Q. Cheng, F. P. Booy, J. F. Conway, S. Curry, C. N. Hiremath, S. K. Tsang, A. C. Steven, and J. M. Hogle.** 2000. Molecular tectonic model of virus structural transitions: the putative cell entry states of poliovirus. *J. Virol.* **74:**1342–1354.
22. **Beneduce, F., A. Ciervo, Y. Kusov, V. Gauss-Müller, and G. Morace.** 1999. Mapping of protein domains of hepatitis A virus 3AB essential for interaction with 3CD and viral RNA. *Virology* **264:**410–421.
23. **Beneduce, F., A. Ciervo, and G. Morace.** 1997. Site-directed mutagenesis of hepatitis A virus protein 3A: ef-

fects on membrane interaction. *Biochim. Biophys. Acta Bio-Membr.* **1326:**157–165.
24. **Berridge, M. J.** 1987. Inositol lipids and cell proliferation. *Biochim. Biophys. Acta* **907:**33–45.
25. **Bienz, K., D. Egger, and L. Pasamontes.** 1987. Association of polioviral proteins of the P2 genomic region with the viral replication complex and virus-induced membrane synthesis as visualized by electron microscopic immunocytochemistry and autoradiography. *Virology* **160:**220–226.
26. **Bienz, K., D. Egger, and T. Pfister.** 1994. Characteristics of the poliovirus replication complex. *Arch. Virol.* **136**(Suppl. 9)**:**147–157.
27. **Bienz, K., D. Egger, T. Pfister, and M. Troxler.** 1992. Structural and functional characterization of the poliovirus replication complex. *J. Virol.* **66:**2740–2747.
28. **Bienz, K., D. Egger, Y. Rasser, and W. Bossart.** 1980. Kinetics and location of poliovirus macromolecular synthesis in correlation to virus-induced cytopathology. *Virology* **100:**390–399.
29. **Bienz, K., D. Egger, Y. Rasser, and W. Bossart.** 1983. Intracellular distribution of poliovirus proteins and the induction of virus-specific cytoplasmic structures. *Virology* **131:**39–48.
30. **Bienz, K., D. Egger, M. Troxler, and L. Pasamontes.** 1990. Structural organization of poliovirus RNA replication is mediated by viral proteins of the P2 genomic region. *J. Virol.* **64:**1156–1163.
31. **Bienz, K., D. Egger, and D. A. Wolff.** 1973. Virus replication, cytopathology, and lysosomal enzyme response of mitotic and interphase Hep-2 cells infected with poliovirus. *J. Virol.* **11:**565–574.
32. **Bolten, R., D. Egger, R. Gosert, G. Schaub, L. Landmann, and K. Bienz.** 1998. Intracellular localization of poliovirus plus- and minus-strand RNA visualized by strand-specific fluorescent in situ hybridization. *J. Virol.* **72:**8578–8585.
33. **Bossart, W., and K. Bienz.** 1979. Virus replication, cytopathology, and lysosomal enzyme response in enucleated HEp-2 cells infected with poliovirus. *Virology* **92:**331–339.
34. **Butterworth, B. E., E. J. Shimshick, and F. H. Yin.** 1976. Association of the polioviral RNA polymerase complex with phospholipid membranes. *J. Virol.* **19:**457–466.
35. **Caliguiri, L. A., and I. Tamm.** 1968. Action of guanidine on the replication of poliovirus RNA. *Virology* **35:**408–417.
36. **Caliguiri, L. A., and I. Tamm.** 1969. Membranous structures associated with translation and transcription of poliovirus RNA. *Science* **166:**885–886.
37. **Caliguiri, L. A., and I. Tamm.** 1970. Characterization of poliovirus-specific structures associated with cytoplasmic membranes. *Virology* **42:**112–122.
38. **Caliguiri, L. A., and I. Tamm.** 1970. The role of cytoplasmic membranes in poliovirus biosynthesis. *Virology* **42:**100–111.
39. **Caliguiri, L. A., and I. Tamm.** 1973. Guanidine and 2-(α-hydroxybenzyl)benzimidazole (HBB): selective inhibitors of picornavirus multiplication, p. 257–294. *In* W. Carter (ed.), *Selective Inhibitors of Viral Function.* CRC Press, Cleveland, Ohio.
40. **Camarasa, M. J., P. Fernández-Resa, M. T. García-Lopez, F. G. de las Heras, P. P. Méndez-Castrillón, B. Alarcón, and L. Carrasco.** 1985. Uridine 5′-diphosphate glucose analogues. Inhibitors of protein glycosylation that show antiviral activity. *J. Med. Chem.* **28:**40–46.
41. **Carrasco, L.** 1978. Membrane leakiness after viral infection and a new approach to the development of antiviral agents. *Nature* **272:**694–699.
42. **Carrasco, L.** 1981. Modification of membrane permeability induced by animal viruses early in infection. *Virology* **113:**623–629.
43. **Carrasco, L.** 1994. Picornavirus inhibitors. *Pharmacol. Ther.* **64:**215–290.
44. **Carrasco, L.** 1995. Modification of membrane permeability by animal viruses. *Adv. Virus Res.* **45:**61–112.
45. **Carrasco, L., and J. L. Castrillo.** 1987. The regulation of translation in picornavirus-infected cells, p. 115–146. *In* L. Carrasco (ed.), *Mechanisms of Viral Toxicity in Animal Cells.* CRC Press, Boca Raton, Fla.
46. **Carrasco, L., M. J. Otero, and J. L. Castrillo.** 1989. Modification of membrane permeability by animal viruses. *Pharmacol. Ther.* **40:**171–212.
47. **Carrasco, L., L. Perez, A. Irurzun, J. Lama, F. Martinez-Abarca, P. Rodriguez, R. Guinea, J. L. Castrillo, M. A. Sanz, and M. J. Ayala.** 1993. Modification of membrane permeability by animal viruses, p. 283–305. *In* L. Carrasco, N. Sonenberg, and E. Wimmer (ed.), *Regulation of Gene Expression in Animal Viruses.* Plenum Press, London, United Kingdom.
48. **Carrasco, L., and A. E. Smith.** 1976. Sodium ions and the shut-off of host cell protein synthesis by picornaviruses. *Nature* **264:**807–809.
49. **Carrasco, L., and D. Vazquez.** 1983. Viral translation inhibitors, p. 279–296. *In* F. E. Hahn (ed.), *Antibiotics VI.* Springer-Verlag, Berlin, Germany.
50. **Castrillo, J. L., and L. Carrasco.** 1985. Increased inhibition of cellular RNA synthesis by α-amanitin during entry of viruses into animal cells. *FEMS Microbiol. Lett.* **26:**221–225.
51. **Castrillo, J. L., and L. Carrasco.** 1986. The inhibition of nucleic acid synthesis in encephalomyocarditis virus-infected L929 cells: effects on nucleoside transport. *Mol. Cell. Biochem.* **71:**53–60.
52. **Castrillo, J. L., and L. Carrasco.** 1987. Adenovirus late protein synthesis is resistant to the inhibition of translation induced by poliovirus. *J. Biol. Chem.* **262:**7328–7334.
53. **Castrillo, J. L., D. Vanden-Berghe, and L. Carrasco.** 1986. 3-Methylquercetin is a potent and selective inhibitor of poliovirus RNA synthesis. *Virology* **152:**219–227.
54. **Chang, Y. S., C. L. Liao, C. H. Tsao, M. C. Chen, G. I. Liu, L. K. Chen, and Y. L. Lin.** 1999. Membrane permeabilization by small hydrophobic nonstructural proteins of Japanese encephalitis virus. *J. Virol.* **73:**6257–6264.
55. **Cho, M. W., N. Teterina, D. Egger, K. Bienz, and E. Ehrenfeld.** 1994. Membrane rearrangement and vesicle induction by recombinant poliovirus 2C and 2BC in human cells. *Virology* **202:**129–145.
56. **Choy, P. C., H. B. Paddon, and D. E. Vance.** 1980. An increase in cytoplasmic CTP accelerates the reaction catalyzed by CTP:phosphocholine cytidylyltransferase in poliovirus-infected HeLa cells. *J. Biol. Chem.* **255:**1070–1073.
57. **Ciervo, A., F. Beneduce, and G. Morace.** 1998. Polypeptide 3AB of hepatitis A virus is a transmembrane protein. *Biochem. Biophys. Res. Commun.* **249:**266–274.
58. **Clark, M. E., and A. Dasgupta.** 1990. A transcriptionally active form of TFIIIC is modified in poliovirus-infected HeLa cells. *Mol. Cell. Biol.* **10:**5106–5113.
59. **Clark, M. E., P. M. Lieberman, A. J. Berk, and A. Dasgupta.** 1993. Direct cleavage of human TATA-binding protein by poliovirus protease 3C in vivo and in vitro. *Mol. Cell. Biol.* **13:**1232–1237.
60. **Collins, F. D., and W. K. Roberts.** 1972. Mechanism of mengo virus-induced cell injury in L cells: use of inhibitors of protein synthesis to dissociate virus-specific events. *J. Virol.* **10:**969–978.

61. **Contreras, A., and L. Carrasco.** 1979. Selective inhibition of protein synthesis in virus-infected mammalian cells. *J. Virol.* **29:**114–122.
62. **Cornatzer, W. E., W. Sandstrom, and R. G. Fischer.** 1961. The effect of poliomyelitis virus type I (Mahoney strain) on the phospholipid metabolism of the HeLa cell. *Biochim. Biophys. Acta* **49:**414–415.
63. **Cotten, M., E. Wagner, K. Zatloukal, S. Phillips, D. T. Curiel, and M. L. Birnstiel.** 1992. High-efficiency receptor-mediated delivery of small and large (48 kilobase gene constructs using the endosome-disruption activity of defective or chemically inactivated adenovirus particles. *Proc. Natl. Acad. Sci. USA* **89:**6094–6098.
64. **Cruciani, R. A., J. L. Barker, M. Zasloff, H. Chen, and O. Colamonici.** 1991. Antibiotic magainins exert cytolytic activity against transformed cell lines through channel formation. *Proc. Natl. Acad. Sci. USA* **88:**3792–3796.
65. **Cuconati, A., A. Molla, and E. Wimmer.** 1998. Brefeldin A inhibits cell-free, de novo synthesis of poliovirus. *J. Virol.* **72:**6456–6464.
66. **Cuconati, A., W. K. Xiang, F. Lahser, T. Pfister, and E. Wimmer.** 1998. A protein linkage map of the P2 nonstructural proteins of poliovirus. *J. Virol.* **72:**1297–1307.
67. **Dales, S., H. J. Eggers, I. Tamm, and G. E. Palade.** 1965. Electron microscopic study of the formation of poliovirus. *Virology* **26:**379–389.
68. **Dales, S., and R. M. Franklin.** 1962. A comparison of the changes in fine structure of L cells during single cycles of viral multiplication, following their infection with the viruses of mengo and encephalomyocarditis. *J. Cell. Biol.* **14:**281–302.
69. **Dever, T. E., M. J. Glynias, and W. C. Merrick.** 1987. GTP-binding domain: three consensus sequence elements with distinct spacing. *Proc. Natl. Acad. Sci. USA* **84:**1814–1818.
70. **Doedens, J., L. A. Maynell, M. W. Klymkowsky, and K. Kirkegaard.** 1994. Secretory pathway function, but not cytoskeletal integrity, is required in poliovirus infection. *Arch. Virol.* **136**(Suppl. 9)**:**159–172.
71. **Doedens, J. R., T. H. Giddings, Jr., and K. Kirkegaard.** 1997. Inhibition of endoplasmic reticulum-to-Golgi traffic by poliovirus protein 3A: genetic and ultrastructural analysis. *J. Virol.* **71:**9054–9064.
72. **Doedens, J. R., and K. Kirkegaard.** 1995. Inhibition of cellular protein secretion by poliovirus proteins 2B and 3A. *EMBO J.* **14:**894–907.
73. **Echeverri, A., R. Banerjee, and A. Dasgupta.** 1998. Amino-terminal region of poliovirus 2C protein is sufficient for membrane binding. *Virus Res.* **54:**217–223.
74. **Echeverri, A. C., and A. Dasgupta.** 1995. Amino terminal regions of poliovirus 2C protein mediate membrane binding. *Virology* **208:**540–553.
75. **Egberts, E., P. B. Hackett, and P. Traub.** 1977. Alteration of the intracellular energetic and ionic conditions by mengovirus infection of Ehrlich ascites tumor cells and its influence on protein synthesis in the midphase of infection. *J. Virol.* **22:**591–597.
76. **Egger, D., L. Pasamontes, R. Bolten, V. Boyko, and K. Bienz.** 1996. Reversible dissociation of the poliovirus replication complex: functions and interactions of its components in viral RNA synthesis. *J. Virol.* **70:**8675–8683.
77. **Etchinson, D., and E. Ehrenfeld.** 1973. Comparison of replication complexes synthesizing poliovirus RNA. *Virology* **111:**33–46.
78. **Etchinson, D., and E. Ehrenfeld.** 1980. Viral polypeptides associated with the RNA replication complex in poliovirus-infected cells. *Virology* **107:**135–143.
79. **Farnham, A. E., and W. Epstein.** 1963. The influence of encephalomyocarditis (EMC) virus infection of potassium transport in L cells. *Virology* **21:**436–447.
80. **Fernández-Puentes, C., and L. Carrasco.** 1980. Viral infection permeabilizes mammalian cells to protein toxins. *Cell* **20:**769–775.
81. **Fiscus, W. G., and W. C. Schneider.** 1966. The role of phospholipids in stimulating phosphorylcholine cytidylyltransferase activity. *J. Biol. Chem.* **241:**3324–3330.
82. **Flanagan, J. F.** 1965. Hydrolytic enzymes in KB cells infected with poliovirus and herpes simplex virus. *J. Bacteriol.* **91:**789–797.
83. **Fradkin, L. G., S. K. Yoshinaga, A. J. Berk, and A. Dasgupta.** 1987. Inhibition of host cell RNA polymerase III-mediated transcription by poliovirus: inactivation of specific transcription factors. *Mol. Cell. Biol.* **7:**3880–3887.
84. **Fraenkel-Conrat, H., and R. R. Wagner.** 1984. Cytopathic effects of viruses: a general survey, p. 1–64. *In* H. Fraenkel-Conrat and R. R. Wagner (ed.), *Comprehensive Virology. Viral Cytopathology*, vol. 19. Plenum Press, New York, N.Y.
85. **Frankel, G., Y. Lorch, P. Karlik, and A. Friedmann.** 1987. Fractionation of Theiler's virus-infected BHK 21 cell-homogenates: isolation of virus-induced membranes. *Virology* **158:**452–455.
86. **Fuchs, P., and A. Kohn.** 1983. Changes induced in cell membranes adsorbing animal viruses, bacteriophages, and colicins. *Curr. Top. Microbiol. Immunol.* **102:**57–99.
87. **Giachetti, C., S.-S. Hwang, and B. L. Semler.** 1992. *cis*-Acting lesions targeted to the hydrophobic domain of a poliovirus membrane protein involved in RNA replication. *J. Virol.* **66:**6045–6057.
88. **Gilbert, V. E.** 1963. Enzyme release from tissue cultures as an indicator of cellular injury by viruses. *Virology* **21:**609–616.
89. **Girard, M., and D. Baltimore.** 1967. The poliovirus replication complex: site for synthesis of poliovirus RNA. *J. Mol. Biol.* **24:**59–74.
90. **Giraudo, A., E. Beck, K. Strebell, P. Mello, J. Torre, E. Scodeller, and I. Bergmann.** 1990. Identification of a nucleotide deletion in parts of polypeptide 3A in two independent attenuated Aphthovirus strains. *Virology* **177:**780–783.
91. **Godman, G. C., R. A. Rifkind, C. Howe, and H. M. Rose.** 1964. A description of ECHO 9 virus infection in cultured cells. I. The cytopathic effect. *Am. J. Pathol.* **44:**1–27.
92. **Godman, G. C., R. A. Rifkind, R. B. Page, C. Howe, and H. M. Rose.** 1964. A description of ECHO 9 virus infection in cultured cells. II. Cytochemical observations. *Am. J. Pathol.* **44:**215–245.
93. **Golini, F., B. L. Semler, A. J. Dorner, and E. Wimmer.** 1980. Protein-linked RNA of poliovirus is competent to form an initiation complex of translation in vitro. *Nature* **287:**600–603.
94. **González, M. E., and L. Carrasco.** 1998. The human immunodeficiency virus type 1 Vpu protein enhances membrane permeability. *Biochemistry* **37:**13710–13719.
95. **González, M. E., F. Martínez-Abarca, and L. Carrasco.** 1990. Flavonoids: potent inhibitors of poliovirus RNA synthesis. *Antivir. Chem. Chemother.* **1:**203–209.
96. **Gosert, R., D. Egger, and K. Bienz.** 2000. A cytopathic and a cell culture adapted hepatitis A virus strain differ in cell killing but not in intracellular membrane rearrangements. *Virology* **266:**157–169.
97. **Guinea, R., and L. Carrasco.** 1990. Phospholipid biosynthesis and poliovirus genome replication, two coupled phenomena. *EMBO J.* **9:**2011–2016.
98. **Guinea, R., and L. Carrasco.** 1991. Effects of fatty acids on lipid synthesis and viral RNA replication in poliovirus-infected cells. *Virology* **185:**473–476.

99. Guinea, R., and L. Carrasco. 1994. Influenza virus M2 protein modifies membrane permeability in *E. coli* cells. *FEBS Lett.* **343:**242–246.
100. Guinea, R., A. Lopez-Rivas, and L. Carrasco. 1989. Modification of phospholipase C and phospholipase A2 activities during poliovirus infection. *J. Biol. Chem.* **264:**21923–21927.
101. Hadaschik, D., M. Klein, H. Zimmermann, H. J. Eggers, and B. Nelsen-Salz. 1999. Dependence of echovirus 9 on the enterovirus RNA replication inhibitor 2-(α-hydroxybenzyl)-benzimidazole maps to nonstructural protein 2C. *J. Virol.* **73:**10536–10539.
102. Heinz, B. A., and L. M. Vance. 1995. The antiviral compound enviroxime targets the 3A coding region of rhinovirus and poliovirus. *J. Virol.* **69:**4189–4197.
103. Heinz, B. A., and L. M. Vance. 1996. Sequence determinants of 3A-mediated resistance to enviroxime in rhinoviruses and enteroviruses. *J. Virol.* **70:**4854–4857.
104. Hinz, R. W., G. Barski, and W. Bernhard. 1962. An electron microscopic study of the development of the encephalomyocarditis (EMC) virus propagated in vitro. *Exp. Cell Res.* **26:**571–586.
105. Holsey, C., E. J. J. Cragoe, and C. N. Nair. 1990. Evidence for poliovirus-induced cytoplasmic alkalinization in HeLa cells. *J. Cell. Physiol.* **142:**586–591.
106. Holsey, C., and C. N. Nair. 1993. Poliovirus-induced intracellular alkalinization involves a proton ATPase and protein phosphorylation. *J. Cell. Physiol.* **155:**606–614.
107. Hope, D. A., S. E. Diamond, and K. Kirkegaard. 1997. Genetic dissection of interaction between poliovirus 3D polymerase and viral protein 3AB. *J. Virol.* **71:**9490–9498.
108. Hotham-Iglewski, B., and E. H. Ludwig. 1966. Effect of cortisone on activation of lysosomal enzymes resulting from mengovirus infection in L-929 cells. *Biochem. Biophys. Res. Commun.* **22:**181–186.
109. Huber, M., K. Watson, C. M. Carthy, K. Klinger, B. M. McManus, and R. Kandolf. 2000. Cleavage of RasGAP and phosphorylation of mitogen-activated protein kinase in the course of coxsackievirus B3 replication. *J. Virol.* **73:**3587–3594.
110. Irurzun, A., J. Arroyo, A. Alvarez, and L. Carrasco. 1995. Enhanced intracellular calcium concentration during poliovirus infection. *J. Virol.* **69:**5142–5146.
111. Irurzun, A., L. Perez, and L. Carrasco. 1992. Involvement of membrane traffic in the replication of poliovirus genomes: effects of brefeldin A. *Virology* **191:**166–175.
112. Irurzun, A., L. Perez, and L. Carrasco. 1993. Enhancement of phospholipase C activity during poliovirus infection. *J. Gen. Virol.* **74:**1063–1071.
113. Irurzun, A., S. Sanchez-Palomino, I. Novoa, and L. Carrasco. 1995. Monensin and nigericin prevent the inhibition of host translation by poliovirus, without affecting p220 cleavage. *J. Virol.* **69:**7453–7460.
114. Jamil, H., Z. M. Yao, and D. E. Vance. 1990. Feedback regulation of CTP:phosphocholine cytidylyltransferase translocation between cytosol and endoplasmic reticulum by phosphatidylcholine. *J. Biol. Chem.* **265:**4332–4339.
115. Jecht, M., C. Probst, and V. Gauss-Müller. 1998. Membrane permeability induced by hepatitis A virus proteins 2B and 2BC and proteolytic processing of HAV 2BC. *Virology* **252:**218–227.
116. Jezequel, A. M., and J. W. Steiner. 1966. Some ultrastructural and histochemical aspects of coxsackie virus-cell interactions. *Lab. Invest.* **15:**1055–1083.
117. Joachims, M., and D. Etchison. 1992. Poliovirus infection results in structural alteration of a microtubule-associated protein. *J. Virol.* **66:**5797–5804.
118. Johnson, K., and P. Sarnow. 1991. Three poliovirus 2B mutants exhibit noncomplementable defects in viral RNA amplification and display dosage-dependent dominance over wild-type poliovirus. *J. Virol.* **65:**4341–4349.
119. Kirkegaard, K. 1992. Genetic analysis of picornavirus. *Curr. Opin. Genet. Dev.* **2:**64–70.
120. Kliewer, S., and A. Dasgupta. 1988. An RNA polymerase II transcription factor inactivated in poliovirus-infected cells copurifies with transcription factor TFIID. *Mol. Cell. Biol.* **8:**3175–3182.
121. Kliewer, S., C. Muchardt, R. Gaynor, and A. Dasgupta. 1990. Loss of a phosphorylated form of transcription factor CREB/ATF in poliovirus-infected cells. *J. Virol.* **64:**4507–4515.
122. Koch, F., and G. Koch. 1985. Morphological alterations of the host cell as an essential basis for poliovirus replication, p. 227–266. In *The Molecular Biology of Poliovirus*. Springer Verlag, Vienna, Austria.
123. Krausslich, H. G., C. Holscher, Q. Reuer, J. Harber, and E. Wimmer. 1990. Myristoylation of the poliovirus polyprotein is required for proteolytic processing of the capsid and for viral infectivity. *J. Virol.* **64:**2433–2436.
124. Kusov, Y., and V. Gauss-Müller. 1999. Improving proteolytic cleavage at the 3A/3B site of the hepatitis A virus polyprotein impairs processing and particle formation, and the impairment can be complemented in *trans* by 3AB and 3ABC. *J. Virol.* **73:**9867–9878.
125. Kusov, Y. Y., C. Probst, M. Jecht, P. D. Jost, and V. Gauss-Muller. 1998. Membrane association and RNA binding of recombinant hepatitis A virus protein 2C. *Arch. Virol.* **143:**931–944.
126. Kyte, J., and R. F. Doolittle. 1982. A simple method for displaying the hydropathic character of a protein. *J. Mol. Biol.* **157:**105–132.
127. Lacal, J. C., and L. Carrasco. 1982. Relationship between membrane integrity and the inhibition of host translation in virus-infected mammalian cells. Comparative studies between encephalomyocarditis virus and poliovirus. *Eur. J. Biochem.* **127:**359–366.
128. Lama, J., and L. Carrasco. 1992. Expression of poliovirus nonstructural proteins in *Escherichia coli* cells. Modification of membrane permeability induced by 2B and 3A. *J. Biol. Chem.* **267:**15932–15937.
129. Lama, J., and L. Carrasco. 1995. Mutations in the hydrophobic domain of poliovirus protein 3AB abrogate its permeabilizing activity. *FEBS Lett.* **367:**5–11.
130. Lama, J., and L. Carrasco. 1996. Screening for membrane-permeabilizing mutants of the poliovirus protein 3AB. *J. Gen. Virol.* **77:**2109–2119.
131. Lama, J., R. Guinea, F. Martinez-Abarca, and L. Carrasco. 1992. Cloning and inducible synthesis of poliovirus nonstructural proteins. *Gene* **117:**185–192.
132. Lama, J., A. V. Paul, K. S. Harris, and E. Wimmer. 1994. Properties of purified recombinant poliovirus protein 3AB as substrate for viral proteinases and as a cofactor for RNA polymerase $3D^{pol}$. *J. Biol. Chem.* **269:**66–70.
133. Lama, J., M. A. Sanz, and L. Carrasco. 1998. Genetic analysis of poliovirus protein 3A: characterization of a non-cytopathic mutant virus defective in killing Vero cells. *J. Gen. Virol.* **79:**1911–1921.
134. Lenk, R., and S. Penman. 1979. The cytoskeletal framework and poliovirus metabolism. *Cell* **16:**289–301.
135. Li, J. P., and D. Baltimore. 1988. Isolation of poliovirus 2C mutants defective in viral RNA synthesis. *J. Virol.* **62:**4016–4021.
136. Li, J. P., and D. Baltimore. 1990. An intragenic revertant of a poliovirus 2C mutant has an uncoating defect. *J. Virol.* **64:**1102–1107.

137. **Lopez-Rivas, A., J. L. Castrillo, and L. Carrasco.** 1987. Cation content in poliovirus-infected HeLa cells. *J. Gen. Virol.* **68:**335–342.
138. **Lykidis, A., I. Baburina, and S. Jackowski.** 1999. Distribution of CTP:phosphocholine cytidylyltransferase (CCT) isoforms. Identification of a new CCTbeta splice variant. *J. Biol. Chem.* **274:**26992–27001.
139. **Lykidis, A., K. G. Murti, and S. Jackowski.** 1998. Cloning and characterization of a second human CTP:phosphocholine cytidylyltransferase. *J. Biol. Chem.* **273:**14022–14029.
140. **Martín-Belmonte, F., J. A. López-Guerrero, L. Carrasco, and M. A. Alonso.** 2000. The amino-terminal nine amino acid sequence of poliovirus capsid VP4 protein is sufficient to confer N-myristoylation and targeting to detergent-insoluble membranes. *Biochemistry* **39:**1083–1090.
141. **Mattern, C. F. T., and W. A. Daniel.** 1965. Replication of poliovirus in HeLa cells: electron microscopic observations. *Virology* **26:**646–663.
142. **Maynell, L. A., K. Kirkegaard, and M. W. Klymkowsky.** 1992. Inhibition of poliovirus RNA synthesis by brefeldin A. *J. Virol.* **66:**1985–1994.
143. **Meldolesi, J., P. Volpe, and T. Pozzan.** 1988. The intracellular distribution of calcium. *TINS* **11:**449–452.
144. **Miroff, G., W. E. Cornatzer, and R. G. Fischer.** 1957. The effect of poliomyelitis virus type I (Mahoney strain) on the phosphorus metabolism of the HeLa cells. *J. Biol. Chem.* **228:**255–262.
145. **Mirzayan, C., and E. Wimmer.** 1994. Biochemical studies on poliovirus polypeptide 2C: evidence for ATPase activity. *Virology* **199:**176–187.
146. **Modalsli, K., G. Bukholm, S. O. Mikalsen, and M. Degre.** 1992. Coxsackie B1 virus-induced changes in cell membrane-associated functions are not responsible for altered sensitivity to bacterial invasiveness. *Arch. Virol.* **124:**321–332.
147. **Molla, A., S. K. Jang, A. V. Paul, Q. Reuer, and E. Wimmer.** 1992. Cardioviral internal ribosomal entry site is functional in a genetically engineered dicistronic poliovirus. *Nature* **356:**255–257.
148. **Molla, A., A. V. Paul, and E. Wimmer.** 1991. Cell-free, de novo synthesis of poliovirus. *Science* **254:**1647–1651.
149. **Molla, A., A. V. Paul, and E. Wimmer.** 1993. Effects of temperature and lipophilic agents on poliovirus formation and RNA synthesis in a cell-free system. *J. Virol.* **67:**5932–5938.
150. **Morace, G., G. Pisani, F. Beneduce, M. Divizia, and A. Panà.** 1993. Mutations in the 3A genomic region of two cytopathic strains of hepatitis A virus isolated in Italy. *Virus Res.* **28:**187–194.
151. **Moscufo, N., J. Simons, and M. Chow.** 1991. Myristoylation is important at multiple stages in poliovirus assembly. *J. Virol.* **65:**2372–2380.
152. **Mosser, A. G., L. A. Caliguiri, A. S. Scheid, and I. Tamm.** 1972. Chemical and enzymatic characteristics of cytoplasmic membranes of poliovirus-infected HeLa cells. *Virology* **47:**30–38.
153. **Mosser, A. G., L. A. Caliguiri, and I. Tamm.** 1972. Incorporation of lipid precursors into cytoplasmic membranes of poliovirus-infected HeLa cells. *Virology* **47:**39–47.
154. **Nair, C. N.** 1981. Monovalent cation metabolism and cytopathic effects of poliovirus-infected HeLa cells. *J. Virol.* **37:**268–273.
155. **Nair, C. N.** 1984. Na^+ and K^+ changes in animal virus-infected HeLa cells. *J. Gen. Virol.* **65:**1135–1138.
156. **Neufeld, K. L., O. C. Richards, and E. Ehrenfeld.** 1991. Expression and characterization of poliovirus proteins $3B^{VPg}$, $3C^{pro}$, and $3D^{pol}$ in recombinant baculovirus-infected *Spodoptera frugiperda* cells. *Virus Res.* **19:**173–188.
157. **Nozawa, C. M., and K. Apostolov.** 1982. Increase in the saturation of C18 fatty acids induced by coxsackie B6 virus in Vero cells. *Virology* **120:**247–250.
158. **Nugent, C. I., K. L. Johnson, P. Sarnow, and K. Kirkegaard.** 1999. Functional coupling between replication and packaging of poliovirus replicon RNA. *J. Virol.* **73:**427–435.
159. **Núñez-Montiel, O., J. Weibel, and V. Vitelli-Flores.** 1961. Electronic study of the cytopathology of echovirus infection in cultivated cells. *J. Biophys. Biochem. Cytol.* **11:**457–467.
160. **Paul, A. V., A. Molla, and E. Wimmer.** 1994. Studies of a putative amphipathic helix in the N-terminus of poliovirus protein 2C. *Virology* **199:**188–199.
161. **Paul, A. V., A. Schultz, S. E. Pincus, S. Oroszlan, and E. Wimmer.** 1987. Capsid protein VP4 of poliovirus is N-myristoylated. *Proc. Natl. Acad. Sci. USA* **84:**7827–7831.
162. **Paul, A. V., J. H. van Boom, D. Filippov, and E. Wimmer.** 1998. Protein-primed RNA synthesis by purified poliovirus RNA polymerase. *Nature* **393:**280–284.
163. **Penman, S.** 1965. Stimulation of the incorporation of choline in poliovirus-infected cells. *Virology* **25:**148–152.
164. **Penman, S., Y. Becker, and J. E. Darnell.** 1964. A cytoplasmic structure involved in the synthesis and assembly of poliovirus components. *J. Mol. Biol.* **8:**541–555.
165. **Penman, S., and D. Summers.** 1965. Effects on host cell metabolism following synchronous infection with poliovirus. *Virology* **27:**614–620.
166. **Perez, L., and L. Carrasco.** 1991. Cerulenin—an inhibitor of lipid synthesis—blocks vesicular stomatitis virus RNA replication. *FEBS Lett.* **280:**129–133.
167. **Perez, L., R. Guinea, and L. Carrasco.** 1991. Synthesis of Semliki Forest virus RNA requires continous lipid synthesis. *Virology* **183:**74–82.
168. **Pfister, T., D. Egger, and K. Bienz.** 1995. Poliovirus subviral particles associated with progeny RNA in the replication complex. *J. Gen. Virol.* **76:**63–71.
169. **Pfister, T., K. W. Jones, and E. Wimmer.** 2000. A cysteine-rich motif in poliovirus protein $2C^{ATPase}$ is involved in RNA replication and binds zinc in vitro. *J. Virol.* **74:**334–343.
170. **Pfister, T., and E. Wimmer.** 1999. Characterization of the nucleoside triphosphatase activity of poliovirus protein 2C reveals a mechanism by which guanidine inhibits poliovirus replication. *J. Biol. Chem.* **274:**6992–7001.
171. **Pincus, S. E., D. C. Diamond, E. A. Emini, and E. Wimmer.** 1986. Guanidine-selected mutants of poliovirus: mapping of point mutations to polypeptide 2C. *J. Virol.* **57:**638–646.
172. **Pincus, S. E., H. Rohl, and E. Wimmer.** 1987. Guanidine-dependent mutants of poliovirus: identification of three classes with different growth requirements. *Virology* **157:**83–88.
173. **Pincus, S. E., and E. Wimmer.** 1986. Production of guanidine-resistant and -dependent poliovirus mutants from cloned cDNA: mutations in polypeptide 2C are directly responsible for altered guanidine sensitivity. *J. Virol.* **60:**793–796.
174. **Pisani, G., F. Beneduce, V. Gauss-Müller, and G. Morace.** 1995. Recombinant expression of hepatitis A virus protein 3A: interaction with membranes. *Biochem. Biophys. Res. Commun.* **211:**627–638.
175. **Plagemann, P. G. W., P. H. Cleveland, and M. A. Shea.** 1970. Effect of mengovirus replication on choline me-

tabolism and membrane formation in Novikoff hepatoma cells. *J. Virol.* **6:**800–812.
176. **Plotch, S. J., and O. Palant.** 1995. Poliovirus protein 3AB forms a complex with and stimulates the activity of the viral RNA polymerase, 3D^{pol}. *J. Virol.* **69:**7169–7179.
177. **Polatnick, J., and S. H. Wool.** 1982. Localization of foot-and-mouth disease-RNA synthesis on newly formed cellular smooth membranous vacuoles. *Arch. Virol.* **71:**207–215.
178. **Rangel, S. R., C. Grief, E. E. Da Silva, A. M. de Filippis, and M. Taffarel.** 1998. Ultrastructural and immunocytochemical study on the infection of enterovirus 71 (EV71) in rhabdomyosarcoma (RD) cells. *J. Submicrosc. Cytol. Pathol.* **30:**71–75.
179. **Rice, J. M., and D. A. Wolff.** 1975. Phospholipase in the lysosomes of Hep-2 cells and its release during poliovirus infection. *Biochim. Biophys. Acta* **381:**17–21.
180. **Rodríguez, P. L., and L. Carrasco.** 1993. Poliovirus protein 2C has ATPase and GTPase activities. *J. Biol. Chem.* **268:**8105–8110.
181. **Rodríguez, P. L., and L. Carrasco.** 1995. Poliovirus protein 2C contains two regions involved in RNA binding activity. *J. Biol. Chem.* **270:**10105–10112.
182. **Rothberg, P. G., T. J. Harris, A. Nomoto, and E. Wimmer.** 1978. O4-(5′-uridylyl)tyrosine is the bond between the genome-linked protein and the RNA of poliovirus. *Proc. Natl. Acad. Sci. USA* **75:**4868–4872.
183. **Rubinstein, S. J., and A. Dasgupta.** 1989. Inhibition of rRNA synthesis by poliovirus: specific inactivation of transcription factors. *J. Virol.* **63:**4689–4696.
184. **Rubinstein, S. J., T. Hammerle, E. Wimmer, and A. Dasgupta.** 1992. Infection of HeLa cells with poliovirus results in modification of a complex that binds to the rRNA promoter. *J. Virol.* **66:**3062–3068.
185. **Sandoval, I. V., and L. Carrasco.** 1997. Poliovirus infection and expression of the poliovirus protein 2B provoke the disassembly of the Golgi complex, the organelle target for the antipoliovirus drug Ro-090179. *J. Virol* **71:**4679–4693.
186. **Sanghera, J. S., and D. E. Vance.** 1989. Stimulation of CTP:phosphocholine cytidylyltransferase and phosphatidylcholine synthesis by calcium in rat hepatocytes. *Biochim. Biophys. Acta* **1003:**284–292.
187. **Sanz, M. A., L. Pérez, and L. Carrasco.** 1994. Semliki Forest virus 6K protein modifies membrane permeability after inducible expression in *Escherichia coli* cells. *J. Biol. Chem.* **269:**12106–12110.
188. **Sarnow, P., S. J. Jacobson, and L. Najita.** 1990. Poliovirus genetics. *Curr. Top. Microbiol. Immunol.* **161:**155–188.
189. **Schaefer, A., J. Kuhne, R. Zibirre, and G. Koch.** 1982. Poliovirus-induced alterations in HeLa cell membrane functions. *J. Virol.* **44:**445–449.
190. **Schaefer, A., R. Zibirre, P. Kabus, J. Kuhne, and G. Koch.** 1982. Alterations in plasma-membrane functions after poliovirus infection. *Biosci. Rep.* **2:**613–615.
191. **Schiffer, M., and A. B. Edmundson.** 1967. Use of helical wheels to represent the structures of proteins and to identify segments with helical potential. *Biophys. J.* **7:**121–135.
192. **Schlegel, A., T. H. Giddings, M. S. Ladinsky, and K. Kirkegaard.** 1996. Cellular origin and ultrastructure of membranes induced during poliovirus infection. *J. Virol.* **70:**6576–6588.
193. **Semler, B. L., C. W. Anderson, R. Hanecak, L. F. Dorner, and E. Wimmer.** 1982. A membrane-associated precursor to poliovirus VPg identified by immunoprecipitation with antibodies directed against a synthetic heptapeptide. *Cell* **28:**405–412.

194. **Semler, B. L., R. J. Kuhn, and E. Wimmer.** 1988. Replication of the poliovirus genome, p. 23–49. *In* E. Domingo, J. J. Holland, and P. Ahlquist (ed.), *RNA Genetics*, vol. I. *RNA-Directed Virus Replication*. CRC Press, Boca Raton, Fla.
195. **Shimizu, H., M. Agoh, Y. Ahog, H. Yoshida, K. Yoshii, T. Yoneyama, A. Hagiwara, and T. Miyamura.** 2000. Mutations in the 2C region of poliovirus responsible for altered sensitivity to benzimidazole derivatives. *J. Virol.* **74:**4146–4154.
196. **Skinner, M. S., S. Halperen, and J. C. Harkin.** 1968. Cytoplasmic membrane-bound vesicles in echovirus 12-infected cells. *Virology* **36:**241–253.
197. **Takeda, N., R. J. Kuhn, C. F. Yang, T. Takegami, and E. Wimmer.** 1986. Initiation of poliovirus plus-strand RNA synthesis in a membrane complex of infected HeLa cells. *J. Virol.* **60:**43–53.
198. **Takeda, N., C. F. Yang, R. J. Kuhn, and E. Wimmer.** 1987. Uridylylation of the genome-linked protein of poliovirus in vitro is dependent upon an endogenous RNA template. *Virus Res.* **8:**193–204.
199. **Takegami, T., R. J. Kuhn, C. W. Anderson, and E. Wimmer.** 1983. Membrane-dependent uridylylation of the genome-linked protein VPg of poliovirus. *Proc. Natl. Acad. Sci. USA* **80:**7447–7451.
200. **Takegami, T., B. L. Semler, C. W. Anderson, and E. Wimmer.** 1983. Membrane fractions active in poliovirus RNA replication contain VPg precursor polypeptides. *Virology* **128:**33–47.
201. **Tershak, D. R.** 1984. Association of poliovirus proteins with the endoplasmic reticulum. *J. Virol.* **52:**777–783.
202. **Teterina, N. L., K. Bienz, D. Egger, A. Gorbalenya, and E. Ehrenfeld.** 1997. Induction of intracellular membrane rearrangements by HAV proteins 2C and 2BC. *Virology* **237:**66–77.
203. **Teterina, N. L., A. E. Gorbalenya, D. Egger, K. Bienz, and E. Ehrenfeld.** 1997. Poliovirus 2C protein determinants of membrane binding and rearrangements in mammalian cells. *J. Virol.* **71:**8962–8972.
204. **Thacore, H., and D. A. Wolff.** 1968. Activation of isolated lysosomes by poliovirus-infected cell extracts. *Nature* **218:**1063–1064.
205. **Tolskaya, E. A., L. I. Romanova, M. S. Kolesnikova, A. P. Gmyl, A. E. Gorbalenya, and V. I. Agol.** 1994. Genetic studies on the poliovirus 2C protein, an NTPase. A plausible mechanism of guanidine effect on the 2C function and evidence for the importance of 2C oligomerization. *J. Mol. Biol.* **236:**1310–1323.
206. **Tosteson, M. T., and M. Chow.** 1997. Characterization of the ion channels formed by poliovirus in planar lipid membranes. *J. Virol.* **71:**507–511.
207. **Totsuka, A., and Y. Moritsugu.** 1999. Hepatitis A virus proteins. *Intervirology* **42:**63–68.
208. **Towner, J. S., T. V. Ho, and B. L. Semler.** 1996. Determinants of membrane association for poliovirus protein 3AB. *J. Biol. Chem.* **271:**26810–26818.
209. **Toyoda, H., C. F. Yang, N. Takeda, A. Nomoto, and E. Wimmer.** 1987. Analysis of RNA synthesis of type 1 poliovirus by using an in vitro molecular genetic approach. *J. Virol.* **61:**2816–2822.
210. **Traub, P.** 1987. The effect of mengovirus infection on lipid synthesis in cultured Erlich ascites tumour cells. *Lipids* **22:**95–103.
211. **Troxler, M., D. Egger, T. Pfister, and K. Bienz.** 1992. Intracellular localization of poliovirus RNA by in situ hybridization at the ultrastructural level using single-stranded riboprobes. *Virology* **191:**687–697.
212. **Van Kuppeveld, F. J. M., J. M. D. Galama, J. Zoll, and W. J. G. Melchers.** 1995. Genetic analysis of a hydro-

phobic domain of coxsackie B3 virus protein 2B: a moderate degree of hydrophobicity is required for a *cis*-acting function in viral RNA synthesis. *J. Virol.* **69:**7782–7790.

213. Van Kuppeveld, F. J. M., J. M. D. Galama, J. Zoll, P. J. J. C. Van den Hurk, and W. J. G. Melchers. 1996. Coxsackie B3 virus protein 2B contains a cationic amphipathic helix that is required for viral RNA replication. *J. Virol.* **70:**3876–3886.

214. Van Kuppeveld, F. J. M., J. G. J. Hoenderop, R. L. L. Smeets, P. H. G. M. Willems, H. B. P. M. Kijkman, J. M. D. Galama, and W. J. G. Melchers. 1997. Coxsackievirus protein 2B modifies endoplasmic reticulum membrane and plasma membrane permeability and facilitates virus release. *EMBO J.* **16:**3519–3532.

215. Van Kuppeveld, F. J. M., W. J. G. Melchers, K. Kirkegaard, and J. R. Doedens. 1997. Structure-function analysis of coxsackie B3 virus protein 2B. *Virology* **227:**111–118.

216. Van Kuppeveld, F. J. M., P. J. J. C. Van den Hurk, W. van der Vliet, J. M. D. Galama, and W. J. G. Melchers. 1997. Chimeric coxsackie B3 virus genomes that express hybrid coxsackievirus-poliovirus 2B proteins: functional dissection of structural domains involved in RNA replication. *J. Gen. Virol.* **78:**1833–1840.

217. Van Kuppeveld, F. J. M., P. J. J. C. van der Hurk, J. Zoll, J. M. D. Galama, and J. G. Melchers. 1996. Mutagenesis of the coxsackie B3 virus 2B/2C cleavage site: determinants of processing efficiency and effects on viral replication. *J. Virol.* **70:**7632–7640.

218. **Vance, D. E., and S. L. Pelech.** 1984. Enzyme translocation in the regulation of phosphatidylcholine biosynthesis. *Trends Biochem. Sci.* **9:**17–20.

219. **Vance, D. E., E. M. Trip, and H. B. Paddon.** 1980. Poliovirus increases phosphatidylcholine biosynthesis in HeLa cells by stimulation of the rate-limiting reaction catalyzed by CTP:phosphocholine cytidylyltransferase. *J. Biol. Chem.* **255:**1064–1069.

220. **Vance, L. M., N. Moscufo, M. Chow, and B. A. Heinz.** 1997. Poliovirus 2C region functions during encapsidation of viral RNA. *J. Virol.* **71:**8759–8765.

221. **Vázquez, D., M. Barbacid, and L. Carrasco.** 1974. Inhibitors of mammalian protein synthesis. *Hamatol. Bluttransfus.* **14:**327–340.

222. **Wang, Y., J. I. S. MacDonald, and C. Kent.** 1993. Regulation of CTP:phosphocholine cytidylyltransferase in HeLa cells. Effect of oleate on phosphorylation and intracellular localization. *J. Biol. Chem.* **268:**5512–5518.

223. **Wang, Y., T. D. Sweitzer, P. A. Weinhold, and C. Kent.** 1993. Nuclear localization of soluble CTP:phosphocholine cytidylyltransferase. *J. Biol. Chem.* **268:**5899–5904.

224. **Weber, S., H. Granzow, F. Weiland, and O. Marquardt.** 1996. Intracellular membrane proliferation in *E. coli* induced by foot-and-mouth disease virus 3A gene products. *Virus Genes* **12:**5–14.

225. **Wimmer, E.** 1972. Sequence studies of poliovirus RNA. I. Characterization of the 5′-terminus. *J. Mol. Biol.* **68:**537–540.

226. **Wimmer, E., C. U. T. Hellen, and X. Cao.** 1993. Genetics of poliovirus. *Annu. Rev. Genet.* **27:**353–436.

227. **Xiang, W., A. Cuconati, A. V. Paul, X. Cao, and E. Wimmer.** 1995. Molecular dissection of the multifunctional poliovirus RNA-binding protein 3AB. *RNA* **1:**892–904.

228. **Yao, Z., H. Jamil, and D. E. Vance.** 1990. Choline deficiency causes translocation of CTP:phosphocholine cytidylyltransferase from cytosol to endoplasmic reticulum in rat liver. *J. Biol. Chem.* **265:**4326–4331.

229. **Young, D. C., D. M. Tuschell, and J. B. Flanegan.** 1985. Poliovirus RNA-dependent RNA polymerase and host cell protein synthesize product RNA twice the size of poliovirion RNA in vitro. *J. Virol.* **54:**256–264.

230. **Zeichhardt, H., K.-O. Habermehl, and W. Diefenthal.** 1982. Modification and exploitation of a poliovirus-induced membrane complex by superinfecting ME virus. *J. Gen. Virol.* **55:**265–274.

231. **Zeichhardt, H., J. R. Schlehofer, K. Wetz, H. Hampl, and K.-O. Habermehl.** 1982. Mouse Elberfeld (ME) virus determines the cell surface alterations when mixedly infecting poliovirus-infected cells. *J. Gen. Virol.* **58:**417–428.

PATHOGENICITY

Clinical Significance, Diagnosis, and Treatment of Picornavirus Infections

HARLEY A. ROTBART

28

The picornaviruses are a diverse group of human viral pathogens that together comprise the most common causes of infections of humans in the developed world. Within the picornavirus family are three well-known groups of human pathogens—the human rhinoviruses (HRVs), the enteroviruses (EVs) (including polioviruses, coxsackieviruses, and echoviruses), and the hepatoviruses (including hepatitis A). Hepatitis A, which differs significantly from the others genomically and clinically, is reviewed elsewhere in this text. This chapter will focus on the rhinoviruses and enteroviruses.

RHINOVIRUSES

The HRVs include more than 100 serotypes in two main groups based on their cellular receptors. HRVs cause about one-half of all common colds (58), the leading cause of acute infectious morbidity worldwide. The common cold results in 25 million days of missed work each year in the United States, a similar number of days of missed school, and approximately the same number of visits to physicians each year (90). The incidence of the common cold is, on average, 5 to 7 episodes per year in children and 2 to 3 episodes per year in adults (90).

Common colds and related syndromes are the most frequent reasons for antibiotic use in the United States (26, 70). This excessive use undoubtedly contributes to the increasing prevalence of antibiotic resistance in pathogenic bacteria and emphasizes the need for effective prophylaxis and treatment of HRV infections.

Transmission of HRV infections is most efficient by direct, hand-to-hand contact, although aerosolization also occurs and may result in person-person spread; the nasal cavity is the primary site of inoculation and initiation of infection (90). Three-quarters of all infections are symptomatic. The major risk factor for HRV infection appears to be contact with young children. HRVs are epidemic in fall and spring, but infections occur year-round.

HRVs are now also known to directly or indirectly cause numerous upper respiratory ailments in addition to the common cold (Table 1). In addition, HRV infections cause lower respiratory tract disease in select populations (Table 1).

Clinical Manifestations

The usual incubation period of HRV colds is 1 to 3 days. Rhinorrhea, nasal stuffiness, and sneezing are the commonest symptoms; other typical manifestations include sore or scratchy throat, facial pressure, headache, cough, hoarseness, and less often, malaise, chills, or feverishness (34). Sore throat tends to be the first symptom, and runny nose the most bothersome (7). Significant fever is very uncommon in adults and should suggest an alternative diagnosis. Infants and young children have fever more often and may show only mucous nasal discharge. Red, sometimes macerated nostrils and glassy nasal mucosa are also typically present, but examination is primarily useful to exclude other diagnoses. Cough usually persists until the end of the first week but may be protracted in smokers. In a recent study of viral upper respiratory tract infections, the median duration of illness as defined by complete resolution of both respiratory and systemic symptoms was 14 days (F. G. Hayden, H. A. Hassman, T. Coats, et al., Abstr. 39th Intersci. Conf. Antimicrob. Agents Chemother., 1999).

HRV infections are associated with a number of upper and lower respiratory tract complications in both children and adults. Viral respiratory tract infections are the most important predisposing factor to acute otitis media (AOM). Viruses have been detected by culture or antigen assay in 11 to 41% of middle ear fluids from children with AOM (5, 40), and HRV is found in up to 8% of such fluids. By PCR, HRV infection is detectable in 35% of children with AOM, including the presence of HRV RNA in 24% of middle ear fluids (77). In adults, middle ear pressure abnormalities commonly develop during HRV colds (10, 21). Coinfection with HRV and bacteria has been reported to predispose to failure of antibiotic therapy in AOM (74).

Most cases of acute sinusitis thought to result from bacterial disease are secondary to a preceding viral upper respiratory tract infection. Sinus abnormalities are frequently detectable during uncomplicated colds (33). Consequently, distinguishing primary viral rhino-sinusitis from secondary

---

Harley A. Rotbart ■ University of Colorado Health Sciences Center, 4200 E. 9th Avenue, Box C227, Denver, CO 80262.

TABLE 1 Clinical illnesses caused by picornavirus infections

Rhinoviruses
    Upper respiratory tract illness
    Otitis media
    Sinusitis
    Exacerbations of asthma, cystic fibrosis, chronic bronchitis
    Lower respiratory tract illness—infants, elderly, immunocompromised

Enteroviruses
    Nonspecific febrile illnesses
    Upper respiratory tract illness
    Otitis media
    Hemorrhagic conjunctivitis, herpangina, hand-foot-mouth syndrome
    Pleurodynia
    Myocarditis
    Aseptic meningitis
    Encephalitis
    Neonatal sepsis-like syndrome

bacterial sinusitis is clinically difficult. HRV is detectable by culture or PCR in 40% of sinus brushings from patients with acute community-acquired sinusitis (76).

HRV infections are major factors in the induction of acute exacerbations of asthma in adults (69) and in children (46). In a 2-year study of adult asthmatics aged 19 to 46 years, peak expiratory flow rate deteriorations occurred during 27% of respiratory illness episodes, and colds were associated within 71% of documented exacerbations (69). HRVs are the most commonly identified pathogens found in asthma exacerbations and hospitalizations for those aged >2 years (45).

HRV infections are also associated with lower respiratory tract syndromes in other patient populations. In children with cystic fibrosis, picornaviruses were detected in about one-fifth of exacerbations and colds were associated with deterioration in pulmonary function testing (18). Among adults aged 60 to 90 years residing in the community, HRV infection was associated with lower respiratory tract symptoms in 65%; 40% consulted their doctor, and 76% of these received antibiotics (68). The impact of HRVs in elderly people, as measured by those indices, approaches that of influenza (68). Up to 40% of exacerbations in patients with chronic bronchitis may be associated with HRV infections (31). In a nursing home outbreak of respiratory disease due to HRV, all infected patients had upper respiratory symptoms, two-thirds had lower respiratory illness, and 71% had systemic symptoms; among those patients with chronic obstructive pulmonary disease at baseline, all developed severe HRV-associated illness. In infants aged <12 months, HRV infections have been associated with hospitalization for lower respiratory tract illness, particularly bronchiolitis (87), and deterioration in those with bronchopulmonary dysplasia (16). Among infants less than a month in age, one of eight cases of viral pneumonia is due to HRV.

Approximately one-half of all common colds in adults (26) and children (70) result in antibiotic prescriptions in the United States. Twenty-one percent of all antibiotics prescribed in this country are for upper respiratory ailments, mostly due to HRV, which do not require or benefit from antibiotics. At a societal level, this complication of HRV infections may have the greatest long-term adverse impact.

Diagnosis

The diagnosis of HRV infection is primarily clinical. No rapid antigen detection or practical serologic tests exist for HRV infections because of the multiplicity of serotypes. Viral culture takes 3 to 7 days and is of limited clinical use. PCR detection of HRV RNA has been frequently positive in HRV culture-negative samples (25), but currently is only a research tool.

Management

A variety of therapies have emerged and have been tested against HRV infections. These fall into the general categories of specific antiviral therapy, symptomatic treatments, antibiotics, and "alternative" approaches.

Antivirals

A major hurdle to effective antiviral therapy is the unclear importance of ongoing viral replication in symptom pathogenesis after illness onset. The only agent consistently shown to have prophylactic activity against HRV infections is intranasal interferon (6). Interferons are potent, selective mediators of cellular changes that induce a number of antiviral, antiproliferative, and immunological effects, all of which collectively affect host cell susceptibility to picornavirus infection (12, 24, 48, 52–55, 71, 85). The cellular antiviral effects of interferons are mediated through specific receptor-signal transduction pathways. In conjunction with double-stranded RNA, interferons induce the expression of proteins, some of which mediate an antiviral activity. The best described pathways are (i) $2',5'$-adenylate synthetase, (ii) double-stranded RNA-dependent protein kinase, and (iii) the Mx proteins.

The clinical efficacy of intranasal interferon as prophylaxis for HRV colds has been demonstrated in several studies (27, 36, 37, 64, 84). Additional studies demonstrated significant efficacy against naturally acquired HRV infections and against contact spread of HRV within family groups after experimental induction of a natural cold (20, 36). Side effects of interferon included nasal irritation and stuffiness and mucosal ulceration (36, 84).

Administered therapeutically 1 day after experimental HRV infection, intranasal interferon had no effect on development of infection or symptoms but did result in moderate reductions of virus shedding and cold symptoms (38). Additional studies with low-dose intranasal interferon also demonstrated a lack of efficacy in postexposure prophylaxis of HRV infections in families (67). Combinations of intranasal interferon, intranasal ipratropium, and oral naproxen provide significantly greater clinical benefits than monotherapy in experimental colds (30). Such results support the general concept of treating HRV colds with combinations of antiviral and anti-inflammatory drugs.

Capsid-inhibiting compounds block viral uncoating and/or viral attachment to host cell receptors. The resolved three-dimensional structure of picornaviruses (HRV and EV) reveals a "canyon" formed by the junctions of VP1 and VP3. Beneath the canyon lies a "pore" that leads to a hydrophobic pocket into which a variety of diverse hydrophobic compounds can integrate. Although the compounds integrate into a virus capsid via a number of noncovalent, hydrophobic-type interactions, the affinity is high, with constants ranging from 2.0×10^{-8} to 2.9×10^{-7} M (22).

Several hypotheses have been proposed for the mechanism of picornavirus inhibition by compounds that affect the function of the virus capsid. Filling the hydrophobic pocket results in increased stability of the virus, making the virus more resistant to uncoating. The increased stability of the virus-compound complex is evidenced by the resistance to thermal inactivation (78). It is also possible that a degree of capsid flexibility may be required for uncoating, and activity of these compounds within the hydrophobic pocket may reduce this necessary flexibility, inducing a more rigid structure. Alternatively, changes in the conformation of the canyon floor as a result of drug activity within the underlying pocket may affect the attachment of the virus to the host cell receptor (72). It has been shown, however, that such perturbations in the canyon floor do not absolutely correlate with antiviral potency (98, 99). The capsid-inhibiting compounds vary in their spectrum of activity, perhaps as a result of factors such as pocket fit discussed above.

Clinical trials of the "R" series of capsid-binding compounds have been limited to intranasal administration to patients with HRV colds (4, 8, 39). Pirodavir (R77975) and R61837 were efficacious in experimentally induced HRV colds when these drugs were administered intranasally before or after infection, but before onset of symptoms (8, 39); pirodavir required six-times-daily dosing, with efficacy loss at three daily doses (39).

The "WIN" series of compounds has also been clinically evaluated in HRV infections. The first compound of this group to advance to clinical trials was disoxaril (WIN 51711). Disoxaril was moderately active against HRV in vitro (61, 62, 72). The appearance of asymptomatic crystalluria in healthy volunteers prevented further clinical study. Shortening of the aliphatic chain from $n = 7$ to $n = 5$ and adding chlorogroups to the phenyl ring resulted in WIN 54954, which had broad, potent anti-HRV activity (97). Clinical efficacy was assessed in two HRV (rhinovirus 23 and rhinovirus 39) challenge trials (91). Despite administering the compound before infection and achieving serum concentrations above the in vitro minimal inhibitory concentrations, both HRV trials failed to show efficacy of WIN 54954 (91); very low concentrations of the drug were found in nasal wash samples, the site of the experimental infection. WIN 54954 was not further developed for clinical use because of adverse reactions of flushing and rash, possibly related to concomitant alcohol ingestion by study volunteers.

Pleconaril (3-13,5-dimethyl-4-[[(3-methyl-5-isoxazolyl)-propyl]phenyl]-5-(trifluoromethyl)-1,2,4-oxadiazole) is the first of a new generation of metabolically stable capsid function inhibitors. This compound has demonstrated broad spectrum and potent anti-RV activity and is highly orally bioavailable (1, 51, 75; G. L. Kearns, J. S. Bradley, R. F. Jacobs, et al., Abstr. 36th Annu. Infect. Dis. Soc. Am. Meet., abstr. 750, 1998). Pleconaril inhibits viral replication by blocking viral uncoating and viral attachment to host cell receptors (75, 81). Oral pleconaril was protective against experimental coxsackievirus A21 (an EV that behaves biologically like the HRV) upper respiratory infection in volunteers (G. M. Schiff, M. A. McKinlay, and J. R. Sherwood, Proc. 36th Intersci. Conf. Antimicrob. Agents Chemother., abstr. H-43, 1996). In a double-blind, placebo-controlled study of 1,024 adults with viral respiratory infection during the fall rhinovirus season, patients receiving pleconaril recovered from all cold symptoms and returned to overall wellness (measured via a global assessment score) 3.5 days sooner than patients receiving placebo (Hayden et al., 39th ICAAC). Individual symptoms of the cold each resolved 1 to 2 days sooner in the pleconaril-treated patients. There were no differences in adverse events between treatment and placebo groups (Hayden et al., 39th ICAAC). In a recently completed large phase III study of pleconaril in viral respiratory infection, the time to resolution of illness was reduced in all patients from 9.4 to 7.7 days ($P = 0.07$), with greater effect in patients who did not take concomitant cold medications (9.0 to 6.75 days; $P = 0.033$). All picornavirus-infected patients treated with pleconaril experienced improvements in objective measures including mucus production, sleep disturbance, cold medication use, middle ear pressure, and viral shedding (ViroPharma, press release, 4/11/00).

Studies of this drug in other picornavirus diseases (see below) indicate both a clinical and virologic beneficial effect. Studies of HRV exacerbations of asthma and otitis media prevention are under way.

The majority of the HRV serotypes bind to a cellular receptor known as ICAM 1 (intercellular adhesion molecule 1). A soluble form of ICAM 1 has been developed and studied as a potential therapeutic approach to treating the common cold. The mechanism of action is binding of HRV virions and preventing those virions from binding to natural receptors on the surfaces of nasal epithelial cells. The soluble ICAM 1 preparation, called tremacamra, was evaluated in a small placebo-controlled study of experimental HRV infections of human volunteers (93). The tremacamra-treated group experienced reduced symptom incidence and severity as well as reduced mucus production. Significant adverse effects were not seen.

A series of compounds are under development that target the 3C protease of picornaviruses, resulting in inhibition of viral protein synthesis via blocking of viral-specific protein processing (A. K. Patrick, C. Ford, S. Binford, et al., Abstr. 10th Int. Conf. Antivir. Res., p. A75, 1997). Published results are limited to those with tripeptide aldehydes derived from the sequence of a natural 3C cleavage site, Leu-Phe-Gln. Anti-enzyme activity is potent ($K_i = 6$ nM), with high therapeutic indices in vitro. Like the RNA inhibitors discussed above, time of addition with the protease inhibitors is several hours without loss of antiviral activity. Clinical trials in HRV upper respiratory infections have been undertaken, but results are not yet available.

Symptomatic Therapies

Antihistamines have been frequently used for the treatment of common colds, but their usefulness has been the subject of controversy (56). Only first-generation antihistamines (e.g., chlorpheniramine, clemastine), which have anticholinergic and sedating effects, are useful in treating cold-associated rhinorrhea and sneezing (32, 92). Selective, nonsedating second-generation antihistamines (e.g., terfenadine, loratadine) are ineffective (9). The anticholinergic nasal spray ipratropium bromide has been shown to reduce rhinorrhea by 30% in natural colds (35). Corticosteroids do not provide clinically meaningful benefit in HRV colds and may serve to increase viral replication (29). Nonsteroidal anti-inflammatory agents variably benefit cold symptoms but certain ones (e.g., ibuprofen, naproxen) relieve discomfort and systemic symptoms (88).

Antibiotics

Despite their frequent use, no convincing evidence of benefit exists for antibiotic use during colds. A recent meta-analysis (23) found that antibiotic treatment in over 1,500 children did not affect the symptoms of the common cold. A subset of about 20% of cold sufferers are colonized with pathogenic respiratory bacteria (*Streptococcus pneumoniae, Haemophilus influenzae, Moraxella catarrhalis*) and may experience modest symptom benefit and lower rates of subsequent antibiotic use if treated with amoxicillin-clavulanate (47). Noncolonized patients do not benefit, and gastrointestinal intolerance develops fivefold more often in amoxicillin-clavulanate recipients (47). Determination of carriers of pathogenic bacteria is not practical in the office setting and of doubtful clinical value. Antibiotics should be withheld unless secondary bacterial infections are strongly suspected.

"Alternative Therapies"

The ubiquitousness and high annoyance qualities of HRV infections have prompted many unconventional therapies over the years. Among those, "nutritional supplements" like vitamin C, echinacea, zinc, ginseng, and others have dominated the news reports of "breakthroughs." Cold treatments such as these are associated with subjectivity and strong placebo effects, so adequate blinding of studies is essential. It is difficult to draw positive or negative conclusions from many studies because of small sample sizes, limited microbiological support, and differing outcome measures.

The best studied of the nutritional supplements in HRV infections is vitamin C. Since Linus Pauling's 1971 monograph on the subject, 21 placebo-controlled studies have been performed to establish whether vitamin C at a dosage of >1 g/day affects the common cold (41). The data reveal no evidence for reduced incidence of the common cold when taken prophylactically. Each of the studies showed a reduction in either duration or severity of the cold; the magnitude of the effect was on average 23% in all the studies cumulatively, but only 10% in studies with large numbers of patients (41).

A randomized placebo-controlled trial of echinacea in naturally occurring colds found no benefit of that compound in decreasing the incidence, duration, or severity of respiratory illnesses (28). Meta-analyses of clinical trials of zinc gluconate lozenges conclude either that zinc is of no proven value (43, 57) or of some benefit but with excessive side effects that limit the compliance with and utility of that therapy (59).

ENTEROVIRUSES

The EVs include nearly 70 serotypes of closely related pathogens that cause a wide spectrum of illness (Table 1). The paralytic potential of the polioviruses, the prototypic EV, was recognized as early as the 14th century B.C. in Egyptian art. Summer epidemics of paralytic poliomyelitis ravaged the United States through the 1950s. Since the introduction of vaccines in the late 1950s and early 1960s, much of the developed world is now virtually free of poliovirus disease. In many developing countries, eradication programs have made dramatic progress (13, 14).

Control of poliovirus infections in much of the world has turned attention to the nonpolio EVs. It is estimated that between 10 and 15 million people in the United States annually develop symptomatic nonpolio EV infections (Table 1). Most of these patients have nonspecific febrile syndromes often with constitutional and/or respiratory symptoms, with or without rashes (89). The EVs are epidemic every summer and fall, but like HRVs, sporadic infections occur year-round. Transmission of the EV is primarily fecal-oral, facilitated by the acid-stability of the EV and prolonged stool shedding.

Clinical Manifestations

Nonspecific Febrile Illnesses

The majority of symptomatic EV infections in the United States are characterized by minor EV illnesses associated with fever and constitutional symptoms, with or without rashes (89). These illnesses are of clinical significance because they may mimic other diseases including bacterial sepsis, other viral exanthematous diseases, and herpes simplex infections. The patients most affected by this mimicry are young infants in whom differentiation of viral illness from more alarming causes of fever and rash is extremely difficult. One prospective study found that 13% of babies born in the summer months were infected with EVs during the first month of life; 21% of the infected babies were hospitalized for suspected bacterial sepsis and received antibiotics or antiherpes therapy (44). Manifestations include fever, usually ≥39°C, and irritability, lethargy, anorexia, diarrhea, vomiting, rash, and respiratory symptoms. The duration of illness in infants beyond the neonatal period is usually 4 to 5 days.

Respiratory Illnesses

Many EV infections are accompanied by nonspecific, usually mild respiratory illness. A recent review of EV-associated respiratory illnesses found that 46% of cases presented with upper respiratory infections, 13% with respiratory distress/apnea, 13% with pneumonia, 12% with otitis media, and fewer cases with bronchiolitis, wheezing, croup, and pharyngotonsillitis (17). Most EV-associated respiratory illnesses are indistinguishable from those due to other respiratory viruses. Several distinctive syndromes are described below.

After an incubation period of about 24 h, hemorrhagic conjunctivitis is characterized by rapid onset of swelling of the eyelids, with congestion, lacrimation, and pain. Epithelial keratitis is common and transient. Occasional patients develop subconjunctival hemorrhages. In outbreak situations, incidence figures may reach pandemic proportions and neurologic complications, including paralytic polio-like disease, have been reported (94).

The highest incidence of herpangina is among children 1 to 7 years old, but infection has also been described in neonates and adults (73). Abrupt onset of fever associated with a sore throat, dysphagia, and malaise is typical. One-fourth of the patients have vomiting and abdominal pain. Early in the illness, grayish-white vesicles measuring 1 to 4 mm in diameter appear over the posterior portion of the palate uvula, tonsillar pillars, and occasionally on the oropharynx. These vesicles are discrete, surrounded by erythema, and usually number fewer than 20. Symptoms begin to improve in 4 to 5 days, and recovery is usually complete within a week of onset (73).

Hand-foot-mouth syndrome typically occurs among children <4 years of age, but adults are also frequently affected; intrafamilial spread is common. The disease is usually mild, and the onset is associated with a sore throat with or without a low-grade fever (15). Scattered vesicular lesions occur randomly on the oral structures, the pharynx, and the lips; these ulcerate readily, leaving shallow lesions with red areolae. Sparse grayish vesicles (3 to 5 mm in diameter, surrounded by erythema) also appear on the dorsum of the fingers, particularly in periungal areas, and on the margins of heels. Palmar, plantar, and groin lesions may appear. As with hemorrhagic conjunctivitis, massive outbreaks of hand-foot-mouth syndrome have been reported with prominent neurologic and other serious systemic manifestations (42).

Pleurodynia is primarily a disease of muscle masquerading as pleuritic disease, although pleural involvement can occur (49). The onset is abrupt in three-fourths of patients, with the remainder first developing headache and other vague prodromal symptoms of 1 to 10 days' duration. The major symptom is severe paroxysmal pain referred to the lower ribs or the sternum. Fever, headache, cough, anorexia, nausea, vomiting, and diarrhea also occur. The mean duration of the illness is $3^1/_2$ days, varying from 1 to 14 days (49).

Myocarditis

The EVs are among the most commonly identified etiologies of myocarditis, causing between 25 and 35% of cases for which a cause is found (60). Neonates and young infants ($\leq$6 months of age) are particularly susceptible to EV myocarditis (see below), but most cases occur in young adults between the ages of 20 and 39 years. Rigorous exercise and recent respiratory illness are anecdotally associated with many cases of myocarditis. Clinically, myocarditis reflects the extent of the cardiac involvement (60). Symptoms include palpitations and chest pain, often with accompanying fever. Arrhythmias and sudden death reflect conducting system involvement often of very recent onset; congestive heart failure or myocardial infarction-like presentations suggest more extensive myocyte necrosis and longer-standing disease. Pericardial friction rub indicates a myopericarditis. Electrocardiographic findings include an evolution from early-stage S-T segment elevation and T-wave inversion to intermediate-stage normalization to late-stage recurrence of T-wave inversion. Myocardial enzyme elevations are detected in the blood. While most patients recover uneventfully from clinically apparent myocarditis, many have residual electrocardiographic or echocardiographic abnormalities for months to years. Smaller proportions develop congestive heart failure, chronic myocarditis, or dilated cardiomyopathy (60).

Aseptic Meningitis

The severity of EV meningitis varies with host age and immune status (83). Neonates <2 weeks of age are at risk for severe systemic illness (see below), commonly including meningitis or meningoencephalitis. EV meningitis beyond the first 2 weeks of life is rarely associated with severe disease or poor outcome. Onset is usually sudden, and fever of 38 to 40°C occurs in 75 to 100% of patients (83). The fever pattern may be biphasic, appearing first with nonspecific constitutional symptoms and reappearing with the onset of meningeal signs. Headache is nearly always present in adults and children old enough to report it, and photophobia is also common (80). Nuchal rigidity is found in more than half of the patients, particularly in children older than 1 to 2 years of age. Nonspecific manifestations include vomiting, anorexia, rash, diarrhea, cough and pharyngitis, diarrhea, and myalgias. Neurologic abnormalities are unusual. The duration of illness due to EV meningitis is usually about 1 week, but many patients, particularly adults, may have symptoms that persist for 2 or more weeks (80). The prognosis for young children with EV meningitis early in life appears to be good, without long-term sequelae (M. L. Rorabaugh, L. E. Berlin, L. Rosenberg, and J. Modlin, Pediatr. Res. 30:177A, 1992).

Encephalitis

Encephalitis due to the EVs is well documented but uncommon (96). Unlike aseptic meningitis, encephalitis due to EV may have more profound acute disease and long-term sequelae. In contrast to the typical focal disease seen with herpes simplex virus, EVs are usually associated with global encephalitis and generalized neurologic depression. The illness usually begins with a prodrome of fever, myalgias, and upper respiratory symptoms. Onset of central nervous system signs and symptoms is often abrupt, with confusion, weakness, lethargy, drowsiness, and/or irritability. Progression to coma and/or generalized seizures may occur. Focal EV encephalitis is less often reported than global disease but may be underappreciated (66).

Congenital and Neonatal Infections

The infected neonate appears to be at greatest risk for severe disease when illness develops in the first days of life; this pattern suggests possible transplacental acquisition (3). Maternal illness has been reported in 59 to 68% of infected neonates. Fever is ubiquitous, often accompanied by vomiting, anorexia, rash, and/or upper respiratory findings. Neurologic involvement may or may not be associated with signs of meningeal inflammation, including nuchal rigidity and bulging anterior fontanelle. Major systemic manifestations such as hepatic necrosis, myocarditis, and necrotizing enterocolitis may develop. Disseminated intravascular coagulation and other findings of "sepsis" result in an illness that may be indistinguishable from that due to overwhelming bacterial infection. An encephalitic picture with seizures and focal neurologic findings may suggest herpes simplex virus. As many as 2,500 cases of neonatal EV sepsis may occur each year; the incidences of severe morbidity and mortality occurring with perinatal EV infections are not precisely known but may be as high as 74 and 10%, respectively (50, 65). Mortality is typically due to hepatic failure or myocarditis.

Diagnosis

Isolation of EVs in cell culture has been the gold standard for laboratory diagnosis for many years (82). However, no single cell line is optimal for all EV serotypes, and virus isolation requires technical expertise and may be quite labor-intensive. In addition, 25 to 35% of specimens from patients with EV infections will be falsely negative by cell culture.

The most promising development in the detection of EVs has been PCR, which is consistently more sensitive than culture and virtually 100% specific (79). This assay is available from numerous reference laboratories around the country. The most appropriate specimens for testing depend on the syndrome: cerebrospinal fluid for meningitis and encephalitis, serum and urine for neonatal sepsis, throat for respiratory illness. The rapidity of this assay (5 h in some formats), coupled with its high degree of accuracy, has made PCR the test of choice for EV diagnosis at centers that offer it.

Management

Immune Serum Globulin (ISG)

ISG has been used prophylactically and therapeutically against EVs in two patient groups: neonates and immunocompromised hosts. Anecdotal reports of clinical success with maternal serum or plasma, or commercial ISG, against a variety of EV serotypes causing severe neonatal EV disease have been reported; other reports describe progressive disease and death despite such therapy (3). One small controlled study demonstrated reduction of viral titers in babies receiving intravenous ISG preparations subsequently shown to contain high antibody titers to the infecting serotype (2).

Before the availability of intravenous ISG, mixed results were reported with intramuscular and/or intrathecal administration of ISG in patients with antibody deficiency (63). Since patients with known antibody deficiency have begun receiving prophylactic intravenous ISG, the incidence of progressive EV meningoencephalitis has fallen and the clinical profile of patients developing such infections has been modified (95). However, it remains unclear if intravenous ISG has therapeutic efficacy in established EV meningoencephalitis in these patients.

Antivirals

Despite in vitro efficacy, interferons have not been clinically evaluated in EV infections. A series of capsid-binding compounds, the phenoxyl imidazoles, are broad-spectrum inhibitors of EVs and demonstrate therapeutic oral efficacy in animal models (11, 19). Further development of candidate drugs in this series has been discontinued. Disoxaril (discussed in the HRV management section above) was very active against EVs both in vitro and in vivo (61, 62, 72). However, as noted previously, the appearance of asymptomatic crystalluria in healthy volunteers prevented further clinical study. WIN 54954 (see HRV management above) also had broad, potent anti-EV activity in vitro and in vivo (97), including oral therapeutic efficacy in mice. In contrast to the negative effects in HRV trials, WIN 54954 significantly reduced the number and severity of colds experimentally induced by coxsackievirus A21 in human volunteer trials and also significantly reduced nasal mucous discharge, respiratory and systemic symptoms, and viral titers (86). The overall symptomatic attack rate was reduced from 15 of 23 patients in the placebo group to 3 of 27 in the WIN 54954-treated groups ($P = 0.0001$). This study represented the first demonstration of oral efficacy of an anti-EV agent; the differences in results compared with those in the HRV studies using the same compound are enigmatic since the minimal inhibitory concentration for one of the HRV serotypes was identical to that of the coxsackievirus A21 strain used. The fact that EV infections are systemic, usually with a viremic phase, may explain the enhanced EV efficacy of an orally active compound that achieves good blood levels over the effect seen in HRV infections, which are limited to the upper airway where drug distribution may have been insufficient. WIN 54954 was not further developed for clinical use because of adverse reactions, as described above.

Pleconaril (see HRV management above) has broad anti-EV activity as well as anti-HRV activity. Potent systemic activity of pleconaril has been demonstrated in volunteers with experimental coxsackievirus A21 respiratory infections (see above) (Schiff et al., 36th ICAAC) and in compassionate-use treatment of potentially life-threatening EV infections (H. A. Rotbart and the Pleconaril Treatment Registry, Abstr. 36th Annu. Meet. Infect. Dis. Soc. Am., abstr. 791, 1998). In a placebo-controlled trial of pleconaril in 221 pediatric patients with EV meningitis, significant reductions in the total morbidity (composite measurement of all disease symptoms) and global assessment (caregiver's assessment of patient's illness) scores were documented for the overall study population (M. H. Sawyer, X. Saez-Llorenz, C. L. Aviles, et al., Proc. 1999 APS/SPR Meet., 1999). Headache duration was significantly reduced by pleconaril treatment in children older than 8 years. Responses were noted as early as 24 h after initiation of treatment. Viral shedding from the throat, reflecting duration of infection, was also reduced in the pleconaril-treated group compared with placebo (Sawyer et al., APS/SPR Meet., 1999). Pleconaril has also been studied in adult patients with EV meningitis (S. D. Shafran, W. Halota, D. Gilbert, et al., Abstr. 39th Intersci. Conf. Antimicrob. Agents Chemother., 1999) In a double-blind, placebo-controlled trial, 180 patients aged 14 to 65 years received either 200 mg of pleconaril three times per day or placebo. Those receiving pleconaril had a 2-day shorter duration of headache and a 2-day faster resolution of all symptoms of meningitis. Pleconaril-treated patients also returned to work or school 2 days faster (Shafran et al., 39th ICAAC).

Results of phase III studies of pleconaril in viral meningitis have recently been announced (ViroPharma press release, 4/11/00). In adult patients with moderate to severe headache and vomiting at presentation, the time to resolution of headache was reduced by 3 days (from 10 days in the placebo-treated patients to 7 days in pleconaril-treated patients; $P = 0.039$); a parallel reduction was seen in the time to return to work ($P = 0.015$). When the same endpoint was evaluated in the overall adult population (all levels of symptom severity) and in children, statistically significant benefit was not observed.

SUMMARY

The picornaviruses, including EVs and HRVs, are the most common causes of viral illnesses worldwide. Ranging from mild diseases of short duration to severe and potentially life-threatening infections, the picornaviruses have protean clinical presentations. New developments in the rapid diagnosis and therapy of these infections promise to significantly reduce the disease burden and the associated costs to affected individuals and to society.

REFERENCES

1. **Abdel-Rahman, S. M., and G. L. Kearns.** 1999. Single oral dose escalation pharmacokinetics of pleconaril capsules in adults. J. Clin. Pharmacol. **39:**613–618.
2. **Abzug, M. J., H. L. Keyserling, M. L. Lee, M. J. Levin, and H. A. Rotbart.** 1995. Neonatal enterovirus infection: virology, serology, and effects of intravenous immune globulin. Clin. Infect. Dis. **20:**1201–1206.
3. **Abzug, M. J., M. J. Levin, and H. A. Rotbart.** 1993. Profile of enterovirus disease in the first two weeks of life. Pediatr. Infect. Dis. J. **12:**820–824.
4. **Al-Nakib, W., P. G. Higgins, G. I. Barrow, D. A. J. Tyrrell, K. Andries, G. V. Bussche, N. Taylor, and P. A. J. Janssen.** 1989. Suppression of colds in human volunteers challenged with rhinovirus by a new synthetic drug (R61837). Antimicrob. Agents Chemother. **33:**522–525.
5. **Arola, M., O. Ruuskanen, T. Ziegler, J. Mertsola, K. Nanto-Salonen, A. Putto-Laurila, M. K. Viljanen, and P. Halonen.** 1990. Clinical role of respiratory virus infection in acute otitis media. Pediatrics **86:**848–855.
6. **Arruda, E., and F. G. Hayden.** 1995. Clinical studies of antiviral agents for picornaviral infections. In D. J. Jeffries

and E. DeCierrq (ed.), *Antiviral Chemotherapy*. John Wiley & Sons Ltd., New York, N.Y.
7. **Arruda, E., A. Pitkaranta, T. J. Witek, Jr., C. A. Doyle, and F. G. Hayden.** 1997. Frequency and natural history of rhinovirus infections in adults during autumn. *J. Clin. Microbiol.* **35:**2864–2868.
8. **Barrow, G. I., P. G. Higgins, D. A. J. Tyrrell, and K. Andries.** An appraisal of the efficacy of the antiviral R 61837 in rhinovirus infections in human volunteers. *Antivir. Chem. Chemother.* **5:**278–283.
9. **Berkowitz, R. B., and D. G. Tinkelman.** 1987. Evaluation of oral terfenadine for treatment of the common cold. *Am. Rev. Resp. Dis.* **136:**556–560.
10. **Buchman, C. A., W. J. Doyle, D. Skoner, P. Fireman, and J. M. Gwaltney.** 1994. Otologic manifestations of experimental rhinovirus infection. *Laryngoscope* **104:**1295–1299.
11. **Buontempo, P., S. Cox, J. Wright-Minogue, J. L. DeMartino, A. Skelton, E. Ferrari, R. Albin, E. J. Rozhon, V. Girijavallabhan, J. F. Modlin, and J. F. O'Connell.** 1997. SCH 48973: a potent, broad spectrum antienterovirus compound. *Antimicrob. Agents Chemother.* **41:**1220–1225.
12. **Capobianchi, M. R., D. Matteucci, A. Glovannetti, E. Soldaini, M. Bendinei, J. G. Stanton, and F. Dianzani.** 1991. Role of interferon in lethality and lymphoid atrophy induced by coxsackievirus S3 infection in mice. *Virol. Immunol.* **5:**103–110.
13. **Centers for Disease Control and Prevention.** 1996. Progress toward global eradication of poliomyelitis. *Morb. Mortal. Wkly. Rep.* **45:**565–568.
14. **Centers for Disease Control and Prevention.** 1997. Progress toward poliomyelitis eradication—Africa, 1996. *Morb. Mortal. Wkly. Rep.* **46:**321–325.
15. **Cherry, J. D.** 1998. Enteroviruses: coxsackieviruses, echoviruses, and polioviruses, p. 1787–1838. *In* R. D. Feigin and J. D. Cherry (ed.), *Textbook of Pediatric Infectious Diseases*, 4th ed. W. B. Saunders, Philadelphia, Pa.
16. **Chidekel, A. S., A. R. Bazzy, and C. L. Rosen.** 1994. Rhinovirus infection associated with severe lower respiratory tract illness and worsening lung disease in infants with bronchopulmonary dysplasia. *Pediatr. Pulm.* **18:**261–263.
17. **Chonmaitree, T., and L. Mann.** 1995. Respiratory infections, p. 255–270. *In* H. A. Rotbart (ed.), *Human Enterovirus Infections*. ASM Press, Washington, D.C.
18. **Collinson, J., K. G. Nicholson, E. Cancio, J. Ashman, D. C. Ireland, V. Hammersley, J. Kent, and C. O'Callaghan.** 1996. Effects of upper respiratory tract infections in patients with cystic fibrosis. *Thorax* **51:**1115–1122.
19. **Cox, S., P. Buontempo, J. Wright-Minogue, J. L. DeMartino, A. M. Skelton, E. Ferrari, J. Schwartz, E. J. Rozhon, C. C. Linn, V. Girijavallabhan, and J. F. O'Connell.** 1996. Antipicornavirus activity of SCH 47802 and analogues: in vitro and in vivo studies. *Antivir. Res.* **32:**71–79.
20. **Douglas, R. M., B. W. Moore, H. B. Miles, L. M. Davies, N. Graham, P. Ryan, D. Worswick, and J. Albricht.** 1986. Prophylactic efficacy of intranasal alpha A2-interferon against rhinovirus infections in the family setting. *N. Engl. J. Med.* **314:**65–70.
21. **Elkhatieb, A., G. Hipskind, D. Woerner, and F. G. Hayden.** 1993. Middle ear abnormalities during natural rhinovirus colds in adults. *J. Infect. Dis.* **168:**618–621.
22. **Fox, M. P., M. A. McKinlay, G. D. Diana, and F. J. Dutko.** 1991. Binding affinities of structurally related human rhinovirus capsid-binding compounds are related to their activities against human rhinovirus type 14. *Antimicrob. Agents Chemother.* **35:**1040–1047.
23. **Gadomski, A. M.** 1993. Potential interventions for preventing pneumonia among young children: lack of effect of antibiotic treatment for upper respiratory infections. *Pediatr. Infect. Dis. J.* **12:**115–120.
24. **Geniteau-Legendre, M., F. Forestier, A. M. Quero, and A. German.** 1987. Role of interferon, antibodies and macrophages in the protective effect of *Corynebacterium parvum* on encephalomyocarditis virus-induced disease in mice. *Antivir. Res.* **7:**161–167.
25. **Gilbert, L. L., A. Dakhama, B. M. Bone, E. E. Thomas, and R. G. Hegele.** 1996. Diagnosis of viral respiratory tract infections in children by using reverse transcription-PCR panel. *J. Clin. Microb.* **34:**140–143.
26. **Gonzales, R., J. F. Steiner, and M. A. Sande.** 1998. Antibiotic prescribing for adults with colds, upper respiratory tract infections, and bronchitis by ambulatory care physicians. *JAMA* **278:**901–904.
27. **Greenberg, S. B., M. W. Harmon, R. B. Couch, P. E. Johnson, S. Z. Wilson, C. C. Dacso, K. Bloom, and J. Quarles.** 1982. Prophylactic effect of low doses of human leukocyte interferon against infection with rhinovirus. *J. Infect. Dis.* **145:**542–546.
28. **Grimm, W., and H.-H. Muller.** 1999. A randomized controlled trial of the effect of fluid extract of Echinacea Purpurea on the incidence and severity of colds and respiratory infections. *Am. J. Med.* **106:**138–143.
29. **Gustafson, L. M., D. Proud, O. Hendley, F. G. Hayden, and J. M. Gwaltney.** 1996. Oral prednisone therapy in experimental rhinovirus infections. *J. Allergy Clin. Immunol.* **97:**1009–1114.
30. **Gwaltney, J. M., Jr.** 1992. Combined antiviral and antimediator treatment of rhinovirus colds. *J. Infect. Dis.* **166:**776–782.
31. **Gwaltney, J. M., Jr.** 1989. Rhinoviruses, p. 593. *In* A. S. Evans (ed.), *Viral Infection of Humans*. Plenum Press, New York, N.Y.
32. **Gwaltney, J. M., Jr., J. Park, R. A. Paul, D. A. Edelman, R. R. O'Connor, and R. B. Turner.** 1996. Randomized controlled trial of clemastine fumarate for treatment of experimental rhinovirus colds. *Clin. Infect. Dis.* **22:**656–662.
33. **Gwaltney, J. M., Jr., C. D. Phillips, R. D. Miller, and D. K. Riker.** 1994. Computed tomographic study of the common cold. *N. Engl. J. Med.* **330:**25–30.
34. **Gwaltney, J. M., Jr., and R. R. Rueckert.** 1997. Rhinovirus, p. 1025–1047. *In* D. D. Richman, R. J. Whitley, and F. G. Hayden (ed.). *Clinical Virology*. Churchill Livingstone, New York, N.Y.
35. **Hayden, F. G., L. Diamond, P. B. Wood, D. C. Korts, and M. T. Wecker.** 1996. Effectiveness and safety of intranasal ipratropium bromide in common colds. A randomized, double-blind, placebo-controlled trial. *Ann. Intern. Med.* **125:**89–97.
36. **Hayden, F., J. K. Albrecht, D. L. Kaiser, and J. M. Gwaltney.** 1986. Prevention of natural colds by contact prophylaxis with intranasal alpha 2-interferon. *N. Engl. J. Med.* **314:**71–75.
37. **Hayden, F., and J. M. Gwaltney.** 1983. Intranasal interferon alpha2 for prevention of rhinovirus infection and illness. *J. Infect. Dis.* **148:**543–550.
38. **Hayden, F., and J. M. Gwaltney.** 1984. Intranasal interferon-a2 treatment of experimental rhinovirus colds. *J. Infect. Dis.* **150:**174–180.
39. **Hayden, F. G., A. Andries, and P. A. J. Janssen.** 1992. Safety and efficacy of intranasal pirodavir (R77975) in experimental rhinovirus infection. *Antimicrob. Agents Chemother.* **36:**727–732.
40. **Heikkinen, T., M. Thint, and T. Chonmaitree.** 1999. Prevalence of various respiratory viruses in the middle ear during acute otitis media. *N. Engl. J. Med.* **340:**260–264.

41. **Hemila, H.** 1994. Does vitamin C alleviate the symptoms of the common cold: a review of current evidence. *Scand. J. Infect. Dis.* **26:**1–6.
42. **Ho, M., E.-R. Chen, K.-H. Hsu, S. J. Twu, K. T. Chen, S. F. Tsai, J. R. Wang, and S. R. Shih.** 1999. An epidemic of enterovirus 71 infection in Taiwan. *N. Engl. J. Med.* **341:**929–935.
43. **Jackson, J. L., C. Peterson, and E. Lesho.** 1997. A meta-analysis of zinc salts lozenges and the common cold. *Arch. Intern. Med.* **157:**2373–2376.
44. **Jenista, J. A., K. R. Powell, and M. A. Menegus.** 1984. Epidemiology of neonatal enterovirus infection. *J. Pediatr.* **104:**685–690.
45. **Johnston, S. L., P. K. Pattemore, G. Sanderson, S. Smith, M. J. Campbell, L. K. Josephs, A. Cunningham, B. S. Robinson, S. H. Myint, M. E. Ward, D. A. Tyrrell, and S. T. Holgate.** 1996. The relationship between upper respiratory infections and hospital admissions for asthma: a time-trend analysis. *Am. J. Respir. Crit. Care Med.* **154:**654–660.
46. **Johnston, S. L., P. K. Pattemore, G. Sanderson, S. Smith, F. Lampe, and L. Josephs.** 1995. Community study of role of viral infections in exacerbations of asthma in 9–11 year old children. *BMJ* **310:**1225–1229.
47. **Kaiser, L., D. Lew, B. Hirschel, R. Auckenthaler, A. Morabia, A. Heald, P. Benedict, F. Terrier, W. Wunderli, L. Matter, D. Germann, J. Voegeli, and H. Stalder.** 1996. Effects of antibiotic treatment in the subset of common-cold patients who have bacteria in nasopharyngeal secretions. *Lancet* **347:**1507–1510.
48. **Kandolf, R., A. Canu, and P. H. Hofschneider.** 1985. Coxsackie B3 virus can replicate in cultured human foetal heart cells and is inhibited by interferon. *J. Mol. Cell. Cardiol.* **17:**167–181.
49. **Kantor, F. S., and G. D. Hsiung.** 1962. Pleurodynia associated with echo virus type 8. *N. Engl. J. Med.* **266:**661–663.
50. **Kaplan, M. H., S. W. Klein, J. McPhee, and R. G. Harper.** 1983. Group B coxsackievirus infections in infants younger than three months of age: a serious childhood illness. *Rev. Infect. Dis.* **5:**1019–1032.
51. **Kearns, G. L., S. M. Abdel-Rahman, L. P. James, D. L. Blowey, J. D. Marshall, T. G. Wells, R. F. Jacobs, and Pediatric Pharmacology Research Unit Network.** 1999. Single-dose pharmacokinetics of a pleconaril (VP63843) oral solution in children and adolescents. *Antimicrob. Agents Chemother.* **43:**634–638.
52. **Kishimoto, C., C. S. Crumpacker, and W. H. Abelmann.** 1988. Prevention of murine coxsackie B3 viral myocarditis and associated lymphoid organ atrophy with recombinant human leucocyte interferon alpha A/D. *Cardiovasc. Res.* **22:**732–738.
53. **Langford, M. P., J. C. Barber, V. E. Sklar, S. W. Clark III, P. A. Patriarca, I. M. Onarato, M. Yin-Murphy, and G. J. Stanton.** 1985. Virus-specific, early appearing neutralizing activity and interferon production in patients with acute hemorrhagic conjunctivitis. *Curr. Eye Res.* **4:**233–239.
54. **Langford, M. P., R. M. Kadi, J. P. Ganley, and M. Yin-Murphy.** 1988. Inhibition of epidemic isolates of coxsackie virus type A24 by recombinant and natural interferon alpha and interferon beta. *Intervirology* **29:**320–327.
55. **Lopez-Guerrero, J. A., F. X. Pimentel-Muinos, M. Fresno, and M. A. Alonso.** 1990. Role of soluble cytokines on the restricted replication of poliovirus in the monocylic U937 cell line. *Virus Res.* **16:**225–230.
56. **Luks, D., and M. R. Anderson.** 1996. Antihistamines and the common cold. A review and critique of the literature. *J. Gen. Intern. Med.* **11:**240–244.
57. **Macknin, M. L., M. Piedmonte, C. Calendine, J. Janosky, and E. Wald.** 1998. Zinc gluconate lozenges for treating the common cold in children: a randomized controlled trial. *JAMA* **279:**1999–2000.
58. **Makela, M. J., T. Puhakka, O. Ruuskanen, M. Leinonen, P. Saikku, M. Kimpimaki, S. Blomqvist, T. Hyypiä, and P. Arstila.** 1998. Viruses and bacteria in the etiology of the common cold. *J. Clin. Microbiol.* **36:**539–542.
59. **Marshall, S.** 1998. Zinc gluconate and the common cold. Review of randomized controlled trials. *Can. Fam. Phys.* **44:**1037–1042.
60. **Martino, T. A., P. Liu, M. Petric, and M. J. Sole.** 1995. Enteroviral myocarditis and dilated cardiomyopathy: a review of clinical and experimental studies, p. 291–351. *In* H. A. Rotbart (ed.), *Human Enterovirus Infections.* ASM Press, Washington, D.C.
61. **McKinlay, M. A., J. A. Frank, and B. A. Steinberg.** 1986. Use of WIN 51711 to prevent echovirus type 9-induced paralysis in suckling mice. *J. Infect. Dis.* **154:**676–681.
62. **McKinlay, M. A., and B. A. Steinberg.** 1986. Oral efficacy of WIN 51711 in mice infected with human poliovirus. *Antimicrob. Agents Chemother.* **29:**30–32.
63. **McKinney, R. E., Jr., S. L. Katz, and G. M. Wilfert.** 1987. Chronic enteroviral meningoencephalitis in agammaglobulinemic patients. *Rev. Infect. Dis.* **9:**334–356.
64. **Merigan, T., S. Reed, T. Hall, and D. Tyrrell.** 1973. Inhibition of respiratory virus infection by locally applied interferon. *Lancet* **i:**536–567.
65. **Modlin, J. F.** 1986. Perinatal echovirus infection: insights from a literature review of 61 cases of serious infection and 16 outbreaks in nurseries. *Rev. Infect. Dis.* **8:**918–926.
66. **Modlin, J. F., R. Dagan, L. E. Berlin, D. M. Virshup, R. H. Yolken, and M. Menegus.** 1991. Focal encephalitis with enterovirus infections. *Pediatrics* **88:**841–845.
67. **Monto, A. S., S. A. Schwartz, and J. K. Albrecht.** 1989. Ineffectiveness of postexposure prophylaxis of rhinovirus infection with low-dose intranasal alpha 2b interferon in families. *Antimicrob. Agents Chemother.* **33:**387–390.
68. **Nicholson, K. G., J. Kent, V. Hammersley, and E. Gancio.** 1996. Risk factors for lower respiratory complications of rhinovirus infections in elderly people living in the community: prospective cohort study. *BMJ* **313:**1119–1123.
69. **Nicholson, K. G., J. Kent, and D. C. Ireland.** 1993. Respiratory viruses and exacerbations of asthma in adults. *BMJ* **307:**982–986.
70. **Nyquist, A.-C., R. Gonzales, J. F. Steiner, and M. A. Sande.** 1998. Antibiotic prescribing for children with colds, upper respiratory tract infections, and bronchitis. *JAMA* **279:**875–877.
71. **Okada, I., A. Matsumori, Y. Matoba, M. Tominaga, T. Yamada, and C. Kowai.** 1992. Combination treatment with ribavirin and interferon for coxsackievirus B3 replication. *J. Lab. Clin. Med.* **120:**569–573.
72. **Otto, M. J., M. P. Fox, M. J. Fancher, M. F. Huhrt, G. D. Diana, and M. A. McKinlay.** 1985. In vitro activity of WIN 51711, a new broad-spectrum antipicornavirus drug. *Antimicrob. Agents Chemother.* **27:**883–886.
73. **Parrott, R. H., S. Ross, F. G. Burke, and E. C. Rice.** 1951. Herpangina: clinical studies of a specific infectious disease. *N. Engl. J. Med.* **245:**275–280.
74. **Patel, J. A., B. Reisner, N. Vizirinia, M. Owen, T. Chonmaitree, and V. Howie.** 1995. Bacteriological failure of amoxicillin-clavulanate in treatment of acute otitis media caused by nontypeable *Haemophilus influenzae*. *J. Pediatr.* **126:**799–806.
75. **Pevear, D. C., T. M. Tull, M. E. Seipel, and J. M.**

Groarke. 1999. Activity of pleconaril against enteroviruses. *Antimicrob. Agents Chemother.* **43**:2109–2115.

76. Pitkaranta, A., E. Arruda, H. Malmberg, and F. G. Hayden. 1997. Detection of rhinovirus in sinus brushings of patients with acute community-acquired sinusitis by reverse transcription-PCR. *J. Clin. Microbiol.* **35**:1791–1793.

77. Pitkaranta, A., A. Virolainen, J. Jero, E. Arruda, and F. G. Hayden. 1998. Detection of rhinovirus, respiratory syncytial virus, and coronavirus infections in acute otitis media by reverse transcriptase polymerase chain reaction. *Pediatrics* **102**:291–295.

78. Rombaut, B., R. Vrijsen, and A. Boeye. 1985. Comparison of arildone and 3-methylquercetin as stabilizers of poliovirus. *Antivir. Res. Suppl.* **1**:67–73.

79. Rotbart, H. A., A. Ahmed, S. Hickey, R. Dagan, G. H. McCracken, Jr., R. J. Whitley, J. F. Modlin, M. Cascino, J. F. O'Connell, M. A. Menegus, and D. Blum. 1997. Diagnosis of enterovirus infection by polymerase chain reaction of multiple specimen types. *Pediatr. Infect. Dis. J.* **16**:409–411.

80. Rotbart, H. A., P. J. Brennan, K. H. Fife, J. R. Romero, J. A. Griffin, M. A. Mckinlay, and F. G. Hayden. 1998. Enterovirus meningitis in adults. *Clin. Infect. Dis.* **27**:896–898.

81. Rotbart, H. A., J. F. O'Connell, and M. A. McKinlay. 1998. Treatment of human enterovirus infections. *Antivir. Res.* **38**:1–14.

82. Rotbart, H. A. 1995. Enteroviruses, p. 1004–1011. *In* P. R. Murray, E. J. Baron, M. A. Pfaller, F. C. Tenover, and R. H. Yolken (ed.), *Manual of Clinical Microbiology*, 6th ed. ASM Press, Washington, D.C.

83. Rotbart, H. A. 1997. Viral meningitis and the aseptic meningitis syndrome, p. 23–46. *In* W. M. Scheld, R. J. Whitley, and D. T. Durack (ed.), *Infections of the Central Nervous System*, 2nd ed. Lippincott-Raven, Philadelphia, Pa.

84. Samo, T. C., S. B. Greenberg, R. B. Couch, J. Quarles, P. E. Johnson, S. Hook, and M. W. Harmon. 1983. Efficacy and tolerance of intranasal applied recombinant leukocyte A interferon in normal volunteers. *J. Infect. Dis.* **148**:535–542.

85. Sasaki, O., T. Karaki, and J. Imanishi. 1986. Protective effect of interferon on infections with hand, foot and mouth disease virus in newborn mice. *J. Infect. Dis.* **153**:498–502.

86. Schiff, G. M., J. R. Sherwood, E. C. Young, and L. J. Mason. 1992. Prophylactic efficacy of WIN 54954 in prevention of experimental human coxsackievirus A21 infection and illness. *Antivir. Res.* **17**(Suppl.):92.

87. Schmidt, H. J., and R. J. Fink. 1991. Rhinovirus as a lower respiratory pathogen in infants. *Pediatr. Infect. Dis. J.* **10**:700–702.

88. Sperber, S. J., J. O. Hendley, F. G. Hayden, D. K. Riker, J. V. Sorrentino, and J. M. Gwaltney, Jr. 1992. Effects of naproxen on experimental rhinovirus colds. A randomized, double-blind, controlled trial. *Ann. Intern. Med.* **117**:37–41.

89. Strikas, R. A., L. J. Anderson, and R. A. Parker. 1986. Temporal and geographic patterns of isolates of nonpolio enterovirus in the United States, 1970–1983. *J. Infect. Dis.* **153**:346–351.

90. Turner, R. B. 1998. The common cold. *Pediatr. Ann.* **27**:790–795.

91. Turner, R. B., F. J. Dutko, N. H. Goldstein, G. Lockwood, and F. G. Hayden. 1993. Efficacy of oral WIN 54954 for prophylaxis of experimental rhinovirus infection. *Antimicrob. Agents Chemother.* **37**:297–300.

92. Turner, R. B., S. J. Sperber, J. V. Sorrentino, R. R. O'Connor, J. Rogers, A. R. Batouli, and J. M. Gwaltney, Jr. 1997. Effectiveness of clemastine fumarate for treatment of rhinorrhea and sneezing associated with the common cold. *Clin. Infect. Dis.* **25**:824–830.

93. Turner, R. B., M. T. Wecker, G. Pohl, T. J. Witek, E. McNally, R. St. George, B. Winther, and F. G. Hayden. 1999. Efficacy of tremacamra, a soluble intercellular adhesion molecule 1 for experimental rhinovirus infection: a randomized clinical trial. *JAMA* **281**:1797–1804.

94. Wadia, N. H., P. N. Wadia, S. M. Katrak, and V. P. Misra. 1983. A study of the neurological disorder associated with acute hemorrhagic conjunctivitis due to enterovirus 70. *J. Neurol. Neurosurg. Psych.* **46**:599–610.

95. Webster, A. D. B., H. A. Rotbart, T. Warner, P. Rudge, and N. Hyman. 1993. Diagnosis of enterovirus brain disease in hypogammaglobulinemic patients by polymerase chain reaction. *Clin. Infect. Dis.* **17**:657–661.

96. Whitley, R. J., C. G. Cobbs, C. A. Alford, Jr., S. J. Soong, M. S. Hirsch, J. D. Connor, L. Corey, D. F. Hanley, M. Levin, and D. A. Powell. 1989. Diseases that mimic herpes simplex encephalitis. Diagnosis, presentation, and outcome. *JAMA* **262**:234–239.

97. Woods, M. G., G. D. Diana, M. C. Rogge, M. J. Otto, F. J. Dutko, and M. A. McKinlay. 1989. In vitro and in vivo activities of WIN 54954, a new broad-spectrum antipicornavirus drug. *Antimicrob. Agents Chemother.* **33**:2069–2074.

98. Zhang, A., R. G. Nanni, G. F. Arnold, D. A. Oren, T. Li, A. Jacobo-Molkina, R. L. William, G. Kamer, D. A. Rubenstein, Y. Li, E. Rozhon, S. Cox, P. Buontempo, J. O'Connell, J. Schwartz, G. Miller, C. Nash, B. Bauer, R. Versace, A. Ganguly, V. Girijavallabhan, and E. Arnold. 1991. Structure of a complex of human rhinovirus 14 with a water soluble antiviral compound SCH 38057. *J. Mol. Biol.* **230**:857–867.

99. Zhang, A., R. G. Nanni, D. A. Oren, E. J. Rozhon, and E. Arnold. 1992. Three-dimensional structure-activity relationships for antiviral agents that interact with picornavirus capsids. *Semin. Virol.* **3**:453–471.

Determinants of Poliovirus Pathogenesis

MATTHIAS GROMEIER AND AKIO NOMOTO

29

Elucidation of the mechanisms of viral replication strategies that lead to disease are of central interest to virologists and physicians alike. Most commonly, the association with clinical overt disease determines the level of interest an infectious pathogen raises among researchers. That is true also for the picornavirus field, where the accumulation of knowledge is lopsided toward the clinically relevant species, e.g., poliovirus or coxsackie B viruses (CBV), at the expense of species of lesser medical importance (Table 1). Thus, the intricate knowledge of the molecular biology of poliovirus may reflect those aspects of picornavirus replication strategies most closely linked with causation of clinical symptoms.

The field of viral pathogenesis is the most complex area of study in the field of virology. Viral disease is the result of an intricate relationship of an infectious agent with its host. Virtually any step in the viral life cycle can have an effect on pathogenic properties. In addition, conditions encountered within the infected host organism, e.g., host cellular factors required for particle entry (cell external factors = receptors) and/or replication (cell internal factors) frequently play a determining role in the manifestation of viral disease. The status and condition of host defenses can critically alter the susceptibility to infectious disease, and components of the immune system can actively contribute to generate clinical manifestations. Finally, individual hosts may differ regarding their susceptibility to viral disease, presenting predetermining conditions that increase or decrease the likelihood of clinical symptoms in consequence to virus infection.

The multifactorial nature of the viral pathogenic phenotype is difficult to reproduce in experimental systems amenable to scientific investigation. Experimentation in simple in vitro or tissue culture model systems, proven to be most useful in the unraveling of many aspects of picornavirus molecular biology, usually is inadequate to allow any predictions on pathogenic properties. Even experimental animal models frequently are fraught with deficiencies that render the interpretation of experimental results obtained difficult. Throughout the 1950s and 1960s, poliovirus research consumed enormous numbers of primates, which provided the only animal model at the time. Since then, the development of a rodent model for poliomyelitis in mice transgenic for the human poliovirus receptor CD155 (CD155 tg mice) (49, 77) has eliminated the need for primates in most experimental procedures. However, oral infection of CD155 tg mice has been exceedingly inefficient, excluding the crucial enteric phase of the natural history of poliomyelitis (see below) from this convenient animal model.

This review will provide a brief synopsis of the natural history of paralytic poliomyelitis. The following paragraphs will give an overview of the status of research concerning the molecular determinants of the pathogenesis of paralytic poliomyelitis.

NATURAL HISTORY OF PARALYTIC POLIOMYELITIS

Paralytic poliomyelitis is the preponderant clinical manifestation associated with poliovirus infection. The term polio- (Gr. πολιο—gray) -myelitis (Gr. μψελο—marrow) alludes to the pathology of poliovirus central nervous system (CNS) infection that shows lesions limited to the gray matter of the spinal cord (myelon). Susceptibility to poliovirus is highly selective. Damage within the CNS of affected patients or experimentally infected primates is limited to the cranial motor nerve nuclei of the brainstem, the roof nuclei of the cerebellum, and the spinal cord anterior horn (Color Plate 25B, following p. 156). The peculiar predilection of poliovirus for motor neurons gives paralytic poliomyelitis a close resemblance to degenerative disorders of the motoneuronal system, rather than viral CNS infections. Neuronal populations outside the motoneuronal system are never affected by poliovirus, in spite of immediate vicinity to the target of polioviral replication. The restrictive tropism of poliovirus for a defined cellular population within the CNS results in a highly characteristic clinical syndrome dominated by progressive flaccid paralysis. The occurrence of any other neurological signs, e.g.,

---

Matthias Gromeier ■ Department of Microbiology, Duke University Medical Center, Durham, NC 27710. *Akio Nomoto* ■ Department of Microbiology, Graduate School of Medicine, University of Tokyo, Tokyo 113-0033, Japan.

TABLE 1 Picornaviruses, their clinical manifestations, and receptor specificities

Genus	Clusters	Major associated syndromes	Receptor[a]
Enterovirus			
	A		
	Coxsackieviruses A 2, 3, 5, 7, 8, 10, 12, 14, 16	Herpangina, hand-foot-and-mouth disease, respiratory disease, meningitis, polio (CAV7)	ND
	Enterovirus 71	Hand-foot-and-mouth disease, polio	ND
	B		
	Coxsackievirus A9	(see CAV above), polio	$\alpha v \beta 3$
	Coxsackieviruses B1–6	Myocarditis, pleurodynia, meningitis, hand-foot-and-mouth disease, respiratory disease	HCAR, DAF
	Echoviruses 1–9, 11–21, 24, 27, 29–33	Meningitis, encephalitis, pleurodynia, exanthema	VLA-2 ($\alpha 2 \beta 1$) DAF (CD55)
	Enterovirus 69		ND
	C		
	Polioviruses types 1–3	Poliomyelitis	CD155
	Coxsackieviruses A 1, 11, 13, 15, 17, 18–22, 24	Common cold, infantile diarrhea	ICAM-1
	Coxsackieviruses A 24v	Acute hemorrhagic conjunctivitis	ND
	D		
	Enterovirus 70 (68)	Acute hemorrhagic conjunctivitis, polio	DAF (CD55)
	E		
	Bovine enterovirus types 1 and 2	Diarrhea (cattle)	ND
Parechovirus	Echoviruses types 22 and 23	Respiratory disease, encephalitis	ND
Rhinovirus	Major receptor group rhinoviruses (>90 types)	Common cold	ICAM-1
	Minor receptor group rhinoviruses (>10 types)	Common cold	LDL receptor
Hepatovirus	Hepatitis A virus	Hepatitis	HAVcr-1
Aphthovirus	Foot-and-mouth disease virus A12O1	Foot-and-mouth disease (cloven-footed livestock)	$\alpha v \beta 3$ Heparan sulfate
Cardiovirus	Encephalomyocarditis virus	Encephalitis, myocarditis (hoofed livestock)	VCAM-1
	Mengovirus		
	Theiler's murine encephalomyocarditis virus	Encephalomyelitis (mice)	ND
	Vilyuisk virus	Encephalitis	ND

[a]ND, not determined; HCAR, human coxsackievirus B and adenovirus receptor; DAF, decay-accelerating factor; ICAM-1, intercellular adhesion molecule 1; LDL, low-density lipoprotein; HAVcr-1, receptor for hepatitis A virus; VCAM-1, vascular cell adhesion molecule 1.

spasticity or sensory loss, indicates damage to neuronal populations other than medullary/spinal cord motor neurons and rules out the diagnosis of poliomyelitis.

Neurological symptoms are a rare complication of poliovirus infection, occurring in only 1 to 2% of infected individuals. Typically, polioviral infections are limited to a gastrointestinal stage characterized by virus replication within an unknown cellular component of the intestinal epithelium (82) and shedding of virus subsequent to ingestion of infectious particles. Poliovirus infections in the absence of neurological symptoms are usually inapparent.

Bodian (10) noted the occurrence of poliovirus particles in lymphatic organs of the alimentary tract (tonsils, Peyer's patches, deep mesenteric and cervical lymph nodes) to precede viremia. Viremia means entry of virus particles into the bloodstream with dissemination throughout the infected organism. Viremia has been demonstrated to occur after oral infection in a small proportion of human patients as well as in monkeys (9, 82) and is believed to precede neuroinvasion of poliovirus.

The mode of CNS invasion of poliovirus, a step that is a critical determining factor in the pathogenesis of paralytic poliomyelitis, remains a contentious issue. Since only a minority of infected individuals actually develop neurological symptoms, conditions determining passage of the blood-brain barrier and CNS invasion should exert critical influence on the neuropathogenesis of poliomyelitis. Evidence obtained from experimental infections in various laboratory animal species implicated poliovirus to use various routes of entry into the CNS. These include (i) retrograde axonal transport through peripheral nerves, (ii) transport across the blood-brain barrier, and (iii) transport via infected macrophages (Trojan horse mechanism).

(i) Retrograde axonal transport of poliovirus has been induced by intraneural or intramuscular inoculation of virus in primates (10, 12) and CD155 tg mice (79). Transport along peripheral nerves can be demonstrated through dissection of the nerve connecting the virus injection site with the spinal cord. Failure of paralytic symptoms to develop in the injected limb upon peripheral nerve dissection is an indication of disruption of a retrograde axonal transport route in infected animals (12, 33, 70, 79). Retrograde axonal transport has also been identified to be operational in the pathogenesis of provocation poliomyelitis (see "Conditions of the Host" below) and has been suspected to have occurred in a series of cases of iatrogenic poliomyelitis known as the "Cutter incident" (see "Conditions of the Host" below).

All incidences of retrograde axonal transport of poliovirus have been described in conjunction with predisposing risk factors (skeletal muscle trauma in provocation poliomyelitis) or experimental administration (intraneural or intramuscular inoculation) of virus. It is unclear whether entry through peripheral nerves is operational in the absence of predisposing factors and/or oral infection with poliovirus. Theories that poliovirus might enter the CNS through peripheral nerves supplying the gastrointestinal tract, the site of initial viral replication in the infected human organism, have never been confirmed.

(ii) A recent study by Yang et al. (104) investigated the rate of passive transport of poliovirus particles across the blood-brain barrier into the CNS. It was determined that crossing of the blood-brain barrier occurs independently of the cellular receptor for poliovirus, CD155. Much earlier, the presence of poliovirus particles in endothelial cells constituting the blood-brain barrier was interpreted as evidence for poliovirus entering the CNS through its vasculature (7).

Since predisposing factors are absent in the vast majority of cases of poliomyelitis and the passage of the blood-brain barrier occurs at random, the development of neurological symptoms may be a chance phenomenon. Certain conditions known to result in altered permeability of the blood-brain barrier potentially could favor poliovirus neuroinvasion and precipitate poliomyelitis (9). However, direct experimental evidence for such a mechanism is missing.

The observation that the administration of antipoliovirus antibody (passive immunization) at the stage of viremia can prevent poliomyelitis in infected primates (8) indicated a viremic state to be a necessary prelude to neuroinvasion (8, 10). At the culmination of viremia, with titers of circulating poliovirus at their highest, passage of the blood-brain barrier might be determined by the titers of infectious particles within the bloodstream.

(iii) Poliovirus has been shown to replicate within certain types of macrophages that express the human poliovirus receptor CD155 (25). Infected macrophages that shuttle across the blood-brain barrier could introduce poliovirus to the CNS, a mechanism that has been implicated as the mechanism of CNS invasion of neuropathogenic retroviruses ("Trojan horse mechanism"; described for Visna virus [75] and human immunodeficiency virus [HIV] [21]). No experimental data exist that support such a mechanism to account for the neuroinvasion of poliovirus in experimental animals or infected patients.

The pathogenesis of paralytic poliomyelitis is determined at multiple stages. The rate of extraneural replication, either in the gastrointestinal epithelium, lymphatic organs associated with the alimentary tract, or macrophages, the rate of progression toward viremia, the success of neuroinvasion, the efficiency of spread within the CNS, and the rate of intraneural replication will determine the outcome of poliovirus infection. Determinants of the pathogenesis of poliomyelitis are either of viral origin, e.g., noncoding viral sequences, structural or nonstructural viral gene products, or of host origin, e.g., distribution of the cellular receptor and host cell factors required for viral replication. The pathogenesis of poliomyelitis may also be influenced by predisposing factors present within the host at the time of infection.

This enumeration illustrates the multifactorial nature of the pathogenic mechanism of poliomyelitis that is determined by a plethora of unrelated conditions at various levels. To provide a rational account of the relative contributions of a multitude of factors toward a complex phenomenon, this chapter is subdivided into sections dealing with the main parameters of poliovirus neurological disease. Tropism, neurovirulence, and conditions of the host are discussed separately. The strict adherence to useful definitions is required to pry apart the various contributors that, cooperatively, will produce a complex neuropathological and clinical entity such as paralytic poliomyelitis.

DETERMINANTS OF THE PATHOGENESIS OF POLIOMYELITIS

Tropism

Affinity of picornaviruses for specific types of host tissues or cells is determined by the distribution of their cellular binding molecules. Tropism (derived from Gr. τροπο— turning, turning toward) is defined as the affinity of a particular virus species for a population of host cells or a specific host tissue composed of susceptible host cells. Tropism, as used in this review, indicates affinity of viral particles to a specific target independent of the result of their interaction.

Examples of misleading use of the term tropism abound in the scientific literature. Frequently, factors that determine the success of viral propagation within the infected host cell are referred to as "cell-internal determinants of tropism." This terminology is confusing, since the turning toward a specific host cell type is strictly determined by the presence of cellular factors that mediate the binding and uptake of viral particles.

By definition, cell internal determinants cannot partake in tropism, which is the result of the interaction of the viral outer shell with its cellular binding molecule.

CD155 and Poliomyelitis

Poliomyelitis provides a prime example for the determining role of receptor-virus interactions for the expression of a pathogenic phenotype. It is tempting to attribute the unusually specific clinical and histopathological features of paralytic poliomyelitis to the distribution of a critical susceptibility determinant such as a cellular receptor required for particle binding and cell entry (10, 82). Elucidating the role of the poliovirus receptor in the pathogenesis of poliomyelitis, however, has been more difficult than originally anticipated. As a result of numerous investigations of the biology of its receptor, we are beginning to understand how poliovirus's predilection for a specific cellular binding molecule may affect the pathogenesis of a peculiar neurologic disease.

The immunoglobulin superfamily molecule CD155, previously known as the human poliovirus receptor (hPVR), has been isolated as the sole cellular binding molecule conferring susceptibility to poliovirus (59). CD155 is the founding member of a growing subfamily of genes: two poliovirus receptor-related molecules (PRR1 [51], PRR2 [20]) that lack binding affinity for poliovirus have been identified in humans. Interestingly, PRR1 functions as a cellular binding molecule for α-herpesviruses (26). CD155 and its simian counterparts (Table 2) (48) have no homologues outside primates, which explains the restricted natural host range of poliovirus. Rodent relatives of hPRR1 or hPRR2, like their human counterparts, have been demonstrated to lack poliovirus-binding activity (62) (Table 2).

It was proposed that expression of CD155 might be the critical determinant directing poliovirus target tropism toward spinal cord anterior horn motor neurons (reviewed in

TABLE 2 Members of the CD155-related family of genes

Gene	Species	Gene product	Polio binding
CD155	Human	CD155α,δ	+
		CD155β,γ^a	+
hPRR1	Human	hPRR1α,δ (implied)	−
hPRR2	Human	hPRR2α,δ (implied)	−
AGMα1	Simian	sPVRα,δ	+
AGMα2	Simian	sPVRα	+
mPRR1	Murine	mPRR1 (implied)	−
mPRR2	Murine	mPRR2α,β^a	−
mTage4	Murine	mTage4	−

^{a}CD155β,γ and mPRR2β are secreted splice variants.

references 30 and 102). Support for this hypothesis is derived from the following simple considerations based on neuropathological observations in different experimental animal models of poliovirus neuropathogenicity.

Rodents ordinarily resist poliovirus infection due to the absence of CD155 (see above). However, in early attempts to generate a suitable nonprimate animal model for poliomyelitis, researchers observed that naturally occurring serotype 2 poliovirus strains are able to elicit a neurological syndrome after intracerebral inoculation into mice and rats (3). The mouse neurovirulent phenotype was later shown to map to a stretch of amino acid residues forming a protruding structure in the capsid of serotype 2 strains (64). Meanwhile, a "true" rodent model for poliomyelitis was generated when transgenic mouse strains were produced that expressed the human poliovirus receptor CD155 (CD155 tg mice) (49, 77).

Comparison of the neuropathology of poliovirus infection in wild-type mice (lacking the human poliovirus receptor) with CD155 tg mice impressively demonstrated the role of CD155 in the mediation of the specific neuropathogenic properties of poliovirus. CD155 tg mice, upon poliovirus inoculation, develop a neurological syndrome clinically and histopathologically identical to primate poliomyelitis (28, 49, 77) (Color Plate 25B, following p. 156). In sharp contrast, wild-type mice inoculated intracerebrally with serotype 2 poliovirus strains develop a nonspecific panencephalomyelitis characterized by widespread lesions throughout the entire CNS, indiscriminantly affecting all cellular components within that organ (Color Plate 25C) (31). In the spinal cord of infected wild-type mice, undamaged motor neurons had escaped infection despite close proximity to severe lesions affecting the spinal cord (Color Plate 25C, insert). Accordingly, poliovirus-infected wild-type mice developed neurological symptoms atypical for paralytic poliomyelitis (31). This experiment illustrated how expression of a cellular binding molecule can influence a clinical disease syndrome, apparently by directing viral tropism to a certain target host cell type (spinal cord anterior horn motor neurons) and excluding viral replication from others (Color Plate 25A to C).

The occurrence of classical poliomyelitis in CD155 tg mice implies that the distribution of CD155 in neural tissues of these animals must parallel that in humans (28, 49, 77). However, in contrast to humans, where oral infection leads to high levels of viral replication in the gastrointestinal tract, infection of CD155 tg mice by the oral route is exceedingly inefficient. Expression of CD155 has been suspected to be absent from the alimentary tract of CD155 tg mice (77). However, even directing CD155 expression to the gastrointestinal epithelium through the insertion of intestine-specific transcriptional control elements could not rescue gastrointestinal susceptibility of CD155 tg mice (106). These observations point toward conditions imposed by the rodent intestinal physiology to interfere with susceptibility to poliovirus. Partly due to the absence of an animal model, the relationship of receptor expression and virus replication in the alimentary tract remains unclear.

Hypotheses that ascribed poliovirus tropism for motor neurons to expression patterns of CD155 needed validation by demonstrating the distribution of CD155 in humans or transgenic mice to match susceptibility to poliovirus. The detection of CD155 polypeptides has been very difficult due to the very low abundance of these proteins in human tissues (5, 88). Most data on the distribution of CD155 in the human organism are based on Northern blot analyses of CD155-specific message in organ homogenates (49, 77). These experiments revealed the presence of CD155 mRNA in a wide variety of tissue types, most of them resistant to poliovirus infection. The interpretation of these results is problematic for various reasons. One possible explanation is that tissue homogenates are composed of a wide variety of cell types, including tissue-resident macrophages and hematogenous cell types. Rather than organ-specific cell types, macrophages known to express CD155 (25) could be the source of CD155-specific message in organ homogenates used for Northern analyses. Furthermore, it has been shown for the cellular receptor for group B coxsackieviruses, the immunoglobulin superfamily molecule CAR, that the distribution of mRNA in the human organism (95) does not necessarily match expression profiles of its translation product (40). Immunofluorescence analysis of human tissues with anti-CD155 antibodies will finally solve the conundrum.

The scarcity of CD155 polypeptides in adult human tissues suggested the possibility that expression of CD155 is regulated developmentally with highest expression levels occurring before partum. Similarity of CD155 with immunoglobulin superfamily molecules that are associated with neurogenesis in insects (32 and references therein) have prompted studies of the regulation of the CD155 gene during embryonic development in transgenic mice. CD155 promoter activity could be observed in a subset of structures determining the morphogenesis of anterior spinal cord polarity, and the differentiation of motor neurons in particular (32) (Color Plate 26, following p. 156). Activity of the CD155 promoter was highest throughout a brief period of midgestation and rapidly declined towards partum (32).

The temporospatial distribution of CD155 expression has been confirmed in human embryos, where, similar to studies in transgenic mice, expression of CD155 declined steadily after reaching its peak around midgestation. Immunohistochemical assays revealed the presence of CD155 in midgestation human embryos while the same experiment failed to detect CD155 in identical structures of the adult organism (32). The developmental expression pattern of CD155 explains the difficulties encountered when attempts were made to detect CD155 in the postnatal human CNS.

Expression of CD155 within the developing CNS matched the distribution of trans-acting factors known to participate in the regulation of the CD155 gene (87–89). Selective expression of CD155 in anatomical structures giving rise to spinal cord anterior horn motor neurons

(Color Plate 26) explains the restricted target tropism of poliovirus for this cellular component of the CNS (32).

Available evidence summarized above suggests CD155 to be the critical determinant of poliovirus target tropism for spinal cord anterior horn motor neurons. It is believed that expression of CD155 polypeptides in structures of the developing motoneuronal system persists throughout life, albeit at very low levels.

Nonpolio Enterovirus Receptors

A poliomyelitis-like neurological syndrome has been observed to occur after infections with enteroviruses other than polio (e.g., coxsackieviruses A7 and A9 [CAV7 and -9] [27, 98], enterovirus 70 [EV70] [99], enterovirus 71 [EV71] [18]). If CD155 plays a determining role in the selective motor neuron tropism of poliovirus, paralytic poliomyelitis elicited by enteroviruses other than polio is likely to depend on virus binding to this cellular receptor as well. Receptors for the neuropathogenic EV71 and CAV7 have never been identified. Cellular binding molecules identified to mediate infectivity of CAV9 (the $\alpha v \beta 3$ integrin [vitronectin receptor]) (80) and EV70 (decay-accelerating factor [DAF] [CD55]) (45) are known to be not exclusive (97).

Affinity for multiple cellular binding molecules, as seen with several nonpolio enteroviruses, complicates the analysis of the role of enteroviral receptors in the pathogenesis of poliomyelitis. The possible use of multiple receptor molecules by some enterovirus species may reflect the variability of clinical syndromes associated with infection (Table 1). In contrast to poliovirus, which is associated with paralytic poliomyelitis alone, nonpolio enteroviruses known to occasionally cause polio-like neurological complications are responsible for a variety of clinical syndromes that target multiple organ systems (Table 1). For example, EV70 and EV71, frequently identified in cases of nonpolioviral paralytic disease, are responsible for epidemics of acute hemorrhagic conjunctivitis and hand-foot-and-mouth disease, respectively (Table 1) (100, 105).

Experimental evidence for binding of any nonpolio enterovirus to CD155, a plausible explanation for their association with polio-like neurological complications, is currently missing. The close genetic kinship among neuropathogenic enteroviruses raises the possibility that nonpolioviruses acquire affinity for CD155 through adaptive changes in the coding region for their structural proteins, resulting in altered conformation of the viral capsid. This possibility and its epidemiological and evolutionary implications are discussed at length in reference 35.

A precedent for the acquisition of a changed pathogenic phenotype with altered tissue tropism occurred when CAV24, an enteroviral agent of the common cold binding to intercellular adhesion molecule 1 (ICAM-1) (Table 1), emerged as a causative agent of acute hemorrhagic conjunctivitis (CAV24 variant) (39). Hypotheses that this changed pathogenic phenotype relies on a switch in receptor affinity await confirmation. However, the striking change in tissue tropism of CAV24 toward ocular tissues is a compelling argument for altered receptor specificity.

Neurovirulence

All factors that influence the ability of a pathogenic virus to replicate within its target host cell will exert an effect on pathogenesis. It is important, therefore, to distinguish defects with a generalized effect on virus viability from those that selectively affect pathogenic properties of picornaviruses. In other words, only those virulence factors that specifically inhibit virus propagation in host cell types associated with disease manifestations should be considered important for pathogenesis. Factors causing general interference with virus viability will inevitably lead to reduced cytopathogenicity and altered pathogenic phenotypes and, thus, do not represent determinants of pathogenesis in a strict sense. Neurovirulence is defined as the potential for particle propagation in neuronal cells. Opposing tropism as an extracellular parameter of pathogenesis, neurovirulence could be viewed as an intracellular parameter determining the pathogenesis of poliomyelitis.

Research on the molecular biology of poliovirus has identified noncoding sequences as well as several gene products to specifically influence replicative efficiency in target host cells without a concomitant decrease in virus viability. Studies of the genetic basis of poliovirus neurovirulence have spearheaded research of picornavirus pathogenesis, aided by the early introduction of the live attenuated vaccine strains of poliovirus (the Sabin strains) (Fig. 1) (83). The identification of genetic markers for the neurovirulent phenotype followed several strategies: (i) sequence comparison of wild-type neurovirulent polioviruses with derivatives with attenuated neurovirulence, (ii) sequence analysis of revertant vaccine strains isolated from patients with vaccine-associated paralytic poliomyelitis (VAPP), and (iii) comparative assessment of growth characteristics in cell lines representing the target host cell type (neuronal cells).

Comparison of the Sabin strains with their virulent progenitors revealed multiple candidate sequences to influence the neurovirulent phenotype. The apparent multifactorial character of the genetic basis of neurovirulence, a common theme in the study of viral pathogenesis, hampered its elucidation. Preferred experimental approaches in the study of poliovirus neurovirulence, for example, genetic mix-and-matching of attenuated with neurovirulent strains, were inappropriate to address the complexity of the neuropathogenic phenotype. Isolation of individual attenuating loci frequently failed to reveal complementary contributions to the virulent phenotype exerted by separate loci within a single or distant coding regions of the viral genome.

The following sections will discuss experimental evidence for the genetic basis of neurovirulence in the 5' nontranslated region (5' NTR) and the coding regions for the structural and nonstructural proteins of poliovirus.

Determinants of Poliovirus Neurovirulence: the 5' NTR

A variety of observations have implicated noncoding sequences located within the poliovirus 5' NTR in the determination of neuropathogenic properties (reviewed in reference 103). Involvement of the internal ribosomal entry site (IRES) in pathogenesis is not surprising, given the prominent role of this cis-acting genetic element in the virus life cycle, exerting critical functions for translational control (44, 74) and, probably, genome replication (13).

The most reliable evidence for participation of IRES sequence in the determination of a pathogenic phenotype stems from sequence analyses of live attenuated vaccine strains and their neurovirulent revertants isolated from patients with VAPP. These studies revealed point mutations mapping to a confined region of stem-loop domain V in the IRES of PV3(Sabin) to be associated with a reversion to neurovirulence in VAPP patients (Fig. 1) (22). Accordingly, wild-type PV(3) strains engineered to carry the

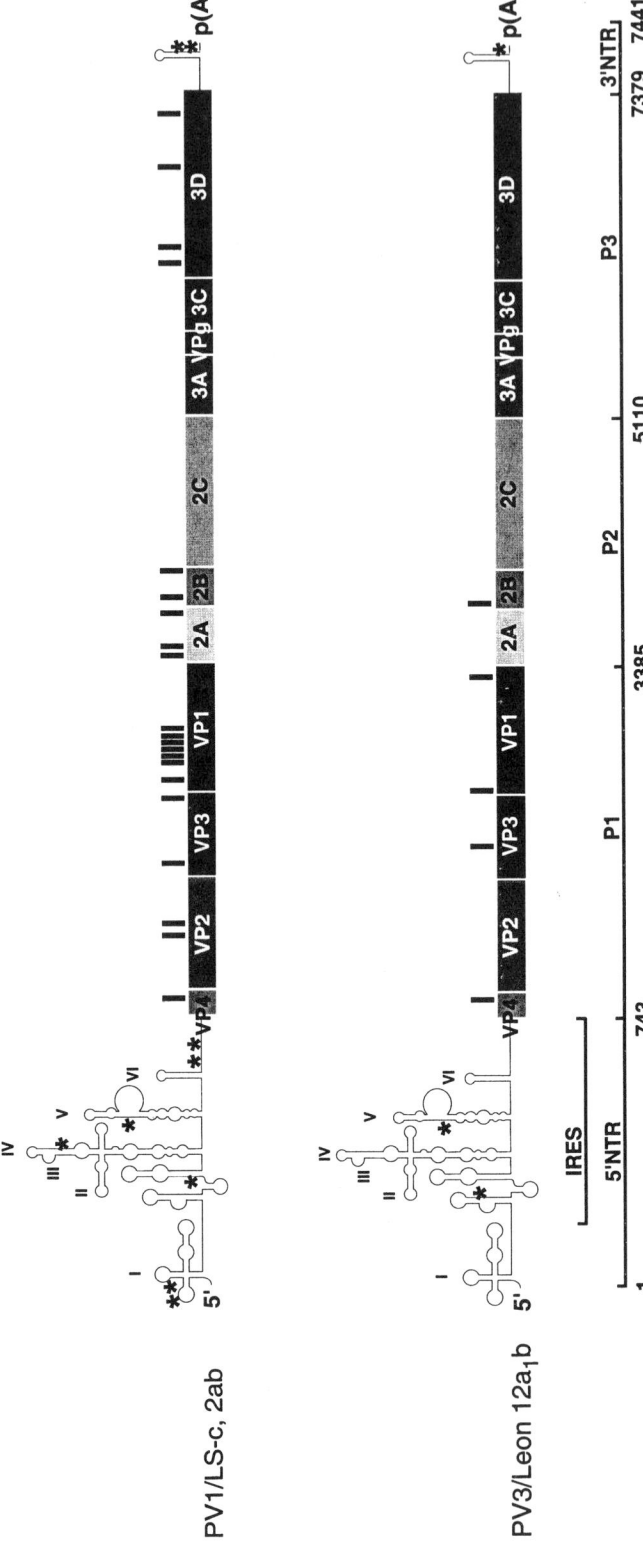

FIGURE 1 Attenuating mutations within the serotype 1 (PV1/LS-c, 2ab) and 3 (PV3/Leon 12a₁b) poliovirus strains of Sabin (83). The general organization of the poliovirus genome is shown below. The positions of the IRES and individual stem-loop domains are indicated by roman numerals atop. Sequence divergence in noncoding regions is indicated by asterisks, mutations in coding regions are shown as vertical bars. PV2(Sabin) is a naturally occurring attenuated strain whose neurovirulent ancestor is not known. PV1(S) is characterized by a large number of mutations within the coding region P1 for the capsid proteins. Both PV1(S) and PV3(S) feature attenuating mutations within stem-loop V of the IRES.

PV3(S) mutation at position 472 in the IRES (Fig. 1) exhibited the neurovirulent phenotype in experimental animals (101).

Since both PV1(S) and PV2(S) feature point mutations in the vicinity of nucleotide 472 of PV3(S) (Fig. 1), a similar role of nucleotide 480 in PV1(S) (46) and nucleotide 481 in PV2(S) (55) has been proposed. Mix-and-match genetics using PV1(S) and its neurovirulent PV1(M) yielded conflicting evidence. Experiments in tissue-cultured cell lines (1), cell extracts (37), and nonprimates (46) clearly implicated the 5' NTR in the attenuation phenotype of PV1(S). Experimental results that challenged this view, as reported by McGoldrick et al. (57), are difficult to reconcile with the extensive evidence for a role of IRES sequences in the neurovirulent phenotype.

The attenuation phenotype of the Sabin strains is evident through impaired growth kinetics in tissue-cultured cell lines of neuronal origin (1, 50). IRES sequences have been shown to be, at least partially, responsible for this cell type-specific growth defect (37, 38). These studies confirmed a neuron-specific functional deficit to be associated with putative attenuating mutations within stem-loop domain V of the poliovirus IRES (37, 38). Mutations within stem-loop domain V may cause destabilization of secondary RNA structure (17, 54, 86). More recent work implicated higher-order structures formed by dual stem-loops V and VI to be influenced by attenuating sequences within IRES stem-loop domain V (29, 37).

Definitive proof for a contribution of IRES sequences to the neurovirulent phenotype stems from IRES recombination studies where rhinoviral IRES sequences have been inserted into a poliovirus backbone (28, 29). Polioviruses whose cognate IRES had been exchanged with its counterpart from human rhinovirus type 2 (HRV2) had lost their ability to propagate in cells of neuronal origin while retaining unabated replicative efficiency within nonneuronal primate cell lines (28). Consequently, polio/rhinovirus IRES recombinants were highly attenuated in CD155 tg mice (28) and nonhuman primates (29). In contrast to the Sabin strains, where attenuation is based on a number of mutations scattered throughout the genome, reduced neurovirulence of polio/rhinovirus IRES chimeras is based on IRES sequences alone (28).

Although sufficient evidence has been accumulated to postulate a contribution of IRES-mediated cell type specificity toward poliovirus neurovirulence, the basic mechanism of tissue-specific IRES function remains to be determined. Possible scenarios include effects of attenuating mutations on higher-order RNA structure that may affect interaction with essential *trans*-activating eukaryotic factors or promote the inhibitory effect of specific neuronal factors. Tissue-specific IRES function is likely to be critically involved also in the pathogenesis of picornaviral disease other than poliomyelitis (e.g., coxsackievirus myocarditis [reviewed in reference 16], cardioviral neuropathogenicity in rodents [76], hepatitis A [84]).

Virulence Factors Determined by Viral Structural Polypeptides

Polypeptides that form the outer shell of enveloped viruses are known to be important determinants of pathogenic features of a wide variety of human pathogenic viruses (e.g., alphaviruses [52], flaviviruses [47], paramyxoviruses [85], murine retroviruses [19], coronaviruses [23], or reoviruses [90]). Picornaviruses exemplify that the capsid of nonenveloped virus species can fulfill a similar role. Participation of the particle outer structures in the determination of pathogenic properties is not surprising, given that these structures determine important parameters influencing the pathogenic phenotype (e.g., spread within the infected host, particle stability, interaction with the cellular receptor, uncoating and conformational rearrangements, immune recognition, or particle assembly). Potent determinants of pathogenic properties have been mapped to the capsid of poliovirus.

Similar to genetic determinants of neurovirulence mapping to the 5' NTR, a role of the capsid in poliovirus neuropathogenicity has been proposed upon sequence comparison of the Sabin strains with their wild-type ancestors. All three Sabin serotypes feature attenuating mutations that are located within the coding region for the structural proteins (71, 79, 101) (Fig. 1). Studies using mix-and-match genetic recombination of capsid regions of PV1(S) with the neurovirulent PV1(M) attributed different levels of importance to the attenuating functions of individual capsid mutations (14, 46, 71). Prediction of the role of individual attenuating mutations mapping to the coding region for the structural proteins of PV1(S) is particularly difficult, due to the large number of such mutations and the possibility of cooperative effects exerted by distant loci. However, it has been shown conclusively in experimental animal studies in CD155 tg mice and nonhuman primates that the entire capsid of PV1(S) is a potent determinant of the attenuation phenotype (28, 71).

Location of capsid mutations in areas known to interact with CD155 (63) or protomer interfaces (24, 61) suggests attenuation to occur through interference with receptor binding (14) or assembly (53), respectively. Mutations that affect virus-receptor interactions would be likely to influence tropism. However, comparative studies of the kinetics of poliovirus receptor binding suggested that, while the viral capsid carries critical determinants of pathogenesis, it is unlikely to interfere with receptor affinity itself (6).

The exact role of capsid mutations in the determination of attenuation of neurovirulence remains to be elucidated. Reduced capsid stability is likely to affect crucial parameters of neuropathogenicity such as neuroinvasion or spread within the CNS. Intracerebral infection of CD155 tg mice is more efficient than intravenous administration of poliovirus, due to the need for passage of the blood-brain barrier in the latter (49, 77). This disparity is much more pronounced in wild-type viruses carrying the capsid of PV1(S), indicating the decreased ability of the Sabin strains to invade the CNS to be caused by attenuating capsid mutations (28). Important steps of the natural history of poliomyelitis, most notably those that lie in between initial replication within the gastrointestinal tract and invasion of the CNS, cannot be reproduced in experimental animal models available at this time. It is therefore impossible to assess the exact role of the viral capsid in the neuroinvasion process.

Determinants of Poliovirus Neurovirulence: the Nonstructural Proteins

A role for nonstructural gene products in the determination of poliovirus neurovirulence has been proposed since it was realized that PV1(S) contains a number of point mutations mapping to the RNA-dependent RNA polymerase $3D^{pol}$ (69). Mutations within the open reading frame of $3D^{pol}$ have been implicated in the determination of the temperature-sensitive (*ts*) phenotype of PV1(S) after serial passages of virus at supraoptimal temperature (17), growth studies in tissue culture (71, 94), and in an in vitro model of 3D^{pol} function (96). A mechanism that could account for temperature sensitivity, and possibly attenuation of PV1(S), has been proposed following the description of protein priming in RNA replication of picornaviruses (72). It was shown that the priming reaction, involving 3D^{pol}, the genome-linked protein VPg (serving as a protein primer), and RNA template, is rendered temperature sensitive through a mutation at nucleotide 6203 in PV1(S) (72, 73).

Mix-and-match genetics aimed to demonstrate a link between the ts phenotype and attenuation of neurovirulence yielded conflicting results (14, 71, 94). It is not known by which mechanism the ts phenotype may relate to the neurovirulent phenotype but in vitro markers of viral growth, such as ts, have been demonstrated to be of little use in the prediction of neurovirulent properties (71). A prominent role of 3D^{pol} in the determination of the attenuation of neuropathogenicity is unlikely, since the serotype 2 and 3 Sabin strains do not contain any mutations within the coding region for 3D^{pol}.

The Composite Nature of the Neurovirulent Phenotype: Why the Sabin Strains Are Safe

The difficult task of poliovirus replicating within the alimentary tract to reach its target within the CNS implies that poliovirus neuropathogenicity can be influenced at multiple stages through various mechanisms. Extraneural determinants of neuropathogenicity, such as invasion of or spread within the CNS, combine with intraneural factors, such as IRES-mediated cell type specificity or the efficiency of genome replication. Without any doubt, the impeccable safety record of the Sabin strains is due to interference with neuropathogenicity simultaneously at various levels (71). Reduced replication rates within the gastrointestinal tract, a potentially reduced neuroinvasion rate, decreased spread within the CNS, and impaired intraneural replication through cell type-specific IRES defects act in concert to emasculate a dangerous neuropathogen.

The Sabin strains are known to revert to a neurovirulent phenotype, even during intestinal replication after oral administration to vaccinees (reviewed in reference 61). Despite their genetic instability, the combined deleterious effect of multiple genetic determinants of attenuation proved to be sufficient to prevent neurological complications in millions of immunized children with a minimal rate of complicating VAPP.

The avid search for single determinants of the attenuation phenotype has met with little success and resulted in a flurry of contradicting reports. The key to the understanding of the neurovirulent phenotype and its attenuation, as Sabin himself reminded molecular biologists early on (see reference 103), lies within the multitude of unrelated determinants affecting the complex process of the pathogenesis of paralytic poliomyelitis on various levels.

Conditions of the Host

It has remained a mystery why neurologic symptoms arising from poliovirus infection only affect a minor proportion of infected individuals. Considering the natural history of poliomyelitis and how difficult it is for virus replicating within the gastrointestinal tract to reach the CNS, it appears tempting to attribute the low rate of neuroinvasion to the inaccessibility of the CNS to enteric viruses. Since the route of poliovirus from the gastrointestinal tract into the CNS has not been determined with certainty, it is unknown exactly how many particles are required to cross the blood-brain barrier to produce clinically overt poliomyelitis and which conditions favor invasion of the CNS.

If we assume that the difficult passage into the CNS largely is responsible for the low incidence of polio among infected individuals, then any condition that would increase the rate of poliovirus entry into the CNS should be considered a risk factor for poliomyelitis. At the height of epidemic poliomyelitis, a frantic search began to identify those factors that may predispose the unfortunate 1 to 2% of infected children likely to develop neurological complications of poliovirus infection. This search has identified a multitude of culprits that might favor neuroinvasion of poliovirus and increase the likelihood of poliomyelitis to occur. The most persistent of these was the popular belief that trivial muscle injury might increase the risk of paralytic poliomyelitis. The commonsense wisdom of concerned parents preceded scientific validation of a phenomenon that was later termed "provocation poliomyelitis." Epidemiological (56, 92) and experimental (9, 10) support for the concept of provocation poliomyelitis followed, and a pathogenic mechanism has been deciphered recently (33, 35). A similar pathogenic mechanism probably has been operational in the pathogenesis of an accumulation of cases of iatrogenic poliomyelitis following administration of improperly prepared Salk poliovirus vaccine (the "Cutter incident") (65–67).

Provocation Poliomyelitis

Provocation poliomyelitis is the term used to describe the phenomenon of increased risk to develop neurological complications due to trivial skeletal muscle injury incurred at the time of poliovirus infection. The elucidation of the pathogenic mechanism of provocation poliomyelitis (33) provides an excellent example of how a specific situation present within the susceptible host at the time of infection can influence pathogenicity.

In the prevaccine era, anecdotal reports had linked the occurrence of paralytic poliomyelitis with physical exertion or trauma incurred at the time of infection. Probably the best known case of polio following trivial skeletal muscle damage was that of Sir Walter Scott, who is said to have suffered from poliomyelitis induced by a fall. These accounts inspired the popular belief that, during polio epidemics, abstinence from physical activity could protect against poliomyelitis. Occasionally, municipal authorities in communities affected by poliovirus epidemics responded by suspending physical education in schools.

The earliest recorded systematic observations describing an association of physical trauma with the neurological complications of poliovirus infection date back to the last century (43). The concept of provocation polio was conceived when epidemiological observations confirmed a heightened incidence of paralytic polio among infant recipients of diphtheria/tetanus/pertussis vaccine, administered by intramuscular inoculation (56). This study was followed by a flurry of similar reports linking the occurrence of paralytic polio to administration of intramuscular injections or strenuous exercise (2, 15, 36, 41, 81, 93). Much later, a similar association accounted for an accumulation of cases of vaccine-related poliomyelitis in children in Romania who had been treated with multiple intramuscular injections at the time of administration of live attenuated poliovirus vaccine (92).

The most reliable accounts of the effect of skeletal muscle injury on the risk to develop polio were obtained from the analysis of large numbers of individuals who received similar forms of trauma, e.g., that stemming from intramuscular administration of vaccines. The effect of less reproducible forms of trauma, for example, strenuous exercise, is more difficult to assess statistically. It is conceivable, however, that a much larger proportion of cases of paralytic poliomyelitis than now assumed can be attributed to favorable conditions produced by skeletal muscle injury.

The clinical hallmark of provocation polio is a striking localization of initial paralytic symptoms to the site where intramuscular inoculation had been administered. The "localization effect" of intramuscular injections (10, 11) directs the site of onset of paralysis to the injected limb and provides clues toward the possible pathogenic mechanism of provocation poliomyelitis (see below).

A number of explanations have been discussed for the increased risk to develop polio associated with intramuscular injections. Contamination of injection supplies or prophylactic agents was excluded as a possible source of poliovirus. Proposed hypotheses centered around two contradicting assumptions: (i) a central effect of skeletal muscle injury and (ii) a peripheral effect of skeletal muscle injury. It was argued that changes in skeletal muscle tissue, induced either by strenuous exercise or trivial trauma, could be reflected by localized alterations in the corresponding areas of the CNS (10, 11, 42). These changes could then either "activate" virus already present within the CNS (42) or favor passage of the blood-brain barrier into the CNS (9, 11).

Although the "central" theory seemed to corroborate analyses of the dissemination of virus and the incubation period of neurological symptoms, the exact nature of the proposed alterations in the CNS has never been determined. Proposals that skeletal muscle injury might induce localized changes in vascular permeability in corresponding segments of the spinal cord have never been substantiated experimentally.

"Peripheral" explanations included those that favored activity of pharmaceutical agents administered via the intramuscular route versus mechanical factors implicating tissue changes induced by trauma or exercise. In later studies, it has been clearly shown that multiple intramuscular injections increase the likelihood of poliomyelitis after oral immunization, irrespective of the nature of the injected agent (92). Localized damage to muscular tissue has been suggested to result in inflammatory changes that might favor intramuscular virus replication or otherwise increase local supply of poliovirus (33, 56). Elevated titers of infectious poliovirus present in the immediate vicinity of peripheral nerve endings that were disrupted by trauma might induce entry into peripheral nerve and subsequent retrograde axonal transport toward the CNS.

The pathogenic mechanism of provocation poliomyelitis was deciphered only very recently through experimental infections of CD155 tg mice that had been treated to mimic the conditions of provocation polio. The hallmark clinical sign of provocation polio, the localization phenomenon, can be reproduced in viremic CD155 tg mice (33) that were treated with multiple intramuscular inoculations (Fig. 2). In animals thus treated (group II in Fig. 2), sciatic nerve dissection prevented the localization phenomenon

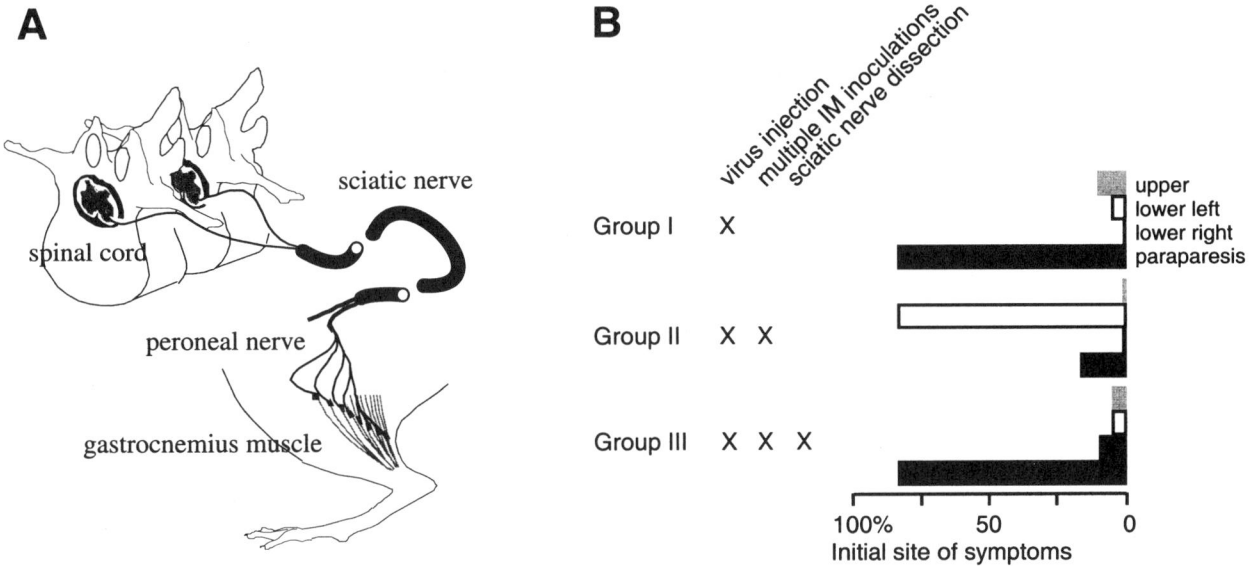

FIGURE 2 The pathogenic mechanism of provocation poliomyelitis. (A) Anatomical representation of the sciatic nerve dissection procedure. Proximal sciatic nerve dissection severs the connection between the gastrocnemius muscle and the spinal cord by interrupting the supplying peripheral nerve. This blocks the retrograde axonal transport route along the peroneal and sciatic nerves into the CNS. (B) The "localization effect" describes the salient clinical feature of provocation poliomyelitis: localization of initial symptoms of paralysis to the injected limb. CD155 tg mice that are infected with poliovirus by the intravenous route develop paraparesis (simultaneous weakness in both lower extremities) at the onset of clinically overt disease (group I). Trivial skeletal muscle trauma in the form of multiple intramuscular (IM) injections diverts initial neurological symptoms to the lower left extremity, where multiple injections had been administered (group II). Dissection of the sciatic nerve abolishes the localization effect, with >70% of infected animals developing initial paraparesis.

characteristic of provocation poliomyelitis (group III in Fig. 2). In addition, the precipitation of paralytic symptoms and accelerated neuroinvasion of poliovirus associated with provocation polio elicited through intramuscular injections in CD155 tg mice also could be reversed by sciatic nerve dissection (33). The sciatic nerve connects the secondary (spinal) motor neuron with its target organ, skeletal muscle in the periphery (Fig. 2). The prevention of clinical signs of provocation polio by severing the connection of injured skeletal muscle with the spinal cord implicates retrograde axonal transport along peripheral nerves to account for provocation poliomyelitis.

Retrograde axonal transport induced by skeletal muscle injury explains the localization phenomenon, because virus entering the CNS through peripheral nerves would destroy those motor neutrons that provide the connection of injured muscle to the spinal cord first. The opening of an alternative route of neuroinvasion may explain the increased incidence of paralytic polio among recipients of trivial skeletal muscle injury. Crossing of the blood-brain barrier as it has been described by Yang et al. (104) can be circumvented by accelerated transport along peripheral nerves. Retrograde axonal transport has been induced in experimental animals by intramuscular (79) or intraneural (12) inoculation of virus before. Experimental evidence from animal studies of provocation poliomyelitis demonstrates that retrograde axonal transport can also be induced by trivial skeletal muscle injury in the presence of viremia (33).

Several mechanisms may be activated by intramuscular injections to promote poliovirus retrograde axonal transport. Upregulation of the expression of the poliovirus receptor CD155 in nerve endings upon peripheral nerve trauma may favor virus uptake. Immunoglobulin superfamily molecules with expression patterns during embryonic development of the CNS are known to be upregulated upon peripheral nerve or spinal cord damage (68, 91). Similarly, upregulation of expression of CD155 in myocytes or macrophages in response to muscle injury may aid local virus replication in skeletal muscle tissue. Elevated titers of virus around the injection site would increase the probability of virus entering peripheral nerves. Physical disruption of peripheral nerves itself may provide the necessary conditions for uptake of poliovirus.

The Cutter Incident

The concept of provocation poliomyelitis, increasing the risk of neurological disease through diversion of the route of neuroinvasion, was confirmed by a tragic series of cases of iatrogenic poliomyelitis. The "Cutter incident" occurred after improperly treated inactivated ("killed") poliovirus vaccine was administered to children. Intramuscular administration to infants of the partially active virus preparation resulted in hundreds of cases of paralytic poliomyelitis. The Cutter incident is the largest and most thoroughly investigated case of adverse reaction to vaccine administration (65).

The Cutter incident features elements implicated in the pathogenesis of provocation poliomyelitis. Children received intramuscular injections that, inadvertently, contained live poliovirus (65–67). Not unexpected, a prominent clinical observation among victims of the Cutter incident was the localization effect originally described with provocation polio (66, 67). Intramuscular inoculation of poliovirus, like in CD155 tg mice (79), was sufficient to divert the "natural" route of neuroinvasion toward retrograde axonal transport.

SUMMARY

Poliovirus, with its uniquely specific pathogenic profile, offers a unique opportunity to understand the relationship between the properties of an infectious agent and its propensity to cause disease. The remarkably limited target tropism of poliovirus for a minute group of inaccessible specialized neurons is produced by a surprising abundance of factors and influences.

We attempted to highlight how binding affinity for a developmentally regulated cell adhesion molecule in the human CNS, cell type-specific IRES function, viral capsid conformation, and physiological state of the infected host cooperatively produce a characteristic neurological condition.

Excellent studies in nonhuman primates in the prevaccine era and recent progress through the advent of genetic engineering and transgenic animal models for human disease have afforded us detailed insight into the pathogenic mechanism of paralytic poliomyelitis. With the global eradication of paralytic poliomyelitis through effective prevention measures imminent, we are beginning to understand the mechanisms of a disease that terrified the world just half a century ago.

REFERENCES

1. **Agol, V. I., S. G. Drozdov, T. A. Ivannikova, M. S. Kolesnikova, M. B. Korolev, and E. A. Tolskaya.** 1989. Restricted growth of attenuated poliovirus strains in cultured cells of a human neuroblastoma. *J. Virol.* **63:**4034–4038.
2. **Anderson, G., and A. Skaar.** 1951. Poliomyelitis occurring after antigen injections. *Pediatrics* **7:**741–759.
3. **Armstrong, C.** 1939. The experimental transmission of poliomyelitis to the eastern cotton rat, *Sigmodon hispidus hispidus*. *Public Health Rep.* **54:**1719–1721.
4. **Bergelson, J. M., J. A. Cunningham, G. Droguett, E. A. Kurt-Jones, A. Krithivas, J. S. Hong, M. S. Horwitz, R. L. Crowell, and R. W. Finberg.** 1997. Isolation of a common receptor for coxsackie B viruses and adenoviruses 2 and 5. *Science* **275:**1320–1323.
5. **Bernhardt, G., J. A. Bibb, J. Bradley, and E. Wimmer.** 1994. Molecular characterization of the cellular receptor for poliovirus. *Virology* **199:**105–113.
6. **Bibb, J. A., G. Witherell, G. Bernhardt, and E. Wimmer.** 1994. Interaction of poliovirus with its cell surface binding site. *Virology* **201:**107–115.
7. **Blinzinger, K., J. Simon, D. Magrath, and L. Boulger.** 1969. Poliovirus crystals within the endoplasmic reticulum of endothelial and mononuclear cells in the monkey spinal cord. *Science* **163:**1336–1337.
8. **Bodian, D.** 1953. Experimental studies on passive immunization against poliomyelitis. III. Passive-active immunization and pathogenesis after virus feeding in chimpanzees. *Am. J. Hyg.* **58:**81–92.
9. **Bodian, D.** 1954. Viraemia in experimental poliomyelitis. II. Viraemia and the mechanism of the "provoking" effect of injections or trauma. *Am. J. Hyg.* **60:**358–370.
10. **Bodian, D.** 1955. Emerging concept of poliomyelitis infection. *Science* **122:**105–108.
11. **Bodian, D.** 1955. Viremia, invasiveness and the influence of injections. *Ann. N.Y. Acad. Sci.* **61:**877–882.
12. **Bodian, D., and H. A. Howe.** 1941. Experimental studies of intraneural spread of poliomyelitis virus. *Bull. Johns Hopkins Hosp.* **68:**248–267.

13. Borman, A. M., F. G. Deliat, and K. M. Kean. 1994. Sequences within the poliovirus internal ribosome entry segment control viral RNA synthesis. *EMBO J.* **13:**3149–3157.
14. Bouchard, M. J., D.-H. Lam, and V. R. Racaniello. 1995. Determinants of attenuation and temperature sensitivity in the type 1 poliovirus Sabin vaccine. *J. Virol.* **69:**4972–4978.
15. Bradford Hill, A., and J. Knowelden. 1950. Inoculation and poliomyelitis. *Br. Med. J.* **II:**1–6.
16. Chapman, N. M., A. I. Ramsingh, and S. Tracy. 1997. Genetics of coxsackievirus virulence. *Curr. Top. Microbiol. Immunol.* **223:**227–258.
17. Christodoulou, C., F. Colbere-Garapin, A. Macadam, L. F. Taffs, S. Marsden, P. Minor, and F. Horaud. 1990. Mapping of mutations associated with neurovirulence in monkeys infected with Sabin 1 poliovirus revertants selected at high temperature. *J. Virol.* **64:**4922–4929.
18. Chumakov, M., M. Voroshilova, L. Shindarov, I. Lavrova, L. Gracheva, G. Koroleva, S. Vasilenko, I. Brodvarova, M. Nikolova, S. Gyurova, M. Gacheva, G. Mitov, N. Ninov, E. Tsylka, I. Robinson, M. Frolova, V. Bashkirtsev, L. Martiyanova, and V. Rodin. 1979. Enterovirus 71 isolated from cases of epidemic poliomyelitis-like disease in Bulgaria. *Arch. Virol.* **60:**329–340.
19. DesGroseillers, L., M. Barette, and P. Jolicoeur. 1984. Physical mapping of the paralysis-inducing determinant of a wild mouse ectropic neurotropic virus. *J. Virol.* **52:**356–363.
20. Eberle, F., P. Dubreuil, M. G. Mattei, E. Devilard, and M. Lopez. 1995. The human PRR21 gene, related to the human poliovirus receptor gene (PVR), is the true homolog of the murine MPH gene. *Gene* **4:**267–272.
21. Eilbott, D. J., N. Peress, H. Burger, D. LaNeve, J. Orenstein, H. E. Gendelman, R. Seidman, and B. Weiser. 1989. Human immunodeficiency virus expression and replication in macrophages in the spinal cords of AIDS patients with myelopathy. *Proc. Natl. Acad. Sci. USA* **86:**3337–3341.
22. Evans, D. M. A., G. Dunn, P. D. Minor, G. C. Schild, A. J. Cann, and J. Almond. 1985. Increased neurovirulence associated with a single nucleotide change in a noncoding region of the Sabin type 3 poliovaccine genome. *Nature* **314:**548–550.
23. Fazakerley, J. K., S. E. Parker, F. Bloom, and M. J. Buchmeier. 1992. The V5A13.1 envelope glycoprotein deletion mutant of mouse hepatitis virus type 4 is neuroattenuated by its reduced rate of spread in the central nervous system. *Virology* **187:**178–188.
24. Filman, D. J., R. Syed, M. Chow, A. J. Macadam, P. D. Minor, and J. M. Hogle. 1989. Structural factors that control conformational transitions and serotype specificity in type 3 poliovirus. *EMBO J.* **8:**1567–1679.
25. Freistadt, M. S., H. B. Fleit, and E. Wimmer. 1993. Poliovirus receptor on human blood cells: a possible extraneural site of poliovirus replication. *Virology* **195:**798–803.
26. Geraghty, R. J., C. Krummenacher, G. H. Cohen, R. J. Eisenberg, and P. G. Spear. 1998. Entry of alphaherpesviruses mediated by poliovirus receptor-related protein 1 and poliovirus receptor. *Science* **280:**1618–1620.
27. Grist, N. R., and E. J. Bell. 1970. Enteroviral etiology of the paralytic poliomyelitis syndrome. *Arch. Environ. Health* **21:**382–387.
28. Gromeier, M., L. Alexander, and E. Wimmer. 1996. Internal ribosomal entry site substitution eliminates neurovirulence in intergeneric poliovirus recombinants. *Proc. Natl. Acad. Sci. USA* **93:**2370–2375.
29. Gromeier, M., B. Bossert, M. Arita, A. Nomoto, and E. Wimmer. 1999. Dual stem loops within the poliovirus internal ribosomal entry site control neurovirulence. *J. Virol.* **73:**958–964.
30. Gromeier, M., H. H. Lu, G. Bernhardt, J. J. Harber, J. A. Bibb, and E. Wimmer. 1995. The human poliovirus receptor. Receptor-virus interaction and parameters of disease specificity. *Ann. N. Y. Acad. Sci.* **753:**19–36.
31. Gromeier, M., H. H. Lu, and E. Wimmer. 1995. Mouse-neurovirulent poliovirus strains cause damage in the central nervous system distinct from poliomyelitis. *Microb. Pathog.* **18:**253–267.
32. Gromeier, M., D. Solecki, D. Patel, and E. Wimmer. Expression of the human poliovirus receptor/CD155 gene during development of the central nervous system: implications for the pathogenesis of poliomyelitis. *Virology* **273:**248–257.
33. Gromeier, M., and E. Wimmer. 1998. Mechanism of injury-provoked poliomyelitis. *J. Virol.* **72:**5056–5060.
34. Gromeier, M., and E. Wimmer. 1999. The relation of prophylactic inoculations to the onset of poliomyelitis. *Rev. Med. Virol.* **9:**219–226.
35. Gromeier, M., E. Wimmer, and A. E. Gorbalenya. 1999. Genetics, pathogenesis and evolution of picornaviruses, p. 287–345. *In* E. Domingo, R. Webster, and J. Holland (ed.), *Origin and Evolution of Viruses*. Academic Press, London, United Kingdom.
36. Guyer, B., A. Bison, J. Gold, M. Brigaud, and M. Aymard. 1980. Infections and paralytic poliomyelitis in tropical Africa. *Bull. WHO* **58:**285–291.
37. Haller, A. A., and B. L. Semler. 1995. Stem-loop structure synergy in binding cellular proteins to the 5' noncoding region of poliovirus RNA. *Virology* **206:**923–934.
38. Haller, A. A., S. R. Stewart, and B. L. Semler. 1996. Attenuation stem-loop lesions in the 5' noncoding region of poliovirus RNA: neuronal cell-specific translation defects. *J. Virol.* **70:**1467–1474.
39. Higgins, P. G., and T. E. Chapman. 1977. Coxsackievirus A24 and acute haemorrhagic conjunctivitis in Sri Lanka. *Lancet* **1:**361.
40. Honda, T., H. Saitoh, M. Masuko, T. Katagiri-Abe, K. Tominaga, I. Kozakai, K. Kobayashi, T. Kumanishi, Y. G. Watanabe, S. Odani, and R. Kuwano. 2000. The coxsackievirus-adenovirus receptor protein as a cell adhesion molecule in the developing mouse brain. *Mol. Brain Res.* **77:**19–28.
41. Horstmann, D. M. 1950. Acute poliomyelitis: relation of physical activity at the time of onset to the course of disease. *JAMA* **142:**236–241.
42. Horstmann, D. M., and J. R. Paul. 1947. The incubation period in human poliomyelitis and its implications. *JAMA* **135:**11–14.
43. Jacobi, M. P. 1886. Infantile spinal paralysis, p. 1113–1164. *In* W. Pepper (ed.), *A System of Medicine by American Authors*, vol. 5.
44. Jang, S. K., H. G. Kraeusslich, M. J. H. Nicklin, G. M. Duke, A. C. Palmenberg, and E. Wimmer. 1988. A segment of the 5' non-translated region of encephalomyocarditis virus RNA directs internal entry of ribosomes during in vitro translation. *J. Virol.* **62:**2636–2643.
45. Karnauchow, T. M., D. L. Tolson, B. A. Harrison, E. Altman, D. M. Lublin, and K. Dimock. 1996. The HeLa cell receptor for enterovirus 70 is decay-accelerating factor (CD55). *J. Virol.* **70:**5143–5152.
46. Kawamura, N., M. Kohara, S. Abe, T. Komatsu, K. Tago, M. Arita, and A. Nomoto. 1989. Determinants in the 5' noncoding region of poliovirus Sabin 1 RNA that influence the attenuation phenotype. *J. Virol.* **63:**1302–1309.
47. Kawano, H., V. Rostapshov, L. Rosen, and C. J. Lai. 1993. Genetic determinants of dengue type 4 virus neurovirulence for mice. *J. Virol.* **67:**6567–6575.

48. Koike, S., I. Ise, Y. Sato, H. Yonekawa, O. Gotoh, and A. Nomoto. 1992. A second gene for the African green monkey poliovirus receptor that has no putative NM-glycosylation site in the functional N-terminal immunoglobulin-like domain. *J. Virol.* **66:**7059–7066.
49. Koike, S., S. Taya, T. Kurata, S. Abe, I. Ise, H. Yonekawa, and A. Nomoto. 1991. Transgenic mice susceptible to poliovirus. *Proc. Natl. Acad. Sci. USA* **88:**951–955.
50. La Monica, N., and V. R. Racaniello. 1989. Differences in replication of attenuated and neurovirulent poliovirus in human neuroblastoma cell lines SH-SY5Y. *J. Virol.* **63:**2357–2360.
51. Lopez, M., F. Eberle, M. G. Mattei, J. Gaert, G. Birg, F. Bardin, C. Maroc, and P. Dubreuil. 1995. Complementary DNA characterization and chromosomal localization of a human gene related to the poliovirus receptor-encoding gene. *Gene* **3:**261–265.
52. Lustig, S., A. Jackson, C. S. Hahn, D. E. Griffin, E. G. Strauss, and J. H. Strauss. 1988. Molecular basis of Sindbis virus neurovirulence in mice. *J. Virol.* **62:**2329–2336.
53. Macadam, A. J., G. Ferguson, C. Arnold, and P. D. Minor. 1991. An assembly defect as a result of an attenuating mutation in the capsid proteins of the poliovirus type 3 vaccine strain. *J. Virol.* **65:**5225–5231.
54. Macadam, A. J., G. Ferguson, J. Burlison, D. Stone, R. Skuce, J. W. Almond, and P. D. Minor. 1992. Correlation of RNA secondary structure and attenuation of Sabin vaccine strains of poliovirus in tissue culture. *Virology* **189:**415–422.
55. Macadam, A. J., S. R. Pollard, G. Ferguson, G. Dunn, R. Skuce, J. W. Almond, and P. D. Minor. 1991. The 5′ non-coding region of the type 2 poliovirus vaccine strain contains determinants of attenuation and temperature sensitivity. *Virology* **181:**451–458.
56. McCloskey, B. P. 1950. The relation of prophylactic inoculations to the onset of poliomyelitis. *Lancet* **i:**659–663.
57. McGoldrick, A., A. J. Macadam, G. Dunn, W. Rowe, J. Burlison, P. D. Minor, J. Meredith, D. J. Evans, and J. W. Almond. 1995. Role of mutations G-480 and C-6203 in the attenuation phenotype of Sabin type 1 poliovirus. *J. Virol.* **69:**7601–7605.
58. Melnick, J. L. 1990. Enteroviruses: polioviruses, coxsackieviruses, echoviruses, and newer enteroviruses, p. 549–605. *In* B. N. Fields and D. M. Knipe (ed.), *Fields Virology.* Raven Press, New York, N.Y.
59. Mendelsohn, C. L., E. Wimmer, and V. R. Racaniello. 1989. Cellular receptor for poliovirus: molecular cloning, nucleotide sequence, and expression of a new member of the immunoglobulin superfamily. *Cell* **56:**855–865.
60. Minor, P. D. 1992. The molecular biology of poliovaccines. *J. Gen. Virol.* **73:**3065–3077.
61. Minor, P. D., G. Dunn, D. M. Evans, D. I. Magrath, A. John, J. Howlett, A. Phillips, G. Westrop, K. Wareham, J. W. Almond, et al. 1989. The temperature sensitivity of the Sabin type 3 vaccine strain of poliovirus: molecular and structural effects of a mutation in the capsid protein VP3. *J. Gen. Virol.* **70:**1117–1123.
62. Morrison, M. E., and V. R. Racaniello. 1992. Molecular cloning and expression of a murine homolog of the human poliovirus receptor gene. *J. Virol.* **66:**2807–2813.
63. Moss, E. G., and V. R. Racaniello. 1991. Host range determinants located on the interior of the poliovirus capsid. *EMBO J.* **5:**1067–1074.
64. Murray, M. G., J. Bradley, X. F. Yang, E. Wimmer, E. G. Moss, and V. R. Racaniello. 1988. Poliovirus host range is determined by a short amino acid sequence in neutralization antigenic site I. *Science* **241:**213–215.
65. Nathanson, N., and A. D. Langmuir. 1963. The Cutter incident. Poliomyelitis following formaldehyde-inactivated poliovirus vaccination in the United States during the spring of 1955. I. Background. *Am. J. Hyg.* **78:**16–28.
66. Nathanson, N., and A. D. Langmuir. 1963. The Cutter incident. Poliomyelitis following formaldehyde-inactivated poliovirus vaccination in the United States during the spring of 1955. II. Relationship of poliomyelitis to Cutter vaccine. *Am. J. Hyg.* **78:**29–60.
67. Nathanson, N., and A. D. Langmuir. 1963. The Cutter incident. Poliomyelitis following formaldehyde-inactivated poliovirus vaccination in the United States during the spring of 1955. III. Comparison of the clinical character of vaccinated and contact cases occurring after use of high rate lots of Cutter vaccine. *Am. J. Hyg.* **78:**61–81.
68. Nieke, J., and M. Schachner. 1985. Expression of the neural cell adhesion molecules L1 and N-CAM and their common carbohydrate epitope 1.2/HNK-1 during development and after transection of the mouse sciatic nerve. *Differentiation* **30:**141–151.
69. Nomoto, A., T. Omata, H. Toyoda, S. Kuge, H. Horie, Y. Kataoka, Y. Genba, Y. Nakano, and N. Imura. 1982. Complete nucleotide sequence of the attenuated poliovirus Sabin 1 strain genome. *Proc. Natl. Acad. Sci. USA* **79:**5793–5797.
70. Ohka, S., W. X. Yang, E. Terada, K. Iwasaki, and A. Nomoto. 1998. Retrograde transport of intact poliovirus through the axon via the fast transport system. *Virology* **250:**67–75.
71. Omata, T., M. Kohara, S. Kuge, T. Komatsu, W. Abe, B. L. Semler, A. Kameda, H. Itoh, M. Arita, E. Wimmer, and A. Nomoto. 1986. Genetic analysis of the attenuation phenotype of poliovirus type 1. *J. Virol.* **58:**348–358.
72. Paul, A., J. A. Mugavero, J. Yin, S. Hobson, S. Schulz, J. H. Van Boom, and E. Wimmer. 2000. Studies on the attenuation phenotype of polio vaccines: poliovirus RNA polymerase derived from Sabin type 1 sequence is temperature sensitive in the uridylylation of VPg. *Virology* **272:**72–84.
73. Paul, A. V., J. H. Van Boom, D. Filipov, and E. Wimmer. 1998. Protein-primed RNA synthesis by purified poliovirus RNA polymerase. *Nature* **393:**280–284.
74. Pelletier, J., and N. Sonenberg. 1988. Internal initiation of translation of eukaryotic mRNA directed by a sequence derived from poliovirus RNA. *Nature* **334:**320–325.
75. Peluso, R., A. Hasase, L. Stowring, M. Edwards, and P. Ventura. 1985. A Trojan horse mechanism for the spread of visna in monocytes. *Virology* **147:**231–236.
76. Pilipenko, E. V., E. G. Viktorova, E. V. Khitrina, S. V. Maslova, N. Jarousse, M. Brahic, and V. I. Agol. 1999. Distinct attenuation phenotypes caused by mutations in the translational starting window of Theiler's murine encephalomyelitis virus. *J. Virol.* **73:**3190–3196.
77. Ren, R., F. Costantini, E. J. Gorgacz, J. J. Lee, and V. R. Racaniello. 1990. Transgenic mice expressing a human poliovirus receptor: a new model for poliomyelitis. *Cell* **63:**353–362.
78. Ren, R., E. G. Moss, and V. R. Racaniello. 1991. Identification of two determinants that attenuated vaccine-related type 2 polioviruses. *J. Virol.* **65:**1377–1382.
79. Ren, R., and V. R. Racaniello. 1992. Poliovirus spreads from muscle to the central nervous system by neural pathways. *J. Infect. Dis.* **166:**747–752.
80. Roivainen, M., L. Piirainen, T. Hovi, I. Virtanen, T. Riikonen, J. Heino, and T. Hyypia. 1994. Entry of coxsackievirus A9 into host cells: specific interactions with alpha v beta 3 integrin, the vitronectin receptor. *Virology* **203:**357–365.

81. **Russell, W. R.** 1947. Poliomyelitis: the preparalytic stage and the effect of physical activity on the severity of paralysis. *Br. Med. J.* **2:**1023.
82. **Sabin, A. B.** 1956. Pathogenesis of poliomyelitis. Reappraisal in the light of new data. *Science* **123:**1151–1157.
83. **Sabin, A. B., and L. Boulger.** 1973. History of Sabin attenuated poliovirus oral live vaccine strains. *J. Biol. Stand.* **1:**115–118.
84. **Schultz, D. E., M. Honda, L. E. Whetter, K. L. McKnight, and S. M. Lemon.** 1996. Mutations within the 5' nontranslated RNA of cell culture-adapted hepatitis A virus which enhance cap-independent translation in cultured African green monkey kidney cells. *J. Virol.* **70:**1041–1049.
85. **Seif, I., P. Coulon, P. E. Rollin, and A. Flamand.** 1985. Rabies virulence: effect on pathogenicity and sequence characterization of rabies virus mutations affecting antigenic site III of the glycoprotein. *J. Virol.* **53:**926–934.
86. **Skinner, M. A., V. R. Racaniello, G. Dunn, J. Cooper, P. D. Minor, and J. W. Almond.** 1989. New model for the secondary structure of the 5' non-coding RNA of poliovirus is supported by biochemical and genetic data that also shows that RNA secondary structure is important in neurovirulence. *J. Mol. Biol.* **207:**379–392.
87. **Solecki, D., G. Bernhardt, M. Lipp, and E. Wimmer.** 2000. Identification of a nuclear respiratory factor-1 binding site within the core promoter of the human poliovirus receptor/CD155 gene. *J. Biol. Chem.* **275:**12453–12462.
88. **Solecki, D., S. Schwarz, E. Wimmer, M. Lipp, and G. Bernhardt.** 1997. The promoters from human and monkey poliovirus receptors. *J. Biol. Chem.* **272:**5579–5586.
89. **Solecki, D., E. Wimmer, M. Lipp, and G. Bernhardt.** 1999. Identification and characterization of the cis-acting elements of the human CD155 gene core promoter. *J. Biol. Chem.* **274:**1791–1800.
90. **Spriggs, D. R., R. T. Bronson, and B. N. Fields.** 1983. Hemagglutinin variants of Reovirus type 3 have altered central nervous system tropism. *Science* **220:**505–507.
91. **Squitti, R., M. E. De Stefano, D. Edgar, and G. Toschi.** 1999. Effects of axotomy on the expression and ultrastructural localization of N-cadherin and neural cell adhesion molecule in the quail ciliary ganglion: an in vivo model of neuroplasticity. *Neuroscience* **91:**707–722.
92. **Strebel, P. M., N. Ion-Nedelcu, A. L. Baughman, R. M. Sutter, and S. L. Cochi.** 1995. Intramuscular injections within 30 days of immunization with oral poliovirus vaccine—a risk factor for vaccine-associated paralytic poliomyelitis. *N. Engl. J. Med.* **332:**500–506.
93. **Sutter, R. W., P. A. Patriarca, A. J. Suleiman, S. Brogan, P. G. Malankar, S. L. Cochi, A. A. Al-Ghassani, and M. S. el-Bualy.** 1992. Attributable risk of DTP (diphtheria and tetanus toxoids and pertussis vaccine) injection in provoking paralytic poliomyelitis during a large outbreak in Oman. *J. Infect. Dis.* **165:**444–449.
94. **Tardy-Panit, M., B. Blondel, A. Martin, F. Tekaia, F. Horaud, and F. Delpeyroux.** 1993. A mutation in the RNA polymerase of poliovirus type 1 contributes to attenuation in mice. *J. Virol.* **67:**4630–4638.
95. **Tomko, R. P., R. Xu, and L. Philipson.** 1997. HCAR and MCAR: the human and mouse cellular receptors for subgroup C adenoviruses and B coxsackieviruses. *Proc. Natl. Acad. Sci. USA* **94:**3352–3356.
96. **Toyoda, H., C. F. Yang, N. Takeda, A. Nomoto, and E. Wimmer.** 1987. Analysis of RNA synthesis of type 1 poliovirus by using an in vitro molecular genetic approach. *J. Virol.* **61:**2816–2822.
97. **Triantafilou, M., K. Triantafilou, K. M. Wilson, Y. Takada, N. Fernandez, and G. Stanway.** 1999. Involvement of beta2-microglobulin and integrin alphavbeta3 molecules the coxsackievirus A9 infectious cycle. *J. Gen. Virol.* **80:**2591–2600.
98. **Voroshilova, M., and M. Chumakov.** 1959. Poliomyelitis-like properties of AB-IV coxsackie A7 group of viruses. *Prog. Med. Virol.* **2:**106–107.
99. **Wadia, N. H., S. M. Katrak, V. P. Misra, P. N. Wadia, K. Miyamura, K. Hashimoto, T. Ogino, T. Hikiji, and R. Kono.** 1983. Polio-like motor paralysis associated with acute hemorrhagic conjunctivitis in an outbreak in 1981 in Bombay, India: clinical and serologic studies. *J. Infect. Dis.* **147:**660–668.
100. **Wang, S. M., C. C. Liu, H. W. Tseng, J. R. Wang, C. C. Huang, Y. J. Chen, Y. J. Yang, S. J. Lin, and T. F. Yeh.** 1999. Clinical spectrum of enterovirus 71 infection in children in southern Taiwan, with an emphasis on neurological complications. *Clin. Infect. Dis.* **29:**184–190.
101. **Westrop, G. D., K. A. Wareham, D. M. A. Evans, G. Dunn, P. D. Minor, D. I. Magrath, F. Taffs, S. Marsden, M. A. Skinner, G. Schild, and J. W. Almond.** 1989. Genetic basis of attenuation of the Sabin type 3 oral poliovirus vaccine. *J. Virol.* **63:**1338–1344.
102. **Wimmer, E., J. J. Harber, J. A. Bibb, M. Gromeier, H. H. Lu, and G. Bernhardt.** 1994. Poliovirus receptors, p. 101–127. *In* E. Wimmer (ed.), *Cellular Receptors for Animal Viruses*. Cold Spring Harbor Laboratory Press, Plainview, N.Y.
103. **Wimmer, E., C. U. T. Hellen, and X. M. Cao.** 1993. Genetics of poliovirus. *Annu. Rev. Genet.* **27:**353–436.
104. **Yang, W.-X., T. Tersaki, K. Shiroki, S. Ohka, J. Aoki, S. Tanabe, T. Nomura, E. Terada, Y. Sugiyama, and A. Nomoto.** 1997. Efficient delivery of circulating poliovirus to the central nervous system independently of poliovirus receptor. *Virology* **229:**421–428.
105. **Yin-Murphy, M.** 1984. Acute hemorrhagic conjunctivitis. *Prog. Med. Virol.* **29:**23–44.
106. **Zhang, S., and V. R. Racaniello.** 1997. Expression of the poliovirus receptor in intestinal epithelial cells is not sufficient to permit poliovirus replication in the mouse gut. *J. Virol.* **71:**4915–4920.

Poliovirus Vaccines: Molecular Biology and Immune Response

P. D. MINOR AND J. ALMOND

30

There are three serotypes of poliovirus defined by their gross serological properties and the cross-protection induced, such that infection with one type does not give solid protection against the other two, but there are also strain differences within a type that affect virulence and to a lesser extent antigenicity. Most infections are silent, but among unimmunized populations the majority of poliomyelitis cases were caused by type 1 poliovirus where about 1% of infections led to disease, followed by type 3 where the incidence was 10-fold less and type 2 where it was even lower.

The pathogenesis of poliomyelitis is central to understanding the effectiveness of the vaccines that are likely to eradicate the wild-type virus from the world over the next few years. The main site of replication of poliovirus is in the intestine, and transmission of infection is normally by the fecal-oral route. Disease occurs when the virus escapes its normal intestinal replication site and infects the central nervous system. It was shown in the 1950s (14) that immunoglobulin can protect against the disease if given before or soon after infection. The appearance of poliomyelitis as a public health problem at the end of the 19th century coincided with improvements in hygiene and is explained by the exposure of infants to infection increasingly later in life when the passive protection of maternal antibody had declined. Individuals unable to mount a humoral immune response are at particular risk of poliomyelitis, and can continue to excrete poliovirus for very long periods. It is, therefore, clear that humoral immunity is central to protection and in practice the effectiveness of polio vaccines in protecting individuals may be judged by the ability to induce serum antibodies. Vaccines must contain a representative of each serotype to be fully effective, but there is very little evidence that the limited antigenic variation observed within a serotype has a major effect on immunity, so that a single strain of each type is likely to be sufficient.

ORIGIN OF VACCINES

The first experimental polio vaccines were produced in the 1930s and consisted of extracts of the spinal cords of infected monkeys extracted and treated to produce one preparation believed to contain only killed virus and another in which the virus was said to be "attenuated"; both preparations caused poliomyelitis in recipients.

The first successful vaccine was the formalin-killed preparation of Salk (also known as inactivated polio vaccine or IPV), which was licensed for human use in the United States in 1955, and resulted in a fall of 90% in the incidence of disease between 1955 and 1962, as shown in Fig. 1. There were difficulties in producing sufficient quantities of the vaccine, however, the type 1 component being particularly problematic, and the inactivation process was a delicate balance between failing to kill the virus, on the one hand, and destroying its antigenicity, on the other. There were also theoretical reasons to believe that a live attenuated vaccine, which would infect the intestine without causing disease, would be more effective and give longer-lasting protection, as it would better imitate naturally acquired immunity. Several different types of live vaccine were developed and given clinical trials, including the type I Cox and Chat strains and the type 3 strain USOL-D-BAC, discussed in more detail later. However, the live oral polio vaccines in general use now, which are both safe and highly effective, are all based on the strains developed by Sabin.

The type 1 strain originated from the archetypal Mahoney strain, passaged through cultures of monkey testes by Li and Schaeffer (20). The type 2 strain originated from an environmental isolate rather than a clinical case, while the type 3 strain originated from a standard laboratory virus isolated from a fatal case in 1937. The passage history of the viruses is given in Fig. 2 (39). The candidate viruses were tested in primates for both attenuation and stability on passage (38). The intraspinal inoculation of Old World monkeys was identified as the most sensitive method for revealing a neurovirulent phenotype, and this was later adopted as part of the safety assessment of vaccines by the World Health Organization. As shown in Fig. 1, the Sabin vaccine strains of polio were introduced in the early 1960s, and the decline in disease incidence initiated by IPV continued. However, there was a small number of residual

---

P. D. Minor ■ Department of Virology, NIBSC, Blanche Lane, South Mimms, Potters Bar, Herts, EN6 3QG, United Kingdom. *J. Almond* ■ Research and Development (France), Aventis Pasteur SA, Campus Merieux, 1541 Ave. Marcel Mérieux, 69280 Marcy-L'Etoile, France.

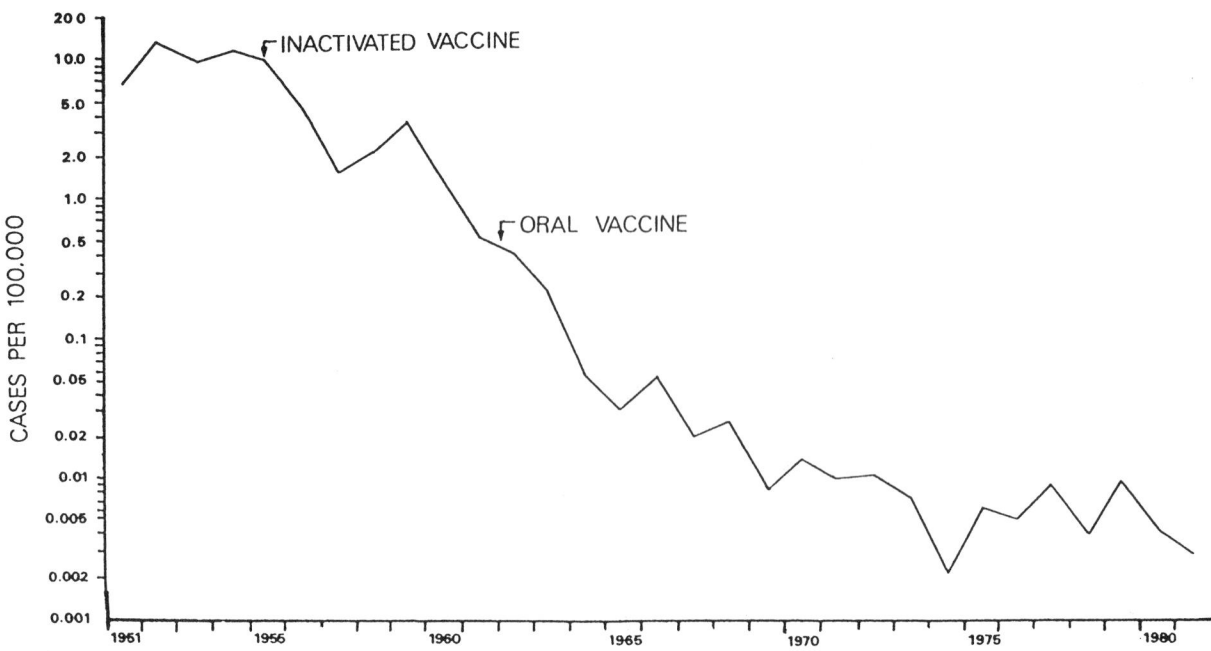

FIGURE 1 Incidence of poliomyelitis in the United States between 1951 and 1980 showing the effect of inactivated and oral (Sabin) vaccine.

cases, and it has been unequivocally shown that at least some are due to the reversion of the vaccines to virulence, the incidence being estimated at 1 per 530,000 primary vaccinees or one per 1.2 million vaccinees overall (32). In contrast to unimmunized populations, type 2 and type 3 are responsible for most vaccine-associated cases, which may occur in recipients or contacts, type 1 making up about 10% of the total.

Studies of the molecular biology of the Sabin live polio vaccines have so far concentrated on their virulence or attenuation for primates or transgenic mice carrying the human receptor for poliovirus where the virus is given directly into the central nervous system or parentally. Infection of humans is usually by the oral route, where different considerations may apply in some circumstances.

THE MOLECULAR BIOLOGY OF THE SABIN VACCINE STRAIN OF POLIOVIRUS

The organization of the poliovirus genome is shown in Fig. 3. It consists of a single strand of positive-sense RNA about 7,500 bases in length in which the 5' end is covalently linked to a virus-encoded protein, VPg, and the 3' end possesses a polyadenylate tail. A long 5' noncoding region of about 750 bases precedes a single large open reading frame translated as a single protein, the polyprotein, which is cleaved as it is translated by virus-encoded proteases (P2A, P3C, and uncleaved P3CD) to give the active proteins involved in virus replication. The structural proteins (VP1–VP4) that form the shell of the virus particle are encoded before the nonstructural proteins (P2A–P2C, P3A–P3D), which are involved in the replication of the viral genome of the poliovirus and subverting the machinery of the host cell to make viral proteins. Because the genome is of positive sense, the RNA is infectious when introduced into cells.

The basis of attenuation or reversion of the Sabin vaccine strains has been studied by comparing the vaccine strain of each serotype with a closely related strain, either the precursor of the vaccine strain or an isolate from a vaccine-associated case of poliomyelitis. The sequence comparisons for the pairs of strains that have been used for the three serotypes are shown in Fig. 4.

Viruses in which segments of genomes were exchanged, or specific mutations introduced, were prepared by manipulation of full-length cDNA copies of the viral genomes, which were then used to recover infectious virus. The type 3 strains that were compared were the Sabin vaccine strain and its virulent precursor Leon (Fig. 2). The number of differences in the sequences of the two strains is surprisingly small (Fig. 4c), but of the 10 seen, only that at position 472 in the 5' noncoding region and that at base 2034, producing an amino acid change at residue 91 of the virus coat protein VP3 from a serine to a phenylalanine, were required to attenuate the virus in an animal model (28). While there were more differences between the Sabin type 2 vaccine strain of poliovirus and the virulent 117 type 2 isolate from a vaccine-associated case (Fig. 4b), only the mutation at residue 481 in the 5' noncoding region and the mutation at base 2908 that produces an amino acid change at residue 143 of the virus coat protein VP1 gave a definite change in the virulence of the virus (23, 35) although the difference at residue 868, producing an alanine to serine change in VP4, might have had a small effect. The effect of the mutation at residue 481 has been disputed (36). The situation with type 1 (Fig. 4a) was more complex. Mutations that caused attenuation included that at residue 480 in the 5' noncoding region, although others in this region seemed to have an effect. Mutations in the structural proteins at amino acid residues 65 of VP4, 225 of VP3, and 106 and 134 of VP1 all had an attenuating effect. No single mutation in any of the nonstructural proteins has been confirmed to have a major effect in changes

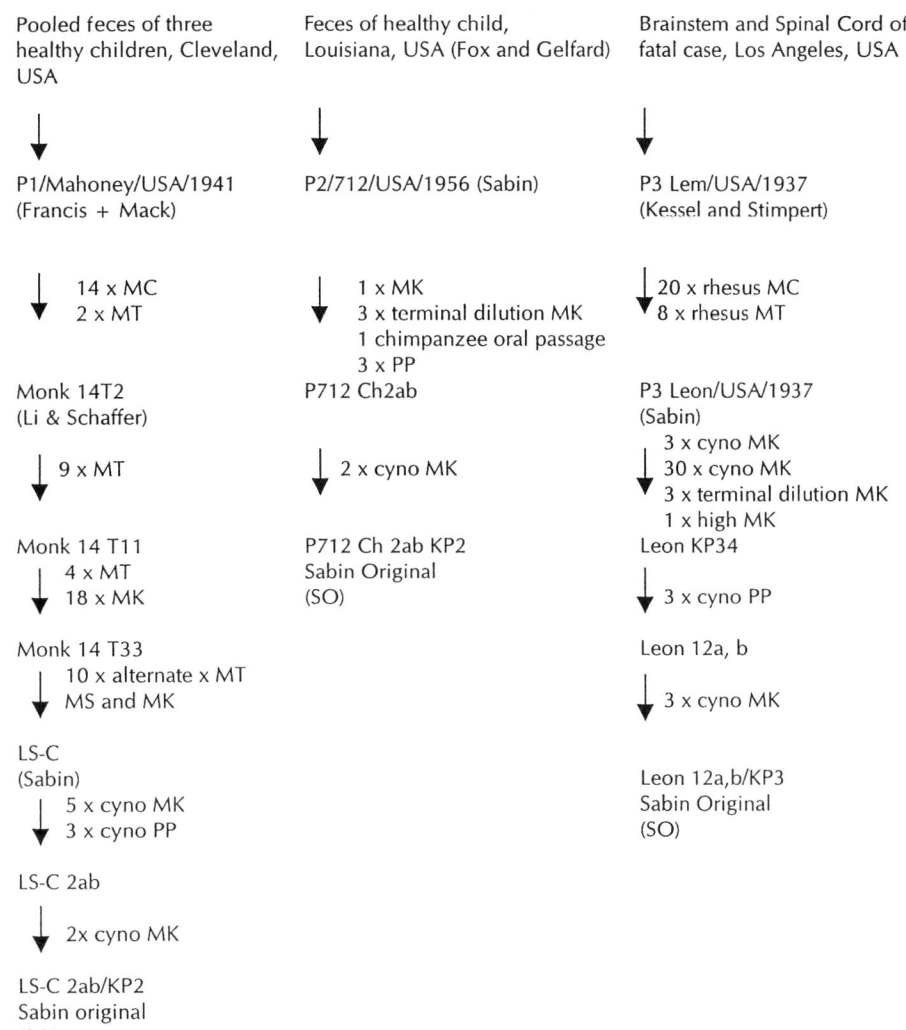

FIGURE 2 Derivation of the Sabin vaccine strains from the original isolates.

of poliovirus virulence for any serotype despite some early findings (6, 8, 26, 33).

If the analysis of the molecular basis of attenuation described here is applicable to human infections, then when isolates of poliovirus from the rare cases of vaccine-associated disease are examined, the mutations implicated in attenuation of the polio vaccine viruses should either revert or be suppressed by mutations at other sites. This has been found to be the case (22, 28). However, the same changes can also be shown to occur in normal vaccinees; in fact, for type 3 and many type 2 strains the vaccine-related poliovirus strains isolated from poliomyelitis cases and from healthy recipients are indistinguishable in their properties (7, 9, 10, 12, 21, 22, 31).

In recipients of poliovaccine who excrete type 3 vaccine strains, the base at position 472 in the 5' noncoding region reverts to the base found in the virulent form within 6 days, and usually by day 3 after vaccination. Individuals typically excrete virus for 5 to 6 weeks following vaccination, and 1% continue for 10 weeks (28). By day 11 postvaccination, the type 3 virus loses all or part of its temperature-sensitive growth phenotype, which can be shown to be due to the

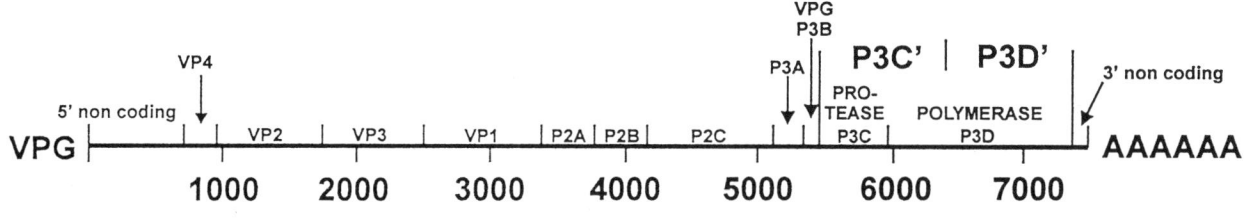

FIGURE 3 Organization of the poliovirus genome.

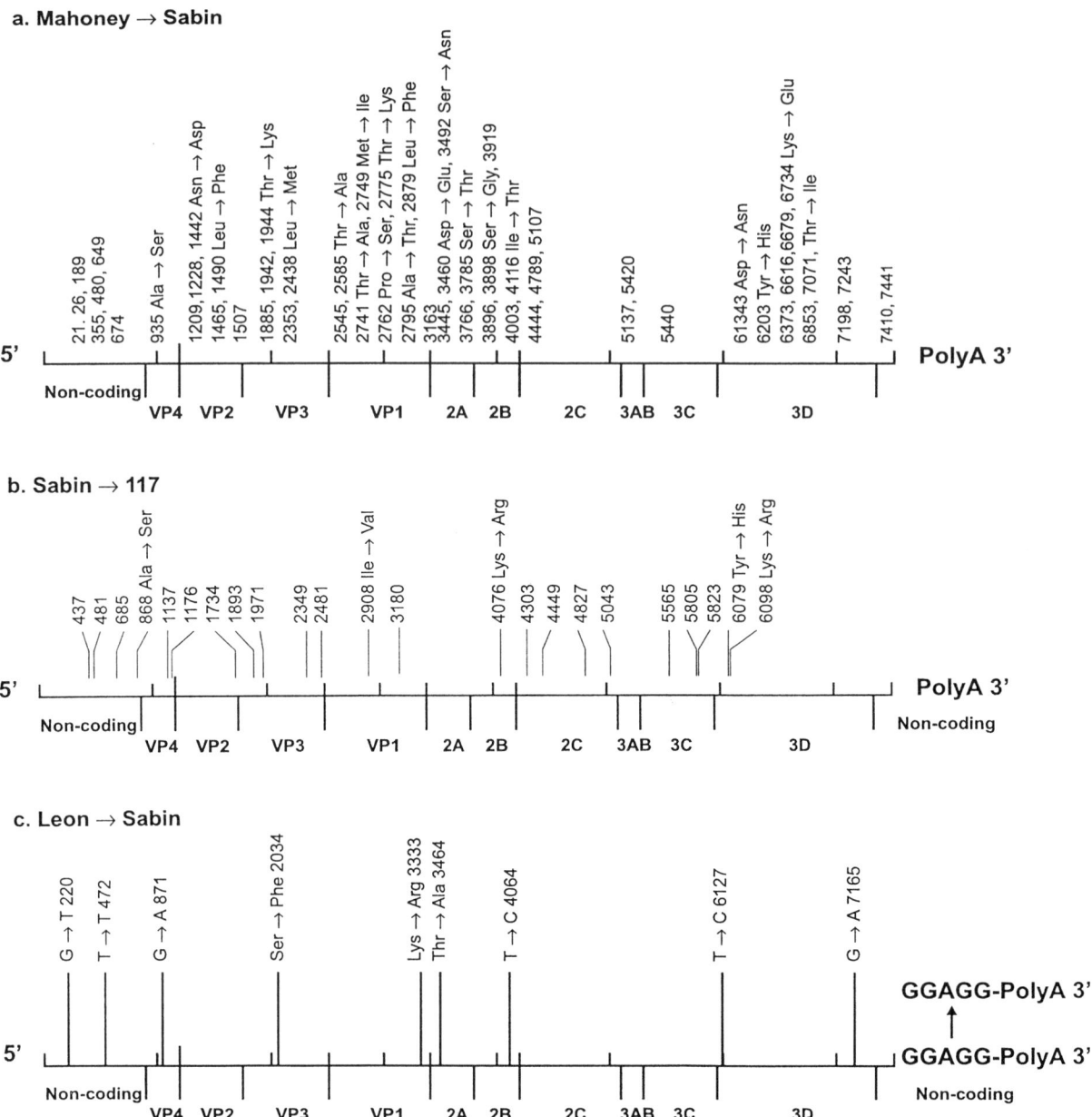

FIGURE 4 Comparison of sequences of strains used in the analysis of the attenuated phenotype of the Sabin vaccine strains. (a) type 1, Mahoney and Sabin type 1; (b) type 2, 117 and Sabin type 2; (c) type 3, Leon and Sabin type 3.

other major attenuating mutation, that at residue 91 of VP3 (22). Moreover, the virus that is excreted is a recombinant in which the structural proteins and a section of the nonstructural proteins derive from type 3 poliovirus and the remainder of the genome derives from either type 2 or type 1. If the recombinant is of the type 3/2 kind and excretion of virus continues, a second recombination event invariably occurs in which the extreme 3' end of the type 2 segment of the recombinant virus is exchanged for that of either type 3 or type 1, leading to a 3/2/3 or a 3/2/1 recombinant, respectively. The probable mechanism involves a recombination event between type 3 and type 2 followed by a second recombination with the product of a cross between type 2 and either type 3 or type 1. These observations imply that growth in the gut selects against some feature of the central part of the vaccine strain type 3 genome and some feature of the extreme 3' end of the vaccine strain type 2 genome, and that the surviving virus escapes whatever selection pressure is applied by removing the offending parts of the genome by recombination. The nature of the selective pressures involved remains unclear. Type 2/3 recombinants have been isolated from vaccine-associated cases of poliomyelitis, but not usually from healthy recipients of polio vaccine (7, 21). Thus, by day 11 the type 3 component has lost the effects of both mutations that have been identified as attenuating the virus and recombined its genome extremely rapidly and precisely. In our experience this occurs in all vaccine recipients who continue to excrete virus after day 11 (28). The type 1 and type 2 strains of poliovirus also evolve rapidly (10). The 5′ noncoding attenuating mutation of type 2 at base 481 is lost at about 7 days postimmunization, slightly later than the corresponding mutation in type 3, and in type 1 the effect of the equivalent mutation (at base 480) is lost in about half of the recipients, sometimes by second-site suppression, as described below. The attenuating mutation in the type 2 strain at residue 143 of VP1 is lost in a significant proportion of isolates from healthy vaccinees. As would be expected if this mutation had an attenuating effect, it is lost from all isolates from vaccine-associated cases of poliomyelitis (23).

The Molecular Consequences of Attenuating and Reverting Changes in the 5′ Noncoding Region of Poliovirus

The 5′ noncoding region of poliovirus is predicted to have a well-defined secondary structure, based in part on computer modeling and in part on the susceptibility of the RNA to chemical and enzymatic treatments (34, 41). In addition, in comparisons of the sequences of different poliovirus strains, when a base difference occurs in a part of the RNA predicted to be in a stem, a compensating difference is found in the base with which it is predicted to pair. This strongly suggests that the structure has a physiological significance in virus growth in the wild as well as in the laboratory. The predicted structure for the 5′ noncoding region of poliovirus is shown schematically in Fig. 5. The mutations associated with attenuation in the 5′ noncoding region of the Sabin vaccine strains of poliovirus occur in the region designated domain V in Fig. 5 and their location is shown in more detail in Fig. 6. The numbering of the nucleotides differs slightly between strains because of deletions and insertions in the sequence before the region shown. The mutations involved in attenuation can all be considered to weaken the base-paired RNA structure. The mutation in type 3 (Fig. 6C) at residue 472 changes a strong G-C base pair to a weaker but still allowed G-U base pair in a stem of three base pairs, and the mutation involved in attenuating the type 1 vaccine strain (Fig. 6A) at residue 480 similarly converts an A-U base pair into a weaker but allowed G-U pair. The structures are therefore weakened without being disrupted. The mutation involved in attenuating the type 2 vaccine strain (Fig. 6B) at residue 481 converts a G into an A and could permit a new base pair to form between residue 481 and residue 511, which would weaken the same structures.

In vaccinees the mutations found in the type 2 and type 3 vaccine strains revert to the wild-type base (9, 12, 31). However, in type 1 only half of vaccinees excrete reverted virus; while most of these involve a direct reversion at base 480 to an A, many may have a change in the base at the complementary position 525, which mutates from a U to a C, so creating a strong G-C base pair between residues 480 and 525. Furthermore, in about 10% of cases neither of these bases changes; instead, the base at residue 476 is mutated to an A to change a mismatched U-U pair to an A-U base pair, resulting in strengthening of the overall structure (9; Minor, unpublished).

The mutations associated with attenuation of the Sabin vaccine strains of poliovirus are all consistent with the predicted RNA structure in so far as none of them introduces a major mismatch into a base-paired stem. The fact that in type 1 mutations that compensate for the effect of the attenuating mutation serve to strengthen the structure although they can occur at a variety of sites is strong evidence that the RNA structure is significant. It also illustrates the variety of ways in which the virus can alter to escape a constraint on its fitness.

It has been shown that the attenuating mutations affect the efficiency of the internal ribosome entry site (IRES) function of the 5′ noncoding region (42–44). Moreover, in vitro studies in neuroblastoma cell lines suggest that the attenuated form of the IRES restricts growth in cells of neural origin (1, 19). Studies on epithelial or fibroblastic cells have shown that the attenuating mutations can produce a temperature-sensitive phenotype that correlates with their attenuating effect and the thermodynamic stability of the structure. The effect is cell specific and can be suppressed in part in primate or human lines but not transgenic mouse lines by mutations in the protease 2A by mechanisms that are not fully understood (24, 37).

The Molecular Consequences of Attenuating and Reverting Changes in the Structural Proteins of the Type 3 Sabin Vaccine Strain

The diversity of ways in which the poliovirus can alter itself is also illustrated by the suppression of the attenuating mutation in the structural proteins of the type 3 Sabin vaccine strain. The attenuating mutation is a serine to phenylalanine change in VP3 and has the effect of introducing a bulky hydrophobic amino acid at the interface between protomeric subunits in the attenuated virus, making the pentamer less stable. The temperature-sensitive growth phenotype so produced is suppressed in most iso-

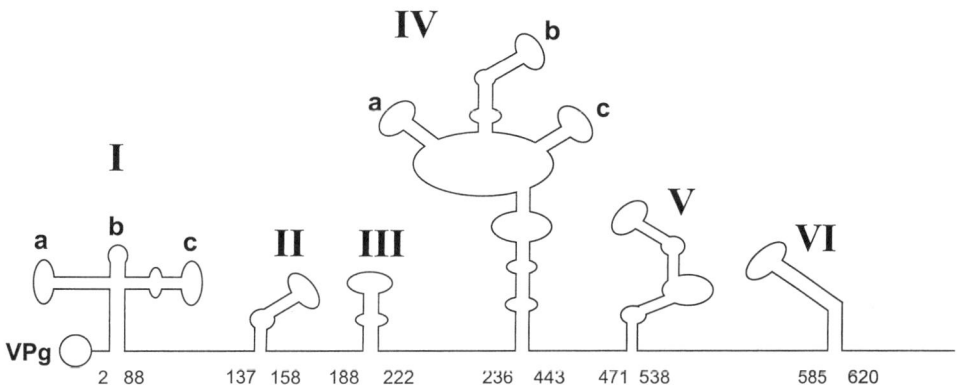

FIGURE 5 Predicted secondary structure of the 5′ noncoding region of the poliovirus genome.

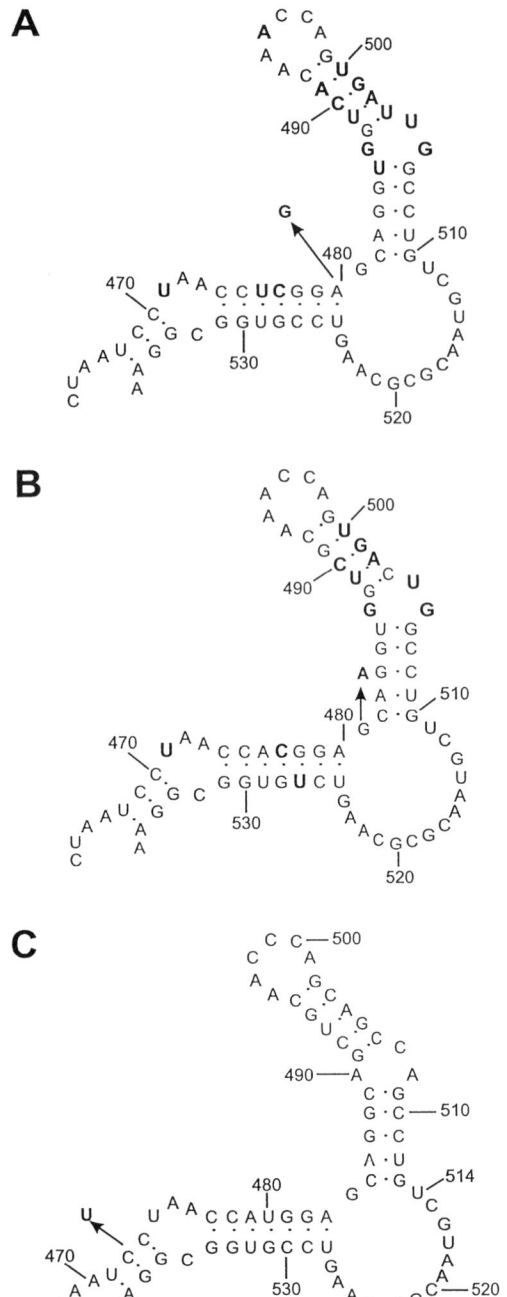

FIGURE 6 Structure of domain V showing mutations involved in the attenuated phenotype of the Sabin vaccine strains (A) type 1, (B) type 2, and (C) type 3.

on the inner surface of the virion away from the protomer interface, in a region that is thought to be involved in the structural transitions involved in the assembly and uncoating of poliovirus, for example, VP1 amino acid 54. The homologous position type 1 is mutated in some receptor site variants. A third kind of mutation suppressing the effect of the mutation at residue 91 involves a substitution in the region that links adjacent pentamers into the viral capsid, for example, in VP2 at residue 18 and VP1 at residue 34. These types of mutation are believed to act by accelerating the transition from pentamers to complete capsid, so compensating for the instability of the pentamers. All of these mutations have been found in poliovirus isolates from both healthy vaccinees and vaccine-associated cases of poliomyelitis. It is of interest that the direct back mutation of residue 91 of VP3 to a serine is relatively rare. It is likely that this preponderance of second-site suppressor mutations is due to the fine-tuning of virus growth to the temperature of the gut, which is 37°C; Leon, the virus that contains a serine and which is the laboratory precursor of the Sabin vaccine strain used in the analyses of virulence and temperature-sensitive growth properties, has a temperature optimum of about 39°C compared with 37°C for the revertants. This illustrates the fact that poliovirus not only has a wide spectrum of ways in which it can revert, but that it can also do so with great specificity, depending on the selection pressures it faces.

ANTIGENIC VARIANTS IN HEALTHY VACCINEES

Early studies with polyclonal sera showed that viruses excreted by vaccinees, particularly type 1 viruses, frequently showed slight changes in antigenicity (27). Monoclonal antibodies can recognize neutralization sites specific for vaccine rather than wild-type strains (27), and the most strain-specific antibodies for any serotype are directed against site 3 (Nag III), composed of sequences from VP3 and VP1. Sequential isolates from vaccinees often acquire point mutations leading to loss of neutralization by antibodies specific for sites 2, 3, and 4 while, in contrast, site 1 is well conserved both in isolates from vaccinees and in wild-type virus of serotypes 2 and 3 (30). It is of interest that site 1 of each of the Sabin vaccine strains contains a protease cleavage site, which, when proteolytically digested, abrogates neutralization by antibodies against that site (27, 30) and the induction of antibodies against it in mice (27, 30). Virus excreted by vaccinees can be shown to be in the cleaved form (30, 31) so that an antibody response directed against it would not be effective against virus in the gut, suggesting that conservation of the cleavage site would be a selective advantage. Site 1 is strongly immunodominant in mice for poliovirus of types 2 and 3 and in at least one case there seemed to be a selection pressure in favor or protease sensitivity in an epidemic strain (30) although this was not always found (16). The conservation of an immunodominant antigenic site not expressed in the gut because of the presence of proteolytic enzymes would help to confine replication to the intestine. Site 1 of type 1 does not seem to be immunodominant in mice, and wild-type strains frequently do not possess a protease cleavage site. Despite the point mutations that arise, the antibody response induced by vaccination is highly cross-reactive, as demonstrated by the efficacy of the available vaccines against poliovirus.

lates obtained from vaccinees more than 11 days postimmunization (28, 31) and most of the amino acid differences between these isolates and the Sabin vaccine strain of type 3 poliovirus from which they derived cluster at the interface between protomers, as might be expected for example at residues 108 and 178 of VP3 or 215 and 265 of VP2 (29). The effect of the amino acid changes is to make it possible for interacting protomers to fit together better, despite the continued presence of the bulky phenylalanine at residue 91 of VP3. However, some mutations are found

LONG-TERM EXCRETION OF POLIOVIRUS BY VACCINEES

In immunocompetent individuals the Sabin vaccine strains of poliovirus replicate for a limited period, usually between a few days and 3 months (3). The cause of the ultimate clearance of the virus infection is not known, although very-long-term excretion can occur in some individuals unable to mount a satisfactory humoral immune response. It has been suggested that viral clearance is related to the development of an immunoglobulin A (IgA) response (40). Several examples of the prolonged excretion of strains of poliovirus by hypogammaglobulinemic patients are documented. Kew et al. (15) described a patient who developed paralysis and from whom type 1 virus was isolated over a period of about 200 days. The patient died 9 years later, and it was not known if the patient was still shedding virus. The strains isolated differed by about 10% from the Sabin type 1 strain, to which they were most closely related, and over the period for which viruses had been isolated, the mean rate of change at third base positions was calculated as 3.4% per year. It was estimated, based on the calculated rate of drift, that the patient had been excreting virus for about 10 years.

Bellmunt et al. (5) described a more extensive study of a paralyzed patient from whom 44 isolates were taken over a 5.5-year period. The sequences of the first and last isolate were determined completely, and it was estimated that the individual excreted virus for at least 10 years.

A study was conducted in 1962 to assess the ability of immune deficient hypogammaglobulinemic patients to mount an immune response to vaccines, including polio vaccine. Patients were given monovalent vaccine preparations and 2 of 30 patients excreted virus for a prolonged period, one excreting type 1 for about 3 years, the other type 3 for about 21 months, although both remained healthy. Isolates from the second patient have been studied in depth (25). Mutations accumulated at a steady rate of 1.28% per year if all mutations over the whole genome were considered, 2.78% per year if synonymous base changes over the whole genome were considered, or 3.4% for just the synonymous base changes in the capsid protein genes. Mutations believed to be significant for virus function continued to appear over the whole period of excretion, highlighting the dynamic status of the virus-host interaction. The occurrence of antigenic variants was of particular interest and occurred at 10-fold lower rate than that in a normal healthy vaccinee. This may have been because of a low-level immune response by the patient or the use of immunoglobulin. The virus excreted was of increased virulence for primates compared with the vaccine strain but less virulent than the wild type seen after 20 months. Adaptation to the gut is therefore not synonymous with neurovirulence. The patient remained healthy and stopped excreting virus after 637 days for reasons that are not clear.

Another instance of a healthy hypogammaglobulinemic patient chronically infected with poliovirus is currently under examination (Minor and Dunn, unpublished data). Isolates were obtained in January 1995 and throughout the remainder of the year, and the patient has been shown to be still shedding virus in April 2000. Moreover, the first isolate, while in the same genetic cluster as the Sabin type 2 vaccine strain, and thus of North American origin, was of the order of 10% different in sequence from the vaccine strain in 1995. While it is known that the individual has been shedding virus for 5 years, it is more likely that it is over 10, based on the extent of genetic drift and consistent with the vaccine history. The virus shed in 1955 has a mutation changing the amino acid at 143 of VP1 from an isoleucine, a reversion of the base at residue 481 in the noncoding region, and a change in VP4. When tested in primates it proved as virulent as 117, the isolate from the vaccine-associated case whose sequence is given in Fig. 2B. The changes and the phenotype are consistent with conclusions on the molecular basis of reversion described above.

In a study of over 100 hypogammaglobulinemic patients attending a clinic in London, United Kingdom, none were found to be shedding poliovirus. In the studies of patients by MacCallum in 1962, only 2 of 30 went on to become long-term excretors. In a study of IgA-deficient patients in Finland, while excretion of virus was more prolonged than in immune competent controls, none of eight excreted for 6 months. Virus excretion can terminate in agammaglobulinemic patients incapable of any humoral response. The reasons for long-term excretion of virus or its termination remain somewhat uncertain.

ALTERNATIVES TO THE SABIN VACCINE STRAINS

The live attenuated poliovirus vaccine strains developed by Sabin are both safe and effective. They cause poliomyelitis in recipients or contacts in rare instances and are able to adapt to the human gut accurately and rapidly. Although they are not considered highly transmissible, there is no reason why they should not become so during the prolonged virus shedding observed in some immune deficient patients. The basis of transmissibility is not understood but might include factors such as the amount of virus excreted and the length of the excretion period. As eradication of wild-type poliovirus is accomplished, the vaccine strains will become one of the main sources of human infection and possible remergence of poliomyelitis. A strain of virus with a completely stable phenotype excreted for a brief period that was still sufficient to immunize the recipient would be valuable, and there have been attempts to develop such strains, based on both classical methods and current understanding of the molecular biology of the virus.

The Sabin vaccine strain of type 3 poliovirus was always regarded as the most problematic; first, because when recovered from vaccine recipients, it can be shown to be of significantly increased virulence for animals (9, 12), due to the rapid reversion or suppression of the mutations that attenuate it, notably that in the 5' noncoding region. Alternative strains were sought in the mid-1960s and one, designated USOL-D-BAC, had particularly promising properties (4, 11), with a high degree of genetic stability on passage in the laboratory or in recipients, coupled with a high immunogenicity and ability to establish itself in the gut. Trials were conducted in a number of countries, including Hungary and Romania. In early 1968, a trial was conducted in Poland in three sites, two of which used USOL-D-BAC and the third the Sabin type 3 strain. At this time Poland used the live Sabin type 1 and type 2 strain, but an inactivated type 3 vaccine because of concerns about the safety of the live Sabin 3 strain. The vaccine recipients responded well and without adverse events, but 4 months later, between March and December 1968, a total of 464 cases were reported in Poznan, close to the site of the trial (18). Several of the strains have been sequenced in whole or part (J. Martin, unpublished data) and are derived from the USOL-D-BAC strain. Changes in the strains from epidemic isolates and from isolates from healthy vaccinees in Poland or other countries showed some common changes in VP1 at residues 191 and 294, but some were found only in isolates from the epidemic cases, including one in the 5' noncoding region at position 26, which strengthened a base-paired structure, and some in the structural proteins. Which of these are associated with an increase in virulence and which reflect the development of a particular genetic lineage as the virus spread through the population are not known. The reason why the largely stable USOL-D-BAC caused an epidemic while the less stable Sabin strain did not is not known. It is possible that the poor transmissibility or infectivity of the Sabin strain compared with that of the USOL strain was a factor. The kinetics and basis of vaccination and virus spread in a population with low immunity to a virus are complex and important for strategies in the cessation of vaccination globally.

The first attempts to produce alternative safer live vaccines than the Sabin strains were based on the Sabin strains themselves (17). The Sabin type 1 strain is the least likely of the three to be implicated in vaccine-associated polio, and it was shown that at least some of the attenuating mutations lie outside the capsid proteins (33) just as it has been shown that some attenuating mutations in the Sabin type 2 and type 3 strains lie within the capsid proteins. The structural proteins of the type 1 Sabin strain were therefore replaced with those of either type 2 or type 3. Batches have been prepared, tested satisfactorily among other things for neurovirulence, and await clinical trial.

A second approach, based on the recognized importance of the 5' noncoding region in the attenuation of the Sabin vaccine strains, has involved the exchange of the 5' IRES plus spacer region of the virulent type 1 Mahoney strain for that of human rhinovirus type 2 retaining the 5' terminal cloverleaf structure required for RNA replication (13). The resulting virus, termed PV1 (RIPO), failed to cause paralysis in transgenic mice when inoculated intracerebrally at a titer of 10^9 PFU. A similar construct based on the Sabin type 1 strain designated PV1 (RIPOS) was similarly highly attenuated. No differences in attenuation were observed between PV1 (RIPO) and PV1 (RIPOS) on intraspinal inoculation of monkeys. Growth of the viruses was severely restricted in neuroblastoma cells, but not in HeLa cells.

Agol et al. (2) reported an analysis of the effect of 5' noncoding elements on the neurovirulence of a mouse pathogenic strain and concluded that a cryptic AUG in the region, designated domain VI in Fig. 5, had a major effect on neurovirulence, which was also reflected in growth in neuroblastoma cells, suggesting a new approach to the design of attenuated poliovirus.

Finally, Macadam et al. (A. J. Macadam, G. Ferguson, D. M. Stone, J. Meredith, J. W. Almond, and P. D. Minor, submitted for publication) described the manipulation of domain V in Fig. 5 and 6C. The rationale was to produce a virus based on the Sabin 3 strain in which reversion was either impossible or difficult. The thermodynamic stability of domain V had been shown to correlate with the degree of temperature sensitivity of growth of the viruses in the African green monkey cell line BGM and also with neurovirulence in animals. The base pairing was, therefore, manipulated by changing G-C, A-U, or G-U base pairs so that the stability was as found in the Sabin strain, but the structure contained no G-U base pairs that could mutate easily to G-C base pairs, increasing the thermostability and virulence. For A-U base pairs to mutate to G-C would require two simultaneous mutations or a mutation to G-U, which would weaken the structure further and therefore make the virus less fit. The resulting strains are extremely stable under in vitro growth conditions where the Sabin type 3 strain reverts completely and as attenuated as the Sabin type 3 strain in animals.

It is not known whether any of the strains described would be satisfactory as immunogens in human recipients, or how stable the phenotype would be in terms of virulence or transmissibility under field conditions.

SUMMARY AND CONCLUSIONS

The live attenuated vaccines developed by Sabin were the result of a meticulous analysis of pathogenesis and genetic stability in animal models, followed by extensive clinical trials. They have proved enormously successful in practical use and are the main instrument for the eradication of wild-type polioviruses. While the molecular basis of the attenuation of the strains or their recovery of a virulent phenotype is well understood for animals, and provides a coherent explanation of their effect in human subjects, their effect in populations is not so clear, particularly with respect to the ultimate mechanism of their clearance from the gut and their poor transmissibility between individuals. These issues assume greater importance as global eradication nears and convincing strategies for stopping vaccination need to be established.

REFERENCES

1. **Agol, V. I., S. G. Drozdou, T. A. Ivannikova, M. S. Kolesnikova, M. B. Kordev, and E. A. Tolskaya.** 1989. Restricted growth of attenuated poliovirus strains in cultured cells of a human neuroblastoma. *J. Virol.* **63:**4034–4308.
2. **Agol, V. I., E. V. Pilipenko, and O. R. Slobodskaya.** 1996. Modification of translational control elements as a new approach to design of attenuated picornavirus strains. *J. Biotechnol.* **44:**119–128.
3. **Alexander, J. P., Jr., H. E. Gary, and M. A. Pallansch.** 1997. Duration of poliovirus excretion and its implications for acute flaccid paralysis surveillance: a review of the literature. *J. Infect. Dis.* **175:**176–182.
4. **Beale, A. J., S. Biberi-Moroeanu, L. R. Boulger, P. N. Burgasov, W. C. Cockburn, M. P. Chumakov, A. De Barbieri, and I. Domok.** 1969. USOL-D-bac (type 3 poliovirus) vaccine studies. *Bull. W. H. O.* **40:**295–300.
5. **Bellmunt, A., G. May, R. Zell, A. Pring, P. Kerblom, V. Vergagen, and A. Heim.** 1999. Evolution of poliovirus type 1 during 5.5 years of prolonged enteral replication in an immunodeficient patient. *Virology* **265:**178–184.
6. **Bouchard, M. J., D. H. Lam, and V. R. Racaniello.** 1995. Determinants of attenuation and temperature sensitivity in the type 1 poliovirus Sabin vaccine. *J. Virol.* **69:**4972–4978.
7. **Cammack, N., A. Phillips, G. Dunn, V. Patel, and P. D. Minor.** 1988. Intertypic genomic rearrangements of poliovirus strains in vaccinees. *Virology* **167:**507–514.
8. **Christodoulou, C., F. Colbere-Garapin, A. Macadam, L. F. Taffs, S. Marsden, P. D. Minor, and F. Horaud.** 1990. Mapping of mutations associated with neurovirulence in monkeys infected with Sabin 1 poliovirus revertants selected at high temperature. *J. Virol.* **64:**4922–4929.

9. Contreras, G., K. Dimmock, J. Furesz, C. Gardell, D. Hazlett, K. Korpinski, G. McCorkle, and L. Wu. 1992. Genetic characterisation of Sabin types 1 and 3 poliovaccine virus following serial passage in the human intestinal tract. *Biologicals* **20:**15–26.
10. Dunn, G., N. T. Begg, N. Cammack, and P. D. Minor. 1990. Virus excretion and mutation by infants following primary vaccination with live oral poliovaccine from two sources. *J. Med. Virol.* **32:**92–95.
11. Elbert, L. B., M. P. Chumakov, N. M. Ralf, G. D. Krutyanshaya, V. P. Grachyov, L. I. Avdeyeva, S. G. Dzagurov, L. A. Grachyova, A. V. Tyufanov, L. B. Tsypkin, and L. I. Ravkina. 1967. Comparative study of two vaccine strains of type 3 poliovirus (USOL-D-bac and Leon 12a1b). *Acta Virol.* **11:**89–99.
12. Evans, D. M., G. Dunn, P. D. Minor, G. C. Schild, A. J. Cann, G. Stanway, J. W. Almond, K. Currey, and J. V. Maizel, Jr. 1985. Increased neurovirulence associated with a single nucleotide change in a non-coding region of Sabin type 3 poliovaccine genome. *Nature* **314:**548–550.
13. Gromeier, M., L. Alexander, and E. Wimmer. 1996. Internal ribosomal entry site substitution eliminates neurovirulence in intergeneric poliovirus recombinants. *Proc. Natl. Acad. Sci. USA* **93:**2370–2375.
14. Hammon, W. M., L. L. Coriell, P. F. Wehrle, and J. Stokes. 1953. Evaluation of Red Cross gammagloblin as a prophylactic agent for poliomyelitis. F. Final report of results based on clinical diagnoses. *JAMA* **151:**1272–1285.
15. Kew, O. M., R. W. Sutter, B. K. Nottay, M. J. McDonough, D. R. Prevols, L. Quick, and M. A. Pallansch. 1998. Prolonged replication of a type 1 vaccine derived poliovirus in an immunodeficient patient. *J. Clin. Microbiol.* **36:**2893–2899.
16. Kinnunnen, L., T. Poyry, and T. Hovi. 1991. Generation of virus genetic lineages during an outbreak of poliomyelitis. *J. Gen. Virol.* **72:**2483–2489.
17. Kohara, M., S. Abe, T. Komatsu, K. Tago, M. Ariata, and A. Nomoto. 1988. A recombinant virus between the Sabin 1 and Sabin 3 vaccine strains of poliovirus as a possible candidate for a new type 3 poliovirus live vaccine strain. *J. Virol.* **62:**2828–2835.
18. Kostrezewski, J., A. Kulesza, and A. Abgarowicz. 1970. The epidemic of type 3 poliomyelitis in Poland in 1968. *Epidem. Rev.* (Warsaw) **24:**89–103.
19. La Monica, N., and V. R. Racaniello. 1989. Difference in replication of attenuated and neurovirulent polioviruses in human neuroblastoma cell line SH-SYSY. *J. Virol.* **63:**2357–2360.
20. Li, C. P., and M. Schaeffer. 1953. Adaptation of type 1 poliovirus to mice. *Proc. Soc. Exp. Biol. Med.* **82:**477–481.
21. Lipskaya, G. Y., A. R. Muzychenko, O. K. Kutilova, S. V. Maslona, M. Equeste, S. G. Drozdov, R. Perez-Beroff, and V. I. Agol. 1991. Frequent isolation of intertypic poliovirus recombinants with serotype 2 specificity from vaccine-associated polio cases. *J. Med. Virol.* **35:**290–296.
22. Macadam, A. J., C. Arnold, J. Howlett, A. John, S. Marsden, F. Taffs, P. Reeve, N. Hamada, K. Wareham, J. Almond, N. Cammack, and P. D. Minor. 1989. Reversion of the attenuated and temperature-sensitive phenotypes of the Sabin type 3 strain of poliovirus in vaccinees. *Virology* **172:**408–414.
23. Macadam, A. J., R. Pollard, G. Ferguson, R. Skuce, D. Wood, J. W. Almond, and P. D. Minor. 1993. Genetic basis of attenuation of the Sabin type 2 vaccine strain of poliovirus in primates. *Virology* **192:**18–26.
24. Macadam, A. J., D. M. Stone, J. W. Almond, and P. D. Minor. 1994. Role for poliovirus protease 2A in cap independent translation. *EMBO J.* **13:**924–927.
25. Martin, J., G. Dunn, R. Hull, V. Patel, and P. D. Minor. 2000. Evolution of the Sabin strain of type 3 poliovirus in an immunodeficient patient during the entire 637-day period of virus excretion. *J. Virol.* **74:**3001–3010.
26. McGoldrich, A., A. J. Macadam, G. Dunn, A. Rowe, J. Burlison, P. D. Minor, J. Meredith, D. J. Evans, and J. W. Almond. 1995. Role of mutations G-480 and C-6203 in the attenuation phenotype of Sabin type 1 poliovirus. *J. Virol.* **69:**7601–7605.
27. Minor, P. D. 1990. Antigenic structure of picornaviruses. *Curr. Top. Microbiol. Immunol.* **161:**121–154.
28. Minor, P. D. 1992. The molecular biology of poliovaccines. *J. Gen. Virol.* **73:**3065–3077.
29. Minor, P. D., G. Dunn, D. M. A. Evans, D. I. Magrath, A. John, J. Howlett, A. Phillips, G. Westrop, K. Wareham, J. W. Almond, and J. M. Hogle. 1989. The temperature sensitivity of the Sabin type 3 vaccine strain of poliovirus: molecular and structural effects of a mutation in the capsid protein VP3. *J. Gen. Virol.* **70:**1117–1123.
30. Minor, P. D., M. Ferguson, A. Phillips, D. I. Magrath, A. Huovilainen, and T. Hovi. 1987. Conservation in vivo of protease cleavage sites in antigenic sites of poliovirus. *J. Gen. Virol.* **68:**1857–1865.
31. Minor, P. D., A. John, M. Ferguson, and J. P. Icenogle. 1986. Antigenic and molecular evolution of the vaccine strain of type 3 poliovirus during the period of excretion by a primary vaccinee. *J. Gen. Virol.* **67:**693–706.
32. Nkowane, B. U., S. G. Wassilak, W. A. Oversteen, K. J. Bart, L. B. Schonberger, A. R. Hinman, and O. M. Kew. 1987. Vaccine associated paralytic poliomyelitis in the United States: 1973 through 1984. *JAMA* **257:**1385–1390.
33. Omata, T., M. Kohara, S. Kuge, T. Komatsu, S. Abe, B. L. Semler, A. Kameda, H. Ithoh, M. Arita, E. Wimmer, and A. Nomoto. 1986. Genetic analysis of the attenuation phenotype of poliovirus type 1. *J. Virol.* **58:**348–358.
34. Pilipenko, E. V., V. Blinov, L. I. Romanova, A. N. Sinyakov, S. V. Maslova, and V. I. Agol. 1989. Conserved structural domains in the 5′ untranslated region of picornaviral genomes. An analysis of the segment controlling translation and neurovirulence. *Virology* **168:**201–209.
35. Ren, R., E. G. Moss, and V. R. Racaniello. 1991. Identification of two determinants that attenuate vaccine-related type 2 polioviruses. *J. Virol.* **65:**1377–1382.
36. Rezapkin, G. V., L. Fan, D. M. Asher, M. R. Fibi, E. M. Dragunsky, and K. M. Chumakov. 1999. Mutations in Sabin 2 strain of poliovirus and stability of attenuation phenotype. *Virology* **258:**152–160.
37. Rowe, A., G. L. Ferguson, P. D. Minor, and A. J. Macadam. 2000. Coding changes in the poliovirus protease 2A compensate for 5′NCR domain V disruptions in a cell-specific manner. *Virology* **269:**284–293.
38. Sabin, A. B. 1955. Characteristics and genetic potentialities of experimentally produced and naturally occurring variants of poliomyelitis virus. *Ann. N. Y. Acad. Sci.* **61:**924–938.
39. Sabin, A. B., and L. R. Boulger. 1973. History of Sabin attenuated poliovirus oral live vaccines. *J. Biol. Stand.* **1:**115–118.
40. Savilahti, E., T. Klemola, B. Carlsson, L. Mellander, M. Stenvik, and T. Hovi. 1988. Inadequacy of mucosal IgM antibodies in selective IgA deficiency: excretion of attenuated polioviruses is prolonged. *J. Clin. Immunol.* **8:**89–94.
41. Skinner, M. A., V. R. Racaniello, G. Dunn, G. Cooper, P. D. Minor, and J. W. Almond. 1989. New model for the secondary structure of the 5′ non-coding RNA of po-

liovirus is supported by biochemical and genetic data that also show that RNA secondary structure is important in neurovirulence. *J. Mol. Biol.* **207:**379–392.

42. **Svitkin, Y., N. Cammack, P. D. Minor, and J. W. Almond.** 1990. Translation deficiency of the Sabin type 3 poliovirus genome: association with an attenuating mutation C472-V. *Virology* **175:**103–109.

43. **Svitkin, Y. V., S. V. Maslova, and V. I. Agol.** 1985. The genomes of attenuated and virulence poliovirus strains differ in their in vitro translation efficiencies. *Virology* **147:**243–252.

44. **Svitkin, Y. V., T. V. Pestova, S. V. Maslova, and V. I. Agol.** 1988. Point mutations modify the response of poliovirus RNA to a translation initiation factor: a comparison of neurovirulent and attenuated strains. *Virology* **166:**394–404.

Immunology of the Coxsackieviruses

NORA M. CHAPMAN, CHARLES J. GAUNTT, AND STEVE TRACY

31

The coxsackieviruses are the best-studied group of nonpolio enteroviruses. Unlike that of the polioviruses, the immune reactions of the human or murine (in models of human disease) hosts of infections by the coxsackieviruses are an important component of the diseases generally induced by these viruses. The six serotypes of group B coxsackieviruses (CVB) and the 23 serotypes of the group A coxsackieviruses (CVA) are etiologic agents of numerous diseases, ranging from a mild flu-like illness to severe diseases with fatal heart or central nervous system involvement (19). Immune responses induced by these viruses are associated with pathologic and protective effects. Among the nonpolio enteroviruses, the immune responses to coxsackievirus B3 (CVB3) and the generation of inflammatory heart disease have been particularly well studied with a variety of CVB3 isolates and inbred strains of mice (21, 36, 66, 89, 156). These murine models have been validated by studies of human myocarditis in which both serology and detection of enteroviral RNA have confirmed enteroviruses as etiologic in this disease (reviewed in references 4 and 97). Studies of CVB3-induced myocarditis have also suggested that there is a pathologic role for autoimmunity induced by this virus. A role for coxsackieviruses in the etiology of pancreatitis and insulin-dependent (type 1) diabetes mellitus is based on serological studies, isolation of the virus from rare acute cases, and the tropism of coxsackieviruses for the pancreas; this association has raised many of the same issues of immune responses and potential virus-induced autoimmunity found in the coxsackievirus-heart disease relationship.

One route of infection of humans by coxsackieviruses is likely to be via the alimentary canal through the Peyer's patches of the gut, which are a common route for entry of enteric bacteria and viruses (52, 112). Polioviruses may use M cells (mucosal epithelial cells) as a route of infection in humans; M cells are associated via their basolateral surface with macrophages and T and B lymphocytes (149). Although coxsackieviruses and polioviruses use different receptors to enter human cells, CVB5 (which can infect pigs) has been shown to bind to lymphoid tissue of porcine ileal explants and replicate in these explants (55, 56). Penetration of this site by coxsackieviruses provides an early exposure of the immune system to viral antigens and may allow coxsackieviruses to infect T and B lymphocytes, in which CVB3 has been shown to replicate (99, 161–163). Viral replication in lymphoid cells present in the blood may account for dissemination of virus throughout the body and result in the infection of organs such as the pancreas and the heart, sites at which pathogenic effects of this infection have been noted, both in humans and in murine models of coxsackievirus disease.

The innate immune defenses are the first to respond to a primary infection; primary effectors of immune defense during a first infection are activated natural killer (NK) cells and macrophages. Decreasing the levels of NK cells in murine models of coxsackievirus infection has been shown to result in a more severe myocarditis induced by CVB3 (40, 41) and CVB4 replication in the pancreas (159), suggesting that NK cells contribute to resistance of virus infection. Assays of NK activity suggest that replication of a coxsackievirus in the mouse or in target fibroblasts in vitro is necessary to stimulate this antiviral activity (40–42). Binding of multiple histocompatibility complex (MHC) class I molecules on the surface of cells by inhibitory receptors on NK cells is necessary for protection against the cytolytic activity of these cells (86). CVB3 has been shown to increase expression of MHC class I on infected cardiac myocytes (144), which might decrease NK activity directed against CVB3-infected cells. However, a pancreotropic CVB4 strain did not increase MHC I expression in acinar cells, suggesting that the correlation of resistance to CVB4-induced pancreatitis with NK activity in mouse strains was unaffected by MHC I protection (159). Indeed, binding of MHC I to one coxsackievirus-derived peptide has been shown to reduce binding of these inhibitory receptors (96), suggesting that coxsackievirus in-

---

Nora M. Chapman and Steve Tracy ■ Department of Pathology and Microbiology, University of Nebraska Medical Center, Omaha, NE 68198-6495. *Charles J. Gauntt* ■ Department of Microbiology, University of Texas Health Science Center at San Antonio, San Antonio, TX 78284-7758.

fection in MHC I-positive cells may increase activity of NK cells toward them, thus limiting the extent of coxsackievirus replication.

Another component of the innate immune defenses is the complement system (14). This system works through a cascade of activation of complement factors to generate antigen phagocytosis, degradation, and display on phagocytes and B cells, release of inflammatory mediators from mast cells and basophils, and cytotoxicity against bacteria and enveloped viruses. Purified CVB3 has been shown to activate the alternative pathway of complement (which is independent of an antigen-antibody interaction), an interaction that may lead to early development of germinal centers wherein CVB3 antigens and RNA are located during a primary infection (1, 2). This virus interaction with C3 may provide rapid formation of germinal centers, even in primary immune responses to coxsackieviruses. Activation of the alternative pathway of the complement system may be dependent on repeated structures found within the surface-exposed residues of the capsid (5). Activation of complement enhances the immunogenicity of antigens and has been shown to enhance B-cell activation, independent of T-cell help (reviewed in reference 14). Thus, early action of this innate immune defense may lead to enhanced adaptive immunity.

How are adaptive immune responses to coxsackieviruses generated? Phagocytic cells take up virus via complement or through phagocytizing virus-infected cells or cell debris and present processed viral peptides to T cells. Evidence from studies using in situ hybridization to detect CVB3 RNA in splenic tissue sections of CVB3-infected mice suggests that not only B lymphocytes, but also follicular dendritic cells in this tissue, are positive for CVB3 RNA (2). The dendritic cells are professional antigen-presenting cells (APCs) and can present viral peptides bound both to MHC class I and class II molecules. Studies in cell cultures of monocytes and B cells have demonstrated the replication of CVB3 (99, 161–163). T cells are activated by recognition of the MHC complex with a foreign antigen when costimulated by an APC. The MHC of the host will affect which epitopes are presented to T cells and, consequently, the extent of activation of T cells. This component of the host immune system can affect the type of immune response to coxsackieviruses and the extent of disease produced by infection (reviewed in reference 36).

Studies of human and murine T-cell responses to a coxsackievirus infection indicate the existence of T-cell epitopes to structural proteins held in common within the enterovirus group (8, 9, 16). The first T-cell epitope of the coxsackieviruses to be recognized is located in the 2C protein and is held in common with other human enteroviruses (10); the predominant lymphocyte population proliferating in response to the 2C epitope was $CD4^+$ T cells. Sites on the CVB3 capsid have been reported, using peptide scanning techniques with virus immunization of mice and measuring the proliferation response of murine lymphocytes in culture to peptides (3, 74, 138). Studies with BALB/c mice and peptides of the largest CVB3 capsid protein, P-1D, identified T-cell epitopes in amino acid (aa) sequences 1–15, 21–35, 79–93, 88–111, 119–133, 129–143, and 199–213 (Fig. 1). The overlap for aa 79–93 and aa 88–111 may identify the 6-amino-acid sequence, AEWVLT, as an essential part of the epitope at this site. Auvinen and colleagues (3) identified peptides in P-1B (aa 159–183) and P-1C (aa 51–75) that contained T-cell epitopes. These studies showed that murine T-cell epitopes overlap or neighbor the neutralizing immunogenic (NIm) sites, an observation that confirms and extends the finding of neighboring or overlapping B- and T-cell epitopes in poliovirus (83, 87; reviewed in reference 156). Studies of regions containing both neutralizing antibody sites and T-cell epitopes of viruses in mice and humans have identified these sequences as likely to generate protective immunity (44, 170).

Human T-cell epitopes of enterovirus capsids were also identified primarily in P-1B and P-1C in a study using in vitro proliferation assays and interferon (IFN)-γ production by peripheral blood mononuclear cells (PBMC) of healthy donors in response to peptides from conserved regions of enterovirus capsid proteins (16). The PBMC of about half of 30 myocarditis patients proliferated, however, in response to CVB3 P-1D peptides aa 41–55, 139–153, 139–253, and 269–283, which neighbor the NIm sites (137). Several antigenic T-cell epitopes were located in poliovirus capsid proteins (44, 83, 87, 94), some of which are cross-reactive with those in other enteroviruses (8). These sites are likely to be influenced by the history of infection of patients with enteroviruses since infections with multiple serotypes are likely and virtually the entire population has been vaccinated for the three poliovirus serotypes.

Studies of murine models of CVB3-induced murine myocarditis have suggested a causative role for the involvement of T cells in enterovirus-associated myocarditis (33, 66, 89, 166). In early work, it was demonstrated that a CVB3 infection induced production of cytolytic T lymphocytes (CTL) that were reactive against both CVB3-infected (69) and uninfected myocytes (67, 68, 70, 166). In addition, transfer of T cells from CVB3-infected mice to uninfected mice generated myocarditis (46). Studies of coxsackievirus infections of mice treated with antibodies to remove specific classes of immune cells or of knockout mice in which essential genes for various immune functions are removed (57, 113; reviewed in references 82 and 90) have demonstrated roles for the various effector cells of the cell-mediated immune response in coxsackievirus-induced inflammatory process. While nude mice (nu^-/nu^-), which lack T cells, have a reduced infiltration of inflammatory cells into the heart upon CVB3 infection (51, 123), CVB3-infected nude mice nonetheless developed myocarditis and had a greater concentration of virus in the heart tissue than CVB3-infected wild-type mice (131, 135). Similar results were observed in nude mice in a CVB1-induced model of polymyositis (169). Later studies using CVB3-inoculated severe combined immunodeficient SCID mice (which lack both B and T cells) demonstrated lethal damage to the heart following infection (23, 76, 158). Studies of CVB3 infection of knockout mice for the CD4 or CD8 T-cell coreceptors, the β chain of the T-cell receptor, and β-microglobulin indicated that these genetic deficiencies correlate with reduced myocarditis but increased cardiac virus titer in heart tissue of some strains (57, 113). As for many other viruses, the immune responses to a coxsackievirus infection are a fine balance between protective effects in clearing virus from the body versus immunopathologic activities (173). When CVB3 can replicate without check, as in SCID mice, eventual necrosis of the myocardium due to virus-induced lysis was found to be more destructive than the effects of a large number of inflammatory lesions in CVB3-infected euthymic mice.

T cells appear in the heart tissues of mice infected with CVB3 at days 4 to 7 postinoculation (42, 63), a time when activation of T cells normally occurs in a primary viral infection. The process of T-cell activation requires the presentation of oligomeric peptides recognized by the T-cell receptor via MHC complexes on APCs. There are two types of MHC molecules; class I MHC is bound by the coreceptor CD8 protein of T cells and class II MHC is bound by the coreceptor CD4. In general, $CD8^+$ cytotoxic T cells act on virus-infected or tumor cells and $CD4^+$ cytotoxic T cells have immunoregulatory functions by inducing apoptosis of MHC class II-presenting cells (reviewed in reference 48). The MHC class I haplotype can affect the extent of coxsackievirus-induced disease, presumably through the presence or lack of presentation of T-cell epitopes likely to be associated with inflammation (71, 120). However, in studies of CVB3-induced murine myocarditis, the non-MHC component of the host genetic background also has a significant effect on the extent of disease (165). Inoculation of mice with CVB3 enhances expression of MHC class I molecules on cardiac myocytes (144), indicating that infected myocytes could interact with $CD8^+$ cells. A study of CVB3-infected mice and three cases of patients with CVB3-associated cardiomyopathy found evidence for a superantigen response; T cells infiltrating the heart showed a restricted T-cell receptor (TCR) β-chain repertoire (92, 145), suggesting the possibility that a non-epitope-driven mechanism for T-cell-dependent inflammation may contribute to disease. Other studies showed similar restriction of the TCR α chain in CVB3-infected mice and cardiomyopathy patients (140, 146), indicating that, rather than a superantigen effect, the skewed TCR repertoire was due to targeting of a specific antigen in the heart. Thus to date, there are no data to provide evidence for superantigen activity in picornavirus-activation of T cells.

$CD4^+$ T cells are primarily associated with T-cell helper activities such as secretion of cytokines, maturation of the B-cell response to antigens, and immunoglobulin (Ig) class switching. Although much emphasis has been given to the cytotoxic activities of T cells in CVB3-induced myocarditis, the majority of the pathogenic T-cell response to CVB3 infection is in fact composed of the $CD4^+$ population (12, 26). Because the MHC binding of T-cell epitopes restricts activation of T cells, MHC class II knockout mice lack activation of $CD4^+$ T cells. In one study of CVB3-induced murine myocarditis that used MHC class II knockout C57BL/6 mice, less severe myocarditis was observed than in wild-type mice, but there was an extended persistence of virus and a significant reduction in production of antiviral neutralizing antibody (88). As in the T-cell-deficient nude and SCID mice, loss of part of the immune function generates a loss of ability to clear the virus infection, although the inflammatory reaction may be reduced. In studies using CD4 knockout mice, CVB3 induced more severe myocarditis in mice with a C57BL/6 background and less severe myocarditis in mice with an A/J background, demonstrating that background strains of these knockouts affect the inflammatory response and the extent to which the immune system can control the virus infection without $CD4^+$ T cells (82). In a study using the CVB4-induced murine pancreatitis model (119), CVB4-inoculated nude and SCID mice had increased viral replication in the pancreas and increased mortality at early stages of disease, but CD4 knockout mice were protected. This work suggests that $CD4^+$ T-cell responses in the pancreas (a tissue which, in intraperitoneally inoculated mice, achieves coxsackievirus titers as high or higher and more rapidly than serum titers observed in viremia) (43, 157) may be essential for survival during early virus-induced disease, but at later times these cells participate in increased inflammatory disease. These two murine models of coxsackievirus disease contrast in both effects of reduced viral clearance and of the component of the T-cell response that contributes to the late inflammatory disease.

Early work suggesting a role for CTL in the pathologic development of myocardial lesions in CVB3-murine models of myocarditis is well established (166). CVB3-challenged knockout mice lacking perforin (the major CTL cytolytic protein) have reductions both in mortality and extent of myocarditis, compared to founder mice of the same strain (38). Treatment of mice with antibody to CD40L and B7-1, respectively, decreased the costimulatory interactions of CD40 and B7-1 on APCs with CD40L and CD28 on T cells, and thus decreased the activated T-cell response, but only reduced the extent of myocarditis in challenged mice (141, 142). The murine strain C57BL/6 is somewhat refractory to CVB3 induction of myocarditis but is susceptible to CVB3-induced death at an early stage. Henke and colleagues (57) showed that C57BL/6 knockout mice deficient for β-microglobulin (a component of MHC class I whose loss prevents presentation of peptide to the $CD8^+$ T cell) demonstrated a greater initial survival to an acute CVB3 infection. Depletion of $CD8^+$ cells from $CD4^+$ knockout mice by antibody treatment increased the cardiac virus titer upon CVB3 inoculation but decreased cardiac inflammation. Henke and colleagues (57) suggested that T cells are critical for protection against the CVB3-induced early stage death and the later development of myocarditis. Opavsky and colleagues (113) studied the response of CD8 knockout mice with an A/J background to a CVB3 infection and found an increase in myocarditis compared to nonknockout littermates. Data from these last two studies again showed that the contribution of the $CD8^+$ cells to myocarditis differs in mice with two different genetic backgrounds. Loss of $CD4^+$ T cells can result in increased survival in the early stage of CVB3-induced myocarditis, but $CD8^+$ T cells are major determinants of later stage development of myocarditis.

$CD4^+$ T-helper cell responses can be skewed to Th1 or Th2 profiles (reviewed in references 66 and 125). The Th1 response is generally characterized by production of IFN-γ, interleukin-2 (IL-2), tissue necrosis factor (TNF), and IgG2a antibodies. The Th2 response is marked by production of IL-4, IL-5, IL-10, transforming growth factor (TGF), and IgG1 antibodies in mice. The predominance of one or the other Th profile in response to virus infection is dependent on the cytokine environment at maturation of the T-helper cells, the type and avidity of the epitopes presented, the type of APC, and the costimulation of T cells by B7-1 (Th1) or B7-2 (Th2). Huber and colleagues demonstrated that a Th1-type response and increased myocarditis correlate in a comparison of infection of BALB/c mice by two CVB3 strains and virus-inoculated male mice or female mice treated with testosterone (73, 75). Seko and colleagues demonstrated that the profile of cytokines expressed by infiltrating cells in the murine heart was of the Th1 type with higher levels of IL-2, IFN-γ, and TNF-α (143). During CVB4-induced murine pancreatitis, late-stage inflammatory disease was enhanced in IL-4 knockout mice, suggesting a role for Th1 responses in this disease as well (119). The human T-cell response to conserved peptides from enterovirus capsid proteins in PBMC nuclear cells from healthy donors is also Th1 (16). The majority

```
P1-B            2005    2016 2134                                              2182     2191      2202
Surface residues             LNN  SSAE GGDSAKEFADKPVASGSNKL       R    Y
PV3 Site 2B                                NAVTSPKRE
                                                    2.3^{a,c,2}
                              2.2^{b,2}             PVASGSNKL.VQRVVYNAGMGVGVGN
                              ATLDNTPSSAELLGGDTAKEFADKPVAS
                E10^{c,1}          2.4^{a,2}                                   E12^{c,1}
                ITLGNSTITTQE       GDTAKEFADKPVASGSNKL                         INLRTNNSATIV
        CVB3-1  -----------        ---N------------S----------------.----------------  ------------
        CVB3-2  -----------        ----------------S----------------.----------------  ------------
        CVB3-3  -----------        ----------------S----------------.----------------  ------------
        CVB1    -----------        SN-N---KF---S---N-RM-T-TE-GTSND-K.--TA-W----------  ------------
        CVB2    -----------        TNKE---LFEK-C-Q-N----TREGPTISKGATD--TA-C----------  ------------
        CVB4    -----------        TNAE-A-AYGD-C--E---S-EQNAAT...GKTA--TA-C----------  ------------
        CVB5    -----------        ---A-K-DQKS-SN-E--NT-.-SQNTT-QT.A.--AN-I----------  ------------
        CVB6    -----------        SN-N-A-LA-D-SA-EV-RQ-TVE-.-N-Q-Q..--TA-H--A---A---  ------------


P1-C            3012    3023 3050           3075    3153     3163
Surface residues             Q   VGEKVNSMEAYQ  P  RSN
                E13^{c,1}    3.1^{b,2}                        E14^{c,1}
                QFLTSDDFQSP  SVVPVQNVGEKVNSMEAYQIPVRSN        HVIWDVGLQSS
        CVB3-1  -----------  -------------------------        --V--------
        CVB3-2  -----------  -------------------------        --I--------
        CVB3-3  -----------  -------------------------        --V--------
        CVB1    -----------  -----N-TDNNV-GLK------Q--        -----------
        CVB2    -----------  ----LN-IQDNLRK-DI-RVQ-S-Q        -----------
        CVB4    -----------  ----IN-LKANLMT----RVQ---T        -----------
        CVB5    -----------  -----N-TEG--S-I-------Q--        -----------
        CVB6    -----------  -----N-TETN--G-D--R---Q--        -----------


2C                      106-111
                        Tracy human and mouse T epitope
                        LEEKGI
        CVB3-1          ------
        CVB3-2          ------
        CVB3-3          ------
        CVB1            ------
        CVB2            ------
        CVB4            ------
        CVB5            ------
        CVB6            ------
```

FIGURE 1 Conservation of amino acid sequence of coxsackieviruses (B group) at sites containing T epitopes, antibody-binding sites, and neutralizing antibody sites. Surface residues are indicated (106). Genbank Accession numbers: CVB1, M16560; CVB2, AF085363; CVB3-1, -2, M88483; CVB3-3, U57056; CVB4, D00149; CVB5, AF105342; CVB6, AF105342. − indicates identical to residue indicated above; . indicates a deletion relative to the peptide sequence; a indicates antibody-binding site; b indicates neutralizing antibody-binding site; c indicates T epitope. 1, reference 16; 2, reference 3; 3, reference 47; 4, reference 74; 5, reference 49; 6, reference 122; 7, reference 15.

population of T cells express the $\alpha\beta$ TCR, but a minority class have the $\gamma\delta$ TCR, and these cells have regulatory effects on the immune response (reviewed in reference 13). In CVB3-induced murine myocarditis, adoptive transfer of murine $\gamma\delta^+$ T cells into mice challenged with a noncardiovirulent CVB3 strain increased the severity of myocarditis (72), whereas depletion of $\gamma\delta^+$ T cells reduced the extent of myocarditis. The likely explanation is that the $\gamma\delta$ T cells lyse the CD4$^+$ Th2 cells (64; reviewed in references 36 and 66). That both the in vitro proliferative T-cell response to enteroviral epitopes in humans (16) and the in vivo response in mice appear to favor a Th1 response leading to inflammatory disease suggests that modifications of the immune response to favor Th2-type responses to a coxsackievirus infection should help ameliorate the inflammatory diseases they induce.

Infection of myocardial cells in culture by CVB3 results in production of cytokines such as IL-1α and β, -6, and -8 and TNF-α (54, 143). CVB3 infection of macrophages results in increased expression of inducible nitric oxide synthase (iNOS) (171). Mice that lack the NOS2 gene have higher titers of CVB3 in heart tissue and more severe myocarditis (171). Treatment of CVB3-infected mice with IL-1 or IL-2 or TNF exacerbated inflammation in heart tissues (75, 85). In general, treating enteroviral disease in mice either with proinflammatory cytokines or with reagents to eliminate cytokines results in increased inflammation (81, 84, 85, 111, 127). In early stages of the infection, some cytokines such as IL-2 may provide some protection, presumably by stimulating immune responses important for eliminating virus-infected cells, but in late stages of the inflammatory disease, administration of cytokines can increase the extent of myocarditis (81). These findings are consistent with the observation that nude or SCID mice can suffer a virus-dependent disease in the absence of T cells (23, 66, 131, 135). Data from studies of CVB3 models of myocarditis using knockout mice indicate a pathologic role for T cells in late-stage inflammatory dis-

```
P-1D             1001           1015  1021           1035  1029           1042  1041           1055  1051           1065
Surface residues
                 VP1-1ᵃ,³,⁴            VP1-3ᵃ,ᶜ,³,⁴         E1ᶜ,¹                VP1-5ᵃ,ᶜ,³           VP1-6ᶜ,⁴
                 GPVEDAITAAIGRVA       GPNNSEAIPALTAAE      PALTAVETGATNPL       QVVPGDTMQTRHVKN      RHVKNYHSRSESTIE
        CVB3-1   ---------------       --T------------      -----A---H-SQV       ----S----------      ---------------
        CVB3-2   ---------------       --T------------      -----A---H-SQV       ----S----------      ---------------
        CVB3-3   ---------------       --T------------      -----A---H-SQV       ---------------      ---------------
        CVB1     ----ESVER-MV---       K-T----S-------      -----A---H-SQV       ----S----------      --------------S--
        CVB2     S---ES-ERS-----       --S------V---V-      -V-------H-SQV       --T-S--------H-      ---H--------SV-
        CVB4     --T-ESVER-M----       --S---Q------V-      ---------H-SQV       --D-S--------H-      ---H--------SV-
        CVB5     --PGE-VER--A---       --V---S--------      -----A---H-SQV       ----A----------      --------------V-
        CVB6     S---G--ER--A---       --T----V-----V-      ---------H-SQV       ----S-N--------      -----------TSV-

                 1069           1083  1074           1093  1083           1089
Surface residues YFTEYE   S G          YFTEYE   S G         KRYAEWV              S G         KRYAE
                                       VP1-9ᶜ,³,⁴
                                       YEN.S..GA..KRYAEWVLT KYSSAESNNLKRYAE
                 VP1-8ᵃ,³               1.3ᶜ,²                                    chimeraᶜ,⁶
                 CRSACVYFTRYKN.S..G    VYFTEYEN.S..GA..KRYAEWVL                   AESNNLKR
        CVB3-1   ---------E-E.-..-     ----------.-..--.-------I-                -N--..GA..-----
        CVB3-2   ---------E---.-..-    ----------.-..--.-------I-                -N--..GA..-----
        CVB3-3   ---------E---.-..-    ----------.-..--.---------                ----..GA..-----
        CVB1     -------YAT-N..N..S    --YAT-N..N..SE...-G-----IN                NN.N...-E..-G---
        CVB2     A-----FY-T-T-.-KNA    -FY-T-T-..KNA-KE-KF-T-KVS                 TN.-KNAAKE-KF-T
        CVB4     ------IYI..-YS-AES    -IYI..KYS-AESNNL-------IN                 ---------------
        CVB5     -------Y-T---.H..-    --Y-T-K-.H..-TDGDNF-Y--IN                 -N.H..GTDGDNF-Y
        CVB6     ---------T---.Q..T    ----T-K-.Q.T-..TN-F-S--I-                 -N.Q..TGATN-F-S

                 1087                 1109  1099          1113  1103          1117  1119                        1152
Surface residues AEWV                                                               T  QQPSTTQ                  PGGPVPD
                                                                                             VP1-14ᶜ,³,⁴
                                                                                             TQNQDAQILTHQIMY
                 1.1ᵃ,ᶜ,²              VP1-8ᵃ,³             CVB4-7ᵇ,⁵            VP1-13ᶜ,³,⁴          VP1-15ᶜ,³
                 AEWVLTPRQAAQ.LRTKLEFFTY  Q.LRRKLEFFTYVRFD  KMEMFTYIRCDMELT      VITSTQQPSTTQNQD      HQIMYVPPGGPVPD
        CVB3-1   ----L-F---V-F-L---       -.------------    -L-F---V-F-L---      ---------------      --------------
        CVB3-2   ----I------.--R-------   -.------------    -L-F---V-F-L---      --------τ------      --------------
        CVB3-3   -----------.--R-------   -.------------    -L-F---V-F-L---      ---------------      --------------
        CVB1     ----INT--V--L--R--.---   -L------.---L---  -L-.---L-F-L---      ----A-E---ATSV--PVQ-Q-----------T
        CVB2     -T-KVSV-----.--R--L---   -.------L---L-C-  -L-L---L---I---      ----A-D---AT-L-VPV--------------E
        CVB4     ----INT--V--.--R-M-M---  -.------M---M---I-C-                  ----H-EM--AT-S-VPVQ--------------
        CVB5     -Y--INT--V--.--R---M---  -.------M---A---  -L-----A-F-L---      ----EQ--I-G--SPV----------------T
        CVB6     -S--I-T--V--.--R---M---  -.------M---L---  -L-----L-F-I---      ----A-DQ--I.S---PVQ-------------T

                 1196                 1214  1219                        1253  1259                     P2A-2
Surface residues WSE SRNGV              N  NN           VNA ST P K     R      L  K        QPSG        TTTRQSITTMTNT
                 1.2ᵃ,ᶜ,²                                 VP1-24ᵃ,³,⁴                                  P1-D/P2-A
                 FSRNGVYGINTLNNM                          IKSTIRIYFKPKHVK                              VP1-28ᵃ,ᶜ,³,⁴
                 VP1-21ᵃ,ᶜ,³,⁴         VP1-23ᵃ,³,⁴         VP1-25ᵃ,ᶜ,³,⁴       VP1-27ᵃ,⁴               TTRQSITTMTNTGA
                 WSEFSRNGVYGINTLNNMG   RHVNAGSTGPIKSTI    PKHVKAWIPRPPRLC     KNVNFQPSGVTTRQ
        CVB3-1   -------------------   ---------------    ---------------     --------------
        CVB3-2   -------------------   ---------------    ---------------     --------------
        CVB3-3   -------------------   ---------------    ---------------     --------------
        CVB1     -TQ----------------   ----EAGQ------V-   ------------V-----  -----N-T------SN---...--
        CVB2     ----RHD----L-------   -----DNP-S-T--V----------------A       N----KITD--EK-D-L--...--
        CVB4     -SN-S-D-I--Y-S-----   ----DS-P-GLT-----------YV-------       -S---DVEA--AE-A-LI-...--
        CVB5     -AK-DKQ-T----------   ----D--P----V--V--------T-V------      G----E-T---ES-TE--A-QT--
        CVB6     -SD--NK-I--L-------   ----GPNPV--T--V---------V-------       RQ---TVT---ES-AN----NT---
```

FIGURE 1 *Continued.*

ease (57, 119). Similar processes may occur in human myocarditis and in human dilated cardiomyopathy, sequela of chronic myocarditis, as high or higher levels of expression of several cytokine genes have been found in endomyocardial biopsy tissue samples relative to that of control heart tissues (132).

How are B cells activated? The B-cell receptor complexed with IgM or IgD (in naive B cells) interacts with antigens and coreceptors. The B cell is then activated via a tyrosine kinase signaling cascade (6). This activation is increased if multiple B-cell receptors are cross-linked by the interaction with the antigen (such as a viral capsid). There can be additional activation provided by helper T cells by direct contact (in particular, by binding of the B-cell CD40 receptor with T-cell CD40L) or by secreting cytokines such as IL-2, -4, and -6, which activate B cells to proliferate and differentiate (115). Coxsackieviruses have been shown to induce strong neutralizing IgM, IgA$_2$, and IgG antibody responses following infections of humans or experimental animals (31).

The normal humoral immune response to an enterovirus infection is a rapid generation of antiviral IgM, followed by antiviral IgA$_2$ and IgG antibodies. An assay that eliminated competition for binding to virus among immunoglobulin classes demonstrated that anticoxsackievirus IgA and IgM were present predominantly in patients with acute enteroviral infections and that IgG3 and IgG1 subclasses dominated the IgG responses to a coxsackievirus infection (155). In mice with a CVB3 infection, IgM is detectable within 3 to 4 days postinoculation and persists for at least 8 days (35). Mice vaccinated with a temperature-sensitive mutant of CVB3 at 1 day of age possessed anti-CVB3 antibodies of both the IgG and IgM classes 4 to 6 weeks later (35). The acute anticoxsackievirus IgM response has fueled the development of tests for coxsackievirus- and enterovirus-specific IgM as an indicator of a recent infection (30, 59, 108, 134, 168). The correlation of higher levels of coxsackievirus- and enterovirus-specific IgM with a variety of diseases has been suggested as proof of a causal relationship between recent enteroviral infection and these diseases; however, many studies have demonstrated persistence of anti-enteroviral IgM (both neutralizing and virus binding) in patients with inflammatory heart disease (25, 107, 153). This correlation is not unexpected, given the higher rate of cross-reactivity seen with enteroviral IgM (93, 101, 116, 121), and the circulation in the human population of a wide variety of enterovirus serotypes increases the potential of detecting an acute immune response to a related virus. This cross-reactivity, by definition not at the NIm sites, could account for some of the differences in IgM titers measured by nonneutralizing assays (enzyme-linked immunosorbent assay [ELISA]) that use different strains of the same coxsackievirus serotype (29). In addition, the presence of enteroviruses in heart tissues of a large proportion of myocarditis patients (reviewed in references 4 and 97) suggests that persistence of enteroviruses might cause such patients to maintain an IgM response (107). These factors may limit the value of using anticoxsackievirus IgM as an indicator of a recent coxsackievirus infection (45).

The humoral immune response, i.e., the production of antibodies, has been shown to be important for protection against enteroviruses in the early stages after infection (31, 89, 156). The importance of the humoral immune response against enterovirus infection is demonstrated by the frequency of chronic enterovirus infection in patients with agammaglobulinemia (103). This disease can be held in check or cured by the use of intravenous immunoglobulin replacement therapy. In the murine model of coxsackievirus-induced myocarditis, administration of neutralizing antibody within 24 h of infection was effective at reducing myocarditis and clearing virus infection more rapidly (22, 39). However, effects other than clearing virus can be seen when immunoglobulins are administered later in infection, as CVB3-induced autoantibodies can have pathogenic effects (32) and nonspecific immunoglobulin therapy can have anti-inflammatory effects (152, 164). Early production of high titers of neutralizing antibody in mice correlated with decreased viremia and less severe myocarditis due to an experimental CVB3 inoculation (165). While numerous experimental studies demonstrate that attenuated viruses (20, 39, 172) or an inactivated virus preparation (28, 139) as well as a subunit vaccine (27) can protect against coxsackievirus-induced disease and speed virus clearance, the extent to which clearance is specifically dependent on induction of a protective antibody response is unknown. Indeed, data from a study in T-cell-deficient nude mice challenged with a CVB3 strain suggested that antibody alone was insufficient to clear the CVB3 infection (131). An interesting test of the value of the antibody response would be antibody reconstitution of the SCID mice with anti-CVB3 murine sera, followed by CVB3 challenge. To have effective protection against high levels of virus replication, neutralizing antibody must be present before or shortly after a CVB3 infection of mice (22, 39, 152, 165). Once infection of cells of the myocardium has occurred, the humoral response alone appears to be relatively ineffective at clearing coxsackievirus from the heart. This could help explain why the high levels of neutralizing antibodies in patients with chronic enteroviral myocarditis have failed to prevent the late-stage disease (53).

NIm sites are amino acid sequences located on the picornavirus capsid to which neutralizing antibodies bind, blocking infection of cells in culture and presumably in vivo. NIm sites are located by identification of altered amino acid sequences in escape mutants, viral isolates capable of replication in the presence of neutralizing antibody, or by induction of neutralizing antibodies in experimental animals via immunization with purified proteins or with synthesized peptides. A definition for neutralization sites in either group A or B coxsackieviruses is not yet at the capsid architectural level achieved for the human rhinovirus and poliovirus serotypes, in which clearly defined sites have been located on the capsid structure (60, 129, 147; reviewed in references 102 and 114). The neutralizing monoclonal antibody (MAb)-binding sites are at surface residues of the capsid (98). Studies of the structural complex of MAbs bound to virus particles or to peptides of capsid sequences indicate that the most complete neutralization reaction correlates with blocking of the binding of the virus particles to the cellular receptor protein, rather than induction of conformational changes in the capsid (58). Sequences involved in NIm sites have been located within structures exposed on the surface of the CVB3 capsid (105, 106). Peptides from CVB3 capsid sequences that are derived from sites in the CVB3 capsid that correspond to the NIm sites of polioviruses and rhinoviruses bind CVB3 antibodies (3), suggesting a similar architectural arrangement. Some of these peptides also are capable of inducing anti-CVB3 neutralizing antibody responses in rabbits (3). As reported for polioviruses, data from studies with neutralizing MAbs to CVB3 that do not bind single proteins or peptides also suggest the existence of neutralizing sites that are discontinuous and cannot easily be studied with synthetic peptides (37, 74). The existence, localization, and contribution to the total neutralizing response of other three-dimensional conformational antigenic epitopes await a comprehensive study using escape mutational analysis based on the structure of the CVB3 virus particle (105, 106).

The definitive localization of NIm sites, generated by analysis of neutralizing antibody-escape mutants and by comparison to a crystallographic structure of the capsid, is lacking in the coxsackieviruses, despite the solved structure of the CVB3 virus particle (105, 106). Other studies have used infection with recombinant viruses to test for generation of neutralizing antibodies in mice. The best evidence of this type was generated using a CVB3:CVB4 chimera in which the CVB4 P-1D (VP1) BC loop was inserted into the corresponding regions of CVB3 (100, 122). This work defined two essential amino acids within this CVB4 loop (aa 84 and 86) that are required for the neutralization of CVB4 in the context of the CVB3 capsid. This site corresponds to the NIm I site on the capsids of the polioviruses (102), in which the P-1D BC loop is prominent on the surface of the fivefold axis of symmetry of both poliovirus and CVB3 capsids (60, 105, 106). In addition, a chimeric CVB3 virus encoding the P-1D BC loops of CVB2 and CVB4 at a site between the P-1D and P2A encoding regions induced neutralizing antibodies against the CVB3 vector and against CVB2 and CVB4 as well (S. Tracy and N. Chapman, unpublished data), indicating that the BC loop region can encode neutralizing antigenic sites outside of the context of the capsid protein itself.

Additional evidence for the identity of NIm sites comes from studies of neutralizing antibodies that were generated against purified proteins and peptides (reviewed in reference 156). Beatrice and colleagues (7) identified sites within P-1B (VP2) of CVB3 using this purified protein to immunize rabbits. Subsequent immunization of rabbits with synthetic peptides derived from the sequence of P-1B, P-1C, or P-1D defined NIm sites in all three of these proteins (3). These peptides, chosen by alignment to the NIm of polioviruses, included the CVB3 P-1D BC loop (aa 74–92), portions (aa 135–163, 159–183, 150–168) of the P-1B EF loop (puff), and a peptide (aa 51–75) within the P-1C knob derived from amino acid sequences located at the surface of the CVB3 virus particle (105, 106). A study of cross-reactivity of antistreptococcal M protein murine MAbs against cardiac myosin identified a set of MAbs that were found to neutralize CVB3 (24). A comparison of the two proteins and the capsid proteins of CVB3 identified a similar sequence bordering the CVB3 P-1D BC loop (aa 84–112) that may contain a site recognized in part by each of the MAbs. One of the neutralizing MAbs was found to bind to two peptides of P-1D (aa 51–65 and 69–83) that border the BC loop (74). Peptides containing sequences of the P-1D C terminus of CVA9 can immunize rabbits to produce neutralizing antibody (117). This region in CVA9 has an extension, in comparison to the other coxsackieviruses, which contains an Arg-Gly-Asp (RGD) motif (17, 18) required for binding of the virus to the integrin receptor in some cell types (124). Another recent study of CVB4 variants that differed in a single amino acid of the P-1D protein, a Met → Thr change at a site in the DE loop in P-1D in a region that corresponds to a part of the conformational epitope NIm 1B in polioviruses, demonstrated a significant increase in neutralizing antibody titers (49). The ability of a peptide (aa 68–82 of P-1D) to block neutralizing antibody in sera of CVB4-immunized mice, coupled with the mutational evidence, indicates that the CVB4 NIm 1B site may include aa 68–78 and aa 129 of P-1D.

The applications of immunoblotting, radioimmunoassays, and ELISA have demonstrated that there are many antibody-binding sites outside of the NIm sites for enteroviruses (3, 15, 47). By using peptides whose sequences were derived from coxsackievirus or enterovirus capsid sequences, numerous amino acid sequences in the CVB3 capsid protein P-1D have been identified that have a high affinity for binding antibodies from sera of immunized animals or seropositive human patients (3, 15, 47). The N-terminal 15 amino acids of P-1D are highly specific for antibodies in sera from rabbits immunized with CVB3 (47). The P-1D aa 21–35 sequence is cross-reactive with sera from rabbits immunized with CVB1, -4, and -6 (47), but a peptide with the P-1D aa 229–243 sequence binds antibodies from sera of rabbits immunized with any of the six CVBs (47). The degree of cross-reactive binding is likely due to the degree of conservation among the enteroviruses for the amino acid sequence at this position of P-1D (Fig. 1). Immunization of rabbits with peptides from P-1D has produced antibodies that identified a common enteroviral linear epitope that is recognized by enterovirus-positive human sera as well: PALTAVETGATNPL (15, 62, 130). The sequence of this peptide overlaps with that of the cross-reactive CVB P-1D aa 21–35 peptide studied by Haarmann and colleagues (47). A similar peptide (PALTAV-ETGHTSQVC) from the CVA9 P-1D sequence also generated antibodies in rabbits capable of binding both CVA9 and CVB4 virus preparations in ELISA (117). In addition to the shared epitopes in structural proteins, peptides derived from the nonstructural proteins, P-2C and P-3D, and recombinant P-2C can induce antibodies that are cross-reactive for the enteroviruses (3, 50). Sites on the N-terminal peptides of capsid protein P-1D are not exposed on the surface of the solved structure of CVB3 (105, 106), confirming the existence of antigenic sites in the virus capsid that are not presented at the surface (101, 121). Such cross-reactive antigens can be exposed by heating or disrupting virions (79). The use of peptides from conserved regions of the enterovirus capsid to screen patients for past coxsackievirus infections (47) should be enhanced by further determination of the extent and location of variation in the conformational epitopes of coxsackievirus capsids within and between serotypes (126).

Autoimmunity has been postulated to play a role in coxsackievirus-induced inflammation (reviewed in reference 37), starting with early studies demonstrating the induction of cytolytic responses to uninfected myocytes in CVB3-induced murine myocarditis (68). Antibodies reactive to cardiac tissues in human myocarditis and dilated cardiomyopathy (95, 136, 150) and cross-reactive antigens between coxsackieviruses and heart tissue have been described (11, 24, 32, 34, 65, 148). Pathogenic reactions can be induced in normal mice with transferred antibodies (32, 37) or lymphocytes (74) from CVB3-inoculated mice. In addition, a peptide of glutamic acid decarboxylase (GAD65) with similarities to a peptide of the 2C region of coxsackieviruses (80) has been found to bind antibodies from patients with type 1 diabetes (61, 91), and T cells from patients with type 1 diabetes proliferate in response to GAD65 and CVB4 P-2C protein (78, 133, 160). The significance of this cross-reactivity is not clear, but these and other serologic data, and the isolation of coxsackievirus from the pancreas of an acute case of diabetes (167) and of a mouse model of CVB-induced diabetes (77, 154), have cumulatively been used to suggest the involvement of coxsackieviruses or other enteroviruses in the induction of type 1 diabetes (118). Autoimmunity can be generated by viruses through antigenic mimicry (cross-reactive epitopes) or by presentation of self-antigens exposed to the immune system through viral and immune system-mediated lysis of host cells, and activation of the response to those antigens in the environment of active inflammation (36, 104, 173). The potential for antigenic mimicry exists in coxsackievirus particles and, in the context of an active antiviral immune response, the potential also exists for presentation of self-antigens in the presence of higher levels of virus-induced cytokines and T-cell costimulation. Cardiac myosin-induced myocarditis (109, 128), a T-cell-mediated disease (151), demonstrates the pathogenic significance of immune reactions to this protein in myocarditis, but whether the coxsackievirus infection induces this self-reactivity through antigenic mimicry or by the lysis of cells to release self-antigens in an inflammatory context is not clear. Whether the pathogenic self-reactivity is due primarily to antibodies or cell-mediated responses is also unclear, although it appears that intact cardiomyocytes are not targets of CTL (110). Murine models of the coxsackievirus-induced disease suggest that while autoreactive antibodies are generated in coxsackievirus infections, the cell-mediated immune response may have greater weight in the generation of pathogenic inflammation in the heart or pancreas.

In conclusion, immune responses against coxsackieviruses have been explored through the use of murine models of virus-induced heart and pancreatic diseases. Although neutralizing antigenic sites on the coxsackievirus particles have not been as well mapped as those for polioviruses and rhinoviruses, studies with peptides have located both antibody-binding sites and T-cell epitopes within the capsid proteins of CVB3, and they map within similar surface regions on virus particles described for other picornaviruses. While the extent of pathology induced by coxsackievirus-mediated lysis in immunodeficient mice can be significant in both cardiac and pancreatic diseases in mice, the importance of the cell-mediated immune response and the induction of apparent autoimmunity in the generation of pathologic damage in human disease is clear. Use of murine models of myocarditis for over 20 years has demonstrated both protective and pathogenic aspects of the immune response to group B coxsackieviruses. The diversity of inbred mouse lines and viral strains leaves the significance of studies to be resolved by comparison with human disease or by a methodical dissection of the immune response to coxsackieviruses generated in the various murine strains.

NOTE ADDED IN PROOF

This chapter was completed in August 2000 and does not review material on the immunology of coxsackieviruses published after this date.

REFERENCES

1. **Anderson, D. R., C. M. Carthy, J. E. Wilson, D. Yang, D. V. Devine, and B. M. McManus.** 1997. Complement component 3 interactions with coxsackievirus B3 capsid proteins: innate immunity and the rapid formation of splenic antiviral germinal centers. *J. Virol.* **71:**8841–8845.
2. **Anderson, D. R., J. E. Wilson, C. M. Carthy, D. Yang, R. Kandolf, and B. M. McManus.** 1996. Direct interactions of coxsackievirus B3 with immune cells in the splenic compartment of mice susceptible or resistant to myocarditis. *J. Virol.* **70:**4632–4645.
3. **Auvinen, P., M. J. Makela, M. Roivainen, M. Kallajoki, R. Vainionpaa, and T. Hyypia.** 1993 Mapping of antigenic sites of coxsackievirus B3 by synthetic peptides. *APMIS* **101:**517–528.
4. **Baboonian, C., M. J. Davies, J. C. Booth, and W. J. McKenna.** 1997. Coxsackie B viruses and human heart disease. *Curr. Top. Microbiol. Immunol.* **223:**31–52.
5. **Bachmann, M. F., and R. M. Zinkernagel.** 1996. Virus structure, antibody response and virus serotypes. *Immunol. Today* **17:**553–558.
6. **Baixeras, E., G. Kroemer, E. Cuende, C. Marquez, L. Bosca, J. E. Ales Martinez, and C. Martinez.** 1993. Signal transduction pathways involved in B-cell induction. *Immunol. Rev.* **132:**5–47.
7. **Beatrice, S. T., M. G. Katze, B. A. Zajac, and R. L. Crowell.** 1980. Induction of neutralizing antibodies by the coxsackievirus B3 virion polypeptide, VP2. *Virology* **104:**426–438.
8. **Beck, M. A., and S. M. Tracy.** 1989. Murine cell-mediated immune response recognizes an enterovirus group-specific antigen(s). *J. Virol.* **63:**4148–4156.
9. **Beck, M. A., and S. M. Tracy.** 1990. Evidence for a group-specific enteroviral antigen(s) recognized by human T cells. *J. Clin. Microbiol.* **28:**1822–1827.
10. **Beck, M. A., S. Tracy, B. A. Coller, N. M. Chapman, G. Hufnagel, J. E. Johnson, and G. Lomonossoff.** 1992. Comoviruses and enteroviruses share a T cell epitope. *Virology* **186:**238–246.
11. **Beisel, K. W., J. Srinivasappa, and B. S. Prabhakar.** 1991. Identification of a putative shared epitope between coxsackie virus B4 and alpha cardiac myosin heavy chain. *Clin. Exp. Immunol.* **86:**49–55.
12. **Blay, R., K. Simpson, K. Leslie, and S. Huber.** 1989. Coxsackievirus-induced disease. CD4+ cells initiate both myocarditis and pancreatitis in DBA/2 mice. *Am. J. Pathol.* **135:**899–907.
13. **Born, W., C. Cady, J. Jones-Carson, A. Mukasa, M. Lahn, and R. O'Brien.** 1999. Immunoregulatory functions of gamma delta T cells. *Adv. Immunol.* **71:**77–144.
14. **Carroll, M. C.** 1998. The role of complement and complement receptors in induction and regulation of immunity. *Annu. Rev. Immunol.* **16:**545–568.
15. **Cello, J., A. Samuelson, P. Stalhandske, B. Svennerholm, S. Jeansson, and M. Forsgren.** 1993. Identification of group-common linear epitopes in structural and nonstructural proteins of enteroviruses by using synthetic peptides. *J. Clin. Microbiol.* **31:**911–916.
16. **Cello, J., O. Strannegard, and B. Svennerholm.** 1996. A study of the cellular immune response to enteroviruses in humans: identification of cross-reactive T cell epitopes on the structural proteins of enteroviruses. *J. Gen. Virol.* **77:**2097–2108.
17. **Chang, K. H., P. Auvinen, T. Hyypia, and G. Stanway.** 1989. The nucleotide sequence of coxsackievirus A9; implications for receptor binding and enterovirus classification. *J. Gen. Virol.* **70:**3269–3280.
18. **Chang, K. H., C. Day, J. Walker, T. Hyypia, and G. Stanway.** 1992. The nucleotide sequences of wild-type coxsackievirus A9 strains imply that an RGD motif in VP1 is functionally significant. *J. Gen. Virol.* **73:**621–626.
19. **Chapman, N., C. Gauntt, and S. Tracy.** 1999. Enteroviruses. *In The Encyclopedia of Life Sciences.* Macmillian Reference Limited, London, United Kingdom.
20. **Chapman, N. M., A. Ragland, J. S. Leser, K. Hofling, S. Willian, B. L. Semler, and S. Tracy.** 2000. A group B coxsackievirus/poliovirus 5′ nontranslated region chimera can act as an attenuated vaccine strain in mice. *J. Virol.* **74:**4047–4056.
21. **Chapman, N. M., A. Ramsingh, and S. Tracy.** 1997. Genetics of coxsackievirus virulence. *Curr. Top. Microbiol. Immunol.* **223:**227–258.
22. **Cho, C. T., K. K. Feng, V. P. McCarthy, and M. F. Lenahan.** 1982. Role of antiviral antibodies in resistance against coxsackievirus B3 infection: interaction between preexisting antibodies and an interferon inducer. *Infect. Immun.* **37:**720–727.
23. **Chow, L. H., K. W. Beisel, and B. M. McManus.** 1992. Enteroviral infection of mice with severe combined immunodeficiency. Evidence for direct viral pathogenesis of myocardial injury. *Lab. Invest.* **66:**24–31.
24. **Cunningham, M. W., S. M. Antone, J. M. Gulizia, B. M. McManus, V. A. Fischetti, and C. J. Gauntt.** 1992. Cytotoxic and viral neutralizing antibodies crossreact with streptococcal M protein, enteroviruses, and human cardiac myosin. *Proc. Natl. Acad. Sci. USA* **89:**1320–1324.
25. **Eggers, H. J., and T. Mertens.** 1986. Persistence of coxsackie B virus-specific IgM. *Lancet* **2:**284.
26. **Estrin, M., and S. A. Huber.** 1987. Coxsackievirus B3-induced myocarditis. Autoimmunity is L3T4$^+$ T helper cell and IL-2 independent in BALB/c mice. *Am. J. Pathol.* **127:**335–341.
27. **Fohlman, J., N. G. Ilback, G. Friman, and B. Morein.** 1990. Vaccination of Balb/c mice against enteroviral mediated myocarditis. *Vaccine* **8:**381–384.
28. **Fohlman, J., K. Pauksen, G. Morein, U. Bjare, N. G. Ilback, and G. Friman.** 1993. High yield production of

an inactivated coxsackie B3 adjuvant vaccine with protective effect against experimental myocarditis. *Scand. J. Infect. Dis. Suppl.* **88:**103–108.
29. **Frisk, G., and H. Diderholm.** 1997. Antibody responses to different strains of coxsackie B4 virus in patients with newly diagnosed type I diabetes mellitus or aseptic meningitis. *J. Infect.* **34:**205–210.
30. **Frisk, G., G. Friman, T. Tuvemo, J. Fohlman, and H. Diderholm.** 1992. Coxsackie B virus IgM in children at onset of type 1 (insulin-dependent) diabetes mellitus: evidence for IgM induction by a recent or current infection. *Diabetologia* **35:**249–253.
31. **Gauntt, C. J.** 1997. Roles of the humoral response in coxsackievirus B-induced disease. *Curr. Top. Microbiol. Immunol.* **223:**259–282.
32. **Gauntt, C. J., H. M. Arizpe, A. L. Higdon, M. M. Rozek, R. Crawley, and M. W. Cunningham.** 1991. Anti-coxsackievirus B3 neutralizing antibodies with pathological potential. *Eur. Heart J.* **12**(Suppl. D)**:**124–129.
33. **Gauntt, C. J., E. K. Godeny, C. W. Lutton, H. M. Arizpe, N. M. Chapman, S. M. Tracy, G. E. Revtyak, A. J. Valente, and M. M. Rozek.** 1989. Mechanism(s) of coxsackievirus-induced acute myocarditis in the mouse, p. 161–182. *In* L. M. de la Maza and E. M. Peterson (ed.), *Medical Virology 8*. Plenum, New York, N.Y.
34. **Gauntt, C. J., A. L. Higdon, H. M. Arizpe, M. R. Tamayo, R. Crawley, R. D. Henkel, M. E. Pereira, S. M. Tracy, and M. W. Cunningham.** 1993. Epitopes shared between coxsackievirus B3 (CVB3) and normal heart tissue contribute to CVB3-induced murine myocarditis. *Clin. Immunol. Immunopathol.* **68:**129–134.
35. **Gauntt, C. J., R. E. Paque, M. D. Trousdale, R. J. Gudvangen, D. T. Barr, G. J. Lipotich, T. J. Nealon, and P. S. Duffey.** 1983. Temperature-sensitive mutant of coxsackievirus B3 establishes resistance in neonatal mice that protects them during adolescence against coxsackievirus B3-induced myocarditis. *Infect. Immun.* **39:**851–864.
36. **Gauntt, C. J., P. Sakkinen, N. R. Rose, and S. A. Huber.** 1998. Picornaviruses: immunopathology and autoimmunity. *In* M. W. Cunningham and R. S. Fujinami (ed.), *Effects of Microbes on the Immune System*. Lippincott-Raven Publishers, Philadelphia, Pa.
37. **Gauntt, C. J., S. M. Tracy, N. Chapman, H. J. Wood, P. C. Kolbeck, A. G. Karaganis, C. L. Winfrey, and M. W. Cunningham.** 1995. Coxsackievirus-induced chronic myocarditis in murine models. *Eur. Heart J.* **16**(Suppl. O)**:**56–58.
38. **Gebhard, J. R., C. M. Perry, S. Harkins, T. Lane, I. Mena, V. C. Asensio, and I. L. Campbell.** 1998. Coxsackievirus B3-induced myocarditis: perforin exacerbates disease, but plays no detectable role in virus clearance. *Am. J. Pathol.* **153:**417–428.
39. **Godeny, E. K., H. M. Arizpe, and C. J. Gauntt.** 1988. Characterization of the antibody response in vaccinated mice protected against coxsackievirus B3-induced myocarditis. *Viral Immunol.* **1:**305–313.
40. **Godeny, E. K., and C. J. Gauntt.** 1986. Involvement of natural killer cells in coxsackievirus B3-induced murine myocarditis. *J. Immunol.* **137:**1695–1702.
41. **Godeny, E. K., and C. J. Gauntt.** 1987. Murine natural killer cells limit coxsackievirus B3 replication. *J. Immunol.* **139:**913–918.
42. **Godeny, E. K., and C. J. Gauntt.** 1987. In situ immune autoradiographic identification of cells in heart tissues of mice with coxsackievirus B3-induced myocarditis. *Am. J. Pathol.* **129:**267–276.
43. **Gomez, R., E. Lascano, and M. Berria.** 1991. Murine acinar pancreatitis preceding necrotizing myocarditis after coxsackievirus B3 inoculation. *J. Med. Virol.* **35:**71–75.
44. **Graham, S., E. C. Wang, O. Jenkins, and L. K. Borysiewicz.** 1993. Analysis of the human T-cell response to picornaviruses: identification of T-cell epitopes close to B-cell epitopes in poliovirus. *J. Virol.* **67:**1627–1637.
45. **Graves, P. M., J. M. Norris, M. A. Pallansch, I. C. Gerling, and M. Rewers.** 1997. The role of enteroviral infections in the development of IDDM: limitations of current approaches. *Diabetes* **46:**161–168.
46. **Guthrie, M., P. A. Lodge, and S. A. Huber.** 1984. Cardiac injury in myocarditis induced by coxsackievirus group B, type 3 in Balb/c mice is mediated by Lyt 2 + cytolytic lymphocytes. *Cell. Immunol.* **88:**558–567.
47. **Haarmann, C. M., P. L. Schwimmbeck, T. Mertens, H. P. Schultheiss, and B. E. Strauer.** 1994. Identification of serotype-specific and nonserotype-specific B-cell epitopes of coxsackie B virus using synthetic peptides. *Virology* **200:**318–389.
48. **Hahn, S., R. Gehri, and P. Erb.** 1995. Mechanism and biological significance of CD4-mediated cytotoxicity. *Immunol. Rev.* **146:**57–79.
49. **Halim, S., and A. I. Ramsingh.** 2000. A point mutation in VP1 of coxsackievirus B4 alters antigenicity. *Virology* **269:**86–94.
50. **Harkonen, T., T. Hovi, and M. Roivainen.** 1997. Expression of coxsackievirus B4 proteins VP0 and 2C in *Escherichia coli* and generation of virus protein recognizing antisera. *J. Virol. Methods* **69:**147–158.
51. **Hashimoto, I., and T. Komatsu.** 1978. Myocardial changes after infection with Coxsackie virus B3 in nude mice. *Br. J. Exp. Pathol.* **59:**13–20.
52. **Hathaway, L. J., and J. P. Kraehenbuhl.** 2000. The role of M cells in mucosal immunity. *Cell Mol. Life Sci.* **57:** 323–332.
53. **Heim, A., I. Grumbach, S. Hake, G. Muller, P. Pring-Akerblom, G. Mall, and H. R. Figulla.** 1997. Enterovirus heart disease of adults: a persistent, limited organ infection in the presence of neutralizing antibodies. *J. Med. Virol.* **53:**196–204.
54. **Heim, A., S. Zeuke, S. Weiss, W. Ruschewski, and I. M. Grumbach.** 2000. Transient induction of cytokine production in human myocardial fibroblasts by coxsackievirus B3. *Circ. Res.* **86:**753–759.
55. **Heinz, B. A., and D. O. Cliver.** 1988. Coxsackievirus-cell interactions that initiate infection in porcine ileal explants. *Arch. Virol.* **101:**35–47.
56. **Heinz, B. A., D. O. Cliver, and B. Donohoe.** 1987. Enterovirus replication in porcine ileal explants. *J. Gen. Virol.* **68:**2495–2499.
57. **Henke, A., S. Huber, A. Stelzner, and J. L. Whitton.** 1995. The role of CD8+ T lymphocytes in coxsackievirus B3-induced myocarditis. *J. Virol.* **69:**6720–6728.
58. **Hewat, E. A., T. C. Marlovits, and D. Blaas.** 1998. Structure of a neutralizing antibody bound monovalently to human rhinovirus 2. *J. Virol.* **72:**4396–4402.
59. **Hillerdal, G., G. Frisk, O. Nettelbladt, and H. Diderholm.** 1992. High frequency of IgM antibodies to coxsackie B virus in sarcoidosis patients and patients with asbestos-related lesions. *Sarcoidosis* **9:**39–42.
60. **Hogle, J. M., and D. J. Filman.** 1989. The antigenic structure of poliovirus. *Philos. Trans. R. Soc. Lond. B. Biol. Sci.* **323:**467–478.
61. **Hou, J., C. Said, D. Franchi, P. Dockstader, and N. K. Chatterjee.** 1994. Antibodies to glutamic acid decarboxylase and P2-C peptides in sera from coxsackie virus B4-infected mice and IDDM patients. *Diabetes* **43:**1260–1266.
62. **Hovi, T., and M. Roivainen.** 1993. Peptide antisera targeted to a conserved sequence in poliovirus capsid VP1 cross-react widely with members of the genus *Enterovirus*. *J. Clin. Microbiol.* **31:**1083–1087.

63. **Huber, S. A.** 1997. Coxsackievirus-induced myocarditis is dependent on distinct immunopathogenic responses in different strains of mice. *Lab. Invest.* **76:**691–701.
64. **Huber, S.A., R. C. Budd, K. Rossner, and M. K. Newell.** 1999. Apoptosis in coxsackievirus B3-induced myocarditis and dilated cardiomyopathy. *Ann. N. Y. Acad. Sci.* **887:**181–190.
65. **Huber, S. A., and M. W. Cunningham.** 1996. Streptococcal M protein peptide with similarity to myosin induces CD4+ T cell-dependent myocarditis in MRL/++ mice and induces partial tolerance against coxsackieviral myocarditis. *J. Immunol.* **156:**3528–3534.
66. **Huber, S. A., C. J. Gauntt, and P. Sakkinen.** 1998. Enteroviruses and myocarditis: viral pathogenesis through replication, cytokine induction, and immunopathogenicity. *Adv. Virus Res.* **51:**35–80.
67. **Huber, S. A., N. Heintz, and R. Tracy.** 1988. Coxsackievirus B-3-induced myocarditis. Virus and actinomycin D treatment of myocytes induces novel antigens recognized by cytolytic T lymphocytes. *J. Immunol.* **141:**3214–3219.
68. **Huber, S. A., L. P. Job, K. R. Auld, and J. F. Woodruff.** 1981. Sex-related differences in the rapid production of cytotoxic spleen cells active against uninfected myofibers during coxsackievirus B-3 infection. *J. Immunol.* **126:**1336–1340.
69. **Huber, S. A., L. P. Job, and J. F. Woodruff.** 1980. Lysis of infected myofibers by coxsackievirus B-3-immune T lymphocytes. *Am. J. Pathol.* **98:**681–694.
70. **Huber, S. A., and P. A. Lodge.** 1984. Coxsackievirus B-3 myocarditis in Balb/c mice. Evidence for autoimmunity to myocyte antigens. *Am. J. Pathol.* **116:**21–29.
71. **Huber, S. A., A. Moraska, and M. Cunningham.** 1994. Alterations in major histocompatibility complex association of myocarditis induced by coxsackievirus B3 mutants selected with monoclonal antibodies to group A streptococci. *Proc. Natl. Acad. Sci. USA* **91:**5543–5547.
72. **Huber, S. A., A. Mortensen, and G. Moulton.** 1996. Modulation of cytokine expression by CD4+ T cells during coxsackievirus B3 infections of BALB/c mice initiated by cells expressing the gamma delta + T-cell receptor. *J. Virol.* **70:**3039–3044.
73. **Huber, S. A., and B. Pfaeffle.** 1994. Differential Th1 and Th2 cell responses in male and female BALB/c mice infected with coxsackievirus group B type 3. *J. Virol.* **68:**5126–5132.
74. **Huber, S., J. Polgar, A. Moraska, M. Cunningham, P. Schwimmbeck, and P. Schultheiss.** 1993. T lymphocyte responses in CVB3-induced murine myocarditis. *Scand. J. Infect. Dis. Suppl.* **88:**67–78.
75. **Huber, S. A., J. Polgar, P. Schultheiss, and P. Schwimmbeck.** 1994. Augmentation of pathogenesis of coxsackievirus B3 infections in mice by exogenous administration of interleukin-1 and interleukin-2. *J. Virol.* **68:**195–206.
76. **Hufnagel, G., N. Chapman, and S. Tracy.** 1995. A noncardiovirulent strain of coxsackievirus B3 causes myocarditis in mice with severe combined immunodeficiency syndrome. *Eur. Heart. J.* **16**(Suppl. O)**:**18–19.
77. **Kang, Y., N. K. Chatterjee, M. J. Nodwell, and J. W. Yoon.** 1994. Complete nucleotide sequence of a strain of coxsackie B4 virus of human origin that induces diabetes in mice and its comparison with nondiabetogenic coxsackie B4 JBV strain. *J. Med. Virol.* **44:**353–361.
78. **Karlsson, M. G., and J. Ludvigsson.** 1998. Peptide from glutamic acid decarboxylase similar to coxsackie B virus stimulates IFN-gamma mRNA expression in Th1-like lymphocytes from children with recent-onset insulin-dependent diabetes mellitus. *Acta Diabetol.* **35:**137–144.
79. **Katze, M. G., and R. L. Crowell.** 1980. Immunological studies of the group B coxsackieviruses by the sandwich enzyme-linked immunosorbent assay (ELISA) and immunoprecipitation. *J. Gen. Virol.* **50:**357–367.
80. **Kaufman, D. L, M. G. Lander, M. Clare-Salzler, M. A. Atkinson, N. K. Maclaren, and A. J. Tobin.** 1992. Autoimmunity to two forms of glutamate decarboxylase in insulin-dependent diabetes mellitus. *J. Clin. Invest.* **89:**283–292.
81. **Kishimoto, C., Y. Kuroki, Y. Hiraoka, H. Ochiai, M. Kurokawa, and S. Sasayama.** 1994. Cytokine and murine coxsackievirus B3 myocarditis. Interleukin-2 suppressed myocarditis in the acute stage but enhanced the condition in the subsequent stage. *Circulation* **89:**2836–2842.
82. **Knowlton, K. U., and C. Badorff.** 1999. The immune system in viral myocarditis: maintaining the balance. *Circ. Res.* **85:**559–561.
83. **Kutubuddin, M., J. Simons, and M. Chow.** 1992. Identification of T-helper epitopes in the VP1 capsid protein of poliovirus. *J. Virol.* **66:**3042–3047.
84. **Lane, J. R., D. A. Neumann, A. Lafond-Walker, A. Herskowitz, and N. R. Rose.** 1991. LPS promotes CB3-induced myocarditis in resistant B10.A mice. *Cell. Immunol.* **136:**219–233.
85. **Lane, J. R., D. A. Neumann, A. Lafond-Walker, A. Herskowitz, and N. R. Rose.** 1992. Interleukin 1 or tumor necrosis factor can promote coxsackie B3-induced myocarditis in resistant B10.A mice. *J. Exp. Med.* **175:**1123–1129.
86. **Lanier, L. L.** 1998. NK cell receptors. *Annu. Rev. Immunol.* **16:**359–393.
87. **Leclerc, C., E. Deriaud, V. Mimic, and S. van der Werf.** 1991. Identification of a T-cell epitope adjacent to neutralization antigenic site 1 of poliovirus type 1. *J. Virol.* **65:**711–718.
88. **Leipner, C., M. Borchers, I. Merkle, and A. Stelzner.** 1999. Coxsackievirus B3-induced myocarditis in MHC class II-deficient mice. *J. Hum. Virol.* **2:**102–114.
89. **Leslie, K., R. Blay, C. Haisch, A. Lodge, A. Weller, and S. Huber.** 1989. Clinical and experimental aspects of viral myocarditis. *Clin. Microbiol. Rev.* **2:**191–203.
90. **Liu, P., J. Penninger, K. Aitken, M. Sole, and T. Mak.** 1995. The role of transgenic knockout models in defining the pathogenesis of viral heart disease. *Eur. Heart J.* **16**(Suppl. O)**:**25–27.
91. **Lonnrot, M., H. Hyoty, M. Knip, M. Roivainen, P. Kulmala, P. Leinikki, H. K. Akerblom, and Childhood Diabetes in Finland Study Group.** 1996. Antibody cross-reactivity induced by the homologous regions in glutamic acid decarboxylase (GAD65) and 2C protein of coxsackievirus B4. *Clin. Exp. Immunol.* **104:**398–405.
92. **Luppi, P., W. A. Rudert, M. M. Zanone, G. Stassi, G. Trucco, D. Finegold, G. J. Boyle, P. Del Nido, F. X. McGowan, Jr., and M. Trucco.** 1998. Idiopathic dilated cardiomyopathy: a superantigen-driven autoimmune disease. *Circulation* **98:**777–785.
93. **Magnius, L. O., L. H. Saleh, T. Vikerfors, and H. Norder.** 1988. A solid-phase reverse immunosorbent test for the detection of enterovirus IgM. *J. Virol. Methods* **20:**73–82.
94. **Mahon, B. P., K. Katrak, and K. H. Mills.** 1992. Antigenic sequences of poliovirus recognized by T cells: serotype-specific epitopes on VP1 and VP3 and cross-reactive epitopes on VP4 defined by using CD4+ T-cell clones. *J. Virol.* **66:**7012–7020.
95. **Maisch, B., E. Bauer, M. Cirsi, and K. Kochsiek.** 1993. Cytolytic cross-reactive antibodies directed against the cardiac membrane and viral proteins in coxsackievirus B3 and B4 myocarditis. Characterization and pathogenetic relevance. *Circulation* **87**(Suppl. 5)**:**IV49–65.
96. **Mandelboim, O., S. B. Wilson, M. Vales-Gomez, H. T. Reyburn, and J. L. Strominger.** 1997. Loading of MHC

I with peptides with P8 K prevents binding of inhibitory receptor. *Proc. Natl. Acad. Sci. USA* **94:**4604–4609.
97. **Martino, T. A., P. Liu, M. Petric, and M. J. Sole.** 1995. Enteroviral myocarditis and dilated cardiomyopathy: a review of clinical and experimental studies, p. 291–351. In H. Rotbart (ed.), *Human Enterovirus Infections*. ASM Press, Washington, D.C.
98. **Mateu, M. G.** 1995. Antibody recognition of picornaviruses and escape from neutralization: a structural view. *Virus Res.* **38:**1–24.
99. **Matteucci, D., M. Paglianti, A. M. Giangregorio, M. R. Capobianchi, F. Dianzani, and M. Bendinelli.** 1985. Group B coxsackieviruses readily establish persistent infections in human lymphoid cell lines. *J. Virol.* **56:**651–654.
100. **McPhee, F., R. Zell, B. Y. Reimann, P. H. Hofschneider, and R. Kandolf.** 1994. Characterization of the N-terminal part of the neutralizing antigenic site I of coxsackievirus B4 by mutation analysis of antigen chimeras. *Virus Res.* **34:**139–151.
101. **Mertens, T., U. Pika, and H. J. Eggers.** 1983. Cross antigenicity among enteroviruses as revealed by immunoblot technique. *Virology* **129:**431–442.
102. **Minor, P. D., M. Ferguson, D. M. Evans, J. W. Almond, and J. P. Icenogle.** 1986. Antigenic structure of polioviruses of serotypes 1, 2 and 3. *J. Gen. Virol.* **67:**1283–1291.
103. **Misbah, S. A., G. P. Spickett, P. C. Ryba, J. M. Hockaday, J. S. Kroll, C. Sherwood, J. B. Kurtz, E. R. Moxon, and H. M. Chapel.** 1992. Chronic enteroviral meningoencephalitis in agammaglobulinemia: case report and literature review. *J. Clin. Immunol.* **12:**266–270.
104. **Mondino, A., A. Khoruts, and M. K. Jenkins.** 1996. The anatomy of T-cell activation and tolerance. *Proc. Natl. Acad. Sci. USA* **93:**2245–2252.
105. **Muckelbauer, J. K., M. Kremer, I. Minor, G. Diana, F. J. Dutko, J. Groarke, D. C. Pevear, and M. G. Rossmann.** 1995. The structure of coxsackievirus B3 at 3.5 A resolution. *Structure* **3:**653–667.
106. **Muckelbauer, J. K., and M. G. Rossmann.** 1997. The structure of coxsackievirus B3. *Curr. Top Microbiol. Immunol.* **223:**191–208.
107. **Muir, P., F. Nicholson, A. J. Tilzey, M. Signy, T. A. English, and J. E. Banatvala.** 1989. Chronic relapsing pericarditis and dilated cardiomyopathy: serological evidence of persistent enterovirus infection. *Lancet* **1:**804–807.
108. **Muir, P., F. Nicholson, S. J. Illavia, T. S. McNeil, J. F. Ajetunmobi, H. Dunn, W. G. Starkey, K. N. Reetoo, N. R. Cary, J. Parameshwar, and J. E. Banatvala.** 1996. Serological and molecular evidence of enterovirus infection in patients with end-stage dilated cardiomyopathy. *Heart* **76:**243–249.
109. **Neu, N., R. Klieber, M. Fruhwirth, and P. Berger.** 1991. Cardiac myosin-induced myocarditis as a model of postinfectious autoimmunity. *Eur. Heart J.* **12**(Suppl. D):117–120.
110. **Neu, N., B. Ploier, and C. Ofner.** 1990. Cardiac myosin-induced myocarditis. Heart autoantibodies are not involved in the induction of the disease. *J. Immunol.* **145:**4094–4100.
111. **Neumann, D. A., J. R. Lane, G. S. Allen, A. Herskowitz, and N. R. Rose.** 1993. Viral myocarditis leading to cardiomyopathy: do cytokines contribute to pathogenesis? *Clin. Immunol. Immunopathol.* **68:**181–190.
112. **Neutra, M. R., A. Frey, and J. P. Kraehenbuhl.** 1996. Epithelial M cells: gateways for mucosal infection and immunization. *Cell* **86:**345–348.
113. **Opavsky, M. A., J. Penninger, K. Aitken, W. H. Wen, F. Dawood, T. Mak, and P. Liu.** 1999. Susceptibility to myocarditis is dependent on the response of alphabeta T lymphocytes to coxsackieviral infection. *Circ. Res.* **85:**551–558.
114. **Page, G. S., A. G. Mosser, J. M. Hogle, D. J. Filman, R. R. Rueckert, and M. Chow.** 1988. Three-dimensional structure of poliovirus serotype 1 neutralizing determinants. *J. Virol.* **62:**1781–1794.
115. **Parker, D. C.** 1993. T cell-dependent B cell activation. *Annu. Rev. Immunol.* **11:**331–360.
116. **Pozzetto, B., O. G. Gaudin, F. R. Lucht, J. Hafid, and A. Ros.** 1990. Detection of immunoglobulin G, M, and A antibodies to enterovirus structural proteins by immunoblot technique in echovirus type 4-infected patients. *J. Virol. Methods* **29:**143–155.
117. **Pulli, T., M. Roivainen, T. Hovi, and T. Hyypia.** 1998. Induction of neutralizing antibodies by synthetic peptides representing the C terminus of coxsackievirus A9 capsid protein VP1. *J. Gen. Virol.* **79:**2249–2253.
118. **Ramsingh, A., N. Chapman, and S. Tracy.** 1997. Coxsackieviruses and diabetes. *Bioessays* **19:**793–800.
119. **Ramsingh, A. I., W. T. Lee, D. N. Collins, and L. E. Armstrong.** 1999. T cells contribute to disease severity during coxsackievirus B4 infection. *J. Virol.* **73:**3080–3086.
120. **Ramsingh, A., J. Slack, J. Silkworth, and A. Hixson.** 1989. Severity of disease induced by a pancreatropic coxsackie B4 virus correlates with the H-2Kq locus of the major histocompatibility complex. *Virus Res.* **14:**347–358.
121. **Reigel, F., F. Burkhardt, and U. Schilt.** 1985. Cross-reactions of immunoglobulin M and G antibodies with enterovirus-specific viral structural proteins. *J. Hyg. (London)* **95:**469–481.
122. **Reimann, B. Y., R. Zell, and R. Kandolf.** 1991. Mapping of a neutralizing antigenic site of coxsackievirus B4 by construction of an antigen chimera. *J. Virol.* **65:**3475–3480.
123. **Robinson, J. A., J. B. O'Connell, L. M. Roeges, E. O. Major, and R. M. Gunnar.** 1981. Coxsackie B3 myocarditis in athymic mice. *Proc. Soc. Exp. Biol. Med.* **166:**80–91.
124. **Roivainen, M., T. Hyypia, L. Piirainen, N. Kalkkinen, G. Stanway, and T. Hovi.** 1991. RGD-dependent entry of coxsackievirus A9 into host cells and its bypass after cleavage of VP1 protein by intestinal proteases. *J. Virol.* **65:**4735–4740.
125. **Romagnani, S.** 1996. Th1 and Th2 in human diseases. *Clin. Immunol. Immunopathol.* **80:**225–235.
126. **Romero, J. R., C. Price, and J. J. Dunn.** 1997. Genetic divergence among the group B coxsackieviruses. *Curr. Top. Microbiol. Immunol.* **223:**97–152.
127. **Rose, N. R., and S. L. Hill.** 1996. The pathogenesis of postinfectious myocarditis. *Clin. Immunol. Immunopathol.* **80:**S92–S99.
128. **Rose, N. R., and S. L. Hill.** 1996. Autoimmune myocarditis. *Int. J. Cardiol.* **54:**171–175.
129. **Rossmann, M. G., E. Arnold, J. W. Erickson, E. A. Frankenberger, J. P. Griffith, H. J. Hecht, J. E. Johnson, G. Kamer, M. Luo, A. G. Mosser, R. R. Rueckert, B. Sherry, and G. Vriend.** 1985. Structure of a human common cold virus and functional relationship to other picornaviruses. *Nature* **317:**145–153.
130. **Samuelson, A., M. Forsgren, B. Johansson, B. Wahren, and M. Sallberg.** 1994. Molecular basis for serological cross-reactivity between enteroviruses. *Diagn. Lab Immunol.* **1:**336–341.
131. **Sato, S., R. Tsutsumi, A. Burke, G. Carlson, V. Porro, Y. Seko, K. Okumura, R. Kawana, and R. Virmani.** 1994. Persistence of replicating coxsackievirus B3 in the

athymic murine heart is associated with development of myocarditic lesions. *J. Gen. Virol.* **75:**2911–2924.

132. **Satoh, M., G. Tamura, I. Segawa, A. Tashiro, K. Hiramori, and R. Satodate.** 1996. Expression of cytokine genes and presence of enteroviral genomic RNA in endomyocardial biopsy tissues of myocarditis and dilated cardiomyopathy. *Virch. Arch.* **427:**503–509.

133. **Schloot, N. C., B. O. Roep, D. R. Wegmann, L. Yu, T. B. Wang, and G. S. Eisenbarth.** 1997. T-cell reactivity to GAD65 peptide sequences shared with coxsackie virus protein in recent-onset IDDM, post-onset IDDM patients and control subjects. *Diabetologia* **40:**332–338.

134. **Schmidt, N. J., R. L. Magoffin, and E. H. Lennette.** 1973. Association of group B coxsackie viruses with cases of pericarditis, myocarditis, or pleurodynia by demonstration of immunoglobulin M antibody. *Infect. Immun.* **8:**341–348.

135. **Schnurr, D. P., Y. Cao, and N. J. Schmidt.** 1984. Coxsackievirus B3 persistence and myocarditis in N:NIH(S) II nu/nu and +/nu mice. *J. Gen. Virol.* **65:**1197–1201.

136. **Schultheiss, H. P., and H. D. Bolte.** 1985. Immunological analysis of auto-antibodies against the adenine nucleotide translocator in dilated cardiomyopathy. *J. Mol. Cell. Cardiol.* **17:**603–617.

137. **Schwimmbeck, P. L., C. Badorff, G. Rohn, K. Schulze, and H. P. Schultheiss.** 1996. The role of sensitized T-cells in myocarditis and dilated cardiomyopathy. *Int. J. Cardiol.* **54:**117–125.

138. **Schwimmbeck, P. L., S. A. Huber, and H. P. Schultheiss.** 1997. Roles of T cells in coxsackievirus B-induced disease. *Curr. Top. Microbiol. Immunol.* **223:**283–303.

139. **See, D. M., and J. G. Tilles.** 1997. Occurrence of coxsackievirus hepatitis in baby rabbits and protection by a formalin-inactivated polyvalent vaccine. *Proc. Soc. Exp. Biol. Med.* **216:**52–56.

140. **Seko, Y., S. Ishiyama, T. Nishikawa, T. Kasajima, M. Hiroe, N. Kagawa, K. Osada, S. Suzuki, H. Yagita, K. Okumura, and Y. Yazaki.** 1995. Restricted usage of T cell receptor V alpha-V beta genes in infiltrating cells in the hearts of patients with acute myocarditis and dilated cardiomyopathy. *J. Clin. Invest.* **96:**1035–1041.

141. **Seko, Y., N. Takahashi, M. Azuma, H. Yagita, K. Okumura, and Y. Yazaki.** 1998. Effects of in vivo administration of anti-B7-1/B7-2 monoclonal antibodies on murine acute myocarditis caused by coxsackievirus B3. *Circ. Res.* **82:**613–618.

142. **Seko, Y., N. Takahashi, M. Azuma, H. Yagita, K. Okumura, and Y. Yazaki.** 1998. Expression of costimulatory molecule CD40 in murine heart with acute myocarditis and reduction of inflammation by treatment with anti-CD40L/B7-1 monoclonal antibodies. *Circ. Res.* **83:**463–469.

143. **Seko, Y., N. Takahashi, H. Yagita, K. Okumura, and Y. Yazaki.** 1997. Expression of cytokine mRNAs in murine hearts with acute myocarditis caused by coxsackievirus B3. *J. Pathol.* **183:**105–108.

144. **Seko, Y., H. Tsuchimochi, T. Nakamura, K. Okumura, S. Naito, K. Imataka, J. Fujii, F. Takaku, and Y. Yazaki.** 1990. Expression of major histocompatibility complex class I antigen in murine ventricular myocytes infected with coxsackievirus B3. *Circ. Res.* **67:**360–367.

145. **Seko, Y., H. Yagita, K. Okumura, and Y. Yazaki.** 1994. T-cell receptor V beta gene expression in infiltrating cells in murine hearts with acute myocarditis caused by coxsackievirus B3. *Circulation* **89:**2170–2175.

146. **Seko, Y., E. Yoshifumi, H. Yagita, K. Okumura, and Y. Yazaki.** 1996. Restricted usage of T-cell receptor V alpha genes in infiltrating cells in murine hearts with acute myocarditis caused by coxsackievirus B3. *J. Pathol.* **178:**330–334.

147. **Sherry, B., A. G. Mosser, R. J. Colonno, and R. R. Rueckert.** 1986. Use of monoclonal antibodies to identify four neutralization immunogens on a common cold picornavirus, human rhinovirus 14. *J. Virol.* **57:**246–257.

148. **Shikhman, A. R., N. S. Greenspan, and M. W. Cunningham.** 1993. A subset of mouse monoclonal antibodies cross-reactive with cytoskeletal proteins and group A streptococcal M proteins recognizes N-acetyl-beta-D-glucosamine. *J. Immunol.* **151:**3902–3913.

149. **Sicinski, P., J. Rowinski, J. B. Warchol, Z. Jarzabek, W. Gut, B. Szczygiel, K. Bielecki, and G. Koch.** 1990. Poliovirus type 1 enters the human host through intestinal M cells. *Gastroenterology* **98:**56–58.

150. **Skylouriotis, P., M. Skylouriotis-Lazarou, S. Natter, R. Steiner, S. Spitzauer, S. Kapiotis, P. Valent, A. M. Hirschl, S. E. Guber, G. Laufer, G. Wollenek, E. Wolner, M. Wimmer, and R. Valenta.** 1999. IgG subclass reactivity to human cardiac myosin in cardiomyopathy patients is indicative of a Th1-like autoimmune disease. *Clin. Exp. Immunol.* **115:**236–247.

151. **Smith, S. C., and P. M. Allen.** 1991. Myosin-induced acute myocarditis is a T cell-mediated disease. *J. Immunol.* **147:**2141–2147.

152. **Takada, H., C. Kishimoto, Y. Hiraoka, and A. Rager-Zisman.** 1995. Therapy with immunoglobulin suppresses myocarditis in a murine coxsackievirus B3 model. Antiviral and anti-inflammatory effects. *Circulation* **92:**1604–1611.

153. **Tilzey, A. J., M. Signy, and J. E. Banatvala.** 1986. Persistent coxsackie B virus specific IgM response in patients with recurrent pericarditis. *Lancet* **1:**1491–1492.

154. **Toniolo, A., T. Onodera, G. Jordan, J. W. Yoon, and A. L. Notkins.** 1982. Virus-induced diabetes mellitus. Glucose abnormalities produced in mice by the six members of the coxsackie B virus group. *Diabetes* **31:**496–499.

155. **Torfason, E. G., M. Pallansch, C. B. Reimer, C. Wickliffe, and H. L. Keyserling.** 1992. Immunoglobulin class and subclass-specific monoclonal antibody sandwich ELISA for the detection of antibodies against coxsackieviruses B, types 1-5. *J. Virol. Methods* **37:**289–303.

156. **Tracy, S., N. M. Chapman, R. Rubocki, and M. Beck.** 1995. The host immune response to enterovirus infections, p. 175–191. *In* H. Rotbart (ed.), *Human Enterovirus Infections.* ASM Press, Washington, D.C.

157. **Tracy, S., K. Hofling, S. Pirruccello, P. H. Lane, S. M. Reyna, and C. J. Gauntt.** 2001. Group B coxsackievirus myocarditis and pancreatitis: connection between viral virulence phenotypes in mice. *J. Med. Virol.* **62:**70–81.

158. **Tu, Z., N. M. Chapman, G. Hufnagel, S. Tracy, J. R. Romero, W. H. Barry, L. Zhao, K. Currey, and B. Shapiro.** 1995. The cardiovirulent phenotype of coxsackievirus B3 is determined at a single site in the genomic 5′ nontranslated region. *J. Virol.* **69:**4607–4618.

159. **Vella, C., and H. Festenstein.** 1992. Coxsackievirus B4 infection of the mouse pancreas: the role of natural killer cells in the control of virus replication and resistance to infection. *J. Gen. Virol.* **73:**1379–1386.

160. **Vreugdenhil, G. R., A. Geluk, T. H. Ottenhoff, W. J. Melchers, B. O. Roep, and J. M. Galama.** 1998. Molecular mimicry in diabetes mellitus: the homologous domain in coxsackie B virus protein 2C and islet autoantigen GAD65 is highly conserved in the coxsackie B-like enteroviruses and binds to the diabetes associated HLA-DR3 molecule. *Diabetologia* **41:**40–46.

161. **Vuorinen, T., R. Vainionpaa, H. Kettinen, and T. Hyypia.** 1994. Coxsackievirus B3 infection in human leukocytes and lymphoid cell lines. *Blood* **84:**823–829.

162. **Vuorinen, T., R. Vainionpaa, R. Vanharanta, and T. Hyypia.** 1996. Susceptibility of human bone marrow

cells and hematopoietic cell lines to coxsackievirus B3 infection. *J. Virol.* **70:**9018–9023.
163. **Vuorinen, T., R. Vainionpaa, J. Heino, and T. Hyypia.** 1999. Enterovirus receptors and virus replication in human leukocytes. *J. Gen. Virol.* **80:**921–927.
164. **Weller, A. H., M. Hall, and S. A. Huber.** 1992. Polyclonal immunoglobulin therapy protects against cardiac damage in experimental coxsackievirus-induced myocarditis. *Eur. Heart J.* **13:**115–119.
165. **Wolfram, L. J., K. W. Beisel, A. Herskowitz, and N. R. Rose.** 1986. Variations in the susceptibility to coxsackievirus B3-induced myocarditis among different strains of mice. *J. Immunol.* **136:**1846–1852.
166. **Woodruff, J.F.** 1980. Viral myocarditis. A review. *Am. J. Pathol.* **101:**425–484.
167. **Yoon, J. W., M. Austin, T. Onodera, and A. L. Notkins.** 1979. Isolation of a virus from the pancreas of a child with diabetic ketoacidosis. *N. Engl. J. Med.* **300:**1173–1179.
168. **Yousef, G. E., E. J. Bell, G. F. Mann, V. Murugesan, D. G. Smith, R. A. McCartney, and J. F. Mowbray.** 1988. Chronic enterovirus infection in patients with postviral fatigue syndrome. *Lancet* **1:**146–150.
169. **Ytterberg, S. R., M. L. Mahowald, and R. P. Messner.** 1987. Coxsackievirus B 1-induced polymyositis. Lack of disease expression in nu/nu mice. *J. Clin. Invest.* **80:**499–506.
170. **Zamorano, P., A. Wigdorovitz, M. Perez-Filgueira, C. Carrillo, J. M. Escribano, A. M. Sadir, and M. V. Borca.** 1995. A 10-amino-acid linear sequence of VP1 of foot and mouth disease virus containing B- and T-cell epitopes induces protection in mice. *Virology* **212:**614–621.
171. **Zaragoza, C., C. Ocampo, M. Saura, M. Leppo, X. Q. Wei, R. Quick, S. Moncada, F. Y. Liew, and C. J. Lowenstein.** 1998. The role of inducible nitric oxide synthase in the host response to coxsackievirus myocarditis. *Proc. Natl. Acad. Sci. USA* **95:**2469–2474.
172. **Zhang, H., P. Morgan-Capner, N. Latif, Y. A. Pandolfino, W. Fan, M. J. Dunn, and L. C. Archard.** 1997. Coxsackievirus B3-induced myocarditis. Characterization of stable attenuated variants that protect against infection with the cardiovirulent wild-type strain. *Am. J. Pathol.* **150:**2197–2207.
173. **Zinkernagel, R. M.** 1997. Virus-induced immunopathology, p. 163–180. *In* N. Nathanson (ed.), *Viral Pathogenesis.* Lippincott-Raven, Philadelphia, Pa.

Pathogenesis of Coxsackievirus B Infections

REINHARD KANDOLF, HANS-CHRISTOPH SELINKA, AND KARIN KLINGEL

32

Enteroviruses of the family *Picornaviridae* have been identified as important etiologic agents of various acute and chronic forms of diseases, including myocarditis, meningoencephalitis, pancreatitis, and insulin-dependent type 1 diabetes (12, 23, 35, 36). Among these viruses especially, coxsackieviruses of group B (CVB) are commonly associated with human viral heart disease. Although the majority of coxsackievirus infections are subclinical, these viruses are capable of producing severe acute myocarditis and may also lead to chronic heart muscle diseases such as chronic myocarditis and dilated cardiomyopathy (24, 34).

Regarding the pathogenesis of enteroviral heart disease there has been uncertainty whether viral cytotoxicity or immune-mediated processes are crucial for organ pathology during acute and persistent heart muscle infection. This review will provide experimental evidence for the decisive role of virus replication in the induction and maintenance of chronic myocardial damage. In addition, the capacity of cellular signal transduction pathways to modulate enterovirus replication as well as CVB receptor interactions and their role in pathogenesis are discussed.

MECHANISMS OF PERSISTENT COXSACKIEVIRUS INFECTION

By establishment of in situ hybridization and polymerase chain reaction in the etiologic diagnosis of viral heart disease, it has been shown that enteroviruses are not only present in the myocardium of patients with acute and chronic myocarditis but also in patients suffering from dilated cardiomyopathy, indicating enterovirus persistence in the human heart (23, 24). The pathogenic concept of a persistent enteroviral infection of the myocardium has been substantiated by the observation of coxsackieviral persistence in different murine models of chronic myocarditis (26, 27, 38). CVB3, typically a cytolytic virus, has been shown to induce a chronic inflammatory heart muscle disease that is consistently associated with viral persistence in A.CA/SnJ (H-2^f), A.BY/SnJ (H-2^b), SWR/J (H-2^q) but not in C57/BL6 (H-2^b) or DBA/1 (H-2^q) mice (26). Resistance to the development of persistent heart muscle infection was found not to be linked to the H-2 haplotype of the host (26).

When the natural course of CVB3-induced myocarditis was followed in permissive A.CA/SnJ mice by in situ hybridization, it has been shown that single myocytes are infected during viremia that replicate the virus prior to invasion of immune cells (Fig. 1A). During acute infection (6 days postinfection [pi]) numerous in situ positive myocytes are observed adjacent to foci of inflammation (Fig. 1B). Around day 12 pi, when the maximum reactive cellular immune response was noted, the number of infected heart muscle cells declines (Fig. 1C), indicating protective effects of the cellular immunity. Thirty days pi the in situ hybridization pattern is characterized by ongoing inflammation in close spatial association with persistently infected myocytes, which revealed a decreased copy number of viral RNA (Fig. 1D).

Regarding molecular mechanisms responsible for myocardial enterovirus persistence, there is evidence that, in addition to host factors, viral determinants contribute to the development of a persistent organ infection. Analysis of persistent myocardial infection by strand-specific in situ hybridization revealed that, in contrast to acute infection, the amount of viral plus-strand RNA appears similar to the amount of minus-strand RNA, indicating that enterovirus persistence is restricted at the level of viral plus-strand RNA (26). Recently, comparable data were obtained in murine CVB1-induced chronic inflammatory myopathy (40). In this model it was suggested that after acute infection a decline of RNA polymerase activity occurs, resulting in a reduced plus-strand RNA synthesis and a corresponding inhibition of strand displacement of the double-stranded replicative form. This double-stranded form is protected from RNA degradation and could thereby promote long-term virus persistence (40).

In addition to myocytes, immune cells have been discovered as important targets of acute and persistent CVB3 infection, providing a noncardiac viral reservoir in the course of the disease (2, 29). By means of a double-labeling

---

Reinhard Kandolf, Hans-Christoph Selinka, and Karin Klingel ■ Department of Molecular Pathology, University Hospital of Tübingen, D-72076 Tübingen, Germany.

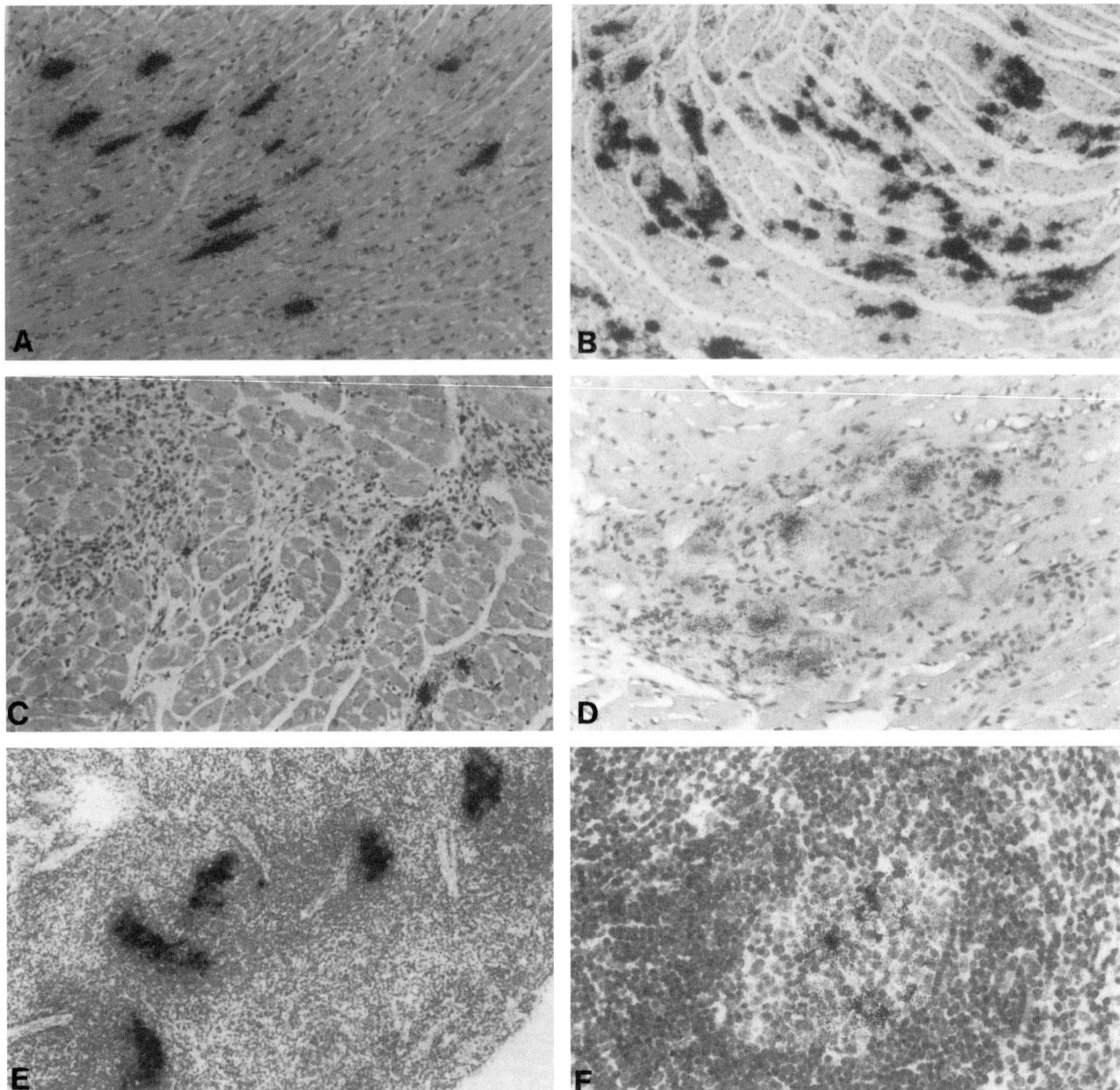

FIGURE 1 Detection of CVB3 RNA in the myocardium of immunocompetent mice (A) 3 days, (B) 6 days, (C) 12 days, and (D) 30 days pi. At any stage of the disease viral RNA is clearly localized to myocytes as detected by radioactive in situ hybridization. In spleens of acutely infected animals, CVB3 RNA-positive cells were primarily observed (E) in the white pulp of follicles whereas at later stages of the infection virus RNA was detected (F) in immune cells within the germinal center.

technique infected spleen cells, which were localized at the periphery of lymph follicles, were mostly identified as B cells (Fig. 1E). Later in disease, the localization of enteroviral RNA revealed a persistent-type of infected B cells within the germinal centers of virus-induced secondary follicles (Fig. 1F). There is evidence for virus replication in lymphoid cells during acute and chronic myocarditis from the detection of the viral minus-strand RNA intermediate in splenic cells, comprising B cells and also certain CD4$^+$ T cells and Mac1$^+$ macrophages (29), and from the induction of virus myocarditis following adoptive transfer of infected splenocytes in SCID mice (M. Hesse et al., submitted for publication).

Cytotoxicity of Coxsackieviruses by Interaction with Distinct Host Cell Proteins

Analyses of early events in enterovirus-infected cells have demonstrated that proteolysis of diverse host cell proteins are due to virus-specific enzymes comprising proteinases 2A^{pro} and 3C^{pro}/3CD^{pro}. Concerning coxsackievirus infection, we found that the CVB3 proteinases 3C^{pro}/3CD^{pro} are capable of inducing cleavage of the p21^{ras}GTPase-activating protein (RasGAP) (16). With regard to the virus-induced "shutoff" of cellular protein synthesis, proteinase 2A^{pro} of CVB3 has been shown to specifically cleave the eukaryotic initiation factor eIF4G (31) and the poly(A)-binding protein (20, 25) (Table 1). In addition, it was recently reported that the CVB3 proteinase 2A^{pro} is directly involved in the destruction of the intracellular architecture of cultured myocytes as well as of myocytes in murine hearts by mediating the cleavage of dystrophin, a large extrasarcomeric cytoskeletal protein (4). The hinge 3 region in human and mouse dystrophin was identified as a direct substrate for the CVB3 proteinase 2A^{pro}, both in vitro and in vivo (3).

To address further mechanisms responsible for target organ injury in enteroviral infection, the course of CVB3 myocarditis was visualized in different immunocompetent mouse strains using in situ hybridization for the detection of viral RNA (26, 27, 29). We found that in all investigated mouse strains CVB3 is capable of inducing acute myocarditis, which is characterized by virus-induced myocytolysis and reactive formation of interstitial mononuclear infiltrates (see Fig. 1B). The pathogenetic significance of direct virus effects in the induction of myocyte injury is indicated by the finding of structural alterations in infected myocytes as early as 3 days pi before T lymphocytes invade the heart muscle. The outstanding role of virus-induced cytopathic effects in CVB3-myocarditis has been further confirmed by the observation of increased myocardial injury in T-cell-deficient mice (21, 38) as well as in mice with severe combined immunodeficiency (10).

To gain further insight into the interplay of virus infection and subcellular structures of heart muscle cells, a high-resolution strand-specific in situ hybridization assay for the detection of viral RNA was established at the electron microscopic level (28). Following the course of infection by this technique, it has been shown that the virus gains access to the myocardium during the viremic phase via the vascular system (Fig. 2A). Early virus replication in myocytes was found to be related with dilation of the sarcoplasmic reticulum in perinuclear regions (Fig. 2B). In the course of myocyte infection, the majority of 5-nm gold particles, visualizing replicating viral RNA of plus-strand polarity, were found in close vicinity with cytoplasmic vacuoles (Fig. 2C, D, E). The observation of prominent cytopathic alterations in close spatial association with viral replication prior to the development of the reactive cellular immune response proves that the loss of host cell integrity is a direct consequence of acute viral replication. Further progression of virus-induced cytopathology in acutely CVB3-infected myocytes is characterized by a dramatic disruption of the cardiomyocyte cytoarchitecture. In the course of myocyte infection viral RNA synthesis was found to be related with histopathologic findings typical for myocyte necrosis, revealing rupture of the plasma membrane and complete destruction of myofilaments associated with aggregated and partially calcified mitochondria (Fig. 2F). According to our previous report (28), persistently infected myocytes in association with chronic inflammatory lesions were detected at the ultrastructural level during chronic myocarditis. Importantly, persistent infection of myocytes was found to be related with morphological changes of the myofibrils. As expected, alterations of the structural integrity in persistently infected myocytes are more subtle compared to those observed in infected myocytes during acute disease, thus reflecting restricted virus replication (26).

To investigate whether persistent coxsackievirus infection interferes with myocyte function, the infectious recombinant CVB3 cDNA (22, 30) was mutated at the VP0 cleavage site from Asn-Ser to Lys-Ala to prevent the formation of infectious virus progeny. In cultured myocytes transfected with the mutated CVB3 cDNA, low-level viral gene expression similar to that observed in the hearts of persistently infected mice was found to induce cytopathic effects, which were indicated by inhibition of cotransfected luciferase reporter gene activity and an increase in release of lactate dehydrogenase from transfected cells (42). From these data it can be concluded that restricted viral replication indeed interferes with myocyte function in the presence of low-level viral protein expression and in absence of cell-mediated immune response.

To further substantiate pathogenic consequences of persistent coxsackievirus infection, transgenic mice were generated that express the replication-restricted CVB3 cDNA mutant exclusively in the heart, driven by the cardiac myocyte-specific myosin light chain-2v (MLC-2v) promoter (13, 32). As expected, heart muscle-specific expression of the CVB3 mutant resulted in the synthesis of viral plus- and minus-strand RNA without formation of infectious virus progeny. Typical morphologic features of transgenic murine hearts, revealing myocardial interstitial fibrosis, hypertrophy, and degeneration of myocytes, were comparable to those observed in hearts of patients with dilated cardiomyopathy. Moreover, similar to pressure overload models of dilated cardiomyopathy, abnormalities in the excitation-contraction coupling as well as dilation of the ventricles were observed (43).

CVB Receptor Interactions and Their Role in Pathogenesis

Since the presence of specific receptor proteins is a major prerequisite for cell and tissue tropism of nonenveloped viruses, the diversity of diseases caused by CVB may also reflect differences in interactions of these viruses with cellular receptors. It has been well documented that CVB may interact with at least two different receptor molecules, the coxsackievirus-adenovirus receptor (CAR), a 46-kDa protein of the immunoglobulin superfamily (5, 41), and decay-accelerating factor (DAF/CD55), a 70-kDa glycosyl-phosphatidylinositol-anchored membrane protein of the family of complement-regulating proteins (6, 39).

Differences in the interactions of various CVB strains with CAR and DAF receptor proteins and their putative influence with regard to pathogenesis were studied by using a hemagglutinating CVB3, designated CVB3-HA, and the nonhemagglutinating cardiotropic strain of CVB3 (37). As depicted in the virus-binding assay in Fig. 3A, infectious

TABLE 1 Cleavage of host cell proteins by coxsackieviral proteinases 2A^{pro}, 3C^{pro}, and 3CD^{pro}

Viral proteinase	Cleavage of:	Reference
2A^{pro}	Eukaryotic initiation factor 4 gamma	31
2A^{pro}	Poly(A)-binding protein	20, 25
2A^{pro}	Dystrophin	4
3C^{pro}	p21^{ras} GTPase-activating protein	16
3CD^{pro}	p21^{ras} GTPase-activating protein	16

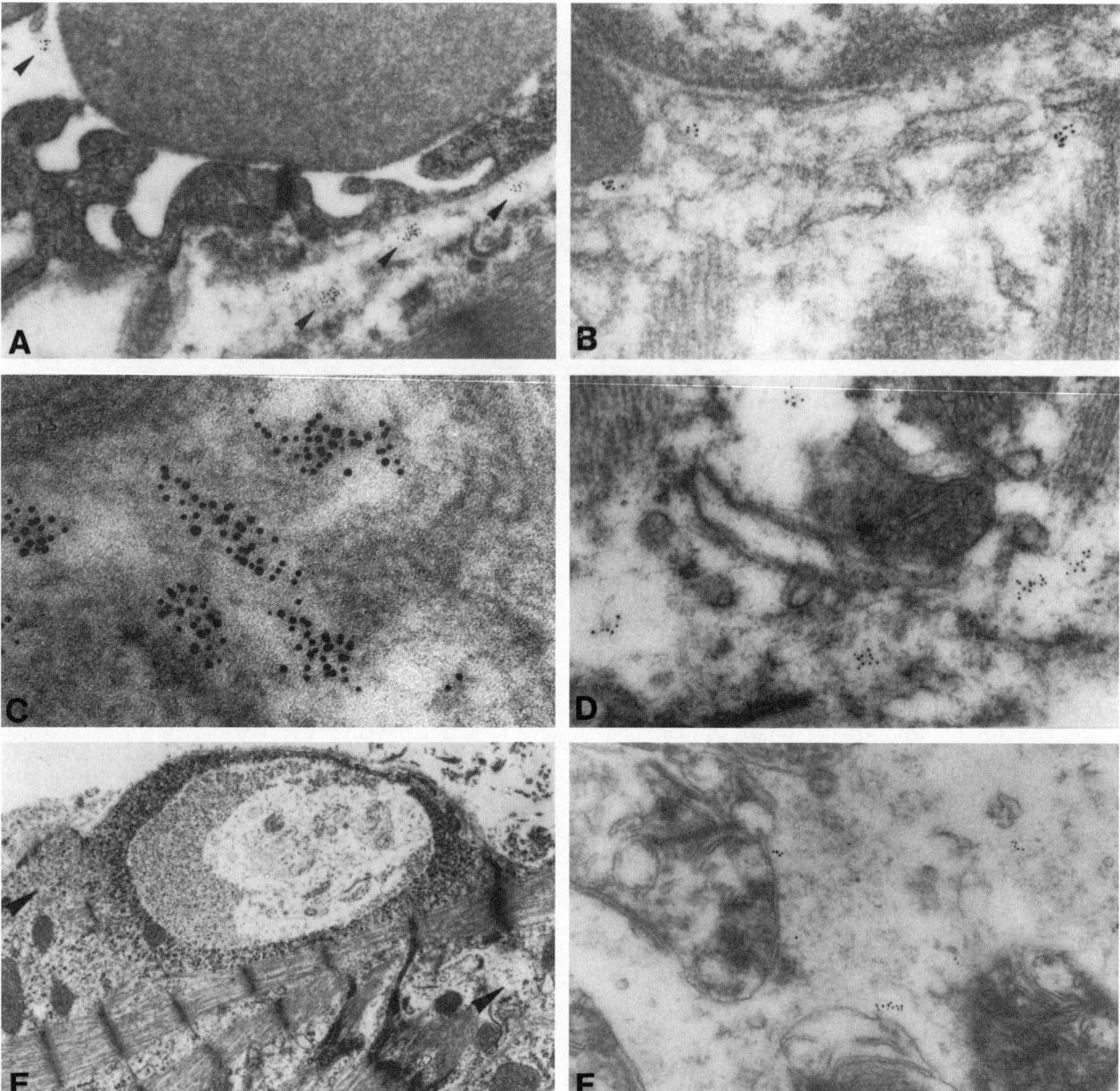

FIGURE 2 Visualization of CVB3 RNA in murine heart muscles by electron microscopic in situ hybridization in the course of virus replication. Following (A) viremia, replicative minus-strand CVB3 RNA was detected (B) in myocytes in close association with sarcoplasmic reticulum. Genomic viral RNA was observed in (C, D) vesiculated regions and (E) virus-induced vacuoles of myocytes. (F) At later stages of acute virus replication viral RNA was found to be related with histopathologic findings typical for myocyte necrosis.

virions of the cDNA-generated CBV3 strain primarily bind to CAR (46 kDa), whereas virions of the hemagglutinating CVB3-HA variant recognize determinants of both DAF (70 kDa) and CAR receptor proteins. Despite clear differences in the binding phenotypes of CVB3 and CVB3-HA, a synergistic inhibitory effect of anti-DAF and anti-CAR antibodies was observed toward infection of HeLa cells with both viruses, supporting the model of preferential interactions of both strains of CVB3 with closely associated DAF and CAR proteins (37). The different binding characteristics of CVB3 and CVB3-HA were also reflected in their cytopathic effects. The hemagglutinating CVB3-HA strain displayed a small plaque phenotype in comparison with the large plaque phenotype of CVB3 (Fig. 3B). However, growth characteristics and virus titers of CVB3-HA were not affected as demonstrated by the comparative analysis of 12-h growth curves of CVB3 and CVB3-HA in various cell lines (Fig. 3C).

In addition, the role of specific receptor and coreceptor proteins for infection with CVB3 and CVB3-HA was investigated with receptor-transfected hamster CHO cells expressing either the CAR protein (CHOCAR cells) or the

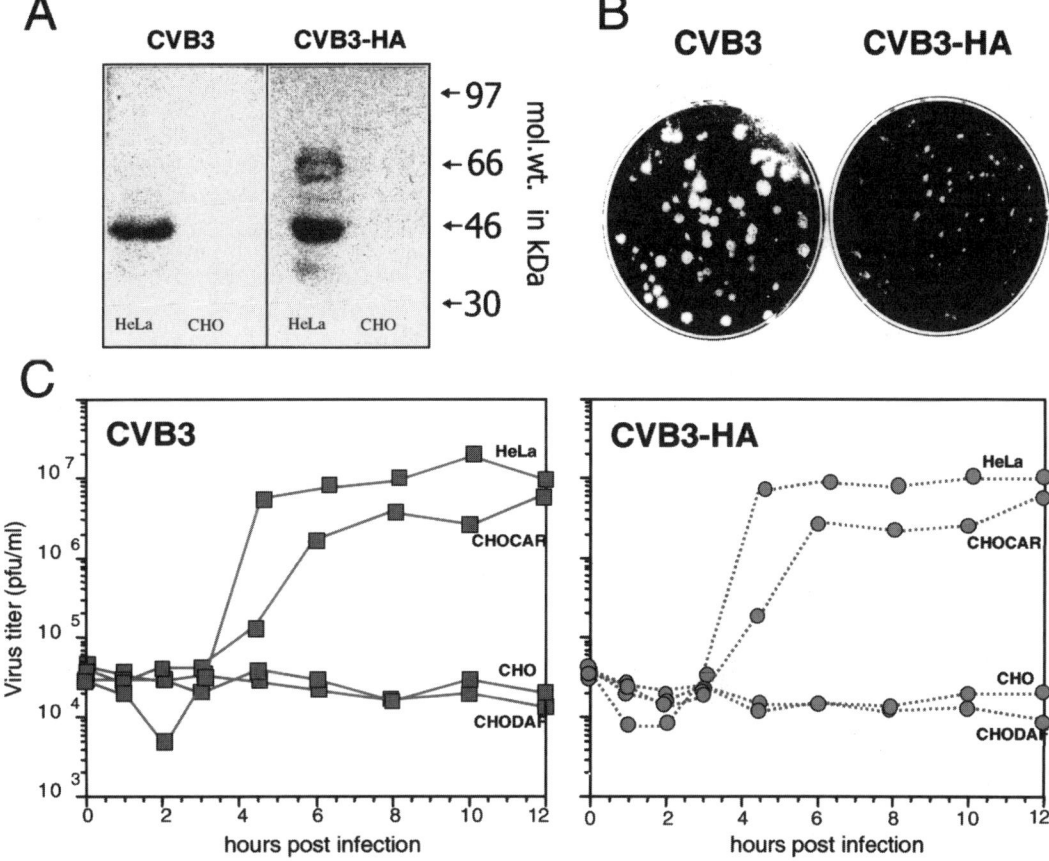

FIGURE 3 Differential interactions of CVB3 variants with host cells. (A) CVB3 and CVB3-HA differ in their interaction with CAR (46 kDa) and DAF (70 kDa). (B) Plaque phenotypes of CVB3 and CVB3-HA on CAR- and DAF-expressing HeLa cells. (C) Growth curves of CVB3 and CVB3-HA in HeLa, CHO, CHOCAR, and CHODAF cells. Despite clear differences in their binding phenotypes and plaque sizes, both CVB3 variants exhibit comparable 12-h growth curves.

DAF receptor protein (CHODAF cells). In contrast to HeLa and CHOCAR cells, which were infected by both virus variants, CHO and CHODAF cells were infected neither by the nonhemagglutinating CVB3 nor by the hemagglutinating CVB3-HA. Despite differences in their binding to these cell lines, both virus variants strictly depend on the CAR receptor protein for initialization of productive infections. However, extension of the binding capacity to the DAF coreceptor protein may also carry an advantage for the virus with regard to pathogenesis. Infection of CHODAF/CAR double-receptor transfectants with CVB3 and CVB3-HA (38a) suggests that simultaneous expression of CAR and DAF receptor proteins may lead to cooperative interactions of both molecules with CVB, as observed with HeLa cells. In this case, initiation of infection is dependent on the additive affinities of CVB to CAR and DAF receptor proteins and may facilitate infection of these cells even by viruses with low affinity to the CAR receptor.

Coxsackievirus-Induced Activation of Cellular Signaling Pathways

Replication of enteroviruses leads to significant modifications in the metabolism of the host cells, predominantly mediated by cleavage of host cell proteins by virus-encoded proteinases $2A^{pro}$, $3C^{pro}$, and $3CD^{pro}$. Preferential targets of the enteroviral proteinase $2A^{pro}$ are proteins involved in the Cap-dependent translation of cellular mRNAs, since enteroviruses employ a Cap-independent mechanism of protein translation.

Importantly, recognition of cellular targets by viral proteinases may be preceded by virus-induced modifications of these proteins. As we have recently shown for CVB and echoviruses, distinct cellular proteins become tyrosine-phosphorylated in the course of enterovirus replication in a time-dependent manner (15). In addition, we found that as early as 2 h pi of HeLa cells with CVB3, the RasGAP, the major down-regulator of $p21^{ras}$, is phosphorylated at its tyrosine residues and is subsequently proteolytically cleaved 5 to 6 h pi, at the maximum of viral protein synthesis. As a consequence of RasGAP cleavage, $p21^{ras}$ is kept in an activated state and initiates activation of the extracellular signal-regulated protein kinase ERK/MAPK pathway of mitogenic signaling in temporal correlation with the appearance of the RasGAP cleavage product (16). Besides activation of ERK/MAPK pathways, physiological and pathological events may result in the activation of two further subgroups of MAPKs, the stress-activated c-Jun amino-terminal kinase JNK/SAPK and the p38/MAPK. All three pathways are finally implicated in mechanisms of transcriptional activation. As demonstrated in Fig. 4, activation of ERK/MAPK but not JNK/SAPK could be measured in CVB3-infected murine hearts 8 days pi. In correlation with the differences in the cardiotropic potential of CVB3 and CVB3-HA, MAPK was found to be less activated in mice infected with the less cardiotropic CVB3-HA variant.

To further analyze the induction of growth-related and stress-activated MAPK pathways, HeLa cells were infected with CVB3 and CVB3-HA, and MAPK activation was monitored by Western blots probed with antibodies specific for the phosphorylated forms of JNK/SAPK, ERK/MAPK, and p38/MAPK (Fig. 5). A mild increase in the expression of p54 JNK/SAPK was observed in the early phase of infection, which rather declined at the time point of maximal virus replication (6 h pi). However, a close temporal correlation was found between activation of ERK1/ERK2 MAPK and viral replication, both of which displayed increased expression levels until reaching the complete cytopathic effect. These results are in accordance with the detection of ERK/MAPK but not JNK/SAPK in CVB3-infected murine hearts 8 days pi. Phosphorylation of p38/MAPK paralleled the activation of ERK/MAPK with a maximum at 6 h pi. As recently suggested for infections with encephalomyocarditis virus, activation of p38/MAPK could be induced by the dsRNA intermediates during enteroviral replication (19).

It is tempting to speculate that activation of preexisting signal transduction pathways by enteroviruses is not only a consequence of accidental cleavage of regulatory proteins

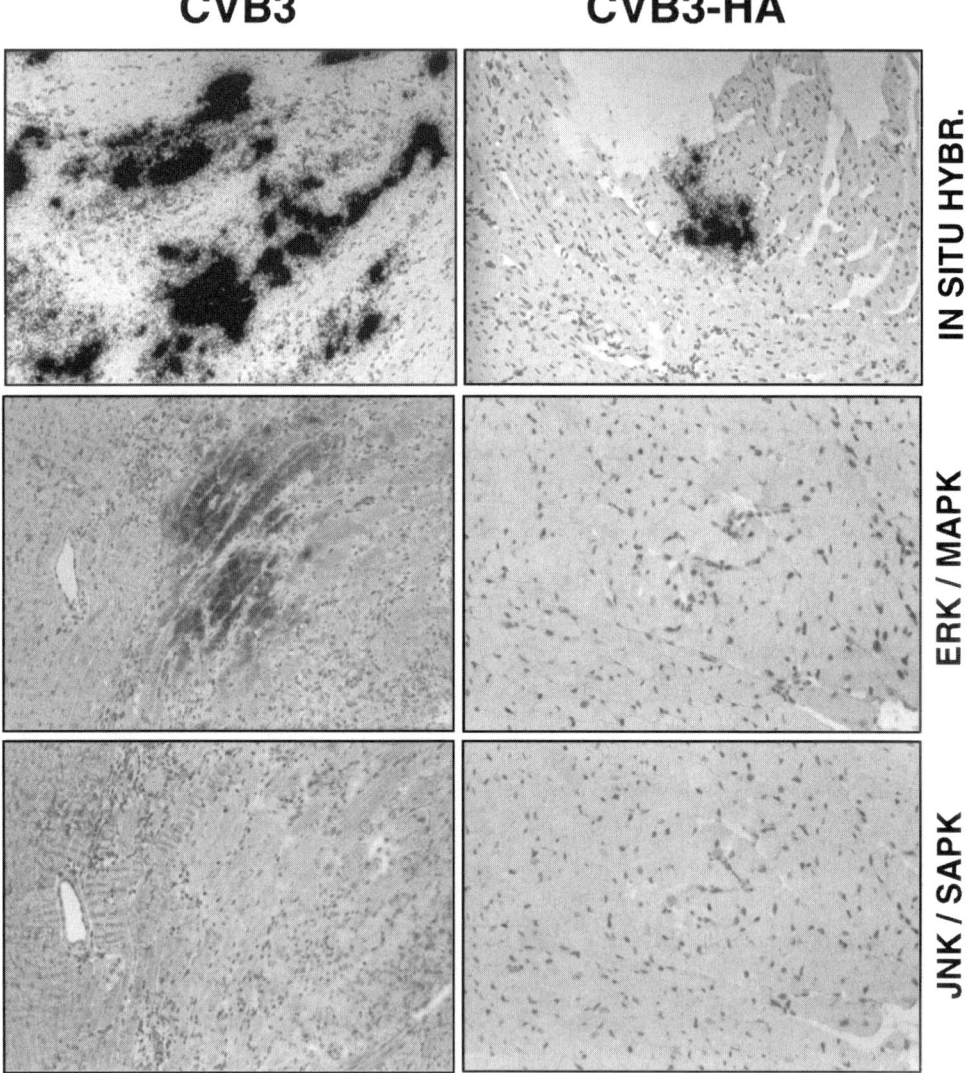

FIGURE 4 In situ detection of CVB3 and virus-induced signaling pathways in murine heart muscle. A.BY/SnJ mice were intraperitoneally infected with CVB3 or CVB3-HA (10^5 PFU) and hearts were analyzed 8 days pi. Differences in the cardiotropism of CVB3 and CVB3-HA are demonstrated by in situ hybridization using a ^{35}S-labeled enterovirus-specific probe (26). Immunohistochemical staining of serial myocardial tissue sections with phospho-ERK/MAPK- and phospho-JNK/SAPK-specific antibodies reveals a close spatial correlation of ERK/MAPK expression and viral replication.

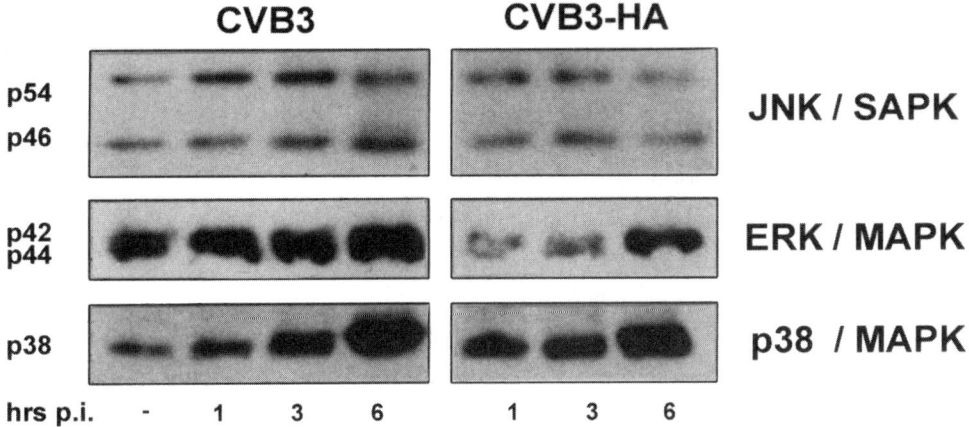

FIGURE 5 Virus-induced activation of MAPK signaling pathways. CVB3- or CVB3-HA-infected (0 to 6 h pi) HeLa cells were subjected to Western blotting using antibodies specific for the phosphorylated forms of JNK/SAPK, ERK/MAPK, and p38/MAPK. Early activation of the proapoptotic JNK/SAPK pathway is temporally followed by activation of the antiapoptotic ERK/MAPK pathway.

but rather intentional to promote virus replication. It has been shown for echovirus 1 that virus replication triggers activation of specific signaling pathways, thus resulting in induction of immediate early genes such as c-jun, junB, and c-fos (17, 18). The importance of the MAPK pathway for control of cell proliferation and survival is highlighted by the various examples of viruses that trigger activation of mitogen-activated protein kinases. There is increasing evidence that stimulation of the MAPK pathways is not only a mechanism employed by tumorigenic viruses like Epstein-Barr virus (11), bovine papillomavirus (33), or adenoviruses (8), but also by enteroviruses (15, 16) and cardioviruses (14, 19). Regarding the infection of cardiac cells by enteroviruses and cardioviruses, activation of MAP kinases may participate in the mobilization of intracellular calcium during virus replication and may thereby contribute to morphological and physiological destruction of infected myocytes.

Moreover, activated MAPKs may be implemented in the regulation of proapoptotic and antiapoptotic factors in CVB-infected cells. In the first few hours of CVB infection, phosphorylation of the JNK/SAPK may lead to increased c-jun activity, which subsequently promotes apoptotic cell death (7, 44). However, during later stages of infection, activation of ERK/MAPK, the key signaling pathway of cell survival, in temporal correlation with viral replication (Fig. 4), may be regarded as a virus-induced protective counterreaction to this early apoptotic process. It was recently reported that cytopathic effect can develop in poliovirus-infected cells due to expression of apoptosis-preventing functions, and competing death programs were suggested to be responsible for the commitment switch from apoptosis to cytopathic effect (1). Caspase activation may not be responsible for the characteristic cytopathic effects following infection of cells with CVB (9). Apoptosis per se seems to be of no value for replicating viruses, and stabilization of the host cell metabolism during infection until completion of the viral replication cycle may be more important for the virus than cell destruction. Further investigations are required to evaluate whether activation of MAPK pathways also plays a role in the switch from acute to persistent CVB infections.

SUMMARY

Enteroviruses, and especially CVB, have been identified as etiologic agents in humans and various experimental murine models of acute myocarditis and chronic heart muscle diseases, indicating enterovirus persistence in the myocardium. Persistent myocardial infection is characterized by restricted viral replication and gene expression in myocytes capable of sustaining chronic inflammation. Viral cytotoxicity was found to be crucial for organ pathology during both acute and persistent infection. In situ hybridization experiments at the cellular and subcellular level have demonstrated that CVB3 replication is associated with severe structural changes of the cardiomyocyte cytoarchitecture at any stage of the disease. In tissue culture experiments and transgenic mice, it has been shown that, in addition to acute viral replication, persistent infection also interferes with myocyte function. Investigations at the molecular level revealed that interference of virus replication with the cellular metabolism is mediated by cleavage of host cell proteins by CVB-encoded proteinases $2A^{pro}$, $3C^{pro}$, and $3CD^{pro}$. Notably, there is also evidence that CVB is able to activate specific cellular signal transduction pathways in the course of infection, thus promoting enteroviral replication. In summary, these data indicate that mutual influences of virus replication and subsequent modifications of the host cell metabolism are crucial for cardiac injury and dysfunction during acute and chronic heart muscle disease.

This work was performed by grants from the Federal Ministry of Education, Science, Research and Technology and the Interdisciplinary Center for Clinical Research (IZKF 01 KS9602) of the Medical Faculty at the University of Tübingen (K. Klingel, R. Kandolf). In addition, the support of the fortune program of the Medical Faculty, University of Tübingen (No. 526-O-1; H.-C. Selinka, R. Kandolf), as well as the Dr. Karl-Kuhn-Stiftung (K. Klingel) is appreciated. We thank Martina Sauter and Sandra Bundschuh for the excellent technical assistance and Peter Rieger, Institute for Pathology, University of Heidelberg, for his support in electron microscopic in situ hybridization. We greatly appreciate the collaboration with the laboratories of Bruce McManus, University of British Columbia, Vancouver, Canada, and Kirk Knowlton, University of California, San Diego, Calif.

REFERENCES

1. Agol, V. I., G. A. Belov, K. Bienz, D. Egger, M. S. Kolesnikova, L. I. Romanova, L. V. Sladkova, and E. A. Tolskaya. 2000. Competing death programs in poliovirus-infected cells: commitment switch in the middle of the infectious cycle. *J. Virol.* **74:**5534–5541.
2. Anderson, D., J. E. Wilson, C. M. Carthy, S. Yang, R. Kandolf, and B. M. McManus. 1996. Direct interaction of coxsackievirus B3 with immune cells in the splenic compartment of mice susceptible or resistant to myocarditis. *J. Virol.* **70:**4632–4645.
3. Badorff, C., N. Berkely, S. Mehrotra, J. W. Talhouk, R. E. Rhoads, and K. U. Knowlton. 2000. Enteroviral protease 2A directly cleaves dystrophin and is inhibited by a dystrophin-based substrate analogue. *J. Biol. Chem.* **275:**11191–11197.
4. Badorff, C., L. Gil-Hwan, B. J. Lamphear, M. E. Martone, K. P. Campbell, R. E. Rhoads, and K. U. Knowlton. 1999. Enteroviral protease 2A cleaves dystrophin: evidence of cytoskeletal disruption in an acquired cardiomyopathy. *Nat. Med.* **5:**320–326
5. Bergelson, J. M., J. A. Cunningham, G. Droguett, E. A Kurt-Jones, A. Krithivas, J. S Hong, M. S Horwitz, R. L. Crowell, and R. W. Finberg. 1997. Isolation of a common receptor for coxsackie B viruses and adenoviruses 2 and 5. *Science* **275:**1320–1323.
6. Bergelson, J. M., J. G. Mohanty, R. L. Crowell, N. F. St. John, D. M Lublin, and R. W. Finberg. 1995. Coxsackievirus B3 adapted to growth in RD cells binds to decay-accelerating factor (CD55). *J. Virol.* **69:**1903–1906.
7. Bossy-Wetzel, E., L. Bakiri, and M. Yaniv. 1997. Induction of apoptosis by the transcription factor c-Jun. *EMBO J.* **16:**1695–1709.
8. Bruder, J. T., and I. Kovesdi. 1997. Adenovirus infection stimulates the Raf/MAPK signaling pathway and induces interleukin-8 expression. *J. Virol.* **71:**398–404.
9. Carthy, C. M., D. J. Granville, K. A. Watson, D. R. Anderson, J. E. Wilson, D. Yang, D. W. Hunt, and B. M. McManus. 1998. Caspase activation and specific cleavage of substrates after coxsackievirus B3-induced cytopathic effect in HeLa cells. *J. Virol.* **72:**7669–7675.
10. Chow, L. H., K. W. Beisel, and B. M. McManus. 1992. Enteroviral infection of mice with severe combined immunodeficiency. Evidence for direct viral pathogenesis of myocardial injury. *Lab. Invest.* **66:**24–31.
11. Fenton, M., and A. J. Sinclair. 1999. Divergent requirements for the MAPK/ERK signal transduction pathway during initial virus infection of quiescent primary B cells and disruption of Epstain-Barr virus latency by phorbol esters. *J. Virol.* **73:**8913–8916.
12. Foulis, A. K., M. A. Farquharson, S. O. Cameron, M. McGill, H. Schönke, and R. Kandolf. 1990. A search for the presence of the enteroviral capsid protein VP1 in pancreases of patients with type 1 (insulin-dependent) diabetes and pancreases and hearts of infants who died of coxsackie viral myocarditis. *Diabetologia* **33:**290–298.
13. Franz, W. M., D. Breves, K. Klingel, G. Brem, P. H. Hofschneider, and R. Kandolf. 1993. Heart-specific targeting of firefly luciferase by myosin-light-chain-2 promoter and developmental regulation in transgenic mice. *Circ. Res.* **73:**629–638.
14. Hirasawa, K., H. S. Jun, H. S. Han, M. L. Zhang, M. D. Hollenberg, and J. W. Yoon. 1999. Prevention of encephalomyocarditis virus-induced diabetes in mice by inhibition of the tyrosine kinase signalling pathway and subsequent suppresssion of nitric oxide production in macrophages. *J. Virol.* **73:**8541–8548.
15. Huber, M., H.-C. Selinka, and R. Kandolf. 1997. Tyrosine phosphorylation events during coxsackievirus B3 replication. *J. Virol.* **71:**595–600.
16. Huber, M., K. A. Watson, H.-C. Selinka, C. M. Carthy, K. Klingel, B. M. McManus, and R. Kandolf. 1999. Cleavage of RasGAP and phosphorylation of mitogen-activated protein kinase in the course of coxsackievirus B3 replication. *J. Virol.* **73:**3587–3594.
17. Huttunen, P., J. Heino, and T. Hyypiä. 1997. Echovirus 1 replication, not only virus binding to its receptor, VLA-2, is required for the induction of cellular immediate-early genes. *J. Virol.* **71:**4176–4180.
18. Huttunen, P., T. Hyypiä, P. Vihinen, L. Nissinen, and J. Heino. 1998. Echovirus 1 infection induces both stress- and growth-activated mitogen-activated protein kinase pathways and regulates the transcription of cellular immediate-early genes. *Virology* **250:**85–93.
19. Iordanov, M. S., J. M. Paranjape, A. Zhou, J. Wong, B. R. Williams, E. F. Meurs, R. H. Silverman, and B. E. Magun. 2000. Activation of p38 mitogen-activated protein kinase and c-Jun NH2-terminal kinase by double-stranded RNA and encephalomyocarditis virus: involvement of Rnase L, protein kinase R, and alternative pathways. *Mol. Cell. Biol.* **20:**617–627.
20. Joachims, M., P. C. van Breugel, and R. E. Lloyd. 1999. Cleavage of poly(A)-binding protein by enterovirus proteases concurrent with inhibition of translation in vitro. *J. Virol.* **73:**718–727.
21. Kandolf, R., D. Ameis, P. Kirschner, A. Canu, and P. H. Hofschneider. 1987. In situ detection of enteroviral genomes in myocardial cells by nucleic acid hybridization: an approach to the diagnosis of viral heart disease. *Proc. Natl. Acad. Sci. USA* **84:**6272–6276.
22. Kandolf, R., and P. H. Hofschneider. 1985. Molecular cloning of the genome of a cardiotropic coxsackie B3 virus: full-length reverse-transcribed recombinant cDNA generates infectious virus in mammalian cells. *Proc. Natl. Acad. Sci. USA* **82:**4818–4822.
23. Kandolf, R., K. Klingel, R. Zell, H.-C. Selinka, U. Raab, W. Schneider-Brachert, and B. Bültmann. 1993. Molecular pathogenesis of enterovirus-induced myocarditis: virus persistence and chronic inflammation. *Intervirology* **35:**140–151.
24. Kandolf, R., M. Sauter, C. Aepinus, J.-J. Schnorr, H.-C. Selinka, and K. Klingel. 1999. Mechanisms and consequences of enterovirus persistence in cardiac myocytes and cells of the immune system. *Virus Res.* **62:**149–158.
25. Kerekatte, V., B. D. Keiper, C. Badorff, A. Cai, K. U. Knowlton, and R. E. Rhoads. 1999. Cleavage of poly(A)-binding protein by coxsackievirus 2A protease in vitro and in vivo: another mechanism for host protein synthesis shutoff. *J. Virol.* **73:**709–717.
26. Klingel, K., C. Hohenadl, A. Canu, M. Albrecht, M. Seemann, G. Mall, and R. Kandolf. 1992. Ongoing enterovirus-induced myocarditis is associated with persistent heart muscle infection: quantitative analysis of virus replication, tissue damage and inflammation. *Proc. Natl. Acad. Sci. USA* **89:**314–318.
27. Klingel, K., and R. Kandolf. 1993. The role of enterovirus replication in the development of acute and chronic heart muscle disease in different immunocompetent mouse strains. *Scand. J. Infect. Dis. Suppl.* **88:**79–85.
28. Klingel, K., P. Rieger, G. Mall, H.-C. Selinka, M. Huber, and R. Kandolf. 1998. Visualization of enteroviral replication in myocardial tissue by ultrastructural in situ hybridization: identification of target cells and cytopathic effects. *Lab. Invest.* **78:**1227–1237.
29. Klingel, K., S. Stephan, M. Sauter, R. Zell, B. M. McManus, B. Bültmann, and R. Kandolf. 1996. Pathogenesis of murine enterovirus myocarditis: virus dissemination and immune cell targets. *J. Virol.* **70:**8888–8895.

30. **Klump, W. M., I. Bergmann, B. C. Müller, D. Ameis, and R. Kandolf.** 1990. Complete nucleotide sequence of infectious coxsackievirus B3 cDNA: two initial 5'uridine residues are regained during plus-strand RNA synthesis. *J. Virol.* **64:**1573–1583.
31. **Lamphear, B. J., R. Yan, F. Yang, D. Waters, H. D. Liebig, H. Klump, E. Kuechler, T. Skern, and R. E. Rhoads.** 1993. Mapping the cleavage site in protein synthesis initiation factor eIF-4 gamma of the 2A proteases from human coxsackievirus and rhinovirus. *J. Biol. Chem.* **268:**19200–19203.
32. **Lee, K. J., R. S. Ross, H. A. Rockman, A. N. Harris, T. X. O'Brien, M. van Bilsen, H. E. Shubeita, R. Kandolf, G. Brem, J. Price, S. M. Evans, H. Zhu, W. M. Franz, and K. R. Chien.** 1992. Myosin light chain-2 luciferase transgenic mice reveal distinct regulatory programs for cardiac and skeletal muscle-specific expression of a single contractile protein gene. *J. Biol. Chem.* **267:**15875–15885.
33. **Martin, P., W. C. Vass, J. T. Schiller, D. R. Lowry, and T. J. Velu.** 1989. The bovine papillomavirus E5 transforming protein can stimulate the transforming activity of EGF and CSF-1 receptors. *Cell* **59:**21–32.
34. **Martino, T., P. Liu, and M. J. Sole.** 1994. Viral infection and the pathogenesis of dilated cardiomyopathy. *Circ. Res.* **74:**182–188.
35. **McManus, B. M., and R. Kandolf.** 1991. Evolving concepts of cause, consequence, and control in myocarditis. *Curr. Opin. Cardiol.* **6:**418–427.
36. **Muir, P., U. Kämmerer, K. Korn, M. N. Mulders, T. Pöyry, B. Weissbrich, R. Kandolf, G. M. Cleator, and A. M. van Loon.** 1998. Molecular typing of enteroviruses: current status and future requirements. *Clin. Microbiol. Rev.* **11:**202–227.
37. **Pasch, A., J.-H. Küpper, A. Wolde, R. Kandolf, and H.-C. Selinka.** 1999. Comparative analysis of virus-host cell interactions of haemagglutinating and non-haemagglutinating strains of coxsackievirus B3. *J. Gen. Virol.* **80:**3153–3158.
38. **Sato, S., R. Tsutsumi, A. Burke, G. Calson, V. Porro, Y. Seko, K. Okumura, R. Kawana, and R. Virmani.** 1994. Persistence of replicating coxsackievirus B3 in the athymic murine heart is associated with development of myocarditic lesions. *J. Gen. Virol.* **7:**2911–2924.
38a. **Selinka, H. C., A. Wolde, A. Pasch, K. Klingel, J. J. Schnorr, J. H. Küpper, A. M. Lindberg, and R. Kandolf.** 2002. Comparative analysis of two coxsackievirus B3 strains: putative influence of virus-receptor interactions on pathogenesis. *J. Med. Virol.* **67:**224–233.
39. **Shafren, D. R., D. T. Williams, and R. D. Barry.** 1997. A decay-accelerating factor-binding strain of coxsackievirus B3 requires the coxsackievirus-adenovirus receptor protein to mediate lytic infection of rhabdomyosarcoma cells. *J. Virol.* **71:**9844–9848.
40. **Tam, P. E., and R. P. Messner.** 1999. Molecular mechanisms of coxsackievirus persistence in chronic inflammatory myopathy: viral RNA persists through formation of a double-stranded complex without associated genomic mutations or evolution. *J. Virol.* **73:**10113–10121.
41. **Tomko, R. P., R. Xu, and L. Philipson.** 1997. HCAR and MCAR: the human and mouse cellular receptors for subgroup C adenoviruses and group B coxsackieviruses. *Proc. Natl. Acad. Sci. USA* **94:**3352–3356.
42. **Wessely, R., A. Henke, R. Zell, R. Kandolf, and K. U. Knowlton.** 1998. Low-level expression of a mutant coxsackieviral cDNA induces a myocytopathic effect in culture: an approach to the study of enteroviral persistence in cardiac myocytes. *Circulation* **98:**450–457.
43. **Wessely, R., K. Klingel, L. F. Santana, N. Dalton, M. Hongo, W. J. Lederer, R. Kandolf, and K. U. Knowlton.** 1998. Transgenic expression of replication-restricted enteroviral genomes in heart muscle induces defective excitation-contraction coupling and dilated cardiomyopathy. *J. Clin. Invest.* **102:**1444–1453.
44. **Xia, Z., M. Dickens, J. Raingeaud, R. J. Davis, and M. E. Greenberg.** 1995. Opposing effects of ERK and JNK-p38 MAP kinase on apoptosis. *Science* **270:**1326–1331.

Hepatitis A Virus Pathogenesis and Attenuation

ROBERT H. PURCELL AND SUZANNE U. EMERSON

33

OVERVIEW AND HISTORICAL PERSPECTIVE

Hepatitis A is believed by some to be an ancient disease (reviewed in reference 141). Outbreaks of hepatitis were common among the military from the 17th to the 20th centuries, leading to the designation of the disease as "campaign jaundice." Outbreaks of hepatitis also occurred among civilians, and in 1912, Cockayne called such epidemics of jaundice "infectious hepatitis" (20). By the 1940s, a second form of hepatitis, with a longer incubation period and association with blood and blood products, was recognized, and in 1947, MacCallum introduced the terms "hepatitis A" for infectious hepatitis and "hepatitis B" for the blood-borne form (90). Volunteer studies in adults and children between the 1950s and 1970s revealed that hepatitis A was transmitted primarily by the fecal-oral route, whereas hepatitis B was transmitted primarily (but not exclusively) by exposure to blood or blood products (67, 80). In 1973, Feinstone et al. first visualized hepatitis A virus (HAV) in the feces of an individual with acute hepatitis A (43). Four years later, Provost and Hilleman recovered and serially passaged HAV in cell culture for the first time, and demonstrated that it had the characteristics of a picornavirus (105, 107).

Ironically, campaign jaundice and many other outbreaks of hepatitis reported before the early decades of the 20th century may not have been caused by HAV at all. The application of sensitive assays to the measurement of antibody to HAV in various populations worldwide revealed that virtually everyone in developing countries was infected with the virus at an early age (before 5 years), when infection is likely to be inapparent. In industrialized countries, widespread infection with HAV diminished in parallel with improved sanitation and public health measures, and this can be localized to the post-World War II era in much of Europe and North America, with southern Europe trailing somewhat behind northern Europe (48, 125). Since HAV infection produces lifelong immunity, it is unlikely that HAV was the cause of many outbreaks of enterically transmitted hepatitis before World War II. Rather, these outbreaks were probably caused by hepatitis E virus (HEV), another enterically transmitted hepatitis virus that remains a common cause of disease in many developing countries but not in industrialized countries (reviewed in reference 108).

CHARACTERISTICS OF HAV

HAV shares many characteristics with the other picornaviruses: it is approximately 28 nm in diameter, is nonenveloped, has a buoyant density in CsCl of 1.32 to 1.34 g/ml, and has a sedimentation coefficient of 156 to 160 (reviewed in reference 69). The HAV genome consists of a single strand of RNA having a small viral protein (VPg) covalently linked to its 5' end and a poly(A) tail at its 3' end. Its 7.5-kb genome is positive sense so the first synthetic event following infection is translation of the single open reading frame into a polyprotein that is processed proteolytically to release functional viral proteins. All primary cleavages are carried out by the virus-encoded 3C proteinase, which is the only proteinase encoded by HAV (82, 92, 117). The VP1/2A junction may not be cleaved directly, but rather VP1 may be released by sequential whittling away of 2A by one or more cellular proteinases (62). The VP4 gene is truncated compared to that of other picornaviruses, and it has not been detected in virions. However, recent evidence indicates that the VP4/VP2 fusion protein is required for pentamer formation and the VP1/2A fusion protein is required for virion formation (102).

Translation of the HAV genome is directed by an internal ribosome entry site (IRES), which is formed from the majority of the 700-plus nucleotides preceding the initiation codon (15, 55). The exact boundaries of the IRES are not known, but the 5' end may be located within the first 151 nucleotides (15, 17, 56) and the 3' end may extend a short distance into the coding region (59).

Replication is not well understood, but extrapolation from studies of poliovirus suggests replication occurs on vesicles formed de novo under the influence of the 2B and 2C proteins (9, 19, 58). The virus gene 3D encodes an

---

Robert H. Purcell and Suzanne U. Emerson ■ Hepatitis Viruses and Molecular Hepatitis Sections, Laboratory of Infectious Diseases, National Institute of Allergy and Infectious Diseases, National Institutes of Health, Bethesda, MD 20892.

RNA-dependent RNA polymerase that replicates the genome. Host cell protein synthesis is not inhibited as it is with poliovirus, and virus egress from cells is inefficient and by an unknown mechanism.

TAXONOMY

HAV was originally classified as enterovirus 72, but subsequent analysis of the sequence of its genome in comparison with newer information about the genomic sequences of other picornaviruses led to its being reclassified in its own genus, Hepatovirus, which it shares with the closely related simian HAVs (96, 113). Surprisingly, avian encephalomyelitis virus was recently shown to be a picornavirus that is most closely related to the HAVs (93).

HOST RANGE

In Vitro

HAV has been very difficult to grow in cell culture. Even under the best conditions replication is relatively inefficient and is dependent on the correct combination of temperature, cell type, and age of cells as well as viral strain. The first successful propagation was of an HAV strain that had been passaged in marmosets prior to inoculation into primary cultures of marmoset liver and into a continuous line of fetal rhesus kidney cells (105). The virus was able to grow in both cultures. Since then various strains of HAV have been grown in primary cultures or established cell lines of primate or human origin (8, 10, 25, 44, 47, 53, 78, 88). Attempts to grow the virus in nonprimate cells have generally failed, but limited replication has been achieved in cultured pig, dolphin, and guinea pig cells (30). Although HAV replication in vitro is basically restricted as to species, it is not as limited by cell type and the hepatotropism so dominant in vivo is not evident in vitro. Thus, even though HAV will replicate in liver cell lines such as PLC/PRF/5 or Huh7 (47, 52), it will also replicate in kidney and lung cells (10, 25, 61, 63, 135). In some cases adaptation to a particular cell is required. The four internationally licensed vaccines are all produced in human diploid cells (5a).

It is not known how HAV enters cells in vivo, nor has the receptor on liver cells been identified. In vitro experiments have implicated calcium as an important component of binding (122, 139). Calcium-dependent binding of ^{125}I-labeled HAV to three permissive cell lines (primate and human) but not to nonpermissive cells (murine) was reported by Stapleton et al. (122). However, although Zajac et al. (139) confirmed the enhancement of binding by calcium, they also reported binding of HAV to three nonpermissive cell lines of mouse or canine origin. These studies both have the caveat that binding was not related to infection and therefore may have been irrelevant to the natural pathway. Bishop et al. (13) used a focus assay to study productive binding of infectious virus to BS-C-1 cells and found that calcium and acidic pH independently increased attachment and reduced rates of virus elution. Calcium reduced the stability of HAV and had a direct effect on the conformation of the viral capsid. Low pH also altered the conformation of the virion (11) and aided scission of VP0, a particle maturation cleavage (12). Two independent groups used recombinant technology and an antibody that blocked binding of HAV to cultured cells to isolate the putative HAV receptor from AGMK cells (74) and from a hybrid marmoset liver-Vero cell line (7, 8). Both groups isolated a class I integral-membrane glycoprotein of unknown natural function. It has characteristics of the mucin-like glycoproteins and the potential to form a lollipop-on-a-stick structure. Although the two proteins were 95% similar in amino acid sequence, the AGMK receptor was smaller and contained 451 amino acids compared to the marmoset-Vero hybrid receptor, which contained 460. Polymorphisms of the receptor were found in different AGMK cell lines (41). The human homologue subsequently isolated from liver and kidney was even smaller and had 359 amino acids and only 79% identity with the AGMK counterpart (42). The gene for the putative receptor in human cells was expressed in all organs analyzed (including liver, small intestine, colon, spleen, kidneys, and testes), with the highest levels of RNA appearing in the kidneys and testes (42). A Cys-rich region and an N-glycosylation site in the cellular receptor were required for HAV binding (128). However, there is no direct evidence that this, or a related, molecule is the receptor actually used in vivo and its presence on so many cell types cannot explain the hepatotropism of HAV.

In Vivo

The host range of HAV is limited to humans and certain species of nonhuman primates (reviewed in reference 69). Probably all of the great and lesser apes are susceptible to human HAV strains, but only chimpanzees bred and raised in captivity are available for study, since all wild apes are endangered and, therefore, legally protected from experimental studies. Other susceptible species include certain species of tamarins and owl monkeys (New World monkeys) and certain species of Old World monkeys, including macaques and African green monkeys. Several outbreaks of hepatitis A among animal handlers could be traced to exposure to asymptomatic infections in nonhuman primates (68). Inoculation of nonhuman primates with HAV is a more sensitive method of detecting wild-type virus than is inoculation of cell cultures.

ANIMAL MODELS OF DISEASE

Tamarin

The first successful transmission of HAV to a laboratory animal was its transmission to tamarins by the late Dr. Friedrich Deinhardt (28, 70). Deinhardt employed Saguinus nigricollis, S. fuscicollis, and S. oedipus in his experiments, but others subsequently found S. mystax and S. labiatis to yield more reproducible results (89, 106). The sensitivity of these latter Saguinus species equals that of chimpanzees (see below) and is probably comparable to that of humans. The typical course of HAV infection in a tamarin is similar to that seen in humans (Fig. 1) and consists of an incubation period of approximately 1 to 8 weeks, depending on the infecting dose (69). Viral replication in the liver, viremia, and fecal shedding occur during the incubation period and usually peak before onset of disease. Antibody (immunoglobulin M [IgM] and IgG) to the virion appears at approximately the time of onset of disease: IgM anti-HAV persists for weeks to months, but IgG anti-HAV usually persists for life. Viremia and fecal shedding generally last for only 2 to 3 weeks but may persist for up to 5 or 6 weeks. Immunity to hepatitis A is thought to be lifelong.

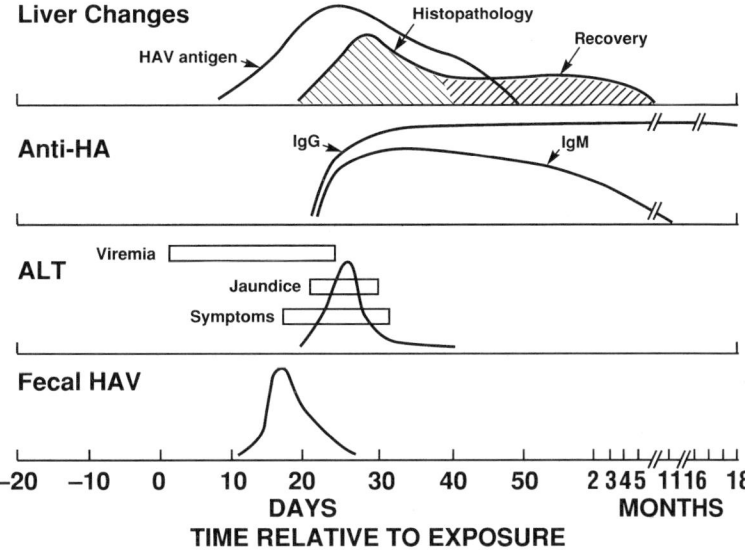

FIGURE 1 Clinical, virologic, and serologic events in a typical case of hepatitis A, as observed in experimentally infected nonhuman primates and confirmed by natural and experimental infections of humans.

Chimpanzee

The typical pattern of HAV infection in a chimpanzee is similar to that seen in tamarins except that the severity of the infection, as measured by biochemical and histologic evidence of hepatitis, is, on average, less. Perhaps that is because infant chimpanzees are often used for these studies: naturally occurring hepatitis A in human infants is usually less severe than in older children and adults (reviewed in reference 65).

Chimpanzees (and tamarins) are much less sensitive to infection with HAV by the oral route than by the intravenous route (Table 1). The reason for this is unclear, nor is it clear whether the relative susceptibility of humans to infection with HAV by the oral versus the intravenous route is similar to that of chimpanzees and tamarins.

Chimpanzees (and tamarins) have been invaluable for the study of wild-type HAV strains that grow sparingly, if at all, in cell culture. These animals have been used to characterize and amplify viruses prior to their adaptation to cell culture (29, 110). More importantly, they have been used to certify the infectivity of cDNA clones derived from wild-type HAV strains (36). This has been achieved by intrahepatic transfection of RNA transcripts of full-length cDNA clones of HAV. Initially, this required a laparotomy to expose the liver for direct inoculation of the RNA transcripts. More recently, the procedure has been achieved by ultrasound-guided percutaneous inoculation (137). This relatively innocuous procedure can be repeated at frequent intervals if necessary to characterize a number of different cDNA clones.

Other

Owl Monkey

Although not used as extensively as tamarins and chimpanzees, owl monkeys have proven to be a useful model for the study of hepatitis A (84). However, many of the studies have been performed with strains of HAV that were originally recovered from owl monkeys, raising a question about the relative susceptibility of these animals to infection with human strains of HAV that have not been adapted to growth in owl monkeys (85).

Old World Monkeys

The susceptibility of Old World monkey species to infection and hepatitis following exposure to HAV has been controversial, but was made more comprehensible by the discovery of simian strains of the virus (4, 98, 113). Whereas human strains of HAV generally produce hepatitis in chimpanzees and tamarins but not Old World monkeys, simian strains often produce hepatitis in Old World monkeys and tamarins but not in chimpanzees (38, 109). Thus, simian HAV recovered from African green monkeys (AGM-27) causes typical viral hepatitis when inoculated into seronegative African green monkeys (38). In contrast, this virus infects but does not cause hepatitis in chimpanzees. Similar results have been obtained in macaque species with simian HAV strains originally recovered from cynomolgus monkeys (5). Nevertheless, these simian HAV/Old World monkey models are useful for studying the biology of HAV infection since these monkeys are more readily available than tamarins or chimpanzees.

PATHOGENESIS OF HEPATITIS A

Virus-Cell Interactions

Natural infection with HAV generally follows oral exposure to contaminated food, water, or fomites and progresses as depicted in Fig. 1 (111). Although an intestinal site of primary replication is presumed to exist, it has never been identified unequivocally and, consequently, the early phase of infection is poorly understood (6, 75, 79, 94). Coproantibodies of the IgA class have been reported in acute hepatitis A, but this has not been confirmed in all studies (87, 138). Regardless, they appear to lack neutralizing ac-

TABLE 1 Relative susceptibility of chimpanzees and tamarins to oral versus intravenous inoculation with hepatitis A virus

Animal	Infectivity titer of HAV pool (SD-11) when administered by indicated route:	
	Oral	Intravenous
Chimpanzee	$10^{4.5}$	$10^{9.0}$
Tamarin	$10^{4.5}$	$10^{9.0}$

tivity (123). In an experimental infection of a chimpanzee, HAV was detected by immunofluorescence in the tonsils at approximately the same time that it was detected in the blood (21). It is not clear, therefore, whether the tonsils represented a primary site of replication, as has been reported for poliovirus, or whether it represented seeding from the liver or seeding from some other site of replication. Similarly, HAV has been detected in the saliva during the acute phase of hepatitis A in a patient (110). However, the titer of HAV in the saliva was 10,000-fold less than that in the serum obtained at the same time and may have represented simply leakage of blood or serum into the oropharynx. Rarely, hepatitis A is transmitted via the blood or blood products; such nonenteric infections produce hepatitis identical to that observed following enteric infection.

HAV enters the hepatocyte via a receptor that is not fully characterized and is believed to replicate by mechanisms similar to those for other picornaviruses. However, at least in cell cultures, HAV does not shut down cellular protein synthesis or cause cytopathic changes in the cells (52) although exceptions have been reported (14). It is, therefore, not clear how HAV exits infected hepatocytes, but large quantities of the virus can be found in the bile during the acute phase of infection (116). The detection of HAV in bile correlates with the finding of HAV in the feces, suggesting that fecal HAV is not the result of replication in the intestine but of transport of HAV from the liver via the bile.

As noted elsewhere, damage to liver cells may be more the result of the host's immune response than the direct effect of the virus on hepatocytes. Histologic changes in the liver are similar to those seen during the acute phase of infection with the other hepatitis viruses (81). In general, histologic changes consist of focal necrosis, Kupffer cell proliferation, apoptotic cells, and ballooning degeneration. Necrosis and mononuclear cell inflammation of the periportal region are more evident than in biopsies from patients with hepatitis B (126).

There may be a heavy infiltration of inflammatory cells, primarily lymphocytes and, less commonly, neutrophils, eosinophils, and plasma cells. Disruption of bile canaliculi may lead to bile retention following liver cell enlargement or necrosis. The severity of acute hepatitis A may range from mild, with focal necrosis, to moderate, with necrosis bridging portal tracts or joining portal areas and central veins, to submassive, with the involvement of the central and middle zones of lobules, to massive, with the involvement of entire lobules. Patients may recover completely or die of fulminant hepatitis, but the vast majority of patients with hepatitis have a mild or moderate case that resolves completely. Hepatitis A never progresses to chronic infection.

Immune Response

Humoral

The humoral immune response is brisk, long-lived, and protective. It is directed largely against the intact virion or empty capsids (95, 137). The principal neutralization epitope appears to be a conformational epitope encompassing amino acid 102 of VP1 and amino acid 70 of VP3: viruses with mutations at these sites and a few other proximate sites can escape neutralization by certain murine monoclonal antibodies directed against the epitope (95, 100, 101). However, these neutralization-escape mutant viruses do not appear to escape from neutralization by polyclonal antisera, suggesting that the antibody-binding site contains multiple epitopes or that other neutralization epitopes also exist (86).

Interestingly, the three simian genotypes of HAV, two recovered from cynomolgus monkeys and the third from an African green monkey, all have identical mutations at residue 70 of VP3 and residue 102 of VP1 to those found in neutralization-escape mutants of human HAV that were generated by growth in the presence of murine monoclonal antibodies (98, 130). Nevertheless, they all react with polyclonal antisera to HAV, and infection with at least one of these (AGM-27, recovered from an African green monkey) can protect against subsequent infection with human HAV (38).

Infection with HAV also stimulates antibody directed against the individual structural peptides of HAV, but these are for the most part not neutralizing (73, 133). Thus, recombinant expressed structural proteins of HAV, although immunogenic, have not been suitable for vaccine development unless they are assembled into capsid-like structures (83).

Infection also stimulates antibody to the nonstructural proteins encoded by the P2 and P3 regions of the HAV genome (73, 114). Best characterized is the immune response to the viral 3C proteinase (124). An immune response to the proteinase was detected by enzyme-linked immunosorbent assay in most chimpanzees experimentally infected with the virus. Although not neutralizing, antibody to the HAV 3C proteinase is useful for differentiating between vaccination with inactivated hepatitis A vaccine and infection.

Cellular

Cell-mediated immunity to HAV has been detected during convalescence from hepatitis A (40, 46, 131, 132). Cytolytic activity of peripheral blood mononuclear cells (PBMCs) against autologous fibroblasts infected with HAV peaked 2 to 3 weeks after onset of jaundice (131). In other studies, lymphocytes were recovered from biopsies of liver obtained during the acute or early convalescent phase of hepatitis A. CD8+ T cells predominated during the acute phase of illness, but CD4+ cells predominated during convalescence (131, 132). Natural killer cells were also detected. The CD8+ T cells killed autologous fibroblasts infected with HAV. These cells also produced interferon gamma.

The role of cell-mediated immunity in the pathogenesis and resolution of HAV infection is unclear. The current hypothesis is that viral hepatitis is both caused and cured by the cytotoxic T lymphocyte (CTL) activity of CD8+ lymphocytes infiltrating the virus-infected liver. Since none of the human hepatitis viruses appears to be truly cytopathogenic, CTL-mediated death of infected hepatocytes by apoptosis has been a plausible explanation for the biochemical and histologic evidence of liver damage seen in acute hepatitis. Such cell death would remove infected hepatocytes from the liver, leading to their replacement by uninfected hepatocytes. However, in acute hepatitis, the vast majority of hepatocytes are infected and efficient removal of these cells by CTL-mediated apoptosis would lead to fulminant hepatitis and death in far more patients than it does. Recent studies of the cell-mediated immune response to hepatitis B virus infection suggest that the principal mechanism of viral clearance is a cytokine-mediated down-regulation of viral replication and, ultimately, clearance of the virus from infected cells (64). CD8$^+$ CTL activity appeared to coincide with biochemical and histologic evidence of hepatitis and not with down-regulation and clearance of viral components. The exact mechanism is still not understood but may be mediated by natural killer cells. Thus, the role of CD8$^+$ CTLs may be more pathogenic than curative.

MOLECULAR BASIS OF ADAPTATION TO IN VITRO REPLICATION

In general, wild-type strains of HAV recovered from clinical cases of acute hepatitis replicate extremely slowly and to low titer in vitro and inoculated cell cultures may require months of incubation before maximum amounts of virus are produced. However, virus that grows more efficiently in cell culture has been obtained, in many cases, by blind serial passage resulting in selection of mutants having an increased capacity for replication in the cells used for passage (1, 10, 25, 47, 63, 135).

However, even those adapted viruses exhibit a prolonged replication cycle in vitro and virus titers do not normally reach a maximum until 3 or more days have passed. The reasons for the inefficient replication are not agreed upon but are postulated to include inefficient uncoating (135), inefficient polyprotein processing (54), sequestration of virion RNA (3), inefficient translation (51, 118, 136), asynchronous replication (18), and down-regulation of viral RNA synthesis (27).

Coincident with this adaptation to cell culture, the virus, in some cases, lost its virulence for primates or humans and acquired an attenuation phenotype (45, 76, 103). Sequence comparisons of the HM-175 wild-type strain of HAV and its attenuated, cell culture-adapted derivative indicated that relatively few mutations were sufficient for adaptation or attenuation (23). Infectious cDNAs of these two strains were assembled and used to construct chimeric viruses, which were first studied to identify the genes responsible for enhanced replication (22, 24, 37). Chimeric viruses were recovered from cells transfected with recombinant chimeric genomes and the replication phenotype in vitro was determined (22, 33). These studies demonstrated that the gene segment encoding 2B and 2C in the P2 region is the most critical for growth of HAV in cell culture (33). The functions of the P2 proteins of HAV are not defined, but they are most likely involved in replication of RNA. The 2B and 2C proteins are localized to a putative replication complex consisting of a tubular-vesicular network that they apparently induce (19, 58). Little is known about the 2B protein of HAV or, for that matter, other picornaviral 2B proteins. It is likely to be a peripheral membrane protein while 2C and 2BC proteins appear to be integral membrane proteins (72). High levels of recombinant 2C and 2BC, but not 2B, proteins induced rearrangement of intracellular membranes into crystalloid ER structures, but similar structures are not seen during normal infection, possibly because of low-level accumulation of nonstructural proteins (127). In another study, expression of recombinant 2B induced the tubular-vesicular network seen in cells infected in vitro with either cytopathogenic or noncytopathogenic strains (58). The 2C protein does have motifs indicative of nucleoside triphosphate (NTP) binding and helicase activity (57) and most likely performs these functions. A single amino acid substitution of valine for alanine in the 2B open reading frame plays a pivotal role in adaptation (33). This mutation is found in many independently adapted strains (23, 60, 97, 99) and can occur very early in the passage series (60). Since overexpression of 2B or 2C increases membrane permeability, it was speculated that 2B might facilitate viral particle release, but the effect of this mutation on permeability has yet to be tested (72). Two mutations in the adjacent 2C gene in combination with the mutation in the 2B gene can permit near maximal growth in FRhK-4 cells. The mechanism for this increased replication is not understood, and interpretation is complicated by the fact that elimination of the mutation(s) in either the 2B or 2C coding region can be at least partially compensated for by inclusion of all other mutations either downstream or upstream of the reverted gene (35).

HAV is normally noncytopathogenic in vitro and infection generally does not result in obvious biochemical perturbation of infected cells (52). However, a few cytopathogenic variants have been isolated that cause rounding of certain cells or induce apoptosis (14). These mutants have generally been selected from persistently infected cell cultures, but they can also be isolated as large "plaque" mutants (52, 97). The cytopathic effect is not dramatic and is influenced by the type of cells and by their condition and age. The cytopathogenic phenotype probably results from more rapid replication. In the best-studied case, mutations responsible for this phenotype are multiple, spread across the genome, and required in aggregate. Thus, unique mutations in the 2B and 2C genes as well as additional mutations in the 5′ untranslated region (UTR) and P3 regions are required for cytopathogenicity (140).

In addition to strains of HAV isolated from humans, four strains have been isolated from captive monkeys (4, 16, 98). The strain isolated from an owl monkey was subsequently recovered from humans and probably represents a human strain (16, 71, 77, 115). The three other strains were recovered from macaques or vervets, and their sequences are so divergent that each has been designated a separate genotype (113). The vervet (AGM-27) strain, isolated from a clinically ill African green monkey, has amino acid and nucleotide sequences that differ significantly from those of common human strains (130). These Old World monkey isolates probably represent true simian strains and are of special interest because they differ markedly from human strains in some biological characteristics. Although the AGM-27 virus is virulent for African green monkeys and tamarins and causes severe hepatitis, in contrast to virulent human strains, it did not require adaptation to replicate moderately efficiently in cell cultures (130). The wild-type AGM-27 virus grew in primary African green monkey kidney (AGMK) cells and in a fetal rhesus kidney (FRhK) continuous cell line much better than did wild-type HM-175 but not as well as did the cell culture-adapted human strain. However, unlike the adapted human strain, it did not replicate in CV-1 cells, a continuous line of

African green monkey kidney cells. This inability to grow in a continuous line of cells derived from its natural host is surprising since the wild-type AGM-27 virus was able to grow directly in a continuous human liver cell line (HepG2) that was totally nonpermissive for the adapted human strain, and it also replicated to detectable levels in human lung cells (MRC-5) (39). The products of the 2B and 2C coding region that control growth of human strains of HAV in cell culture appear to have a similar function in AGM-27. However, the adaptive alanine to valine mutation present in the 2B coding region of many human strains is not present in the AGM-27 gene. Whereas the 2C coding regions of HM-175 human wild-type and adapted strains differ by only 4 amino acids, the 2C coding region of AGM-27 contains many mutations compared to that of the human HAV coding region and differs from the wild-type HM-175 protein in 31 of 335 amino acids (129). The amino acid mutations are not evenly distributed but are clustered within the two terminal thirds of the gene, leaving the central third identical to that of HM-175 except for a single amino acid. This central region contains the NTP-binding and helicase motifs and is probably conserved for that reason. HM-175 chimeric viruses containing the 2C coding region of AGM-27 in place of the HM-175 gene had a dramatically reduced ability to replicate in FRhK cells (112). This reduction was partially reversed in intergenic chimeras in which either half of the HM-175 coding region was replaced with the corresponding half of the AGM-27 gene.

Adaptation to one particular cell culture system may not be sufficient to enhance replication in all cell types. For instance, the HM-175 strain of HAV adapted to grow in AGMK cells replicated efficiently in FRhK cells but not in MRC-5 cells until serially passaged in the MRC-5 cells (49). Chimera mapping experiments demonstrated that although mutations in the 2B and 2C open reading frames were required for adaptation in general, cell-specific mutations in the 5' noncoding region were required to expand the host range in some cases (26, 37). Thus, an additional cluster of mutations between bases 124 and 203 is necessary for growth in CV-1 cells (34) and a separate group of four mutations between bases 591 and 687 is critical for replication in MRC-5 cells (49). The most important of these MRC-5 adaptative mutations (base 687) (51) occurred independently in another HM-175 variant but had only a minor role in enhancing growth in BS-C-1 cells (26). Since the MRC-5 host-range mutations occur in a putative stem-loop of the IRES near the initiation translation codon, it may be that they affect the interaction of host cell proteins required for translation.

Experiments in which translation of a reporter gene was controlled by the HAV IRES showed that the rate of translation in MRC-5 cells, but not in BS-C-1 cells, was increased when the IRES contained mutations that were selected during adaptation to MRC-5 cells (51). When the effect of these mutations on viral replication was tested, the MRC-5 mutations significantly increased HAV replication in MRC-5 cells but not in BS-C-1 cells. Because the rate of virus replication was highly correlated with the rate of translation in MRC-5 cells, translation is apparently rate-limiting for virus replication in these cells. Therefore, in this case, host-range adaptation probably occurred through selection of mutations that increased translation, most likely by altering interactions with MRC-5 cell-specific components. However, inefficient translation is not a universal explanation for the slow growth of HAV in cell culture since in more permissive cells such as BS-C-1, a correlation between replication and translation of HAV was not observed (51). The question must be asked, however, whether the host cell-range effect might provide an explanation for the hepatotropism of HAV in vitro. Although HAV will grow in nonliver cells in culture, translation of HAV in a reticulocyte lysate was stimulated by addition of rat liver cell extract, supporting the possibility that hepatotropism reflects enhanced translation rather than something such as receptor selection (56).

MOLECULAR BASIS OF VIRULENCE AND ATTENUATION

Since adaptation of HM-175 to efficient growth in cell culture resulted in attenuation (as it has also for other strains), many of the same chimeric viruses that were used to map determinants of growth in cell culture were used to map determinants of virulence for nonhuman primates. Initially, chimeric viruses recovered from transfection of cultured cells were titered and known quantities were inoculated into S. mystax tamarins. The intravenous route was required because oral inoculation is inefficient and requires too much virus to be practical (Table 1). Later, to avoid the potential selection in cell culture of more rapidly growing mutants from a slowly growing population, in vitro transcribed RNAs were transfected directly into the liver of the animal (36). One caveat is that both the intravenous inoculation and the intrahepatic transfection bypass any primary replication site that might be critical for natural infection. Therefore, these studies assess only the ability of the virus to infect hepatocytes and to cause disease.

Virulence determinants of the HM-175 strain for tamarins mapped to the 2C coding regions and to two mutations close to the VP1/2A junction (32). Therefore, the function of the 2C protein impacts both replication in cultured cells and virulence in vivo although it is not known if the same mutations affect both phenotypes. In contrast, there is no evidence that the mutation in the 2B protein, which is so critical in vitro, has a discernible effect in vivo. Rather, two mutations affecting the 2A protein, the first in the 2A coding region itself and the second at the VP1/2A junction, are implicated. The 2A protein of HAV is not a proteinase as it is for poliovirus. Recent data suggest it plays a role in particle morphogenesis (102). During primary polyprotein processing, 2A protein is cleaved only at its carboxy terminus to yield a VP1/2A intermediate called PX (2). Assembly of P1 proteins into pentameric viral intermediates apparently requires 2A (102) and empty capsids contain VP1/2A (102). The 2A portion appears to be nibbled away by a host proteinase during particle maturation (62). If 2A is required for particle assembly, it is somewhat perplexing that the mutation in 2A that attenuates the virus for tamarins does not appear to inhibit virus particle formation as reflected by spread in vitro. Surprisingly, deletion of 10 to 15 amino acids (~15%) from the central portion of 2A leads to a small plaque phenotype in vitro and the virus is still able to infect tamarins and cause disease (66). The VP1/2A and 2C genes appear to contribute about equally to virulence, and intermediate hepatitis is observed if either VP1/2A or 2C is from an attenuated virus (32).

Mutations in the 5' UTR have not been found to play a significant role in attenuation. Deletion of a pyrimidine-rich tract from the 5' UTR of HAV affected neither growth in vitro nor virulence for tamarins (119, 120) whereas a comparable deletion in a murine picornavirus markedly attenuated that virus (31). HAV containing 5' UTR mutations that had been selected during cell culture adaptation of the HM-175 strain elicited lower serum liver enzyme levels than did wild-type virus, but the extent of virus excretion or liver pathology was not diminished (50).

In general, the level of virus shedding in the feces parallels that of serum liver enzyme levels, suggesting that the severity of hepatitis may simply reflect the level of viral replication in the liver (32). Although studies are not complete, there appears to be a dichotomy between ability to replicate in vivo and in vitro: those mutants that replicate most efficiently in cell culture replicate to the lowest levels in tamarins and chimpanzees and are the most attenuated. In general, mutants that form small plaques in vitro are more virulent than those that form large plaques.

APPLICATION TO VACCINE DEVELOPMENT

Because hepatitis A vaccines are based on the immunogenicity of intact virions, an appreciation (or at least an application) of the molecular basis for efficient growth in cell culture or of attenuation has been necessary for the development of such vaccines. All current hepatitis A vaccines commercially available and internationally licensed were developed by adaptation to, and serial passage in, vaccine-acceptable cell cultures and are inactivated (5a). The cell culture of choice for inactivated vaccines has been MRC-5 cells (human diploid fibroblast cells). As noted above, certain mutations in the 5' UTR of the HM-175 strain of HAV were necessary before the virus could grow in these cells. Interestingly, this strain of HAV grows at 35°C but not 37°C in MRC-5 cells, but at both temperatures in most continuous kidney cell lines of monkey origin.

Live attenuated hepatitis A vaccines have also been developed, but they have not been licensed for commercial application in the United States (45, 76, 91, 103). These vaccines also have been developed by isolation and blind serial passage in cells. The most promising candidate vaccines have been grown in primary or continuous monkey kidney cells. However, virtually all primary monkey kidney cells are contaminated with simian viruses and therefore not useful for vaccine propagation. Most continuous monkey kidney cell lines are also not licensed for vaccine use (certain lots of Vero cells are an exception, but some of the best candidate vaccine strains of HAV grow inefficiently in these cells). Unfortunately, adaptation of HAV to growth in MRC-5 cells usually results in overattenuation of the virus for primates, including humans (104, 121). In this case, attenuation probably cannot be separated from enhanced growth in vitro and the availability of practical live, attenuated HAV vaccines must probably await the certification and licensing for vaccine use of more permissive kidney cell lines.

REFERENCES

1. **Anderson, D. A., S. A. Locarnini, B. C. Ross, A. G. Coulepis, B. N. Anderson, and I. D. Gust.** 1987. Single-cycle growth kinetics of hepatitis A virus in BSC-1 cells, p. 497–507. *In* M. A. Brinton and R. R. Rueckert (ed.), *Positive Strand RNA Viruses*. Alan R Liss, New York, N.Y.
2. **Anderson, D. A., and B. C. Ross.** 1990. Morphogenesis of hepatitis A virus: isolation and characterization of subviral particles. *J. Virol.* **64:**5284–5289.
3. **Anderson, D. A., B. C. Ross, and S. A. Locarnini.** 1988. Restricted replication of hepatitis A virus in cell culture: encapsidation of viral RNA depletes the pool of RNA available for replication. *J. Virol.* **62:**4201–4206.
4. **Andzhaparidze, A. G., M. S. Balayan, A. P. Savinov, Y. A. Kazachkov, and I. P. Titova.** 1987. Spontaneous hepatitis, similar to hepatitis A in African green monkeys. *Vopr. Virusol.* **6:**681–686.
5. **Andzhaparidze, A. G., Y. A. Kazachkov, M. S. Balayan, Y. Y. Kusov, and V. F. Poleschuk.** 1987. Hepatitis A in *Macaca fascicularis* and *Macaca arctoides* infected with the YuM-55 strain of hepatitis A virus. *Vopr. Virusol.* **2:**440–448.
5a. **Anonymous.** 2000. Hepatitis A vaccines. *Wkly. Epidemiol. Rec.* **75(5):**38–44.
6. **Asher, L. V., L. N. Binn, T. L. Mensing, R. H. Marchwicki, R. A. Vassell, and G. D. Young.** 1995. Pathogenesis of hepatitis A in orally inoculated owl monkeys (*Aotus trivirgatus*). *J. Med. Virol.* **47:**260–268.
7. **Ashida, M., and C. Hamada.** 1997. Molecular cloning of the hepatitis A virus receptor from a simian cell line. *J. Gen. Virol.* **78:**1565–1569.
8. **Ashida, M., H. Hara, H. Kojima, T. Kamimura, F. Ichida, and C. Hamada.** 1989. Propagation of hepatitis A virus in hybrid cell lines derived from marmoset liver and Vero cells. *J. Gen. Virol.* **70:**2487–2494.
9. **Bienz, K., D. Egger, and L. Pasamontes.** 1987. Association of polioviral proteins of the P2 genomic region with the viral replication complex and virus-induced membrane synthesis as visualized by electron microscopic immunocytochemistry and autoradiography. *Virology* **160:**220–226.
10. **Binn, L. N., S. M. Lemon, R. H. Marchwicki, R. R. Redfield, N. L. Gates, and W. H. Bancroft.** 1984. Primary isolation and serial passage of hepatitis A virus strains in primate cell cultures. *J. Clin. Microbiol.* **20:**28–33.
11. **Bishop, N. E.** 1999. Conformational changes in the hepatitis A virus capsid in response to acidic conditions. *J. Med. Microbiol.* **48:**443–450.
12. **Bishop, N. E.** 1999. Effect of low pH on the hepatitis A virus maturation cleavage. *Acta Virol.* **43:**291–296.
13. **Bishop, N. E., and D. A. Anderson.** 1997. Early interactions of hepatitis A virus with cultured cells: viral elution and the effect of pH and calcium ions. *Arch. Virol.* **142:**2161–2178.
14. **Brack, K., W. Frings, A. Dotzauer, and A. Vallbracht.** 1998. A cytopathogenic, apoptosis-inducing variant of hepatitis A virus. *J. Virol.* **72:**3370–3376.
15. **Brown, E. A., S. P. Day, R. W. Jansen, and S. M. Lemon.** 1991. The 5' nontranslated region of hepatitis A virus: secondary structure and elements required for translation in vitro. *J. Virol.* **65:**5828–5838.
16. **Brown, E. A., R. W. Jansen, and S. M. Lemon.** 1989. Characterization of a simian hepatitis A virus (HAV): antigenic and genetic comparison with human HAV. *J. Virol.* **63:**4932–4937.
17. **Brown, E. A., A. J. Zajac, and S. M. Lemon.** 1994. In vitro characterization of an internal ribosomal entry site (IRES) present within the 5' nontranslated region of hepatitis A virus RNA: comparison with the IRES of encephalomyocarditis virus. *J. Virol.* **68:**1066–1074.
18. **Cho, M. W., and E. Ehrenfeld.** 1991. Rapid completion of the replication cycle of hepatitis A virus subsequent to reversal of guanidine inhibition. *Virology* **180:**770–780.
19. **Cho, M. W., N. Teterina, D. Egger, K. Bienz, and E. Ehrenfeld.** 1994. Membrane rearrangement and vesicle induction by recombinant poliovirus 2C and 2BC in human cells. *Virology* **202:**129–145.
20. **Cockayne, E. A.** 1912. Catarrhal jaundice, sporadic and epidemic, and its relation to acute yellow atrophy of the liver. *Q. J. Med.* **6:**1–28.

21. **Cohen, J. I., M. Feinstone, and R. H. Purcell.** 1989. Hepatitis A virus infection in a chimpanzee: duration of viremia and detection of virus in saliva and throat swabs. *J. Infect. Dis.* **160:**887–890.
22. **Cohen, J. I., B. Rosenblum, S. M. Feinstone, J. Ticehurst, and R. H. Purcell.** 1989. Attenuation and cell culture adaptation of hepatitis A virus (HAV): a genetic analysis with HAV cDNA. *J. Virol.* **63:**5364–5370.
23. **Cohen, J. I., B. Rosenblum, J. R. Ticehurst, R. J. Daemer, S. M. Feinstone, and R. H. Purcell.** 1987. Complete nucleotide sequence of an attenuated hepatitis A virus: comparison with wild-type virus. *Proc. Natl. Acad. Sci. USA* **84:**2497–2501.
24. **Cohen, J. I., J. R. Ticehurst, S. M. Feinstone, B. Rosenblum, and R. H. Purcell.** 1987. Hepatitis A virus cDNA and its RNA transcripts are infectious in cell culture. *J. Virol.* **61:**3035–3039.
25. **Daemer, R. J., S. M. Feinstone, I. D. Gust, and R. H. Purcell.** 1981. Propagation of human hepatitis A virus in African green monkey kidney cell culture: primary isolation and serial passage. *Infect. Immun.* **32:**388–393.
26. **Day, S. P., P. Murphy, E. A. Brown, and S. M. Lemon.** 1992. Mutations within the 5' nontranslated region of hepatitis A virus RNA which enhance replication in BS-C-1 cells. *J. Virol.* **66:**6533–6540.
27. **de Chastonay, J., and G. Siegl.** 1987. Replicative events in hepatitis A virus-infected cells. *Virology* **157:**68–75.
28. **Deinhardt, F., A. W. Holmes, R. B. Capps, and H. Popper.** 1967. Studies on the transmission of human viral hepatitis to marmoset monkeys. I. Transmission of disease, serial passages, and description of liver lesions. *J. Exp. Med.* **125:**673–688.
29. **Dienstag, J. L., S. M. Feinstone, R. H. Purcell, J. H. Hoofnagle, L. F. Barker, W. T. London, H. Popper, J. M. Peterson, and A. Z. Kapikian.** 1975. Experimental infection of chimpanzees with hepatitis A virus. *J. Infect. Dis.* **132:**532–545.
30. **Dotzauer, A., S. M. Feinstone, and G. Kaplan.** 1994. Susceptibility of nonprimate cell lines to hepatitis A virus infection. *J. Virol.* **68:**6064–6068.
31. **Duke, G. M., J. E. Osorio, and A. C. Palmenberg.** 1990. Attenuation of mengo virus through genetic engineering of the 5' noncoding poly(C) tract. *Nature (London)* **343:**474–476.
32. **Emerson, S. U.** 1997. Hepatitis A virus: molecular basis for replication in vitro and virulence in vivo, p. 19–21. *In* M. Rizzetto, R. H. Purcell, J. L. Gerin, and G. Verme (ed.), *Proceedings of IX Triennial International Symposium on Viral Hepatitis and Liver Disease*. Edizoni Minerva Medica, Turin, Italy.
33. **Emerson, S. U., Y. K. Huang, C. McRill, M. Lewis, and R. H. Purcell.** 1992. Mutations in both the 2B and 2C genes of hepatitis A virus are involved in adaptation to growth in cell culture. *J. Virol.* **66:**650–654.
34. **Emerson, S. U., Y. K. Huang, C. McRill, M. Lewis, M. Shapiro, W. T. London, and R. H. Purcell.** 1992. Molecular basis of virulence and growth of hepatitis A virus in cell culture. *Vaccine* **10**(Suppl. 1):S36–S39.
35. **Emerson, S. U., Y. K. Huang, and R. H. Purcell.** 1993. 2B and 2C mutations are essential but mutations throughout the genome of HAV contribute to adaptation to cell culture. *Virology* **194:**475–480.
36. **Emerson, S. U., M. Lewis, S. Govindarajan, M. Shapiro, T. Moskal, and R. H. Purcell.** 1992. cDNA clone of hepatitis A virus encoding a virulent virus: induction of viral hepatitis by direct nucleic acid transfection of marmosets. *J. Virol.* **66:**6649–6654.
37. **Emerson, S. U., C. McRill, B. Rosenblum, S. Feinstone, and R. H. Purcell.** 1991. Mutations responsible for adaptation of hepatitis A virus to efficient growth in cell culture. *J. Virol.* **65:**4882–4886.
38. **Emerson, S. U., S. A. Tsarev, S. Govindarajan, M. Shapiro, and R. H. Purcell.** 1996. A simian strain of hepatitis A virus, AGM-27, functions as an attenuated vaccine for chimpanzees. *J. Infect. Dis.* **173:**592–597.
39. **Emerson, S. U., S. A. Tsarev, and R. H. Purcell.** 1991. Biological and molecular comparisons of human (HM-175) and simian (AGM-27) hepatitis A viruses. *J. Hepatol.* **13**(Suppl. 4):S144–S145.
40. **Fasel-Felley, J., L. R. Overby, and P. C. Frei.** 1986. A specific immune response to purified HA antigen (HAAg) demonstrated by leukocyte migration inhibition in patients recovering from viral hepatitis A. *J. Hepatol.* **2:**237–244.
41. **Feigelstock, D., P. Thompson, P. Mattoo, and G. G. Kaplan.** 1998. Polymorphisms of the hepatitis A virus cellular receptor 1 in African green monkey kidney cells result in antigenic variants that do not react with protective monoclonal antibody 190/4. *J. Virol.* **72:**6218–6222.
42. **Feigelstock, D., P. Thompson, P. Mattoo, Y. Zhang, and G. G. Kaplan.** 1998. The human homolog of HAV cr-1 codes for a hepatitis A virus cellular receptor. *J. Virol.* **72:**6621–6628.
43. **Feinstone, S. M., A. Z. Kapikian, and R. H. Purcell.** 1973. Hepatitis A: detection by immune electron microscopy of a viruslike antigen associated with acute illness. *Science* **182:**1026–1028.
44. **Flehmig, B.** 1980. Hepatitis A-virus in cell culture. I. Propagation of different hepatitis A-virus isolates in a fetal rhesus monkey kidney cell line (Frhk-4). *Med. Microbiol. Immunol.* **168:**239–248.
45. **Flehmig, B., R. F. Mauler, G. Noll, E. Weinmann, and J. P. Gregersen.** 1988. Progress in the development of an attenuated, live hepatitis A vaccine, p. 87–90. *In* A. J. Zuckerman (ed.), *Viral Hepatitis and Liver Disease*. Alan R Liss, New York, N.Y.
46. **Fleischer, B., S. Fleischer, K. Maier, K. H. Wiedmann, M. Sacher, H. Thaler, and A. Vallbracht.** 1990. Clonal analysis of infiltrating T lymphocytes in liver tissue in viral hepatitis A. *Immunology* **69:**14–19.
47. **Frösner, G. G., F. Deinhardt, R. Scheid, V. Gauss-Müller, N. Holmes, V. Messelberger, G. Siegl, and J. J. Alexander.** 1979. Propagation of human hepatitis A virus in a hepatoma cell line. *Infection* **7:**303–305.
48. **Frösner, G., H. Willers, R. Müller, D. Schenzle, F. Deinhardt, and W. Höpken.** 1978. Decrease in incidence of hepatitis A infections in Germany. *J. Clin. Study Treat. Infect.* **6:**259–260.
49. **Funkhouser, A. W., R. H. Purcell, E. D'Hondt, and S. U. Emerson.** 1994. Attenuated hepatitis A virus: genetic determinants of adaptation to growth in MRC-5 cells. *J. Virol.* **68:**148–157.
50. **Funkhouser, A. W., G. Raychaudhuri, R. H. Purcell, S. Govindarajan, R. Elkins, and S. U. Emerson.** 1996. Progress toward the development of a genetically engineered attenuated hepatitis A virus vaccine. *J. Virol.* **70:**7948–7957.
51. **Funkhouser, A. W., D. Schultz, S. M. Lemon, R. H. Purcell, and S. U. Emerson.** 1999. Hepatitis A virus translation is rate-limiting for virus replication in MRC-5 cells. *Virology* **254:**268–278.
52. **Gauss-Müller, V., and F. Deinhardt.** 1984. Effect of hepatitis A virus infection on cell metabolism in vitro. *Proc. Soc. Exp. Biol. Med.* **175:**10–15.
53. **Gauss-Müller, V., G. G. Frösner, and F. Deinhardt.** 1981. Propagation of human hepatitis A virus in human embryo fibroblasts. *J. Med. Virol.* **7:**233–239.
54. **Gauss-Müller, V., K. von der Helm, and F. Deinhardt.**

1984. Translation in vitro of hepatitis A virus RNA. *Virology* **137**:182–184.
55. Glass, M. J., X.-Y. Jia, and D. F. Summers. 1993. Identification of the hepatitis A virus internal ribosome entry site: in vivo and in vitro analysis of bicistronic RNAs containing the HAV 5' noncoding region. *Virology* **193**:842–852.
56. Glass, M. J., and D. F. Summers. 1993. Identification of a *trans*-acting activity from liver that stimulates hepatitis A virus translation in vitro. *Virology* **193**:1047–1050.
57. Gorbalenya, A. E., V. M. Blinov, A. P. Donchenko, and E. V. Koonin. 1989. An NTP-binding motif is the most conserved sequence in a highly diverged monophyletic group of proteins involved in positive strand RNA viral replication. *J. Mol. Evol.* **28**:256–268.
58. Gosert, R., D. Egger, and K. Bienz. 2000. A cytopathic and a cell culture adapted hepatitis A virus strain differ in cell killing but not in intracellular membrane rearrangements. *Virology* **266**:157–169.
59. Graff, J., and E. Ehrenfeld. 1998. Coding sequences enhance internal initiation of translation by hepatitis A virus RNA in vitro. *J. Virol.* **72**:3571–3577.
60. Graff, J., C. Kasang, A. Normann, M. Pfisterer-Hunt, S. M. Feinstone, and B. Flehmig. 1994. Mutational events in consecutive passages of hepatitis A virus strain GBM during cell culture adaptation. *Virology* **204**:60–68.
61. Graff, J., A. Normann, S. M. Feinstone, and B. Flehmig. 1994. Nucleotide sequence of wild-type hepatitis A virus GBM in comparison with two cell culture-adapted variants. *J. Virol.* **68**:548–554.
62. Graff, J., O. C. Richards, K. M. Swiderek, M. T. Davis, F. Rusnak, S. A. Harmon, X.-Y. Jia, D. F. Summers, and E. Ehrenfeld. 1999. Hepatitis A virus capsid protein VP1 has a heterogeneous C terminus. *J. Virol.* **73**:6015–6023.
63. Gregersen, J.-P., S. Mehdi, and R. Mauler. 1988. Adaptation of hepatitis A virus to high titre growth in diploid and permanent cell cultures. *Med. Microbiol. Immunol.* **177**:91–100.
64. Guidotti, L. G., R. Rochford, J. Chung, M. Shapiro, R. H. Purcell, and F. V. Chisari. 1999. Viral clearance without destruction of infected cells during acute HBV infection. *Science* **284**:825–829.
65. Hadler, S. C. 1991. Global impact of hepatitis A virus infection changing patterns, p. 14–20. *In* F. B. Hollinger, S. M. Lemon, and H. S. Margolis (ed.), *Viral Hepatitis and Liver Disease*. Williams & Wilkins, Baltimore, Md.
66. Harmon, S. A., S. U. Emerson, Y. K. Huang, D. F. Summers, and E. Ehrenfeld. 1995. Hepatitis A viruses with deletions in the 2A gene are infectious in cultured cells and marmosets. *J. Virol.* **69**:5576–5581.
67. Havens, W. P., Jr. 1947. The etiology of infectious hepatitis. *JAMA* **134**:653–655.
68. Hillis, W. D. 1961. An outbreak of infectious hepatitis among chimpanzee handlers at a United States Air Force base. *Am. J. Hyg.* **73**:316–328.
69. Hollinger, F. B., and J. R. Ticehurst. 1996. Hepatitis A virus, p. 735–782. *In* B. N. Fields, D. M. Knipe, P. M. Howley, R. M. Chanock, J. L. Melnick, T. P. Monath, B. Roizman, and S. E. Straus (ed.), *Field's Virology*. Lippincott-Raven Publishers, Philadelphia, Pa.
70. Holmes, A. W., L. Wolfe, F. Deinhardt, and M. E. Conrad. 1971. Transmission of human hepatitis to marmosets: further coded studies. *J. Infect. Dis.* **124**:520.
71. Jansen, R. W., G. Siegl, and S. M. Lemon. 1991. Molecular epidemiology of human hepatitis A virus, p. 58–62. *In* F. B. Hollinger, S. M. Lemon, and H. S. Margolis (ed.), *Viral Hepatitis and Liver Disease*. Williams & Wilkins, Baltimore, Md.
72. Jecht, M., C. Probst, and V. Gauss-Muller. 1998. Membrane permeability induced by hepatitis A virus proteins 2B and 2BC and proteolytic processing of HAV 2BC. *Virology* **252**:218–227.
73. Jia, X. Y., D. F. Summers, and E. Ehrenfeld. 1992. Host antibody response to viral structural and nonstructural proteins after hepatitis A virus infection. *J. Infect. Dis.* **165**:273–280.
74. Kaplan, G., A. Totsuka, P. Thompson, T. Akatsuka, Y. Moritsugu, and S. M. Feinstone. 1996. Identification of a surface glycoprotein on African green monkey kidney cells as a receptor for hepatitis A virus. *EMBO J.* **16**:4282–4296.
75. Karayiannis, P., M. J. McGarvey, M. A. Fry, and H. C. Thomas. 1998. Detection of hepatitis A virus RNA in tissues and faeces of experimentally infected tamarins by cDNA-RNA hybridisation, p. 117–120. *In* A. J. Zuckerman (ed.), *Viral Hepatitis and Liver Disease*. Alan R Liss, New York, N.Y.
76. Karron, R. A., R. Daemer, J. Ticehurst, E. D'Hondt, H. Popper, K. Mihalik, S. Phillips, S. Feinstone, and R. H. Purcell. 1988. Studies of prototype live hepatitis A virus vaccines in primate models. *J. Infect. Dis.* **157**:338–345.
77. Khanna, B., J. E. Spelbring, B. L. Innis, and B. H. Robertson. 1992. Characterization of a genetic variant of human hepatitis A virus. *J. Med. Virol.* **36**:118–124.
78. Kojima, H., T. Shibayama, A. Sato, S. Suzuki, F. Ichida, and C. Hamada. 1981. Propagation of human hepatitis A virus in conventional cell lines. *J. Med. Virol.* **7**:273–286.
79. Krawczynski, K. K., D. W. Bradley, B. L. Murphy, J. W. Ebert, T. E. Anderson, I. L. Doto, A. Nowoslawski, W. Duermeyer, and J. E. Maynard. 1981. Pathogenetic aspects of hepatitis A virus infection in enterally inoculated marmosets. *Am. J. Clin. Pathol.* **76**:698–706.
80. Krugman, S., J. P. Giles, and J. Hammond. 1967. Infectious hepatitis: evidence for two distinctive clinical epidemiological and immunological types of infection. *JAMA* **200**:365–373.
81. Kryger, P., and P. Christoffersen. 1983. Liver histopathology of the hepatitis A virus infection: a comparison with hepatitis B and non-A, non-B. *J. Clin. Pathol.* **36**:650–654.
82. Kusov, Y. Y., W. Sommergruber, M. Schreiber, and V. Gauss-Müller. 1992. Intermolecular cleavage of hepatitis A virus (HAV) precursor protein P1-P2 by recombinant HAV proteinase 3C. *J. Virol.* **66**:6794–6796.
83. LaBrecque, F. D., D. R. LaBrecque, D. Klinzman, S. Perlman, J. B. Cederna, P. L. Winokur, J. Q. Han, and J. T. Stapleton. 1998. Recombinant hepatitis A virus antigen: improved production and utility in diagnostic assays. *J. Clin. Microbiol.* **36**:2014–2018.
84. LeDuc, J. W., S. M. Lemon, C. M. Keenan, R. R. Graham, R. H. Marchwicki, and L. N. Binn. 1983. Experimental infection of the New World owl monkey (*Aotus trivirgatus*) with hepatitis A virus. *Infect. Immun.* **40**:766–772.
85. Lemon, S. M., J. W. LeDuc, L. N. Binn, A. Escajadillo, and K. G. Ishak. 1982. Transmission of hepatitis A virus among recently captured Panamanian owl monkeys. *J. Med. Virol.* **10**:25–36.
86. Lemon, S. M., and B. H. Robertson. 1993. Current perspectives in the virology and molecular biology of hepatitis A virus. *Semin. Virol.* **4**:285–295.
87. Locarnini, S. A., A. G. Coulepis, J. Kaldor, and I. D. Gust. 1980. Coproantibodies in hepatitis A: detection by enzyme-linked immunosorbent assay and immune electron microscopy. *J. Clin. Microbiol.* **11**:710–716.
88. Locarnini, S. A., A. G. Coulepis, E. G. Westaway, and I. D. Gust. 1981. Restricted replication of human hepatitis A virus in cell culture: intracellular biochemical studies. *J. Virol.* **37**:216–225.

89. **Lorenz, D., L. Barker, D. Stevens, M. Peterson, and R. Kirschstein.** 1970. Hepatitis in the marmoset: *Saguinus mystax*. *Proc. Soc. Exp. Biol. Med.* **135:**348–354.
90. **MacCallum, F. O.** 1947. Homologous serum jaundice. *Lancet* **2:**691–692.
91. **Mao, J. S., D. X. Dong, H. Y. Zhang, N. L. Chen, X. Y. Zhang, H. Y. Huang, R. Y. Xie, T. J. Zhou, Z. J. Wan, Y. Z. Wang, Z. H. Hu, Y. Y. Cao, H. M. Li, and C. M. Cue.** 1989. Primary study of attenuated live hepatitis A vaccine (H2 strain) in humans. *J. Infect. Dis.* **159:**621–624.
92. **Martin, A., N. Escriou, S.-F. Chao, M. Girard, S. M. Lemon, and C. Wychowski.** 1995. Identification and site-directed mutagenesis of the primary (2A/2B) cleavage site of the hepatitis A virus polyprotein: functional impact on the infectivity of HAV RNA transcripts. *Virology* **213:**213–222.
93. **Marvil, P., N. J. Knowles, A. P. Adrian Mockett, P. Britton, T. D. K. Brown, and D. Cavanagh.** 1999. Avian encephalomyelitis virus is a picornavirus and is most closely related to hepatitis A virus. *J. Gen. Virol.* **80:**653–662.
94. **Mathiesen, L. R., J. Drucker, D. Lorenz, J. A. Wagner, R. J. Gerety, and R. H. Purcell.** 1978. Localization of hepatitis A antigen in marmoset organs during acute infection with hepatitis A virus. *J. Infect. Dis.* **138:**369–377.
95. **Mattioli, S., L. Imberti, R. Stellini, and D. Primi.** 1995. Mimicry of the immunodominant conformation-dependent antigenic site of hepatitis A virus by motifs selected from synthetic peptide libraries. *J. Virol.* **69:**5294–5299.
96. **Minor, P.** 1995. Picornaviridae, p. 329–336. In F. A. Murphy, C. M. Fauquet, D. H. L. Bishop, S. A. Ghabrial, A. W. Jarvis, G. P. Martelli, M. A. Mayo, and M. D. Summers (ed.), *Virus Taxonomy. Classification and Nomenclature of Viruses. Sixth Report of the International Committee on Taxonomy of Viruses*. Springer-Verlag, Vienna, Austria.
97. **Morace, G., G. Pisani, F. Beneduce, M. Divizia, and A. Panà.** 1993. Mutations in the 3A genomic region of two cytopathic strains of hepatitis A virus isolated in Italy. *Virus Res.* **28:**187–194.
98. **Nainan, O. V., H. S. Margolis, B. H. Robertson, M. Balayan, and M. A. Brinton.** 1991. Sequence analysis of a new hepatitis A virus naturally infecting cynomolgus macaques (*Macaca fascicularis*). *J. Gen. Virol.* **72:**1685–1689.
99. **Paul, A. V., H. Tada, K. von der Helm, T. Wissel, R. Kiehn, E. Wimmer, and F. Deinhardt.** 1987. The entire nucleotide sequence of the genome of human hepatitis A virus (isolate MBB). *Virus Res.* **88:**153–171.
100. **Ping, L. H., R. W. Jansen, J. T. Stapleton, J. I. Cohen, and S. M. Lemon.** 1988. Identification of an immunodominant antigenic site involving the capsid protein VP3 of hepatitis A virus. *Proc. Natl. Acad. Sci. USA* **85:**8281–8285.
101. **Ping, L. H., and S. M. Lemon.** 1992. Antigenic structure of human hepatitis A virus defined by analysis of escape mutants selected against murine monoclonal antibodies. *J. Virol.* **66:**2208–2216.
102. **Probst, C., M. Jecht, and V. Gauss-Muller.** 1999. Intrinsic signals for the assembly of hepatitis A virus particles. *J. Biol. Chem.* **274:**4527–4531.
103. **Provost, P. J., R. P. Bishop, R. J. Gerety, M. R. Hilleman, W. J. McAleer, E. M. Scolnick, and C. E. Stevens.** 1986. New findings in live, attenuated hepatitis A vaccine development. *J. Med. Virol.* **20:**165–176.
104. **Provost, P. J., E. A. Emini, J. A. Lewis, and R. J. Gerety.** 1988. Progress toward the development of a hepatitis A vaccine, p. 83–86. In A. J. Zuckerman (ed.), *Viral Hepatitis and Liver Disease*. Alan R Liss, New York, N.Y.
105. **Provost, P. J., and M. R. Hilleman.** 1979. Propagation of human hepatitis A virus in cell culture in vitro. *Proc. Soc. Exp. Biol. Med.* **160:**213–221.
106. **Provost, P. J., V. M. Villarejos, and M. R. Hilleman.** 1977. Suitability of the Rufiventer marmoset as a host animal for human hepatitis A virus. *Proc. Soc. Exp. Biol. Med.* **155:**283–286.
107. **Provost, P. J., B. S. Wolanski, W. J. Miller, O. L. Ittensohn, W. J. McAleer, and M. R. Hilleman.** 1975. Physical, chemical and morphologic dimensions of human hepatitis A virus strain CR326. *Proc. Soc. Exp. Biol. Med.* **148:**532–539.
108. **Purcell, R. H.** 1996. Hepatitis E virus, p. 2831–2843. In B. N. Fields, D. M. Knipe, P. M. Howley, R. M. Chanock, J. L. Melnick, T. P. Monath, and B. Roizman, et al. (ed.), *Field's Virology*. Raven Press, Ltd., New York, N.Y.
109. **Purcell, R. H., and J. L. Dienstag.** 1978. Experimental hepatitis A virus infection, p. 3–12. In T. Oda (ed.), *Hepatitis Viruses*. University of Tokyo Press, Tokyo, Japan.
110. **Purcell, R. H., S. M. Feinstone, J. R. Ticehurst, R. J. Daemer, and B. M. Baroudy.** 1984. Hepatitis A virus, p. 9–22. In G. N. Vyas, J. L. Dienstag, and J. H. Hoofnagle (ed.), *Viral Hepatitis and Liver Disease*. Grune & Stratton, Orlando, Fla.
111. **Purcell, R. H., J. H. Hoofnagle, J. Ticehurst, and J. L. Gerin.** 1989. Hepatitis viruses, p. 957–1065. In N. J. Schmidt and R. W. Emmons (ed.), *Diagnostic Procedures for Viral, Rickettsial and Chlamydial Infections*. American Public Health Association, Washington, D.C.
112. **Raychaudhuri, G., S. Govindarajan, M. Shapiro, R. H. Purcell, and S. U. Emerson.** 1998. Utilization of chimeras between human (HM-175) and simian (AGM-27) strains of hepatitis A virus to study the molecular basis of virulence. *J. Virol.* **72:**7467–7475.
113. **Robertson, B. H., R. W. Jansen, B. Khanna, A. Totsuka, O. V. Nainan, G. Siegl, A. Widell, H. S. Margolis, S. Isomura, K. Ito, T. Ishizu, Y. Moritsugu, and S. M. Lemon.** 1992. Genetic relatedness of hepatitis A virus strains recovered from different geographic regions. *J. Gen. Virol.* **73:**1365–1377.
114. **Robertson, B. H., X.-Y. Jia, H. Tian, H. S. Margolis, D. F. Summers, and E. Ehrenfeld.** 1993. Antibody response to nonstructural proteins of hepatitis A virus following infection. *J. Med. Virol.* **40:**76–82.
115. **Robertson, B. H., B. Khanna, O. V. Nainan, and H. S. Margolis.** 1991. Genetic variation of wild-type hepatitis A isolates, p. 54–58. In F. B. Hollinger, S. M. Lemon, and H. S. Margolis (ed.), *Viral Hepatitis and Liver Disease*. Williams & Wilkins, Baltimore, Md.
116. **Schulman, A. N., J. L. Dienstag, D. R. Jackson, J. H. Hoofnagle, R. J. Gerety, R. H. Purcell, and L. F. Barker.** 1976. Hepatitis A antigen particles in liver, bile, and stool of chimpanzees. *J. Infect. Dis.* **134:**80–84.
117. **Schultheiss, T., Y. Y. Kusov, and V. Gauss-Müller.** 1994. Proteinase 3C of hepatitis A virus (HAV) cleaves the HAV polyprotein P2-P3 at all sites including VP1/2A and 2A/2B. *Virology* **198:**275–281.
118. **Schultz, D. E., M. Honda, L. E. Whetter, K. L. McKnight, and S. M. Lemon.** 1996. Mutations within the 5′ nontranslated RNA of cell culture-adapted hepatitis A virus which enhance cap-independent translation in cultured African green monkey kidney cells. *J. Virol.* **70:**1041–1049.
119. **Shaffer, D. R., E. A. Brown, and S. M. Lemon.** 1994. Large deletion mutations involving the first pyrimidine-rich tract of the 5′ nontranslated RNA of hepatitis A virus define two adjacent domains associated with distinct replication phenotypes. *J. Virol.* **68:**5568–5578.

120. Shaffer, D. R., S. U. Emerson, P. C. Murphy, S. Govindarajan, and S. M. Lemon. 1995. A hepatitis A virus deletion mutant which lacks the first pyrimidine-rich tract of the 5' nontranslated RNA remains virulent in primates after direct intrahepatic nucleic acid transfection. *J. Virol.* **69:**6600–6604.
121. Sjogren, M. H., R. H. Purcell, K. McKee, L. Binn, P. Marcarthy, J. Ticehurst, S. Feinstone, J. Caudill, A. See, C. Hoke, W. Bancroft, and E. D'Hondt. 1992. Clinical and laboratory observations following oral or intramuscular administration of a live attenuated hepatitis A vaccine candidate. *Vaccine* **10**(Suppl. 1):S135–S137.
122. Stapleton, J. T., J. Frederick, and B. Meyer. 1991. Hepatitis A virus attachment to cultured cell lines. *J. Infect. Dis.* **164:**1098–1103.
123. Stapleton, J. T., J. W. LeDuc, L. N. Binn, and S. M. Lemon. 1987. Lack of neutralizing activity in fecal extracts following experimental hepatitis A virus (HAV) infection in man and owl monkeys. *J. Med. Virol.* **21:**17A.
124. Stewart, D. R., T. S. Morris, R. H. Purcell, and S. U. Emerson. 1997. Detection of antibodies to the nonstructural 3C proteinase of hepatitis A virus. *J. Infect. Dis.* **176:**593–601.
125. Szmuness, W., J. L. Dienstag, R. H. Purcell, E. J. Harley, C. E. Stevens, and D. C. Wong. 1976. Distribution of antibody to hepatitis A antigen in urban adult populations. *N. Engl. J. Med.* **295:**755–759.
126. Teixeira, M. R., Jr., I. V. D. Weller, A. Murray, M. Bamber, H. C. Thomas, S. Sherlock, and P. J. Scheuer. 1982. The pathology of hepatitis A in man. *Liver* **2:**53–60.
127. Teterina, N. L., K. Bienz, D. Egger, A. E. Gorbalenya, and E. Ehrenfeld. 1997. Induction of intracellular membrane rearrangements by HAV proteins 2C and 2BC. *Virology* **237:**66–77.
128. Thompson, P., J. Lu, and G. G. Kaplan. 1998. The cys-rich region of hepatitis A virus cellular receptor 1 is required for binding of hepatitis A virus and protective monoclonal antibody 190/4. *J. Virol.* **72:**3751–3761.
129. Tsarev, S. A., S. U. Emerson, and M. S. Balayan. 1991. Sequence of simian AGM-27 strain of hepatitis A virus determined from polymerase chain reaction (PCR), p. 64–65. *In* F. B. Hollinger, S. M. Lemon, and H. S. Margolis (ed.), *Viral Hepatitis and Liver Disease.* Williams & Wilkins, Baltimore, Md.
130. Tsarev, S. A., S. U. Emerson, M. S. Balayan, J. Ticehurst, and R. H. Purcell. 1991. Simian hepatitis A virus (HAV) strain AGM-27: comparison of genome structure and growth in cell culture with other HAV strains. *J. Gen. Virol.* **72:**1677–1683.
131. Vallbracht, A., P. Gabriel, K. Maier, F. Hartmann, H. J. Steinhardt, C. Muller, A. Wolf, K. H. Manncke, and B. Flehmig. 1986. Cell-mediated cytotoxicity in hepatitis A virus infection. *Hepatology* **6:**1308–1314.
132. Vallbracht, A., K. Maier, Y. D. Stierhof, K. H. Wiedmann, B. Flehmig, and B. Fleischer. 1989. Liver-derived cytotoxic T cells in hepatitis A virus infection. *J. Infect. Dis.* **160:**209–217.
133. Wang, C.-H., S.-Y. Tschen, U. Heinricy, M. Weber, and B. Flehmig. 1996. Immune response to hepatitis A virus capsid proteins after infection. *J. Clin. Microbiol.* **34:**707–713.
134. Weitz, M., B. Finkel-Jimenez, and G. Siegl. 1991. Empty hepatitis A virus particles in vaccines, p. 104–110. *In* F. B. Hollinger, S. M. Lemon, and H. S. Margolis (ed.), *Viral Hepatitis and Liver Disease.* Williams & Wilkins, Baltimore, Md.
135. Wheeler, C. M., H. A. Fields, C. A. Schable, W. J. Meinke, and J. E. Maynard. 1986. Adsorption, purification, and growth characteristics of hepatitis A virus strain HAS-15 propagated in fetal rhesus monkey kidney cells. *J. Clin. Microbiol.* **23:**434–440.
136. Whetter, L. E., S. P. Day, O. Elroy-Stein, E. A. Brown, and S. M. Lemon. 1994. Low efficiency of the 5' nontranslated region of hepatitis A virus RNA in promoting cap-independent translation in permissive monkey kidney cells. *J. Virol.* **68:**5253–5263.
137. Yanagi, M., M. St. Claire, M. Shapiro, S. U. Emerson, R. H. Purcell, and J. Bukh. 1998. Transcripts of a chimeric cDNA clone of hepatitis C virus genotype 1b are infectious in vivo. *Virology* **244:**161–172.
138. Yoshizawa, H., Y. Itoh, S. Iwakiri, F. Tsuda, S. Nakano, Y. Miyokawa, and M. Mayumi. 1980. Diagnosis of type A hepatitis by fecal IgA antibody against hepatitis A antigen. *Gastroenterology* **78:**114–118.
139. Zajac, A. J., E. M. Amphlett, D. J. Rowlands, and D. V. Sangar. 1991. Parameters influencing the attachment of hepatitis A virus to a variety of continuous cell lines. *J. Gen. Virol.* **72:**1667–1675.
140. Zhang, H., S.-F. Chao, L.-H. Ping, K. Grace, B. Clarke, and S. M. Lemon. 1995. An infectious cDNA clone of a cytopathic hepatitis A virus: genomic regions associated with rapid replication and cytopathic effect. *Virology* **212:**686–697.
141. Zuckerman, A. J. 1976. Twenty-five centuries of viral hepatitis. *Rush-Presbyterian-St. Luke's Med. Bull. Perspectives in Viral Hepatitis* **15:**57–82.

Pathogenesis of Theiler's Murine Encephalomyelitis Virus-Induced Disease

RAYMOND P. ROOS

34

HISTORY

Strains of Theiler's murine encephalomyelitis virus (TMEV) were first isolated by Max Theiler at the Rockefeller Foundation during his investigations of yellow fever virus vaccine. The GDVII strain of TMEV was named because this isolate was the seventh made by George, Theiler's technician, from an uninoculated mouse that was found to be diseased (paralyzed). A subsequent isolate was called TO, referring to Theiler's original.

Early investigations showed that TMEV was a picornavirus causing subclinical enteric infection and rare paralysis in mouse colonies. This clinical picture resembled poliovirus so that TMEV became known as "mouse poliovirus." The early interest in this virus as a model for human poliomyelitis disappeared when scientists adapted human poliovirus to mice. In the 1950s, Daniels and colleagues described a chronic progressive demyelinating disease caused by DA, another TMEV strain (10). Interest in TMEV was renewed with the recognition that the demyelinating disease induced by DA and similar strains of TMEV resembled multiple sclerosis (30, 35). Studies of TMEV were facilitated by the availability of a reliable supply of TMEV-free mice made possible through serological screening of mice. In addition, tissue culture passage of demyelinating strains of TMEV was found to attenuate the early gray matter disease following inoculation of highly virulent brain tissue-derived TMEV; the use of tissue culture passed virus allowed one to study the late white matter disease in a large group of survivors.

THE TWO SUBGROUPS OF TMEV AND THEIR DISEASE PHENOTYPE

Strains of TMEV are classified on the basis of genome organization and sequence as members of the Theilovirus species of the cardiovirus genus in the family of *Picornaviridae*. There is about 50% nucleotide sequence identity between TMEV and mengovirus, a member of the encephalomyocarditis virus species of cardioviruses. However, in contrast to other cardioviruses, TMEV has no poly(C) tract in the 5' untranslated region (5' UTR). In addition, TMEV strains differ from other cardioviruses with respect to serological relationships as well as acid-lability in the presence of 0.1 M chloride ion.

TMEV strains fall into two groups on the basis of differences in their biological activities (Table 1). Strains of the GDVII subgroup, GDVII and FA, are highly virulent and produce an acute disease that resembles poliomyelitis. Weanling mice inoculated intracerebrally with as little as 1 PFU of GDVII strain develop decreased activity, weight loss, and ruffled fur with progressive flaccid paralysis of the lower limbs. Mice usually die in days to a couple of weeks from an encephalomyelitis with prominent pathology in the gray matter of the cerebral hemispheres, hippocampus, brainstem, and spinal cord. Death of the mouse is presumably related to involvement of the brainstem and the subsequent failure of the cardiovascular and respiratory systems. The neuropathological findings include microglial proliferation and neuronaphagia and destruction of the anterior horn cells of the spinal cord, the same motor neurons that are targeted in poliomyelitis. The reason that the cerebellum is spared is unknown. Viral antigen and RNA are localized to regions with histopathology. Titers of GDVII virus increase to levels of approximately 10^8 PFU/g of tissue. Attenuation of GDVII virus may lead to persistence of the virus in the central nervous system of survivors (E. Viktorova, E. Pilipenko, S. Guest, and R. P. Roos, unpublished data).

In contrast to GDVII strains, TO subgroup strains such as DA and BeAn (Table 1) do not kill weanling mice but produce a biphasic disease. Inoculated mice initially manifest a flaccid paralysis or fail to show any signs, especially if the virus stock is tissue-culture passed. Animals sacrificed within this period have histopathological evidence of an encephalomyelitis that peaks about 10 to 12 days postinoculation (dpi). The gray matter of the hippocampus, brainstem, and spinal cord is infiltrated with inflammatory mononuclear cells and microglial cells. As is the case with GDVII subgroup strains, the anterior horn cells of the spinal cord show evidence of neuronaphagia with microglial

---

Raymond P. Roos ■ Department of Neurology, University of Chicago Medical Center, Chicago, IL 60637.

TABLE 1 Phenotypic differences between TMEV subgroups

Phenotype	TO subgroup strains (DA, BeAn, TO, WW, Yale, etc.)	GDVII subgroup strains (GDVII, FA)
Neurovirulence (50% lethal dose)	−(>10^6 PFU)	++(1 PFU)
Persistent infection, restricted virus expression	+	−
Early disease (neuronal)	+	+
Late disease (white matter demyelination)	+	−

proliferation. Quite remarkably, the inflammation that was initially found in the hippocampus is usually completely cleared by 3 weeks postinoculation. At this time, an inflammatory demyelinating disease develops, almost exclusively present in the spinal cord, that peaks at about 6 weeks and continues for the life of the mouse. Inflammatory cells, especially microglial cells, infiltrate the white matter of the spinal cord, which is demyelinated with a general preservation of axons, i.e., this is a true primary demyelinating process. Animals with this pathology have decreased activity, spastic lower limbs, a waddling gait, and urinary incontinence.

Following inoculation, titers of DA virus peak at about 5 dpi and then fall to low levels that persist for the life of the mouse. The virus primarily persists in microglia and less so in oligodendrocytes in the central nervous system (6, 37). The expression of TO subgroup strains is said to be restricted during the second phase of the disease since there is relatively little detectable virus and viral antigen at this time. The persistence of virus—as well as an immune response—is necessary for demyelination to occur (see "The Immune Response in TMEV Infections" below). In summary, weanling mice inoculated with DA develop an inflammatory gray matter disease of the brain and spinal cord that is replaced within 3 weeks postinoculation by a chronic inflammatory demyelinating disease associated with a low level and restricted expression of persistent virus.

The genetics of the host are important in determining whether a mouse strain is susceptible to the late demyelinating disease. For example, the major histocompatibility complex (MHC) H-2 class I is important in susceptibility since certain inbred strains of mice are susceptible to TMEV-induced demyelination while others are resistant. The H-2 complex is presumably important because a class I-dependent $CD8^+$ cytolytic T cell clears virus in resistant mice, preventing virus persistence and subsequent demyelination (11, 34). At least two genes in the region of the interferon (IFN)-γ gene as well as the myelin basic protein gene are also important in susceptibility (1).

There are several other noteworthy differences between GDVII and TO subgroup strains: (i) GDVII subgroup strains have a larger plaque size on BHK-21 cells than TO subgroup strains. (ii) Neutralizing monoclonal antibodies (MAbs) may be subgroup-specific so that some MAbs may be able to neutralize TO subgroup strains but not GDVII subgroup strains and vice versa (46); these studies suggest that there are differences between the structure of the capsid proteins in the two subgroups. (iii) Electron microscopic studies have demonstrated that TO subgroup strains tend to be more membrane-associated than GDVII subgroup strains, whereas crystalline arrays of virions are more frequently seen with infections with GDVII subgroup strains than TO subgroup strains (12).

THE VALUE OF THE TMEV MODEL

The study of the TMEV system is an especially valuable one for molecular pathogenesis studies for the following reasons: infectious TMEV clones are available, easing preparation of recombinant or mutated viruses; many of the TMEV neutralizing MAb sites (46, 60) and T-cell epitopes, both ones that stimulate $CD4^+$ helper T cells as well as $CD8^+$ cytolytic T cells, are known (5, 11, 67); the three-dimensional crystal structure of three TMEV strains has been solved (18, 40, 41); the experimental and natural host for TMEV, the mouse, is easily manipulated and well studied immunologically and genetically; and the phenotype of TO subgroup strains is unusual compared to other picornaviruses, viz., virus persistence, restricted virus expression, and immune-mediated demyelination. In addition, the white matter disease induced by TO subgroup strains serves as an excellent experimental model for multiple sclerosis. Both disease processes have a similar inflammatory demyelinating disease pathology that appears to be mediated by immune factors. An identification of the determinants for TMEV-induced disease may be valuable to better understand picornavirus biology, normal central nervous system function, and viral- and nonviral-induced central nervous system disease (e.g., multiple sclerosis).

GENOME ORGANIZATION

The TMEV genome has approximately 8,100 nucleotides (nt) of positive-sense RNA. As is the case with all picornaviruses, TMEV contains a long 5′ UTR (1,065 nt in the case of DA strain) that precedes an AUG used to initiate translation of a polyprotein from one long open reading frame (Fig. 1). The polyprotein is sequentially cleaved into structural and nonstructural proteins. The 3C protease carries out most of these cleavages (56), as is true with other picornaviruses. The TMEV 2A, like 2A of mengovirus, is a polypeptide that mediates a primary cleavage between LP12A and 2BCP3 (56). Studies with encephalomyocarditis virus (EMCV), a non-Theiler's cardiovirus, have demonstrated that an amino acid sequence located at the carboxyl end of 2A is conserved among the cardioviruses (including TMEV) and aphthoviruses and cleaves at the 2A and 2B site (19).

An L coding region is found in cardioviruses as well as aphthoviruses. In contrast to aphthoviruses where L is a protease that cleaves itself from the polyprotein, L of cardioviruses is not a protease but of unknown function; potential clues to the function of the TMEV L protein may be its acidic nature and the fact that it binds zinc (8). Mutagenesis studies of the TMEV L have shown that this gene product is necessary for growth in the mouse central nervous system and for spread of the virus in cultured L929 cells (29). A recent study reported that "leaderless" GDVII

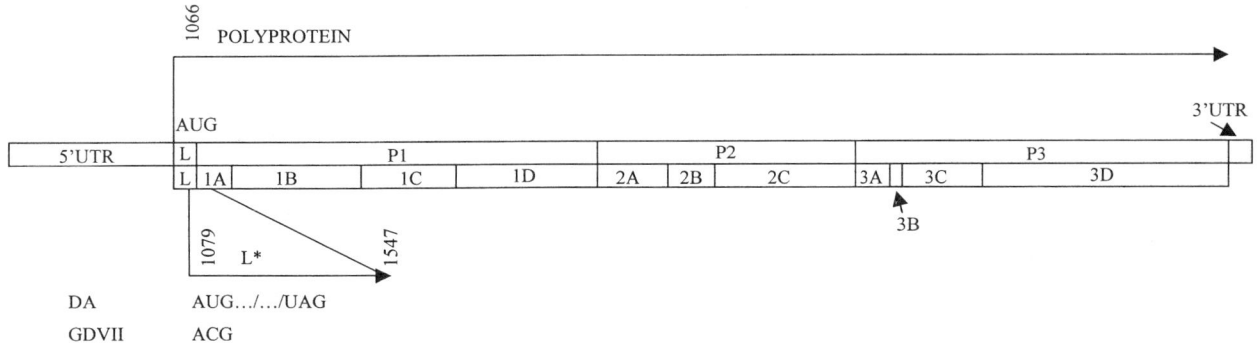

FIGURE 1 The TMEV single-stranded RNA of approximately 8,100 nucleotides. The 5' UTR precedes the polyprotein coding region, which has the leader (L) coding region as its most amino terminus; a 3' UTR is at the 3' end of the genome. The genomic region of P1 is divided into 1A, 1B, 1C, and 1D coding regions, which synthesize, respectively, the structural proteins VP4, VP2, VP3, and VP1. P2 (which includes 2A, 2B, 2C, and 2D) and P3 (which includes 3A, 3B, 3C, and 3D) encode various nonstructural proteins. The polyprotein's initiation codon is at nucleotide 1066, while the initiation codon for L* in the case of the DA strain of TMEV is at nucleotide 1079. There is a stop codon (UAG) for L* at nucleotide 1547. The GDVII strain of TMEV has an ACG rather than an AUG in the position corresponding to the DA L* initiation codon, so GDVII fails to synthesize L*.

virus has a defect in virus assembly in L929 cells, perhaps related to failure in the myristoylation of VP4 because of a change in the conformation of P1 (due to the absence of L) (2).

A cis-acting signal in the viral genome has been found to be required for replication of a number of picornaviruses. In the case of TMEV, this cis replication element (CRE) is contained in a 130-nt stretch (nt 1511 to 1638) in the VP2 coding region (39). The CRE is very similar to and functionally interchangeable with a region in VP2 of mengovirus. The mechanism by which the CRE functions is unknown.

The three sequenced strains of TMEV, GDVII, DA, and BeAn, have a sequence identity of over 90% at the nucleotide level and approximately 95% at the predicted amino acid level (50, 51). Interestingly, the degree of sequence difference between DA and BeAn is similar to that between DA (or BeAn) and GDVII despite the fact that they belong to different TMEV subgroups, suggesting that the determinants for subgroup-specific biological activities are relatively few in number. Although the sequence differences are dispersed throughout the genome, they tend to be more frequent in regions that have been shown to represent targets for neutralizing MAbs.

HOST CELL SHUTOFF, VIRAL PROTEIN TRANSLATION, AND THE L* PROTEIN

The 5' UTR contains an internal ribosome entry site (IRES), beginning at approximately nt 500 and ending between nt 1043 and 1053, which is used for the cap-independent translation of the polyprotein (3). TMEV induces a shutoff of host cell cap-dependent translation by an unclear mechanism. There is no evidence of cleavage of eIFG by 2A (as is the case for enteroviruses) or the leader (as is the case for aphthoviruses) (38). Studies suggest that EMCV induces dephosphorylation of 4E-BP1 and that this dephosphorylated form of 4E-BP1 sequesters eIF4E into an inactive eIF4E-4E-BP1 complex, thereby in-

hibiting eIF4E-eIF4G interaction (17). It is unclear whether this dephosphorylation also occurs in the case of TMEV infection and whether it is the only cause for host cell shutoff.

One remarkable and unique feature of the TO subgroup strains is that an 18-kDa protein, L*, is synthesized out of frame with the polyprotein of TMEV from an initiation codon at nt 1079, 13 nt downstream from the polyprotein's AUG (9, 29). In contrast to the TO subgroup strains, GDVII subgroup strains have an ACG rather than an AUG corresponding to the nt 1079 position, and therefore do not synthesize L*. Several other picornaviruses have an initiation codon downstream from the polyprotein AUG; however, these alternatively initiated proteins are in frame with the polyprotein, i.e., these viruses synthesize both a truncated as well as a full-length polyprotein in vitro (e.g., hepatitis A virus and EMCV) or in vivo (e.g., foot-and-mouth disease virus) (27, 58, 63).

L* is initiated within the L coding region and terminates within the 1A coding region (Fig. 1). Interestingly, the third nucleotide position of the codons of L is relatively conserved among TMEV strains so that the amino acid sequence of L* (that is within the L coding region) is more similar than L among TMEV strains. These data suggest that L* has an important function, presumably related to TO subgroup-specific functions, such as virus persistence and demyelination, since L* is only synthesized by TO subgroup strains. In fact, our studies demonstrated that virus that fails to synthesize L* does not persist or demyelinate (9). Recent data suggest that L* inhibits an antivirus cytolytic T-cell response (33) and therefore allows virus to avoid immunological clearance in order to persist (see "The Immune Response in TMEV Infections" below); demyelination presumably occurs as a result of the virus persistence and the associated immune response.

What regulates ribosomal initiation at nt 1079, the L* AUG, rather than nt 1066, the polyprotein AUG? Studies have shown that the spacing of the L* AUG from the IRES in the case of the BeAn strain affects the efficiency of

TMEV translation initiation; initiation of translation at the BeAn L* AUG increased (and translation of the polyprotein AUG decreased) following deletion of 4 to 11 nt in the region between the IRES and the polyprotein AUG (52). Our investigations with DA showed that translation initiation at the polyprotein start codon affects utilization of the L* AUG, i.e., mutation of the polyprotein AUG leads to increased utilization of the L* AUG (66). These studies suggested that to initiate translation of L*, ribosomes normally travel from the IRES to the polyprotein AUG before they pass on to the L* AUG, rather than jumping directly from the IRES to nt 1079. The results were most consistent with "leaky scanning," in which ribosomes that first land on the polyprotein's mutated AUG do not initiate there but continue downstream to initiate at the L* AUG and carry out synthesis of L*.

We also found that the efficiency of translation initiation at the L* AUG depends on the cellular milieu, presumably because cell-specific factors bind the viral RNA. The ratio of L* synthesis to VP2 synthesis varied in rabbit reticulocyte lysate versus BHK-21 cells and also in different tissue-culture cell types. In addition, transcripts derived from DA/GDVII chimeric cDNA constructs that substitute the corresponding part of GDVII for a segment of DA from nt 659 to 1B or from nt 934 to 1B synthesized levels of L* in vitro that were similar to those seen with in vitro translation of wild-type DA; however, levels of L* were extremely low in BHK-21 cells infected with virus derived from these same chimeric cDNAs (66). These results suggest that interactions of host cell-specific factors with the DA RNA genome affect the efficiency of L* translation initiation and that these host cell factors may be more available in reticulocyte lysates than in BHK-21 cells.

We suspect that the cell-specific factors that regulate the usage of the polyprotein versus L* AUG for translation initiation determine whether the central nervous system infection is a productive one or one with a restricted virus expression. We hypothesize that early after DA infection (during the first phase of disease), ribosomes in infected neuronal cells initiate translation primarily at the polyprotein AUG, with the subsequent synthesis of the polyprotein that is cleaved into capsid and nonstructural proteins leading to large amounts of infectious virus. In contrast, late after infection (during the white matter demyelinating phase), ribosomes in infected microglial cells, which are the major reservoir for virus during the persistent infection (37), initiate translation primarily at the L* AUG, leading to a restricted infection (since an increased utilization of the L* AUG for translation initiation leads to a decreased use of the polyprotein AUG, with a resultant decrease in synthesis of the polyprotein and of the capsid proteins that are cleaved from it).

We hypothesize that certain cells have factors that bind the viral RNA and determine how much synthesis of the polyprotein versus L* occurs. Our recent data (52a) suggest that the efficiency of translation initiation of the GDVII and DA polyprotein depends on the binding of polypyrimidine tract binding protein (PTB) and a neural cell-enriched form of PTB (nPTB) (53), as well as binding of canonical initiation factors to the IRES. The sites of binding of PTB and nPTB on the TMEV IRES correspond to some PTB-binding sites previously identified in the case of EMCV (28). The presence of PTB and nPTB binding sites in GDVII affects neurovirulence (see "Pathogenesis Studies of Recombinants" below).

THE TMEV CELL RECEPTOR

The TMEV receptor has not yet been identified. The receptor is believed to bind to a "pit"-like structure seen on X-ray crystallographic studies of the virion. Data from TMEV mutagenesis studies support the importance of the pit in binding TMEV to the cell receptor (20).

There is evidence that TO subgroup strains bind a sialyl moiety and the protein surface of the receptor while GDVII subgroup strains only bind the protein surface of the receptor (68). Recent crystallographic studies have been performed on DA virus bound to sialyllactose, a mimic of the sialic acid moiety (69). The ligand was found to bind to a pocket on the cell surface that is composed primarily of amino acid residues from VP2 puff B near the VP1 loop 2 and the VP3 carboxyl terminus. The sialic acid-binding site is about 15 Å from the pit, the putative cell receptor-binding site. The importance of sialic acid binding to virus entry is further supported by studies that showed that a variant of DA that has enhanced binding to L929 cells has mutations in the VP2 puff B or VP1 loop 2 (26); this region is also one that has been found important in disease pathogenesis (24) (see "Pathogenesis Studies of Recombinants" below).

APOPTOSIS

As has been observed with other picornaviruses, TMEV induces apoptosis of some cell types. TMEV-induced apoptosis is a result of virus infection since virus that is inactivated by UV-irradiation fails to induce apoptosis (25). There are multiple cell types in which apoptosis is triggered, including neurons and oligodendrocytes in the central nervous system, and cultured mouse macrophage cell lines (64). The GDVII strain is much more efficient at inducing apoptosis than the DA strain. Our studies demonstrated that L* has an antiapoptotic effect in mouse macrophage cell lines, suggesting than at least part of the reason that GDVII is more proapoptotic than DA is because it lacks the L* protein (16). Apoptosis seems more likely to occur in cells that are relatively nonpermissive to the virus, perhaps explaining why the GDVII strain has an increased apoptotic activity coupled with a decreased replicative capacity in mouse macrophage cell lines compared to DA (61).

PATHOGENESIS STUDIES OF RECOMBINANTS ENGINEERED BETWEEN MEMBERS OF THE TO AND GDVII SUBGROUP

The availability of infectious clones of strains from each of the two subgroups of TMEV provided the opportunity to prepare chimeric cDNAs and subsequently to generate recombinant viruses. These constructs have been used to identify determinants for the subgroup-specific differences in biological activity, especially neurovirulence, demyelinating activity, and virus persistence.

The GDVII Capsid Is Important for TMEV Neurovirulence

Studies showed that recombinant virus (called GD1B-2A/DA) that has a substitution of a segment of GDVII for the corresponding region of the DA genome that runs from the middle of the 1B coding region to the middle of 2A is neurovirulent (14). There was a slight increase in neurovirulence with the additional substitution of the GDVII 5′ UTR for that of DA. An analysis of the pathology of the different recombinant viruses suggested that death was correlated with elevated levels of virus and the presence of viral antigen within the brainstem and gray matter of the spinal cord.

These studies demonstrated that the capsid proteins of GDVII are critical for neurovirulence. In other words, conversion of the DA virus to neurovirulence could be accomplished by replacement of DA capsid with GDVII capsid sequences. Our studies also indicated that multiple regions of the GDVII genome (e.g., the 5′ UTR) also contribute to the enhanced neurovirulence of GDVII, although they have a relatively minor effect. This redundancy is not unexpected since it is likely that GDVII virus, under evolutionary pressure, developed varied determinants to kill a mouse.

Mutation of PTB (nPTB) Binding Sites in the IRES Attenuates GDVII

Our recent study identified a number of PTB (nPTB) binding sites in the GDVII IRES (52a). Data showed a correlation between nPTB binding, stimulation of 48S complex formation, and neurovirulence. More specifically, a mutation of a PTB (nPTB) binding site in the GDVII IRES led to attenuation of the virus's neurovirulence with relative maintenance of its growth in BHK-21 cells. These attenuated mutants had a decrease in binding of nPTB that was more severe than that of PTB at one or more of the nonmutated PTB (nPTB) binding sites. The more prominent loss in nPTB binding correlated with a more significant decrease in 48S complex formation following addition of nPTB than PTB. The results provided an explanation for attenuation of the mutant viruses, since the mutant virus would be predicted to have inefficient translation initiation and therefore less growth in neural cells in the central nervous system (because there is less PTB) than in tissue culture cells (where there is more PTB); the presence of nPTB in the central nervous system failed to compensate for the defect in translation initiation of the mutant viruses, presumably because of the decrease in nPTB binding to the mutated IRES. These results demonstrate that cell type-specific proteins can regulate viral RNA translation and virus-induced disease.

Both the DA and GDVII Capsid Can Lead to Virus Persistence and Demyelination

Chimeric cDNA studies allowed us to address the question as to whether the reason that wild-type GDVII virus fails to persist or demyelinate is because animals die of a lethal neuronal disease before the white matter disease is manifest. We found that demyelination can occur when one replaces any part of the DA genome with the corresponding segment from the GDVII genome (13). The vigorous demyelination seen with GD1B-2A/DA virus also indicated that replacement of half of VP2 and all of VP3 and VP1 with GDVII sequence does not impair demyelinating activity or the capacity of the virus to persist. It is likely that multiple viral genetic determinants are responsible for persistence and demyelinating activity, and that some may be unique to TO subgroup strains.

The results of these studies were at odds with those of Brahic and colleagues, who reported that the presence of DA VP1 was necessary and sufficient for demyelination and that recombinant virus that had a replacement of this coding region with the corresponding GDVII sequence failed to demyelinate or persist (62). Further investigations compared GD1B-2A/DA (which demyelinated and persisted, and which was constructed in the Roos lab) with Brahic's chimera R4 (which was thought to be an identical recombinant virus to GD1B-2A/DA, but did not persist or demyelinate) (23). Sequencing studies showed that R4 contained a mutation from Asn to Lys at VP2 position 141. Interestingly, this amino acid mutation was present in Brahic's original parental infectious DA clone (i.e., in the DA "backbone") and was not in the GDVII segment that had been substituted into the DA genome in the case of chimera R4. Amino acid residue 141 of VP2 is located at the tip of the EF loop in the VP2 puff on the rim of the depression spanning the twofold axis of the capsid. These results demonstrated that interactions between the TMEV 1B-2C segment and VP2 141 are important in determining the capacity of the virus to persist and demyelinate. A similar conclusion about the importance of a conformational determinant involving homologous sequences in both the VP2 puff and VP1 loop regions to virus persistence was found in other studies of intratypic TMEV recombinants (36). In addition, further studies by Brahic and colleagues demonstrated that VP2-141 is important in the tropism of the virus and its spread from the brain to the spinal cord (22).

The above data suggest that the GDVII strain has determinants for virus persistence, but that wild-type GDVII is so virulent that there are no survivors. We hypothesized that attenuated GDVII might persist. Recent studies have shown that GDVII virus with varied mutations in PTB-binding sites in the 5′ UTR is attenuated and does persist (Viktorova et al., unpublished). Preliminary results indicate that this attenuated virus does not demyelinate, perhaps because the DA virus capsid proteins are essential for demyelination: DA virions may bind cells that are critical for induction of the white matter disease and that are not bound by GDVII. It is obvious that attenuation of GDVII is not sufficient for virus persistence, and it is clear that one can so markedly attenuate the virus that it grows poorly and is unable to persist. An extreme example of an attenuated GDVII mutant that is unable to persist is leaderless GDVII virus, which is unable to grow in the central nervous system and therefore cannot persist (7). It is also clear that persistence of TMEV, at least certain GDVII mutants, can occur in the absence of L*.

Shortcomings of Chimeric cDNA Studies

The redundancy of determinants important for the biological activity of TMEV can complicate the interpretation of chimeric cDNA studies. The interpretation can be further complicated because certain recombinant viruses that are prepared may be compromised with respect to growth because of disruptions in the assembly of the virion capsid, RNA replication, receptor binding, or viral protein processing (31, 54). In some cases the disruptions are so significant that the constructs can be noninfectious. An example of difficulties that can be seen with these studies can be appreciated by examining results of studies of a recombinant virus (GD1B-2C/DA) that contains a sequence of GDVII that runs from 1B to 2C substituted into the DA genome. We found that the GD1B-2C segment was important for neurovirulence since GD1B-2C/DA virus caused lethal neuronal disease in mice. However, viruses that contained separate substitutions of GD1B-2A or GD2A-2C into DA were not neurovirulent (31). Interactions between GDVII genes or gene products that are critical for neurovirulence were presumably disrupted in these two attenuated constructs.

The shortcomings of the intratypic TMEV chimeric cDNA studies seem to be more apparent than in the case of similar studies with wild-type and vaccine strains of poliovirus. This is presumably the case because the evolutionary divergence of GDVII and TO subgroup strains is far greater than the differences in the poliovirus genome that occurred as a result of Sabin's passage. The substantial differences between the GDVII and TO subgroup strains are the most likely reason that interactions of the genome segments from GDVII and TO subgroup strains may even create somewhat new phenotypes in recombinant viruses.

THE IMMUNE RESPONSE IN TMEV INFECTIONS

The Immune Response against TMEV

Certain strains of mice ($H-2^{s,q,r,v,f,p}$) are susceptible to TO subgroup strain-induced demyelination while others are resistant ($H-2^{b,d,k}$). The resistant strains of mice develop an initial gray matter encephalitis that is cleared while the susceptible mouse strains develop a persistent infection with chronic inflammatory demyelinating disease. Several studies have reported that virus-specific cytolytic T cells play a critically important role in early clearance of the virus and that resistant, but not susceptible, mouse strains mount an MHC H-2D-restricted virus-specific cytolytic response (11, 34). The cytolytic response is primarily directed against a peptide from VP2 positions 121 to 130 (5). The cytolytic response is perforin-dependent, as demonstrated by the finding that perforin-deficient C57BL/6 mice, which are normally resistant and clear DA virus, die from an encephalomyelitis between 12 and 18 dpi with high levels of viral RNA (44).

Although susceptible mouse strains inoculated with wild-type DA virus fail to generate an antivirus cytolytic response, susceptible mouse strains infected with a mutant of DA virus that does not synthesize L* (but has no change in the amino acid sequence of the polyprotein) clear virus and develop little if any demyelination. These findings suggested that L* might inhibit the antivirus cytolytic response following inoculation of DA wild-type virus into susceptible strains of mice. Subsequent studies showed that L* inhibits the MHC H-2K-restricted virus-specific cytolytic response in the central nervous system of susceptible strains of mice (Table 2) (33). The inhibition of an H-2K-restricted virus-specific cytolytic response presumably allows virus to persist in and subsequently demyelinate susceptible strains of mice.

There are other antivirus defenses of the host besides the cytolytic response. A vigorous B-cell response is seen in animals infected with TMEV (48). In addition, neutralizing antibody directed against the virus can increase survival of the infected mouse, e.g., passive administration of neutralizing MAb in athymic mice leads to increased survival and decreased virus spread (15). The neutralizing sites of the MAbs that have been mapped on the basis of sequencing neutralizing MAb-resistant viruses correspond to regions known to be neutralization sites in the case of other picornaviruses. Some of the MAbs are conformation-dependent, including one that has VP2-141, -143, and -173 as part of a neutralization site on all TMEV strains. Other MAbs are conformation-independent, including sites localized to VP1-101 and VP1-268 on TO subgroup strains (49, 60). In some cases mutant viruses have been produced that are resistant to the neutralizing MAbs, and some of the MAb-resistant DA viruses are no longer able to demyelinate. For example, virus that has a mutation in VP1-268 (57, 70) has a change in disease phenotype and is no longer able to persist or to demyelinate (60). We suspect that the change in disease phenotype is because the loops of the capsid protein that correspond to the neutralization sites are also ones that border the pit, which is the putative receptor-binding site of the virion; therefore, a mutation of the neutralization epitope may lead to a disturbance in cell receptor binding. Recent data also suggested that immunologic mechanisms associated with the CD4-mediated host immune response are also involved in the altered phenotype of these mutant viruses (55a).

There have been a number of investigations of the cytokine and chemokine response that is present during TMEV infections (4, 21, 43, 59). Generally, a Th1 cytokine response has been found during the late demyelinating disease in susceptible but not resistant strains of mice. A Th2 cytokine response was seen in some mouse strains but did not necessarily correlate with susceptibility or resistance. IFN-γ is important for resistance to TMEV-induced demyelination as evidenced by the finding that resistant mouse strains develop demyelinating lesions after treatment with antibody to IFN-γ (55). A variety of chemokines, including MIP-1α, RANTES, MCP-1, C10, IP-10, and MIP-1β, have been found to be expressed during GDVII and DA infection.

TABLE 2 The cytolytic response, L*, and susceptibility

Mouse strain	Virus	Virus-specific MHC class I restriction (7 dpi)		Persistent virus (45 dpi)	Myelin loss (45 dpi)
		H-2K	H-2D		
B6, B10 ($H-2^b$, *resistant*)	DA without L*	+	+	−	−
	Wild-type DA	−	+	−	−
B10.S, SJL/J ($H-2^s$, *susceptible*)	DA without L*	+	−	−	−
	Wild-type DA	−	−	+	+

Immunological Contributors to TO Subgroup Strain-Induced Demyelination

The white matter lesions induced by TO subgroup strains resemble plaques seen in the central nervous system of patients with multiple sclerosis, a presumed autoimmune disease. In addition, the immune system is believed to mediate the pathology in both diseases. Therefore, it is hoped that investigations of TMEV-induced demyelination may provide insights into the pathogenesis of multiple sclerosis. Unfortunately, an understanding of TMEV demyelination still remains out of reach—a humbling thought when one realizes how simplified this disease is compared to the complexities of multiple sclerosis.

Miller and colleagues have emphasized the importance of $CD4^+$ T cells in mediating the TO subgroup strain late demyelinating disease (42, 65). The first phase of the demyelination is believed to be carried out by a delayed-type hypersensitivity reaction and T-cell proliferation mediated by a $CD4^+$ class II restricted T-cell response that has an immunodominant epitope localized to VP1 233–250 or VP2 74–86, and an additional T-cell epitope on VP3 24–37 (67). The presence of this response and its intensity are correlated with the development of demyelination and susceptibility of mouse strains to the white matter disease. These investigators have emphasized that a Th1 response against viral antigen with secondary macrophage recruitment mediates the white matter disease by means of a "bystander" mechanism of myelin damage, e.g., macrophages release proteases that can lead to the breakdown of myelin (42, 65). In the later phase of the demyelinating disease myelin damage occurs by "epitope spreading," a situation in which an initiating antigenic epitope leads to a widening immune response directed against other antigenic epitopes on the same molecule or a different molecule. In the case of TO strain-induced demyelination, epitope spreading has been found after day 50, when new populations of T cells appear with varying myelin peptides as epitope targets (e.g., different peptides of proteolipid protein of myelin and myelin oligodendrocyte glycoprotein) (42). No investigators have found reproducible evidence of antigenic mimicry in which autoreactive T cells cross-react with a viral epitope.

The importance of $CD4^+$ T cells in the late white matter disease needs to be allied with compelling data from the Rodriguez lab demonstrating the importance of both $CD4^+$ and $CD8^+$ T cells to the demyelination (32, 45, 47). For example, the Rodriguez lab showed that C.B-17-*scid* mice develop severe encephalitis and death within a few weeks postinoculation; C.B-17-*scid* fail to demonstrate demyelination by the time they die even though congenic C.B-17 mice have evidence of demyelination at this same time; and adoptive transfer of nonimmune spleen cells from BALB/c mice into the *scid* mice (following depletion of either $CD4^+$ T cells or $CD8^+$ T cells prior to inoculation) leads to severe demyelination (and virus persistence). These studies suggested that either $CD4^+$ T cells or $CD8^+$ T cells are capable of inducing demyelinating disease. Additional studies have demonstrated that DA virus can demyelinate mice that are deficient in MHC-II molecules, which are generally required for a $CD4^+$ T-cell response (47), and that susceptible PLJ mice that lack $CD4^+$ T cells develop more demyelination than wild-type PLJ mice. Although Rodriguez and colleagues have identified a cytolytic response that is present 45 dpi with DA and appears to foster the white matter disease, the antigenic target of this response remains unknown (32).

TOPICS FOR FUTURE INVESTIGATIONS

There are many remaining questions of special interest to investigators of TMEV. The identity of the TMEV receptor, or what are probably TMEV receptors, is likely to help clarify the pathogenesis of TMEV-induced central nervous system disease. In addition, the identification of cell-specific RNA-binding proteins that affect translation and regulate the synthesis of L* versus the polyprotein is also likely to help in the understanding of picornaviral gene expression and TMEV disease pathogenesis. Continuing investigations of molecular determinants of virus persistence and demyelination as well as the mechanism by which the immune system contributes to the demyelination must remain main goals. It may be that future studies will benefit from investigations that involve mice with an inducible knockout of a specific arm of the immune system.

REFERENCES

1. **Aubagnac, S., M. Brahic, and J. F. Bureau.** 1999. Viral load and a locus on chromosome 11 affect the late clinical disease caused by Theiler's virus. *J. Virol.* **73:**7965–7971.
2. **Badshah, C., M. A. Calenoff, and K. Rundell.** 2000. The leader polypeptide of Theiler's murine encephalomyelitis virus is required for the assembly of virions in mouse L cells. *J. Virol.* **74:**875–882.
3. **Bandyopadhyay, P. K., C. Wang, and H. L. Lipton.** 1992. Cap-independent translation by the 5′ untranslated region of Theiler's murine encephalomyelitis virus. *J. Virol.* **66:**6249–6256.
4. **Begolka, W. S., C. L. Vanderlugt, S. M. Rahbe, and S. D. Miller.** 1998. Differential expression of inflammatory cytokines parallels progression of central nervous system pathology in two clinically distinct models of multiple sclerosis. *J. Immunol.* **161:**4437–4446.
5. **Borson, N. D., C. Paul, X. Lin, W. K. Nevala, M. A. Strausbauch, M. Rodriguez, and P. J. Wettstein.** 1997. Brain-infiltrating cytolytic T lymphocytes specific for Theiler's virus recognize H2Db molecules complexed with a viral VP2 peptide lacking a consensus anchor residue. *J. Virol.* **71:**5244–5250.
6. **Brahic, M., W. G. Stroop, and J. R. Baringer.** 1981. Theiler's virus persists in glial cells during demyelinating disease. *Cell* **26:**123–128.
7. **Calenoff, M. A., C. S. Badshah, M. C. Dal Canto, H. L. Lipton, and M. K. Rundell.** 1995. The leader polypeptide of Theiler's virus is essential for neurovirulence but not for virus growth in BHK cells. *J. Virol.* **69:**5544–5549.
8. **Chen, H. H., W. P. Kong, and R. P. Roos.** 1995. The leader peptide of Theiler's murine encephalomyelitis virus is a zinc-binding protein. *J. Virol.* **69:**8076–8078.
9. **Chen, H. H., W. P. Kong, L. Zhang, P. L. Ward, and R. P. Roos.** 1995. A picornaviral protein synthesized out of frame with the polyprotein plays a key role in a virus-induced immune-mediated demyelinating disease. *Nat. Med.* **1:**927–931.
10. **Daniels, J. B., A. M. Pappenheimer, and S. Richardson.** 1952. Observation on encephalomyelitis of mice (DA strain). *J. Exp. Med.* **96:**517–535.
11. **Dethlefs, S., M. Brahic, and E. L. Larsson-Sciard.** 1997. An early, abundant cytotoxic T-lymphocyte response against Theiler's virus is critical for preventing viral persistence. *J. Virol.* **71:**8875–8878.
12. **Friedmann, A., and H. Lipton.** 1980. Replication of Theiler's murine encephalomyelitis viruses in BHK21 cells: an electron microscopic study. *Virology* **101:**389–398.

13. **Fu, J., M. Rodriguez, and R. P. Roos.** 1990. Strains from both Theiler's virus subgroups encode a determinant for demyelination. *J. Virol.* **64:**6345–6348.
14. **Fu, J. L., S. Stein, L. Rosenstein, T. Bodwell, M. Routbort, B. L. Semler, and R. P. Roos.** 1990. Neurovirulence determinants of genetically engineered Theiler viruses. *Proc. Natl. Acad. Sci. USA* **87:**4125–4129.
15. **Fujinami, R. S., A. Rosenthal, P. W. Lampert, A. Zurbriggen, and M. Yamada.** 1989. Survival of athymic (nu/nu) mice after Theiler's murine encephalomyelitis virus infection by passive administration of neutralizing monoclonal antibody. *J. Virol.* **63:**2081–2087.
16. **Ghadge, G. D., L. Ma, S. Sato, J. Kim, and R. P. Roos.** 1998. A protein critical for a Theiler's virus-induced immune system-mediated demyelinating disease has a cell type-specific antiapoptotic effect and a key role in virus persistence. *J. Virol.* **72:**8605–8612.
17. **Gingras, A. C., Y. Svitkin, G. J. Belsham, A. Pause, and N. Sonenberg.** 1996. Activation of the translational suppressor 4E-BP1 following infection with encephalomyocarditis virus and poliovirus. *Proc. Natl. Acad. Sci. USA* **93:**5578–5583.
18. **Grant, R. A., D. J. Filman, R. S. Fujinami, J. P. Icenogle, and J. M. Hogle.** 1992. Three-dimensional structure of Theiler's virus. *Proc. Natl. Acad. Sci. USA* **89:**2061–2065.
19. **Hahn, H., and A. C. Palmenberg.** 1996. Mutational analysis of the encephalomyocarditis virus primary cleavage. *J. Virol.* **70:**6870–6875.
20. **Hertzler, S., M. Luo, and H. L. Lipton.** 2000. Mutation of predicted virion pit residues alters binding of Theiler's murine encephalomyelitis virus to BHK-21 cells. *J. Virol.* **74:**1994–2004.
21. **Hoffman, L. M., B. T. Fife, W. S. Begolka, S. D. Miller, and W. J. Karpus.** 1999. Central nervous system chemokine expression during Theiler's virus-induced demyelinating disease. *J. Neurovirol.* **5:**635–642.
22. **Jarousse, N., L. Fiette, R. A. Grant, J. M. Hogle, A. McAllister, T. Michiels, C. Aubert, F. Tangy, M. Brahic, and C. Pena Rossi.** 1994. Chimeric Theiler's virus with altered tropism for the central nervous system. *J. Virol.* **68:**2781–2786.
23. **Jarousse, N., R. A. Grant, J. M. Hogle, L. Zhang, A. Senkowski, R. P. Roos, T. Michiels, M. Brahic, and A. McAllister.** 1994. A single amino acid change determines persistence of a chimeric Theiler's virus. *J. Virol.* **68:**3364–3368.
24. **Jarousse, N., C. Martinat, S. Syan, M. Brahic, and A. McAllister.** 1996. Role of VP2 amino acid 141 in tropism of Theiler's virus within the central nervous system. *J. Virol.* **70:**8213–8217.
25. **Jelachich, M. L., and H. L. Lipton.** 1996. Theiler's murine encephalomyelitis virus kills restrictive but not permissive cells by apoptosis. *J. Virol.* **70:**6856–7861.
26. **Jnaoui, K., and T. Michiels.** 1999. Analysis of cellular mutants resistant to Theiler's virus infection: differential infection of L929 cells by persistent and neurovirulent strains. *J. Virol.* **73:**7248–7254.
27. **Kaminski, A., M. T. Howell, and R. J. Jackson.** 1990. Initiation of encephalomyocarditis virus RNA translation: the authentic initiation site is not selected by a scanning mechanism. *EMBO J.* **9:**3753–3759.
28. **Kolupaeva, V. G., C. U. Hellen, and I. N. Shatsky.** 1996. Structural analysis of the interaction of the pyrimidine tract-binding protein with the internal ribosomal entry site of encephalomyocarditis virus and foot-and-mouth disease virus RNAs. *RNA* **2:**1199–1212.
29. **Kong, W. P., and R. P. Roos.** 1991. Alternative translation initiation site in the DA strain of Theiler's murine encephalomyelitis virus. *J. Virol.* **65:**3395–3399.
30. **Lehrich, J. R., B. G. Arnason, and F. H. Hochberg.** 1976. Demyelinative myelopathy in mice induced by the DA virus. *J. Neurolog. Sci.* **29:**149–160.
31. **Liang, Z., A. Senkowski, B. Shim, and R. P. Roos.** 1993. Chimeric cDNA studies of Theiler's murine encephalomyelitis virus neurovirulence. *J. Virol.* **67:**4404–4408.
32. **Lin, X., L. R. Pease, P. D. Murray, and M. Rodriguez.** 1998. Theiler's virus infection of genetically susceptible mice induces central nervous system-infiltrating CTLs with no apparent viral or major myelin antigenic specificity. *J. Immunol.* **160:**5661–5668.
33. **Lin, X., R. P. Roos, L. R. Pease, P. Wettstein, and M. Rodriguez.** 1999. A Theiler's virus alternatively initiated protein inhibits the generation of H-2K-restricted virus-specific cytotoxicity. *J. Immunol.* **162:**17–24.
34. **Lin, X., N. R. Thiemann, L. R. Pease, and M. Rodriguez.** 1995. VP1 and VP2 capsid proteins of Theiler's virus are targets of H-2D-restricted cytotoxic lymphocytes in the central nervous system of B10 mice. *Virology* **214:**91–99.
35. **Lipton, H. L.** 1975. Theiler's infection in mice: an unusual biphasic disease process leading to demyelination. *Infect. Immun.* **11:**1147–1155.
36. **Lipton, H. L., and M. L. Jelachich.** 1997. Molecular pathogenesis of Theiler's murine encephalomyelitis virus-induced demyelinating disease in mice. *Intervirology* **40:**143–152.
37. **Lipton, H. L., G. Twaddle, and M. L. Jelachich.** 1995. The predominant virus antigen burden is present in macrophages in Theiler's murine encephalomyelitis virus-induced demyelinating disease. *J. Virol.* **69:**2525–2533.
38. **Lloyd, R. E., M. J. Grubman, and E. Ehrenfeld.** 1988. Relationship of p220 cleavage during picornavirus infection to 2A proteinase sequencing. *J. Virol.* **62:**4216–4223.
39. **Lobert, P. E., N. Escriou, J. Ruelle, and T. Michiels.** 1999. A coding RNA sequence acts as a replication signal in cardioviruses. *Proc. Natl. Acad. Sci. USA* **96:**11560–11565.
40. **Luo, M., C. He, K. S. Toth, C. X. Zhang, and H. L. Lipton.** 1992. Three-dimensional structure of Theiler murine encephalomyelitis virus (BeAn strain). *Proc. Natl. Acad. Sci. USA* **89:**2409–2413.
41. **Luo, M., K. S. Toth, L. Zhou, A. Pritchard, and H. L. Lipton.** 1996. The structure of a highly virulent Theiler's murine encephalomyelitis virus (GDVII) and implications for determinants of viral persistence. *Virology* **220:**246–250.
42. **Miller, S. D., C. L. Vanderlugt, W. S. Begolka, W. Pao, R. L. Yauch, K. L. Neville, Y. Katz-Levy, A. Carrizosa, and B. S. Kim.** 1997. Persistent infection with Theiler's virus leads to CNS autoimmunity via epitope spreading. *Nat. Med.* **3:**1133–1136.
43. **Murray, P. D., K. Krivacic, A. Chernosky, T. Wei, R. M. Ransohoff, and M. Rodriguez.** 2000. Biphasic and regionally-restricted chemokine expression in the central nervous system in the Theiler's virus model of multiple sclerosis. *J. Neurovirol.* **6**(Suppl. 1):S44–S52.
44. **Murray, P. D., D. B. McGavern, X. Lin, M. K. Njenga, J. Leibowitz, L. R. Pease, and M. Rodriguez.** 1998. Perforin-dependent neurologic injury in a viral model of multiple sclerosis. *J. Neurosci.* **18:**7306–7314.
45. **Murray, P. D., K. D. Pavelko, J. Leibowitz, X. Lin, and M. Rodriguez.** 1998. CD4(+) and CD8(+) T cells make discrete contributions to demyelination and neurologic disease in a viral model of multiple sclerosis. *J. Virol.* **72:**7320–7329.
46. **Nitayaphan, S., M. M. Toth, and R. P. Roos.** 1985. Neutralizing monoclonal antibodies to Theiler's murine encephalomyelitis viruses. *J. Virol.* **53:**651–657.

47. Njenga, M. K., K. D. Pavelko, J. Baisch, X. Lin, C. David, J. Leibowitz, and M. Rodriguez. 1996. Theiler's virus persistence and demyelination in major histocompatibility complex class II-deficient mice. *J. Virol.* **70:** 1729–1737.
48. Ohara, Y., and R. Roos. 1987. The antibody response in Theiler's virus infection: new perspectives on multiple sclerosis. *Prog. Med. Virol.* **34:**156–179.
49. Ohara, Y., A. Senkowski, J. L. Fu, L. Klaman, J. Goodall, M. Toth, and R. P. Roos. 1988. Trypsin-sensitive neutralization site on VP1 of Theiler's murine encephalomyelitis viruses. *J. Virol.* **62:**3527–3529.
50. Ohara, Y., S. Stein, J. L. Fu, L. Stillman, L. Klaman, and R. P. Roos. 1988. Molecular cloning and sequence determination of DA strain of Theiler's murine encephalomyelitis viruses. *Virology* **164:**245–255.
51. Pevear, D. C., J. Borkowski, M. Calenoff, E. Rozhon, and H. L. Lipton. 1987. Analysis of the complete nucleotide sequence of the picornavirus Theiler's murine encephalomyelitis virus (TMEV) indicates that it is closely related to the cardioviruses. *J. Virol.* **61:**1507–1516.
52. Pilipenko, E. V., A. P. Gmyl, S. V. Maslova, G. A. Belov, A. N. Sinyakov, M. Huang, T. D. Brown, and V. I. Agol. 1994. Starting window, a distinct element in the cap-independent internal initiation of translation on picornaviral RNA. *J. Molec. Biol.* **241:**398–414.
52a. Pilipenko, E. V., E. G. Viktorova, S. T. Guest, V. I. Agol, and R. P. Roos. 2001. Cell-specific proteins regulate viral RNA translation and virus-induced disease. *EMBO J.* **20:**6899–6908.
53. Polydorides, A. D., H. J. Okano, Y. Y. Yang, G. Stefani, and R. B. Darnell. 2000. A brain-enriched polypyrimidine tract-binding protein antagonizes the ability of Nova to regulate neuron-specific alternative splicing. *Proc. Natl. Acad. Sci. USA* **97:**6350–6355.
54. Pritchard, A. E., K. Jensen, and H. L. Lipton. 1993. Assembly of Theiler's virus recombinants used in mapping determinants of neurovirulence. *J. Virol.* **67:**3901–3907.
54a. Ransohoff, R. M., T. Wei, K. D. Pavelko, J.-C. Lee, P. D. Murray, and M. Rodriguez. 2002. Chemokine expression in the central nervous system of mice with a viral disease resembling multiple sclerosis: roles of CD4$^+$ and CD8$^+$ T cells and viral persistence. *J. Virol.* **76:**2217–2224.
55. Rodriguez, M., K. Pavelko, and R. L. Coffman. 1995. Gamma interferon is critical for resistance to Theiler's virus-induced demyelination. *J. Virol.* **69:**7286–7290.
55a. Rodriguez, M., R. P. Roos, D. McGavern, L. Zoecklein, K. Pavelko, H. Sang, and X. Lin. 2000. The CD4-mediated immune response is critical in determining the outcome of infection using Theiler's viruses with VP1 capsid protein point mutations. *Virology* **275:**9–19.
56. Roos, R. P., W. P. Kong, and B. L. Semler. 1989. Polyprotein processing of Theiler's murine encephalomyelitis virus. *J. Virol.* **63:**5344–5353.
57. Roos, R. P., S. Stein, M. Routbort, A. Senkowski, T. Bodwell, and R. Wollmann. 1989. Theiler's murine encephalomyelitis virus neutralization escape mutants have a change in disease phenotype. *J. Virol.* **63:**4469–4473.
58. Sangar, D. V., S. E. Newton, D. J. Rowlands, and B. E. Clarke. 1987. All foot and mouth disease virus serotypes initiate protein synthesis at two separate AUGs. *Nucleic Acids Res.* **15:**3305–3315.
59. Sato, S., S. L. Reiner, M. A. Jensen, and R. P. Roos. 1997. Central nervous system cytokine mRNA expression following Theiler's murine encephalomyelitis virus infection. *J. Neuroimmunol.* **76:**213–223.
60. Sato, S., L. Zhang, J. Kim, J. Jakob, R. A. Grant, R. Wollmann, and R. P. Roos. 1996. A neutralization site of DA strain of Theiler's murine encephalomyelitis virus important for disease phenotype. *Virology* **226:**327–337.
61. Takata, H., M. Obuchi, J. Yamamoto, T. Odagiri, R. P. Roos, H. Iizuka, and Y. Ohara. 1998. L* protein of the DA strain of Theiler's murine encephalomyelitis virus is important for virus growth in a murine macrophage-like cell line. *J. Virol.* **72:**4950–4955.
62. Tangy, F., A. McAllister, and M. Brahic. 1991. Determinants of persistence and demyelination of DA strain of Theiler's virus are found only in VP1 gene. *J. Virol.* **63:** 1101–1106.
63. Tesar, M., S. A. Harmon, D. F. Summers, and E. Ehrenfeld. 1992. Hepatitis A virus polyprotein synthesis initiates from two alternative AUG codons. *Virology* **186:** 609–618.
64. Tsunoda, I., C. I. Kurtz, and R. S. Fujinami. 1997. Apoptosis in acute and chronic central nervous system disease induced by Theiler's murine encephalomyelitis virus. *Virology* **228:**388–393.
65. Vanderlugt, C. L., W. S. Begolka, K. L. Neville, Y. Katz-Levy, L. M. Howard, T. N. Eagar, J. A. Bluestone, and S. D. Miller. 1998. The functional significance of epitope spreading and its regulation by co-stimulatory molecules. *Immunol. Rev.* **164:**63–72.
66. Yamasaki, K., C. C. Weihl, and R. P. Roos. 1999. Alternative translation initiation of Theiler's murine encephalomyelitis virus. *J. Virol.* **73:**8519–8526.
67. Yauch, R. L., J. P. Palma, H. Yahikozawa, C. S. Koh, and B. S. Kim. 1998. Role of individual T-cell epitopes of Theiler's virus in the pathogenesis of demyelination correlates with the ability to induce a Th1 response. *J. Virol.* **72:**6169–6174.
68. Zhou, L., X. Lin, T. J. Green, H. L. Lipton, and M. Luo. 1997. Role of sialyloligosaccharide binding in Theiler's virus persistence. *J Virol.* **71:**9701–9712.
69. Zhou, L., Y. Luo, Y. Wu, J. Tsao, and M. Luo. 2000. Sialylation of the host receptor may modulate entry of demyelinating persistent Theiler's virus. *J. Virol.* **74:** 1477–1485.
70. Zurbriggen, A., C. Thomas, M. Yamada, R. P. Roos, and R. S. Fujinami. 1991. Direct evidence for amino acid 101 of VP1 for central nervous system disease in Theiler's murine encephalomyelitis virus infection. *J. Virol.* **65:**1929–1937.

Persistent Infections by Picornaviruses

FLORENCE COLBÈRE-GARAPIN, ISABELLE PELLETIER, AND LAURENT OUZILOU

35

Viral persistence is currently one of the main public health problems. It depends on specific virus and host factors and particularly on the capacity of the virus to escape the immune defense. Antigenic variation, suppression of the expression of cellular molecules required for immune recognition, interference with antiviral cytokines, and immune tolerance are all among the factors that contribute to viral persistence. Certain cells such as those of the immune system and cells partially protected from the immune system, like neural cells, are preferential targets for persistence. The emergence of viral mutants, which is a common feature of persistent infections, may contribute to persistence in several ways. Some picornaviruses establish persistent infections in their natural animal hosts, while others are suspected to be responsible for chronic human diseases. The involvement of very common viruses in rare human pathologies is difficult to demonstrate, particularly when infectious virus is not easily recovered from the infected host. The in vivo and in vitro models briefly presented here shed some light on the capacity of these viruses to cause chronic infections and/or disease. They are also valuable tools for elucidating the various molecular mechanisms of persistent viral infections.

PICORNAVIRUS INFECTIONS IN VIVO WITH PERSISTING VIRION PRODUCTION

Theiler's Murine Encephalomyelitis Virus

Theiler's murine encephalomyelitis virus (TMEV) is related to the *Cardiovirus* genus. The GDVII strain is highly neurovirulent and causes fatal acute encephalitis, whereas most strains, like Daniels (DA), BeAn, and Theiler's original (TO) strains, cause a biphasic disease (for reviews, see references 62, 79). The early phase corresponds to a mild encephalomyelitis, mostly of the gray matter, during which the virus replicates mainly in neurons of the brain and spinal cord. The second phase is a chronic demyelinating disease of white matter tracts in the spinal cord of susceptible mice. TMEV pathogenesis will not be addressed here, since it is the subject of chapter 34 in this volume; this review will focus on the aspects relating to virus persistence. TMEV persistence appears to be required for immune-mediated demyelination (62). During the chronic phase, the number of infected cells is always low (16), there are only small amounts of capsid proteins in infected cells, and viral RNA replication seems to be blocked at the minus-strand RNA synthesis step (22).

There is over 90% sequence identity between the highly virulent GDVII strain, which does not persist in surviving animals (62), and persistent strains, like BeAn or DA. One of the main strategies used to identify the viral determinants of TMEV persistence has been to construct recombinant viruses. A chimeric DA/GDVII virus with a genome encoding 30 amino acids of the L protein, the entire capsid, and 27 amino acids of protein 2A from the DA strain produced a persistent infection in susceptible mice (72). The inverse chimeric virus was not able to persist, even though it was able to infect the white matter (72). These results strongly suggested that the capsid carries important determinants of persistence and demyelination. This was confirmed by studying a chimera, in which the regions encoding the capsid protein VP1 and a small portion of protein 2A came from GDVII and the rest of the genome from the DA strain. This chimeric virus did not persist in the central nervous system (CNS) of immunocompetent SJL/J mice (47). However, this virus persisted in the gray matter of the brain of BALB/c *nu/nu* mice, in neurons, and never reached the white matter of the spinal cord. Zurbriggen et al. (116) constructed and characterized a point mutant of the DA virus with a Thr to Ile change at amino acid 101 of VP1. Spread, replication, and persistence of this mutant virus in the CNS were markedly lower than those of the parental persistent DA strain (116). This and other studies provide evidence that loop II of VP1 is one factor determining DA virus growth, spread, and/or persistence in the CNS (111). A DA mutant with an insertion between positions 102 and 103 of VP1 resulted in a strain that induced demyelination, but it was limited to small areas and was observed later than that caused by the DA strain. Mutation

---

Florence Colbère-Garapin, Isabelle Pelletier, and Laurent Ouzilou ■ Groupe de Génétique Virale-Unité NRSN, Département de Virologie, Institut Pasteur, 25, rue du Dr Roux, 75724 Paris Cedex 15, France.

of residue 268 of VP1, which is near the putative receptor binding site, attenuated DA-induced demyelination (106).

The comparison of the phenotype of similar DA-derived chimeras constructed in two laboratories, having part of VP2, VP3, and VP1 and part of the 2A protein from the virulent strain, revealed the importance of residue 141 of VP2 ($VP2_{141}$) in cell tropism and persistence (48). Residue $VP2_{141}$ is at the rim of a depression between the arms of the star-shaped plateau believed to contain the receptor binding site (68). It is, therefore, possible that the role of residue $VP2_{141}$ in persistence may involve a receptor-mediated effect. Although the Asn to Lys substitution at amino acid position 141 of VP2 is required for the chimeric virus to persist, the Asn residue at this postion is present in the DA strain of the Pasteur Institute that is persistent (48). Thus, both Asn and Lys residues are compatible with persistence, although the Lys residue is required for persistence in a particular capsid context. Furthermore, another DA mutant with an Asn at position $VP2_{141}$ persists but does not induce significant white matter disease, indicating that there may be persistence with little or no demyelination (105). A DA mutant with a Thr to Phe substitution at position 173 of VP2, which is in the same neutralization site as $VP2_{141}$, fails to persist or to induce significant demyelination (105). Therefore, a modification of interactions of the virus and its receptor is most probably important in TMEV persistence (105).

There have been fewer studies on the capsid determinants of persistence for the other persistent strains than for DA. However, the analysis of the phenotype of GDVII/BeAn recombinants confirmed the involvement of the leader-capsid sequences in persistence and suggested that a conformational determinant requiring homologous sequences in both the VP2 puff and VP1 loop regions might underlie persistence (1). In addition, residue 244 of VP1, which is part of a predominant T-cell epitope, has been described as being important for persistence of the BeAn strain of TMEV (55).

The most significant structural differences between neurovirulent and persistent strains are at sites that may influence binding to cellular receptors. It now appears that the capsid structure, having a crucial importance, will have to be considered in terms of dynamic interactions rather than simply in terms of isolated amino acid residues.

Interestingly, it was found a few years ago that the genomes of all the persistent strains sequenced contain an alternate open reading frame in the L region, in addition to the large open reading frame (75). The corresponding protein L* is translated from an initiation codon 13 nucleotides downstream from the polyprotein initiating AUG (45). L* is associated with membranes and has antiapoptotic activity in macrophage cells. It may play a critical role in virus persistence (45). It has been proposed that L* could foster virus persistence in macrophages in two ways. The antiapoptotic activity of L* could play a role in inhibiting the virus-specific cytolytic T-cell response, or alternatively, it could inhibit the apoptosis of macrophages, thereby allowing widespread infection of these cells with the subsequent elimination of these antigen-presenting cells at a time critical for effective viral clearance (45). A cell-type-specific use of the two initiation codons could determine the balance between the synthesis of L*, leading to virus persistence, and that of the polyprotein and capsid proteins, target for the cytolytic T-cell response, leading to virus clearance (45).

The fact that the acute phase of the disease involves the gray matter while the chronic phase involves the white matter of the CNS strongly suggests that TMEV persistence depends on a particular cell tropism of TO strains. Lipton and colleagues (64) have shown that the predominant virus antigen load is in macrophages during the demyelinating disease (Table 1). The virus may persist in these phagocytic cells by active virus replication (64). In vitro, the GDVII strain significantly inhibited cellular protein synthesis and did not actively replicate in a macrophage-like cell line, whereas the persistent DA strain induced little if any shutoff and productively infected the cells (85). Interestingly, a key determinant for the cell-type-specific restriction of virus growth in a murine macrophage-like cell line is the L* protein of TO subgroup strains (108).

In contrast to the neurovirulent GDVII strain, the persistent DA strain infects glial cells at the beginning of the disease (5). During the chronic phase of DA infection, viral genomes are still present in glial cells (16) (Table 1). The TMEV capsid plays a role in the cell tropism of persistent strains, since a Lys at position $VP2_{141}$ of a DA/GDVII chimeric virus increases its ability to infect the white matter (48). It has been proposed that myelin as a structure might be needed for the virus to persist (79), since C3H mice homozygous for either the shiverer mutation (a deletion in the myelin basic protein gene) or the rumpshaker mutation (point mutation in the proteolipid protein gene) are completely resistant (13).

Zhou et al. (115) have shown that sialyllactose reduced BeAn replication in BHK-21 cells by blocking cellular attachment, but it did not reduce GDVII replication. These investigators proposed a model in which BeAn has both susceptible and nonsusceptible receptors. BeAn binds to sialic acid on a nonsusceptible receptor, and this traps the virus and slows down its spread. In contrast, GDVII does not bind to sialic acid and the selective binding of this virus to its receptor makes this infection much more efficient (115). Cellular clones of the murine L929 cells, susceptible to DA strain infection but with a decreased susceptibility to the GDVII strain, have been isolated (49). The characterization of these clones suggested that neurovirulent and persistent viruses use partly distinct pathways for both entry into cells and replication.

TABLE 1 Persistent picornavirus infection with virus production in vivo

Virus (genus)	Host	Site of persistence	Maximal length of virus production	References
TMEV (Cardiovirus)	Mouse	CNS (macrophages, glial cells)	Lifelong	16, 64
FMDV (Aphthovirus)	Cloven-hoofed animals	Pharynx? (epithelial cells?)	18 months	43
PV (Enterovirus)	Immunodeficient person	Intestine, CNS	≥10 years	9, 29, 54, 69

Susceptibility or resistance to Theiler's virus persistence depends on numerous murine genes both in and outside the major histocompatibility complex (MHC) (4, 17). Genetic and immunological aspects of the chronic disease have been reviewed elsewhere (79). Host factors involved in TMEV persistence will only be briefly summarized here.

The humoral response to TMEV limits viral spread during persistent infection (101), but it is not sufficient to cure susceptible mice (62). Within the H-2 complex, susceptibility has been mapped to the D region (23, 98, 99), which controls viral persistence (6, 63, 79). The b haplotype confers resistance, which is dominant; the q haplotype confers susceptibility; and haplotypes d, k, and s are associated with intermediate levels of susceptibility (reviewed in reference 79). This suggested that $CD8^+$ cytotoxic T lymphocytes (CTL) limit viral multiplication and prevent the persistent infection. Indeed, an early and efficient CTL response ensures recovery rather than viral persistence (33, 58). The genes encoding the T-cell receptor are good candidates for the control of persistence; however, the direct involvement of the Tcrb locus itself has not been demonstrated.

Each of the T-cell subsets makes a discrete and nonredundant contribution to protection from viral persistence. Indeed, genetic depletion of either $CD8^+$ or $CD4^+$ T cells from resistant B6 mice resulted in viral persistence (82). $CD4^+$ lymphocytes help antibody production by B cells at early times postinfection (pi) and by other mechanisms contribute to control viral replication. First, MHC class II-restricted Th1 T cells are directed to virus epitopes, then T cells specific for myelin epitopes are primed via epitope spreading, resulting in the damage to myelin (77). Nonetheless, TMEV persists in MHC class II-deficient mice from the resistant H2b background (40, 83). Interferon (IFN)-α/β controls the early infection of neurons and IFN-γ plays an important role in limiting the late persistent infection (39).

Thus, a tremendous amount of work has been done to understand viral persistence and the chronic demyelinating disease caused by the persistent strains of TMEV in susceptible mice. Although many results have been obtained, the way by which the virus propagates within the murine CNS and escapes the host defenses is not yet fully elucidated.

Foot-and-Mouth Disease Virus

Foot-and-mouth disease virus (FMDV) is an aphthovirus that naturally infects cloven-hoofed animals. After recovery from an acute infection, animals occasionally become carriers of the virus, which can then be isolated from throat fluids (43). Cows vaccinated with attenuated FMDV strains can also become inapparent carriers of the virus, even in the presence of neutralizing antibodies. Up to 9 months pi, antisense FMDV RNA can be detected in the pharynx of persistently infected cattle, suggesting that the pharynx is a site of virus persistence (94), and virus has been recovered from the esophageal pharyngeal area of the animals up to 18 months pi (43) (Table 1). FMDV sequences have been detected in spleen, lung, larynx, tonsils, pancreas, liver, esophagus, and white blood cells more than 2 years after infection of bovids, even when virus isolation was no longer possible (12). Indeed, although FMDV may persist in ruminants for extended periods, virus production can be temporary, in vivo as in vitro (30). Little is known about the factors that allow FMDV persistence in vivo.

Poliovirus and Other Enteroviruses in Immunodeficient Individuals

In humans, agammaglobulinemic individuals infected with an enterovirus (EV) may develop chronic meningitis or meningoencephalitis lasting many years, often with a fatal outcome (73). During the infection of a child with severe combined immunodeficiency, genetically related echovirus 30 variants coexisted over a 22-month period (8). Immunodeficient children may also develop chronic progressive poliomyelitis following vaccination with live attenuated strains of poliovirus (PV) (29). Molecular studies of isolates from several individuals with primary immune deficiency disorders indicate that PV vaccine strains may persist in the gastrointestinal tract, accumulate mutations involved in neurovirulence, and be excreted for as long as 10 years (9, 54). The administration of gammaglobulins to these patients can protect them from the pathologies due to PV persistence but does not necessarily cure the persistent PV infection (78). Recently, Sabin 3-derived PV strains isolated from a hypogammaglobulinemic patient who excreted virus for almost 2 years without symptoms of poliomyelitis were studied in detail (69). The rate of nucleotide substitution of these isolates was similar to that of circulating wild-type PV. The Sabin 3-derived isolates displayed a branched phylogenetic tree, presumably because the virus was colonizing different sites in the gastrointestinal tract. All Sabin 3-derived strains tested were more neurovirulent than Sabin 3 (69). These studies indicate that PV persistence in immunodeficient persons will probably complicate the worldwide eradication of PV.

PICORNAVIRUS INFECTIONS IN VIVO WITH PERSISTING VIRAL RNA

Coxsackieviruses

EV and, in particular, coxsackieviruses (CV) are suspected to be responsible for chronic diseases in humans several years after the acute infection (3, 80). CV may contribute to the pathogenesis of cardiomyopathies by a mechanism based on the cleavage of dystrophin by protease 2A (7). In developed countries, acute myocarditis is commonly associated with infections by B group CV (CVB), and some of the cases may evolve into a chronic form such as dilated cardiomyopathy. High titers of CVB neutralizing antibodies, persistent anti-CVB IgM antibodies, and the detection of EV RNA in sequential biopsy samples of myocardial tissue are suggestive of a persistent EV infection (reviewed in reference 80). However, virus isolation during these chronic diseases remains exceptional. In addition, EV have been implicated in the pathogenesis of polymyositis and the chronic fatigue syndrome. It is also possible that CV play a role in the development of insulin-dependent diabetes mellitus (type 1) (113), but in this case a persistent viral infection is not necessarily involved in the pathogenesis of the chronic disease.

Murine models have been developed with CVB3 to elucidate the relationship between virus persistence and chronic enteroviral heart disease. It would be valuable to know whether myocardial lesions are directly caused by viral replication, as proposed by Klingel and colleagues (56), or indirectly, by autoimmune mechanisms, as proposed by others (66). Note that the two mechanisms are not mutually exclusive and/or may vary with the mouse strain. In susceptible mice, there is evidence that myocytes are infected during viremia and that the virus spreads directly from cell to cell (56). After the episode of acute myocarditis, the number of infected cells and the copy number of viral RNA molecules per cell decreased. Infectious virus could no longer be recovered 15 days pi, but 30 days pi, persisting viral RNA was still found in the hearts of inbred mouse strains A.CA/SnJ, A.BY/SnJ, and SWR/J (but not in DBA/1J mice). The development of persistent heart muscle infection was not found to be linked to the H-2 haplotype of the mouse (56). In susceptible A.CA/SnJ mice, about 0.01% of myocardial cells were found to be infected 30 days pi. Whenever myocardial inflammatory lesions were observed at late disease stages, they were consistently associated with infected myocardial cells, suggesting a direct relationship between viral replication and ongoing heart lesions (56). Interestingly, 30 days pi, the amount of plus-strand RNA was not higher than that of minus-strand RNA in myocardial cells of infected mice, indicating that viral replication was limited. Capsid protein synthesis was also decreased. These results indicate that CVB3 can induce a persistent infection in the heart of susceptible mouse strains and that host determinants play a role in the development of the chronic disease. Interrelationships between virus replication and myocardial damage in persistent cardiac infection have been confirmed in several mouse strains (2).

In addition to heart muscle cells, lymphoid cells from spleen and lymph nodes of susceptible SWR/J mice were persistently infected by CVB3, while those of resistant DBA/1 mice, which do not develop chronic myocarditis, were cured following the acute infection. Therefore, in susceptible SWR/J mice infected with CVB3, lymphoid cells may be a virus reservoir and contribute to virus dissemination (56). Virus could be recovered from spleens up to 18 days pi, and during the late stage of the disease (42 days pi), viral RNA was detected in B cells. In addition to B lymphocytes, viral RNA-positive macrophages were detected during chronic disease (57). Plus- and minus-strand viral RNAs were consistently detected in heart and splenic tissues during chronic myocarditis (57).

In A/J mice inoculated with CVB3, viral genome has not been detected in the myocardium of all mice with chronic ongoing myocarditis. An autoimmune mechanism involved in the persistent inflammation would be consistent with the detection of heart myosin autoantibodies in some CVB3-infected mice (95).

Virus variants of the Tucson strain of CVB1 can induce chronic inflammatory myopathy and polymyositis in susceptible mice such as CD1 Swiss (109). Double-stranded CVB RNA persists in muscle for extended periods (109), but the role of CVB RNA persistence in these diseases is still debatable.

Poliovirus

In immunocompetent individuals, PV excretion generally stops a few weeks after infection. However, many survivors of poliomyelitis (10 to 50%), particularly in North America, develop the postpoliomyelitis syndrome (PPS) after decades of clinical stability. PPS includes a variety of neuromuscular symptoms. Several nonexclusive hypotheses have been proposed to explain PPS, and one of these is PV persistence (28). Intrathecal synthesis of IgM antibodies to PV was specifically detected in PPS patients (60, 107). Furthermore, PV or enterovirus sequences have been specifically detected in the cerebrospinal fluid of PPS patients by three independent laboratories (60, 61, 81). However, no infectious PV has ever been recovered from the cerebrospinal fluid of PPS patients, and the etiology of the PPS syndrome remains uncertain (74).

Using a murine model, Miller (76) has shown that a wild-type strain of PV that is neurovirulent in mice can persist for more than 2 months in the CNS of surviving animals. These results were confirmed in another study, in which PV persistence in the murine brain was demonstrated for 45 days in 3% of inoculated BALB/c mice and 43% of inoculated mice treated with antithymocyte serum (50). During persistence, genetic changes occurred in the genome of viruses isolated from the CNS of paralyzed and nonparalyzed animals (102). Interestingly, PV persistence was demonstrated even in the case of an attenuated PV infection, both in control and in cyclophosphamide-treated mice, although the frequency was much higher in the immunosuppressed mice (50). More recently, Destombes and colleagues (32) have shown that PV can persist in the spinal cord of immunocompetent mice for at least 12 months postparalysis. Infectious PV could not be recovered from homogenates of spinal cord from paralyzed mice, but PV particles were detected in the cytoplasm of motoneurons in the area of the lesion (32).

IN VITRO AND EX VIVO MODELS

TMEV and Encephalomyocarditis Virus

Compared to the number of studies on TMEV persistence in vivo, there have been few studies dealing with the establishment of persistent TMEV infections in vitro. Nevertheless, persistent TMEV infections have been established in murine L929 cells (100) and in a glioma cell line (88). Cerebrovascular endothelial cells from susceptible and resistant mice can also be persistently infected by TMEV (104).

Encephalomyocarditis virus (EMCV), another cardiovirus, establishes persistent infections in human erythroleukemic K562 cells (87). There was coevolution of small-plaque virus variants and cells resistant to superinfection associated with establishment of persistence (87). In the promonocytic U937 cell line, highly cytolytic EMCV infection was shifted to persistent infection as a result of repression of the expression of the double-stranded RNA-dependent protein kinase: a deficiency of this enzyme resulted in a delay in EMCV-induced apoptosis, allowing establishment of persistent infection (112).

FMDV

Early studies showed that FMDV can persist in primary cultures. A model of BHK-21 cells persistently infected with FMDV has been developed and studied extensively (30). Ten to 30 h pi, infected cells displayed cytopathic effects (CPE) but some of them survived. Initially, infectious titers were comparable to those of a lytic infection but then decreased gradually. IFN levels were low, suggesting that IFN is not involved. The viruses in infected cells rapidly became genetically heterogeneous. At late passages, FMDV RNA synthesis decreased. Spontaneous curing of cell cultures was observed, and the cured cells had an increased and specific resistance to superinfection by the parental FMDV strain.

Interestingly, it was in the case of FMDV that it was first demonstrated that the critical element in initiating viral persistence may be the capacity of cells to vary genetically (Fig. 1). The genetic changes appeared very shortly after infection and the degree of resistance to

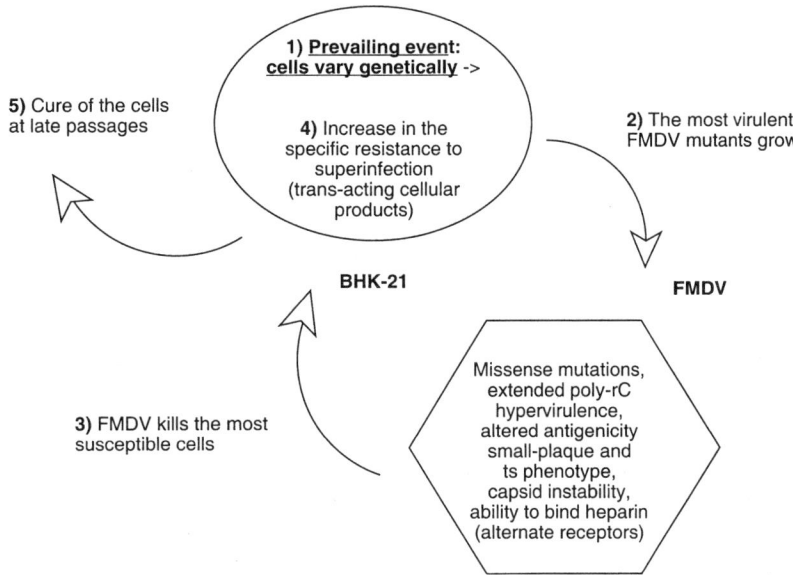

FIGURE 1 Principal events in the persistent FMDV infection of BHK-21 cells. The graph summarizes the data presented in several articles (30, 31, 34, 37, 38, 70, 103). ts, temperature sensitive.

FMDV of carrier cells increased with the passage number of infected cultures. The resistance to superinfection was a stable genetic trait, which seemed to be mediated by *trans*-acting cellular products (31, 70).

FMDV variants produced by carrier cultures differ from the parental FMDV strain (C-S8c1) by several phenotypic characters: small-plaque phenotype, temperature sensitivity, and less stable virions. The FMDV quasispecies selected during the establishment of persistence had a high level of genetic heterogeneity and became hypervirulent for BHK-21 cells (70). Diez et al. (34) studied the capsid-encoding region of an FMDV variant, selected after 100 passages in the carrier cells. Interestingly, this mutant had fixed several unique amino acids and has an extended polyribocytidylate tract in the 5′ untranslated region (38). In population replacement experiments, Saiz and Domingo (103) found that the initial persisting virus was always dominant in persistently infected cells, except when virulent viruses were used for the challenge. These results led to a new idea: hypervirulence can confer a selective advantage on a mutant virus in interaction with a population of partially resistant cells. Escarmis et al. (37) further characterized the FMDV mutants generated a few days after infection of partially permissive BHK cells (previously persistently infected and then cured). Interestingly, the FMDV mutants able to overcome the resistance of these modified BHK cells reproducibly acquired the ability to bind heparin and to infect wild-type Chinese hamster ovary cells.

Therefore, in the course of FMDV persistence in cell culture, a coevolution of host cells and the resident virus was observed (Fig. 1). The prevailing event ensuring cell survival during initiation of persistence was the rapid variation of the cells, and this was followed by the selection of increasingly virulent FMDV mutants. This model is worth comparing with that of epithelial cells, the natural targets of FMDV in susceptible animals: epithelial cells divide and are replaced rapidly. In vivo, it is possible that cell variation makes a large contribution to FMDV persistence (70).

Human Hepatitis A Virus

Human hepatitis A virus (HAV) is typically responsible for an acute infection in humans, whereas infection of susceptible primate cells in vitro leads to an inapparent, persistent infection (110). In persistently infected human embryo fibroblasts, subculture of cells with HAV-immune serum did not reduce the number of infected cells, whereas the addition of exogenous IFN cured the cells (110). In persistently infected green monkey kidney cells, replication of antigenic variants was favored (59). The absence of host cell shutoff is probably a main cause of this type of persistent infection. However, other factors may also contribute (59, 84).

Echoviruses

A model of echovirus 6 (EV6) persistence has been developed in cloned human amnion WISH cells (46). In contrast to the FMDV/BHK-21 model described above, WISH cells persistently infected by EV6 had a morphology and growth pattern indistinguishable from those of uninfected cells, and all cell clones produced virus (46). Persistently infected (PI-P) cells did not exhibit IFN antiviral activity, and the steady-state infection could not be cured by treating cells with an excess of neutralizing antibodies. About one-third of PI-P cells scored as infectious centers, and viral antigens were produced by most of the cells. Large amounts of defective virus were produced by these cells. However, these noninfectious viruses were not interferent (46). The precursor VP0 of VP2 and VP4 was not processed during persistent infection (97). Wild-type EV6 attached to the persistently infected cells, but the entry of the viral genome into the cell was blocked at a subsequent step (97).

The replication rate of the persistent viral RNA was low, suggesting that genomic regions involved in replication may be important in viral persistence (96). There were 13 differences between the nucleotide sequences of the P3 region of the wild-type and persistent (PI) strains of EV6.

TABLE 2 Poliovirus persistence in human cell lines

Cell line	Origin	Factors involved in persistence	References
IMR-32	Neuronal, neuroblastoma	Cellular determinants; PVR and other factors	24, 90
HEp-2	Epidermoid carcinoma, larynx	Viral determinants; multiplicity of infection	35, 36, 92
HeLa	Epitheloid carcinoma, cervix	Intracellular factors and down-regulation of PVR	53
K562	Erythroblastoid leukemia	Little or no shutoff of host protein synthesis	65
NB 103	Lymphoid (B cells)	Small percentage of permissive cells	21

A recombinant cDNA carrying PI sequences encoding the majority of the 3C protease, the 3D polymerase along with the 3' noncoding region of the persistent genome, and wild-type EV6 sequences in the 5' part of the genome was infectious. The cell line transfected with this cDNA synthesized and released transmissible nonlytic virus particles. Viral determinants of EV6 persistence in WISH cells mapped in the P3 genomic region, most likely in the sequence encoding the 3D polymerase. However, one cannot exclude the possibility that in PI-P cells, the large amounts of particles defective for the VP0 cleavage and some cellular determinants are also involved.

Another very different model of echovirus persistence was developed with EV1, in murine 3T3 cells expressing the EV1 human receptor, human very late antigen 2 (VLA-2, $\alpha 2\beta 1$), or its $\alpha 2$ subunit only (114). All EV1-infected $\alpha 2$-3T3 cells produced infectious virus but remained viable, and host cell translation was not inhibited. Persistently infected cultures produced infectious virus for months. Further studies will be required to elucidate the mechanisms of this persistent infection, and two hypotheses have been proposed: modified signals normally transduced by the EV1 receptor could be involved in the resistance of the 3T3 transformants to cell lysis; or alternatively, the 3T3 transformants could be more resistant to the changes in cell membrane permeability normally resulting in CPE (114).

Coxsackieviruses

Persistent infections have been established with most serotypes of CVB in human lymphoid cell lines (71). A model that may be relevant to chronic myocarditis is the persistent infection of human myocardial fibroblasts (51). The permissiveness of human vascular endothelial cells by CVBs has been investigated by Conaldi and colleagues (26), who found that CVB3 and -5 caused persistent infection in these cells. It is possible that the production of IFN-β by these cells plays an important role in the establishment of the infection. In addition, persistently infected cells released tumor necrosis factor alpha, which exerts negative ionotropic effects on cardiac myocytes (26).

CVBs induce different effects in different types of cultured human renal cells, and interestingly, CVB1, -3, -4, and -5 established persistent infections in glomerular mesangial cells, which failed to develop CPE (25). The persistent infection induced the synthesis of factors important for the progression from glomerular inflammation to glomerulosclerosis, and CVB impaired the phagocytic and contractile activity of mesangial cells. These results suggest that CVB infections may be associated with progressive renal injury (25).

CVB3 can infect human insulin-containing beta cells (113). A model of persistent infection by CVB4 has been developed in rat insulinoma cells, but insulin production by these cells was not altered (41).

Poliovirus

Several models of persistent PV infection have been developed (Table 2). Cell killing of human blood cell lines by PV depends on their differentiation stage (86). A persistent low-grade replication of virus was observed in several human lymphoid cell lines (21). The virus produced by persistently infected cells differs from that of the inoculum by several phenotypic properties (21). Presumably, a very small fraction of PV-susceptible cells is continuously recruited from among refractory cells. This situation is quite different from that of various human erythroblastoid K562 cell strains. With one of them, cells could be persistently infected, and there was little or no shutoff of host cell protein synthesis (65). Most of these infected cells scored as infectious centers and could not be cured by incubation with PV-neutralizing antibodies (65). In these cells, however, after hemin-induced differentiation, the outcome of infection became more lytic (11).

We found that PV can induce a persistent infection in two human neuronal cell lines, derived from neuroblastomas (24). After a crisis period, the neuroblastoma IMR-32 cells reached confluence and CPE disappeared despite continuous virus production. Persistently infected cells were obtained with the three serotypes of PV and with both virulent and attenuated strains. During the first weeks of infection, viral antigen was detected in almost all cells of persistently infected cultures, and 5 to 25% of the cells liberated virions. The neuronal origin of the infected cells was confirmed by the detection of human neurofilaments. Persistently infected cells were resistant to superinfection

FIGURE 2 Simplified models of persistent PV infection in neuroblastoma IMR-32 cells (star shapes) and HEp-2 cells (large hexagons). The majority of PV strains (small white hexagons) are able to establish persistent infections in IMR-32 cells (24). Virus and cell coevolution occurs, leading to the selection of PVpi (small black hexagons). PVpi and PV mutants carrying particular PVpi determinants are able to establish persistent infections in HEp-2 cells (35, 36, 91, 92). During the establishment of persistent PV infection, cellular factors are of crucial importance in the IMR-32 cell model, whereas viral determinants play the principal role in the HEp-2 cell model (93).

35. Persistent Infections by Picornaviruses ■ 443

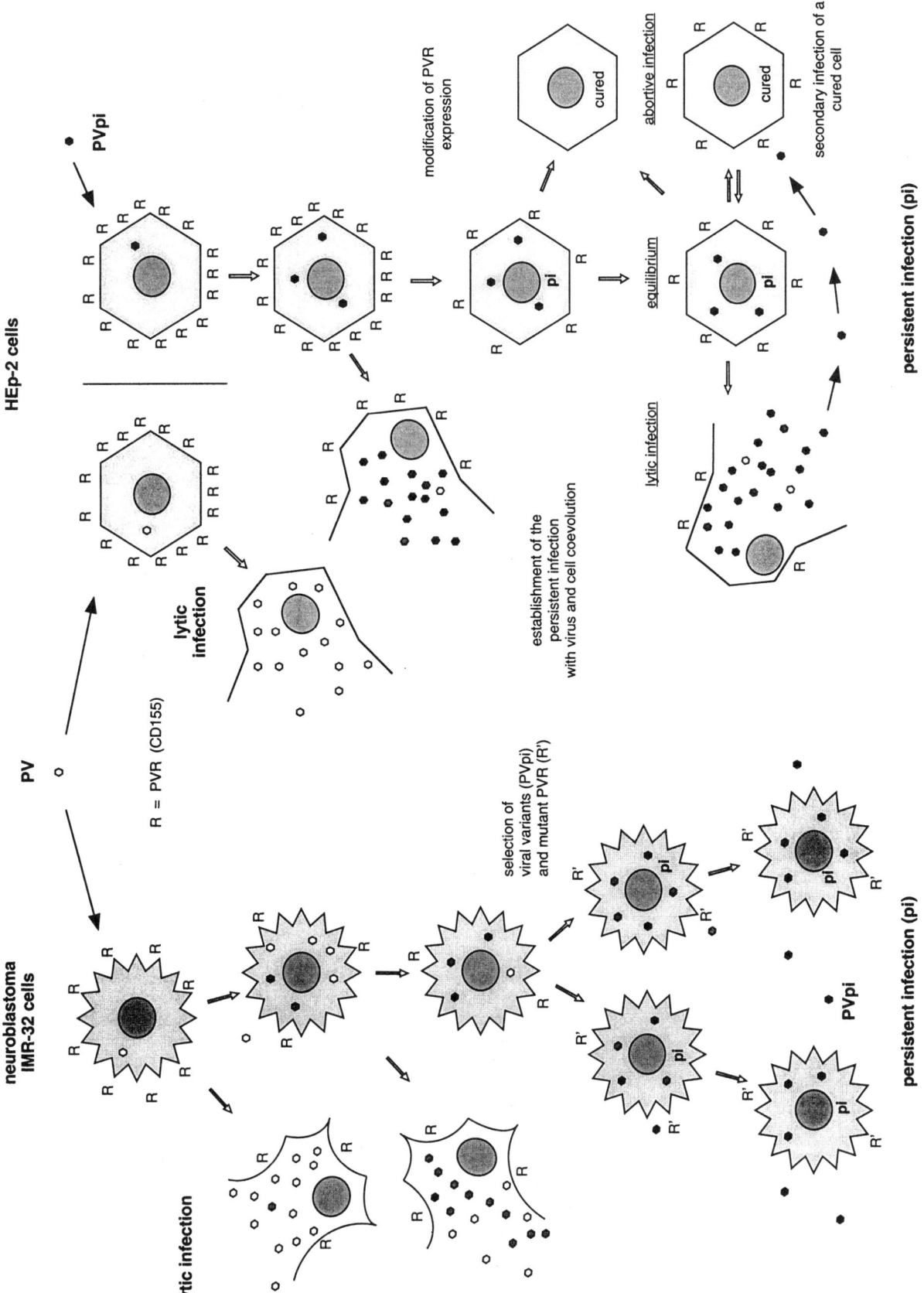

by many strains of PV, but not to CVB3. The synthesis of IFN-α and -β was not detected in persistently infected IMR-32 cells (24). We have recently found that mutant PV receptors are expressed in persistently PV-infected IMR-32 cells (90). These mutant PV receptors conferred on murine LM cells partial resistance to PV-induced lysis, suggesting that they contribute to persistence.

In IMR-32 cells persistently infected by PV, mutant viruses, named PVpi, were rapidly selected (91) (Fig. 2). The majority of missense mutations selected during a persistent PV infection of neuroblastoma cells map in the regions encoding capsid proteins (15). Many missense mutations as well as silent mutations were repeatedly selected in independent infections. The silent mutations may play a role in the structure of viral RNA and in RNA-protein interactions. Mutations were selected in the first weeks after infection at particular nucleotide positions, suggesting that there is a strong selective pressure in human neuroblastoma cells (20). The positions of modified amino acid residues on the structure of the PV capsid suggested that several of these mutations affect the early steps of the PV cycle. In agreement with this, four of five determinants present in the capsid proteins of a PVpi deriving from the wild-type Mahoney strain conferred to this strain the capacity to infect the murine motor neurons (27).

Thus, PVpi have a phenotype very different from that of the parental strains and, in particular, have a modified cell tropism. Moreover, they are able to infect HEp-2c cells persistently in the absence of any viral inhibitor. The establishment of a persistent infection in HEp-2c cells depends on two factors of crucial importance: the PV strain and the multiplicity of infection (MOI) (14). The latter must generally be lower than 10^{-1} 50% infective dose (ID_{50}) per cell, and even lower than 10^{-4} ID_{50} per cell for PV mutants differing from the lytic strains by only very few mutations. Similarly, the establishment of a persistent infection in HeLa cells by human rhinovirus 2 also depends on the MOI (44).

As in a model of HeLa cells persistently infected by PV (52), the maintenance of the persistent PV infection in HEp-2c cells correlated with the selection of cells in which PV multiplication was restricted (14). HEp-2c cultures could be cured spontaneously, or by growing them at 39°C, or by prolonged cultivation in a medium containing a mixture of PV-neutralizing antibodies. Nevertheless, the virus or its genome could remain intracellular for 10 days (14). As in the case of persistent infections by FMDV (70), the phenotype of the cured cells proved to be heterogeneous. Some cell clones were highly resistant to PV superinfection and had a very low level of PV receptor expression, while others were susceptible to superinfection (19) (Fig. 2). The results obtained with the cell clones studied in greater detail suggested that in HEp-2c cells there is an equilibrium between an abortive and a lytic infection and that the stability of this equilibrium depends on the expression of a host factor involved in the PV cycle (14).

Since tumor cell lines do not always reflect the pathways of in vivo infections, we investigated the possibility of establishing persistent PV infections in primary cultures of human brain cells. In these cells, the pattern of virus production was similar to that of neuroblastoma cells (89). Some mutations were repeatedly selected, and most interestingly, mutations modifying residues 95 of VP1 ($VP1_{95}$) and 142 of VP2 ($VP2_{142}$) in the Mahoney genome were identical to those selected in neuroblastoma cells, suggesting that common neural factors were responsible for this selection. During the first days of infection, cells permitting PV multiplication belonged to both the neuronal and glial lineage, while 2 weeks after infection, infected surviving cells mostly expressed markers of the neuronal lineage. At this time, the majority of infected cells expressed a marker of early commitment to the neuronal lineage. Some infected cells expressed a marker of postmitotic neurons, and therefore were probably young postmitotic neurons (89). This result is in agreement with PV being able to persist in the postmitotic motoneurons of patients who have survived poliomyelitis.

We have started to study the molecular mechanisms of PV persistence in HEp-2c cells because this cell model can be used for both lytic and persistent PV strains, allowing the identification of viral determinants involved in persistence. When HEp-2c cells were infected at an MOI of 10^{-2} ID_{50} per cell, PVpi mutations from both VP1 and VP2 together conferred the persistent phenotype to a recombinant between a type 1 PVpi and its parental lytic strain (18). Then, in a more precise study, we identified two determinants conferring the persistent phenotype to the Sabin 1 strain: one was a His to Tyr substitution at amino acid residue $VP2_{142}$, the other was Val to Ile substitution at amino acid $VP1_{160}$. Both are on the capsid surface. In fact, each of these determinants could confer the persistent phenotype to the Sabin 1 strain if an MOI as low as 10^{-4} ID_{50} per cell was used, but a mutant carrying both determinants established persistent infections in HEp-2c cells with a greater efficiency (92). A parallel study with a type 3 PVpi derived from the wild-type Leon strain led to the identification of two other capsid determinants involved in persistence in HEp-2c cells (36). In this case, the first is internal (Leu residue at position $VP2_{13}$) and the second is on the surface of the capsid in neutralization antigenic site 3a (Asn residue at position $VP1_{290}$). Both these determinants modify the cell tropism of the corresponding point mutants (36).

The type 1 and type 3 determinants involved in persistence confer to the virus a greater heat stability and also improve the efficiency of virus adsorption onto the receptor. They modify, although differently, the conformational transitions induced by the receptor following adsorption, as well as the efficiency of elution of viral particles from the receptor (36, 92). The conformational transitions induced by the receptor normally lead to the formation of A particles, which have lost VP4 and have a lower sedimentation coefficient than virions in sucrose gradient (135S instead of 160S) (10, 42, 67). A particles are considered to be a marker of the conformational modifications of the capsid during the early steps of infection. Surprisingly, the PV3 Leon-derived point mutant carrying the Asn residue at position $VP1_{290}$ and the double mutant carrying both type 3 determinants underwent unique conformational changes in the capsid upon interaction with host cells expressing the receptor, such that the sedimentation coefficient of the particle was 147S (35, 36). In contrast to the 135S particles, which are only formed at temperatures higher than 32°C, the 147S particles can be formed at 0°C (93). Another difference between the 135S and 147S particles is that the 147S have not been produced upon heating in a hypotonic buffer containing calcium, in the absence of receptor (35). It would be particularly interesting to know whether the 147S particles are a normally occurring but usually highly transitory uncoating intermediate, as we have recently proposed (36, 93), or abortive particles that form upon contact between a particular mutant PV and the receptor. These particles are currently being characterized in our laboratory.

CONCLUSIONS

It is clear from the studies briefly summarized above that many picornaviruses can establish persistent infections either in vivo or in vitro, or both. The use of animal models has revealed that severe disease can result from such infections. Furthermore, some of these animal models can be used as models for human pathologies (TMEV/multiple sclerosis). Other persistent infections have a veterinary importance with huge economic implications (FMDV). Moreover, new problems are becoming apparent, like that of PV persistence in the intestine of immunodeficient individuals, which will increase the difficulty of eradicating PV worldwide. Persistent picornavirus infections are valuable models for understanding complicated pathologies resulting from persistent viral infections. The various persistent picornavirus infections show some common features, like the coevolution of cells and virus, but it remains evident that there is a great diversity of mechanisms involved in persistent infections. Investigations with several models, therefore, provide complementary data, and the use of diverse models will be valuable. Much remains to be done.

We thank Prof. M. Brahic and Dr. B. Blondel for critical reading of the manuscript. The work from our group was supported by grants from the Pasteur Institute and from the Association Française contre les Myopathies (contract no. 6495).

REFERENCES

1. **Adami, C., A. E. Pritchard, T. Knauf, M. Luo, and H. L. Lipton.** 1998. A determinant for central nervous system persistence localized in the capsid of Theiler's murine encephalomyelitis virus by using recombinant viruses. *J. Virol.* **72:**1662–1665.
2. **Andreoletti, L., D. Hober, P. Becquart, S. Belaich, M. C. Copin, V. Lambert, and P. Wattre.** 1997. Experimental CVB3-induced chronic myocarditis in two murine strains: evidence of interrelationships between virus replication and myocardial damage in persistent cardiac infection. *J. Med. Virol.* **52:**206–214.
3. **Andreoletti, L., D. Hober, C. Decoene, M. C. Copin, P. E. Lobert, A. Dewilde, C. Stankowiac, and P. Wattre.** 1996. Detection of enteroviral RNA by polymerase chain reaction in endomyocardial tissue of patients with chronic cardiac diseases. *J. Med. Virol.* **48:**53–59.
4. **Aubagnac, S., M. Brahic, and J. F. Bureau.** 1999. Viral load and a locus on chromosome 11 affect the late clinical disease caused by Theiler's virus. *J. Virol.* **73:**7965–7971.
5. **Aubert, C., and M. Brahic.** 1995. Early infection of the central nervous system by the GDVII and DA strains of Theiler's virus. *J. Virol.* **69:**3197–3200.
6. **Azoulay, A., M. Brahic, and J. F. Bureau.** 1994. FVB mice transgenic for the H-2Db gene become resistant to persistent infection by Theiler's virus. *J. Virol.* **68:**4049–4052.
7. **Badorff, C., G. H. Lee, B. J. Lamphear, M. E. Martone, K. P. Campbell, R. E. Rhoads, and K. U. Knowlton.** 1999. Enteroviral protease 2A cleaves dystrophin: evidence of cytoskeletal disruption in an acquired cardiomyopathy. *Nat. Med.* **5:**320–326.
8. **Bailly, J. L., M. Chambon, C. Henquell, J. Icart, and H. Peigue-Lafeuille.** 2000. Genomic variations in echovirus 30 persistent isolates recovered from a chronically infected immunodeficient child and comparison with the reference strain. *J. Clin. Microbiol.* **38:**552–557.
9. **Bellmunt, A., G. May, R. Zell, P. Pring-Akerblom, W. Verhagen, and A. Heim.** 1999. Evolution of poliovirus type I during 5.5 years of prolonged enteral replication in an immunodeficient patient. *Virology* **265:**178–184.
10. **Belnap, D. M., D. J. Filman, B. L. Trus, N. Cheng, F. P. Booy, J. F. Conway, S. Curry, C. N. Hiremath, S. K. Tsang, A. C. Steven, and J. M. Hogle.** 2000. Molecular tectonic model of virus structural transitions: the putative cell entry states of poliovirus. *J. Virol.* **74:**1342–1354.
11. **Benton, P. A., D. J. Barret, R. L. Matts, and R. E. Lloyd.** 1996. The outcome of poliovirus infections in K562 cells is cytolytic rather than persistent after hemin-induced differentiation. *J. Virol.* **70:**5525–5532.
12. **Bergmann, I. E., V. Malirat, P. Auge de Mello, and I. Gomes.** 1996. Detection of foot-and-mouth disease viral sequences in various fluids and tissues during persistence of the virus in cattle. *Am. J. Vet. Res.* **57:**134–137.
13. **Bihl, F., C. Pena-Rossi, J. L. Guenet, M. Brahic, and J. F. Bureau.** 1997. The shiverer mutation affects the persistence of Theiler's virus in the central nervous system. *J. Virol.* **71:**5025–5030.
14. **Borzakian, S., T. Couderc, Y. Barbier, G. Attal, I. Pelletier, and F. Colbère-Garapin.** 1992. Persistent poliovirus infection: establishment and maintenance involve distinct mechanisms. *Virology* **186:**398–408.
15. **Borzakian, S., I. Pelletier, V. Calvez, and F. Colbère-Garapin.** 1993. Precise missense and silent point mutations are fixed in the genomes of poliovirus mutants from persistently infected cells. *J. Virol.* **67:**2914–2917.
16. **Brahic, M., and W. G. Stroop.** 1981. Theiler's virus persists in glial cells during demyelinating disease. *Cell* **26:**123–128.
17. **Bureau, J. F., X. Montagutelli, F. Bihl, S. Lefebvre, J. L. Guenet, and M. Brahic.** 1993. Mapping loci influencing the persistence of Theiler's virus in the murine central nervous system. *Nat. Genet.* **5:**87–91.
18. **Calvez, V., I. Pelletier, S. Borzakian, and F. Colbère-Garapin.** 1993. Identification of a region of the poliovirus genome involved in persistent infection of HEp-2 cells. *J. Virol.* **67:**4432–4435.
19. **Calvez, V., I. Pelletier, T. Couderc, N. Pavio-Guédo, B. Blondel, and F. Colbère-Garapin.** 1995. Cell clones cured of persistent poliovirus infection display selective permissivity to the wild-type poliovirus strain Mahoney and partial resistance to the attenuated Sabin 1 strain and Mahoney mutants. *Virology* **212:**309–322.
20. **Calvez, V., I. Pelletier, N. Guédo, S. Borzakian, T. Couderc, B. Blondel, and F. Colbère-Garapin.** 1995. Persistent poliovirus infection: development of new models with cell lines, p. 370–373. *In* M. C. Dalakas, H. Bartfeld, and L. T. Kurland (ed.), *The Post-Polio Syndrome*, vol. 753. The New York Academy of Sciences, New York, N.Y.
21. **Carp, R. I.** 1981. Persistent infection of human lymphoid cells with poliovirus and development of temperature-sensitive mutants. *Intervirology* **15:**49–56.
22. **Cash, E., M. Chamorro, and M. Brahic.** 1988. Minus-strand RNA synthesis in the spinal cords of mice persistently infected with Theiler's virus. *J. Virol.* **62:**1824–1826.
23. **Clatch, R. J., R. W. Melvold, S. D. Miller, and H. L. Lipton.** 1985. Theiler's murine encephalomyelitis virus (TMEV)-induced demyelinating disease in mice is influenced by the H-2D region: correlation with TMEV spe-

cific delayed-type hypersensitivity. *J. Immunol.* **135:**1408–1414.
24. **Colbère-Garapin, F., C. Christodoulou, R. Crainic, and I. Pelletier.** 1989. Persistent poliovirus infection of human neuroblastoma cells. *Proc. Natl. Acad. Sci. USA* **86:**7590–7594.
25. **Conaldi, P. G., L. Biancone, A. Bottelli, A. de Martino, G. Camussi, and A. Toniolo.** 1997. Distinct pathogenic effects of group B coxsackieviruses on human glomerular and tubular kidney cells. *J. Virol.* **71:**9180–9187.
26. **Conaldi, P. G., C. Serra, A. Mossa, V. Falcone, F. Basolo, G. Camussi, A. Dolei, and A. Toniolo.** 1997. Persistent infection of human vascular endothelial cells by group B coxsackieviruses. *J. Infect. Dis.* **175:**693–696.
27. **Couderc, T., N. Guédo, V. Calvez, I. Pelletier, J. Hogle, F. Colbère-Garapin, and B. Blondel.** 1994. Substitutions in the capsids of poliovirus mutants selected in human neuroblastoma cells confer on the Mahoney type 1 strain a phenotype neurovirulent in mice. *J. Virol.* **68:**8386–8391.
28. **Dalakas, M. C.** 1986. New neuromuscular symtoms in patients with old poliomyelitis: a three year follow-up study. *Eur. Neurol.* **25:**381–387.
29. **Davis, L. E., D. Bodian, D. Price, I. Butler, and J. H. Vickers.** 1977. Chronic progressive poliomyelitis secondary to vaccination of an immunodeficient child. *N. Engl. J. Med.* **297:**241–245.
30. **de la Torre, J. C., M. Davila, F. Sobrino, J. Ortin, and E. Domingo.** 1985. Establishment of cell lines persistently infected with foot-and-mouth disease virus. *Virology* **145:**24–35.
31. **de la Torre, J. C., E. Martinez-Salas, J. Diez, and E. Domingo.** 1989. Extensive cell heterogeneity during persistent infection with foot-and-mouth disease virus. *J. Virol.* **63:**59–63.
32. **Destombes, J., T. Couderc, D. Thiesson, S. Girard, S. G. Wilt, and B. Blondel.** 1997. Persistent poliovirus infection in mouse motoneurons. *J. Virol.* **71:**1621–1628.
33. **Dethlefs, S., M. Brahic, and E. L. Larsson-Sciard.** 1997. An early, abundant cytotoxic T-lymphocyte response against Theiler's virus is critical for preventing viral persistence. *J. Virol.* **71:**8875–8878.
34. **Diez, J., M. Davila, C. Escarmis, M. G. Mateu, J. Dominguez, J. J. Perez, E. Giralt, J. A. Melero, and E. Domingo.** 1990. Unique amino acid substitutions in the capsid proteins of foot-and-mouth disease virus from a persistent infection in cell culture. *J. Virol.* **64:**5519–5528.
35. **Duncan, G., and F. Colbère-Garapin.** 1999. Two determinants in the capsid of a persistent type 3 poliovirus exert different effects on mutant virus uncoating. *J. Gen. Virol.* **80:**2601–2605.
36. **Duncan, G., I. Pelletier, and F. Colbère-Garapin.** 1998. Two amino acid substitutions in the type 3 poliovirus capsid contribute to the establishment of persistent infection in HEp-2c cells by modifying virus-receptor interactions. *Virology* **241:**14–29.
37. **Escarmis, C., E. C. Carrillo, M. Ferrer, J. F. Garcia Arriaza, N. Lopez, C. Tami, N. Verdaguer, E. Domingo, and M. T. Franze-Fernandez.** 1998. Rapid selection in modified BHK-21 cells of a foot-and-mouth disease virus variant showing alterations in cell tropism. *J. Virol.* **72:**10171–10179.
38. **Escarmis, C., M. Toja, M. Medina, and E. Domingo.** 1992. Modifications of the 5′ untranslated region of foot-and-mouth disease virus after prolonged persistence in cell culture. *Virus Res.* **26:**113–125.
39. **Fiette, L., C. Aubert, U. Muller, S. Huang, M. Aguet, M. Brahic, and J. F. Bureau.** 1995. Theiler's virus infection of 129Sv mice that lack the interferon alpha/beta or interferon gamma receptors. *J. Exp. Med.* **181:**2069–2076.
40. **Fiette, L., M. Brahic, and C. Pena-Rossi.** 1996. Infection of class II-deficient mice by the DA strain of Theiler's virus. *J. Virol.* **70:**4811–4815.
41. **Frank, J. A., Jr., E. V. Schmidt, R. E. Smith, and C. M. Wilfert.** 1986. Persistent infection of rat insulinoma cells with coxsackie B4 virus. *Arch. Virol.* **87:**143–150.
42. **Fricks, C. E., and J. M. Hogle.** 1990. Cell-induced conformational change in poliovirus: externalization of the amino terminus of VP1 is responsible for liposome binding. *J. Virol.* **64:**1934–1945.
43. **Gebauer, F., J. C. de la Torre, I. Gomes, M. G. Mateu, H. Barahona, B. Tiraboschi, I. Bergmann, P. A. de Mello, and E. Domingo.** 1988. Rapid selection of genetic and antigenic variants of foot-and-mouth disease virus during persistence in cattle. *J. Virol.* **62:**2041–2049.
44. **Gercel, C., K. B. Mahan, and V. V. Hamparian.** 1985. Preliminary characterization of persistent infection of HeLa cells with human rhinovirus type 2. *J. Gen. Virol.* **66:**131–139.
45. **Ghadge, G. D., L. Ma, S. Sato, J. Kim, and R. P. Roos.** 1998. A protein critical for a Theiler's virus-induced immune system-mediated demyelinating disease has a cell type-specific antiapoptotic effect and a key role in virus persistence. *J. Virol.* **72:**8605–8612.
46. **Gibson, J. P., and V. F. Righthand.** 1985. Persistence of echovirus 6 in cloned human cells. *J. Virol.* **54:**219–223.
47. **Jarousse, N., L. Fiette, R. A. Grant, J. M. Hogle, A. McAllister, T. Michiels, C. Aubert, F. Tangy, M. Brahic, and C. P. Rossi.** 1994. Chimeric Theiler's virus with altered tropism for the central nervous system. *J. Virol.* **68:**2781–2786.
48. **Jarousse, N., C. Martinat, S. Syan, M. Brahic, and A. McAllister.** 1996. Role of VP2 amino acid 141 in tropism of Theiler's virus within the central nervous system. *J. Virol.* **70:**8213–8217.
49. **Jnaoui, K., and T. Michiels.** 1999. Analysis of cellular mutants resistant to Theiler's virus infection: differential infection of L929 cells by persistent and neurovirulent strains. *J. Virol.* **73:**7248–7254.
50. **Jubelt, B., S. L. Ropka, S. J. Goldfarb, and J. L. Janavs.** 1989. Anti-thymocyte serum delays clearance of poliovirus from the mouse central nervous system. *J. Neuroimmunol.* **22:**223–232.
51. **Kandolf, R., A. Canu, and P. A. Hofschneider.** 1985. Coxsackie B3 virus can replicate in cultured human foetal heart cells and is inhibited by interferon. *Mol. Cell. Cardiol.* **17:**167–181.
52. **Kaplan, G., A. Levy, and V. R. Racaniello.** 1989. Isolation and characterization of HeLa cell lines blocked at different steps in the poliovirus life cycle. *J. Virol.* **63:**43–51.
53. **Kaplan, G., and V. R. Racaniello.** 1991. Down regulation of poliovirus receptor RNA in HeLa cells resistant to poliovirus infection. *J. Virol.* **65:**1829–1835.
54. **Kew, O. M., R. W. Sutter, B. K. Nottay, M. J. McDonough, D. R. Prevots, L. Quick, and M. A. Pallansch.** 1998. Prolonged replication of a type 1 vaccine-derived poliovirus in an immunodeficient patient. *J. Clin. Microbiol.* **36:**2893–2899.
55. **Kim, B. S., R. L. Yauch, Y. Y. Bahk, J. A. Kang, M. C. Dal Canto, and C. K. Hall.** 1998. A spontaneous low-pathogenic variant of Theiler's virus contains an amino acid substitution within the predominant VP1(233-250) T-cell epitope. *J. Virol.* **72:**1020–1027.
56. **Klingel, K., C. Hohenadl, A. Canu, M. Albrecht, M. Seemann, G. Mall, and R. Kandolf.** 1992. Ongoing en-

terovirus-induced myocarditis is associated with persistent heart muscle infection—quantitative analysis of virus replication, tissue damage, and inflammation. *Proc. Natl. Acad. Sci. USA* **89:**314–318.
57. **Klingel, K., S. Stephan, M. Sauter, R. Zell, B. M. McManus, B. Bultman, and R. Kandolf.** 1996. Pathogenesis of murine enterovirus myocarditis: virus dissemination and immune cell targets. *J. Virol.* **70:**8888–8895.
58. **Larsson-Sciard, E. L., S. Dethlefs, and M. Brahic.** 1997. In vivo administration of interleukin-2 protects susceptible mice from Theiler's virus persistence. *J. Virol.* **71:**797–799.
59. **Lemon, S. M., P. C. Murphy, P. A. Shields, L. H. Ping, S. M. Feinstone, T. Cromeans, and R. W. Jansen.** 1991. Antigenic and genetic variation in cytopathic hepatitis A virus variants arising during persistent infection: evidence for genetic recombination. *J. Virol.* **65:**2056–2065.
60. **Leon-Monzon, M. E., and M. C. Dalakas.** 1995. Detection of poliovirus antibodies and poliovirus genome in patients with the post-polio syndrome. *Ann. N. Y. Acad. Sci.* **753:**208–218.
61. **Leparc-Goffart, I., J. Julien, F. Fuchs, I. Janatova, M. Aymard, and H. Kopecka.** 1996. Evidence of presence of poliovirus genomic sequences in cerebrospinal fluid from patients with postpolio syndrome. *J. Clin. Microbiol.* **34:**2023–2026.
62. **Lipton, H. L., and M. L. Jelachich.** 1997. Molecular pathogenesis of Theiler's murine encephalomyelitis virus-induced demyelinating disease in mice. *Intervirology* **40:**143–152.
63. **Lipton, H. L., R. Melvold, S. D. Miller, and M. C. Dal Canto.** 1995. Mutation of a major histocompatibility class I locus, H-2D, leads to an increased virus burden and disease susceptibility in Theiler's virus-induced demyelinating disease. *J. Neurovirol.* **1:**138–144.
64. **Lipton, H. L., G. Twaddle, and M. L. Jelachich.** 1995. The predominant virus antigen burden is present in macrophages in Theiler's murine encephalomyelitis virus-induced demyelinating disease. *J. Virol.* **69:**2525–2533.
65. **Lloyd, R. E., and M. Bovee.** 1993. Persistent infection of human erythroblastoid cells by poliovirus. *Virology* **194:**200–209.
66. **Lodge, P. A., M. Herzum, J. Olszewski, and S. A. Huber.** 1987. Coxsackievirus B3 myocarditis. Acute and chronic forms of the disease caused by different immunopathogenic mechanisms. *Am. J. Pathol.* **128:**455–463.
67. **Lonberg-Holm, K. L., L. B. Gosser, and J. J. Kauer.** 1975. Early alteration of poliovirus in infected cells and its specific inhibition. *J. Gen. Virol.* **27:**329–342.
68. **Luo, M., K. S. Toth, L. Zhou, A. Pritchard, and H. L. Lipton.** 1996. The structure of a highly virulent Theiler's murine encephalomyelitis virus (GDVII) and implications for determinants of viral persistence. *Virology* **220:**246–250.
69. **Martin, J., G. Dunn, R. Hull, V. Patel, and P. D. Minor.** 2000. Evolution of the Sabin strain of type 3 poliovirus in an immunodeficient patient during the entire 637-day period of virus excretion. *J. Virol.* **74:**3001–3010.
70. **Martin-Hernandez, A. M., E. C. Carrillo, N. Sevilla, and E. Domingo.** 1994. Rapid cell variation can determine the establishment of a persistent viral infection. *Proc. Natl. Acad. Sci. USA* **91:**3705–3709.
71. **Matteucci, D., M. Paglianti, A. M. Giangregorio, M. R. Capobianchi, F. Dianzani, and M. Bendinelli.** 1985. Group B coxsackieviruses readily establish persistent infections in human lymphoid cell lines. *J. Virol.* **56:**651–654.
72. **Mc Allister, A., F. Tanguy, C. Aubert, and M. Brahic.** 1990. Genetic mapping of the ability of Theiler's virus to persist and demyelinate. *J. Virol.* **64:**4252–4257.
73. **McKinney, R. E., Jr., S. L. Katz, and C. M. Wilfert.** 1987. Chronic enteroviral meningoencephalitis in agammaglobulinemic patients. *Rev. Infect. Dis.* **9:**334–356.
74. **Melchers, W., M. de Visser, P. Jongen, A. van Loon, R. Nibbeling, P. Oostvogel, D. Willemse, and J. Galama.** 1992. The postpolio syndrome: no evidence for poliovirus persistence. *Ann. Neurol.* **32:**728–732.
75. **Michiels, T., N. Jarousse, and M. Brahic.** 1995. Analysis of the leader and capsid coding regions of persistent and neurovirulent strains of Theiler's virus. *Virology* **214:**550–558.
76. **Miller, J. R.** 1981. Prolonged intracerebral infection with poliovirus in asymptomatic mice. *Ann. Neurol.* **9:**590–596.
77. **Miller, S. D., C. L. Vanderlugt, W. S. Begolka, W. Pao, R. L. Yauch, K. L. Neville, Y. Katz-Levy, A. Carrizosa, and B. S. Kim.** 1997. Persistent infection with Theiler's virus leads to CNS autoimmunity via epitope spreading. *Nat. Med.* **3:**1133–1136.
78. **Minor, P. D.** 1999. Poliovirus vaccination: current understanding of poliovirus interactions in humans and implications for the eradication of poliomyelitis. *Expert Rev. Molec. Med.* **23:**1–17.
79. **Monteyne, P., J. F. Bureau, and M. Brahic.** 1997. The infection of mouse by Theiler's virus: from genetics to immunology. *Immunol. Rev.* **159:**163–176.
80. **Muir, P.** 1992. The association of enteroviruses persistence with chronic heart disease. *Rev. Med. Virol.* **2:**9–18.
81. **Muir, P., F. Nicholson, M. K. Sharief, E. J. Thompson, N. J. Cairns, P. Lantos, G. T. Spencer, H. J. Kaminski, and J. E. Banatvala.** 1995. Evidence for persistent enterovirus infection of the central nervous system in patients with previous paralytic poliomyelitis. *Ann. N. Y. Acad. Sci.* **753:**219–232.
82. **Murray, P. D., K. D. Pavelko, J. Leibowitz, X. Lin, and M. Rodriguez.** 1998. CD4(+) and CD8(+) T cells make discrete contributions to demyelination and neurologic disease in a viral model of multiple sclerosis. *J. Virol.* **72:**7320–7329.
83. **Njenga, M. K., K. D. Pavelko, J. Baisch, X. Lin, C. David, J. Leibowitz, and M. Rodriguez.** 1996. Theiler's virus persistence and demyelination in major histocompatibility complex class II-deficient mice. *J. Virol.* **70:**1729–1737.
84. **Nuesch, J. P., M. Weitz, and G. Siegl.** 1993. Proteins specifically binding to the 3' untranslated region of hepatitis A virus RNA in persistently infected cells. *Arch. Virol.* **128:**65–79.
85. **Obuchi, M., Y. Ohara, T. Takegami, T. Murayama, H. Takada, and H. Iizuka.** 1997. Theiler's murine encephalomyelitis virus subgroup strain-specific infection in a murine macrophage-like cell line. *J. Virol.* **71:**729–733.
86. **Okada, Y., G. Toda, H. Oka, A. Nomoto, and H. Yoshikura.** 1987. Poliovirus infection of established human blood cell lines: relationship between the differentiation stage and susceptibility or cell killing. *Virology* **156:**238–245.
87. **Pardoe, I. V., K. K. Grewal, M. Pah Baldeh, J. Hamid, and A. T. H. Burness.** 1990. Persistent infection of K562 cells by encephalomyocarditis virus. *J. Virol.* **64:**6040–6044.
88. **Patick, A. K., E. L. Oleszak, J. L. Leibowitz, and M. Rodriguez.** 1990. Persistent infection of a glioma cell line generates a Theiler's virus variant which fails to induce demyelinating disease in SJL/J mice. *J. Gen. Virol.* **71:**2123–2132.
89. **Pavio, N., M.-H. Buc-Caron, and F. Colbère-Garapin.** 1996. Persistent poliovirus infection of human fetal brain cells. *J. Virol.* **70:**6395–6401.

90. **Pavio, N., T. Couderc, S. Girard, J.-Y. Sgro, B. Blondel, and F. Colbère-Garapin.** 2000. Expression of mutated poliovirus receptors in human neuroblastoma cells persistently infected with poliovirus. *Virology* **274:**331–342.
91. **Pelletier, I., T. Couderc, S. Borzakian, E. Wyckoff, R. Crainic, E. Ehrenfeld, and F. Colbère-Garapin.** 1991. Characterization of persistent poliovirus mutants selected in human neuroblastoma cells. *Virology* **180:**729–737.
92. **Pelletier, I., G. Duncan, and F. Colbère-Garapin.** 1998. One amino acid change on the capsid surface of poliovirus Sabin 1 allows the establishment of persistent infections in HEp-2c cell cultures. *Virology* **241:**1–13.
93. **Pelletier, I., G. Duncan, N. Pavio, and F. Colbère-Garapin.** 1998. Molecular mechanisms of poliovirus persistence: key role of capsid determinants during the establishment phase. *Cell. Mol. Life Sci.* **54:**1385–1402.
94. **Prato Murphy, M. L., R. F. Meyer, C. Mebus, A. A. Schudel, and M. Rodriguez.** 1994. Analysis of sites of foot and mouth disease virus persistence in carrier cattle via the polymerase chain reaction. *Arch. Virol.* **136:**299–307.
95. **Rabausch-Starz, I., A. Schwaiger, K. Grunewald, H. K. Muller-Hermelink, and N. Neu.** 1994. Persistence of virus and viral genome in myocardium after coxsackievirus B3-induced murine myocarditis. *Clin. Exp. Immunol.* **96:**69–74.
96. **Righthand, V. F.** 1991. Transmission of viral persistence by transfection of human cultured cells with RNA of a persistent strain of echovirus 6. *Microb. Pathog.* **11:**57–65.
97. **Righthand, V. F., and R. V. Blackburn.** 1989. Steady-state infection by echovirus 6 associated with nonlytic viral RNA and an unprocessed capsid polypeptide. *J. Virol.* **63:**5268–5275.
98. **Rodriguez, M., and C. S. David.** 1995. H-2 Dd transgene suppresses Theiler's virus-induced demyelination in susceptible strains of mice. *J. Neurovirol.* **1:**111–117.
99. **Rodriguez, M., J. Leibowitz, and C. S. David.** 1986. Susceptibility to Theiler's virus-induced demyelination. Mapping of the gene within the H-2D region. *J. Exp. Med.* **163:**620–631.
100. **Roos, R. P., O. C. Richards, J. Green, and E. Ehrenfeld.** 1982. Characterization of a cell culture persistently infected with the DA strain of Theiler's murine encephalomyelitis virus. *J. Virol.* **43:**1118–1122.
101. **Rossi, C. P., E. Cash, C. Aubert, and A. Coutinho.** 1991. Role of the humoral immune response in resistance to Theiler's virus infection. *J. Virol.* **65:**3895–3899.
102. **Rozhon, E. J., A. K. Wilson, and B. Jubelt.** 1984. Characterization of genetic changes occurring in attenuated poliovirus 2 during persistent infection in mouse central nervous systems. *J. Virol.* **50:**137–144.
103. **Saiz, J. C., and E. Domingo.** 1996. Virulence as a positive trait in viral persistence. *J. Virol.* **70:**6410–6413.
104. **Sapatino, B. V., A. D. Petrescu, B. A. Rosenbaum, R. Smith, J. A. Piedrahita, and C. J. Welsh.** 1995. Characteristics of cloned cerebrovascular endothelial cells following infection with Theiler's virus. II. Persistent infection. *J. Neuroimmunol.* **62:**127–135.
105. **Sato, S., L. Zhang, J. Kim, J. Jakob, R. A. Grant, R. Wollmann, and R. P. Roos.** 1996. A neutralization site of DA strain of Theiler's murine encephalomyelitis virus important for disease phenotype. *Virology* **226:**327–337.
106. **Senkowski, A., B. Shim, and R. P. Roos.** 1995. The effect of Theiler's murine encephalomyelitis virus (TMEV) VP1 carboxyl region on the virus-induced central nervous system disease. *J. Neurovirol.* **1:**101–110.
107. **Sharief, M. K., R. Hentges, and M. Ciardi.** 1991. Intrathecal immune response in patients with the post-polio syndrome. *N. Engl. J. Med.* **325:**749–755.
108. **Takata, H., M. Obuchi, J. Yamamoto, T. Odagiri, R. P. Roos, H. Iizuka, and Y. Ohara.** 1998. L* protein of the DA strain of Theiler's murine encephalomyelitis virus is important for virus growth in a murine macrophage-like cell line. *J. Virol.* **72:**4950–4955.
109. **Tam, P. E., and R. P. Messner.** 1999. Molecular mechanisms of coxsackievirus persistence in chronic inflammatory myopathy: viral RNA persists through formation of a double-stranded complex without associated genomic mutations or evolution. *J. Virol.* **73:**10113–10121.
110. **Vallbracht, A., L. Hofmann, K. G. Wurster, and B. Flehmig.** 1984. Persistent infection of human fibroblasts by hepatitis A virus. *J. Gen. Virol.* **65:**609–615.
111. **Wada, Y., I. J. McCright, F. G. Whitby, I. Tsunoda, and R. S. Fujinami.** 1998. Replacement of loop II of VP1 of the DA strain with loop II of the GDVII strain of Theiler's murine encephalomyelitis virus alters neurovirulence, viral persistence, and demyelination. *J. Virol.* **72:**7557–7562.
112. **Yeung, M. C., D. L. Chang, R. E. Camantigue, and A. S. Lau.** 1999. Inhibitory role of the host apoptogenic gene PKR in the establishment of persistent infection by encephalomyocarditis virus in U937 cells. *Proc. Natl. Acad. Sci. USA* **96:**11860–11865.
113. **Yoon, J.** 1990. The role of viruses and environmental factors in the induction of diabetes. *Curr. Top. Microbiol. Immunol.* **164:**95–123.
114. **Zhang, S., and V. R. Racaniello.** 1997. Persistent echovirus infection of mouse cells expressing the viral receptor VLA-2. *Virology* **235:**293–301.
115. **Zhou, L., X. Lin, T. J. Green, H. L. Lipton, and M. Luo.** 1997. Role of sialyloligosaccharide binding in Theiler's virus persistence. *J. Virol.* **71:**9701–9712.
116. **Zurbriggen, A., C. Thomas, M. Yamada, R. P. Roos, and R. S. Fujinami.** 1991. Direct evidence of a role for amino acid 101 of VP-1 in central nervous system disease in Theiler's murine encephalomyelitis virus infection. *J. Virol.* **65:**1929–1937.

CELL-FREE SYNTHESIS AND CELL-FREE GENETICS OF POLIOVIRUS

Cell-Free Genetics of Poliovirus

ROHIT DUGGAL

36

For years it has been the endeavor of researchers to be able to mimic viral multiplication events outside cells. This has been particularly true for plus-strand RNA viruses, starting with the successful detection of RNA replication with the replicase enzyme of the coliphage Qβ (1) and minus-strand synthesis for the plant virus brome mosaic virus (7). Imitation of particle morphogenesis in experiments using viral RNA and purified capsid protein for the plant virus tobacco mosaic virus (8) generated virus particles in cell-free conditions. However, it was still not feasible to carry out the complete life cycle of viruses in vitro that culminated in the synthesis of infectious viral particles. Thus, in 1991, when Molla et al. (12) demonstrated the successful in vitro synthesis of poliovirus starting with poliovral RNA, it was a major achievement. Theoretically, one could now dissect all the events of the life cycle of this RNA virus in the "test tube." In this chapter discussions will center on two processes of the poliovral life cycle that were successfully reproduced in the cell-free system, recombination and complementation. First, recombination, the components of the cell-free recombination system, and the alteration of crossover sites by temperature will be discussed, and then the inadvertently discovered phenomenon of complementation will be presented.

CELL-FREE RECOMBINATION

The cell-free system has a limitation in that it works best when either viral RNA (extracted from purified poliovirus particles) or efficiently replicating in vitro-synthesized transcripts are used in conjunction with the HeLa extract (3). To observe and study recombination in the cell-free system it was imperative to use genetic markers that did not impair replication to a larger extent, markers that were present on relatively separated loci and generated phenotypes in recombinants that could be exploited to separate the parents from the recombinant molecules. In the Wimmer laboratory, a chimeric poliovirus [PV1(RIPO)] had been generated that had the internal ribosomal entry site (IRES) replaced with that of human rhinovirus type 2 (HRV2). This chimeric poliovirus had an unusual property: it could grow like wild type in cells of the epithelial lineage, e.g., HeLa, but grew poorly in neuronal cells (6). Resistance to guanidine hydrochloride (Gua-HCl) has been used extensively as a marker for studying recombination. Hence, Wimmer suggested using the IRES and resistance to Gua-HCl (g^r, N179G) as markers and PV1(RIPO) carrying the g^r mutation [PV1(RIPO)g^r] with wild-type poliovirus [PV1(M)g^s] as the parents (Fig. 1A and B). The conditions used for selecting recombinants were growth in neuronal cells, SK-N-MC, in the presence of 2 mM of Gua-HCl. These conditions would prevent the growth of the parental viruses but would enable the recombinants to grow. Transcripts of PV1(RIPO)g^r were used to transfect HeLa cells and the subsequently produced virions were purified concomitantly with wild-type virus on cesium chloride gradients. RNA extracted from these purified viruses was used to program cell-free reactions.

To prove that recombination had indeed occurred in the cell-free system, several controls were used. These experiments showed that only when the two parental RNAs were coreplicated, recombinants were generated. When the parental RNAs were used to program cell-free reactions separately and then plated together under the selection conditions or the RNAs alone were plated under the selection conditions, no recombinants were produced. The former control addressed the issue that the cell-free recombinants did not arise by coinfection followed by recombination of parental viruses produced in the cell-free reactions. The latter ruled out the possibility that the cell-free recombinants arose by cotransfection followed by recombination of the parental RNAs present in the cell-free reactions.

Determination of Crossover Sites and Frequency of Recombination

To analyze the recombinants, recombinant plaques were amplified once under the selection conditions (Fig. 1D) and the reverse transcriptase PCR (RT-PCR) product sequenced to confirm the presence of the g^r mutation and subjected to restriction analysis. The fact that PV1(M)g^s virus was derived from the wild-type viral isolate and PV1(RIPO)g^r virus from in vitro-synthesized transcripts of

---

Rohit Duggal ■ Agouron Pharmaceuticals, San Diego, CA 92121.

a modified cDNA clone gave us the opportunity to exploit the presence of restriction sites present only on PV1(RIPO)g^r that could be used for mapping the crossover sites. The restriction analyses indicated that the crossover sites for all the recombinants were between the SacI and StuI sites (Fig. 1). To determine the frequency of recombination, it was important to determine the yield of the parental viruses in extracts programmed by the parental RNAs. To facilitate this, the reaction volumes were scaled up and each reaction was split into three fractions and plated on SK-N-MC cells to determine the yield of PV1(M)g^s, on HeLa cells with 2 mM of Gua-HCl to determine the yield of PV1(RIPO)g^r, and on SK-N-MC cells with 2 mM of Gua-HCl to determine the yield of the recombinants. The frequency of recombination was found to be 10^{-4}. An interesting observation of this analysis was the high yield of PV1(RIPO)g^r parent, which we believe is due to complementation by the PV1(M)g^s genome. This phenomenon will be discussed in more detail below. In a similar study of cell-free recombination, a higher recombination frequency between 10^{-2} and 10^{-3} was obtained (14). This latter study employed RT-PCR to detect recombinants instead of selecting them. The higher frequency could be due to the inclusion of recombinants that were not viable.

Effect of Gua-HCl on Cell-Free Recombination

When Gua-HCl was added to the cell-free recombination reactions, it resulted in a significant reduction of recom-

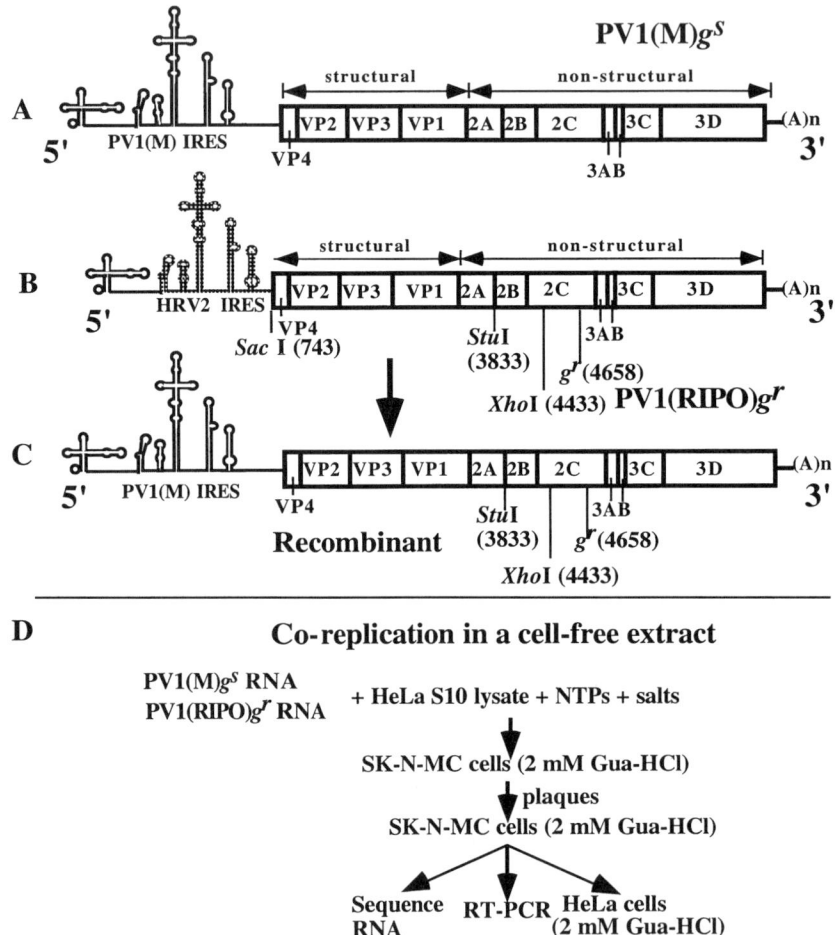

FIGURE 1 Schematic representation of the parental molecules used in the recombination study and the resulting recombinant. PV1(M)g^s viral RNA (A) is the wild-type poliovirus RNA and PV1(RIPO)g^r (B) is the RNA of the chimeric poliovirus PV1(RIPO) that contains the mutation for guanidine resistance (g^r) starting at nucleotide 4658. The sphere at the end represents the genome-linked nonstructural protein (VPg) at the 5' terminus. 3' to the VPg is the cloverleaf-like structure that contains the promoter for plus-strand synthesis. The stem-loop structures 3' to the cloverleaf-like structure represent the IRES for poliovirus (solid lines) or HRV2 (broken lines). For both RNAs 3' to the IRESs are the open reading frames of poliovirus followed by the 3' nontranslated region (line) and the poly(A) tail. The restriction sites that are present on the cDNA of PV1(RIPO)g^r only are shown. (C) The recombinant molecule that originated through a crossover event between the SacI and StuI restriction sites. (D) The scheme for studying polioviral recombination in the cell-free system. SK-N-MC cells are a line of neuroblastoma cells, and Gua-HCl is guanidine hydrochloride.

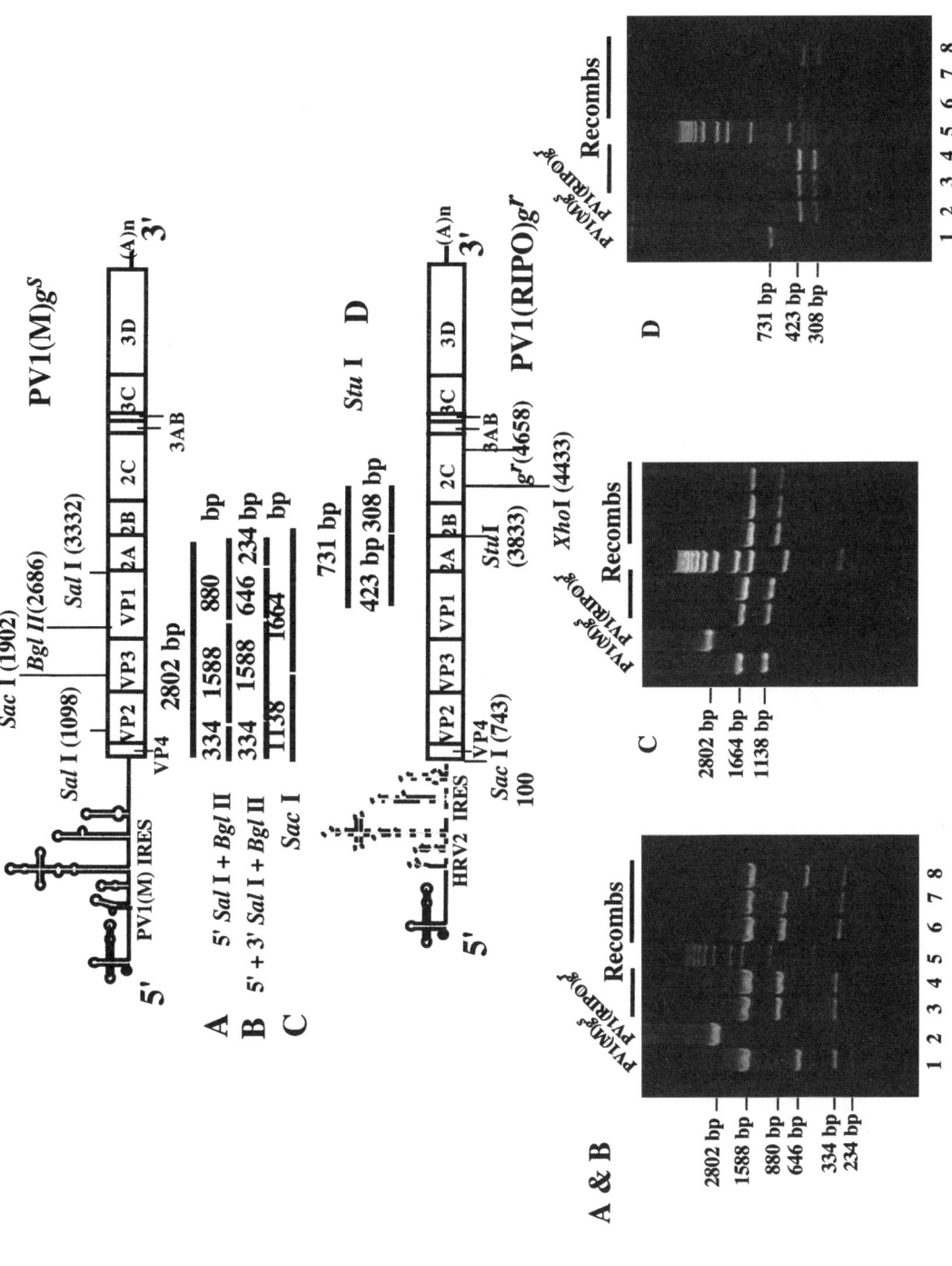

FIGURE 2 Mapping of crossover sites for five representative recombinants that were generated in the poliovirus cell-free system. The genome representation for wild-type poliovirus, PV1(M)g^s with the four new silent restriction sites, and that of PV1(RIPO)g^r with previous restriction sites, and the marker for Gua-HCl resistance (g^r) are shown. Below the genome representation are agarose gels showing RT-PCR products of the parents [PV1(M)g^s and PV1(RIPO)g^r] and five recombinants after being digested with restriction enzymes SalI and BglII (A and B), with restriction enzyme SacI (C), and with restriction enzyme StuI (D). All the gels shown are 0.8% agarose gels. Lane 5 in A and B, C, and D is DNA molecular weight marker. Sizes of the bands are indicated on the side. Reprinted from reference 4 with permission.

binants (only one out of six reactions gave a single recombinant plaque). This observation is significant because it may provide insights into the mechanism of recombination. It has been elegantly shown by Kirkegaard and Baltimore (9) that recombination occurs via strand switching during minus-strand synthesis. In the cell-free system described here, it would mean that minus-strand synthesis would initiate on the PV1(RIPO)g^r parent and cross over to PV1(M)g^s RNA after acquiring the mutation for guanidine resistance (Fig. 1). The other possibility, though unlikely due to the rarity of the event, would be a double crossover event that initiated on PV1(M)g^s RNA switched to PV1(RIPO)g^r RNA and back to PV1(M)g^s RNA. Yet another possibility would be crossover during plus-strand synthesis that had initiated on the PV1(M)g^s parent and switched over to the PV1(RIPO)g^r to acquire the mutation for Gua-HCl resistance. Circumstantial evidence to support the last mechanism would be the effect of Gua-HCl when introduced in the cell-free recombination system. While PV1(M)g^s RNA replicates to high titers in the cell-free system, PV1(RIPO)g^r replicates poorly. Introducing Gua-HCl into the cell-free recombination system would shut down replication of the PV1(M)g^s parent, and if recombination resulted from strand switching during plus-strand synthesis that had initiated on the PV1(M)g^s parent, there would be a substantial decrease in recombination (which we observed). However, it is also quite possible that the complementation provided by the PV1(M)g^s parent

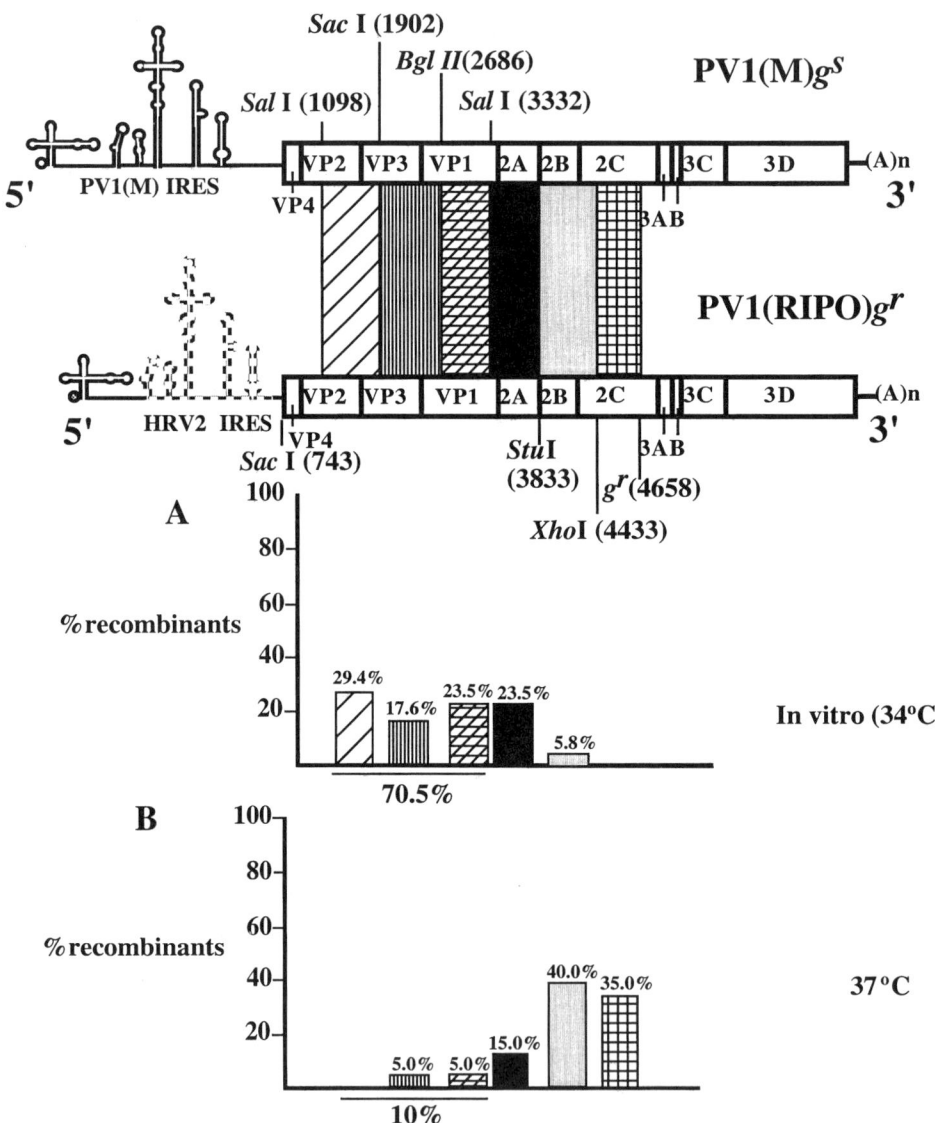

FIGURE 3 Pattern of crossover of the recombinants obtained in the cell-free system at 34°C and after recombination in vivo at 37°C. The six different regions of crossover as defined by the new restriction sites on PV1(M)g^s and the previously existing restriction sites on PV1(RIPO)g^r are shown by six differently shaded columns between the two genomes. The columns in the bar graphs represent the percentage of the total recombinants generated in the cell-free system at 34°C (A) and in vivo at 37°C (B). Reprinted from reference 4 with permission.

could make the PV1(RIPO)g^r replicate more efficiently and that could result in crossover events mainly during minus-strand synthesis.

Further Mapping of Crossover Junctions and Comparison of In Vitro and In Vivo Recombinants

To define the region in which strand switching occurred, four new restriction sites were created in the structural protein region (starting from VP2 to VP1) (Fig. 2) of PV1(M)g^s (4). The restriction sites were created by altering the codons but not the amino acids encoded at these positions. Purified viral RNA from this new virus was used in the cell-free recombination reactions with PV1(RIPO)g^r RNA at 34°C. The RNA of the recombinants was amplified by RT-PCR and digested with restriction enzymes. The analyses for five representative recombinants are shown in Fig. 2.

To compare the crossover patterns of these recombinants generated in vitro with those of recombinants produced in vivo, HeLa cells were coinfected at 37°C with PV1(M)g^s and PV1(RIPO)g^r at equal multiplicities of infection (4). Mapping of crossover sites for the in vivo recombinants gave a pattern very different from those generated in vitro at 34°C (Fig. 3), with only 10% of the recombinants crossing over in the structural protein region in vivo at 37°C compared to 70.5% of the in vitro recombinants. This was surprising, and when the temperature for in vivo recombination was lowered to 34°C, the pattern of

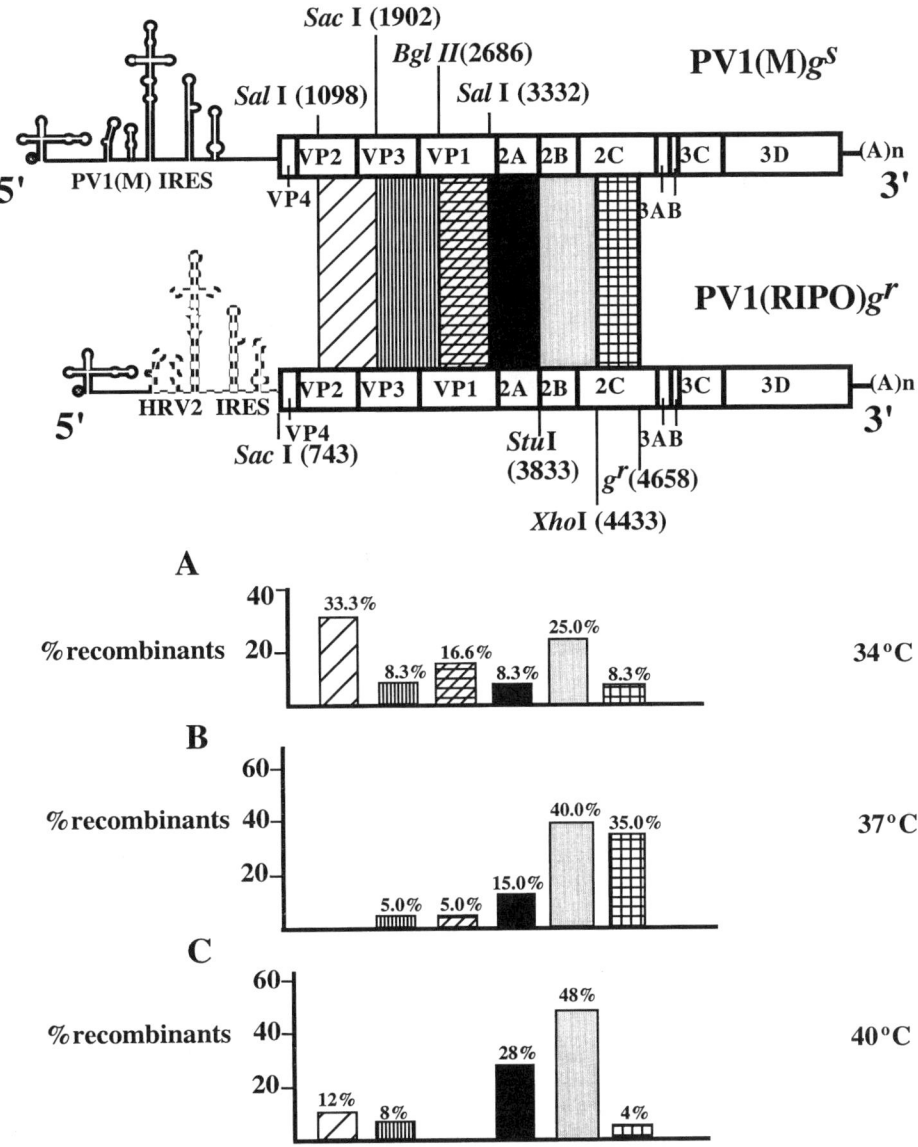

FIGURE 4 Pattern of crossover of the recombinants obtained in vivo at three different temperatures. The six different regions of crossover as defined by the new restriction sites on PV1(M)g^s and the previously existing restriction sites on PV1(RIPO)g^r are shown by six differently shaded columns. The columns in the bar graphs represent the percentage of the total recombinants generated in vivo at (A) 34°C, (B) 37°C, and (C) 40°C. Reprinted from reference 4 with permission.

recombination in the structural protein region resembled that of the one obtained for recombinants generated in vitro at 34°C (compare Fig. 3A with Fig. 4A).

Effect of Temperature in Poliovirus Recombination and Possible Role for Secondary Structure

To examine how temperatures higher than 37°C might alter the pattern of recombination further, HeLa coinfections with PV1(RIPO)g^r and PV1(M)g^s were carried out at 40°C (4). The pattern of recombination changed further compared to that at 37°C (Fig. 4). The crossover pattern of the recombinants obtained at 40°C was similar to that at 37°C but quite different from those recovered in vivo at 34°C and from the cell-free system (Fig. 4). Especially pronounced was the fraction of recombinants obtained in the region of crossover between the StuI and XhoI sites. At 34°C about 25% of in vivo recombinants crossed over in this region, at 37°C the percentage of total in vivo recombinants went up to 40%, and at 40°C about 50% of the total recombinants crossed over in this region.

The 600-nucleotide region between the StuI and XhoI restriction sites was folded by using the mfold program of Michael Zucker (http://128.252.122.176/~zuker/rna/). The secondary structure was generated for four tempera-

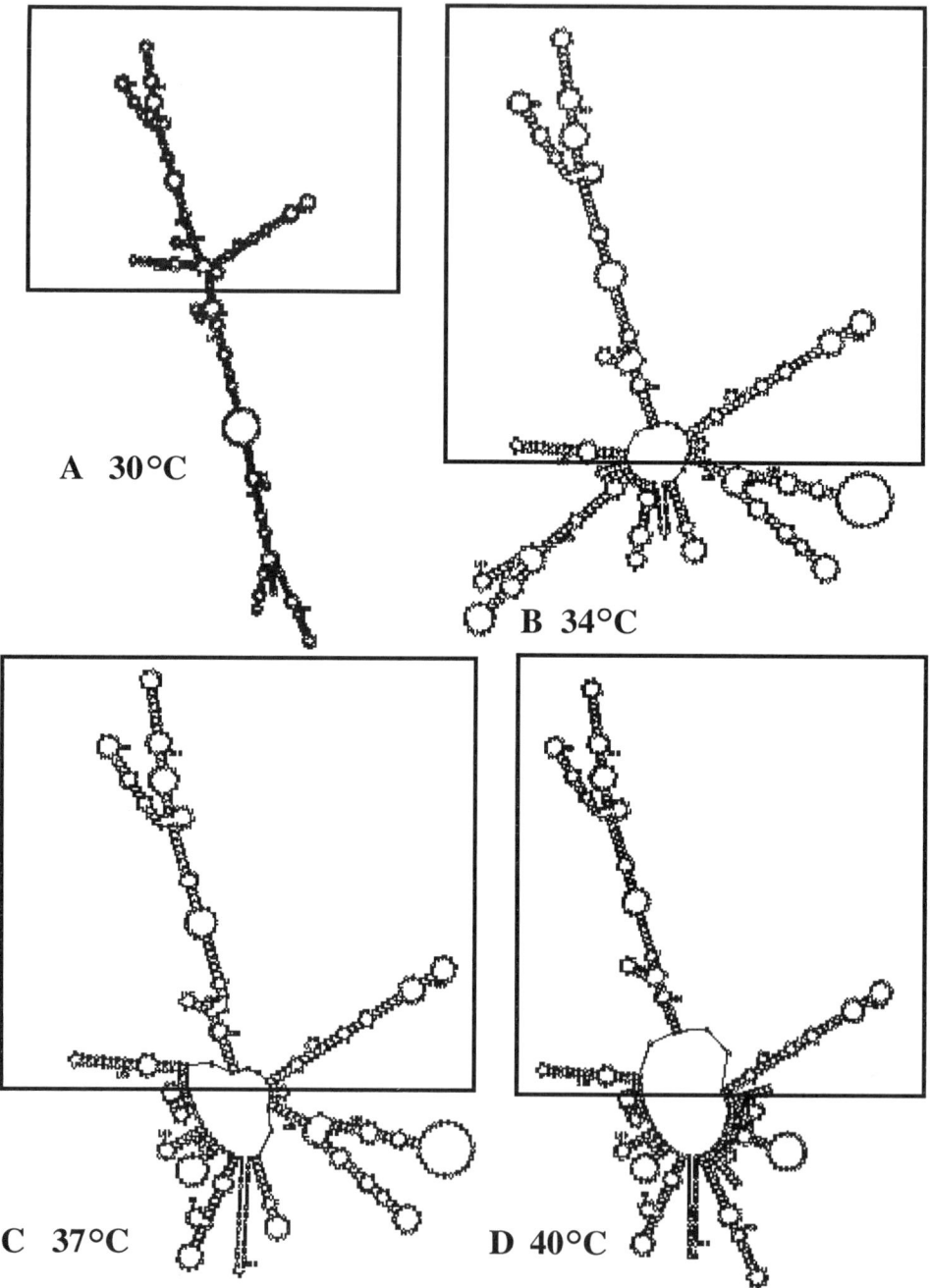

FIGURE 5 Secondary structure of the StuI-XhoI region at (A) 30°C, (B) 34°C, (C) 37°C, and (D) 40°C.

tures of 30, 34, 37, and 40°C (Fig. 5). As is evident from the secondary structures in Fig. 5, the folding patterns at the four different temperatures are different. However, there seems to be a conservation of three stem-loop structures at all four temperatures (shown by boxed regions in Fig. 5) while the rest of the structure opens up with an increase in temperature. One reason that no preference for crossover sites exists at lower temperatures could be that at those temperatures other stem-loop structures, in addition to the three identified by boxes in Fig. 5, could also exist that could cause crossover events to occur at other regions of the genomic RNA. But at elevated temperatures of 40°C some of the secondary structures might not be stable and the dominant structures could be the three stem-loop structures, resulting in a strong tendency for crossover to occur at the three stem-loop structures.

Studies involving intertypic poliovirus recombination have suggested a role for RNA secondary structure and a preference for crossover to occur in loop regions of stem-loop structures (15). A similar observation was reported for recombinants of foot-and-mouth disease virus, where the crossover sites were found to be located in regions of RNA that had a tendency to have strong secondary structure (16). Structure-specific determination of crossover sites has also been identified in subviral RNAs of the plant virus turnip crinkle virus (2).

The details of how RNA secondary structure could force recombination to occur are still not known. In a model

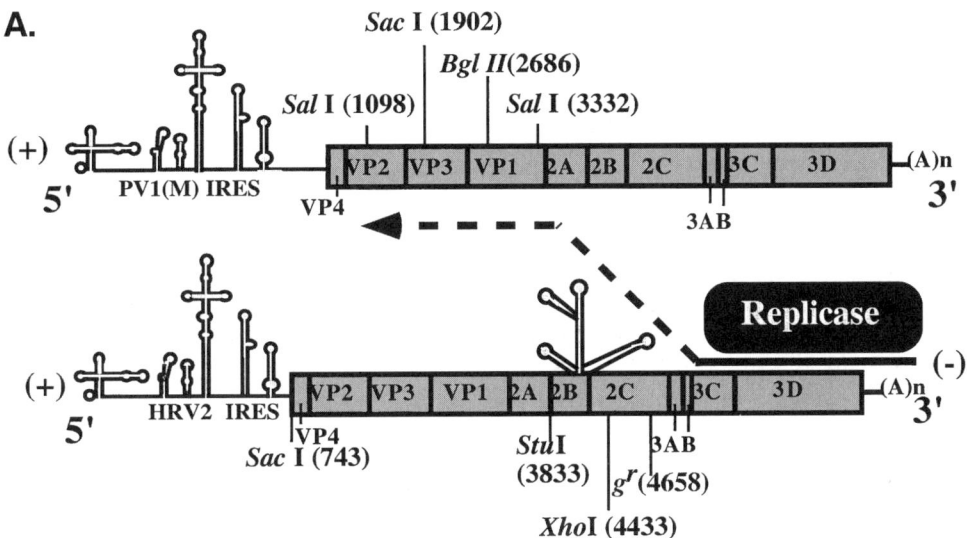

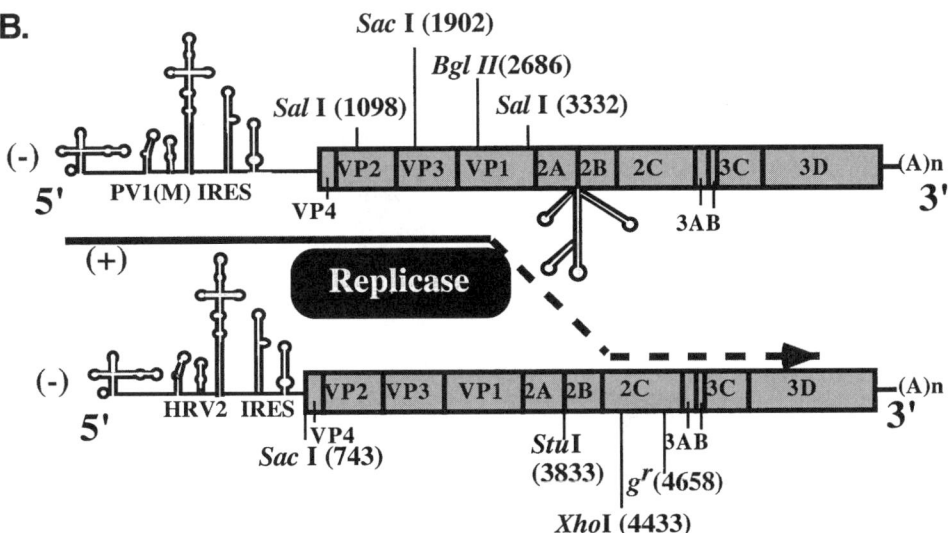

FIGURE 6 Possible models for recombination based on the presence of the secondary structure in the 2BC region and the inclusion of Gua-HCl in the cell-free recombination system. (A) The established mechanism of strand switching during minus-strand synthesis that is facilitated by the secondary structure. (B) A possible mechanism of strand switching during plus-strand synthesis if the secondary structure also exists in the minus orientation. This mechanism draws support from the observation that very few recombinants were recovered during cell-free recombination in the presence of Gua-HCl.

proposed by Romanova et al. (13), the formation of intermolecular duplexes between regions that normally have secondary structure was proposed to be responsible for providing an obstacle for the replicase complex to make it switch strands and continue polymerization of nucleotides on the acceptor strand. It is also possible that the secondary structures identified in Fig. 5 exist in plus as well as minus strands of polioviral RNAs (Fig. 6). The secondary structures contain long stems that could potentially prove difficult to separate and force the replicase to switch templates (Fig. 6). Alternatively, these polioviral stem-loop structures could be responsible for determining crossover sites by binding viral or host proteins that could provide the necessary signals for crossover to occur. Indeed, a report by Goodfellow et al. (5) that describes the discovery of an internal stem-loop structure that acts as a *cis*-acting signal for replication in the poliovirus 2C region provides evidence for a role for stem-loop structures present in the coding region of poliovirus. The presence of internal stem-loop structures that function in replication and other viral processes could be a unifying feature among picornaviruses, since similar structures have been identified in the capsid region of HRV14 (11) and cardioviruses (10).

CELL-FREE COMPLEMENTATION

During our studies on cell-free recombination, we found that the replication of PV1(RIPO)g^r RNA could be complemented by PV1(M)g^s RNA to yield infectious virus 3 orders of magnitude higher than when no PV1(M)g^s RNA was present in the reaction mixture (3). The PV1(M)g^s RNA and PV1(RIPO)g^r RNA used for these recombination studies were isolated from cesium chloride-purified poliovirions. To analyze the complementation phenomenon further we employed two RNA transcripts generated from the poliovirus cDNA [encoding PV1(M)g^s] by in vitro transcription by linearizing at the *Eco*RI (RI) or *Pvu*I restriction sites present downstream of the genome-encoded poly(A) tail (Fig. 7). While the RI linearized transcript carries 3 extra nonviral bases 3' to the poly(A) tail, the *Pvu*I transcript has 626 nonviral nucleotides downstream of the poly(A) tail. Interestingly, these two types of polioviral transcripts were found to have different abilities of replication in the cell-free system (4). Reactions programmed with the *Pvu*I transcripts (PVM txpt. PvuI) produced only a few virus particles, whereas the RI transcript (PVM txpt. RI) produced virus titers only 2 orders of magnitude lower than RNA from cesium chloride-purified poliovirions (PVM vRNA) (Fig. 7), which has the authentic 3' end. To determine the effects of the two types of RNA transcripts on the complementation of replication of PV1(RIPO)g^r RNA, the virion-purified PV1(RIPO)g^r RNA was coincubated with either of the two types of RNA transcripts in the cell-free system. The yield of PV1(RIPO)g^r was then assayed on HeLa cells in the presence of Gua-HCl. The *Pvu*I transcript complemented PV1(RIPO)g^r replication very poorly whereas the RI transcript provided much better complementation, with 1,000 ng of this transcript complementing PV1(RIPO)g^r replication to levels very similar to 600 ng of PVM viral RNA

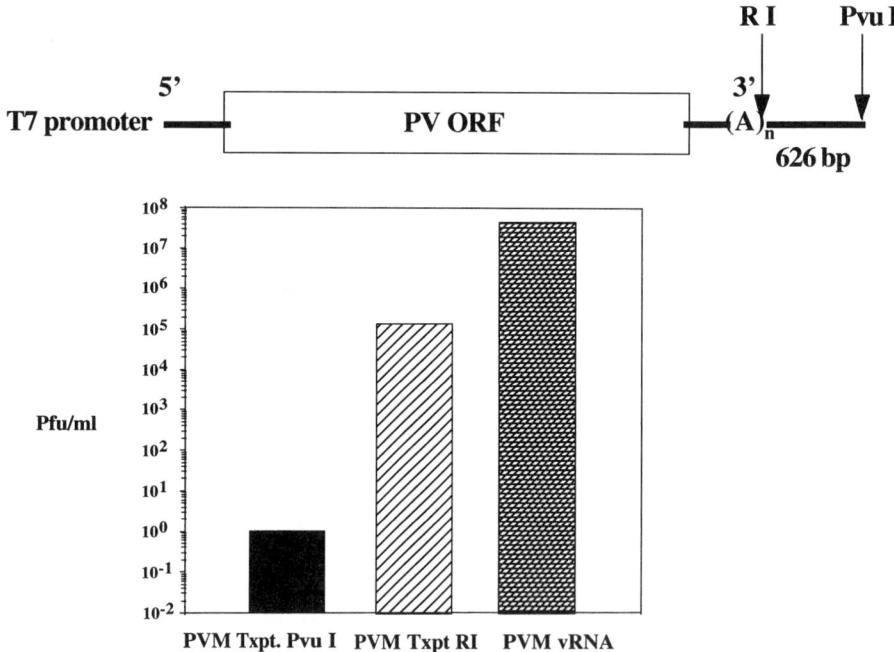

FIGURE 7 A comparison of replication of two different in vitro-synthesized polioviral transcripts with that of virion-purified RNA in the cell-free system. The polioviral cDNA is depicted on top of the bar chart. The polioviral open reading frame (ORF) is shown as an open box and the lines on either side represent the 5' and 3' nontranslated regions. The two restriction sites used for linearizing the cDNA for carrying out runoff transcription, the *Eco*RI site (adds 3 extra nonviral bases) and *Pvu*I (adds 626 nonviral bases), are shown. In the bar graph the three columns represent the RNAs and the polioviral titers ($\log_{10}$ PFU/ml). Reprinted from reference 4 with permission.

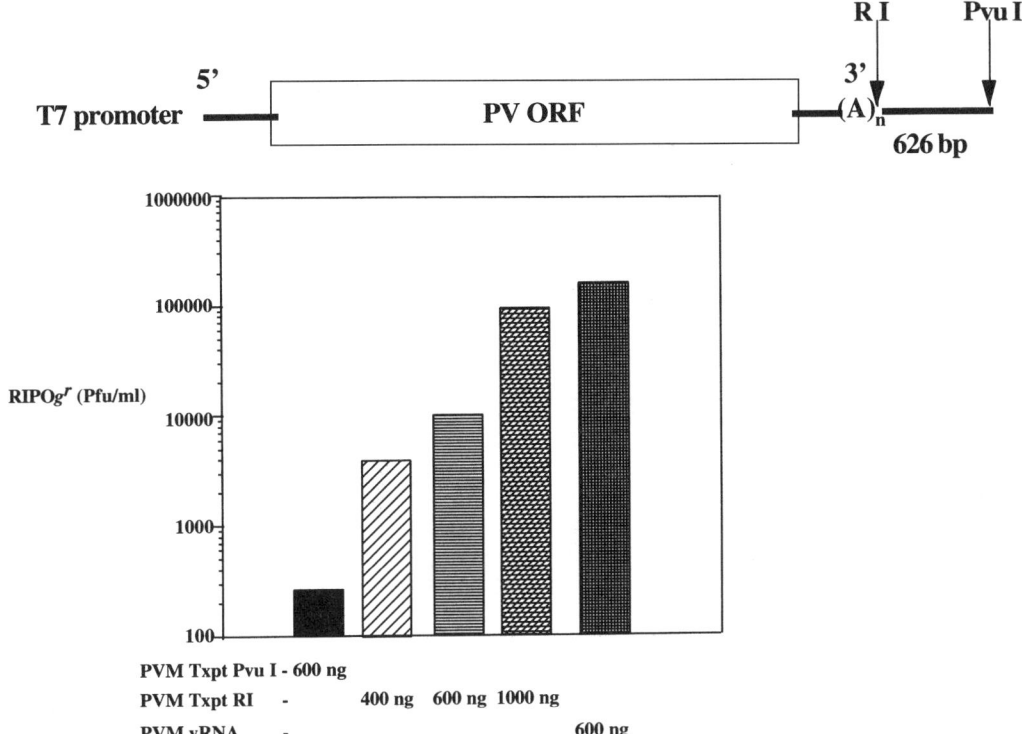

FIGURE 8 The ability of a polioviral RNA to complement the replication of PV1(RIPO)g^r RNA depends on its capacity to replicate in the cell-free system. The poliovirus cDNA is depicted on top of the bar chart. The poliovirus open reading frame (ORF) is shown as an open box, and the lines on either side represent the 5' and 3' nontranslated regions. The two restriction sites used for linearizing the cDNA for carrying out runoff transcription, the EcoRI site (adds 3 extra nonviral bases) and PvuI (adds 626 nonviral bases), are shown. In the bar graph the columns represent the various amounts of polioviral transcript RNAs and viral RNA (along the x axis) that complement the replication of PV1(RIPO)g^r, shown in terms of virus titer ($\log_{10}$ PFU/ml) along the y axis. The yield of PV1(RIPO)g^r in the absence of coreplicating wild-type polioviral RNA is 10^2 PFU/ml (3). Reprinted from reference 4 with permission.

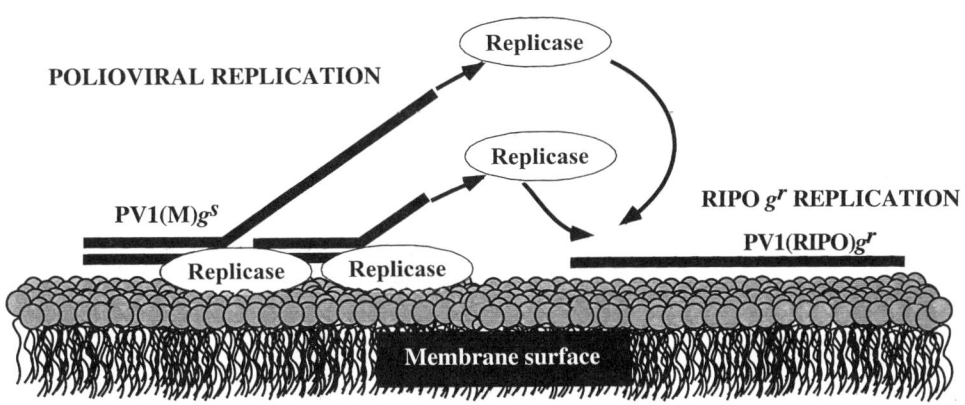

FIGURE 9 A model for complementation in the cell-free system. This model tries to explain a requirement for replication for complementation to occur. Since virion-purified polioviral RNA can replicate efficiently and RIPOg^r cannot, it is possible that the translational products (that form the replicase) from PV1(M)g^s RNA during or soon after replication could be the molecules responsible for complementing the poor replication of PV1(RIPO)g^r RNA.

(Fig. 8). These data suggest that complementation in the cell-free system is dependent on the replication ability of the complementing RNA molecule. Complementation does not appear to be due to different efficiencies by which these transcripts direct protein synthesis in the cell-free system. We have previously observed that poorly replicating polioviral molecules due to the genotype of the RNA (3) or due to the inhibition of 2 mM of Gua-HCl (12) produced equal amounts of protein compared to wild-type polioviral RNA in the cell-free system. However, it is possible that there is complementation at the translation level, but it happens during or soon after replication (Fig. 9). In such a scenario, the complementing molecule [PV1(M)g^s RNA] would replicate in close proximity to the complemented molecule [PV1(RIPO)g^r RNA]. Protein synthesis from the complementing molecule, either during replication or from nascently synthesized RNA molecules, could complement replication of the poorly replicating molecule. In such a situation, it could be likely that certain polioviral proteins carry out complementation only in association with the replicating form or intermediate of poliovirus RNA replication.

Very interestingly, complementation of the type seen in the cell-free system is not observed during coinfection of HeLa cells with PV1(M)g^s and PV1(RIPO)g^r. PV1(RIPO)g^r by itself replicates quite well in vivo and is amplified to titers only an order of magnitude lower than those of wild-type poliovirus. Therefore, it is possible that complementation occurs in vivo, but the high level of replication of PV1(RIPO)g^r masks the complementation that might occur during the coinfection by the two parental viruses.

CONCLUSIONS

The development of a cell-free system for poliovirus has given an opportunity to study different aspects of the life cycle of this virus in a test tube, starting from translation, then replication, ending in virus particle morphogenesis. In this system everything is confined to cell-free conditions, and there is no amplification observed as seen with cell-cell spread in an in vivo infection. This results in reduced viral multiplication and an increased sensitivity to programming the system with RNAs that have slight replication-defective phenotypes. However, this sensitivity can be used to discover phenomena such as complementation and to identify the effects of mutations that are not detected in the in vivo system.

REFERENCES

1. **Blumenthal, T., and G. G. Carmichael.** 1979. RNA replication: function and structure of Qbeta-replicase. *Annu. Rev. Biochem.* **48:**525–548.
2. **Cascone, P. J., T. F. Haydar, and A. E. Simon.** 1993. Sequences and structures required for recombination between virus-associated RNAs. *Science* **260:**801–805.
3. **Duggal, R., A. Cuconati, M. Gromeier, and E. Wimmer.** 1997. Genetic recombination of poliovirus in a cell-free system. *Proc. Natl. Acad. Sci. USA* **94:**13786–13791.
4. **Duggal, R., and E. Wimmer.** 1999. Genetic recombination of poliovirus in vitro and in vivo: temperature-dependent alteration of crossover sites. *Virology* **258:**30–41.
5. **Goodfellow, I., Y. Chaudhry, A. Richardson, J. Meredith, J. W. Almond, W. Barclay, and D. J. Evans.** 2000. Identification of a cis-acting replication element within the poliovirus coding region. *J. Virol.* **74:**4590–4600.
6. **Gromeier, M., L. Alexander, and E. Wimmer.** 1996. Internal ribosomal entry site substitution eliminates neurovirulence in intergeneric poliovirus recombinants. *Proc. Natl. Acad. Sci. USA* **93:**2370–2375.
7. **Hardy, S. F., T. L. German, L. S. Loesch-Fries, and T. C. Hall.** 1979. Highly active template-specific RNA-dependent RNA polymerase from barley leaves infected with brome mosaic virus. *Proc. Natl. Acad. Sci. USA* **76:**4956–4960.
8. **Hiebert, E., J. B. Bancroft, and C. E. Bracker.** 1968. The assembly in vitro of some small spherical viruses, hybrid viruses, and other nucleoproteins. *Virology* **34:**492–508.
9. **Kirkegaard, K., and D. Baltimore.** 1986. The mechanism of RNA recombination in poliovirus. *Cell* **47:**433–443.
10. **Lobert, P. E., N. Escriou, J. Ruelle, and T. Michiels.** 1999. A coding RNA sequence acts as a replication signal in cardioviruses. *Proc. Natl. Acad. Sci. USA* **96:**11560–11565.
11. **McKnight, K. L., and S. M. Lemon.** 1998. The rhinovirus type 14 genome contains an internally located RNA structure that is required for viral replication. *RNA* **4:**1569–1584.
12. **Molla, A., A. V. Paul, and E. Wimmer.** 1991. Cell-free, de novo synthesis of poliovirus. *Science* **254:**1647–1651.
13. **Romanova, L. I., V. M. Blinov, E. A. Tolskaya, E. G. Viktorova, M. S. Kolesnikova, E. A. Guseva, and V. I. Agol.** 1986. The primary structure of crossover regions of intertypic poliovirus recombinants: a model of recombination between RNA genomes. *Virology* **155:**202–213.
14. **Tang, R. S., D. J. Barton, J. B. Flanegan, and K. Kirkegaard.** 1997. Poliovirus RNA recombination in cell-free extracts. *RNA* **3:**624–633.
15. **Tolskaya, E. A., L. I. Romanova, V. M. Blinov, E. G. Viktorova, A. N. Sinyakov, M. S. Kolesnikova, and V. I. Agol.** 1987. Studies on the recombination between RNA genomes of poliovirus: the primary structure and nonrandom distribution of crossover regions in the genomes of intertypic poliovirus recombinants. *Virology* **161:**54–61.
16. **Wilson, V., P. Taylor, and U. Desselberger.** 1988. Crossover regions in foot-and-mouth disease virus (FMDV) recombinants correspond to regions of high local secondary structure. *Arch. Virol.* **102:**131–139.

Poliovirus RNA Replication and Genetic Complementation in Cell-Free Reactions

DAVID J. BARTON, B. JOAN MORASCO, LUCIA EISNER SMERAGE, AND JAMES B. FLANEGAN

37

Poliovirus RNA replicates in membrane-associated replication complexes in the cytoplasm of infected cells (11–15, 17). Virion RNA contains a covalently linked 5′-terminal protein, VPg, a 3′-terminal poly(A) tail, and a single open reading frame that encodes the viral polyprotein (20, 28, 43). Virion RNA contains cis-active sequences that regulate viral RNA stability, translation, and replication. These cis-active sequences, in combination with trans-active viral and cellular proteins, regulate the translation and replication of poliovirus RNA. To understand the molecular basis of viral RNA replication, these cis-active sequences must be identified and functionally characterized.

CELL-CULTURE AND RECONSTITUTED SYSTEMS

Cell-culture systems permissive for poliovirus replication have been used to investigate viral protein synthesis and RNA replication (16, 19). Cells can be simultaneously infected and then characterized relative to virus attachment, penetration, uncoating, protein synthesis, RNA replication, virus assembly, and release (40). During the course of the infection cycle, a significant overlap develops between the translation and replication steps because of their mutual interdependence. Therefore, the amplification of viral RNA in infected cells occurs in a circular pathway involving iterative steps of translation and RNA replication. The inhibition of either step significantly affects the other and complicates the analysis of the regulatory mechanisms controlling virus replication. Reconstituted in vitro replication assays have also been used to study poliovirus replication. Reactions containing purified proteins and RNAs have been useful for conducting a detailed biochemical analysis of polymerase elongation rates (47), nucleotide misincorporation rates (51, 52), template-primer requirements (3, 31, 54), and the uridylylation of VPg (36, 38). The primary disadvantage of this approach is that it has not been possible to reconstitute authentic replication complexes that synthesize infectious virus and negative- and positive-strand RNAs linked to VPg.

Coupled In Vitro Translation-RNA Replication Reactions

Many of the limitations associated with the above approaches can now be overcome by using HeLa S10 extracts programmed with poliovirion RNA (4, 5, 32, 33). These reactions support the translation of the input RNA, the formation of membrane-associated replication complexes, the synthesis of VPg-pUpU, VPg-linked viral RNA, and the assembly of infectious virus. Since the cell-free replication reactions contain saturating concentrations of the input RNA, translation starts at maximum rates at time zero and is not dependent on the synthesis of new viral mRNA. Viral protein synthesis and RNA replication can be measured by pulse-labeling with labeled amino acid and nucleotide substrates, respectively. At 30°C, there is a linear increase in viral protein synthesis during the first 6 h (4). Viral RNA synthesis follows and is observed from 4 to 12 h, with maximum rates of synthesis between 6 and 8 h (4). The labeled RNA detected in these reactions is predominantly positive-strand RNA and is covalently linked to VPg. Infectious virus can be detected as early as 6 h and reaches maximum titers ($\sim 10^7$ PFU/ml) by about 12 h in these reactions (4). Therefore, translation, RNA replication, and virus assembly follow a linear and sequential pathway in these reactions.

Synchronous RNA Replication

By using a reversible inhibitor of poliovirus RNA replication, it is possible to synchronize viral RNA replication (6). Adding 2 mM of guanidine HCl to HeLa S10 translation-RNA replication reactions specifically inhibits the initiation of negative-strand synthesis without affecting

---

B. Joan Morasco, Lucia Eisner Smerage, and James B. Flanegan ■ Department of Biochemistry and Molecular Biology, College of Medicine, University of Florida, Gainesville, FL 32610-0245.　David J. Barton ■ Department of Biochemistry and Molecular Biology, College of Medicine, University of Florida, Gainesville, FL 32610-0245, and Department of Microbiology and Molecular Biology Program, University of Colorado Health Sciences Center, Denver, CO 80262.

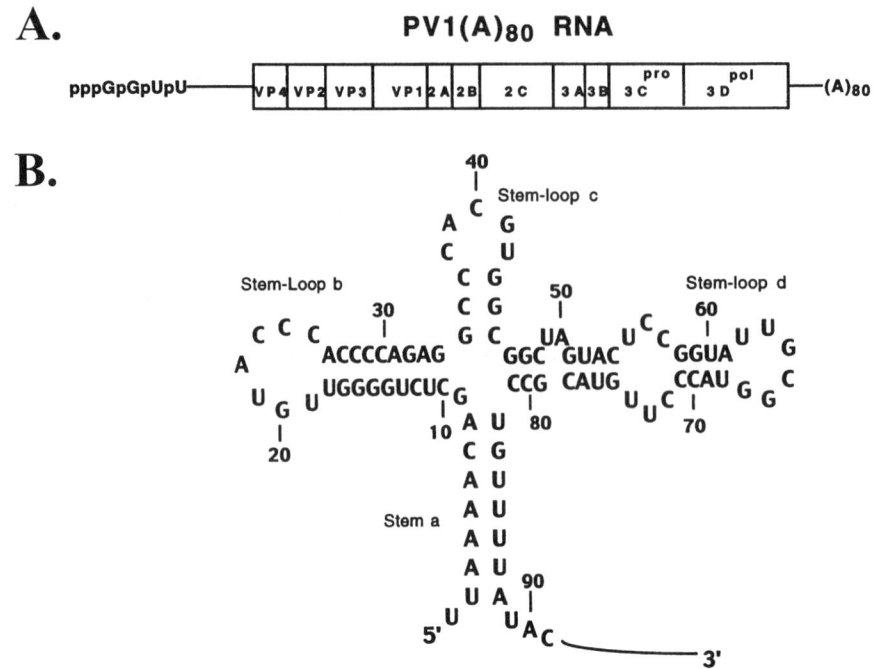

FIGURE 1 Diagram of poliovirus RNAs. (A) T7PV1(A)$_{80}$ RNA. (B) 5' Cloverleaf structure. Modified from reference 10 by permission of Oxford University Press.

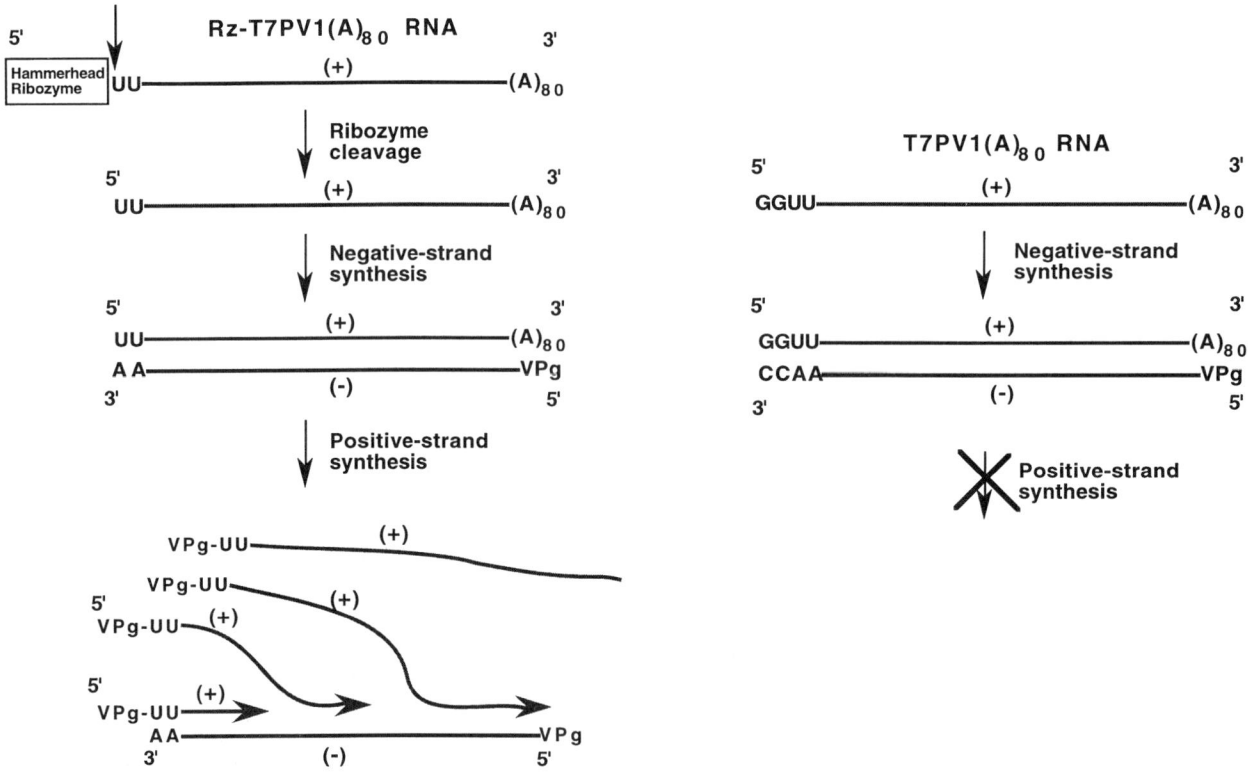

FIGURE 2 Diagrams of negative- and positive-strand RNA synthesis using poliovirus RNA transcripts. (Left panel) Rz-T7PV1(A)$_{80}$ transcript RNA with 5' hammerhead ribozyme (Rz-RNA) undergoes autocatalytic cleavage to form (+) strand viral RNA with correct 5'-terminal sequence. This RNA is copied to form (−) strand RNA in replicative form (RF) RNA intermediate. The negative-strand RNA serves as a template for multiple rounds of VPg-UU primed (+) strand RNA synthesis. This results in the synthesis of replicative-intermediate RNA and ss (+) strand RNA. (Right panel) T7PV1(A)$_{80}$ transcript RNA containing two nonviral 5' guanine nucleotides (GG-RNA) is copied to form (−) strand RNA in RF RNA intermediate. The synthesis of (+) strand RNA, however, is inhibited below detectable levels.

viral protein synthesis. Therefore, preinitiation RNA replication complexes can be isolated from translation-replication reactions containing guanidine. The removal of guanidine from the preinitiation complexes results in the synchronous initiation and synthesis of negative-strand RNA (6). This is immediately followed by the asymmetric synthesis of positive-strand RNA and infectious virus. Therefore, negative- and positive-strand RNAs are synthesized in a temporally separate and sequential manner by preinitiation complexes. Under defined conditions at 37°C, negative strands are synthesized from 0 to 18 min and positive strands are synthesized from 18 to 36 min (6). Therefore, it is possible to directly measure the sequential synthesis of negative- and positive-strand RNA. This assay is of significant practical importance since RNA synthesis inhibitors, as well as conditional and lethal mutations of the virus, can be tested for their specific effect on individual steps in the RNA replication cycle. For example, by using this general approach, it was possible to show that guanidine HCl completely inhibited negative-strand initiation but had no effect on negative-strand elongation or the initiation or elongation of positive-strand RNA (6).

Specific Synthesis of Negative- and Positive-Strand Viral RNAs

As described above, both negative- and positive-strand RNAs are synthesized by preinitiation complexes formed with poliovirion RNA (6). In comparison, preinitiation complexes formed with bacteriophage T7 transcripts of poliovirus RNA were limited to the synthesis of negative-strand RNA (8, 9, 26). This was confirmed by using a one-dimensional RNase T1 fingerprint analysis of the labeled product RNAs. Both negative- and positive-strand RNAs were synthesized with virion RNA (6), but only negative-strand RNA was synthesized with transcript RNA (6). The transcript RNA contains two nonviral 5'-terminal GMP nucleotides that are required for efficient transcription by T7 polymerase (Fig. 1 and 2). The presence of the two extra Gs has no effect on negative-strand synthesis but inhibits positive-strand RNA synthesis below detectable levels (Fig. 2, right panel). To overcome this limitation, T7 transcripts of poliovirus RNA that contain the correct 5'-terminal sequence can be prepared using a self-cleaving 5' ribozyme (Rz) (Fig. 2, left panel) (26). In contrast to the 5' GG-RNA transcript, the 5' Rz-RNA transcript supports the synthesis of both negative- and positive-strand RNA (Fig. 2, left panel). This was demonstrated by characterizing the labeled RNAs synthesized by preinitiation complexes formed with GG-RNA transcript, Rz-RNA transcript, and poliovirus RNA. Electrophoresis of these labeled RNAs on a nondenaturing agarose gel showed that full-length positive-strand RNA was only synthesized in reactions containing Rz-RNA transcript and virion RNA (Fig. 3, lanes 2 and 3). As expected, negative-strand RNA in the form of replicative-intermediate (RI) and replicative-form (RF) RNAs was synthesized in all three reactions (Fig. 3). These results have been confirmed by characterizing the labeled RNAs in time-course reactions using denaturing gels. The same amount of negative-strand RNA was synthesized with all three RNA templates during the first 20 min, but positive-strand RNA was only synthesized from 20 to 40 min in the Rz-RNA and the virion RNA reactions (data not shown). Therefore, by using both the GG-RNA and the Rz-RNA it is possible to accurately quantitate negative-strand and positive-strand synthesis. The ability to synthesize mutant GG-RNA and Rz-RNA transcripts is

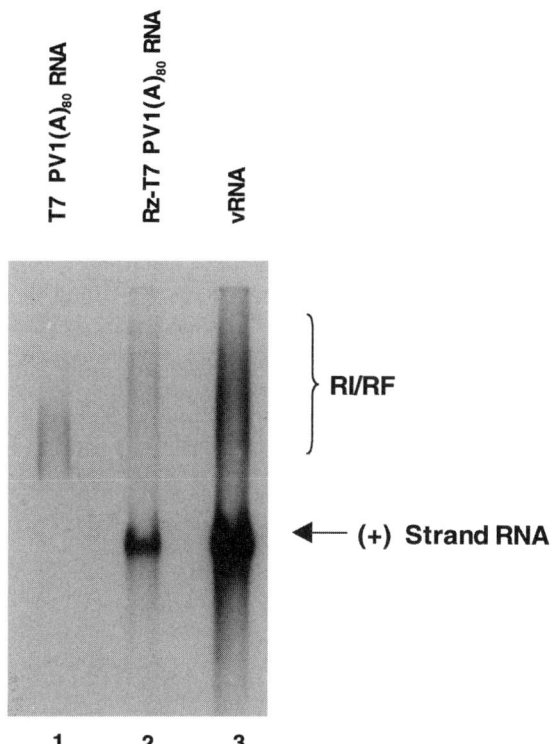

FIGURE 3 Two nonviral 5' Gs in T7PV1(A)$_{80}$ transcript RNA inhibit positive-strand RNA synthesis. Nondenaturing agarose gel electrophoresis of ^{32}P-labeled viral RNAs synthesized in 60-min reactions containing preinitiation replication complexes formed with either poliovirion RNA or the transcript RNAs indicated. Positions of (+) strand RNA and RI/RF RNAs in gel are shown above. See diagrams in Fig. 2 for additional information.

proving to be extremely valuable in ongoing studies to characterize the molecular basis of viral RNA recombination and replication.

In Vitro Complementation: Identification of Viral Protein Precursors Required for Replication

In previous studies, we characterized an RNA-negative temperature-sensitive mutation, 3D-M394T (7). This mutation inhibited the initiation of negative- and positive-strand synthesis but not the elongation of preformed nascent chains. In preinitiation replication complexes formed with 3D-M394T mutant RNA, negative-strand RNA synthesis was normal at 34°C (Fig. 4, lane 1) but was inhibited at 39°C (Fig. 4, lane 2). To determine if the 3D-M394T mutant RNA could be complemented in vitro, we isolated preinitiation complexes from HeLa S10 translation-replication reactions that contained both the mutant RNA and a helper RNA (RNA2). Efficient complementation was observed at the nonpermissive temperature in the presence of the helper RNA (Fig. 4, lane 3). To determine if cotranslation was required for efficient complementation, we cotranslated the mutant and helper RNAs for decreasing amounts of time in reactions where the total translation time was held constant. Cotranslation with the helper RNA for periods less than 2 h resulted in a sharp drop in the replication of 3D-M394T mutant RNA at 39°C (Fig. 4, lanes 3 to 8). These results and others showed that efficient complementation in the HeLa S10 translation-replication reaction requires cotranslation with helper RNA. Similar results were obtained characterizing mutations in other viral replication proteins (data not shown). Therefore, a complementing wild-type (wt) protein must be provided during the time when viral RNA replication complexes are being assembled. Once the complexes are assembled, there does not appear to be a dynamic exchange of mutant and wt proteins. This may explain why it is difficult to complement some mutant proteins in infected cells (34, 45) even though high concentrations of the complementing protein are eventually synthesized at late infection times.

The processing of the viral polyprotein results in the formation of the individual viral proteins (Fig. 1A) along with stable intermediates in the processing pathway (27). To determine if precursors of 3D^{pol} were required to complement the 3D-M394T mutation, we used the in vitro complementation assay described above. For this assay, modified viral helper RNA transcripts were engineered to express 3D^{pol} and its precursors 3CD, P3, and P23. The results of these assays showed that the 3D-M394T mutation was efficiently rescued in trans by 3CD, P3, and P23 but not by 3D^{pol} itself (18). Since 3CD was also formed by proteolytic processing of P3 and P23, 3CD appears to be the minimal 3D^{pol} precursor capable of complementing the 3D-M394T mutation. This suggests that functional RNA replication complexes are originally formed with 3CD and that 3D^{pol} is derived by proteolytic processing of 3CD within preinitiation RNA replication complexes. Similar results with a 3A mutation were previously reported by Towner et al. (46). In this case, the authors found that a 3A-F69H mutation was not complemented in HeLa S10 translation-replication reactions when wt 3AB was provided in trans. Complementation was only observed when the mutant RNA was cotranslated with a wt P3-expressing helper RNA. These authors also suggested that 3AB may be delivered to the replication complex in the form of a precursor protein rather than the mature viral protein itself.

In Vitro Complementation: Identification of cis-Active RNA Sequences

To expand the utility of the in vitro complementation assay, we designed experiments to determine if all of the viral replication proteins could be provided in trans to support the replication of mutant RNA templates. We engineered two transcript RNAs (DJB2 and DJB15) that contained large out-of-frame deletions in the polyprotein coding sequence (Fig. 5A). To determine if these RNAs would serve as functional templates for negative-strand synthesis, preinitiation complexes were formed in reactions containing one of the mutant RNAs and a helper RNA (RNA2). The results of these experiments showed that both mutant RNAs were functional templates for negative-strand synthesis in the presence of the helper RNA (Fig. 5B). Therefore, all of the viral replication proteins can be provided in trans in these experiments, which allows for the identification of the cis-active sequences required for the replication of viral RNA templates. Our results to date using the in vitro complementation assay indicate that the 5′ cloverleaf, the 3′ nontranslated region (NTR), and the

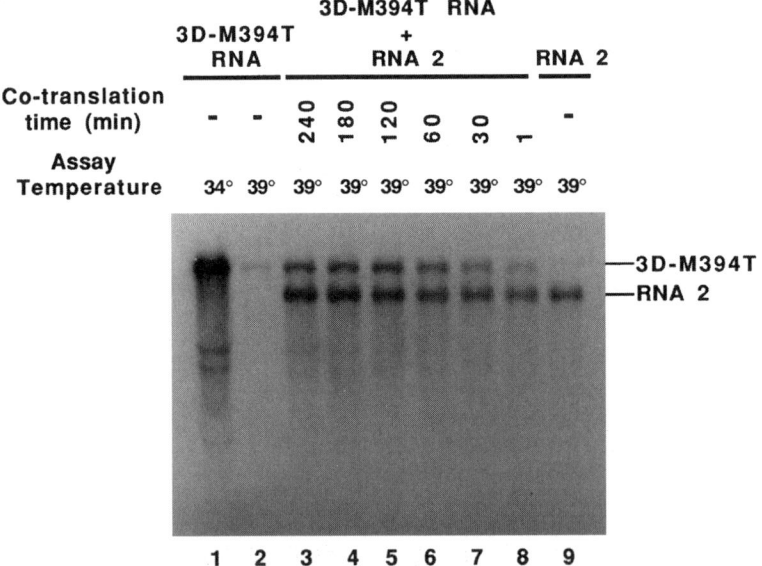

FIGURE 4 Complementation of 3D-M394T mutation requires cotranslation with helper RNA. RNA synthesis was assayed at 34 and 39°C in preinitiation RNA replication complexes isolated from HeLa S10 translation-replication reactions containing 3D-M394T RNA and/or RNA2 (a subgenomic replicon helper RNA) as indicated. The total translation time for each reaction was 4 h. For complementation, the reactions containing 3D-M394T RNA and RNA2 were mixed and cotranslated for the times indicated. For cotranslation times of less than 4 h, reactions containing each RNA were incubated separately for the appropriate amount of time before mixing. Labeled RNA was characterized by electrophoresis on a denaturing agarose gel and detected by autoradiography. The positions of 3D-M394T RNA and RNA2 are indicated.

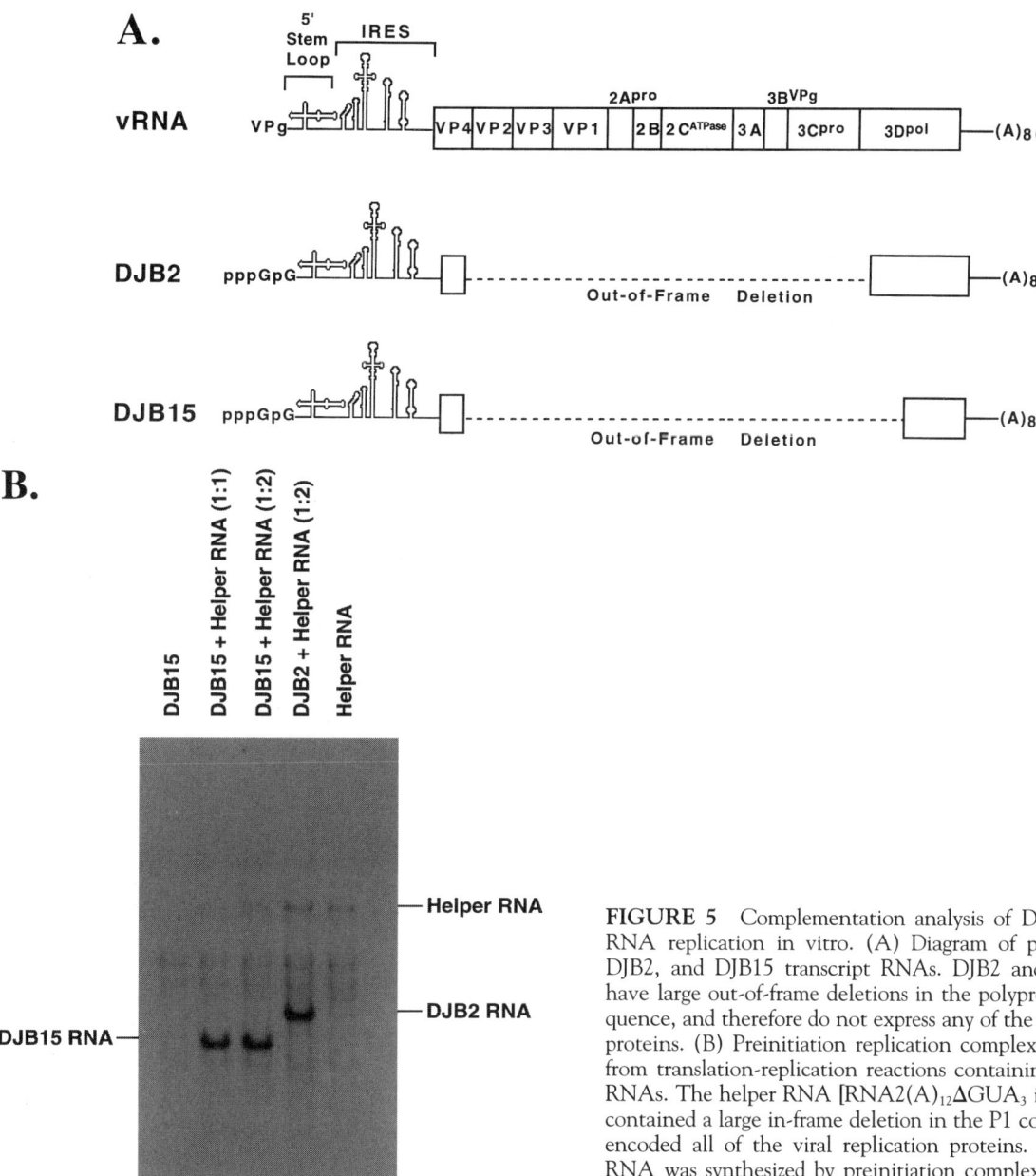

FIGURE 5 Complementation analysis of DJB2 and DJB15 RNA replication in vitro. (A) Diagram of poliovirus RNA, DJB2, and DJB15 transcript RNAs. DJB2 and DJB15 RNAs have large out-of-frame deletions in the polyprotein coding sequence, and therefore do not express any of the viral replication proteins. (B) Preinitiation replication complexes were isolated from translation-replication reactions containing the indicated RNAs. The helper RNA [RNA2(A)$_{12}\Delta$GUA$_3$ in reference 10], contained a large in-frame deletion in the P1 coding region and encoded all of the viral replication proteins. Negative-strand RNA was synthesized by preinitiation complexes incubated at 37°C for 30 min. Radiolabeled negative-strand product RNAs were analyzed on denaturing agarose gels as previously described.

poly(A) tail are the minimum sequences required for negative-strand synthesis. The conserved stem-loop structure in the 2C coding region that was recently reported to be a cis-active replication element (CRE) in poliovirus-infected cells (22, 38) was not required for negative-strand synthesis by preinitiation complexes (Fig. 5B). The entire 2C coding sequence was deleted from the DJB2 and DJB15 RNAs used in these experiments. This suggests that either the 2C CRE is not required for negative-strand synthesis or the 2C CRE in the helper RNA was able to function in trans in the in vitro assays. Additional studies are required to investigate these observations, but it is clear that there is a fundamental difference between the 5' cloverleaf (see next section) and the 2C CRE relative to being required components of the template RNA during negative-strand synthesis in vitro.

5' Cloverleaf Is a cis-Active RNA Stability and Replication Element

Previous studies have shown that the 5' cloverleaf plays an important role in viral RNA replication. Disrupting this structure inhibits viral RNA replication in infected cells and disrupts its association with viral and cellular proteins in binding assays (1, 2, 53, 55). It has been proposed that the 5' cloverleaf forms a ribonucleoprotein (RNP) complex that functions in trans during the initiation of positive-strand RNA synthesis (1). To investigate the role of the 5' cloverleaf in negative-strand synthesis, we determined

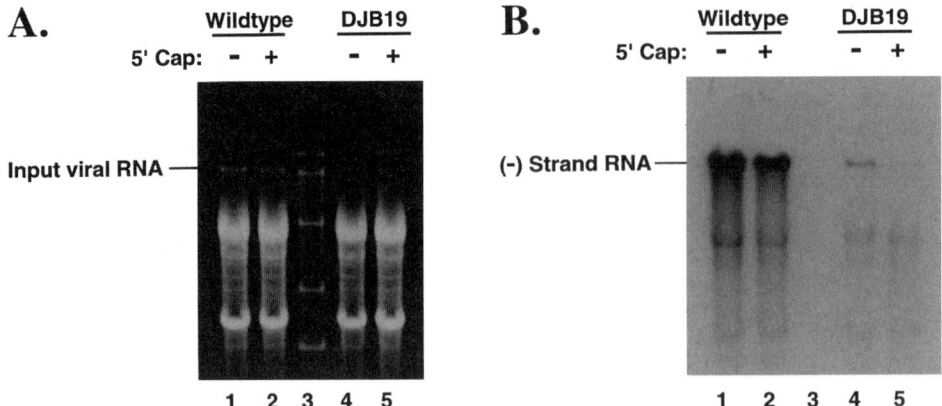

FIGURE 6 Effect of 5' cloverleaf mutation on RNA stability and negative-strand synthesis. DJB19 transcript RNA contains a four-nucleotide insertion in the 5' cloverleaf structure following nucleotide 66 (see Fig. 1). PV1(A)$_{80}$ RNA (wild type) and DJB19 RNA were transcribed in vitro with and without a 5' cap. The stability of these RNAs and their ability to support negative-strand synthesis were measured in reactions containing preinitiation complexes. The reactions were incubated at 37°C for 30 min, and the total RNA and the labeled product RNAs were analyzed by denaturing agarose gel electrophoresis as described (10). (A) The total RNA within the gel was stained with ethidium bromide and visualized with UV light. The position of the input viral RNA in the gel is indicated. (B) Labeled negative-strand product RNAs were detected in the gels by autoradiography. The position of negative-strand RNA in the gel is indicated. The results shown here were derived from results originally published in the *EMBO Journal* (10).

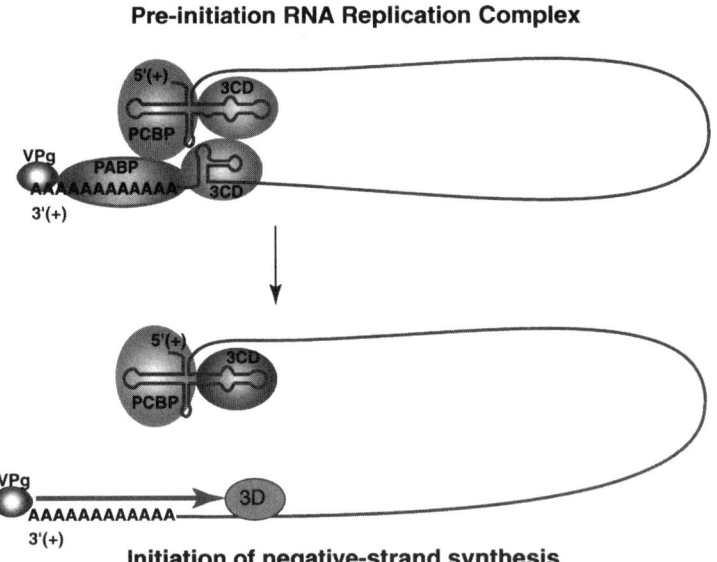

FIGURE 7 Model of circular RNP complex used for the initiation of negative-strand RNA synthesis. PABP, PCBP, and viral proteins 3CD and VPg are proposed to interact with each other and the 5' and 3' ends of the viral RNA to form a circular RNP complex. Negative-strand synthesis initiates by the elongation of a VPg primer by the viral polymerase 3D^{pol} to form a nascent negative strand. Additional viral and cellular proteins, proteolytic processing of viral protein precursors, and cellular membranes are also required for negative-strand initiation but for clarity are not depicted in this model. See text for additional details. This is a modified version of a model originally published in the *EMBO Journal* (10).

how cloverleaf mutations affected negative-strand synthesis in preinitiation RNA replication complexes (10). Results of these experiments showed that 5' cloverleaf mutations dramatically diminished RNA stability and negative-strand RNA synthesis. A four-nucleotide deletion at nucleotide 66 in the 5' cloverleaf (Fig. 1B) resulted in a dramatic destabilization of the mutant RNA and completely inhibited negative-strand synthesis. A four-nucleotide insertion at the same site (designated as DJB19 in our studies) resulted in a partial destabilization of the mutant RNA (Fig. 6A, lane 4), and strongly inhibited negative-strand synthesis (Fig. 6B, lane 4). Since the instability of DJB19 RNA could indirectly inhibit negative-strand synthesis, capped RNA transcripts were prepared and characterized for stability and negative-strand synthesis. The presence of a 5' cap had no effect on the stability or replication of wt RNA transcripts (Fig. 6A and 6B). The presence of a 5' cap fully restored the stability of DJB19 RNA (Fig. 6A, lane 5) but did not restore the ability of this mutant RNA to serve as a template for negative-strand synthesis (Fig. 6B, lane 5). Therefore, capped DJB19 RNA was stable and translated normally, but negative-strand synthesis was severely inhibited.

These results and others led to the conclusion that the 5' cloverleaf is multifunctional, being required for both RNA stability and for the initiation of negative-strand synthesis. Poliovirus RNA, unlike most cellular mRNAs, is not capped and yet is relatively stable in infected cells and HeLa cell extracts. VPg may play a role in protecting the viral RNA from degradation, but it is rapidly removed from input virion RNA by a cellular unlinking activity. Therefore, the 5' cloverleaf, most likely in the form of an RNP complex, appears to be primarily responsible for protecting viral RNAs from rapid degradation by cellular nucleases. Because of the initial lag in the synthesis of viral proteins in infected cells and in cell extracts, the 5' RNP complex would initially contain only cellular proteins. Poly(rC)-binding proteins (PCBP) are known to bind to the 5' cloverleaf (21, 35). PCBP in association with other cellular proteins may be responsible for controlling the initial stability of viral RNA. PCBP (also described as αCP) in coordination with poly(A)-binding protein (PABP) is known to mediate the stability of α-globin mRNA. As discussed below, it is possible that a similar interaction helps mediate viral RNA stability and the formation of a circular RNP complex (Fig. 7).

Circular Model for Negative-Strand Initiation

The results of recent studies indicate that the 5' cloverleaf is required for the initiation of negative-strand synthesis (10, 25, 44). In addition, the 3' NTR and poly(A) tail are required for efficient negative-strand synthesis (8, 25, 29, 30, 37, 39, 42, 48). Therefore, we and others have proposed that poliovirus RNA forms a circular RNP complex that results in the direct interaction between the 5' and 3' ends of the viral genome (10, 25) (Fig. 7). This model is similar to existing models for cellular mRNA translation that also involve the formation of circular complexes (24, 41). It is possible that temporally dynamic circular RNP complexes could mediate viral RNA stability, the switch from translation to replication, and the initiation of negative-strand RNA synthesis. The precise composition of RNP complexes mediating interactions between the 5' and 3' ends of viral RNA remains hypothetical and the composition obviously changes as viral RNP complexes mature into preinitiation RNA replication complexes. A significant step of viral replication is the transition from viral mRNA translation to viral RNA replication. Indeed, ribosomes translating poliovirus mRNA inhibit negative-strand RNA synthesis (9). Therefore accumulating viral replication proteins may displace translation initiation factors within the temporally dynamic circular RNP complexes, precluding continued translation initiation. The elongation of previously initiated ribosomes would ultimately lead to the clearance of ribosomes from virion RNA templates. Once the viral mRNA is cleared of translating ribosomes, it could then serve as a template for negative-strand synthesis. 3CD is known to bind to both ends of poliovirus RNA (1, 21, 23, 53). PCBP and PABP are known to bind to each other and to the 5' and 3' ends of viral RNA, respectively (49, 50). Therefore, a homodimer of 3CD binding to both ends of the RNA and an RNA-dependent interaction between PCBP and PABP may help circularize viral RNA within preinitiation RNA replication complexes (Fig. 7). The initiation of negative-strand synthesis should disrupt the circular orientation of the RNP complex and preclude the initiation of additional rounds of negative-strand synthesis. This would limit negative-strand synthesis and help establish the asymmetric mode of replication that favors the synthesis of positive-strand RNA. Although few details are known about the initiation of positive-strand synthesis, it is reasonable to assume that the 5' cloverleaf plays a central role in this process as previously proposed (1, 23). Therefore, the 5' cloverleaf appears to be a multifunctional cis-active structure that plays a role in regulating the stability, translation, and replication of poliovirus RNA. It seems likely that this general mechanism is used by other picornaviruses and positive-strand RNA viruses to ensure the specific and efficient replication of their genomes.

We thank Brian O'Donnell for excellent technical assistance. This work was supported by Public Health Service grants AI 15539 and AI 32123 and D. J. Barton was supported by Public Health Service grants AI 07110 and AI 42189 from the National Institute of Allergy and Infectious Diseases.

REFERENCES

1. **Andino, R., G. E. Rieckhof, P. L. Achacoso, and D. Baltimore.** 1993. Poliovirus RNA synthesis utilizes an RNP complex formed around the 5'-end of viral RNA. *EMBO J.* **12:**3587–3598.
2. **Andino, R., G. E. Rieckhof, and D. Baltimore.** 1990. A functional ribonucleoprotein complex forms around the 5' end of poliovirus RNA. *Cell* **63:**369–380.
3. **Baron, M. H., and D. Baltimore.** 1982. In vitro copying of viral positive strand RNA by poliovirus replicase. Characterization of the reaction and its products. *J. Biol. Chem.* **257:**12359–12366.
4. **Barton, D. J., E. P. Black, and J. B. Flanegan.** 1995. Complete replication of poliovirus in vitro: preinitiation RNA replication complexes require soluble cellular factors for the synthesis of VPg-linked RNA. *J. Virol.* **69:**5516–5527.
5. **Barton, D. J., and J. B. Flanegan.** 1993. Coupled translation and replication of poliovirus RNA in vitro: synthesis of functional 3D polymerase and infectious virus. *J. Virol.* **67:**822–831.
6. **Barton, D. J., and J. B. Flanegan.** 1997. Synchronous replication of poliovirus RNA: initiation of negative-strand RNA synthesis requires the guanidine-inhibited activity of protein 2C. *J. Virol.* **71:**8482–8489.
7. **Barton, D. J., B. J. Morasco, L. Eisner Smerage, P. S. Collis, S. E. Diamond, M. J. Hewlett, M. A. Merchant,**

B. J. O'Donnell, and J. B. Flanegan. 1996. Poliovirus RNA polymerase mutation 3D-M394T results in a temperature-sensitive defect in RNA synthesis. *Virology* **217:** 459–469.

8. Barton, D. J., B. J. Morasco, and J. B. Flanegan. 1996. Assays for poliovirus polymerase, 3D^{pol}, and authentic RNA replication in HeLa S10 extracts. *Methods Enzymol.* **275:**35–57.

9. Barton, D. J., B. J. Morasco, and J. B. Flanegan. 1999. Translating ribosomes inhibit poliovirus negative-strand RNA synthesis. *J. Virol.* **73:**10104–10112.

10. Barton, D. J., B. J. O'Donnell, and J. B. Flanegan. 2001. 5′ cloverleaf in poliovirus RNA is a *cis*-acting replication element required for negative-strand synthesis. *EMBO J.* **20:**1439–1448.

11. Bienz, K., D. Egger, and L. Pasamontes. 1987. Association of polioviral proteins of the P2 genomic region with the viral replication complex and virus-induced membrane synthesis as visualized by electron microscopic immunocytochemistry and autoradiography. *Virology* **160:** 220–226.

12. Bienz, K., D. Egger, and T. Pfister. 1994. Characteristics of the poliovirus replication complex. *Arch. Virol. Suppl.* **9:**147–157.

13. Bienz, K., D. Egger, T. Pfister, and M. Troxler. 1992. Structural and functional characterization of the poliovirus replication complex. *J. Virol.* **66:**2740–2747.

14. Caliguiri, L. A., and I. Tamm. 1969. Membranous structures associated with translation and transcription of poliovirus RNA. *Science* **166:**885–886.

15. Caliguiri, L. A., and I. Tamm. 1970. Characterization of poliovirus-specific structures associated with cytoplasmic membranes. *Virology* **42:**112–122.

16. Darnell, J. E., L. Levintow, M. M. Thoren, and J. L. Hooper. 1961. The time course of synthesis of poliovirus RNA. *Virology* **13:**271–279.

17. Egger, D., N. Teterina, E. Ehrenfeld, and K. Bienz. 2000. Formation of the poliovirus replication complex requires coupled viral translation, vesicle production, and viral RNA synthesis. *J. Virol.* **74:**6570–6580.

18. Eisner Smerage, L. 1998. Poliovirus RNA replication: separation of initiation and elongation functions of the viral polymerase using a cell-free system. Ph.D. dissertation. University of Florida, Gainesville.

19. Enders, J. F., T. H. Weller, and F. C. Robbins. 1949. Cultivation of the Lansing strain of poliomyelitis virus in cultures of various human embryonic tissues. *Science* **109:** 85–87.

20. Flanegan, J. B., R. F. Petterson, V. Ambros, M. J. Hewlett, and D. Baltimore. 1977. Covalent linkage of a protein to a defined nucleotide sequence at the 5′-terminus of virion and replicative intermediate RNAs of poliovirus. *Proc. Natl. Acad. Sci. USA* **74:**961–965.

21. Gamarnik, A. V., and R. Andino. 1997. Two functional complexes formed by KH domain containing proteins with the 5′ noncoding region of poliovirus RNA. *RNA* **3:**882–892.

22. Goodfellow, I., Y. Chaudhry, A. Richardson, J. Meredith, J. W. Almond, W. Barclay, and D. J. Evans. 2000. Identification of a *cis*-acting replication element within the poliovirus coding region. *J. Virol.* **74:**4590–4600.

23. Harris, K. S., W. Xiang, L. Alexander, W. S. Lane, A. V. Paul, and E. Wimmer. 1994. Interaction of poliovirus polypeptide 3CD^{pro} with the 5′ and 3′ termini of the poliovirus genome: identification of viral and cellular cofactors needed for efficient binding. *J. Biol. Chem.* **269:** 27004–27014.

24. Hentze, M. W. 1997. eIF4G: a multipurpose ribosome adaptor? *Science* **275:**500–501.

25. Herold, J., and R. Andino. 2001. Poliovirus RNA replication requires genome circularization through a protein-protein bridge. *Mol. Cell* **7:**581–591.

26. Herold, J., and R. Andino. 2000. Poliovirus requires a precise 5′ end for efficient positive-strand RNA synthesis. *J. Virol.* **74:**6394–6400.

27. Lawson, M. A., and B. L. Semler. 1992. Alternate poliovirus nonstructural protein processing cascades generated by primary sites of 3C proteinase cleavage. *Virology* **191:**309–320.

28. Lee, Y. F., A. Nomoto, B. M. Detjen, and E. Wimmer. 1977. A protein covalently linked to poliovirus genome RNA. *Proc. Natl. Acad. Sci. USA* **74:**59–63.

29. Melchers, W. J. G., J. G. J. Hoenderop, H. J. Bruins Slot, C. W. A. Pleij, E. V. Pilipenko, V. I. Agol, and J. M. D. Galama. 1997. Kissing of the two predominant hairpin loops in the coxsackie B virus 3′ untranslated region is the essential structural feature of the origin of replication required for negative-strand RNA synthesis. *J. Virol.* **71:**686–696.

30. Mirmomeni, M. H., P. J. Hughes, and G. Stanway. 1997. An RNA tertiary structure in the 3′ untranslated region of enteroviruses is necessary for efficient replication. *J. Virol.* **71:**2363–2370.

31. Mirzayan, C., and E. Wimmer. 1994. Biochemical studies on poliovirus polypeptide 2C: evidence for ATPase activity. *Virology* **199:**176–187.

32. Molla, A., A. V. Paul, and E. Wimmer. 1991. Cell-free, de novo synthesis of poliovirus. *Science* **254:**1647–1651.

33. Molla, A., A. V. Paul, and E. Wimmer. 1993. Effects of temperature and lipophilic agents on poliovirus formation and RNA synthesis in a cell-free system. *J. Virol.* **67:** 5932–5938.

34. Novak, J. E., and K. Kirkegaard. 1994. Coupling between genome translation and replication in an RNA virus. *Genes Dev.* **8:**1726–1737.

35. Parsley, T. B., J. S. Towner, L. B. Blyn, E. Ehrenfeld, and B. L. Semler. 1997. Poly (rC) binding protein 2 forms a ternary complex with the 5′-terminal sequences of poliovirus RNA and the viral 3CD proteinase. *RNA* **3:** 1124–1134.

36. Paul, A. V., E. Rieder, D. W. Kim, J. H. van Boom, and E. Wimmer. 2000. Identification of an RNA hairpin in poliovirus RNA that serves as the primary template in the in vitro uridylylation of VPg. *J. Virol.* **74:**10359–10370.

37. Pilipenko, E. V., K. Poperechny, S. V. Maslova, W. J. G. Melchers, H. J. Bruins Slot, and V. I. Agol. 1996. Cis-element, oriR, involved in the initiation of (−) strand poliovirus RNA: a quasi-globular multi-domain RNA structure maintained by tertiary ('kissing') interactions. *EMBO J.* **15:**5428–5436.

38. Rieder, E., A. V. Paul, D. W. Kim, J. H. van Boom, and E. Wimmer. 2000. Genetic and biochemical studies of poliovirus *cis*-acting replication element cre in relation to VPg uridylylation. *J. Virol.* **74:**10371–10380.

39. Rohll, J. B., D. H. Moon, D. J. Evans, and J. W. Almond. 1995. The 3′ untranslated region of picornavirus RNA: features required for efficient genome replication. *J. Virol.* **69:**7835–7844.

40. Roizman, B. 1990. Multiplication of viruses: an overview, p. 87–94. *In* B. N. Fields (ed.), *Virology*. Raven Press, New York, N.Y.

41. Sachs, A. B., P. Sarnow, and M. W. Hentze. 1997. Starting at the beginning, middle, and end: translation initiation in eukaryotes. *Cell* **89:**831–838.

42. Sarnow, P., H. D. Bernstein, and D. Baltimore. 1986. A poliovirus temperature-sensitive RNA synthesis mutant in a noncoding region of the genome. *Proc. Natl. Acad. Sci. USA* **83:**571–575.

43. Spector, D. H., and D. Baltimore. 1974. Requirement of

3'-terminal poly(A) for the infectivity of poliovirus RNA. *Proc. Natl. Acad. Sci. USA* **71:**2983–2987.

44. **Teterina, N. L., D. Egger, K. Bienz, D. M. Brown, B. L. Semler, and E. Ehrenfeld.** 2001. Requirements for assembly of poliovirus replication complexes and negative-strand RNA synthesis. *J. Virol.* **75:**3841–3850.

45. **Teterina, N. L., W. D. Zhou, M. W. Cho, and E. Ehrenfeld.** 1995. Inefficient complementation activity of poliovirus 2C and 3D proteins for rescue of lethal mutations. *J. Virol.* **69:**4245–4254.

46. **Towner, J. S., M. M. Mazanet, and B. L. Semler.** 1998. Rescue of defective poliovirus RNA replication by 3AB-containing precursor polyproteins. *J. Virol.* **72:**7191–7200.

47. **Van Dyke, T. A., R. J. Rickles, and J. B. Flanegan.** 1982. Genome-length copies of poliovirion RNA are synthesized in vitro by the poliovirus RNA-dependent RNA polymerase. *J. Biol. Chem.* **257:**4610–4617.

48. **Wang, J., J. M. Bakkers, J. M. Galama, H. J. Bruins Slot, E. V. Pilipenko, V. I. Agol, and W. J. Melchers.** 1999. Structural requirements of the higher order RNA kissing element in the enteroviral 3'UTR. *Nucleic Acids Res.* **27:**485–490.

49. **Wang, Z., N. Day, P. Trifillis, and M. Kiledjian.** 1999. An mRNA stability complex functions with poly(A)-binding protein to stabilize mRNA in vitro. *Mol. Cell. Biol.* **19:**4552–4560.

50. **Wang, Z., and M. Kiledjian.** 2000. The poly(A)-binding protein and an mRNA stability protein jointly regulate an endoribonuclease activity. *Mol. Cell. Biol.* **20:**6334–6341.

51. **Ward, C. D.** 1993. Ph.D. thesis. University of Florida, Gainesville.

52. **Ward, C. D., M. A. Stokes, and J. B. Flanegan.** 1988. Direct measurement of the poliovirus RNA polymerase error frequency in vitro. *J. Virol.* **62:**558–562.

53. **Xiang, W., K. S. Harris, L. Alexander, and E. Wimmer.** 1995. Interaction between the 5'-terminal cloverleaf and 3AB/3CD^{pro} of poliovirus is essential for RNA replication. *J. Virol.* **59:**3658–3667.

54. **Young, D. C., G. J. Tobin, and J. B. Flanegan.** 1987. Characterization of product RNAs synthesized in vitro by poliovirus RNA polymerase purified by chromatography on hydroxylapatite or poly(U) Sepharose. *J. Virol.* **61:**611–614.

55. **Zhao, W. D., F. C. Lahser, and E. Wimmer.** 2000. Genetic analysis of a poliovirus/hepatitis C virus (HCV) chimera: interaction between the poliovirus cloverleaf and a sequence in the HCV 5' nontranslated region results in a replication phenotype. *J. Virol.* **74:**6223–6226.

GLOBAL ERADICATION OF POLIOVIRUS

Global Eradication of Poliovirus: History and Rationale

WALTER R. DOWDLE AND STEPHEN L. COCHI

38

Disease eradication is the ultimate achievement in public health. Global eradication brings health equity and social justice and frees scarce resources for other purposes (2, 6). Knowledge gained from the unsuccessful eradication initiatives against yellow fever, malaria, and yaws contributed to the successful eradication of smallpox in 1977 (17, 18), which, in turn, influenced the current eradication initiatives for guinea worm and polio.

Polio meets the biological criteria for an eradicable disease. An effective intervention (vaccine) is available to interrupt agent transmission, tools are available to detect levels of infection leading to agent transmission, and humans are essential for the life cycle of the agent (16, 29). On the other hand, there are major qualifiers. Oral polio vaccine (OPV), although inexpensive and easy to deliver, is less than fully effective in areas of the world where the incidence of polio is highest (31). Poliovirus is highly transmissible, with only 1 of every 100 to 1,000 infections among susceptible individuals resulting in clinically recognizable disease. The tools for agent detection and characterization are laboratory-based and relatively complex, as described in chapter 39 in this volume. Also to be addressed are the critical issues of national and international health priorities and political will (3, 11). The eradication of polio presents far greater challenges than that of smallpox. In 1988, when the World Health Assembly (WHA) adopted the resolution of global polio eradication by the year 2000 (47), skeptics abounded. They still do.

The origins of the ambitious 1988 resolution extend back through nearly three decades and involve many people and numerous events. To do justice to them all would not be possible in the allotted space of a chapter. However, the major factors that may have most influenced the events leading to the resolution were Albert Sabin, smallpox eradication, Brazil, the 1983 International Symposium on Poliomyelitis Control, the Pan American Health Organization (PAHO), Rotary International, and the Declaration of Talloires.

ALBERT B. SABIN

The origin of global eradication of poliomyelitis is conventionally attributed to Albert Sabin and his colleagues in the frequently quoted and often reprinted 1960 report on the effects of rapid mass OPV immunization in Toluca, Mexico (41). Sabin and others (33) had previously recognized that the practice of feeding children three vaccine types separately at intervals of 4 to 6 weeks, regarded as optimal during the cold months of the year in temperate climates, had little effect in developing countries in subtropical or tropical climates. Such programs failed to effectively immunize a considerable proportion of vaccinated children and had minimal influence on the circulation of wild poliovirus. They attributed these findings to vaccine interference by enteric viruses, common in areas with climatic and hygienic conditions favoring sustained fecal-oral transmission.

Toluca was a city of 100,000, described by Sabin as paying an average price of 14 paralytic cases per year for naturally acquired immunity. Trivalent oral polio vaccine was fed en masse to all children less than 11 years of age, followed 12 weeks later by a second dose of trivalent vaccine in a subgroup of children who remained serologically negative. The rationale was that the three types of vaccine strains would be implanted in the largest number of children and further disseminated in the community by nature. The strategy worked. The authors concluded that feeding trivalent OPV on two brief occasions at an interval of 6 to 8 weeks to all children under 4 or 5 years was a rational initial approach to the eradication of poliomyelitis. This strategy serves as the foundation of today's global polio eradication initiative.

Whether Sabin and colleagues used the term "eradication" in the national, regional, or global context is unclear. Equally unclear is whether at that time he envisioned eradication of the virus itself. Whatever was meant, capitalizing on the Toluca success was not destined to follow immediately. Conducting a single mass campaign in a small city is

---

Walter R. Dowdle ■ World Health Organization, The Task Force for Child Survival and Development, Suite 400, 750 Commerce Dr., Decatur, GA 30030. **Stephen L. Cochi** ■ Vaccine Preventable Disease Eradication Division, National Immunization Program, Centers for Disease Control and Prevention, 1600 Clifton Rd., MS/E-05, Atlanta, GA 30333.

challenging. Expanding to multiyear campaigns at national, regional, and global levels requires far greater commitment and resources.

Many countries mounted mass OPV campaigns in the decade that followed, including the United States, Japan, and several Eastern and Western European countries. With a few exceptions (such as Hungary and Romania), the purpose of these campaigns was to jump start protection against polio, with the policy of routine childhood immunization to follow thereafter. Cuba is the only country that initially adopted and retained the Sabin strategy until the present day (28). For the better part of 40 years, Cuba has relied essentially on two annual mass campaigns for children less than 4 years of age in lieu of routine immunization.

Cuba eliminated wild poliovirus shortly after the strategy was introduced, but the Cuban model failed to be adopted elsewhere in the world. Its success was explained away with arguments that Cuba was an island with good hygiene standards, minimal contact with countries of endemicity, and a communist form of government, which made it uniquely capable of mobilizing its citizens.

Nevertheless, impressed by Cuba's success, Sabin and Horstmann in 1968 recommended a similar program to that of PAHO for other countries in the Americas (39). Nothing happened. Sabin made similar recommendations over a number of years to Brazil but lamented that nothing had happened there as well, until 1980. The program that began in Brazil in 1980 was based on the Sabin principles but had equally strong roots in the successful smallpox eradication program of a decade earlier.

SMALLPOX ERADICATION

The global eradication of smallpox began in 1966 in response to the WHA resolution to eradicate smallpox by 1976. Under evolving World Health Organization (WHO) leadership, strong central coordination, and support of member states, the last case of naturally occurring smallpox was recorded in Somalia in 1977. The formal declaration of eradication was issued by an independent WHO commission in 1980 (18).

For the many who had worked with the program over the 11-year period, this was a day of great pride and a profound sense of achievement. The announcement received media coverage as a major milestone in international cooperation, an unprecedented public health accomplishment, and a model for the future. But in many sectors of the international public health community this great achievement was either given lip service or altogether ignored. For many, smallpox eradication would be a fluke in the annals of public health. No other infectious diseases were thought to share the unique characteristics that made it possible to eradicate smallpox: clinically apparent disease; low agent transmissibility; and an effective, inexpensive, and easily administered vaccine. For others, the smallpox program represented the worst of a military style, externally goal-driven, vertical program, the likes of which should never again be permitted. The prevailing thinking in international public health had moved on to locally organized and decentralized horizontal programs of sustainable, integrated primary health care (22). The 1978 Alma-Ata (Kazhakstan) International Conference on Primary Health Care, which declared the goal of health for all by the year 2000, promised there would never again be another vertical program like smallpox eradication to divert attention from primary health care (48).

But the public health legacies of smallpox eradication, like its humanitarian accomplishments, were not to be so easily dismissed. Lessons learned from the program deeply influenced the thinking of participating public health workers and had a lasting effect on national and international public health practices, and WHO's Expanded Program on Immunization (EPI) became one of the legacies (22). In many developing countries, the young professionals who had received their basic public health training in the smallpox program became the public health leaders in later years. The eradication of smallpox had proven the value of program goals based on disease outcome rather than service coverage. It had introduced the concept of timely disease surveillance and use of such information to guide public health strategy and ensure effective and efficient use of resources. It had created alliances between local and national public health practitioners, resulting in a personal public health network that provided an environment for working together in the years to come. The smallpox eradication program had strongly influenced the public health practices of Brazil.

BRAZIL

Understanding the path taken by this developing tropical country to control polio is key to understanding the evolution of the global eradication initiative. The account given here is primarily from the writings of Joao Baptista-Risi, Jr. (4, 5), a former member of the smallpox eradication team and a major force in shaping the program in Brazil.

The first polio immunization campaign in Brazil was launched in 1961. In the absence of a national immunization authority, polio control was a state responsibility, attendant with the usual problems of irregular purchasing and distribution of vaccine in a huge country with varying degrees of development, high birth rates, and extensive internal migration. Under this undirected policy, immunization against polio became, in effect, a practice restricted to those who could afford it or who had access to it. Predictably, poliomyelitis became a disease predominantly of the lower socioeconomic classes, those with no access to health services or routine vaccination facilities. There was no national reporting system until 1969, and, even then, reporting compliance varied widely by state and geographic area.

In 1971, Brazil created a National Poliomyelitis Control Program (NPCP) to overcome the inequities of the previous immunization policies. The NPCP strategy was based on the Sabin principles of mass campaigns (three times a year) for all children 3 months to 5 years of age, irrespective of their previous vaccination status. While providing overall guidance, the federal government delegated to the states such decisions as when and how campaigns were to be conducted. Success was measured by vaccination coverage. Sustainability of NPCP became a question even after the second year, primarily because of the decentralized nature of the program. States often worked at cross-purposes, schedules were not established clearly, mass media communications were lacking, and surveillance was inadequate to guide program strategy.

Before corrections could be enacted, NPCP was replaced in 1973 by the newly formed National Immunization Program (NIP), which was designed to integrate all activities for control of vaccine-preventable diseases. NIP became largely a service-based public health practice.

Childhood vaccines were viewed as the attraction for people to seek regular health care. In 1975, a federal vaccination law made polio immunization compulsory for all children under the age of 1 year. Despite these well-meaning efforts, sporadic polio epidemics continued.

About this time, Baptista-Risi began to build a national polio surveillance system that included systematic reporting of suspected polio cases, confirmation of clinical diagnoses, field investigations, and the collection of specimens for laboratory analysis. A network of six laboratories was established, coordinated by Fundacao Oswaldo Cruz, Rio de Janeiro, under the leadership of Herman Schatzmayr, who had performed a similar function for the smallpox eradication program. This newly implemented laboratory-based national polio surveillance system revealed that polio was highly endemic throughout the country, over 85% of the cases were under 5 years of age, and 90% of them had never been vaccinated. Major epidemics in several regions of Brazil in 1979 confirmed the inadequacy of the vaccination strategy of the time and led to public announcements that changes must be made.

Baptista-Risi, who at that time was the National Secretary for Basic Health Activities, proposed returning to the mass vaccination strategy, incorporating the lessons learned from NCPC, which had been abandoned in 1973. The plan was to introduce coordinated, widely promoted, countrywide national immunization days twice a year for all children under 5 years of age and to involve all existing governmental and societal mechanisms. The rationale for coordinated mass immunization was simple; they had already tried everything else.

The first national immunization day was launched on Saturday, 14 June 1980, with 17.5 million children immunized. The second was on Saturday, 16 August. Unlike in Cuba, where children were vaccinated in their homes, children in Brazil were brought to designated vaccination posts. Mobile teams visited homes only in sparsely populated rural areas.

The Brazilian program was highly successful (4). Over the next few years, it achieved extraordinary coverage in remote locations and in high-risk communities, resulting in a sharp drop in polio cases. In 1983, only 45 cases of polio were confirmed, the lowest ever reported. Brazil's success and pioneering efforts demonstrated to the world that annual mass campaigns were feasible in large, developing, noncommunist countries.

THE 1983 INTERNATIONAL SYMPOSIUM ON POLIOMYELITIS CONTROL

Although the 1980 declaration of smallpox eradication may have come at a time when popular international public health thinking was moving away from vertical programs, for some it still brought to the forefront the potential for eradication of other infectious diseases. At the request of DeWitt Stetten, senior scientific advisor, National Institutes of Health, the Fogarty International Center sponsored a small conference on the eradication of infectious diseases shortly after smallpox eradication had been declared. Measles, polio, and yaws emerged from the conference as the three most likely candidates for eradication (1). In 1983, the Fogarty International Center sponsored an International Symposium on Poliomyelitis Control at PAHO, the first meeting of its kind since 1960.

This symposium is often said to be the beginning of the global polio eradication initiative. Such conclusions are difficult to glean from the written reports. Despite encouragement for mass immunization in India (26) and striking results from the strategy in Brazil (4), Cuba (37), and Mexico (19), the overall tone of the symposium was not eradication friendly. In fact, there was very little discussion devoted to eradication per se. As the title suggests, most of the discussion focused on improved control. Even Sabin never mentioned the word "eradication" (39). He stressed that the main problem in controlling polio in most countries was "administrative, not immunologic" (38) and pressed for mass campaigns in developing nations, assisted by WHO's EPI. WHA had approved EPI in 1974. It began operations in 1977, dedicated to reaching infants and young children in developing countries with six basic vaccines (BCG, OPV, diphtheria-pertussis-tetanus, and measles) through improved routine immunization (22). EPI did not see mass campaigns as its role (23).

Several speakers supported eventual elimination (10, 21), but, overall, the opposition to a vertical global program was strong, particularly by the WHO representatives (23, 36, 44). This was not surprising, given the declaration of the 1978 Alma-Ata conference. Some viewed even EPI as being inconsistent with the Alma-Ata principles, because it continued to be operated in some countries as a vertical program.

Polio, it was said, could never be considered a priority health program for most of the poorer countries, given the toll taken by measles, malaria, gastroenteritis, and other diseases of childhood (44). Further concern was expressed that the resources required for mass campaigns would deprive general health services of staff, support, and budgetary allocations. The campaign approach as a long-term strategy was "... politically unattractive, administratively difficult, and economically extravagant" (36).

The view was expressed that "its control requires a long-term program that may outlive the humanitarian impulse. The most appropriate context for poliomyelitis control, from the point of view of the efficient use of limited resources and the assurance of continuing political support, is the primary health care program" (36). These and the previous comments failed for the most part to recognize Sabin and his colleagues' 1960 conclusions that control of polio in most developing tropical countries could be accomplished only through mass immunization.

Frederick Robbins, Nobel laureate, who, at the time of the symposium, was president of the Institute of Medicine in the United States, authored the summary (35). He recommended, in brief, that each country should develop its own program to achieve control and WHO should assist in planning, conducting, and evaluating such programs, with the eventual goal to incorporate polio vaccination into routine health care services. He added, however, that special campaigns for polio vaccination should not be discouraged. They can be used to increase private and public motivation and help develop a public health infrastructure.

He concluded by stating, "... it would appear that a practical and potentially feasible goal is worldwide control of paralytic poliomyelitis within this century, but global eradication as the ultimate goal should not be abandoned." PAHO found this to be encouraging.

PAHO

PAHO has been an influential and highly respected force in Latin American public health since its inception in 1902, providing strong leadership in addressing many of the pressing infectious disease challenges in Latin America and the Caribbean. PAHO also has served as the WHO Regional Office for the Americas since 1947.

At the time of the International Conference on Poliomyelitis Control in 1983, PAHO, along with other WHO regions, was exploring strategies to meet the goal of universal childhood immunization by 1990 (13). Carlyle Guerra de Macedo was the newly elected director of PAHO, a Brazilian, and a strong proponent of childhood immunization. Ciro de Quadros was chief, EPI, since its formation by PAHO in 1978. Also a Brazilian, he had extensive smallpox eradication experience in Brazil and Africa and firsthand knowledge of the progress of polio elimination in Brazil. They were convinced, in direct contrast to most views expressed at the Polio Conference, that vertical programs would strengthen, not weaken, overall development of immunization and health services and systems, particularly disease surveillance. They saw polio eradication as the "banner disease" to revitalize interest in achieving the elusive childhood immunization goal.

Meanwhile in Brazil, a new government had assumed power, with the avowed intent to discontinue all vertical programs, including mass campaigns. This latest threat to the mass immunization strategy was averted by the persuasive powers of Baptista-Risi and his colleagues and knowledge of PAHO's interest in modeling the regional program based on the Brazilian experience.

On 14 May 1985, in Washington, D.C., de Macedo announced the goal of polio eradication in the Americas by the year 1990 (30). The fact that the announcement was made during the time of the WHA in Geneva did not go unnoticed. de Quadros assumed the responsibility for implementing the polio eradication initiative in the Americas. Along with the assignment came no money, ongoing civil wars and unrest, and little evidence of political will. At the same time, Rotary International was searching for a global target to be achieved by the centennial of its founding in 1905. Sabin, who had continued to push for polio elimination (40), suggested polio eradication (13).

ROTARY INTERNATIONAL

In 1985, Rotary International launched a 20-year crusade to help eradicate polio worldwide by 2005. The polio campaign was in addition to its strong community commitment. Rotary was uniquely suited for this global task, with nearly 1.5 million business and professional members in nearly 30,000 clubs located in 155 countries. During the 1970s, Rotary had supported immunization programs in several South American and African countries under its Health, Hunger, and Humanity Program, but polio eradication was on a greater scale than any volunteer program previously undertaken (49).

Initially, Rotary set out to raise $120 million from its membership and other sources. Two years later they had raised more than twice the target. They wisely used the funds to supplement, leverage, and directly support crucial eradication activities. At least $500 million will have been provided by Rotary by the year 2005. However, the real value of Rotary's early involvement in the eradication campaign in the Americas, and since, cannot be measured in dollars alone. In 27 countries in Latin America and the Caribbean, Rotarians worked with PAHO and UNICEF as advocates, mediators, and community and national leaders. They opened doors in areas where governments were not welcome or trusted. They publicized mass campaigns, mobilized communities, provided vaccine cold chain equipment, staffed immunization posts, and administered vaccine. They facilitated immunizations across borders and in areas of civil unrest. They provided aprons for vaccinators, banners for immunization booths, and equipment for individual laboratories. Rotarians from countries experienced in polio eradication strategies assisted fellow Rotarians in countries that were just beginning.

To be sure, the individual countries in the Americas bore 80% of the eradication costs and provided most of the human resources, but Rotary's active commitment and involvement energized and added legitimacy to national programs and mobilized communitywide participation in a manner that few governments could do alone. With so many Rotarians acting on the belief that polio eradication was a dream that could be realized, there was no turning back.

THE 1988 DECLARATION OF TALLOIRES

The basic strategy for global eradication evolved under PAHO leadership during the first few years of the program in the Americas. Vaccine cold chains were established or strengthened. OPV National Immunization Days (NIDs) were conducted in addition to routine childhood immunizations. House-to-house immunizations were undertaken to reach children in areas at high risk of continuing virus transmission. "Mop-up" campaigns were initiated to focus on areas with persistent virus transmission. Uniform case definitions and surveillance standards were developed. Over 20,000 surveillance units were established throughout the region (14). In collaboration with the Centers for Disease Control and Prevention (CDC), in Atlanta, a regionwide poliovirus laboratory network was set up to isolate and characterize poliovirus in stool specimens from cases of acute flaccid paralysis (32). Within 2 years after beginning the eradication initiative in the Americas, routine childhood immunization had greatly increased and the number of polio cases had decreased dramatically. Global eradication of polio was being discussed openly (24).

The remarkable reduction in polio cases in the Americas in such a short time strongly influenced the agenda for the 10–12 March 1988 meeting in Talloires, France, organized by William Foege and sponsored by the Task Force for Child Survival and Development, Atlanta. Among the 60 participants at the meeting were Baptista-Risi and de Quadros, who made the case for eradication. Others included Jim Grant, executive director, UNICEF; Halfdan Mahler, director general, WHO; Ralph Henderson, director, EPI, WHO; and Donald Henderson, dean, Johns Hopkins School of Hygiene and Public Health. The outcome of the meeting was the Declaration of Talloires, where the first on an impressive list of recommendations was the call for global eradication of polio by the year 2000 (42).

Jim Grant was a strong supporter of polio eradication. Halfdan Mahler, who had for the past 10 years carried the WHO banner in opposition to vertical public health programs, changed his position at Talloires. He concluded that vertical programs such as immunization, control of diarrheal diseases, and family planning could serve as "messenger RNA" for the insertion of low-cost, effective, and equitable measures into the vector of primary health care (45). Two months later, Mahler placed polio eradication on the agenda for the May 1988 WHA meeting.

POST-1988 WHA RESOLUTION TO ERADICATE POLIO BY THE YEAR 2000

At the time of the 1988 WHA resolution, paralytic polio was endemic in 125 countries on 5 continents, with an estimated 350,000 cases occurring annually. Polio was still endemic in eight countries in Central and South America. It was a daunting challenge. Kew and Pallansch review eradication strategies and current progress in chapter 39.

Like the slogan "Health for all by the year 2000," which emerged from the Alma-Ata conference in 1978, many in international public health, including WHO staff, believed that polio eradication was one more impossible dream that would be given lip service for awhile and eventually abandoned. Few were supportive. Many were skeptical. Many were publicly opposed.

Indeed, not much happened on the global front during the remainder of 1988. The initiative lost its major supporter within WHO when Mahler completed his final term as Director General that same year. The incoming director general, Hiroshi Nakajima, showed little enthusiasm for polio eradication. But polio eradication was different from other forgotten resolutions. Its strengths were built on the unflagging conviction of Rotary International, a few determined and capable key individuals inside and outside WHO, and the successful technical and funding partnerships that had already been put in place in the American Region.

In 1990, the World Summit for Children in New York (Jim Grant's last major appearance before his death) endorsed the goal of polio eradication. In 1991, the last indigenous polio case in the Americas was detected in Peru. These two events gave the initiative a major boost.

In 1991, CDC initiated an annual joint technical meeting with WHO on polio eradication. By 1995 the meeting had grown from a handful to nearly 100 participants, consisting of CDC and WHO technical staff and representatives of other organizations. In 1996, the venue for the annual meeting was shifted to the Geneva headquarters of an invigorated WHO. Participation increased in size and diversity.

Leadership in the remaining five WHO regions was key to advancing global polio eradication and increasing childhood immunization. Earliest to begin were countries of the Western Pacific Region (WPR), spurred on by the unfortunate nationwide epidemics in China in 1989 and 1990, when about 10,000 children were paralyzed. High routine coverage rates with three doses of OPV had failed to prevent multiprovince outbreaks (53). WPR began planning for eradication in 1990 with assistance from CDC, the government of Japan, and PAHO. China launched its first NID in December 1993, followed by a second round a month later. A total of 83 million children were immunized in each of the two rounds (43).

In August 1994, an Independent International Certification Commission on Poliomyelitis Eradication declared virus transmission interrupted in the Americas (7). The legacy of the polio eradication initiative in the Americas was impressive. A large cadre of epidemiologists had been trained, a network of virology laboratories had been built, all countries had improved their capacity for health planning, immunization management systems had been established, and a comprehensive Hemisphere-wide surveillance system had been placed in operation. The entire health sector had benefited from the added prestige of a successful program. The national and regional Interagency Coordinating Committee concept, pioneered by PAHO and operational in each country, also proved to be a crucial model for all of the other regions to manage diverse sources of extra budgetary funding.

The Polio Eradication Initiative has grown into a true global partnership, implemented by a broad coalition spearheaded by WHO, Rotary International, CDC, and UNICEF. The coalition includes national governments; private foundations such as the United Nations Foundation and Bill and Melinda Gates Foundation; the World Bank; donor governments (e.g., Australia, Belgium, Canada, Denmark, Finland, Germany, Italy, Japan, United Kingdom, and United States); and corporate partners (e.g., Aventis Pasteur and De Beers). Volunteers in developing countries also play a key role, with an estimated 10 million participating in NIDs in 1999.

POSTERADICATION ISSUES

When it became increasingly likely in the mid-1990s that global polio eradication could become reality, attention began to turn to posteradication issues. In March 1998, a technical consultative group was convened by WHO in Geneva to review posteradication issues. The group recommended that vaccination with OPV should stop and that with inactivated polio vaccine (IPV) can stop when there is sufficient assurance of the global eradication of wild polioviruses, suitable laboratory containment of the remaining stocks of wild polioviruses, and evidence that vaccine-derived poliovirus will only circulate for a limited period in the postimmunization era (50).

Certification of Global Eradication

The process of global certification of polio eradication follows the smallpox example and the polio model pioneered by the American Region in 1990 to 1994 (7, 34). An independent national committee submits documentation to its Regional Commission that it is free of indigenous polio. When satisfied with the evidence submitted by all member countries, the commission certifies the region as polio-free. When all regions of the world are certified as free of wild poliovirus transmission after at least 3 years of adequate surveillance and wild viruses in laboratories can be documented as appropriately contained, the Global Commission will certify the world as polio-free (51).

Laboratory Containment

Successful containment requires the reasons to be clear and compelling, the risks to justify the biosafety measures, and the goals to be realistic. Absolute containment cannot be ensured. Questions of intentional or unintentional transmission of poliovirus from the laboratory to the community will always remain. But effective containment, that is, prevention of inadvertent transmission, is a realistic goal.

In 1999, WHO published the *Global Action Plan for Laboratory Containment of Wild Polioviruses* (52). This stepwise plan is linked to the three major phases of eradication. The first step toward containment consists of national surveys of all laboratories that might possess wild poliovirus infectious (defined as stocks, specimens from polio patients, and products of research) or potentially infectious materials (defined as throat, fecal, or environmental specimens collected for any purpose at a time and at a geographical location where polio was endemic). The purpose of the survey is to encourage disposal of all unneeded materials and establish a national inventory of laboratories that retain such materials. Laboratories on the inventory will be kept informed of progress and notified 1 year after the last polio case to implement biosafety measures appropriate for the materials being stored and procedures performed. Risks are highest in virology laboratories working with products of poliovirus replication and lowest in nonvirology laboratories working with potentially infectious materials. Decisions on posteradication immunization strategies directly affect final containment requirements. When OPV immunization stops, increasingly stringent standards will be required over a period of years to effectively reduce the risk of unintentional release.

Stopping Immunization

As with smallpox eradication, one of the anticipated major benefits of polio eradication is the cessation of immunization. Unlike the live smallpox (vaccinia) vaccine strain, Sabin OPV strains commonly spread from vaccinees to close nonimmune contacts and are genetically unstable, regaining certain wild virus characteristics upon replication in the human gut. The former offers the advantage of attaining maximum benefit from the vaccine. The latter has the disadvantage of rare adverse neurological consequences in highly immune populations.

Continuous person-to-person circulation of vaccine-derived polioviruses (VDPV) in poorly immunized polio-free populations may lead to sufficient genetic changes to assume characteristic wild poliovirus neurovirulence and transmissibility. Retrospective evidence suggests that circulating (feral) VDPV type 2 may have caused polio 10 or more years ago for limited periods in Egypt (9). The polio outbreak on the island of Hispaniola in late 2000 and early 2001 extends these findings to feral VDPV type 1 (8, 27). However, observations in Cuba and elsewhere over the past 40 years suggest that circulation of OPV strains in well-immunized populations cease about 3 months after the last NID. Whether these observations apply to well-immunized populations in environments biologically favoring transmission is unknown (15, 20, 25).

Adding further to the complexity of stopping immunization are the rare immunocompromised individuals who may shed OPV-derived viruses for a prolonged period. Nearly a dozen such persons have been identified worldwide over the last 38 years. Some have stopped spontaneously, but some have shed vaccine-derived poliovirus up to 10 years or more (46).

The strategy for stopping immunization must both maximize the benefits and minimize the risks (12, 46). Strategies currently under consideration include (i) global and/or regional "pulse" immunization campaigns with OPV to maintain high levels of immunity and prevent circulation of VDPV until synchronized global discontinuation of OPV or (ii) gradually replacing OPV with IPV for routine immunization worldwide to achieve cessation of all OPV, followed by cessation of IPV. Each is associated with specific advantages (financial benefits for OPV discontinuation) and disadvantages (cost of switching to IPV) and inherent uncertainties (risk of continued poliovirus circulation in certain populations or prolonged virus replication in immunodeficient persons). A research agenda coordinated by WHO addresses these remaining questions and issues. Nevertheless, several generalities are already clear. Unprecedented collaboration among countries, regions, and indeed the entire world will be required to implement a global OPV discontinuation strategy. Manufacturers will need sufficient lead time to produce adequate quantities of IPV. The financial implication for either of these strategies must be carefully considered. Whatever the strategy, contingency plans and stockpiles of OPV (and possibly IPV) will be required in the event an outbreak of polio may occur postcessation of vaccination.

CONCLUSION

The rationale for supporting the polio eradication initiative differs for different proponents. For Brazil and other developing American countries, the rationale for adopting nationwide mass OPV immunization to eliminate polio was simply that all other strategies had failed. For PAHO, and later WHO, mass immunization against polio offered a regional and global public health promise and a vehicle for improving other childhood immunization rates and strengthening primary health care. For Rotary International, polio eradication was a great humanitarian effort, with achievable goals worthy of support by its worldwide membership. For developed country partners, the eradication initiative was justified on humanitarian and eventual cost-savings grounds. For developing countries of endemicity, polio eradication offered a tangible achievement in public health and a promise for the future. These diverse motivations brought strength to the initiative. However, the rationale expounded by Sabin remains the roots of the initiative. The only way to fully control poliomyelitis in the developing tropical world with limited health infrastructure is to interrupt virus transmission through mass OPV immunization. Global eradication is a natural outcome.

The authors thank Ciro de Quadros, Olen Kew, and Mark Pallansch for their critical reviews and helpful comments.

REFERENCES

1. **Anonymous.** 1982. Can infectious diseases be eradicated? A report on the International Conference on the Eradication of Infectious Diseases. *Rev. Infect. Dis.* **4:**912–983.
2. **Aylward, R. B., H. F. Hull, S. L. Cochi, R. W. Sutter, J. M. Olive, and B. Melgaard.** 2000. Disease eradication as a public health strategy: a case study of poliomyelitis eradication. *Bull. W. H. O.* **78:**285–297.
3. **Aylward, R. B., H. F. Hull, C. A. de Quadros, J. M. Olive, and B. Melgaard.** 1998. Disease eradication initiatives and general health services: ensuring common principles lead to mutual benefits, p. 61–74. *In* W. R. Dowdle and D. R. Hopkins (ed.), *The Eradication of Infectious Diseases.* John Wiley and Sons, New York, N.Y.
4. **Baptista-Risi, J.** 1984. The control of poliomyelitis in Brazil. *Rev. Infect. Dis.* **6**(Suppl. 2)**:**S400–S403.
5. **Baptista-Risi, J.** 1997. Poliomyelitis in Brazil, p. 159–179. *In* T. M. Daniel and F. C. Robbins (ed.), *Polio.* University of Rochester Press, Rochester, N.Y.
6. **Centers for Disease Control and Prevention.** 1993. Recommendations of the International Task Force for Disease Eradication. *Morb. Mortal. Wkly. Rep.* **42:**1–38.
7. **Centers for Disease Control and Prevention.** 1994. Certification of poliomyelitis eradication in the Americas. *Morb. Mortal. Wkly. Rep.* **43:**720–722.
8. **Centers for Disease Control and Prevention.** 2000. Outbreak of poliomyelitis—Dominican Republic and Haiti, 2000. *Morb. Mortal. Wkly. Rep.* **49:**1094–1103.
9. **Centers for Disease Control and Prevention.** 2001. Circulation of a type 2 vaccine-derived poliovirus—Egypt, 1982–1993. *Morb. Mortal. Wkly. Rep.* **50:**41–51.

10. **Chin, J.** 1984. Can paralytic poliomyelitis be eliminated? *Rev. Infect. Dis.* **6**(Suppl. 2):S581–S585.
11. **Cochi, S. L., C. A. de Quadros, S. Dittmann, S. Foster, J. Galvez Tan, F. Grant, J. M. Olive, H. Pigman, C. Taylor, and K. A. Wang.** 1998. Group report: what are the societal and political criteria for disease eradication? p. 157–175. *In* W. R. Dowdle and D. R. Hopkins (ed.), *The Eradication of Infectious Diseases.* John Wiley and Sons, New York, N.Y.
12. **Cochi, S. L., R. W. Sutter, O. M. Kew, M. Pallansch, and W. R. Dowdle.** 1997. *A Decision Tree for Stopping Polio Immunization.* EPI/POLIO/TECH.97/WP18. The World Health Organization, Geneva, Switzerland.
13. **de Quadros, C. A.** 1997. Onwards towards victory, p. 181–198. *In* T. M. Daniel and F. C. Robbins (ed.), *Polio.* University of Rochester Press, Rochester, N.Y.
14. **de Quadros, C. A., B. S. Hersh, J. M. Olive, J. K. Andrus, C. M. da Silveira, and P. A. Carrasco.** 1997. Eradication of wild poliovirus from the Americas: acute flaccid paralysis surveillance, 1988–1995. *J. Infect. Dis.* **175**(Suppl. 1):S37–S42.
15. **Dove, A. W., and V. R. Racaniello.** 1997. The polio eradication effort: should vaccine eradication be next? *Science* **277**:779–780.
16. **Dowdle, W. R., and M. E. Birmingham.** 1997. The biologic principles of poliovirus eradication. *J. Infect. Dis.* **175**(Suppl. 1):S286–S292.
17. **Fenner, F., A. Hall, and W. R. Dowdle.** 1998. What is eradication? p. 3–17. *In* W. R. Dowdle and D. Hopkins (ed.), *The Eradication of Infectious Diseases.* John Wiley and Sons, New York, N.Y.
18. **Fenner, F., D. A. Henderson, I. Arita, A. Jezek, and I. Ladnyi.** 1988. *Smallpox and Its Eradication.* The World Health Organization, Geneva, Switzerland.
19. **Fernandez de Castro, J.** 1984. Mass vaccination against poliomyelitis in Mexico. *Rev. Infect. Dis.* **6**(Suppl. 2):S397–S399.
20. **Fine, P. E., and I. A. Carneiro.** 1999. Transmissibility and persistence of oral polio vaccine viruses: implications for the global poliomyelitis eradication initiative. *Am. J. Epidemiol.* **150**:1001–1021.
21. **Gregg, M. B.** 1984. Paralytic poliomyelitis can be eliminated. *Rev. Infect. Dis.* **6**(Suppl. 2):S577–S580.
22. **Henderson, D. A.** 1998. Eradication: lessons from the past. *Bull. W. H. O.* **76**(Suppl. 2):17–21.
23. **Henderson, R. H.** 1984. The expanded programme on immunization of the World Health Organization. *Rev. Infect. Dis.* **6**(Suppl. 2):S475–S479.
24. **Hinman, A. R., W. H. Foege, C. A. de Quadros, P. A. Patriarca, W. A. Orenstein, and E. W. Brink.** 1987. The case for global eradication of poliomyelitis. *Bull. W. H. O.* **65**:835–840.
25. **Hull, H. F., and R. B. Aylward.** 1997. Ending polio immunization. *Science* **277**:780.
26. **John, T. J.** 1984. Poliomyelitis in India: prospects and problems of control. *Rev. Infect. Dis.* **6**:S438–S441.
27. **Kew, O. M., V. Morris-Glasgow, M. Landaverde, C. Burns, J. Shaw, Z. Garib, J. Andre, E. Blackman, C. Freeman, J. Jorba, R. W. Sutter, G. Tambini, L. Venczel, C. Pedreira, F. Laender, H. Shimizu, T. Yoneyama, T. Miyamura, H. van der Avoort, M. Oberste, D. Kilpatrick, S. L. Cochi, M. Pallansch, and C. A. de Quadros.** Outbreak of poliomyelitis in Hispaniola associated with circulating type 1 vaccine-derived poliovirus. *Science* **296**:356–359.
28. **Mas, L. P.** 1999. Eradication of poliomyelitis in Cuba: a historical perspective. *Bull. W. H. O.* **77**:681–687.
29. **Ottesen, E., W. R. Dowdle, F. Fenner, K.-O. Habermehl, T. J. John, M. Koch, G. Medley, A. Muller, S. Ostroff, and H. Zeichhardt.** 1998. Group report: how is eradication to be defined and what are the biological criteria? p. 47–59. *In* W. R. Dowdle and D. Hopkins (ed.), *The Eradication of Infectious Diseases: Dahlem Workshop Reports.* John Wiley, New York, N.Y.
30. **Pan American Health Organization.** 1985. Director announces campaign to eradicate poliomyelitis from the Americas. *Bull. Pan Am. Health Organ.* **19**:213–215.
31. **Patriarca, P. A., P. F. Wright, and T. J. John.** 1991. Factors affecting the immunogenicity of oral poliovirus vaccine in developing countries: review. *Rev. Infect. Dis.* **13**:926–939.
32. **Pinheiro, F. P., O. M. Kew, M. H. Hatch, C. M. da Silveira, and C. A. de Quadros.** 1997. Eradication of wild poliovirus from the Americas: wild poliovirus surveillance—laboratory issues. *J. Infect. Dis.* **175**(Suppl. 1):S43–S49.
33. **Plotkin, S., and H. Koproski.** 1959. *Epidemiologic Studies of Safety and Efficacy of Vaccination with CHAT Strain of Attenuated Poliovirus in Leopoldville, Belgian Congo, in Live Poliovirus Vaccines.* Scientific publication no. 44. Pan American Sanitary Bureau, Washington, D.C.
34. **Robbins, F. C., and C. A. de Quadros.** 1997. Certification of the eradication of indigenous transmission of wild poliovirus in the Americas. *J. Infect. Dis.* **175**(Suppl. 1):S281–S285.
35. **Robbins, F. C.** 1984. Summary and recommendations. *Rev. Infect. Dis.* **6**(Suppl. 2):S596–S600.
36. **Robinson, D.** 1984. Political, administrative, and economic resources for the control of poliomyelitis. *Rev. Infect. Dis.* **6**(Suppl. 2):S586–S588.
37. **Rodriguez, C. R.** 1984. Cuba: mass polio vaccination program, 1962–1982. *Rev. Infect. Dis.* **6**(Suppl. 2):S408–S412.
38. **Sabin, A. B.** 1980. Vaccination against poliomyelitis in economically underdeveloped countries. *Bull. W. H. O.* **58**:141–157.
39. **Sabin, A. B.** 1984. Strategies for elimination of poliomyelitis in different parts of the world with use of oral poliovirus vaccine. *Rev. Infect. Dis.* **6**(Suppl. 2):S391–S396.
40. **Sabin, A. B.** 1985. Oral poliovirus vaccine: history of its development and use and current challenge to eliminate poliomyelitis from the world. *J. Infect. Dis.* **151**:420–436.
41. **Sabin, A. B., M. Ramos-Alvarez, J. Alvarez-Amezquita, W. Pelon, R. Michaels, I. Spigland, M. Koch, J. Barnes, and J. Rhim.** 1960. Live, orally given poliovirus vaccine: effects of rapid mass immunization on population under conditions of massive enteric infections with other viruses. *JAMA* **173**:1521–1626.
42. **Task Force for Child Survival and Development.** 1988. *Protection of the World's Children: an Agenda for the 1990s.* Task Force for Child Survival and Development, Atlanta, Ga.
43. **Wang, K., L. B. Zhang, M. W. Otten, Jr., X. L. Zhang, C. Yasuo, R. Z. Zhang, T. Xu, X. Liu, M. Liu, Q. L. Li, J. J. Yu, and Z. Wang.** 1997. Status of the eradication of indigenous wild poliomyelitis in the People's Republic of China. *J. Infect. Dis.* **175**(Suppl. 1):S105–S112.
44. **Ward, N. A.** 1984. Practicalities of a global poliomyelitis control program. *Rev. Infect. Dis.* **6**(Suppl. 2):S591–S593.
45. **Warren, K. S.** 1988. Conference: Protecting the world's children, an agenda for the 1990s. *Lancet* **i**:659–659.
46. **Wood, D. J., R. W. Sutter, and W. R. Dowdle.** 2000. Stopping poliovirus vaccination after eradication: issues and challenges. *Bull. W. H. O.* **78**:347–357.
47. **World Health Assembly.** 1988. Global eradication of poliomyelitis by the year 2000: resolution of the 41st World Health Assembly. Resolution WHA 41.28. World Health Organization, Geneva, Switzerland.

48. **World Health Organization.** 1978. *Primary Health Care: Report of the International Conference on Primary Health Care.* World Health Organization, Geneva, Switzerland.
49. **World Health Organization.** 1997. *Polio: the Beginning of the End.* World Health Organization, Geneva, Switzerland.
50. **World Health Organization.** 1998. *Global Eradication of Poliomyelitis: Report of the Meeting on the Scientific Basis for Stopping Polio Immunization.* WHO/EPI/GEN/98.12. World Health Organization, Geneva, Switzerland.
51. **World Health Organization.** 1998. *Global Eradication of Poliomyelitis: Report of the Third Meeting of the Global Commission for the Certification of the Eradication of Polio.* WHO/EPI/GEN/98.12. World Health Organization, Geneva, Switzerland.
52. **World Health Organization.** 1999. *WHO Global Action Plan for Laboratory Containment of Wild Polioviruses.* WHO/V&B/99.32. World Health Organization, Geneva, Switzerland.
53. **Yang, B., J. Zhang, M. W. Otten, Jr., K. Kusumoto, T. Jiang, R. Zhang, L. Zhang, and K. A. Wang.** 1995. Eradication of poliomyelitis: progress in the People's Republic of China. *Pediatr. Infect. Dis. J.* **14:**308–314.

*Molecular Biology of Picornaviruses*
Editors, B. L. Semler and E. Wimmer
©2002 ASM Press, Washington, DC 20036-2904

The Mechanism of Poliovirus Eradication

OLEN M. KEW AND MARK A. PALLANSCH

39

Fifty years ago, polio was endemic throughout the world (47). Children everywhere faced odds of ~1 in 200 of being paralyzed for life following a poliovirus infection. The first major step toward the conquest of polio was the introduction in 1955 of the injectable inactivated polio vaccine (IPV) of Salk and Youngner (49). Widespread use of IPV in developed countries sharply decreased the incidence of polio in those settings (47, 49), but IPV was much more challenging to administer in developing countries. In 1961, the live, attenuated oral polio vaccine (OPV) of Sabin was licensed for use in the United States and other countries (54). OPV has several logistic and biological advantages over IPV, including ease of administration by oral route, lower cost, and the ability to induce intestinal immunity capable of effectively blocking person-to-person spread of poliovirus in an immune population (54). OPV was initially used in mass immunization campaigns in both developed (e.g., the "Sabin Oral Sundays" campaigns of 1962 in the United States) and developing countries. By 1963, Cuba became the first country to eliminate polio through the comprehensive use of OPV in mass campaigns (17). By the late 1960s, polio had nearly disappeared in most developed countries (54), but the disease persisted widely in the developing world.

Systematic international efforts to eradicate polio from the developing world began in the Americas in 1985, when the Pan American Health Organization (PAHO) declared a target date of 1990 for the eradication of polio throughout the Americas (45). Feasibility of the PAHO goal had been demonstrated by the effectiveness of the mass OPV campaign approach in Cuba and Brazil (51). In view of the rapid progress attained in the Americas, the World Health Assembly resolved in 1988 to eradicate polio worldwide by the year 2000 (62). A detailed account of the origins of polio eradication is presented in chapter 38 of this volume.

CURRENT PROGRESS TOWARD POLIO ERADICATION

At the time of the World Health Assembly Resolution, wild polioviruses were circulating unabated in much of the developing world, with an estimated 350,000 paralytic polio cases occurring in >125 endemic countries in 1988 (65). By the end of 2001, poliovirus endemicity was restricted to <15 countries, and the total number of polio cases worldwide was estimated from comprehensive surveillance to be <1,000, a reduction of >99% in 13 years (65) (Fig. 1). Wild poliovirus type 2 was last detected in October 1999 in Uttar Pradesh, India (11). Wild poliovirus type 3 was detected in only five countries (Afghanistan, India, Nigeria, Pakistan, and Somalia) in 2001. Wild poliovirus type 1 was detected in the same five countries and in nine others (Angola, Bulgaria [importation], Ethiopia, Egypt, Georgia [importation], Mauritania, Niger, Sudan, and Zambia) (65). Since 1988, immunization has spared an estimated 8 million children worldwide from paralytic poliomyelitis (54). Regular updates on the progress toward global polio eradication are posted on the World Health Organization (WHO) web site, http://www.polio-eradication.org/.

Two WHO Regions have been certified free of indigenous wild poliovirus circulation, the Americas in 1994 (last indigenous case: Peru, 1991) (7), and the Western Pacific Region in 2000 (last indigenous case: Cambodia, 1997) (9). Certification of the European Region (last indigenous case: Turkey, 1998) is likely to occur in 2002 (65). Wild poliovirus circulation is highly localized to parts of northern India in the Southeast Asia Region, but is still more widespread in the African and Eastern Mediterranean Regions (65) (Fig. 1 and 2).

BASIC STRATEGY FOR POLIO ERADICATION

The basic strategy of polio eradication rests on four main pillars: (i) high routine immunization coverage of infants with OPV, (ii) supplementary OPV immunization through National Immunization Days (NIDs) and Subnational Immunization Days (SNIDs), (iii) sensitive surveillance for poliovirus, and (iv) targeted door-to-door "mop-up" OPV immunization in areas of focal transmission. Routine immunization is provided throughout the year according to

---

Olen M. Kew ■ Division of Viral and Rickettsial Diseases, National Center for Infectious Diseases, Centers for Disease Control and Prevention, 1600 Clifton Rd., Mailstop G-10, Atlanta, GA 30333. *Mark A. Pallansch* ■ Division of Viral and Rickettsial Diseases, National Center for Infectious Diseases, Centers for Disease Control and Prevention, 1600 Clifton Rd., Mailstop G-17, Atlanta, GA 30333.

481

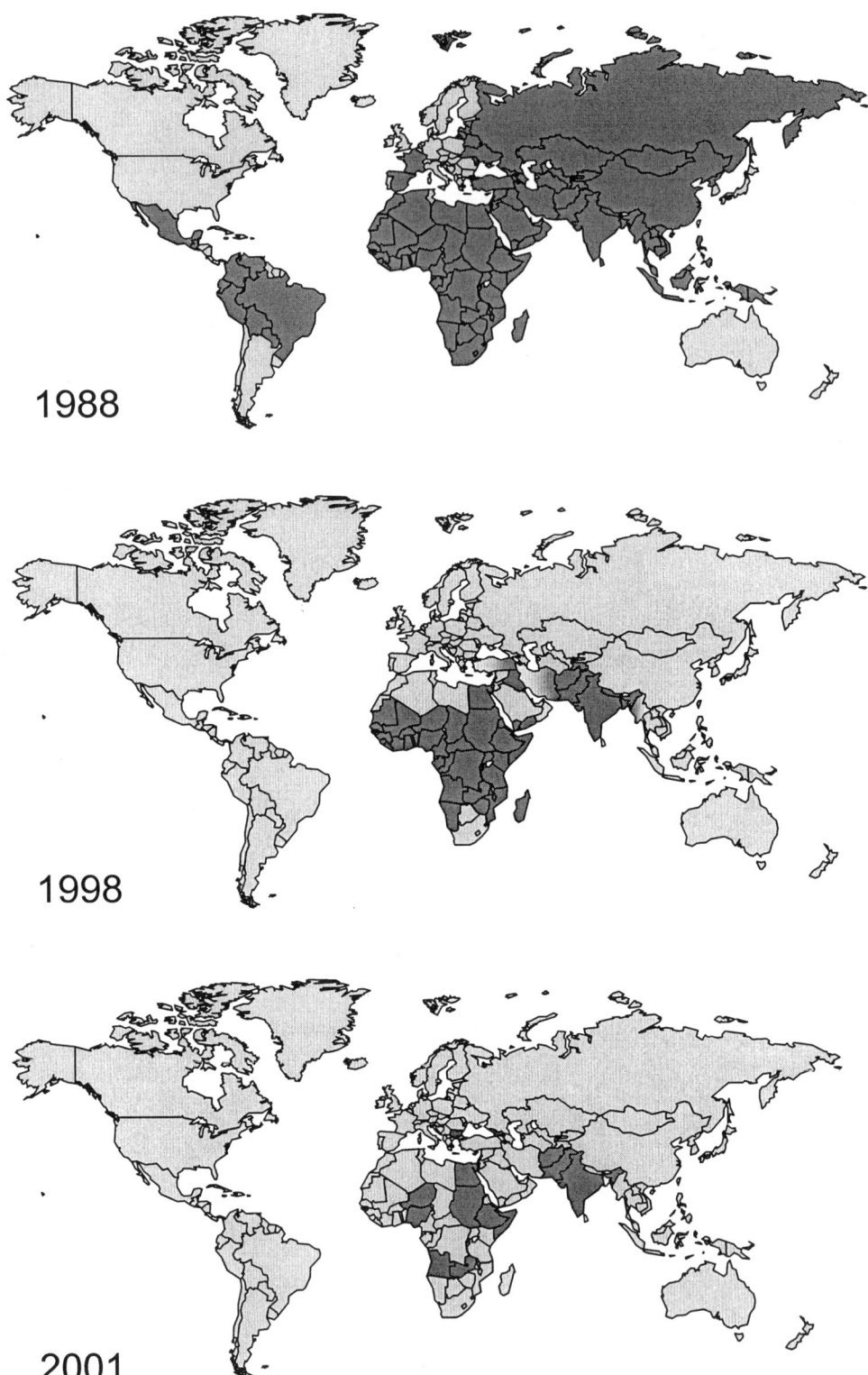

FIGURE 1 Countries with indigenous wild poliovirus circulation (shaded) in 1988, 1998, and 2001.

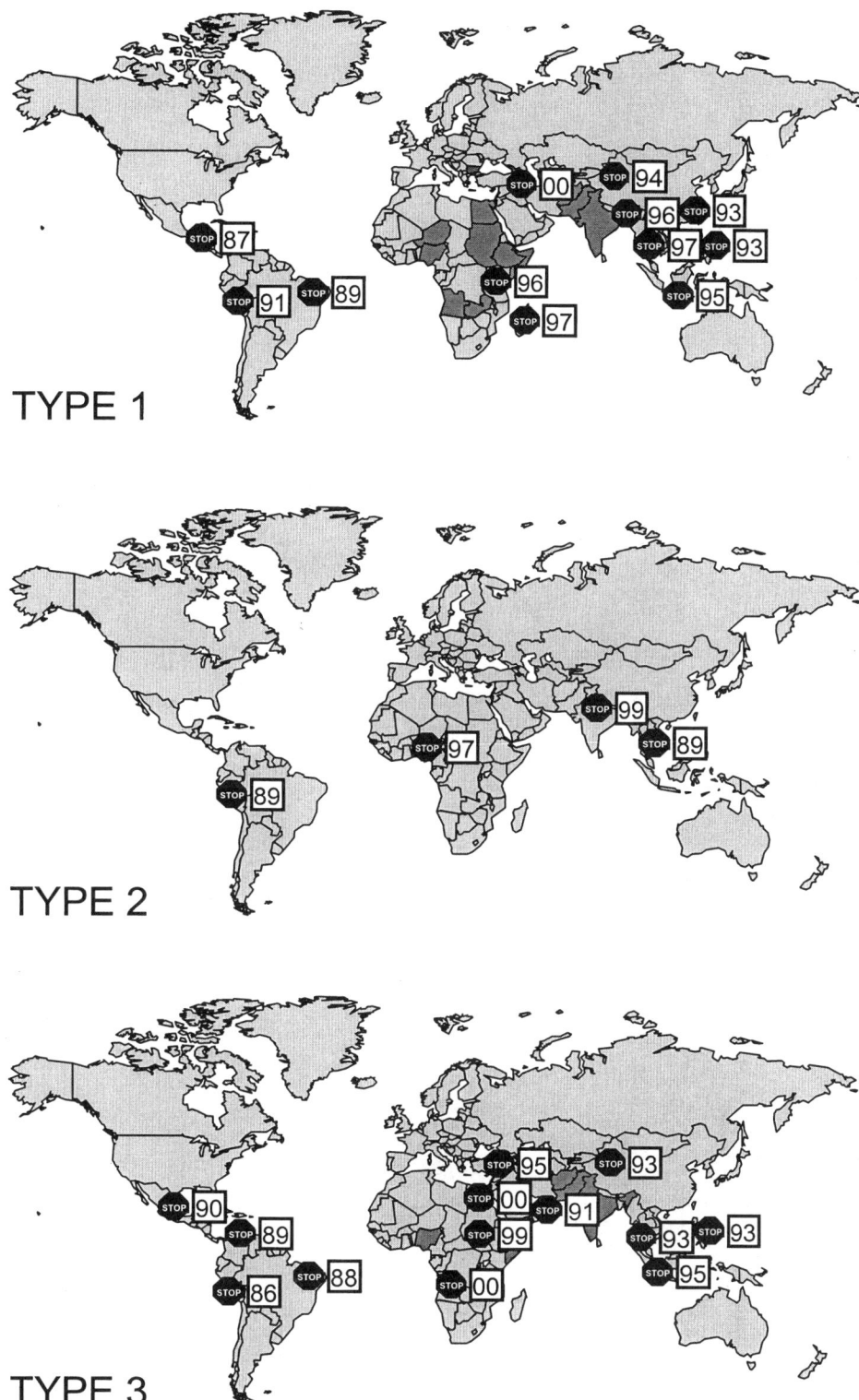

FIGURE 2 Progressive eradication of wild poliovirus genotypes, 1988 to 2001. Stop signs indicate the year and location where the last isolate was obtained for each extinct genotype.

the age of the child. However, very high rates of routine OPV immunization are required to block poliovirus circulation in areas having high population densities, large birth cohorts, poor hygiene and sanitation, and tropical climates (23, 46, 51, 54). In such areas, the density of susceptible nonimmune children (including newborns) may be very high, contacts with infected individuals may be frequent, the efficiency of poliovirus transmission is high, and the duration of the peak poliovirus/enterovirus transmission season is prolonged. Under such conditions, routine OPV coverage rates exceeding 90% may be insufficient to block poliovirus circulation (23, 54). Such rates are currently unattainable through routine immunization in the least developed countries. However, high-quality supplementary immunization in the form of NIDs and SNIDs has succeeded in raising population immunity rates above the thresholds required to block poliovirus transmission. The biological rationale for this approach is that high levels of population immunity can be synchronously induced during the low poliovirus transmission season (winter months), when the fewest chains of transmission sustain poliovirus endemicity. NIDs are usually conducted through at least two successive rounds spaced about a month apart. Continuation of NID or SNID rounds into the spring months may be needed in highly endemic areas to sustain high levels of population immunity and to delay or eliminate the onset of the peak transmission season. When population immunity rises, the frequency of productive contacts between infected and susceptible individuals falls below the threshold critical for continued propagation of chains of transmission, and circulation stops.

Supplementary immunization is the mainstay of polio eradication in developing countries (65), not only because of its biological advantages, but also because of logistical advantages and the potential for excellent community outreach. In 2001, approximately 575 million children in 94 countries received ~2 billion doses of OPV through supplementary immunization. In the winter of 2001–2002, nearly 150 million children received OPV in two rounds of NIDs in India. In west and central Africa, 80 million children were immunized in NIDs synchronized across 16 countries in what was the largest public health activity in the history of that continent (64).

High-quality NIDs and SNIDs, especially when coupled with high levels of routine immunization, can achieve the eradication of indigenous wild polioviruses in less than 3 years, even in areas where the environmental conditions for poliovirus circulation are very favorable (such as in southern China, Indonesia, and Bangladesh). Immunization strategies are driven by poliovirus surveillance, which is used to guide the intensified SNIDs and mop-up campaigns to the reservoir communities where the chains of poliovirus transmission continue to survive and propagate.

POLIOVIRUS SURVEILLANCE

Surveillance for wild polioviruses has two arms: (i) acute flaccid paralysis (AFP) case investigations and (ii) virologic studies of polioviruses obtained from clinical specimens. AFP surveillance by itself is neither highly specific nor highly sensitive for detecting individual wild poliovirus infections (2). The background rate of AFP from etiologies other than wild poliovirus infection (including Guillain-Barré syndrome, transverse myelitis, and transient [or occasionally permanent] paralyses associated with nonpolio enterovirus infections) is at least 1 case per 100,000 persons <15 years of age (2, 23, 44, 54). Therefore, the detection of an AFP case does not necessarily indicate infection with wild poliovirus. Virologic analysis of clinical specimens is needed to investigate the possible etiologic role of wild polioviruses.

The sensitivity of AFP surveillance to detect most wild poliovirus infections is limited because only ~0.5% of nonimmune children infected with wild poliovirus show signs of AFP (2, 23, 44, 54). In populations with higher levels of immunity, AFP cases may appear in fewer than 1 of 10,000 wild poliovirus infections (50). Regardless of these limitations, all effectively performing AFP surveillance systems are able, over time, to detect endemic poliovirus circulation in a population. In situations where effective AFP surveillance is difficult to achieve, supplementary surveillance activities, such as sampling community contacts of AFP cases, stool surveys of healthy children, or environmental sampling, may be implemented in suspected high-risk areas to increase sensitivity for detecting wild polioviruses (40, 42, 50, 55, 57).

The importance of surveillance increases with each stage of polio eradication. At the current advanced stage, it is essential to identify all remaining community reservoirs sustaining wild poliovirus circulation so that they may be targeted for supplementary immunization activities. At present, the key surveillance questions are as follows: (i) How can we identify reservoir communities? (ii) What are the virologic links between infections or cases? (iii) How do we know when wild poliovirus eradication has been achieved? (iv) Is there any residual poliovirus circulation associated with vaccine-derived polioviruses (VDPVs)? These questions have been addressed through the integration of AFP surveillance, standard virologic methods, and detailed molecular and phylogenetic analysis of poliovirus isolates, an approach described as molecular epidemiology.

POLIOVIRUS SURVEILLANCE METHODS

The laboratory tools of poliovirus surveillance are well developed. A global network of 147 formally accredited and highly competent poliovirus laboratories has been established by WHO to apply these tools in support of polio eradication (15). Standard methods for poliovirus isolation in cultured cells (63) have been enhanced by the use of recombinant murine cells expressing the poliovirus receptor (28, 48). Polioviruses can be distinguished from nonpolio enteroviruses either by using standard typing assays (63) or by PCR using poliovirus group-specific (35) or serotype-specific (34) primer sets. Intratypic differentiation (ITD) of poliovirus isolates (testing whether they are vaccine related or wild) is performed throughout the global network using one antigenic and one molecular method (15). The standard antigenic ITD method uses an enzyme-linked immunosorbent assay system with preparations of highly specific cross-adsorbed antisera (58, 59). The molecular ITD methods use genotype-specific nucleic acid probes (18, 19), genotype-specific PCR primers (37, 66, 67), or PCR coupled to analysis of restriction fragment length polymorphism (3).

The purpose of ITD is to screen out poliovirus isolates that are closely related (>99% VP1 sequence identity) to the Sabin OPV strains and are unlikely to be of current epidemiologic importance. The remaining poliovirus isolates are either wild polioviruses or atypical VDPVs. Since the beginning of 2001, network laboratories routinely sequence the complete VP1 region of any wild poliovirus isolated from an AFP case. Analysis of the full ~900-nucleotide VP1 region is performed in order to obtain the degree of phylogenetic resolution necessary to reconstruct individual chains of transmission, as is currently needed to distinguish among local endemic reservoirs (53). The sequencing windows may be widened to the complete poliovirus genome in order to increase resolution (30, 39). Sequence relationships are generally summarized in the form of phylogenetic trees (Fig. 3 through 5).

THE POLIOVIRUS MOLECULAR CLOCK

Polioviruses are among the most rapidly evolving viruses known. This rapid evolution permits the patterns of poliovirus transmission to be followed with precision (39, 53). Several factors combine to determine the overall rates of virus evolution. These include the replicase error rates, the virus population size and growth rate, the frequency of genetic bottlenecks, the intensity of selective forces, and the existence of mechanisms for genetic exchange (21). Error rates for the poliovirus replicase have been estimated to be 10^{-4} to 10^{-5} per site per replication (20, 22, 60), very close to the error catastrophe threshold for the poliovirus genome (27). Nucleotide substitutions (~90% of which in the coding region are to synonymous codons) accumulate at an overall rate of 10^{-2} substitutions per site per year and at ~3×10^{-2} substitutions per year at synonymous sites (4, 24, 31, 33, 39, 41). Evolution rates appear to be similar across serotypes and between wild and vaccine-derived polioviruses. Interestingly, the bottlenecks driving the rapid evolution of polioviruses appear also to occur during replication in the human intestine (in addition to that during person-to-person transmission) (6, 36). They also appear to be largely independent of immune selection, as evolution rates are similar during prolonged replication in immunodeficient patients (4, 33, 41) and during widespread circulation (24, 30, 31, 39).

Many poliovirus clinical isolates are recombinants (6, 26, 30, 38, 39). Heterotypic recombinants are frequently isolated from vaccinees given trivalent OPV (6, 26, 38). All wild polioviruses probably have a recent history of recombination, because frequent genetic exchange with other species C enteroviruses and (vaccine-derived) polioviruses appears to be typical of circulating polioviruses (30, 32, 39; H.-M. Liu, D.-P. Zheng, L.-B. Zhang, O. M. Kew, and M. A. Pallansch, presented at the American Society for Virology, Ft. Collins, Colo., abstr. W34-6, 2000). Crossovers appear to be most common in the noncapsid region, less common in the 5′-untranslated region (25), and rare within the capsid region (presumably because of structural constraints) (39).

Molecular clock data have been used to estimate the dates of the common ancestors to wild (39, 53) and vaccine-derived (4, 30, 33) poliovirus isolates. Phylogenetic relationships inferred from the pattern of fixation of nucleotide substitutions may be confirmed by the detection of common recombination breakpoints among related viruses (30, 39).

THE REMAINING POLIOVIRUS RESERVOIRS

The global distribution of wild poliovirus genotypes has been reviewed (29, 31). Poliovirus eradication has achieved the elimination of individual lineages (equivalent to chains of transmission), different genotypes (groups of related lineages sharing >85% nucleotide sequence identity), and probably wild poliovirus type 2 (11). Most of the genotypes found in 1988 appear now to be extinct (Fig. 2).

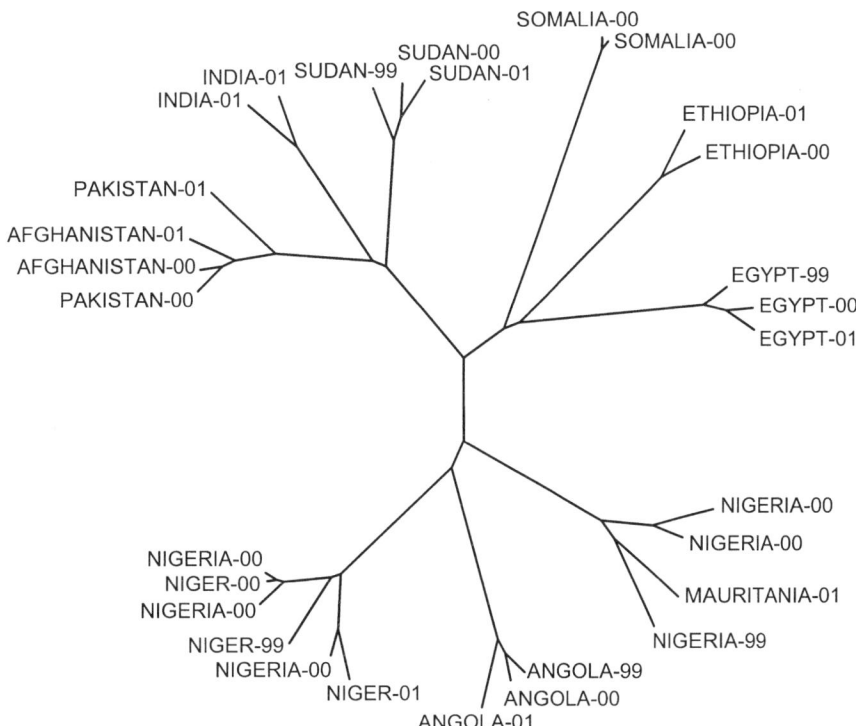

FIGURE 3 Trees of VP1 sequence relationships among representative isolates of surviving type 1 poliovirus genotypes.

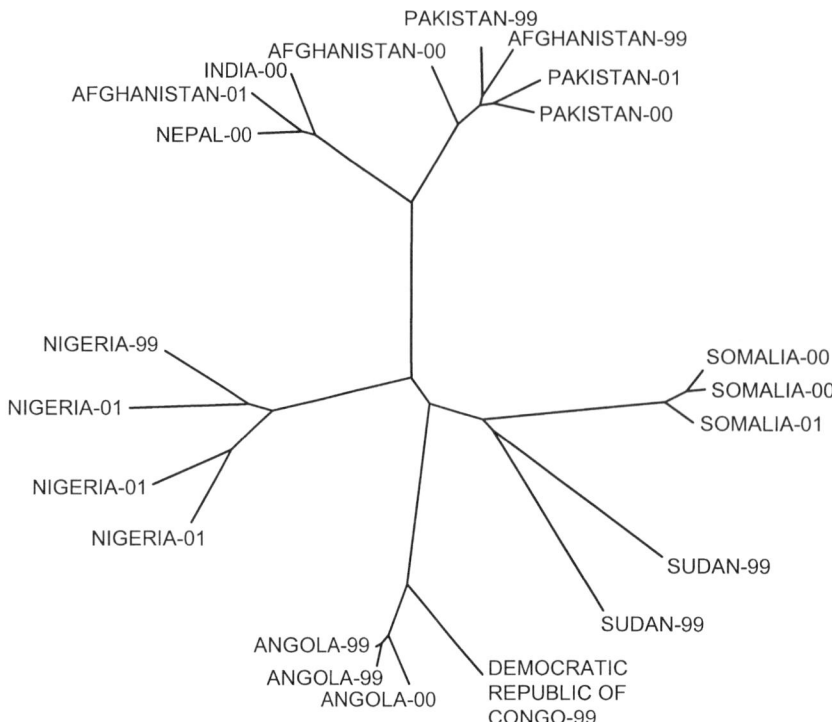

FIGURE 4 Trees of VP1 sequence relationships among representative isolates of surviving type 3 poliovirus genotypes.

The remaining wild poliovirus reservoirs are localized to areas with pockets of low OPV coverage and where demographic and environmental conditions favor poliovirus circulation. During the peak months of poliovirus circulation (summer through fall in many areas), virus spreads from the reservoir communities (where poliovirus circulation is sustained throughout the year) to adjacent nonreservoir indicator communities (where the density of nonimmune susceptible children can support some poliovirus circulation during the peak transmission season). Within a country or region, it is important to identify and target reservoir communities for intensified SNIDs and mop-up campaigns.

Molecular epidemiologic methods are routinely used to help identify reservoir communities (65). This has led to a refinement in the concept of virus importation, which in previous usage referred to virus transmission across political boundaries. Indeed, many importations over long distances have been documented (31). However, reservoirs and their associated indicator communities frequently overlap international borders (Fig. 3 to 5) (68), underscoring the importance of regional synchronization of NIDs. Even more important are the patterns of importation from reservoir communities to indicator communities within a country. Effective intervention in the reservoir communities, especially during the low transmission season, prevents the subsequent spread to indicator communities.

High vaccine coverage rates must be maintained in polio-free countries to prevent reestablishment of polio endemicity. In recent years, wild poliovirus has been imported into Iran from Afghanistan and Pakistan (multiple importations), from India to China in 1999 (16), from Angola to the Cape Verde Islands in 2000 (8), and from the subcontinent to Bulgaria (13) and Georgia in 2001 (Fig. 5). Polio cases associated with these importations have revealed pockets of unimmunized children in the new host areas, prompting local immunization responses. However, by far the most effective response is to eliminate the source reservoirs.

DETECTING GAPS IN AFP SURVEILLANCE

Gaps in vaccine coverage are frequently signaled by the appearance of polio cases. However, weak immunization programs are often accompanied by weak surveillance, such that polio cases are missed. One indication of inadequate surveillance is a detection rate for AFP cases below the target rate 1 per 100,000 persons <15 years of age. However, local gaps in surveillance may be difficult to detect from aggregate AFP data. Molecular epidemiologic methods open a new avenue for detecting gaps in polio surveillance. In areas with good surveillance, poliovirus isolates representing frequent sampling of a single chain of transmission are typically closely related (usually >99.5% VP1 sequence identity among the closest relatives). These closely related viruses are represented on phylogenetic trees as short branch connections between sequences (30, 53). Long branch connections between isolate sequences indicate missing information. If the virus was imported, the missing information may be recovered from the sequence relationships among viruses from the source reservoir (31). However, in other circumstances, no closely related viruses can be found, and the recent virologic history of the isolate lineage is indeterminate. For example, gaps in surveillance in southern Egypt were inferred from the sequence data, as indigenous type 3 isolates in 1999 appeared as "orphan lineages" on phylogenetic trees, and the closest relatives were isolated nearly 3 years earlier.

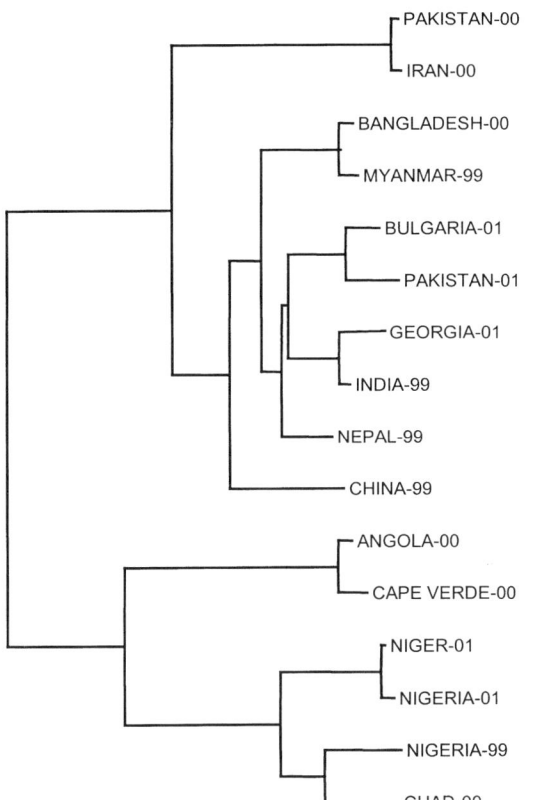

FIGURE 5 Trees showing long-range importation and cross-border transmission of wild type 1 poliovirus lineages, 1999 to 2001. The VP1 sequence of the Bulgaria isolate was kindly provided by Lucia Fiore.

MONITORING LABORATORY PERFORMANCE

Performance within the WHO Global Laboratory Network is reviewed by an annual accreditation process (15). Various supplementary approaches are implemented to monitor ongoing laboratory performance. A serious challenge to the integrity of poliovirus surveillance data is the occurrence of poliovirus contamination of cultures. Very high workloads in several network laboratories increase the risk of contamination. Fortunately, sequence analysis can usually distinguish contaminants from true clinical isolates. Contaminants are easily recognized when they are standard wild reference strains, such as Mahoney, MEF-1, or Saukett (Sabin strain contaminants are of little current programmatic importance), but are more difficult to recognize when they are the wild polioviruses indigenous to a country or community. However, when wild polioviruses isolated at different times and locations have identical VP1 sequences, contamination is suspected, as such sequence identities are inconsistent with the rapid rate of evolution of poliovirus genomes. If the surveillance question is crucial, the sequencing window may be expanded to increase confidence in the observed genetic relationships. At the advanced stages of polio eradication, laboratory contamination could have severe programmatic consequences if unrecognized, prompting the diversion of resources into unnecessary immunization campaigns mobilizing large populations and costing millions of dollars, as well as potentially delaying certification of a Region as polio free.

DIRECT DETECTION OF WILD POLIOVIRUS CIRCULATION

The detection sensitivity of AFP surveillance is limited by the paralytic attack rates of wild polioviruses as well as the efficiency in identifying paralyzed children in a population. The paralytic case-to-infection ratio in unimmunized populations is highest for wild type 1 polioviruses (~1 case per 200 infections), intermediate for wild type 3 polioviruses (~1 per 1,200), and lowest for wild type 2 polioviruses (<1 per 2,500) (43). The efficiency of the AFP surveillance system is the result of the significant enrichment of the population from whom clinical specimens are obtained. This effectiveness is evident when one considers that even though more than 700 million children are living in countries with AFP surveillance, all areas of endemic poliovirus circulation in the world have been identified by testing "only" 50,000 specimens each year. However, in small populations and over short periods of time, it is possible to miss low levels of virus circulation because the expected number of AFP cases due to poliovirus infection will be small. Because of these limitations, several approaches have been taken to improve diagnostic sensitivities, particularly in areas where AFP surveillance is suspected to be weak.

One approach has been to sample healthy contacts of AFP cases, a form of targeted community survey. However, at advanced stages of eradication, most AFP cases are not associated with wild poliovirus infections, and little additional sensitivity is obtained by this approach outside of high-risk communities (2). An alternative approach is to screen directly for wild poliovirus circulation in high-risk communities, either through stool surveys of healthy children or virologic analysis of community wastewater.

Environmental and community surveillance has been routinely used in several countries to monitor wild poliovirus circulation. For example, studies during the 1984 epidemic in Finland revealed that up to 100,000 people were infected with wild type 3 poliovirus, although only 10 clinical cases were reported (50). Community and environmental surveillance in coastal Colombia in 1991 found a high rate (8%) of wild type 1 poliovirus carriage among healthy children and the prevalence of closely related viruses in community wastewater (55). In the Netherlands, wild poliovirus type 3 was recovered from river water sampled 3 weeks before the onset of the 1992 epidemic (57). Wild type 3 poliovirus was isolated in the following year from healthy members of a community in western Canada known to have had close contact with the Dutch outbreak community (42). In each study, sequence analysis of the isolates confirmed the close links between the AFP cases and the subclinical infections.

Intensive environmental surveillance has been implemented in Israel and Gaza (40, 53), Mumbai, India, and southern Egypt (14). In Israel, periodic outbreaks of subclinical wild poliovirus infections have been detected by wastewater sampling (40), along with an unusual type 2 VDPV (52). Sequence analysis of the wild poliovirus isolates traced their origin to reservoir communities in a neighboring country. Similarly, wild polioviruses recently isolated from wastewater in Mumbai are closely related to viruses found in known reservoir communities elsewhere in India (J. M. Deshpande, personal communication). A special environmental study at 10 sampling sites in seven governorates of southern Egypt was initiated in 2000 to supplement AFP surveillance. Wild poliovirus type 1 was found at every site, and a very high-resolution view was obtained of poliovirus circulation along multiple chains of transmission (14), prompting an urgent reassessment of immunization and AFP surveillance activities in Egypt.

POTENTIAL PERSISTENCE OF VACCINE-DERIVED POLIOVIRUSES

When immunologically normal individuals are infected with poliovirus, the period of excretion is typically 3 to 4 weeks (1). Short excretion times and high rates of OPV coverage normally limit the spread of OPV-derived polioviruses to close contacts of the vaccine recipients (5, 23). This is reflected in the high VP1 sequence similarities (>99%) between vaccine-derived isolates (described as "Sabin-like") obtained from the large majority of patients with AFP from whom polioviruses are isolated. However, the sequence properties of some VDPV isolates are suggestive of prolonged replication of the vaccine virus. Two categories of atypical VDPV isolates have been described. The first category (iVDPV isolates) have been isolated from immunodeficient patients with defects in antibody production (4, 33, 61). Some iVDPV isolates have substitutions in as many as 10% of VP1 nucleotide positions, suggesting that some chronic infections with iVDPVs may persist for as long as 10 years (33, 61). There is no current evidence of spread of iVDPVs from chronically infected persons to the wider community (61).

Recently, polio outbreaks associated with circulating vaccine-derived poliovirus (cVDPV) have been recognized in three different parts of the world. In Egypt, type 2 cVDPV was isolated from polio patients during the years 1988 to 1993 (10). The rate and pattern of VP1 divergence from the Sabin type 2 OPV strain suggested that all lineages were derived from a single OPV infection that occurred around 1985. Phylogenetic analysis showed that the cVDPVs circulated widely in Egypt along several independent chains of transmission. In Hispaniola (Haiti and the Dominican Republic), an outbreak of 21 confirmed cases (including two fatal cases) in 2000–2001 was associated with type 1 cVDPV (30). A more limited outbreak, associated with an independent lineage of type 1 cVDPV, occurred in the Philippines in 2001 (12). The common risk factors for cVDPV circulation were major gaps in OPV coverage, environmental conditions favoring poliovirus spread, and the prior eradication of the corresponding serotype of indigenous wild poliovirus.

The occurrence of iVDPVs and cVDPVs appears to be rare. The small number of chronic iVDPV excretors have been found only in middle- or high-income industrialized countries (56, 61). Long-term poliovirus carriers have not been found in less developed countries, presumably because the survival rates of immunodeficient individuals in these countries are very low. Moreover, most chronic poliovirus excretors in developed countries spontaneously stop shedding or die of complications from their immunodeficiency (56). Because an increasing number of highly developed countries have switched to IPV, the chances for the occurrence of new iVDPV infections have decreased.

Intensive, worldwide poliovirus surveillance for cVDPV isolates has not identified any other cVDPV outbreaks. In response to the three documented outbreaks, immunization program managers in all countries have been alerted to the importance of maintaining high polio vaccine coverages. NIDs have been recommended for a number of nonendemic countries in order to restore high levels of population immunity. In essence, the WHO Polio Eradication Initiative has clearly recognized that it is currently fighting poliovirus circulation on two fronts, as it must prevent the emergence of cVDPVs while at the same time eliminating the last pockets of wild poliovirus circulation (56, 65).

"ENDGAME" CHALLENGES

The top priority for polio eradication is to complete the task of eradicating all wild polioviruses. The chief obstacles to that goal are primarily managerial and social and present challenges similar to those already surmounted by the program in many other countries. There is a growing consensus that the primary goal of wild poliovirus eradication will soon be achieved. In 1998, WHO began to address the complex issues of the now imminent posteradication era. The key issues are (i) certification of global polio eradication, (ii) containment of laboratory stocks of polioviruses, (iii) maintenance of sensitive AFP and poliovirus surveillance, (iv) options for stopping OPV use worldwide, (v) the prospects of continued circulation of VDPVs, and (vi) establishment of emergency stockpiles of OPV (56, 65; chapter 38, this volume). These important issues are explored further in chapter 38.

CONCLUSIONS

The Polio Eradication Initiative of WHO is the largest and most complex public health endeavor in human history. Its progress can be measured by the >99% reduction in the incidence of polio cases since 1988, the apparent eradication of wild poliovirus type 2, the localization of poliovirus circulation to a few reservoir countries, the extinction of most poliovirus genotypes since 1988, and the protection of the large majority of the world's children from polio. However, the ultimate success of the Initiative is measured by the strictest of criteria: the permanent cessation of all poliovirus circulation. This long-sought goal now appears within reach. Much remains to be done, particularly in developing an effective strategy for maintaining indefinitely a worldwide polio-free status. Although the task is not yet finished, it is not too early to consider the legacy of polio eradication. Beyond the obvious health and cost benefits of eradicating a disease that has afflicted children for over 3 millennia (47), polio eradication has raised the standards of public health performance worldwide. Hundreds of millions of children are immunized against polio every year. NIDs are synchronized across many countries. Conflicts are suspended during NIDs. Populations who have never before received health services are sought out and immunized. AFP surveillance conforms to the same high uniform standards. A global network of highly proficient virology laboratories performs comprehensive poliovirus surveillance. The tools of virology, molecular biology, and evolutionary biology are widely used in the laboratory network. The integrated virologic and epidemiologic findings are used to drive the program. Certification will be based upon solid, objective, scientific evidence.

Polio eradication has had a positive impact on other public health initiatives, especially on the broader Expanded Program on Immunization. Coverage rates for other vaccine-preventable diseases have risen sharply in recent years. Once polio is eradicated, the next step will be to further accelerate efforts to control, and possibly eradicate, measles. A new cohort of skilled epidemiologists and virologists will be available to apply the lessons learned from polio eradication to other disease control initiatives. The challenge for the global polio eradication team in this relay for improved global health is to be sure that the baton is passed securely to the next team.

We thank the virologists of the WHO Global Polio Laboratory Network for sharing their poliovirus isolates with us, and our colleagues in our own laboratories for their dedicated efforts to characterize poliovirus isolates from all parts of the world. We thank Larry Anderson, Steve Cochi, Walter Dowdle, David Featherstone, Chris Maher, Ray Sanders, and Roland Sutter for helpful discussions.

REFERENCES

1. **Alexander, J. P., Jr., H. E. Gary, Jr., and M. A. Pallansch.** 1997. Duration of poliovirus excretion and its implications for acute flaccid paralysis surveillance: a review of the literature. *J. Infect. Dis.* **175**(Suppl. 1):S176–S182.
2. **Andrus, J. K., C. de Quadros, J. M. Olivé, and H. F. Hull.** 1992. Screening of cases of acute flaccid paralysis for poliomyelitis eradication: ways to improve specificity. *Bull. W.H.O.* **70**:591–596.
3. **Balanant, J., S. Guillot, A. Candréa, F. Delpeyroux, and R. Crainic.** 1991. The natural genomic variability of poliovirus analyzed by a restriction fragment polymorphism assay. *Virology* **184**:645–654.
4. **Bellmunt, A., G. May, R. Zell, P. Pring-Akerblom, W. Verhagen, and A. Heim.** 1999. Evolution of poliovirus type I during 5.5 years of prolonged enteral replication in an immunodeficient patient. *Virology* **265**:178–184.
5. **Benyesh-Melnick, M., J. L. Melnick, W. E. Rawls, I. Wimberley, J. Barrera-Oro, E. Ben-Porath, and V. Rennick.** 1967. Studies on the immunogenicity, communicability, and genetic stability of oral poliovaccine administered during the winter. *Am. J. Epidemiol.* **86**:112–136.
6. **Cammack, N. J., A. Phillips, G. Dunn, V. Patel, and P. D. Minor.** 1989. Intertypic genomic rearrangements of poliovirus strains in vaccinees. *Virology* **167**:507–514.
7. **Centers for Disease Control and Prevention.** 1994. Certification of poliomyelitis eradication—the Americas, 1994. *Morb. Mortal. Wkly. Rep.* **43**:720–722.
8. **Centers for Disease Control and Prevention.** 2000. Public health dispatch: outbreak of poliomyelitis—Cape Verde, 2000. *Morb. Mortal. Wkly. Rep.* **49**:1070.
9. **Centers for Disease Control and Prevention.** 2001. Public health dispatch: certification of poliomyelitis eradication—Western Pacific Region, October 2000. *Morb. Mortal. Wkly. Rep.* **50**:1–3.
10. **Centers for Disease Control and Prevention.** 2001. Circulation of a type 2 vaccine-derived poliovirus—Egypt, 1982–1993. *Morb. Mortal. Wkly. Rep.* **50**:41–42, 51.
11. **Centers for Disease Control and Prevention.** 2001. Apparent global interruption of wild poliovirus type 2 transmission. *Morb. Mortal. Wkly. Rep.* **50**:222–224.
12. **Centers for Disease Control and Prevention.** 2001. Public health dispatch: acute flaccid paralysis associated with circulating vaccine-derived poliovirus—Philippines, 2001. *Morb. Mortal. Wkly. Rep.* **50**:874–875.
13. **Centers for Disease Control and Prevention.** 2001. Imported wild poliovirus causing poliomyelitis—Bulgaria, 2001. *Morb. Mortal. Wkly. Rep.* **50**:1033–1035.
14. **Centers for Disease Control and Prevention.** 2002. Progress toward poliomyelitis eradication—Egypt, 2001. *Morb. Mortal. Wkly. Rep.* **51**:305–307.
15. **Centers for Disease Control and Prevention.** 2002. Laboratory surveillance for wild poliovirus and vaccine-derived polioviruses, 2000–2001. *Morb. Mortal. Wkly. Rep.* **51**:369–371.
16. **Chiba, Y., H. Murakami, M. Kobayashi, H. Shimizu, H. Yoshida, T. Yoneyama, T. Miyamura, J. Yu, and L. Zhang.** 2000. A case of poliomyelitis associated with infection of wild poliovirus in Qinghai Province, China, in October 1999. *Jpn. J. Infect. Dis.* **53**:135–136.
17. **Cruz, R. R.** 1984. Cuba: mass polio vaccination program, 1962–1982. *Rev. Infect. Dis.* **6**(Suppl. 2):S408–S412.
18. **De, L., B. K. Nottay, C.-F. Yang, B. P. Holloway, M. A. Pallansch, and O. Kew.** 1995. Identification of vaccine-related polioviruses by hybridization with specific RNA probes. *J. Clin. Microbiol.* **33**:562–571.
19. **De, L., C.-F. Yang, E. da Silva, J. Boshell, P. Cáceres, J. R. Gómez, M. Pallansch, and O. Kew.** 1997. Genotype-specific RNA probes for the direct identification of wild polioviruses by blot hybridization. *J. Clin. Microbiol.* **35**:2834–2840.
20. **de la Torre, J. C., C. Giachetti, B. L. Semler, and J. J. Holland.** 1992. High frequency of single-base transitions and extreme frequency of precise multiple-base reversion mutations in poliovirus. *Proc. Natl. Acad. Sci. USA* **89**:2531–2535.
21. **Domingo, E., and J. J. Holland.** 1997. RNA virus mutations and fitness for survival. *Annu. Rev. Microbiol.* **51**:151–178.
22. **Drake, J. W.** 1993. Rates of spontaneous mutation among RNA viruses. *Proc. Natl. Acad. Sci. USA* **90**:4171–4175.
23. **Fine, P. E. M., and I. A. M. Carneiro.** 1999. Transmissibility and persistence of oral polio vaccine viruses: implications for the global poliomyelitis eradication initiative. *Am. J. Epidemiol.* **150**:1001–1021.
24. **Gavrilin, G. V., E. A. Cherkasova, G. Y. Lipskaya, O. M. Kew, and V. I. Agol.** 2000. Evolution of circulating wild poliovirus and of vaccine-derived poliovirus in an immunodeficient patient: a unifying model. *J. Virol.* **74**:7381–7390.
25. **Georgescu, M.-M., F. Delpeyroux, and R. Crainic.** 1995. Tripartite genome organization of a natural type 2 vaccine/nonvaccine recombinant poliovirus. *J. Gen. Virol.* **76**:2343–2348.
26. **Georgescu, M. M., F. Delpeyroux, M. Tardy-Panit, J. Balanant, M. Combiescu, A. A. Combiescu, S. Guillot, and R. Crainic.** 1994. High diversity of poliovirus strains isolated from the central nervous system from patients with vaccine-associated paralytic poliomyelitis. *J. Virol.* **68**:8089–8101.
27. **Holland, J. J., E. Domingo, J. C. de la Torre, and D. A. Steinhauer.** 1990. Mutation frequencies at defined codon sites in vesicular stomatitis virus and poliovirus can be increased only slightly by chemical mutagenesis. *J. Virol.* **64**:3960–3962.
28. **Hovi, T., and M. Stenvik.** 1994. Selective isolation of poliovirus in recombinant murine cell line expressing the human poliovirus receptor gene. *J. Clin. Microbiol.* **32**:1366–1368.
29. **Kew, O. M., L. De, C.-F. Yang, B. K. Nottay, E. da Silva, and M. A. Pallansch.** 1993. The role of virologic surveilance in the global initiative to eradicate poliomyelitis, p. 215–246. *In* E. Kurstak (ed.), *Control of Virus Diseases*, 2nd ed. Marcel Dekker, New York, N.Y.
30. **Kew, O. M., V. Morris-Glasgow, M. Landaverde, C. Burns, J. Shaw, Z. Garib, J. André, E. Blackman, C. J. Freeman, J. Jorba, R. Sutter, G. Tambini, L. Venczel, C. Pedreira, F. Laender, H. Shimizu, T. Yoneyama, T. Miyamura, H. van der Avoort, M. S. Oberste, D. Kilpatrick, S. Cochi, M. Pallansch, and C. de Quadros.** 2002. Outbreak of poliomyelitis in Hispaniola associated with circulating type 1 vaccine-derived poliovirus. *Science* **296**:356–359.
31. **Kew, O. M., M. N. Mulders, G. Y. Lipskaya, E. E. da Silva, and M. A. Pallansch.** 1995. Molecular epidemiology of polioviruses. *Semin. Virol.* **6**:401–414.
32. **Kew, O. M., M. A. Pallansch, B. K. Nottay, R. Rico-Hesse, L. De, and C.-F. Yang.** 1990. Genotypic relation-

ships among wild polioviruses from different regions of the world, p. 357–365. *In* M. A. Brinton and F. X. Heinz (ed.), *New Aspects of Positive-Strand RNA Viruses.* American Society for Microbiology, Washington, D.C.

33. **Kew, O. M., R. W. Sutter, B. Nottay, M. McDonough, D. R. Prevots, L. Quick, and M. Pallansch.** 1998. Prolonged replication of a type 1 vaccine-derived poliovirus in an immunodeficient patient. *J. Clin. Microbiol.* **36:** 2893–2899.

34. **Kilpatrick, D. R., B. Nottay, C.-F. Yang, S.-J. Yang, E. da Silva, S. Peñaranda, M. Pallansch, and O. Kew.** 1998. Serotype-specific identification of polioviruses by PCR using primers containing mixed-base or deoxyinosine residues at positions of codon degeneracy. *J. Clin. Microbiol.* **36:**352–357.

35. **Kilpatrick, D. R., B. Nottay, C.-F. Yang, S.-J. Yang, M. N. Mulders, B. P. Holloway, M. A. Pallansch, and O. M. Kew.** 1996. Group-specific identification of poliovirus by PCR using primers containing mixed-base or deoxyinosine residues at positions of codon degeneracy. *J. Clin. Microbiol.* **34:**2990–2996.

36. **Kinnunen, L., A. Huovilainen, T. Pöyry, and T. Hovi.** 1990. Rapid molecular evolution of wild type 3 poliovirus during infection in individual hosts. *J. Gen. Virol.* **71:** 317–324.

37. **Lipskaya, G. Y., E. A. Chervonskaya, G. I. Belova, S. V. Maslova, T. N. Kutateladze, S. G. Drozdov, M. N. Mulders, M. A. Pallansch, O. M. Kew, and V. I. Agol.** 1995. Geographic genotypes (geotypes) of poliovirus case isolates from the former Soviet Union: relatedness to other known poliovirus genotypes. *J. Gen. Virol.* **76:**1687–1699.

38. **Lipskaya, G. Y., A. R. Muzychenko, O. K. Kutitova, S. V. Maslova, M. Equestre, S. G. Drozdov, R. Perez Bercoff, and V. I. Agol.** 1991. Frequent isolation of intertypic poliovirus recombinants with serotype 2 specificity from vaccine-associated polio cases. *J. Med. Virol.* **35:** 290–296.

39. **Liu, H.-M., D.-P. Zheng, L.-B. Zhang, M. S. Oberste, M. A. Pallansch, and O. M. Kew.** 2000. Molecular evolution of a type 1 wild-vaccine poliovirus recombinant during widespread circulation in China. *J. Virol.* **74:** 11153–11161.

40. **Manor, Y., R. Handsher, T. Halmut, M. Neuman, A. Bobrov, H. Rudich, A. Vonsover, L. Shulman, O. Kew, and E. Mendelson.** 1999. Detection of poliovirus circulation by environmental surveillance in the absence of clinical cases in Israel and the Palestinian Authority. *J. Clin. Microbiol.* **37:**1670–1675.

41. **Martín, J., G. Dunn, R. Hull, V. Patel, and P. D. Minor.** 2000. Evolution of the Sabin strain of type 3 poliovirus in an immunodeficient patient during the entire 637-day period of virus excretion. *J. Virol.* **74:**3001–3010.

42. **Mulders, M. N., A. M. van Loon, H. G. A. M. van der Avoort, J. H. J. Riemerink, A. Ras, T. M. Bestebroer, M. A. Drebot, O. M. Kew, and M. P. G. Koopmans.** 1995. Molecular characterization of the wild poliovirus type 3 epidemic in the Netherlands (1992–93). *J. Clin. Microbiol.* **33:**3252–3256.

43. **Nathanson, N., and J. R. Martin.** 1970. The epidemiology of poliomyelitis: enigmas surrounding its appearance, epidemicity, and disappearance. *Am. J. Epidemiol.* **110:**672–692.

44. **Pallansch, M. A., and R. P. Roos.** 2001. Enteroviruses: polioviruses, coxsackieviruses, echoviruses, and newer enteroviruses, p. 723–775. *In* D. M. Knipe, P. M. Howley, D. E. Griffin, R. A. Lamb, M. A. Martin, B. Roizman, and S. E. Strauss (ed.), *Fields Virology*, 4th ed. Lippincott Williams and Wilkins, Philadelphia, Pa.

45. **Pan American Health Organization.** 1985. Director announces campaign to eradicate poliomyelitis from the Americas by 1990. *Bull. PAHO* **19:**21–35.

46. **Patriarca, P. A., R. W. Sutter, and P. M. Oostvogel.** 1997. Outbreaks of paralytic poliomyelitis, 1976–1995. *J. Infect. Dis.* **175:**S165–S172.

47. **Paul, J. R.** 1971. *A History of Poliomyelitis.* Yale University Press, New Haven, Conn.

48. **Pipkin, P. A., D. J. Wood, V. R. Racaniello, and P. D. Minor.** 1993. Characterisation of L cells expressing the human poliovirus receptor for the specific detection of polioviruses in vitro. *J. Virol. Methods* **41:**333–340.

49. **Plotkin, S. A., A. Murdin, and E. Vidor.** 1999. Inactivated polio vaccine, p. 345–363. *In* S. A. Plotkin and W. A. Orenstein (ed.), *Vaccines*, 3rd ed. The W.B. Saunders Co., Philadelphia, Pa.

50. **Pöyry, T., M. Stenvik, and T. Hovi.** 1988. Viruses in sewage waters during and after a poliomyelitis outbreak and subsequent nationwide oral poliovirus vaccination campaign in Finland. *Appl. Environ. Microbiol.* **54:**371–374.

51. **Risi, J. B.** 1984. The control of poliomyelitis in Brazil. *Rev. Infect. Dis.* **6**(Suppl. 2):S400–S403.

52. **Shulman, L., J. Manor, R. Handsher, F. Delpeyroux, M. McDonough, T. Halmut, I. Silberstein, J. Alfandari, J. Quay, T. Fisher, J. Robinov, O. Kew, R. Crainic, and E. Mendelson.** 2000. Molecular and antigenic characterization of a highly evolved derivative of the type 2 oral poliovaccine strain isolated from sewage in Israel. *J. Clin. Microbiol.* **38:**3729–3734.

53. **Shulman, L. M., R. Handsher, S.-J. Yang, C.-F. Yang, J. Manor, A. Vonsover, Z. Grossman, M. Pallansch, E. Mendelson, and O. M. Kew.** 2000. Resolution of the pathways of poliovirus type 1 transmission during an outbreak. *J. Clin. Microbiol.* **38:**945–952.

54. **Sutter, R. W., S. L. Cochi, and J. L. Melnick.** 1999. Live attenuated poliovirus vaccine, p. 364–408. *In* S. A. Plotkin and W. A. Orenstein (ed.), *Vaccines*, 3rd ed. The W.B. Saunders Co., Philadelphia, Pa.

55. **Tambini, G., J. K. Andrus, E. Marques, J. Boshell, M. Pallansch, C. A. de Quadros, and O. M. Kew.** 1993. Direct detection of wild poliovirus transmission by stool surveys of healthy children and analysis of community wastewater. *J. Infect. Dis.* **168:**1510–1514.

56. **Technical Consulting Group to the World Health Organization on the Global Eradication of Poliomyelitis.** 2002. "Endgame" issues for the Global Polio Eradication Initiative. *Clin. Infect. Dis.* **34:**72–77.

57. **van der Avoort, H. G., J. H. Reimerink, A. Ras, M. N. Mulders, and A. M. van Loon.** 1995. Isolation of epidemic poliovirus from sewage during the 1992–3 type 3 outbreak in The Netherlands. *Epidemiol. Infect.* **114:**481–491.

58. **van der Avoort, H. G. A. M., B. P. Hull, T. Hovi, M. A. Pallansch, O. M. Kew, R. Crainic, D. J. Wood, M. N. Mulders, and A. M. van Loon.** 1995. A comparative study of five methods of intratypic differentiation of polioviruses. *J. Clin. Microbiol.* **33:**2562–2566.

59. **van Wezel, A. L., and A. G. Hazendonk.** 1979. Intratypic serodifferentiation of poliomyelitis virus by strain-specific antisera. *Intervirology* **11:**2–8.

60. **Wimmer, E., C. U. Hellen, and X. Cao.** 1993. Genetics of poliovirus. *Annu. Rev. Genet.* **27:**353–436.

61. **Wood, D. J., R. W. Sutter, and W. R. Dowdle.** 2000. Stopping poliovirus vaccination after eradication: issues and challenges. *Bull. W.H.O.* **78:**347–357.

62. **World Health Assembly.** 1998. Polio eradication by the year 2000 Resolution 41.28. World Health Organization, Geneva, Switzerland.

63. **World Health Organization.** 1997. Manual for the virologic investigation of poliomyelitis. (WHO/EPI/GEN/97.1.) World Health Organization, Geneva, Switzerland.
64. **World Health Organization.** 2001. Global polio eradication of poliomyelitis: report of the sixth meeting of the Global Technical Consultative Group for Poliomyelitis Eradication. (WHO/V&B/01.32.) World Health Organization, Geneva, Switzerland.
65. **World Health Organization.** 2002. Progress towards the global eradication of poliomyelitis, 2001. *Wkly. Epidemiol. Rec.* **77:**98–107.
66. **Yang, C.-F., L. De, B. P. Holloway, M. A. Pallansch, and O. M. Kew.** 1991. Detection and identification of vaccine-related polioviruses by the polymerase chain reaction. *Virus Res.* **20:**159–179.
67. **Yang, C.-F., L. De, S.-J. Yang, J. R. Gómez, J. R. Cruz, B. P. Holloway, M. A. Pallansch, and O. M. Kew.** 1992. Genotype-specific *in vitro* amplification of sequences of the wild type 3 polioviruses from Mexico and Guatemala. *Virus Res.* **24:**277–296.
68. **Yoshida, H., J. Li, T. Yoneyama, K. Yoshii, H. Shimizu, T. H. Nguyen, K. Toda, T. L. Nguyen, V. T. Phan, T. Miyamura, and A. Hagiwara.** 1997. Two major strains of type 1 wild poliovirus circulating in Indochina. *J. Infect. Dis.* **175:**1233–1237.

Index

A

A (altered) particle, in poliovirus replication, 73, 75, 80
2A proteinase, see Proteinases, 2A
3A proteinase, activity of, 189t
3AB proteinase, activity of, 189t
Accessory factors, for viral receptors, 63t, 65
Acute bee paralysis virus, proteinases of, 216, 218f
Adaptive immune response, to coxsackieviruses, 392
Aggregation, in virus-antibody neutralization, 44
Aichi virus
  internal ribosomal entry sites of, 160
  nucleotide preferences of, 152–153
  serotypes of, 18t
Alphaviruses, antibody interactions with, 46
Altered particle, in poliovirus replication, 73, 75
Alternative therapies, for rhinovirus infections, 360
Animal models, hepatitis A, 416–417, 417f, 418t, 419
Antiapoptotic activity, genomic determinants of, 133–134
Antibiotics, see Antiviral agents
Antibody(ies)
  coxsackievirus, 395–396
  hepatitis A virus, 417–418
  neutralizing, virus interactions, 31, 46–47; see also Rhinovirus(es), antibody interactions
Antigen(s)
  evolution of, 289–290
  foot-and-mouth disease virus, 51–58
  picornavirus, taxonomy based on, 19–20
  variability of, 270
Antigen-presenting cells, in coxsackievirus response, 392
Antigenic intratypic differentiation, of polioviruses, 484
Antihistamines, for rhinovirus infections, 359
Antiviral agents
  action of, on poliovirus, 75
  based on loss of infectivity, 292
  capsid-binding, 32–34, 34f,
  for enterovirus infections, 362
  evolution and, 291–292
  resistance to
    evolution of, 287–288
    variability in, 270
  for rhinovirus infections, 358–360
Aphthovirus(es), see also specific viruses
  genome of, 20f, 21, 21t
    alignments of, 150
    overall design of, 128, 128f
    polyprotein processing determinants in, 131
    replication determinants in, 132
    translation determinants in, 129
  in host cell translation shutoff, 302, 303
  infections due to, clinical manifestations of, 63t, 368t
  internal ribosomal entry sites of
    cellular RNA-binding proteins and, 179–180
    structure of, 160, 162
  nucleotide preferences of, 151
  proteinases of, 188f
    2A, 189, 213–223
    in primary cleavage, 199, 200f, 213–223
  receptors for, 32, 63t, 368
  replication of, cis-acting RNA elements in, 231
  serotypes of, 18t
  similarity plots of, 150–151, 152f
  structures of, 28t, 30–31
  taxonomy of, see Taxonomy
APK pathways, activation of, by coxsackieviruses, 409–411, 410f, 411f
Apoptosis
  vs. cytopathy, 247
  genomic determinants of, 133–134, 135
  Theiler's murine encephalomyelitis virus inducing, 430
Aseptic meningitis, enterovirus, 361, 362
Asthma, exacerbation of, in rhinovirus infections, 358
ATP, hydrolysis of, in virus translation, 173, 174t, 175–176
Attenuation
  hepatitis A virus, 419–421
  poliovirus, Sabin strains, 382–386
  viral evolution for, 290–291
Autocatalytic cleavage, in polyprotein processing, genomic determinants of, 131
Autoimmunity, coxsackieviruses and, 397–398
Avian encephalomyelitis-like virus
  nucleotide preferences of, 152
  serotypes of, 18t
Avian encephalomyelitis virus
  evolution of, 291
  hepatitis A virus resembling, 416

B

B lymphocytes, response of
  to coxsackievirus, 395–396
  to Theiler's murine encephalomyelitis virus, 432
2B proteinase
  activity of, 189t, 190
  in replication, 228
3B proteinase, activity of, 189t
Basal transcription factor, inactivation of, by poliovirus, 322–325, 323f–326f
BeAn strain, Theiler's murine encephalomyelitis virus, persistence of, 437–438
Black beetle virus, structure of, 29t
Blood-brain barrier, poliovirus penetration of, 368–369
Bodian, D., poliomyelitis research of, 8–9
Bovine enterovirus
  infections due to, clinical manifestations of, 368t
  internal ribosomal entry sites of, 162
  nucleotide preferences of, 151
  serotypes of, 18t
  structure of, 28t
Brazil, poliovirus eradication in, 474–476
Brome mosaic virus, structure of, 29t
Bronchitis, chronic, exacerbation of, in rhinovirus infections, 358
Burnet, Frank M., on poliovirus strains, 8

C

2C/2BC proteinase
  activity of, 189t, 190–191
  in replication, 228–229
2C proteinase, activity of, 189t, 190–191
3C proteinases, see Proteinases, 3C
Calcium, in hepatitis A virus cell entry, 416
Campaign jaundice, 415
Canonical initiation factors, in internal ribosomal entry site activity, 172–177, 174f, 174t, 176f
Canyon hypothesis, of neutralizing antibody interaction, 32f, 43, 46–47
  rhinovirus, 85–86,
Cap-binding protein, in protein synthesis, 302, 302f
Capsid proteins
  structures of, 27, 29, 30f, 31f
  synthesis of, genomic determinants of, 134
  taxonomy based on, 21
CAR (coxsackie-adenovirus receptor), 62f, 63t, 64–66, 66t, 108–110, 108f
Cardiomyopathy
  coxsackievirus, 393, 439–440
  enterovirus, 361
Cardiovirus(es), see also Encephalomyocarditis virus (EMCV); Theiler's murine encephalomyelitis virus
  genome of, 20f, 21, 21t
    alignments of, 150
    overall design of, 128, 128f
    polyprotein processing determinants in, 131
    replication determinants in, 132
    translation determinants in, 129
  in host cell translation shutoff, 302
  infections due to, clinical manifestations of, 63t, 368t
  internal ribosomal entry sites of
    cellular RNA-binding proteins and, 179–180
    structure of, 160, 162
  nucleotide preferences of, 154
  proteinases of, 188f
    2A, 189, 213–223
    in primary cleavage, 199, 200f, 213–223
  receptors for, 368
    clinical manifestations and, 63t, 368t
    interactions with, 32
  replication of, cis-acting RNA elements in, 231, 233
  serotypes of, 18t
  similarity plots of, 150–151, 153f
  structures of, 28t, 30–31
  taxonomy of, see Taxonomy
CD55 (decay accelerating factor), as viral receptor, 61, 62f, 63t, 64–66
  coxsackievirus, 107–110, 108f, 407–409, 409f
  echovirus, 110
  enterovirus, 371
CD59, as viral receptor accessory, 65, 111
CD155, as viral receptor, 62–63, 62f, 63t, 65–67, 66t
  gene family of, 369–370, 370t
  poliovirus, 369–371, 370t, 376
3CD proteinase, see Proteinases, 3CD
Cell(s), host, see Host cell(s)

Cell culture
  coxsackievirus, 442
  echovirus, 441–442
  enterovirus, 361
  foot-and-mouth disease virus, 440–441, 441f
  hepatitis A virus, 416, 419–420, 441
  poliovirus, 442, 442t, 443f, 444–445
Cell-free systems, for poliovirus study, see Poliovirus(es), cell-free systems for
Cell membranes
  P2 protein action on, 190–191
  permeability of, 337–339, 338f
  replication effects on, 247–250, 248f, 249f, 337–354
    early, 337, 338f
    glycoprotein processing, 338f, 341–342, 343f
    intracellular membranous vesicle proliferation, 338f, 339, 340f–341f, 342–344
    late, 337–342, 338f, 340f–342f
    lipase activity changes, 341, 342f
    lipid composition changes, 339–341
    permeability enhancement, 337–339, 338f
    proteins involved in, 338f, 344–348, 345f–348f
    schematic representation of, 337, 338f
    vesicular trafficking inhibition, 338f, 341–342, 343f
Cellular immune response
  to hepatitis A virus, 418–419
  to Theiler's murine encephalomyelitis virus, 432–433, 433t, 439
Centers for Disease Control, poliovirus eradication program, 476, 477
Charcot, J. M., on poliomyelitis neuropathology, 4–5
Chat strain, poliovirus, 381
Chemokines, in Theiler's murine encephalomyelitis virus infections, 432
Chimeras, 277
Chimpanzee model
  for hepatitis A, 416, 417f, 418t
  for poliovirus, 8–9
Chronic obstructive pulmonary disease, exacerbation of, in rhinovirus infections, 358
Chymotrypsin, vs. 3C proteinase, 203–204
Cleavage
  of initiation factors, 302f, 303–306, 304f
  by poliovirus, 313–320, 315f–317f
  in polyprotein processing
    cellular proteins, 200, 202–203, 202t
    genomic determinants of, 131
    of host substrates, 192–193
    primary, 199, 213–223
      mechanism of, 217, 219
      mutagenic analysis of, 216
      in nonpicornaviruses, 215f, 216–217, 218f
      proteinase hypothesis of, 217
      sequences in, 213–216, 214f, 215f
      structural aspects of, 217
      substrate hypothesis of, 217
      translational model for, 219–222, 220f
    secondary, 199–200, 201f
Cloverleaf structure, in replication, 231, 231t, 232f, 233–234
CLUSTAL algorithm, for genomic sequence alignment, 150
Common cold, rhinovirus, 357–360
Comoviruses, structures of, 29t, 30f, 31f

Complement system, activation of, in coxsackievirus infections, 392
Complementation, 275–276, 458–469, 458f, 459f
  in genetic analysis, 276
  in poliovirus replication, 458–460, 458f, 459f, 461–469
    cis-active RNA sequence identification in, 464–465, 465f, 466f, 467
    negative-strand synthesis in, 462f, 463, 463f, 467
    positive-strand synthesis in, 462f, 463, 463f
    precursor identification in, 463–464, 464f
    synchronous RNA replication in, 461, 463
    translation-replication reactions in, 461
Complexity, evolution and, 291
Conformational changes, in virus-antibody neutralization, 44–45
Congenital infections, enterovirus, 361–362
Conjunctivitis, enterovirus, 360
Cowpea chlorotic mottle virus, structure of, 27, 29t
Cowpea mosaic virus, replication of, translation coupling with, 234
Cowpea mottle virus, structure of, 29t
Cox strain, poliovirus, 381
Coxsackie-adenovirus receptor (CAR), 62f, 63t, 64–66, 66t, 108–110, 108f
  pathogenesis and, 407–409, 409f
Coxsackievirus(es)
  cell culture of, 442
  cellular signaling pathway activation by, 409–411, 410f, 411f
  chimeras of, 277
  evolution of, 291–292
  genome of, anti-host determinants in, 134
  in host cell translation shutoff, 302–306
  host range of, 270
  in host substrate cleavage, 202, 202t
  immune response to, 391–403
    adaptive, 392
    antigen-presenting cells in, 392
    autoimmunity and, 397–398
    B lymphocytes in, 395–396
    complement system activation, 392
    natural killer cells in, 391–392
    NIm sites in, 396–397
    T lymphocytes in, 392–395, 393f–395f
  infections due to
    adaptive immune responses in, 392
    antigen-presenting cells in, 392
    autoimmune aspects of, 397–398
    B-lymphocyte responses in, 395–396
    clinical manifestations of, 368t
    complement system in, 392
    diabetes mellitus in, 391, 397
    humoral immune responses in, 395–396
    myocarditis in, 391–398, 405–411, 406f, 404t, 408f–411f, 439–440
    natural killer cells in, 391–392
    NIm sites in, 396–397
    pancreatic effects of, 391, 397
    persistent, 405–411, 406f, 404t, 408f–411f, 439–440
    routes of, 391
    spectrum of, 391
    T-lymphocyte responses in, 392–395, 393f–395f
  internal ribosomal entry sites of, 162
  NIm sites of, 396–397
  pathogenicity of, variability of, 271

  proteinases of, host cell interactions with, 406–407, 407t, 409–411, 410f, 411f
  proteins of, host cell membrane effects of, 344
  receptors for, 61, 64–65, 368
    accessory factors for, 65
    attachment sites for, 65–66, 66t
    clinical manifestations and, 63t
    group A, 110
    group B, 107–110, 108f
    interactions with, 32
    multiple, 109–110
    paralytic disease and, 371
    pathogenesis and, 67, 407–409, 409f
    types of, 62, 62f, 64–65
    virus structure and, 109
  replication of
    cell membrane alterations in, 247
    cis-acting RNA elements in, 233
    host cell intracellular membranous vesicle proliferation in, 339
    host cell lipid alterations in, 341
    host cell membrane effects of, 337–338, 344
    intracellular membrane proliferation in, 342
    proteins involved in, 231t
  resistance in, 287
  serotypes of, 391
  structures of, 28t, 109
Coxsackievirus B, infections due to, pathogenesis of, 405–411, 406f, 404t, 408f–411f
CREB (cyclic AMP-responsive element binding protein), cleavage of, 202, 202t
cre (2C) element, in replication, 232f, 233
Cricket paralysis virus
  proteinases of, 216, 218f
  structure of, 27
Cuba, poliovirus eradication in, 474
Cucumber mosaic virus, structure of, 29t
Culture, see Cell culture
Cutter incident, 376
Cyclic AMP-responsive element binding protein (CREB), cleavage of, 202, 202t, 325–327, 327f
Cytokeratin, cleavage of, 202, 202t, 306
Cytokines
  in coxsackievirus infections, 393–394
  in intercellular adhesion molecule 1 expression, 85–86
Cytolytic T lymphocytes, response of, to hepatitis A virus, 418–419
Cytopathy, 247
  genomic determinants of, 135
  host cell cleavage in, 200, 202–203, 202t
Cytoplasmic eosinophilic paranuclear mass, in replication, 247, 248f
Cytoskeletal proteins, cleavage of, in host cell translation shutoff, 306

D

3D proteinase, activity of, 189t
DA strain, Theiler's murine encephalomyelitis virus, 428, 428t, 431, 437–438
Data bases, for viral genomes, 149–150
de Macedo, Guerra, in poliovirus eradication program, 476
de Quadros, Ciro, in poliovirus eradication program, 476
Decay accelerating factor (CD55), as viral receptor, 61, 62f, 63t, 64–66
  coxsackievirus, 107–110, 108f, 407–409, 409f

echovirus, 110
enterovirus, 371
Declaration of Talloires (1988), on poliovirus eradication, 476
Deletion/insertion genomes, 271
Demyelination, in Theiler's murine encephalomyelitis virus infection, 428, 428t, 431–433
DI (deletion/insertion) genomes, 271
Diabetes mellitus, in coxsackievirus infections, 391, 397
Disoxaril
   for enterovirus infections, 362
   for rhinovirus infections, 359
DNA, protein-primed, synthesis of, vs. picornavirus RNA synthesis, 241–242, 241f
Drosophila C virus, proteinases of, 216, 218f
Drummond, D., on poliomyelitis, 5–6
Duchenne de Boulogne, G. B. A., on poliomyelitis, 4
Dynamin, receptors for, 73
Dystrophin, cleavage of, 202, 202t, 306

E

Echinacea, for rhinovirus infections, 360
Echovirus(es)
   cell culture of, 441–442
   infections due to
      clinical manifestations of, 368t
      persistent, 441–442
   receptors for, 63t, 65, 108f, 110–111, 368
   replication of
      cis-acting RNA elements in, 233
      host cell intracellular membranous vesicle proliferation in, 339
      intracellular membrane proliferation in, 342
   structure of, 28t
eIF4GIase, 315–318, 315f–317f
eIFs (initiation factors)
   cleavage of, 200, 202, 202t, 302f, 303–306, 304f
      by poliovirus, 313–320, 315f–317f
   in internal ribosomal entry site activity, 164–165, 172–177, 174f, 174t, 176f
Encephalitis, enterovirus, 361
Encephalomyocarditis virus (EMCV)
   evolution of, 291
   genome of
      vs. other picornaviruses, 137
      translation determinants in, 129–130
   infections due to
      clinical manifestations of, 368t
      persistent, 440
   internal ribosomal entry sites of, 234
      canonical initiation factors and, 174t, 175–176, 176f
      cellular RNA-binding proteins and, 179–180
      mechanism of action of, 165–166
      structure of, 161f, 162, 163
   nucleotide preferences of, 152
   P3 proteins of, 229
   polypeptides of, 228
   proteinases of, 216
   receptors for, 63t, 67, 368
   replication of
      cis-acting RNA elements in, 233, 234
      host cell intracellular membranous vesicle proliferation in, 339
      host cell lipid alterations in, 339
      host cell membrane permeability enhancement in, 337
      internal ribosomal entry sites in, 234
      intracellular membrane proliferation in, 342
   proteins involved in, 231t
   RNA polymerase of, evolution of, 288
   serotypes of, 18t
   similarity plots of, 150–151
   translation of, historical perspective of, 159
Enders, John, on poliovirus tissue culture, 9–10
Enterovirus(es), see also specific viruses
   antigens of, 19
   cell culture of, 361
   complementation of, 275–276
   genome of, 20f, 21, 21t
      alignments of, 150
      anti-host determinants in, 133
      vs. other picornaviruses, 137
      plasticity of, 274
      replication determinants in, 131–132
      translation determinants in, 129
   in host cell translation shutoff, 302–306
   infections due to, 360–362
      clinical manifestations of, 358t, 360–361, 368t
      diagnosis of, 361
      epidemiology of, 360
      persistent, 439
      treatment of, 361–362
   interactions with other viruses, 275–276
   internal ribosomal entry sites of
      canonical initiation factors and, 172, 177
      cellular RNA-binding proteins and, 177–179
      structure of, 160, 162
   nucleotide preferences of, 151–152, 154
   pathogenicity of, variability of, 271
   PCR detection of, 361
   proteinases of, 188f, 214f
      2A, 188–189, 228
      in cleavage, 199, 200, 200f
   proteins of, host cell membrane effects of, 344
   receptors for, 63t, 66t, 67, 368
      paralytic disease and, 371
   replication of
      cis-acting RNA elements in, 231, 233
      host cell intracellular membranous vesicle proliferation in, 339
      host cell membrane effects of, 344
      resistance in, 270
   serotypes of, 18t
   similarity plots of, 150–151, 152f
   structures of, 28t
   taxonomy of, see Taxonomy
Enterovirus 70, receptors for, paralytic disease and, 371
Enterovirus 71, receptors for, paralytic disease and, 371
Environmental control and trafficking, genomic determinants of, 132–133
Equine rhinitis A virus
   nucleotide preferences of, 152
   serotypes of, 18t
Equine rhinitis B virus
   nucleotide preferences of, 152
   serotypes of, 18t
Equine rhinovirus, evolution of, 291
Eradication
   poliovirus, see Poliovirus(es), eradication of
   smallpox, 474
Erbovirus
   genome of, 20f, 21, 21t
   serotypes of, 18t
   taxonomy of, see Taxonomy
ERK/MAPK pathway, activation of, by coxsackieviruses, 409–411, 410f, 411f
Eukaryotic initiation factors, see Initiation factors
Evolution, 285–298; see also specific viruses
   antibody effects on, 287–288
   antigenic site coevolution with receptor-recognition sites, 289–290
   antiviral strategies and, 292
   complexity and, 291
   drug effects on, 287–288
   error frequencies in, 287–289
   genomic aspects of, 137–138, 274–275
   high mutation rates in, 289–292
   of host cell tropism, 290–291
   long-term, 287
   measurement of, 288–289
   memory and, 291–292
   overview of, 285
   proofreading activity in, 286
   protein replacements in, 290–291
   quasispecies in, 286–287, 291–292
   rate of, 274
   regulatory region replacements in, 290–291
   structure conservation in, 29
   taxonomy based on, 21–23
   vs. viral reproduction cycle length, 274
   of virulence, 290–291
Exercise, provocation poliomyelitis in, 374–376, 375f

F

Fab-virus complexes, in antibody interactions, 42–44, 42t, 43t
Fever, in enterovirus infections, 360
Fitness
   gains or losses of, 286
   variability of, 270
Flexner, S., on poliomyelitis, 7
FMDVs, see Foot-and-mouth disease virus(es)
Foot-and-mouth disease virus(es), 51–58
   antibody interactions with, 45–46
   antigens of
      discovery of, 51–52
      structures of, 52–55, 53f, 54f
      vaccine preparation and, 52
      variability of, 52, 270
   arginine-glycine-aspartic acid sequence of, in cell binding, 116–117
   cell culture of, 440–441, 441f
   economic significance of, 115
   evolution of, 274, 285, 289–291
   genome of
      anti-host determinants in, 133
      essential vs. nonessential elements of, 136
      vs. other picornaviruses, 137, 138
      plasticity of, 274
      polyprotein processing determinants in, 131
      translation determinants in, 130
   in host cell translation shutoff, 303–305, 304f
   host range of, 118–119, 119t, 270
   in host substrate cleavage, 202, 202t
   infections due to
      clinical manifestations of, 368t
      persistent, 438, 439–441, 441f
   interactions with other viruses, 275
   internal ribosomal entry sites of
      canonical initiation factors and, 172

Foot-and-mouth disease virus(es), internal ribosomal entry sites of (continued)
    structure of, 162, 163
    as virulence determinant, 165
  L protein of, 187–188
    in host substrate cleavage, 192
    structure of, 208–209
  nucleotide preferences of, 152
  polypeptides of, 228
  proteinases of, see also L protein
    in cellular protein cleavage, 200
    in primary cleavage, 213–214, 214f, 215f, 216
    in secondary cleavage, 199–200
    structures of, 203t
  proteins of, host cell membrane effects of, 344, 348
  quasispecies of, memory in, 291–292
  receptors for, 115–123, 118–119, 119t, 368
    alternative, 118–119, 119t
    binding of, 56, 116–117
    clinical manifestations and, 63t
    early studies of, 115–116, 116f
    integrins as, 117–119
    interactions of, 56
    pathogenesis and, 67
    types of, 62, 65
  replication of
    cell membrane alterations in, 247
    host cell intracellular membranous vesicle proliferation in, 339
    host cell lipid alterations in, 339
    host cell membrane effects of, 344, 348
    intracellular membrane proliferation in, 342
  resistance in, 288
  serotypes of, 18t, 19, 115
    discovery of, 51–52
    structures of, 55–56, 55f
    variation in, 52
  similarity plots of, 151, 152f
  structures of, 31, 55–56, 55f
  vaccines for, practical considerations with, 52
  virulence of, 290–291
    alteration of, 118–119, 119t
  VPg proteins of, 229

G

Gastrointestinal disorders, in poliomyelitis, 368
GDVII strain, Theiler's murine encephalomyelitis virus, 427–431, 428t, 437–438
GenBank, 149
Genetics
  overview of, 269–284
    chimeras, 277
    genetic analysis, 276–277
    genome variability, 271–275, 272f, 273f
    milestones, 269
    phenotype variability, 270–271
    replicons, 277
    vectors, 277
    viral interactions, 275–276
  taxonomy based on, 21, 22f
Genome(s), picornavirus, 127–155; see also specific viruses
  alignments of, 150
  coding organization of, 138
  complexity of, 291
  data base for, 149–150
  determinants of
    anti-host offense and defense, 133–134

antiapoptotic activity, 133–134
autocatalytic cleavages, 131
cleavage sites, 131
elongation, 130
encapsidation signals, 134
environmental control and trafficking, 132–133
immune response modulation, 134
intracellular structural and environmental changes, 132–133
macromolecular shutoff, 133
maturation cleavage, 134–135
polyprotein processing, 130–131
proteinases, 131
replication, 131–132
RNA internalization, 135–136
termination, 130
translation, 128–130
virion assembly, 134–135
virion release, 135
essential vs. nonessential elements in, 136
evolutionary aspects of, 137–138, 274–275
functional coordination in, 136
historical studies of, 127–128
interactions among, 275–276
vs. nonpicornavirus genomes, 137–138
nucleotide preferences in, 151–154, 154f
overall design of, 128, 128f
phenotypes and, 136–137
plasticity of, 273–274
point mutations in, 271
proteins encoded in, 187, 188f
rearrangements of, 271–273, 272f, 273f
replication of, see Replication
similarity plots of, 150–151, 152f–153f
taxonomy based on, 20–21, 20f
variability of, 271–275, 272f, 273f
variation of, 137
Global eradication, of poliovirus, see Poliovirus(es), eradication of
Glycophorin A, as viral receptor, 61, 63t
Glycoprotein processing, in host cell membranes, replication effects on, 338f, 341–342, 343f
Guanidine hydrochloride, as viral inhibitor, 270
  resistance to, 287

H

Hand-foot-mouth syndrome, enterovirus, 360–361
Headache, enterovirus, 361
Heine, Jacob, on infantile paralysis, 3–4
Heparan sulfate, as viral receptor, 63t, 64, 65, 118
Hepatitis, infectious, see Hepatitis A virus, infections due to
Hepatitis A virus
  antibodies to, 417–418
  attenuation of, 419–421
  cell culture of, 419–420, 441
  cell interactions with, 417–418
  characteristics of, 415–416
  evolution of, 290
  genome of, 415–416
    anti-host determinants in, 133
    mutations in, 419–421
    polyprotein processing determinants in, 131
    replication determinants in, 132
    translation determinants in, 129
    virion assembly determinants in, 134–135
    virion release determinants in, 135

  host range of, 270, 416
  immune response to, 418–419
  infections due to, 415–425
    animal models of, 416–417, 417f, 418t, 419–420
    clinical manifestations of, 368t
    epidemiology of, 415
    historical perspective of, 415
    pathogenesis of, 417–419
    pathology of, 418
    persistent, 441
    spectrum of, 418
  internal ribosomal entry sites of, 160, 161f, 415
    adjacent sequences affecting, 164
    canonical initiation factors and, 172, 174t, 177
  nucleotide preferences of, 152–154
  P3 proteins of, 229
  polypeptides of, 228
  proteinases of, structures of, 203–206, 203t, 204t, 205f
  proteins of, host cell membrane effects of, 346, 348
  receptors for, 368
    clinical manifestations and, 63t
    types of, 62f, 64, 65
  replication of, 415–420
    cell membrane alterations in, 247
    cis-acting RNA elements in, 233
    host cell membrane effects of, 346, 348
    proteins involved in, 231t
  resistance in, 288
  serotypes of, 18t, 19
  strains, 419–420
  taxonomy of, 416
  translation of, 415
  transmission of, 415
  vaccines for, 421
  virulence of, molecular basis of, 420–421
Hepatitis B virus, transmission of, 415
Hepatitis C virus
  evolution of, 285
  genome of, 291
  internal ribosomal entry sites of, canonical initiation factors and, 172, 174t
  RNA polymerase of, structure of, 255–256
Hepatocytes, hepatitis A virus entry into, 417–418
Hepatoviruses, see also Hepatitis A virus
  genome of, 20f, 21, 21t, 150
  infections due to, clinical manifestations of, 368t
  internal ribosomal entry sites of, 160, 161f, 162
  nucleotide preferences of, 151
  proteinases of, in primary cleavage, 199, 200f
  receptors for, 368
  replication of, cis-acting RNA elements in, 231
  serotypes of, 18t
  similarity plots of, 150–151, 152f, 153f
  taxonomy of, see Taxonomy
Herpangina, enterovirus, 360
Hidden Markov model, for genomic sequence alignment, 150
Histone H3, cleavage of, 202, 202t
Historical perspective, of poliomyelitis, 3–14
HMMER program, for genomic sequence alignment, 150
Horstmann, Dorothy, on viremia in poliomyelitis, 9

Host cell(s), see also Host cell shutoff
  attachment to, in virus-antibody neutralization, 45
  destruction of, cleavage in, 200, 202–203, 202t
  entry of, calcium in, 416
  hepatitis A virus interactions with, 417–418
  internal changes of, genomic determinants of, 132–133
  intracellular membranous vesicle proliferation in, 338f, 339, 340f–341f, 342–344
  membranes of, see Cell membranes
  poliovirus entry of, see Poliovirus(es), cell entry by
  proteins of, in viral replication, 229–231, 231t
  structure of, after infection, 247, 248f
  subcellular fractions of, RNA synthesis in, 249–250, 249f
  tropism of, evolution and, 290–291
  variability of, 270
  virus action on, 200, 202–203, 202t
Host cell shutoff, 200, 202, 202t
  cell membrane alterations in, see Cell membranes, replication effects on
  transcription, poliovirus in, see Poliovirus(es), in host cell transcription shutoff
  translation, 301–311
    initiation factor cleavage in, 303–306, 304f
    initiation of protein synthesis and, 301–302, 302f
Host defenses, suppression of, genomic determinants of, 133–134
Host factors, in poliomyelitis severity, 374–376, 375f
Human immunodeficiency virus
  evolution of, 285, 286
  RNA polymerase of, 255
Humoral immune response
  to coxsackievirus, 395–396
  to hepatitis A virus, 418
  to Theiler's murine encephalomyelitis virus, 432, 439
2-(α-Hydroxybenzyl)-imidazole, resistance to, 287
Hypogammaglobulinemia, poliovirus excretion in, after vaccination, 387, 439

I

Immune globulin(s), enterovirus, 361–362
Immune response
  to coxsackievirus, 391, 392, 395–396
  to hepatitis A virus, 418–419
  to Theiler's murine encephalomyelitis virus, 432–433, 433t, 439
Immunization, see Vaccine(s)
Immunodeficiency
  enterovirus persistence in, 439
  poliovirus excretion in, after vaccination, 387, 439
Immunoglobulin(s), in coxsackievirus infections, 395–396
Immunoglobulin G, viral receptors resembling, 65–66, 66t
Independent International Certification Commission, for poliovirus eradication, 477
Infantile paralysis, see Poliomyelitis
Infectious flacherie virus, proteinases of, 216, 218f
Infectious hepatitis, see Hepatitis A virus, infections due to
Influenza virus
  antibody interactions with, 46
  cell entry of, 71
Initiation factors
  cleavage of, 192–193, 200, 202, 202t, 302f, 303–306, 304f
    by poliovirus, 313–320, 315f–317f
  in internal ribosomal entry site activity, 164–165, 172–177, 174f, 174t, 176f
Injury, muscle, provocation poliomyelitis in, 374–376, 375f
Innate immune response, to coxsackieviruses, 391–392
Insect picornaviruses
  proteinases of, 214f, 216, 218f
  structures of, 27, 28t
Integrins, as viral receptors, 61–62, 62f, 65, 66
  coxsackievirus, 109, 110
  enterovirus, 371
  foot-and-mouth disease virus, 117–119
Intercellular adhesion molecule 1
  soluble preparation of, for rhinovirus infections, 359
  as viral receptor, 61–63, 62f, 63t, 65–67, 66t
    coxsackievirus, 108f, 110
    echovirus, 108f
    rhinovirus, 85–91
      complex formation, 86–90, 87t, 88f, 90f
      mechanisms of, 89–90, 90f
      structural aspects of, 85–86, 86f
      specificity of, 87–89
      stimulation of, 85–86
      structure of, 85–86, 86f, 97
Intercellular adhesion molecule 2, vs. intercellular adhesion molecule 1, 87–88
Interference, among picornaviruses, 276
Interferon(s), for rhinovirus infections, 358
Interferon-γ, in coxsackievirus infections, 393
Interleukin(s), in coxsackievirus infections, 393–394
Internal ribosomal entry site(s) (IRES)
  aphthovirus, cellular RNA-binding proteins and, 179–180
  boundaries of, 162
  canonical initiation factors and, 172–177, 174f, 174t, 176f
  cardiovirus, cellular RNA-binding proteins and, 179–180
  cellular RNA-binding proteins and, 177–180, 179f
  classes of, 160, 161f
  common sequence motifs in, 162
  discovery of, 172
  domains of, trans-action of, 165
  efficiency of, sequences affecting, 163–164
  encephalomyocarditis virus
    canonical initiation factors and, 174t, 175–176, 176f
    cellular RNA-binding proteins and, 179–180
  enterovirus
    canonical initiation factors and, 172, 177
    cellular RNA-binding proteins and, 177–179
  essential domains of, 162
  foot-and-mouth disease virus, canonical initiation factors and, 172
  hepatitis A virus, 172, 174t, 177, 415
  hepatitis C virus, 172, 174t
  historical perspective of, 159–160, 160f, 171, 172
  mechanism of action of, 164–165
  in non-picornaviruses, 160
  pestivirus, 172, 174t
  in picornavirus genome, 128–130
  poliovirus
    canonical initiation factors and, 177
    discovery of, 172
    in replication, 234
  rhinovirus
    canonical initiation factors and, 172, 177
    cellular RNA-binding proteins and, 177–179, 179f
  structures of, 160–163, 161f
    adjacent sequences affecting, 163–164
    higher order, 163
  Theiler's murine encephalomyelitis virus, 180, 431
  translation initiation factor recruitment by, 164–165
  types of, 302
  as virulence determinant, 165–166
Internal ribosomal entry site-specific translation factors, in picornavirus genome, 130
International Conference on Poliomyelitis Control (1983), 476
International Symposium on Poliomyelitis Control (1988), 475
IRES, see Internal ribosomal entry site(s)

J

Jaundice, campaign, 415
JNK/SAPK pathway, activation of, by coxsackieviruses, 409–411, 410f, 411f
Joffroy, A., on poliomyelitis, 4–5

K

Kling, C., on poliomyelitis, 7
Kobuvirus
  genome of, 20f, 21, 21t
  internal ribosomal entry sites of, 160
  serotypes of, 18t
  taxonomy of, see Taxonomy

L

L protein
  action of, 187–188, 188f, 189t
  in cellular protein cleavage, 302–306, 302f, 304f
  in host cell translation shutoff, 302–306, 302f, 304f
  in host substrate cleavage, 192, 202t
  in P protein recognition, 208–209
  vs. papain, 208
  structure of, 187–188, 203t, 208–209
  substrate binding to, 208
L* protein
  action of, 189t
  Theiler's murine encephalomyelitis virus, 428–430, 429f
La protein, in internal ribosomal entry site activity, 177
Landsteiner, K., on poliomyelitis etiology, 6–7
Leader protein, see L protein
Leon strain, poliovirus, 382, 383f, 384f
Lipase action, in host cells, viral replication effects on, 341, 342f
Lipid alterations, in host cells, in viral replication, 339–341, 342f

Liver, hepatitis A virus effects on, 418
Low density lipoprotein receptor (LDLR), 61, 64
  rhinovirus
    identification of, 94–95
    minireceptor type, 98–100, 98f–100f
    regulation of, 95, 96f
    structural requirements for, 97–100, 97f–100f
  superfamily of, 95–96, 95f, 96f
Low density lipoprotein receptor-related protein (LRP), 66, 96
LS-C 2ab strain, poliovirus, 383f
Lymph nodes, coxsackievirus persistence in, 440

M

Macnamara, Jean, on poliovirus strains, 8
Macromolecular synthesis, suppression of, genomic determinants of, 133
Macrophages, poliovirus proliferation in, 369
Mahoney strain, poliovirus, 381, 383f, 384f
MAP-70 protein, as viral receptor accessory, 65
Medin, K. O., on poliomyelitis clinical impact, 5–6
Memory, evolution and, 291–292
Mengovirus
  genome of
    early studies of, 127
    replication determinants in, 132
    virion assembly determinants in, 134
  host range of, 270
  infections due to, clinical manifestations of, 368t
  proteinases of, 214f
  receptors for, 368
  replication of
    cell membrane alterations in, 247
    cis-acting RNA elements in, 232f, 233
    host cell intracellular membranous vesicle proliferation in, 339
    host cell lipid alterations in, 339–341
    host cell membrane permeability enhancement in, 337–338
    intracellular membrane proliferation in, 342
  resistance in, 288
  structure of, 28t
  vs. Theiler's murine encephalomyelitis virus, 427
Meningitis, enterovirus, 361, 362, 439
Meningoencephalitis, enterovirus, 439
β-Microglobulin, as viral receptor accessory, 65, 111
Microtubule-associated protein 4, cleavage of, 202, 202t, 314
Molecular clock data, for polioviruses, 485
Monk strain, poliovirus, 383f
Monkey model, of hepatitis A, 417, 419–420
Monoclonal antibody-resistant mutations, 287–288
Mouse hepatitis virus, replication of, translation coupling with, 234
Muller's ratchet, in evolution, 274
Multiple sclerosis, Theiler's murine encephalomyelitis virus infection resembling, 428, 428t, 431–433
Multiplicity-of-infection passages, in viral replication, 271
Muscle injury, provocation poliomyelitis in, 374–376, 375f

Mutation(s)
  evolution and, 274–275; see also Evolution
  frequencies of, 285–292
  hepatitis A virus, 419–421
  mapping of, 276
  measurement of, 288–289
  monoclonal antibody-resistant, 287–288
  in mutational analysis, 276
  neutral, 274
  point, 271
  poliovirus, 274, 371, 372f, 373–374
    RNA polymerase, 261, 261t
  rates of, 285–292
Myocarditis, see also Theiler's murine encephalomyelitis virus
  coxsackievirus, 439–440
    immunology of, 391–398
    pathogenesis of, 404t, 405–411, 406f, 408f–411f
  enterovirus, 361

N

National Immunization Days, for poliovirus eradication, 476, 477, 481, 484
National Poliomyelitis Control Program, Brazil, 474–475
Natural killer cells, in coxsackievirus response, 391–392
Necrosis, liver, in hepatitis A, 418
Nectins, in poliovirus replication, 71
Neonatal infections, enterovirus, 361–362
Neurologic disorders, in poliomyelitis, 368–369, 371–374, 372f
Neurovirulence
  polioviruses, 371–374, 372f
  Theiler's murine encephalomyelitis virus, 430–431, 437–438
Neutralizing antibodies
  coxsackievirus, 396
  virus interactions with, 31, 46–47, see also Rhinovirus(es), antibody interactions with
Neutralizing immunogenic sites, of viruses, 39, 40f, 43
NIm sites, coxsackievirus, 396–397
Nonreplicative rearrangements, 272f, 273

O

Octamer-binding protein, cleavage of, in host cell shutoff, 326–327, 328f
Oral cavity, enterovirus infections of, 360–361
oriI, in replication, 233
oriR, in replication, 233, 274
Otitis media
  enterovirus, 360
  rhinovirus, 357
Ovarian vitellogenin/very low density lipoprotein receptor, 96

P

p38/MAPK pathway, activation of, by coxsackieviruses, 409–411, 410f, 411f
p53 protein, cleavage of, in host cell shutoff, 325–327, 328f
P1 proteins, 190, 191f
P2 proteins, 190, 191f
  host cell membrane effects of, 344–346, 345f–347f
  in replication, 228–229, 249, 250
P3 proteins, 191–192
  host cell membrane effects of, 346–348, 348f

  in replication, 229, 230t, 249
Pan American Health Organization, poliovirus eradication program of, 475–476
Pancreas, coxsackievirus effects on, 391, 397
Papain, vs. L protein, 208
Parechovirus(es)
  genome of, 20f, 21, 21t
    alignments of, 150
    translation determinants in, 129
  infections due to, clinical manifestations of, 368t
  internal ribosomal entry sites of, 160, 162
  nucleotide preferences of, 152, 154
  proteinases of, in primary cleavage, 199, 200f
  receptors for, clinical manifestations and, 63t
  serotypes of, 18t
  similarity plots of, 150–151, 153f
  taxonomy of, see Taxonomy
Pathogenicity, see also specific viruses
  variability of, 271
PCR, see Polymerase chain reaction
Permeability, of host cell membranes, in viral replication, 337–339, 338f
Persistent infections, 437–448
  coxsackievirus, 405–411, 406f, 404t, 408f–411f, 439–440
  echovirus, 441–442
  encephalomyocarditis virus, 440
  enterovirus, 439
  foot-and-mouth disease virus, 438t, 439–441, 441f
  hepatitis A virus, 441
  poliovirus, 384–387, 438t, 439, 440, 442, 443f, 442t, 444–445, 488
  Theiler's murine encephalomyelitis virus, 437–439, 438t, 440
Pestivirus, internal ribosomal entry sites of, canonical initiation factors and, 172, 174t
Pettersson, A., on poliomyelitis, 7
Pharyngitis, enterovirus, 360–361
Phenotypes, viral
  genetic basis of, 136–137
  variability of, 270–271
Philanthropic organizations, for poliomyelitis research, 8
Phospholipase action, in host cells, viral replication effects on, 341, 342f
Phylogeny, 21–23
  of polioviruses, 484–485, 485f–486f
Physalis mottle virus, structure of, 29t
Picornavirus(es), see also specific viruses
  interactions among, 275–276
  structures of, 27–38, 28t–29t
  taxonomy of, see Taxonomy
Picornavirus Sequence Database, 149
Pirodavir, for rhinovirus infections, 359
Plant comoviruses, structures of, 29t
Plasticity, genome, 273–274
Pleconaril
  for enterovirus infections, 362
  mechanism of action of, 32–34, 34f
  for rhinovirus infections, 359
Pleurodynia, enterovirus, 361
PLOTSIMILARITY program, 150–151, 152f–153f
Pneumonia, enterovirus, 360
Pocket factor
  drug resistance and, 287
  in receptor interactions, 32, 33, 33f, 34f, 44
Polio Eradication Initiative, organizations involved in, 477

Poliomyelitis, *see also* Poliovirus(es)
  clinical manifestations of, 3–6, 368t
  epidemiology of, 10, 360
    in early 20th century, 6
    vaccine effects on, 381, 382f
  historical perspective
    epidemiology of, 10
    molecular virology, 10–11
    mouse virus adaptation, 8–10
    old records, 3–8
    philanthropic organizations, 8
    vaccine development, 10
  natural history of, 367–369
  neuropathology of, 4–5
  paralytic, natural history of, 367–369
  pathogenesis of, 7–8, 369–376
    CD155 in, 369–371, 370t
    host conditions and, 374–376, 375f
    neurovirulence in, 371–374, 372f
    nonpolio enterovirus receptors in, 371
    nonstructural proteins in, 373–374
    structural polypeptides in, 373
    tropism in, 369–371, 370t
  pathophysiology of, 381
  persistent, 384–387, 438t, 439, 440, 442, 443f, 442t, 444–445, 488
  provocation, 374–376, 375f
  rodent model for, 370
  susceptibility to, 367
  vaccine-related, 376, 387
  vaccines for, *see* Poliovirus(es), vaccines for
Poliovirus(es)
  antibody interactions with, 46–47
  antigenic variability of, 270
  antiviral agent effects on, 75
  attenuation of, 290–291
  in blood, 9
  blood-brain barrier penetration by, 368–369
  cell culture of, 442, 442t, 443f, 444–445
  cell entry by
    empty capsid assembly intermediate in, 76–78
    intermediates for, 78, 79f, 80
    model for, 80–81
    A particle and, 73, 75
    site of, 73
    structural alterations during, 73
    virion structure and, 76, 77f
    virus-receptor complex in, 78–79
  cell-free systems for, 451–469
    complementation, 458–469, 458f, 459f
    recombination studies, 451–458, 452f–457f
  Chat strain, 381
  chimeras of, 277
  complementation of, 275–276
  Cox strain, 381
  discovery of, 6–7
  eradication of, 473–491, 481
    in Brazil, 474–476
    certification of, 477
    in Cuba, 474
    current programs toward, 481, 482f, 483f
    Declaration of Talloires (1988), 476
    endgame challenges in, 488
    evolutionary aspects of, 485
    International Symposium (1983) on, 475
    laboratory containment and, 477–478
    laboratory performance monitoring in, 487
    mop-up campaigns in, 481
    National Immunization Days in, 476, 477, 481, 484
    Pan American Health Organization and, 475–476
    posteradication issues in, 477–478
    remaining reservoirs for, 485–486
    Rotary International in, 476
    routine immunization coverage in, 481, 484
    Sabin role in, 473–474
    smallpox eradication model and, 474
    stopping immunization after, 478
    strategy for, 481, 484
    Subnational Immunization Days for, 481, 484
    surveillance after, 484–488, 485f–487f
    World Health Assembly goals for, 477
  error frequencies of, 288–289
  evolution of, 274, 288–289, 290, 485
  excretion of, after vaccination, 384–387
  fitness variability of, 270
  genome of, 382, 383f, 384f
    anti-host determinants in, 133–134
    data base for, 149
    early studies of, 127–128
    environmental control and trafficking determinants in, 132–133
    mutations in, 371, 372f, 373–374
    plasticity of, 274
    polyprotein processing determinants in, 131
    replication determinants in, 131
    structure of, 227, 228f
    translation determinants in, 129
    virion assembly determinants in, 134
    virion release determinants in, 135
  in host cell transcription shutoff, 321–335
    activated transcription factor cleavage and inactivation in, 325–327, 327f, 328f
    basal transcription factor inactivation in, 322–325, 323f–326f
    cleavage in, 322–325, 323f–326f
    proteinase 3C in, 325–327, 327f, 328f
    RNA polymerase I in, 323f, 329–330, 331f
    RNA polymerase II in, 323f, 322, 323f
    RNA polymerase III in, 323f, 327–329, 329f, 330f
    SnRNA and, 330–331, 332f
    unanswered questions concerning, 331–333, 332t
  in host cell translation shutoff, 302–306, 313–320, 315f–317f
  host range of, 270
  in host substrate cleavage, 202, 202t
  importation of, 486
  indigenous wild circulation of, 481, 482f, 483f
  infections due to, *see* Poliomyelitis
  interactions with other viruses, 275–276
  internal ribosomal entry sites of, 201f
    adjacent sequences affecting, 163
    canonical initiation factors and, 177
    pathogenicity and, 373
    structure of, 161f, 162
  laboratory containment of, 477–478
  Leon strain, 382, 383f, 384f
  life cycle of
    complementation, 458–469, 458f, 459f
    recombination, 451–458, 452f–457f
  LS-C 2ab strain, 383f
  Mahoney strain, 381, 383f, 384f
  molecular clock data for, 485
  molecular virology of, 10–11
  Monk strain, 383f
  mouse strain, 8
  mutations of, 271, 274
  neurovirulence of, 371–374, 372f
  nonstructural proteins of
    pathogenicity and, 373–374
    in replication, 227–229, 230t
  nucleotide preferences of, 152
  P2 proteins of, 190–191
  P3 proteins of, 191–192, 229–230t
  pathogenicity of, variability of, 271
  phenotypes of, 137
  phylogeny of, 484–485, 485f–486f
  proliferation of, in macrophages, 369
  proteinases of
    3C, 189–190
    in host substrate cleavage, 192
    in secondary cleavage, 199–200
    structures of, 203–207, 203t, 204t, 205f, 207f
  proteins of, host cell membrane effects of, 344–348, 345f–347f
  receptors for, 71–83, 368
    adaptation to, 270
    attachment sites for, 65–66, 66t
    cell entry pathway for, 80–81
    cell entry site for, 73
    clinical manifestations and, 63t
    interactions with, 32, 71, 74f
    pathogenesis and, 67, 369–371, 370t
    in replication cycle, 71, 73, 74f, 76
    significance of, 66
    structures of, 74f, 76–80, 77f, 79f
    types of, 62f
  recombination among, 276
  regions certified virus-free, 481, 482f, 483f
  replication of, 71, 73, 74f, 75, 80, 255–267
    cell-free systems for, 451–469
    cellular proteins in, 229–231, 231t
    cis-acting RNA elements for, 231, 232f, 233–234
    complementation, 458–469, 458f, 459f
    complex formation in, 250–251
    in crude complexes, 235
    DNA vs. RNA, 241–242, 241f
    extraneural, 369
    host cell glycoprotein alterations in, 342, 343f
    host cell intracellular membranous vesicle proliferation in, 339, 340f–341f
    host cell lipid alterations in, 339–341
    host cell membrane effects of, 337–338, 344–348, 345f–347f
    internal ribosomal entry sites in, 234
    membrane alterations in, 247, 248f, 250
    membranous structures for, 234
    pathway for, 227, 228f
    proteins involved in, 231t
    recombination studies, 451–458, 452f–457f
    synthesis products of, 234–235
    translation coupling with, 234
    vesicle formation in, 248–250, 248f, 249f
    viral proteins for, 227–229, 230t
  reservoirs of, 485–486
  resistance in, 287–288
  retrograde axonal transport of, 368–369, 376
  RIPO and RIPOS strains, 388
  RNA polymerases of, 255–267
    action of, 235
    evolution of, 288
    functional analysis of, 261–262, 263t

Poliovirus(es), RNA polymerases of (*continued*)
  in host cell transcription shutoff, 322–325, 323f–326f, 327–330, 329f–331f
  kinetic constants of, 262, 263t
  mutations of, 261, 261t
  oligomerization of, 256–257, 258t, 259f
  properties of, 229, 230t
  replication complex of, 257, 259–264
  ribavirin action and, 292
  structure of, 255–256, 258t
  thermodynamic constants of, 262, 263t
Sabin strains of, *see* Sabin strains, poliovirus
serotypes of, 18t, 19
similarity plots of, 152f
strains, 8
structural polypeptides of
  pathogenicity and, 373
  in replication, 227–229, 230t
structures of, 28t, 31f, 72f–73f, 76, 77f
  in cell entry, 73, 79–80, 79f
surveillance for
  acute flaccid paralysis cases, 484, 486–488
  clinical specimen studies in, 484
  direct detection in, 487–488
  gaps in, 486
  importance of, 484
  laboratory performance monitoring in, 487
  methods for, 484–485, 485f–487f
taxonomy of, *see* Taxonomy
tissue culture of, 9–10
translation of, historical perspective of, 159
transmission of, eradication program and, 478
Trojan horse transport mechanism for, 368–369
tropism of, 369–371, 370t
USOL-D-BAC strain, 387–388
vaccines for, 381–390, *see also* Poliovirus(es), eradication of
  alternatives to, 387–388
  attenuation for, 290–291
  Cutter incident and, 376
  discontinuation of, 477–478
  early work on, 10
  immune response to, 386–387
  origin of, 381–382, 382f, 383f
  paralytic disease from, 371
  poliomyelitis epidemiology and, 381, 382f
  Sabin strain for, *see* Sabin strains, poliovirus
  Salk (inactivated, IPV), 381, 382f
  in Toluca, Mexico, study, 473–474
  virus excretion due to, 383–384, 386–387, 439
VPg proteins of, 229
Poliovirus receptor-related molecules, 369
Poly(A) binding protein
  cleavage of, 202, 202t, 314
  in internal ribosomal entry site activity, 164
  in replication, 230–231, 233
Poly(A) tails, in internal ribosomal entry site activity, 164
Poly(C) binding protein, in internal ribosomal entry site activity, 163–164
Poly(rC) binding protein
  in internal ribosomal entry site activity, 178–180, 179f
  in replication, 230

Polymerase, poliovirus, *see* Poliovirus(es), RNA polymerases of
Polymerase chain reaction, for enterovirus detection, 361
Polypeptides
  pathogenicity and, 373
  in replication, 227–229, 230t
Polyproteins
  processing of, *see also* Proteinases
    genomic determinants of, 130–131
    translation and, 302–307, 304f
  structures of, 199–203, 200f, 201f, 202f
Polypyrimidine tract binding (PTB) protein, in internal ribosomal entry site activity, 178–180, 179f
  mutations of, 431
Popper, E., on poliomyelitis etiology, 6–7
Porcine enteroviruses
  nucleotide preferences of, 151
  serotypes of, 18t
Porcine teschovirus
  nucleotide preferences of, 152
  serotypes of, 18t
Postpoliomyelitis syndrome, 440
Primary cleavage, *see* Cleavage, in polyprotein processing, primary
Proofreading-repair activity, in replication, 286
Protein(s)
  synthesis of, initiation of, 301–302, 302f
  in viral structure, 30–31, 31f
Proteinases, *see also specific viruses*
2A
  active site of, 207
  activity of, 188–190, 189t, 192, 217, 219–222, 220f
  vs. 3C proteinase, 206–207, 207f
  in cellular protein cleavage, 200, 201f, 202, 202t, 302–306, 302f, 304f
  cleavage specificity of, 305–306
  mutagenic analysis of, 216
  nonpicornavirus, 215f, 216–217, 218f
  P protein residue interactions with, 207–208
  in primary cleavage, 213–223
  ribosome interactions with, 219, 221
  structure of, 188–189, 203t, 206–208, 207f, 217, 305–306
  substrate specificity of, 207
3A, activity of, 189t
3AB, activity of, 189t
2B
  activity of, 190
  in replication, 228
3B, activity of, 189t
2C, activity of, 189t, 190–191
2C/2BC
  activity of, 189t, 190–191
  in replication, 228–229
3C, 189–190
  in activated transcription factor cleavage, 325–327, 327f, 328f
  active sites of, 204–205
  activity of, 188f, 189–190, 189t
  in basal transcription factor inactivation, 322–325, 323f–326f
  vs. chymotrypsin, 203–204
  in host substrate cleavage, 202t
  in P protein residue recognition, 205–206
  properties of, 230t
  in replication, 230t
  RNA binding site of, 206
  sequence alignment of, 203–204, 204t, 205f

  structure of, 189–190, 203–206, 203t, 204t, 205f
  substrate binding by, 205
3CD
  activity of, 189t, 190, 191f
  cloverleaf complex with, 231, 233
  properties of, 230t
  cleavage by
    host substrates, 192–193
    primary, *see* Cleavage, in polyprotein processing, primary
    secondary, 199–200, 201f
3D, activity of, 189t
  genomic determinants of, 131
  in host cell transcription shutoff, poliovirus, *see* Poliovirus(es), in host cell transcription shutoff
  in host substrate cleavage, 192–193
L protein, *see* L protein
substrates for
  nonstructural polypeptide products, 188f, 190–192
  structural polypeptide products, 188f, 190, 191f
Proteolytic processing, *see also* Proteinases
  host substrate cleavage in, 192–193
  substrates for
    nonstructural polypeptide products, 188f, 190–192, 227–229, 230t
    structural polypeptide products, 188f, 190, 191f
Provocation poliomyelitis, 374–376, 375f

Q

Quality control, in picornavirus genome, 138
Quasispecies, evolution of, 286–287, 291–292

R

Rash, in enterovirus infections, 360
Rearrangements, genome, 271–273, 272f, 273f
Receptor(s), viral, 368t
  accessory factors for, 63t, 65
  aphthovirus, 63t, 368t
  attachment sites on, 65–66, 66t
  cardiovirus, 32, 63t, 368t
  competition for, 276
  coxsackievirus, *see* Coxsackievirus(es), receptors for
  definition of, 61
  echovirus, 63t, 65, 108f, 110–111, 368t
  encephalomyocarditis virus, 63t, 67, 368t
  enterovirus, 63t, 67, 368t
  evolution of, 289–290
  foot-and-mouth disease virus, *see* Foot-and-mouth disease virus(es), receptors for
  hepatitis A virus, 62f, 63t, 64, 368t
  interactions with, structures involved in, 31–32, 32f, 33f
  molecules serving as, 61–62, 62f, 63t, 64
  multiple, 109–110
  number of per virus, 64–65
  overview of, 61–69, 62f, 63t, 66t
  paralytic disease and, nonpolio enteroviruses, 371
  parechovirus, 63t
  pathogenesis and, 67
  poliovirus, *see* Poliovirus(es), receptors for
  rhinovirus, *see* Rhinovirus(es), receptors for
  significance of, 66
  taxonomy based on, 18–19

Theiler's murine encephalomyelitis virus, 368t, 430
Receptor-associated protein, 96
Recombination
　in genetic analysis, 276–277
　between picornaviruses, 276
　in poliovirus replication, 451–458, 452f
　　cell-free systems for, 451–458, 452f–457f
　　crossover sites in, 451–452, 455–456, 453f–455f
　　frequency of, 451–452
　　guanidine hydrochloride effects on, 452, 454–455
　　temperature effects on, 456–458, 456f, 457f
Red clover mottle virus, structure of, 29t
Replication, 227–246; see also specific viruses
　cell membrane alterations in, see Cell membranes, replication effects on
　cellular proteins in, 229–231, 231t
　cis-acting RNA elements for, 231, 232f, 233–234
　complex of, 250–251
　in crude complexes, 235
　DNA vs. RNA, 241–242, 241f
　evolution in, see Evolution
　genomic determinants of, 131–132
　host cells in, 247–253
　　cleavage of, 200, 202–203, 202t
　　destruction of, 247
　　membrane alterations in, 247–250, 248f, 249f
　　vesicles formation in, 248–250, 248f, 249f
　membranous structures for, 234
　model for, 235–241, 236f, 237f, 239f
　multiplicity-of-infection passages in, 271
　pathway for, 227, 228f
　proofreading-repair activity in, 286
　proteinases in, see Proteinases
　synthesis products of, 234–235
　translation coupling with, 234
　viral proteins for, 227–229, 230t
Replicative rearrangements, 272–273, 272f, 273f
Replicons, 277
Resistance, to virus inhibitors
　evolution of, 287–288
　variability of, 270
Respiratory disorders, enterovirus, 360
Retrograde axonal transport, of polioviruses, 368–369, 376
Rhinovirus(es)
　antibody interactions with, 39–49
　　antibody strength and, 49, 40f, 41
　　canyon hypothesis of, 46–47
　　crystal structure of, 42–44, 43t
　　Fab-virus complexes in, 42–44, 42t, 43t
　　in vitro versus in vivo, 45–46
　　mechanisms of, 44–45
　　profiles of, 39, 40f, 41
　　pseudo-atomic models of, 42, 42t
　　structural analysis of, 41–42
　antigenic variability of, 270
　evolution of, 291
　genome of, 20f, 21, 21t
　　alignments of, 150
　　anti-host determinants in, 133
　　vs. other picornaviruses, 137
　　replication determinants in, 132
　　translation determinants in, 129
　　virion assembly determinants in, 134

　in host cell translation shutoff, 302–306, 304f
　in host substrate cleavage, 202, 202t
　infections due to
　　clinical manifestations of, 357–358, 358t, 368t
　　diagnosis of, 358
　　epidemiology of, 357
　　treatment of, 358–360
　internal ribosomal entry sites of, 234
　　canonical initiation factors and, 172, 177
　　cellular RNA-binding proteins and, 177–179, 179f
　　structure of, 160, 162
　major group of, receptor interactions of, 85–91
　minor group of
　　definition of, 85
　　receptor interactions of, 93–105
　nucleotide preferences of, 151, 152, 154
　P3 proteins of, 229
　proteinases of, 188f, 214f
　　2A, 188–189, 228
　　in cellular protein cleavage, 200
　　in primary cleavage, 199, 200f
　　in secondary cleavage, 200
　　structures of, 203–204, 203t, 204t, 205f, 206–208, 207f
　receptors for, 368
　　attachment sites for, 65–66, 66t
　　clinical manifestations and, 63
　　identification of, 93–97, 94f–96f
　　interactions with, 32
　　major group, 85–91
　　minor group, 93–105
　　open questions involving, 100–101
　　pathogenesis and, 67
　　significance of, 66
　　structures of, 72f–73f, 97–100, 97f–100f
　replication of
　　cell membrane alterations in, 247
　　cis-acting RNA elements in, 231, 232f, 233–234
　　host cell membrane permeability enhancement in, 337
　　internal ribosomal entry sites in, 234
　　plus-strand RNA synthesis in, 237
　　proteins involved in, 231t
　resistance in, 270, 287
　RNA polymerase of, 229
　serotypes of, 18t
　similarity plots of, 150–151, 152f
　structures of, 28t
　taxonomy of, see Taxonomy
　VPg proteins of, 229
Ribavirin, RNA polymerase activity and, 292
RIPO and RIPOS strains, poliovirus, 388
RNA
　folding of, prediction of, 162–163
　internal ribosomal entry sites of, see Internal ribosomal entry site(s)
　internalization of, genomic determinants of, 135–136
　replication of, see Replication
　synthesis of
　　error-prone, 285–292
　　genomic determinants of, 131–132
　　minus-strand, 236–239, 236f, 237f
　　plus-strand, 239, 239f, 241
　　products of, 234–235
　　protein 3A in, 346–348, 348f
　translation of, see Internal ribosomal entry site(s); Translation

RNA-binding proteins, cellular, in internal ribosomal entry site activity, 177–180, 179f
RNA polymerase(s)
　evolution of, 288
　mutations of, 271
　poliovirus, see Poliovirus(es), RNA polymerases of
　in rearrangements, 272
　in replication, 227
Robbins, Frederick
　on poliovirus eradication, 475
　on poliovirus tissue culture, 9–10
Rosette formation, formation of, 249–250, 249f
Ross River virus, antibody interactions with, 46
Rotary International, in poliovirus eradication program, 476
Rotaviruses, proteinases of, 214f, 216, 218f

S

Sabin, Albert B.
　on poliovirus eradication, 473–474
　on poliovirus pathogenesis, 7–8
Sabin strains, poliovirus
　alternatives to, 387–388
　attenuated, 382–383, 384f–386f, 385–386
　derivation of, 383f
　molecular biology of, 382–386, 383f–386f
　persistent excretion of, 437–439
　safety of, 371, 372f, 373–374, 381–382
　vaccine efficacy and, 382f
Salk (inactivated, IPV) vaccine, for poliovirus, 381, 382f
Satellite tobacco mosaic virus, structure of, 27
Serotypes, picornavirus, taxonomy based on, 18t, 19–20
Sesbania mosaic virus, structure of, 29t
Shannon entropies, 291
Signaling pathways, activation of, by coxsackieviruses, 409–411, 410f, 411f
Simian immunodeficiency virus, evolution of, 285
Similarity plots, of picornaviruses, 150–151, 152f–153f
Sinusitis, in rhinovirus infections, 357–358
Skin lesions, enterovirus, 360–361
Smallpox, eradication of, 474
SnRNA transcription, 330–331, 332f
Southern bean mosaic virus, structure of, 29t, 30f
Spleen, coxsackievirus persistence in, 440
Stabilization, virion, in virus-antibody neutralization, 44
Streptomyces griseus protease B, structure of, 204–207, 204t
Structures, picornavirus, 27–38, 28t–29t; see also *specific viruses and components*
　antiviral compound binding to, 32–34, 34f
　assembly of, 29–30
　capsid, 27, 29, 30f, 31f
　evolution of, 29
　neutralizing antibody interactions and, 31
　proteins, 30–31, 31f
　receptor interactions with, 31–32, 32f, 33f
Subnational Immunization Days, for poliovirus eradication, 481, 484
Swine vesicular disease virus, evolution of, 291

T

T lymphocytes, response of
　to coxsackieviruses, 392–395, 393f–395f
　to hepatitis A virus, 418–419

T lymphocytes, response of (*continued*)
  to Theiler's murine encephalomyelitis virus, 432–433, 433t, 439
Talloires, France, Declaration of (1988), on poliovirus eradication, 476
Tamarin model, of hepatitis A, 416–417, 417f, 418t
TATA-binding protein, cleavage of, 202, 202t, 314
Taxonomy, 17–24, 18t
  basis for
    antigenic properties, 19–20
    evolution, 21–23
    genetic relationships, 21, 22f
    genome organization, 20–21, 20f, 21t
    pathogenesis, 17–19
  hepatitis A virus, 416
  problems in, 23
Template switching (replicative rearrangement), 272–273, 272f, 273f
Teschovirus
  genome of, 20f, 21, 21t, 150
  serotypes of, 18t
  similarity plots of, 150–151, 153f
  taxonomy of, *see* Taxonomy
Theiler's murine encephalomyelitis virus
  apoptosis induced by, 430
  BeAn strain, persistence of, 437–438
  DA strain, 428, 428t, 431
    persistence of, 437–438
  evolution of, 289
  GDVII strain, 427–431, 428t, 437–438
  genome of, 428–429, 429f
    anti-host determinants in, 134
    vs. other picornaviruses, 137
    translation determinants in, 129
  host cell shutoff by, 429–430
  infections due to
    animal models of, 428
    clinical manifestations of, 368t
    historical perspective of, 427
    immune response in, 432–433, 433t
    pathogenesis of, 430–431
    persistent, 437–439, 438t, 440
    phenotypes of, 427–428, 428t
  internal ribosomal entry sites of
    binding site mutations in, 431
    cellular RNA-binding proteins and, 180
    mechanism of action of, 166
    as virulence determinant, 165
  L protein of, 188
  L* protein of, 428–430
  nucleotide preferences of, 152
  pathogenicity of, variability of, 271
  phenotypes of, 137
  polypeptides of, 228
  polypyrimidine tract binding sites of, mutation of, 431
  protein of, translation of, 429–430
  proteinases of, 213
  receptors for, 368, 430
  replication of
    cell membrane alterations in, 247
    cis-acting RNA elements in, 232f, 233
    host cell intracellular membranous vesicle proliferation in, 339

TO (Theiler's original) strain, 427–428, 428t, 430–433, 437–438
  structure of, 28t
  subgroups of, 427–428, 428t
  susceptibility to, 431–433, 433t, 439
  virulence factors in, 430–431, 437–438
Theilovirus, serotypes of, 18t
Thosea asigna virus, proteinases of, 216, 218f
Tissue culture, poliovirus, 9–10
TMEV, *see* Theiler's murine encephalomyelitis virus
TO (Theiler's original) strain, Theiler's murine encephalomyelitis virus, 427–428, 428t, 430–433, 437–438
Tobacco etch virus, replication of, translation coupling with, 234
Tobacco ringspot virus, structure of, 29t
Tomato bushy stunt virus, structure of, 29t, 30f
Transcription, host cell, proteinase effects on, 321–335
Transcription factor(s), in host cell transcription shutoff, 322, 323f, 327–330, 329f, 330f
Transcription factor IIIC, cleavage of, 202, 202t
Transcriptional activator Oct-1, cleavage of, 202, 202t
Translation
  canonical initiation factors in, 164–165, 172–177, 174f, 174t, 176f
  genomic determinants of, 128–130
  historical perspective of, 159–160, 160f, 171
  host cell shutoff of
    poliovirus, 313–320
    proteinase-mediated, 301–311, 302f, 304f
  internal ribosomal entry sites in, *see* Internal ribosomal entry site(s)
  replication coupled with, 234
  Theiler's murine encephalomyelitis virus protein, 429–430
Tremacamra, for rhinovirus infections, 359
Tropism
  host cell, evolution and, 290–291
  polioviruses, 369–371, 370t
Trypanosoma, proteinases of, 214f, 216–217, 218f
Tumor necrosis factor-α
  in coxsackievirus infections, 393–394
  inhibition of, genomic determinants of, 134
Turnip yellow mosaic virus, structure of, 29t

U

Underwood, Michael, on poliomyelitis, 3
unr gene, in internal ribosomal entry site activity, 178, 179f
USOL-D-BAC strain, poliovirus, 387–388

V

Vaccine(s)
  foot-and-mouth disease viruses, 52
  hepatitis A virus, 421

poliovirus, *see* Poliovirus(es), vaccines for
viral evolution for, 290–291
Variability, of phenotypes, 270–271
Vascular cell adhesion molecule, as viral receptor, 61, 62, 62f, 63t
  coxsackievirus, 108f
  echovirus, 108f, 110
Vectors, 277
Very-low-density lipoprotein receptor, 62f, 64
  binding site of, 99–100
  expression of, 96–98
  structure of, 95, 95f, 96
Vesicles, formation of, in replication, 248–250, 248f, 249f, 338f, 339, 340f–341f, 342–344
Vilyuisk virus
  infections due to, 368t
  receptors for, 368
Virions
  assembly of, genomic determinants of, 134–135
  release of, genomic determinants of, 135
Viroporins, 338f, 339, 344
Virulence factors
  evolution and, 290–291
  foot-and-mouth disease virus, 118–119, 119t, 165
  hepatitis A virus, 420–421
  internal ribosomal entry sites as, 165–166
  polioviruses, 371–374, 372f
  Theiler's murine encephalomyelitis virus, 165, 430–431, 437–438
  variability of, 271
Vitamin C, for rhinovirus infections, 360
Vitronectin, as viral receptor, 65, 371
VPg protein
  in replication, 228f
  structure of, 230
Vulpian, A., on poliomyelitis, 4–5

W

Weller, Thomas, on poliovirus tissue culture, 9–10
Wernstedt, W., on poliomyelitis, 7
White matter disease, Theiler's murine encephalomyelitis virus, 428, 428t, 431–433
Wickman, I., on poliomyelitis epidemiology, 6
WIN compounds
  for enterovirus infections, 362
  resistance to, 287
  for rhinovirus infections, 359
World Health Assembly, poliovirus eradication goals of, 477
World Health Organization, poliovirus eradication activities of
  Expanded Program on Immunization, 474, 475
  leadership, 477
World Summit for Children (1990), on poliovirus eradication, 477

Z

Zinc, for rhinovirus infections, 360